The Hospital Addiction Medicine Handbook

The Hospital Addiction Medicine Handbook

Edited by

Melissa B. Weimer, DO, MCR

Associate Professor of Medicine and Epidemiology; Medical Director of the Yale Addiction Medicine Consult Service, Program in Addiction Medicine; Associate Program Director of the Yale Addiction Medicine Fellowship Program
Yale School of Medicine
Yale School of Public Health
New Haven, Connecticut

Susan L. Calcaterra, MD, MPH, MS

Director, Addiction Consultation Service University of Colorado
Associate Professor of Medicine
Department of Medicine
University of Colorado Anschutz Medical Campus
Aurora, Colorado

Wolters Kluwer

Philadelphia • Baltimore • New York • London
Buenos Aires • Hong Kong • Sydney • Tokyo

Acquisitions Editor: James Sherman
Development Editor: Ariel S. Winter
Editorial Coordinator: Abirami Balakrishnan
Marketing Manager: Janet Feeney
Production Project Manager: Matthew West
Manager, Graphic Arts and Design: Stephen Druding
Art Director, Illustration: Jennifer Clements
Manufacturing Coordinator: Margie Orzech
Prepress Vendor: Aptara, Inc.

9 8 7 6 5 4 3 2 1

Printed in Mexico

Cataloging in Publication data available on request from publisher.

ISBN-13: 978-1-9752-5447-6

shop.lww.com

QUADM0626

Dedication

"Dedicated to our patients who inspire us daily.
In remembrance of Samantha, Tracy, Andrea, and Tom,
whose experiences with addiction shone a light on the urgent
need to expand addiction services in health systems."

Contributors

Soraya Azari, MD
Clinical Professor
Department of Medicine
San Francisco Department of Public Health
San Francisco, California

Paxton Bach, MD, MSc
Clinical Assistant Professor
Department of Medicine
University of British Columbia
Vancouver, British Columbia

Stephen Baldassarri, MD, MHS
Assistant Professor of Medicine
Department of Internal Medicine
Yale School of Medicine
New Haven, Connecticut

Cecily M. Barber, MD, MPH
Assistant Professor
Department of Obstetrics and Gynecology
Boston University Chobanian & Avedisian School of Medicine
Boston Medical Center
Boston, Massachusetts

Emily E. Beahm, MSW, LCSW
Senior Social Worker
VA Butler Healthcare's Housing and Urban Development
Butler, Pennsylvania

Olivia Berger, PharmD
Clinical Pharmacy Specialist
Planning Department
Johns Hopkins Bayview Medical Center
Baltimore, Maryland

Alia Bodnar, MD
Physician, Assistant Professor of Medicine
Department of Medicine, Divisions of Addiction and General Internal Medicine
Johns Hopkins School of Medicine
Baltimore, Maryland

Lindsay A. Bowman, PharmD
Clinical Pharmacy Specialist
Department of Pharmacy
The John Hopkins Hospital
Baltimore, Maryland

Megan E. Buresh, MD
Associate Professor
Department of Medicine
Johns Hopkins School of Medicine
Baltimore, Maryland

Susan L. Calcaterra, MD, MPH, MS
Director, Addiction Consultation Service University of Colorado
Associate Professor of Medicine
Department of Medicine
University of Colorado Anschutz Medical Campus
Aurora, Colorado

Deepa R. Camenga, MD, MHS
Associate Professor
Department of Emergency Medicine, Pediatrics, Public Health
Yale School of Medicine
New Haven, Connecticut

Arianna Campbell, DMSc, MPH, PA-C
Physician Assistant
Department of Emergency Medicine and Addiction Psychiatry
VA Northern California Healthcare System
Mather, California

Carolyn A. Chan, MD, MHS
Assistant Professor of Medicine
Department of Psychiatry and Behavioral Neuroscience, Department of Internal Medicine
University of Cincinnati College of Medicine
Cincinnati, Ohio

Alyssa Cheng, DO
Addiction medicine Fellow
Department of Internal Medicine
Yale School of Medicine
New Haven, Connecticut

Julie W. Childers, MD, MS, FAAHPM, FASAM
Professor of Medicine
Section of Palliative Care and Medical Ethics
Division of General Internal Medicine
Department of Medicine
University of Pittsburgh School of Medicine and University of Pittsburgh Medical Center
Pittsburgh, Pennsylvania

Shawn M. Cohen, MD
Assistant Professor
Department of Internal Medicine
Yale School of Medicine
New Haven, Connecticut

Itai Danovitch, MD
Professor
Department of Psychiatry and Behavioral Neurosciences
Cedars-Sinai Medical Center
Los Angeles, California

Brittany Dennis, MBBS, PhD
Assistant Professor
Department of Medicine
University of British Columbia
Vancouver, British Columbia

Gail D'Onofrio, MD, MS
Albert E. Kent Professor of Emergency Medicine
Department of Emergency Medicine
Department of Public Health
Yale Schools of Medicine and Public Health
New Haven, Connecticut

Honora Englander, MD
Professor of Medicine
Department of Medicine
Oregon Health & Science University
Portland, Oregon

Sarah Follman, MD
Postdoctoral Fellow
Department of Emergency Medicine
Yale School of Medicine
New Haven, Connecticut

Sheria Y. Francis, MSW
Department of Mental Health
Perry Point VA Medical Center
Perry Point, Maryland

O. Trent Hall, DO
Assistant Professor
Department of Psychiatry
The Ohio State University
Columbus, Ohio

Miriam T.H. Harris, MD, MSc
Assistant Professor
Department of Medicine
Boston University Chobanian & Avedisian School of Medicine
Boston Medical Center
Boston, Massachusetts

Erica Heiman, MD
Assistant Professor
Department of Internal Medicine
Yale School of Medicine
New Haven, Connecticut

Andrew Herring, MD
Physician Chief of Addiction Medicine
Emergency Medicine
Highland General Hospital
Oakland, California

Thomas R. Hickey, MD
Assistant Professor
Anesthesiology Department
Yale School of Medicine
New Haven, Connecticut

Stephen Holt, MD, MS
Associate Professor of Medicine
Department of Internal Medicine
Yale School of Medicine
New Haven, Connecticut

Ilana Hull, MD, MSc
Assistant Professor of Medicine
Division of General Internal Medicine
Department of Medicine
University of Pittsburgh School of Medicine and University of Pittsburgh Medical Center
Pittsburgh, Pennsylvania

Michael A. Incze, MD, MSEd
Associate Professor
Internal Medicine
University of Utah
Salt Lake City, Utah

Raagini Jawa, MD, MPH
Assistant Professor of Medicine
Department of Medicine
Center for Research on Healthcare
University of Pittsburgh School of Medicine
Assistant Professor of Public Health
Department of Behavioral and Community Health Sciences
University of Pittsburgh School of Public Health
Pittsburgh, Pennsylvania

Sivabalaji Kaliamurthy, MD
Physician
Department of Psychiatry
Children's National/Howard University
Washington, DC

Ximena A. Levander, MD, MCR
Assistant Professor
Department of Medicine
Oregon Health & Science University
Portland, Oregon

Josh Luftig, PA-C
Co-Founder
BRIDGE
Public Health Institute
Oakland, California

Ethan Manelin, MD, PhD
Assistant Professor
General Internal Medicine
Boston University Chobanian & Avedisian School of Medicine
Boston Medical Center
Boston, Massachusetts

Laura R. Marks, MD, PhD
Assistant Professor
Division of Infectious Diseases
Department of Medicine
Washington University School of Medicine
St. Louis, Missouri

Madeline McCrary, MD
Assistant Professor
Division of Infectious Diseases
Department of Medicine
Washington University School of Medicine
St. Louis, Missouri

Phaedra Moore, BA
Certified Addiction Recovery Coach
Department of Obstetrics and Gynecology
Boston University Chobanian & Avedisian School of Medicine
Boston Medical Center
Boston, Massachusetts

Kenneth L. Morford, MD
Associate Professor of Medicine
Department of Internal Medicine
Yale School of Medicine
New Haven, Connecticut

Reed A. Nerness, MD
Hospice and Palliative Care and Addiction Medicine Fellow
Division of General Internal Medicine
Department of Medicine
University of Pittsburgh Medical Center
Pittsburgh, Pennsylvania

Max Jordan Nguemeni, MD, MS
Assistant Professor in Residence
Department of Medicine
University of California Los Angeles
Los Angeles, California

Linda Peng, MD
Assistant Professor
Department of General Internal Medicine, Section of Addiction Medicine
Oregon Health & Science University
Portland, Oregon

Molly M. Perri, MD, MAT
Assistant Professor
Department of Family and Community Medicine
University of Illinois College of Medicine Rockford
Rockford, Illinois

Alyssa F. Peterkin, MD
Assistant Professor of Medicine
Department of Medicine
Boston University Chobanian & Avedisian School of Medicine
Boston Medical Center
Boston, Massachusetts

Erica Kirsten Rapp, MD
Assistant Professor of Psychiatry
Denver Health Medical Center
Department of Psychiatry
University of Colorado Anschutz Medical Center
Aurora, Colorado

Payel Jhoom Roy, MD, MSc
Associate Professor of Medicine
Division of General Internal Medicine
Department of Medicine
University of Pittsburgh School of Medicine
and University of Pittsburgh Medical Center
Pittsburgh, Pennsylvania

Margaret Shang, MD, MS
Assistant Professor of Medicine and Pediatrics
Division of General Internal Medicine
Department of Medicine
Division of General Academic Pediatrics
Department of Pediatrics
University of Pittsburgh School of Medicine
and University of Pittsburgh Medical Center
Pittsburgh, Pennsylvania

Eleasa Sokolski, MD
Assistant Professor of Medicine and Psychiatry
General Internal Medicine & Geriatrics, Section
of Addiction Medicine
Oregon Health & Science University
Portland, Oregon

Kento Sonoda, MD
Associate Professor
Family and Community Medicine
Saint Louis University
St. Louis, Missouri

Leslie Suen, MD, MAS
Assistant Professor
Department of Medicine
University of California San Francisco
San Francisco, California

Dale Terasaki, MD, MPH
Assistant Professor of Medicine
Department of Behavioral Health Services
Denver Health Medical Center
Denver, Colorado

Ashish P. Thakrar, MD, MS
Assistant Professor
Department of Medicine
University of Pennsylvania
Philadelphia, Pennsylvania

Thida Thant, MD
Assistant Professor of Psychiatry
Department of Psychiatry
University of Colorado Anschutz Medical Center
Aurora, Colorado

Kristine E. Torres-Lockhart, MD
Assistant Professor
Department of Medicine
Montefiore Medical Center
Bronx, New York

Elisha M. Wachman, MD
Professor of Pediatrics
Department of Pediatrics
Boston University Chobanian & Avedisian School
of Medicine
Boston Medical Center
Boston, Massachusetts

Melissa B. Weimer, DO, MCR
Associate Professor of Medicine and Epidemiology;
Medical Director of the Yale Addiction Medicine
Consult Service, Program in Addiction Medicine;
Associate Program Director of the Yale Addiction
Medicine Fellowship Program
Yale School of Medicine
Yale School of Public Health
New Haven, Connecticut

Zoe M. Weinstein, MD, MS
Associate Professor
General Internal Medicine
Boston University Chobanian & Avedisian School
of Medicine
Boston, Massachusetts

Beth Williams, AGNP/WHNP
Assistant Professor of Medicine
Division of General Internal Medicine and
Geriatrics
Oregon Health & Science University
Portland, Oregon

Morgan Zipperly, MD, PhD
Resident Physician
Department of Psychiatry
University of Colorado Anschutz Medical Center
Aurora, Colorado

Preface

It was 2015, 5 weeks after my second child was born, when my colleagues at Oregon Health & Science University (OHSU) and I began conversations about how to improve the care of hospitalized patients with substance use disorders (SUD). I distinctly remember sitting on my porch between breastfeeding and infant napping, feeling very tired, but also incredibly energized about the idea of starting a dedicated addiction medicine consultation service at OHSU. I already provided some specialized addiction treatment in the hospital on an ad hoc basis, and it was clear there was a vast need. Those initial porch conversations turned into formalized plans and the creation of The Improving Addiction Care Team (IMPACT) at OHSU. I didn't appreciate it at the time, but that was also the start of my career path in the field of hospital-based addiction treatment and the inspiration for this book.

I transitioned out of my faculty position at OHSU in 2017 to move closer to family on the east coast. I worked in New York for a brief stint and was then recruited to Yale School of Medicine in the fall of 2018. Despite its preeminence in addiction education and research, Yale had limited clinical resources for patients with SUD in the hospital or ambulatory settings at the time. The large health system and its staff, particularly the hospitalist group, identified SUD as a gaping hole in the hospital-based care they provided. My colleagues at Yale knew of OHSU's successful IMPACT team and wanted a similar consultation service at Yale and Yale New Haven Hospital (YNHH). On November 28, 2018, the Yale Addiction Medicine Consult Service (YAMCS) was officially born and saw its first patient at YNHH's Saint Raphael Campus. Since 2018, YAMCS has treated over 14,000 patients and expanded to the York Street Campus and the YNHH Children's Hospital.

Two successful addiction treatment programs across two health systems are not enough to create the change needed to support the care of all hospitalized patients with SUD, however. My dream is that hospital leaders across the United States understand the importance of this work and support their clinicians to offer evidence-based SUD care to all hospitalized patients who need it. That is why sharing my expertise about designing, implementing, growing, and iterating hospital-based SUD care is so critical. I am thrilled to share this knowledge and experience with you and hope you too will be inspired to do this important work.

Let's not sugar-coat it—providing SUD treatment is not always easy. It can be grueling and frustrating. That is why patient stories ground us in the work and remind us why this hospital-based work is so essential. Each book chapter begins with a narrative story that inspired the chapter authors' work caring for hospitalized patients with SUD. The stories are meant to educate and motivate others who provide this care or who hope to change practice in their own health systems.

I have partnered on this book with Dr Susan Calcaterra, Director of the Addiction Medicine Consultation Service at the University of Colorado Hospital. She is a brilliant colleague and friend who I frequently ask for advice on a range of topics from addiction medicine to parenting. She has been a phenomenal co-editor, and I am so greatly appreciative of her exceptional writing, editing, expertise, and collaboration.

Alexis's Story

To emphasize the positive impact hospital-based SUD care can have on patient's lives, let's hear from Alexis (pseudonym), a former patient of mine, in her own words. She surprised me with an email last year to let me and my team know she was doing well (the absolute best email to receive). I was thrilled to hear of her recovery because I had worried about her prognosis. Alexis had undergone three (!!) open heart surgeries for recurrent infective endocarditis, and the last time I saw her, she was struggling with mental health issues and still using opioids and cocaine. I held my breath when she last discharged from the hospital. The last time I saw her, I hugged her and told her, "please take care of yourself." In the following excerpt, Alexis reflects on her journey of addiction and recovery. I also sat down with her and asked her about her experiences in the hospital. My questions are bolded and her answers are italicized. This expert and our conversation is shared with Alexis's expressed permission.

"During my addiction, I experienced a lot of negativity. But it was nothing out of the ordinary because I experienced that my entire life. My parents were in a toxic relationship where negativity and hate just rolled off of people's tongues. We lived in a two-family house where my grandma and grandpa also lived. My family wasn't the kindest—dreams were shut down and my grandma didn't even speak English so communicating was difficult. But, their apartment was my sanctuary, my escape from my parents' fighting and name calling. Growing up, I started to surround myself with people from similar backgrounds trying to escape the problems in their lives.

I'm sure there are many people who think, "why should I care or show kindness to someone who isn't even kind to themselves?" Maybe because that one, two, or three people who show they care and show kindness to someone who has never received it may instill some hope in them. Because the drugs were never the issue. The issue is that people with substance use disorders are trying to escape from whatever it is they are trying to escape from. They don't show kindness to themselves because they don't know how. It's important for people who feel unlovable to know that they have people who care and love them.

I think the "tough love" thing with parents and family doesn't work because where does tough love leave people? It leaves them on the street with people who don't care or love themselves either... and then more trauma occurs."

Tell me about your experiences being hospitalized for endocarditis and receiving addiction treatment.
I think it's great that you have a specialized team for that. I feel like if there wasn't that, I don't think anybody would know much about addiction [in the hospital]. The kindness that you guys had, and the support, was very helpful. Because... it's more difficult when there's nobody [in the hospital] who cares, you know? It's very helpful that there are specific people who care and who are willing to help. I mean, you guys helped me get my surgeries. I'm sure if it wasn't for you guys, I might not have gotten them. I'm really grateful for that. I wish I was more ready [for recovery] at that time.

It's really hard. It's a tricky question because with the addiction, from my experience, you have to be ready. You guys were so great, but if you're not ready, it doesn't matter. But the love, that definitely helps, the support, and just having somebody in your corner, that definitely helps.

Do you think the support the team offered helped you be more ready or do you think nothing we could have done or said would have helped you?
I think it definitely laid some seed in there. It definitely wasn't my [addiction] ending factor, but it definitely helped me. Because even the breath routine you showed me that time I was in the hospital, you helped me a lot. The fact that I didn't want to let you guys down.

And I think [addiction] is so misunderstood. People think, oh, 'How can you have had endocarditis and just go back out and use?' 'You almost lost your life.' And it's like, maybe I was trying to do that.

Trying to lose your life?
I wasn't trying to like "off" myself, but I think I didn't care. I think it would have been easier for me because it's hard getting clean. I think nobody wants to do it because they have to deal with all the stuff they did and they have to deal with all the trauma... because you have trauma that starts the addiction, right? But then throughout your years of addiction, trauma happens due to the lifestyle you live. Then you create this whole big snowball that just keeps rolling and rolling and you have to literally push it up yourself. It's difficult. And I think that's why a lot of people don't get clean because it's hard.

It's upsetting. You wake up and you're like. 'I wasted all this time, what am I going to do, the world didn't stop?'.

The most difficult part of my experience in the hospital was probably having the judgmental people there, you know, the people who really didn't care that much.

How did you know they didn't care?
Maybe I was just sick. Maybe I was just embarrassed. Who knows? But it was something about the way they interacted with you, it felt judgmental. They were short. They wouldn't really be friendly. I had one [nurse who said], "Oh, you're back here again for the same thing."

Just like they're little things that made me feel that way. But I'm also very sensitive so I analyze everything. I'm an overthinker.

How helpful was it to have a hospital team of people who were supporting you?
They're very helpful because when I was in that situation and I was stuck there, it was actually something to look forward to. It was nice that I knew you guys. I knew that you guys cared and you guys did check up on me. Often it was very helpful, and it made the [hospital] stay a lot easier.

I'm glad to hear our care and our conversations were really helpful. Were there other things about being in the hospital that you remember being helpful?
Yeah. Just like you guys helped me with the buprenorphine... I think for me, like seeing the same people every day that I knew, that was helpful for me. And the [medications], like the buprenorphine, that was helpful for a while, you know, if I stuck with it. But I wasn't ready at the time.

If you were advising a hospital that didn't have any addiction services, what would you say is the most essential thing for them to offer?
I think they should add a team that specializes in addiction for sure. Because if people don't understand [addiction], then they can't help.

I think it's good that you guys can help get people into programs and start medications, like buprenorphine and methadone. If you don't have an addiction team in a hospital, how do they help people with addiction? They're just going to send them out with nothing.

For the surgery, you know, what if there was nobody there? And they just had the doctor making the decision. I know there's one doctor my mom said that doesn't even do second surgeries, I would have been screwed. I think it's very important for there to be people who understand and actually care or know more in detail about [addiction]... because most doctors really don't know. They read books but you guys actually know and do research. You guys put more effort into it. I think that definitely helps.

I think it's a testament to our relationship with you because you reached out and let us know you were doing well after you left the hospital. That means so much to us because sometimes people we see don't get better.
Yeah. Of course, I'll always remember you guys because that was a really tough time in my life, especially after my coma. That was... awful. And just having you guys there helped a lot, definitely. It was honestly one of the only things I looked forward to there. You guys also really talked to me. Our conversations weren't just superficial.

What do you think has been most helpful in your recovery. You talked about feeling like a switch went off, but are there other things that have been helpful to you?
To tell you the truth... I think every little piece that I've gone through in the last few years has been helpful. So, my interactions with you guys. Now, maybe it didn't help me right then, but those little seeds all ended up planting and sprouting eventually.

I definitely hit an emotional, physical, and mental bottom. I was in pain emotionally and physically and that was it. I think everything helped me, you know, having supportive people around me. Having [my boyfriend] who had the same goal as me. But also, seeing siblings struggle made me think, 'wow', like, if I was anywhere like 25% as bad as that, 'What am I doing?'. So, I think a number of things helped.

And I don't think tough love helps either because when you don't have anyone, people end up in the hotels. I've seen it because there is a point where I was getting drugs over there and I saw all these people in the New Haven hotels. They're literally living out there. Like just getting high their whole life. And now, seeing that, it's crazy what it has done [to those people].

A lot of people we're seeing have been struggling for a very long time, have no family support, and have been homeless or unhoused. That's a hard life to dig yourself out of, right?
Because New Haven's got real bad [drugs]. The drugs, they're not even the same anymore. They were destroying my arms. It was getting really bad. I think they need to figure out what they're going to do about the dope thing because a lot of people can't get off the dope right now because it's mixed with tranq (xylazine) and other stuff. And the tranq withdrawal is a lot worse than the dope withdrawal. And methadone doesn't help tranq withdrawal. That's the crazy part.

What are you hearing about tranq withdrawal?
Well, I went through it. I was done after that. I did it two or three times, it was really bad. Your body feels like you have muscle aches everywhere. You have hypertension and you need somebody to rub your back when you're going through it. My boyfriend and I were constantly rubbing each other's back because we were so stiff and you're sick times 100. You're getting the cold sweats, hot sweats. And I'm telling you, methadone does not help. It may take the edge off, maybe 5%. It was so awful. For me, it was double the pain, double the suffering. I think maybe that's a reason why a lot of people don't stay [in the hospital] for detox anymore.

That sounds like an awful experience.
[After using it], I think I'd be asleep for an hour. I don't even remember, but I think it was an hour. And then I would get up, and then you instantly get sick again. It doesn't last long.

So, you're constantly doing it. I was to the point where I was doing it, sleeping, waking up, doing it, sleeping, waking up, doing it. Same, like repeating, repeating. But then your arms get all messed up. You blow out every single vein.

I'm so glad you were able to stop that stuff. Is there anything else you think is important to share about addiction or being treated in the hospital?
I think people need to know about endocarditis. Because I don't think a lot of people know about it. I didn't know about it or what happened to the heart. You can literally not even die from an overdose, you can die from endocarditis. In the beginning it feels like you're dope sick. You don't know until it's too late. It's also very important that hospitals get teams like yours.

It's important that people with addiction have access to care also.
Right. And they should have access to care when they need it. So, if they're in the emergency department or the

hospital, or they show up to a clinic, they should have access to it.

Part of what we're trying to do with the book is to help other hospitals know how to implement addiction services so that people like yourself get started on methadone or other treatments and are showed kindness to "plant those seeds", like you said.
Yeah. Helping people know that they can get better, recognizing that it may not happen right then, and planting those seeds. I think it's really important because that helps the person eventually get better. Maybe like having a team to stay in contact with.

Thank you so much for sharing your experience and story. And it's so wonderful to see you doing so well. And it's important for people in health care to know what's essential for hospital-based addiction care.
And I think... if anything, just be kind. [Clinicians in the hospital] don't have to know how to titrate methadone, but they should know how to be kind.

Understand that people have hardships, and you don't know what caused the addiction, what happened in their life that they want to run away from. People with addiction are just so desperate trying not to feel that they're putting themselves in danger and experiencing more pain.

—Melissa B. Weimer

Acknowledgments

To Dr Martha Wunsch and Dr Ingrid Binswanger, who inspired us to pursue careers in addiction medicine and who have supported us throughout our careers as woman in medicine.

To Dr David Fiellin, a tireless mentor and friend who helped bring the dream of this book to a reality.

To our husbands, our steadfast supporters throughout years of medical training and cross country moves for job opportunities. And to our children, who provide us with a glimpse of a future society that is accepting and kind to all people.

To the contributing authors who generously lent their time and expertise to make this book such a tremendous resource.

To the team at Wolters Kluwer who helped assemble and edit this book from word documents to a beautiful book.

Contents

1

Hospital-Based Substance Use Disorder Treatment

Melissa B. Weimer, Susan L. Calcaterra, Zoe M. Weinstein

In 2010, I had a career-changing experience treating Samantha (pseudonym), a 21-year-old woman with opioid use disorder (OUD) and injection-related infective endocarditis. The experience of caring for Samantha opened my eyes to the flaws in our health care system, especially when caring for people who use substances.

I was working as a general internist in an academic primary care clinic, and I held a once-weekly outpatient clinic to treat patients with substance use disorders (SUD). During my clinic session, I received an urgent call from a hospitalist who asked if I would come to the hospital and see Samantha. The hospitalist explained that Samantha underwent urgent valve surgery for infective endocarditis 2 days earlier and the hospital clinicians were struggling with her postoperative pain management. I didn't usually see patients in the hospital unless I was attending on general medicine wards, but I made an exception for my hospitalist colleague. I could hear in her voice that this was a desperate situation; she felt helpless to improve Samantha's care and treat her postoperative pain. Samantha had been ripping out her chest tubes and threatened to leave the hospital prematurely if her pain was not controlled. I left the clinic to meet with Samantha. I, along with my colleague, quickly adjusted Samantha's opioid pain medication to better control her acute pain and provided medications to ensure she had adequate control of opioid withdrawal as she recovered from her valve-replacement surgery. Once her pain improved, she relaxed and agreed to remain in the hospital to treat her infection.

After many visits consulting with Samantha during her hospitalization, I learned that she ran away from home at the age of 16, was living in a van, and her most trusted allies in life were her two dogs. She developed infective endocarditis from injecting opioids and cocaine and was struggling with OUD for the past 5 years. She had never sought treatment for her OUD and wasn't sure if she wanted it now. Understandably, Samantha was very worried about her dogs. She wanted them to come stay with her in the hospital. Despite efforts from her care team, the hospital would not allow the dogs to stay with her, and 2 weeks after her valve surgery, she left the hospital before completing the antibiotic course for her endocarditis. Despite my concerns about her leaving, she did agree to see me in my outpatient clinic in the coming days after she checked on her dogs. When she presented to clinic 2 days later, I was alarmed to see her looking ill and frail. We talked about reinitiating treatment for OUD, and I offered to facilitate her rehospitalization. She declined my offers for both. Five days later she was rehospitalized in severe septic shock and died within 24 hours.

Samantha changed my career and helped change the health system I worked in. Colleagues and I went on to develop a hospital-based addiction medicine consultation service to support patients like Samantha. Samantha helped me realize that our massive and complex health care system was focused only on "treating the symptoms (ie, infective endocarditis), but not the underlying disease of addiction or substance use disorder (SUD)".[1] We could treat patients with 6 weeks of powerful intravenous antibiotics and perform complex surgeries like valve replacement or valve repair, but unless we addressed the underlying life-threatening chronic medical disease of addiction, our patients wouldn't have the chance to truly recover from their illness and prevent future harms.

Health systems must be able to equally address addiction and complex cardiac valve disease, so our patients have the greatest opportunity to recover. Many of the individuals we treat with SUD and infective endocarditis like Samantha are at the beginning of their lives. As their medical team, we are responsible to give them hope for the future by offering evidence-based therapies, just as we would do for any other patient without SUD. My goal is that all patients with infective endocarditis and other SUD-related medical or surgical conditions in all health care systems are offered lifesaving treatment for both their medical or surgical conditions and their SUD. By doing so, hopefully we can keep Samantha's tragic story from being in vain.

—Melissa B. Weimer

Key Points

- **Substance use disorders (SUD) commonly cause medical and surgical complications that require hospitalization.**
- **The hospital is an essential health care setting to treat SUD.**
- **Untreated SUD leads to poor medical and surgical outcomes, prolonged hospitalization, and increased acute care utilization.**
- **Evidence supports the many benefits of hospital-based SUD treatment, including hospital-initiated medications for SUD treatment.**
- **Hospital-based SUD care is an important clinical treatment that all health systems should adopt.**

Substance use and substance use disorders (SUD) frequently cause concomitant medical and surgical conditions that require emergency care or acute hospitalization. In the United States (US), it is estimated that every 1 in 11 emergency department (ED) visits and every 1 in 9 hospitalizations are related to a SUD and these numbers are potentially higher in some geographic areas of the US.[2] From 2016 to 2021, there were more than 4 million annual ED visits for alcohol-related conditions and 2 million annual visits for opioid-related conditions; there were nearly 2 million annual alcohol-related hospitalizations and 1.4 million annual opioid-related hospitalizations in the same time period (Table 1.1).[3] During this time period, substance-related hospitalizations increased by 47% at US Children's hospitals as well.[4] Clinicians in ED and hospital settings are trained to address the complicated medical and surgical conditions that accompany SUD, but they are generally not trained to address the underlying SUD that led to these problems. Not addressing SUD leads to poor outcomes for patients and health care systems.

Definitions of Substance Use, Unhealthy Substance Use, SUD, and Addiction

When discussing substance use and SUD, it is important to define and differentiate the terms. As illustrated in Figure 1.1, most individuals are abstinent or have "low-risk" use of substances. This means that their substance use has limited, if any, impact on their daily life. Some also describe low-risk substance use

TABLE 1.1

Substance Use and SUD Epidemiology at a Glance[3,5–9]

	Tobacco	Alcohol	Opioids	Cannabis	Stimulants[a]
2023 past year substance use estimates (12 and older)	64.4 million (22.7%)	134.7 million (47.5%)	8.9 million (3.1%)	61.8 million (21.8%)	7.6 million (2.7%)
Prevalence of SUD, % of US population (12 and older)	11.6%	10.2%	2.0%	6.8%	1.0%
Estimated annual deaths	447,751	178,000[b]	84,873[c]	NR	66,169[c]
Estimated annual ED visits	Not Reported (NR)	4,274,523	2,149,474	54.2 per 100,000	12.9 per 100,000
Estimated annual hospitalizations	NR	1,987,498	1,400,019	NR	NR

Data are specific to the US.

[a]Includes methamphetamine and cocaine.

[b]2021 data.

[c]2023 data.

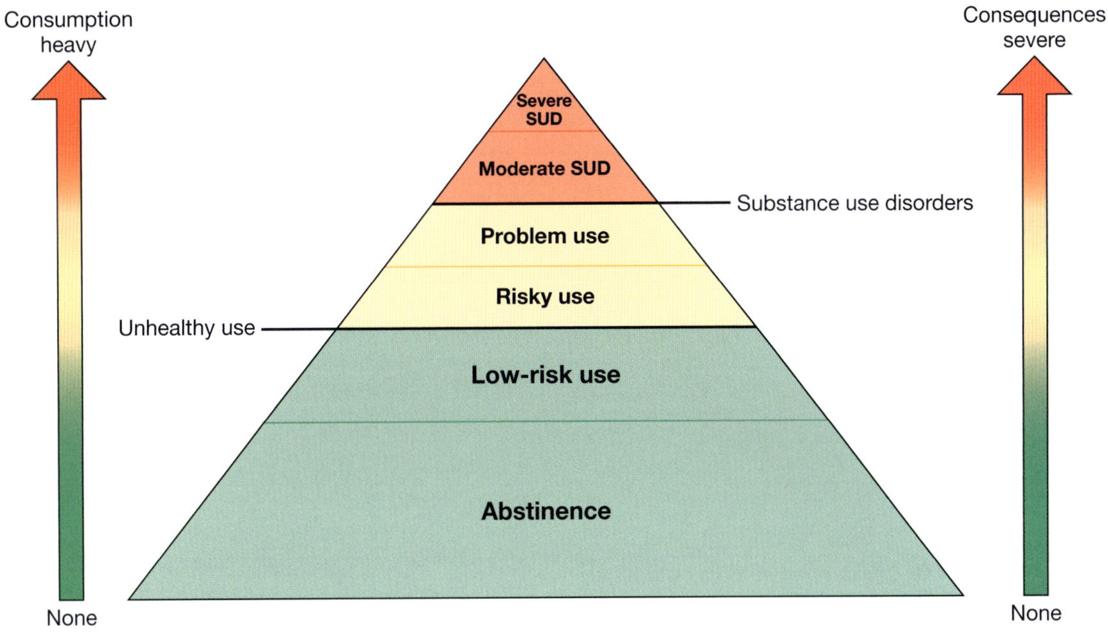

Figure 1.1: Spectrum of substance use.

as "recreational use." Unhealthy substance use affects at least 20% of adults in the general population and more individuals in the hospitalized population.[2] Unhealthy substance use is defined as "any use of alcohol and/or drugs that increases risk of experiencing adverse health consequences, the severity of which generally increases with the amount and frequency of consumption."[10] Unhealthy substance use is inclusive of SUD. For example, while any level of alcohol use has potential to pose health risks, unhealthy alcohol use is defined by the US Health and Human Services Dietary Guidelines for Americans and the National Institute of Alcohol Abuse and Alcoholism as alcohol use that exceeds guideline-recommended limits.[5,10,11] For women aged 21 to 65, the recommended alcohol limit is no more than 3 drinks in a day or 7 drinks in a week.[5,11] For men aged 21 to 65, the recommended alcohol limit is no more than 4 drinks in day or 14 drinks in a week.[5,11] For both men and women over the age of 65, the recommended limit is no more than 3 drinks in a day or 7 drinks in a week.[5,11] Unhealthy substance use for other substances depends on the substance, but in general, any nonprescribed use of substances like opioids, cannabis, tobacco, or stimulants is considered unhealthy.[10] It is generally recognized that as an individual's substance use increases, the social, medical, functional, and psychological consequences related to their substance use also increase.

Terms such as "substance abuse," "substance misuse," "alcoholism," "alcoholic," and "addict" are not clinically accurate terms to describe the medical condition of SUD or people who use substances and should be avoided, both in discussion and in medical documentation. Some patients may continue to use these terms when describing themselves or others, but in clinical settings, clinically accurate terms should be used by clinicians.

In North America, the American Psychiatric Association's Diagnostic and Statistical Manual of Mental Disorders—Fifth Edition ("DSM-5") provides the basis for the diagnosis of SUD.[12] SUD refers to the DSM-5 criteria that are observed in individuals who suffer from the medical disease of addiction.[12] These criteria are divided into four categories: impaired control, social impairment, risky use of substances, and pharmacologic criteria. These 4 categories comprise 11 specific behaviors, signs, and symptoms that occur over a 12-month period in individuals with SUD (Figure 1.2). These identifiable and well-described criteria are the diagnostic basis used to differentiate substance use, unhealthy substance use, and SUD.

Defining and Describing SUD

SUD is categorized by severity levels, from mild to severe, with severity based on the number of symptom criteria endorsed in a 12-month period. Mild SUD refers to the presence of 2 to 3 symptoms; moderate SUD refers to the presence of 4 to 5 symptoms, and severe SUD refers to the presence

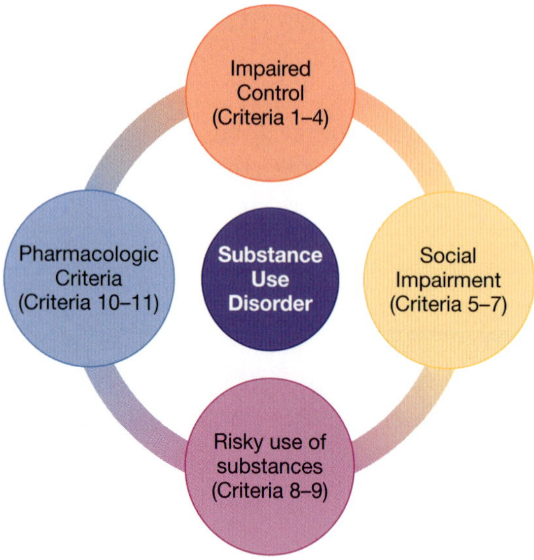

Figure 1.2: The four criteria domains of substance use disorders.[12]

of 6 or more symptoms. As SUD progresses, typically an individual will exhibit more symptoms. OUD refers to a SUD where the disordered substance use is related to an opioid-like morphine, oxycodone, heroin, or nonprescribed high-potency synthetic opioids like fentanyl and fentanyl analogs. SUDs encompass a range of disorders from alcohol use disorder (AUD), tobacco use disorder (TUD), OUD, stimulant use disorder (StUD), benzodiazepine use disorder, and any of the other SUD that cause the symptoms of loss of control of the use of substances, compulsive use of substances, use of substances despite harms, and craving. If an individual has more than one SUD, they would appropriately carry multiple diagnoses for SUD based on their substance use. For example, an individual who uses alcohol, opioids, and stimulants and meets criteria for a SUD in each of these would have all the following diagnoses based on severity of the disorder: AUD, OUD, and StUD. Typically, an individual will be able to identify which one substance is their primary SUD and which are secondary. The term "polysubstance use disorder" is an inaccurate clinical term and should be avoided in clinical documentation.[13]

Defining and Describing Recovery From SUD

The National Institute of Alcohol Abuse and Alcoholism (NIAAA) provides a detailed description of recovery from AUD which may be applied to any other SUD.[14]

Recovery is a process through which an individual pursues both remission from AUD and cessation from heavy drinking. An individual may be considered "recovered" if both remission from AUD and cessation from heavy drinking are achieved and maintained over time. For those experiencing alcohol-related functional impairment and other adverse consequences, recovery is often marked by the fulfillment of basic needs, enhancements in social support and spirituality, and improvements in physical and mental health, quality of life, and other dimensions of well-being. Continued improvement in these domains may, in turn, promote sustained recovery.[14]

In this description, recovery from AUD is not one size fits all and can involve any of the following: complete cessation of alcohol, cessation from heavy use of alcohol, and/or improvements in social, functional, physical, and mental health. This is important because it acknowledges that cessation from substances alone is not the only indicator for recovery from a SUD and some individuals can maintain SUD recovery with low quantity use of substances.

Remission is another term used to describe recovery from SUD and is the descriptive term used in the DSM-5.[12] In the context of SUD, remission means that the patient no longer meets the prior DSM-5 criteria for that SUD. Remission is further categorized based on its duration: "early remission" (3 months to 12 months) and "sustained remission" (12 months or longer). The DSM-5 defines "early remission" as the period of time "after full criteria for [SUD] were previously met, none of the criteria for [SUD] have been met for at least 3 months but for less than 12 months (with the exception that [craving] may be met)."[12] The DSM-5 defines "sustained remission" as the period of time "after full criteria for [SUD] were previously met, none of the criteria for [SUD] have been met any time during a period of 12 months or longer (with the exception that [craving] may be met)."[12] Whenever possible, it is important to include these qualifiers when caring for patients with SUD, not only to recognize and acknowledge the person's recovery and/or remission, but to ensure that the most clinically accurate medical diagnosis is documented in the medical chart.

Distinguishing Addiction and SUD

Addiction is a distinctly different term than SUD and is very commonly used by medical professionals and lay people. In general, it is used to describe more severe forms of SUD. It is not included in the DSM-5 due to its "potentially negative connotation."[12] In this book, the term SUD will be used, but understanding how SUD relates to addiction is important.

Addiction is formally defined by the American Society of Addiction Medicine (ASAM), the leading professional organization representing addiction medicine health professionals, as a medical disease.[15]

American Society of Addiction Medicine

Definition of Addiction[15]

"Addiction is a treatable, chronic medical disease involving complex interactions among brain circuits, genetics, the environment, and an individual's life experiences. People with addiction use substances or engage in behaviors that become compulsive and often continue despite harmful consequences. Prevention efforts and treatment approaches for addiction are generally as successful as those for other chronic diseases."

Addiction is a medical disease that affects the brain reward systems including three central parts of the brain: the basal ganglia involving pathologic habits, the extended amygdala involving negative emotional states, and the prefrontal cortex involving dysfunction in executive function and decision making (Figure 1.3).[16,17] Neurobiologic changes occur in the brains of individuals with addiction and SUD that correlate to the behaviors that are characteristic of SUD such as compulsive use of substances, loss of control of substance use, use of substances despite harms, and substance craving.[16] It is important to note that individuals can develop non–substance involved use disorders as well, including pathologic gambling, food, internet, and sex.[18] In order for a substance or an activity to develop into a use disorder, the behavior must produce a reinforcing stimulus that leads to repetitive and harmful behaviors over time.[19] With cessation of the activity, or substance used, there is a concomitant withdrawal period with cravings and physical symptoms, which are diminished, or fully resolve, with resumption of the activity or substance used.

Brain imaging studies of people with SUD demonstrate characteristic differences compared to people without SUD. Brain circuitry changes of people with SUD progress over time and are observed using functional magnetic resonance imaging (fMRI).[20] fMRI studies show a reduction in activity of dopamine receptors in the brains of people with SUD. Importantly, changes in dopamine receptor activity can remit when people enter into remission via processes like neuroplasticity.[21] As an example, with OUD, regular use of opioids generates intense reactivity to opioid-conditioned cues while also producing tolerance and withdrawal symptoms, hyperalgesia (increased pain), hyperkatifeia (increased sensitivity to negative emotions), and dysphoria.[16] The peak stage of opioid withdrawal depends on the type of opioid used and its associated half-life, that is, oxycodone, where symptoms peak between 1 and 3 days from cessation of use and may last up to a week, versus methadone, where symptoms may not peak until 36 hours after last use and persist up to 14 days or more. In contrast, the experience of postacute withdrawal describes the period of neuroplasticity where dopamine receptors slowly upregulate in response to a dopamine deficit following

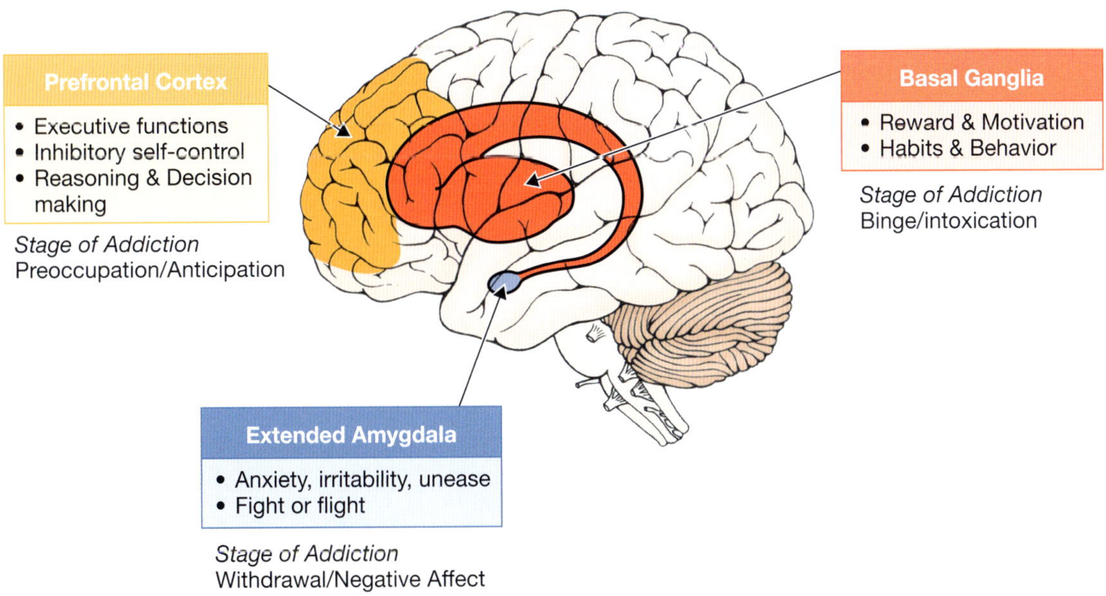

Figure 1.3: Brain regions affected by addiction.

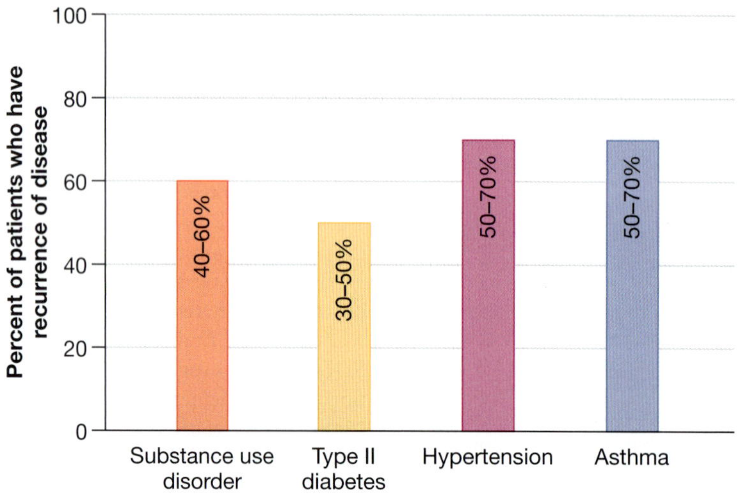

Figure 1.4: The chronic medical disease of SUD compared to other chronic diseases.

cessation of substance use. During the postacute withdrawal period, physical withdrawal symptoms may not be noticeable on physical examination, but patients may report experiencing agitation, depression, poor sleep, and irritability.[22] Supporting patients throughout this period is important to reduce the risk of a return to substance use.

Just like other chronic medical conditions (eg, diabetes, hypertension, and asthma), individuals with SUD can have symptoms of their disease reemerge if treatment is discontinued (Figure 1.4).[23] Unfortunately, some SUD, such as OUD, can be fatal with return to opioid use; therefore, initiation and retention in medication treatment of SUD is vitally important to address this chronic condition.

Risk Factors for SUD Development

People with SUDs have multiple risk factors for the development of SUD, including genetic, biologic, and environmental influences.[16,24,25] One of the greatest risk factors is genetic risk.[16] Other risk factors include male gender, use of any substance, including tobacco in adolescence, mental health conditions, adverse childhood experiences, reduced access to resources like food, shelter and safety, lack of economic opportunity, and social isolation.[16,24,25] In addition, "those whose initial, physiologic responses to alcohol or other drugs are extremely pleasurable will be more likely to repeat the (substance) taking than those whose reaction is neutral or negative."[23] Protective factors against the development of a SUD include education, employment, access to housing, and access to mental health services.[25] Primary prevention efforts like age limits on alcohol and tobacco, sales taxes on alcohol and tobacco, advertising regulations, early intervention programs, education, and drug-free school policies, among others in adolescence are also effective to reduce people's risk of SUD development.[26]

Prevalence of SUD and SUD-Related Mortality in North America

Prevalence of SUD

Worldwide, tobacco, alcohol, cannabis, and stimulants are the four most prevalent substances used.[27] In North America, opioids are more commonly used than stimulants relative to other countries. The higher prevalence of opioid use in North America is related to well-described efforts by pharmaceutical companies to increase the prescription use of opioids in the early 1990s.[28]

In the US, the prevalence of each SUD was historically estimated by the National Survey of Drug Use and Health (NSDUH) which was led by the US Substance Abuse and Mental Health Services Administration (SAMHSA) (Table 1.1).[6] NSDUH was administered to 70,000 randomly selected individuals (aged 12 and older) in the US who agreed to participate in face-to-face or web-based interviews. NSDUH does not include individuals who are not housed or who are incarcerated, therefore it likely underestimates population-based estimates of substance use and SUD. NSDUH asked participants to identify which, if any, of the DSM-5 criteria they experienced during the preceding 12 months. In 2023, 70.5 million people (24.9% of the included population) reported past year use of substances like cannabis, opioids, and cocaine and 48.5 million people (17.1% of the included population) aged 12 or older met criteria for SUD in the past year.[6] NSDUH reports that the most prevalent SUD is TUD, followed by AUD. As many as 64.4 million people report use of tobacco or nicotine products in the past month and 28.9 million people met criteria for AUD in 2023.[6] After tobacco and alcohol, cannabis is the third most commonly used substance both in the US and internationally.[29] Opioids are the fourth most commonly used substance in the US and is reported in 8.9 million people 12 and older: 96.4% related to prescription opioid use and 7.4% related to heroin.[6]

In Canada, the Canadian Substance Use Survey (CSUS) is a biennial survey of Canadians 15 years of age and older. Individuals are recruited by telephone, and youth aged 15 to 19 are offered an incentive for survey completion. In 2023, alcohol and cannabis were the most commonly reported substances used. Heavy alcohol use was reported in 18% of people aged 12 years and older.[30] Opioid use and OUD is also a problem in Canada. There were nearly 51,000 opioid-related deaths in Canada from January 2016 to September 2024.[31]

In Mexico, statistics about SUD are limited.[32] Data from 2008 estimated that 5.5% of the population of people aged 12 to 65 met criteria for AUD, and 0.6% of the population met criteria for "dependence on illicit drugs."[33] Tobacco, cocaine, and cannabis are also widely used in Mexico.[32] Estimates of OUD in Mexico are not reported.[34] Treatment options for SUD are limited in Mexico, and additional statistics are not reported.[34]

SUD-Related Mortality

Other data sources, such as the Centers for Disease Control, capture mortality risks related to substance use in the US (Table 1.1). Tobacco and alcohol are in the top three leading causes of preventable death in the US. From 2020 to 2021, over 178,000 individuals died from alcohol-related causes, which is more than the number of individuals who die from stroke each year.[35] According to data from the US National Center for Health Statistics, overdose deaths related to opioids were as high as 114,000 individuals per year in 2023.[36] More recently, reported opioid overdose deaths are declining.[37] This may be attributed to increased access to naloxone for opioid overdose, greater access to evidence-based treatment, and shifts in the substance supply.[37]

In Canada, alcohol accounts for 15,000 deaths every year.[38] In 2024, nearly 3,800 Canadians died of apparent opioid toxicity (an 11% decrease from 2023), and opioid overdose deaths are highest in British Columbia, Alberta, and Ontario.[31]

A recent study of over 500,000 individuals reported that the adjusted risk of death within 5 years of an ED visit or hospitalization is 30% higher for individuals with AUD, 69% higher for individuals with StUD, 180% higher for individuals with cannabis use disorder, and 118% higher for individuals with OUD.[29]

Prevalence of SUD in the Hospitalized Population

Morbidity and mortality related to substance use and SUD are high compared to other medical conditions, and many individuals with SUD will develop acute medical and surgical conditions that require emergency care or hospital interventions. National estimates of substance-related ED and hospitalizations in the US show relative increases by 30% to 60% over the last 20 years in parallel with increases in US alcohol, opioid, and stimulant-related deaths.[2] Increases have been reported by multiple data sources and publications in all types of substance-related hospital admissions such as alcohol withdrawal, opioid overdose and its complications, trauma related to substance intoxication, infectious endocarditis related to substance use, and stimulant-related cardiac conditions.[3,39–43]

However, alcohol-related hospitalizations drive the majority of acute care utilization in North America. They are approximately 1.5 to 2 times more prevalent than opioid-related hospitalizations in the US and 13 times more prevalent than opioid-related hospitalizations in Canada.[43] In Canada, from 2015 to 2016 there were 77,000 hospitalizations related to alcohol and 45,707 opioid-related overdose hospitalizations from 2016 to 2024. There were more than 187,000 opioid-related ED visits from 2016 to 2024.[31]

It is estimated that from 2014 to 2018, at least 12% of US hospitalizations involved SUD. Some studies report that rates of hospitalizations related to AUD range as high as 19% to 50% and rates of other SUD are 12% to 15%.[44–46] Looking at specific SUD-related conditions, infectious endocarditis related to substance use doubled in incidence from 48 per 10,000 in 2002 to 79 per 10,000 people in 2016.[47] Most hospitals recognize SUD as a "top 5 priority" in their communities on their Community Health Needs Assessment. The Community Health Needs Assessment is a federally required survey that nonprofit hospitals must complete every 3 years to assess the health needs of their communities by gathering input from people who represent broad interests in their communities.[2,48,49]

Characteristics of People Hospitalized With SUD-Related Conditions

SUD-related acute care encounters, including ED encounters and hospitalizations, are more common among men, those experiencing homelessness, and those with Medicaid insurance.[2] SUD-related hospitalizations that involve injury or trauma, overdose or poisoning, and nonpsychiatric mental health evaluation appear to be the most common.[2] Interestingly, frequency of SUD-related ED visits and hospitalizations do not significantly differ between safety-net and non–safety-net settings, indicating that SUD affects all populations.[2] SUD-related hospitalizations can also have longer hospital stays, higher costs, and people with past SUD-related acute care encounters are more likely to be rehospitalized, compared to people without a SUD-related acute care encounter.[44] People with a past SUD-related hospitalization are also at an increased risk of death within 5 years of their hospital discharge.

Cost of SUD-Related Care

Total annual estimated spending on SUD-related medical costs in US hospitals range from $13.2 to 30 billion/year.[50,51] Canadian estimates are as high as $40 billion/year.[38]

In the US in 2020, 36% of Medicaid substance use medical claims were related to alcohol, accounting for more than $129 million in health care dollars spent. One study found that having an AUD, for example, increased health care costs by nearly $15,000 per year per person. Because alcohol-related hospitalizations are more frequent than other SUD-related hospitalizations, they account for the costliest SUD-related ED or hospital care compared to other commonly used substances. In 2017, mental health and SUD-related ED costs were $5.6 million dollars and alcohol-related diagnoses accounted for 22% of these costs. Individuals aged 18 to 64 years old with Medicaid insurance coverage contributed to the highest costs compared to individuals with other types of insurance.[52]

Why Hospitals Should Address and Offer SUD Treatment

As stated before, SUD are medical conditions like mental illness, diabetes, heart disease, and hypertension. Just like other medical conditions, there are certain innate factors that increase risk for the development of these conditions and personal choice can also contribute to the development and treatment of these diseases. The conflict surrounding the conceptualization of SUD as a medical disease versus a moral failing based on poor individual choices is summarized here by Dr Yngvild Olsen, MD, Former Director for the Center for Substance Abuse Treatment at SAMHSA.

"Some dispute the concept of addiction as a disease, pointing to a lack of autonomy and free will perceived as inherent in this framing. At its core, some of the concerns involve the idea of disease itself. Addiction medicine specialists understand that not everyone who uses a substance has a disease. Modern society understands that disease is not just the opposite or absence of health. Importantly, disease definitions do not necessarily equate with full disability, complete loss or lack of individual responsibility or choice, or necessarily purely biologically focused approaches. For some, concepts of disease, spirituality, and religion can, and do, coexist, whether the disease in question is addiction, diabetes, end-stage renal disease, or heart disease. For a person with a chronic disease, accepting, managing, and learning to live with, and despite, their illness requires making choices and acting on one's own behalf. Acknowledging the existence of different viewpoints, an analysis of current definitions of disease finds common criteria: identifiable, characteristic set of signs and symptoms; interruption, cessation, or disorder of a body part, system, or organ structure or function; cause and pathology may be known or unknown and may involve several variables including infection, inflammation, environmental factors, genetics. Current scientific understanding of addiction meets the criteria for disease."[17]

(Reprinted from Olsen Y, with permission from Elsevier.)

The understanding that SUD is a medical disease makes clear the fundamental position that health systems should address and treat it. A decision not to address or treat SUD would be akin to some hospitals choosing not to treat or offer standard medical care to patients who present with hyperglycemia related to diabetes or acute myocardial infarctions related to heart disease. In addition, because the risk of death increases significantly for individuals with SUD who require hospital-based care, hospital-based interventions are necessary to help reduce overall morbidity and mortality related to SUD.[29,53]

SUD is also considered a "disability" by the Americans with Disability Act (ADA) and Rehabilitation Act of 1973.[54] This means that individuals with SUD may not be legally denied medical care based on their disability or use of substances.[54] This legal protection means that withholding certain types of medical care such as screening for unhealthy substance use or providing medications treatments for individuals with SUD could be deemed discriminatory.[54]

Despite these understanding, as well as the recognition that SUD is a "top 5" community need and is a "top 5" contributor to preventable death in the US,

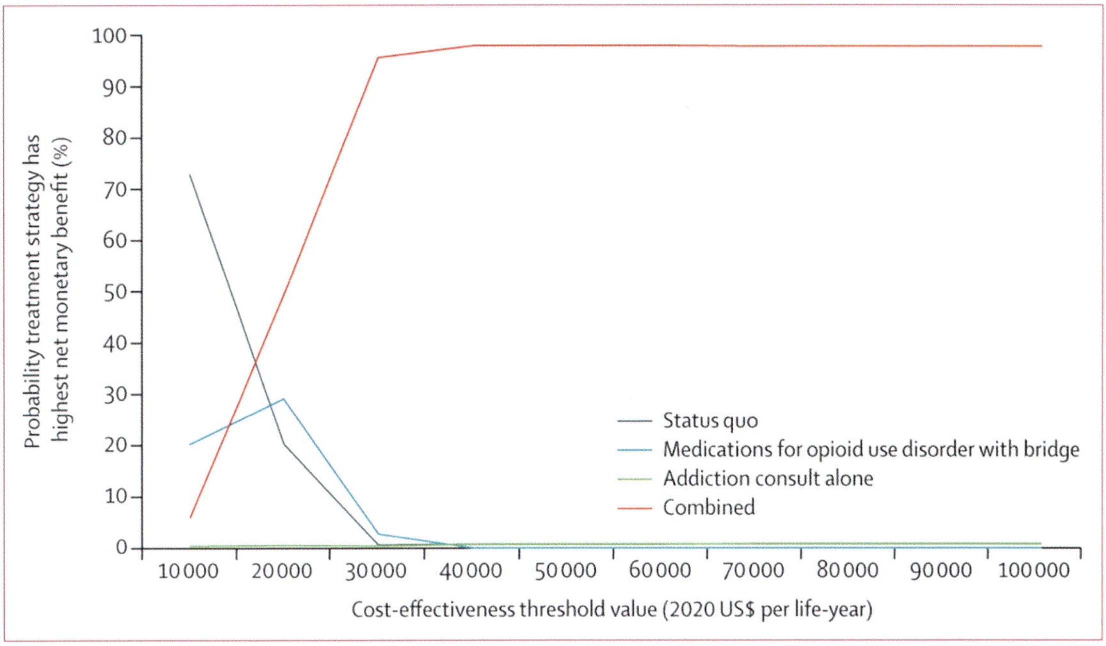

Figure 1.5: Cost effectiveness for hospital-based SUD care. Probabilistic sensitivity analysis of hospital-based SUD care showing that a combined strategy of addiction consultation services and medication treatments reduce overall costs and has a cost-effectiveness threshold of $30,000 per life-year.[57] (© Elsevier.)

health systems have many competing demands for resources. Addressing and treating SUD is not likely to create large profits for health systems, but it is a part of a commitment to their larger mission to serve their communities. Addressing and treating SUD may also offset negative financial impacts historically associated with providing care to hospitalized people who use substances, including longer length of stay, higher readmissions, poorer patient experience, care quality gaps, and staff burnout.[55–57] Cost-effectiveness studies have modeled potential cost savings and life-years gains when hospital-based SUD care services that combine medication treatment and consultation services are provided and have shown these interventions to be cost effective (Figure 1.5).[57]

The idea of hospital-based SUD care may be novel to many health systems. System-specific barriers and facilitators will determine how easily hospital-based SUD care is integrated into the health system. Qualitative research has identified six themes of hospital settings that either promoted or inhibited the development and implementation of addiction consultation services as an example: "stigma and discrimination towards patients with SUD; support from internal (eg, hospital administrators) and external stakeholders; workforce and institutional culture; access to community-based treatment programs (eg, local opioid treatment programs); SUD treatment policies (restrictive or permissive); and financing."[58] The authors noted that "stigma and discrimination is presented as a stand-alone-theme but permeates the five other themes as a broader meta-theme."[58] The authors proposed ways to address these barriers and facilitators to promote the integration of SUD treatment into hospital settings (Figure 1.6) (see Chapter 2).

Current Prevalence of SUD Treatment in Hospital Settings

Despite the high prevalence of SUD-related hospitalizations and high health care costs, few hospitals or health care systems provide direct, hospital-based SUD initiation and treatment services.[59] There could be many reasons for this including fundamental misunderstandings about SUD and its treatment, institutional culture regarding SUD treatment, lack of staffing or SUD treatment workforce, lack of financial resources, misunderstanding about federal or state policies for addiction treatment, or lack of awareness of the importance to prevent future harm.[58] Failure to provide these treatments represents a tremendous missed opportunity and leads to worse patient outcomes compared to hospitals that offer SUD treatment.[57,60] Studies show that in hospitals without integrated SUD treatment, patients are more likely to have untreated substance withdrawal, disruptive behavior, failure to complete medical treatments,

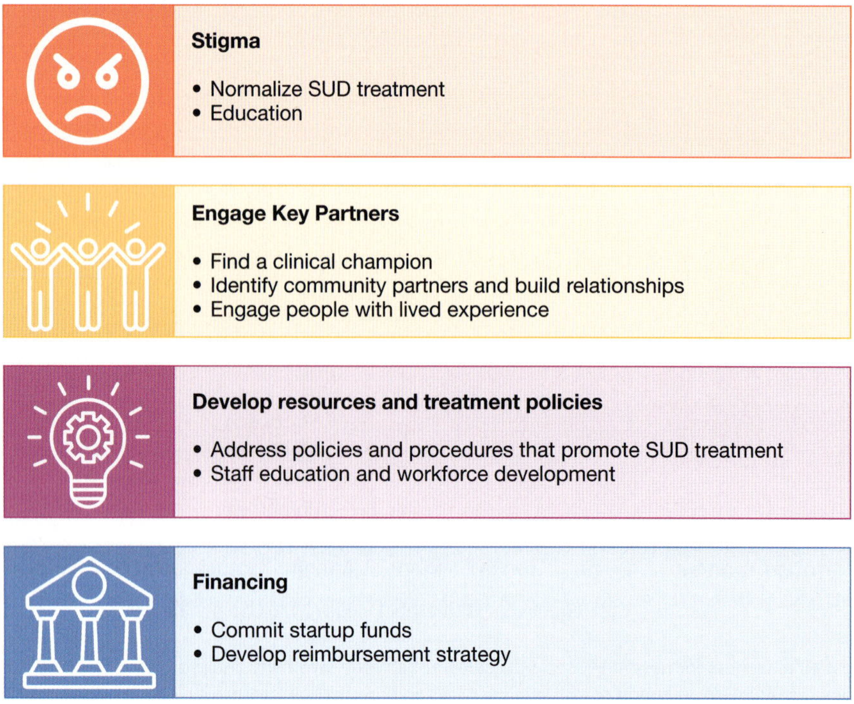

Figure 1.6: Barriers and facilitators for integrating addiction treatment into hospital settings.

leave the hospital prematurely, and have poor overall experiences.[56] Untreated SUD can also cause moral distress and burnout in the clinicians caring for individuals with SUD.[56]

The American Hospital Association (AHA) Annual Survey of Hospitals from 2021 provides the best current estimate of SUD services in hospitals in the US.[59] Out of 6,201 US hospitals, 2,846 (46%) completed the survey. Of the few hospitals that responded to the survey, 67% reported providing SUD screening in the hospital setting and 74% in the ED; 65% reported screening in both settings (Figure 1.7).[59] Fewer respondents reported having an addiction consultation service in their hospital setting (46%) and in their ED setting (34%). Forty-four percent of respondents reported that their hospitals offered addiction consultation services in both the hospital and ED settings.[59] In the survey, the AHA did not provide a definition of an addiction consultation service, nor did they include a description of the services commonly offered by an addiction consultation service. Thus, survey results may over- or underestimate SUD treatment provision across US community hospitals. For example, while 46% of respondents reported that their hospitals provided SUD treatment services, only 37% of respondents reported that their hospitals offered medications for SUD treatment, a well-recognized and essential medical treatment offered by an addiction consultation service.[59] Survey results identified that provision of hospital-based SUD services were higher in metropolitan areas in the northeastern US regions and in hospitals with over 400 beds.[59] Hospital-based SUD services were lowest in the southern US regions, in rural areas, and in areas with a higher proportion of Black individuals.[59] These results are consistent with a study that shows some hospitals have been both prioritizing and implementing hospital-based SUD care from 2015 to 2021 across the US.[48]

Similar data describing community hospital SUD treatment provision in Canada and Mexico are not regularly reported. However, the growth and implementation of hospital-based SUD consultation services across Canadian hospitals are well characterized.[61,62]

In summary, it appears that most hospitals recognize a need to identify unhealthy substance use and SUD and there is a large opportunity for many more hospitals to invest in the resources to adequately address and offer effective SUD treatment.

Hospital-Based SUD Treatment Is Part of the SUD Care Continuum

Treating SUD in the hospital setting was first described in 1976 by Dr Marc Galanter. Dr Galanter established the addiction consultation service at the Bronx Municipal Hospital Center, the principal

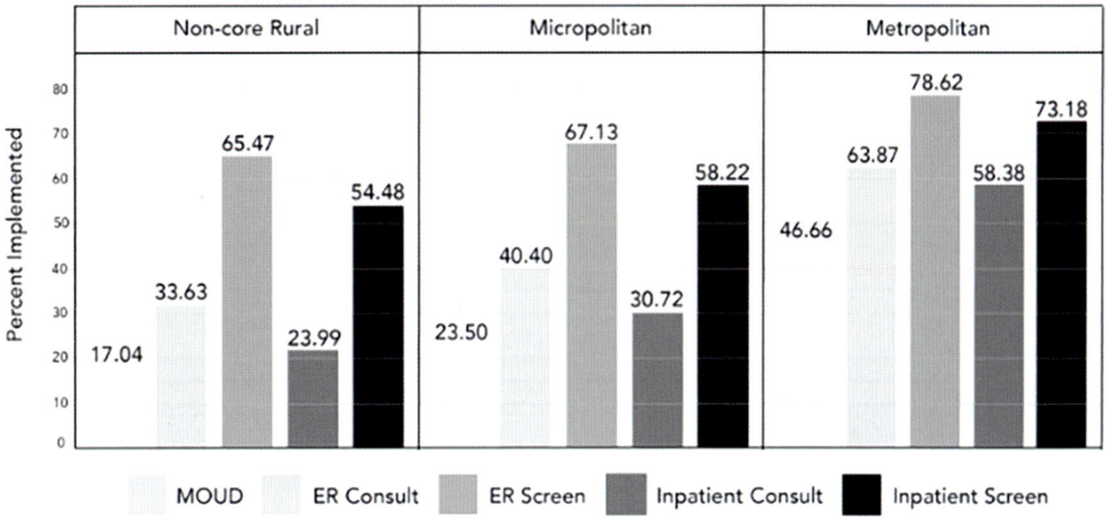

Figure 1.7: Percentage of hospital and ED-based SUD services by type of service provided. (Reprinted from Franz B, Cronin CE, Lindenfeld Z, et al. Rural-urban disparities in the availability of hospital-based screening, medications for opioid use disorder, and addiction consult services. *J Subst Use Addict Treat*. 2024;160:209280, with permission from Elsevier.)

teaching hospital of the Albert Einstein College of Medicine.[63] He recognized that people access care in multiple health care settings, like outpatient clinics, EDs, and medical specialty clinics, among others. Identifying and treating SUD across all health care settings is important to make SUD treatment more accessible and benefit the most people with SUD (Figure 1.8).

Since the 1980s, ASAM has included the hospital setting as a key level of care in the ASAM Criteria, the set of standards and treatment settings for SUD.[64] The "medically managed inpatient care" known as

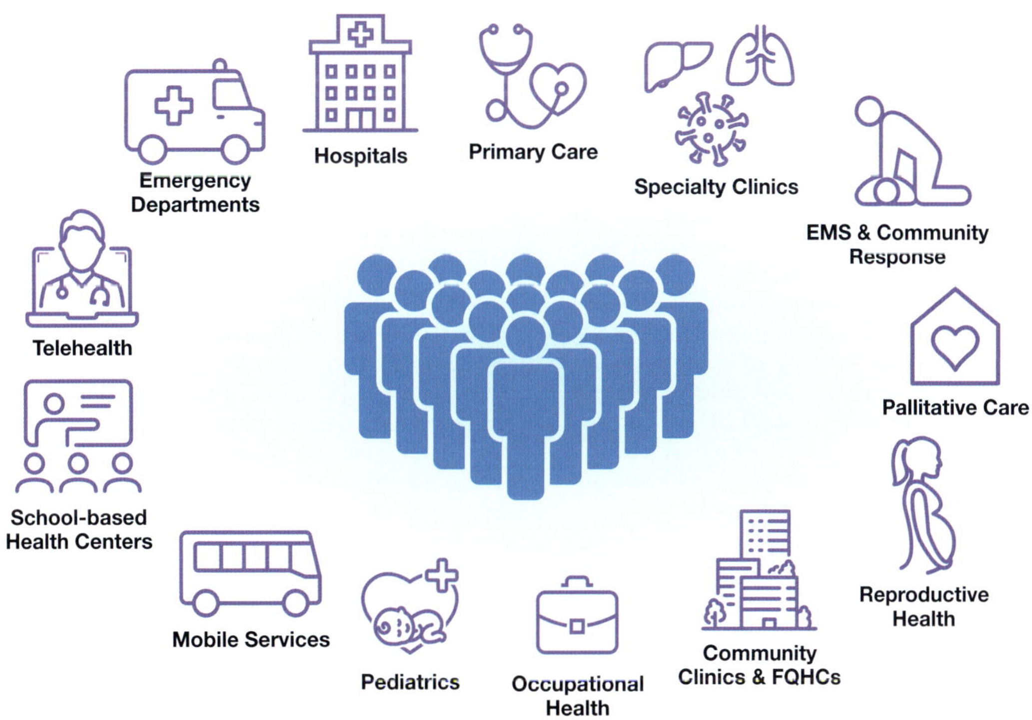

Figure 1.8: Various medical settings where people may access SUD treatment.

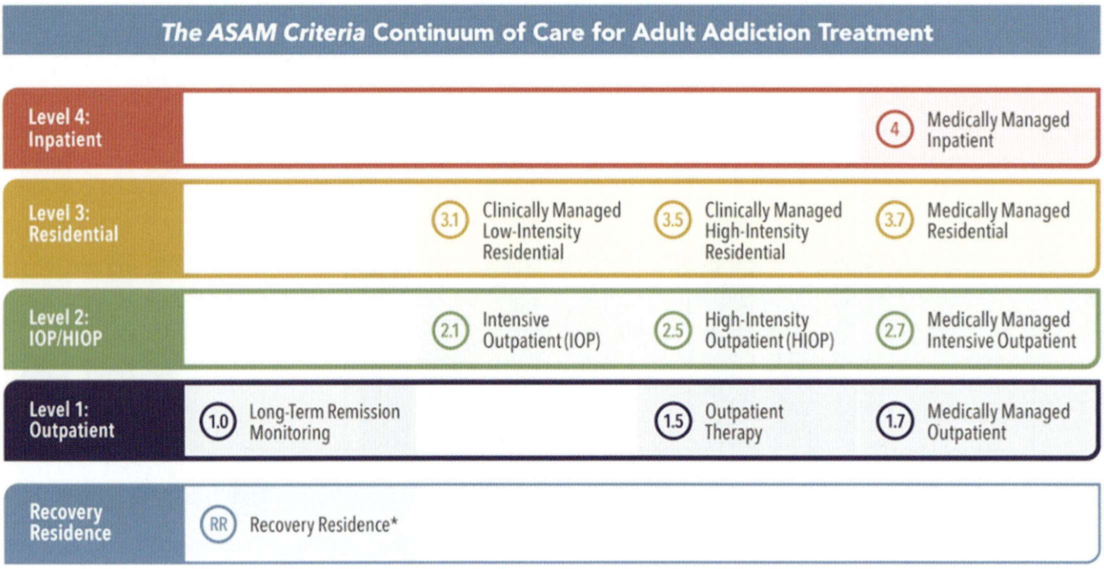

Figure 1.9: ASAM addiction specialty levels of care for adults.[64]

"Level 4" is the highest level of SUD treatment in the ASAM Criteria.[64] ASAM recognizes that people with high biomedical and social needs may require hospital-based SUD care for withdrawal management and initiation of treatment and these services may not be feasible in lower levels of SUD care (Figure 1.9).[64] Unlike ambulatory settings, hospitals are always open and are required by federal laws such as the Emergency Medical Treatment and Labor Act (EMTALA) to evaluate every individual who presents to the hospital regardless of their ability to pay for services.[65] In some communities, it may be easier for patients to access hospital-based services than primary care or specialty care, particularly if the person lacks insurance coverage, or if they have other barriers to care such as a lack of transportation, language barriers, or physical or invisible disabilities. Hospitals have 24 hours of continuous nursing care, daily physician care, and are equipped with advanced medical and surgical interventions, specialty services, and multidisciplinary teams to address acute illness and medical complexity. The close medical observation and environmental safety provided by hospital staff and clinicians are beneficial to individuals with complex medical, mental health, and social needs.

Models of Hospital-Based SUD Care

Over the last 50 years, health systems have developed innovative approaches ranging from simple to complex to address SUD in the hospital and facilitate postdischarge SUD treatment (see Chapter 4).[66,67] Integrated hospital-based SUD treatment services could include different models of care such as the following:

- Universal screening for all individuals presenting to the ED or hospital, followed by treatment initiation for individuals who screen positive
- Consultation models provided by addiction-specific consultation services
- Psychiatry consultation liaison services or individual consultants
- Practice-based models such as SUD treatment provided by general hospital staff
- In-reach SUD consultation models that are community based
- Integrated care pathways for SUD treatment guidance that is provided by hospital clinicians
- Transitional SUD-focused services to connect to ongoing SUD treatment[44,66]

Of the models mentioned, hospital-based SUD care by addiction consultation services have emerged as a robust and effective resource for both patients and hospitals to address the complex needs of hospitalized individuals with SUD. Addiction consultation services are like other specialty consultative services like cardiology or nephrology services. They vary in their service composition, operations, service availability, and financing, but like other specialty consultative services, physician specialty expertise is a core component. For addiction consultation services, physician expertise is generally provided by board-certified addiction medicine, addiction psychiatry, or psychiatry physicians, though other specialties like internal medicine, family medicine, emergency medicine, toxicology, anesthesia, and palliative care may also be involved, depending on their level of experience. Access to specialty physicians is recognized as an essential part of hospital care provision due to the complexity of medical and surgical conditions related to different disease states or organ systems among hospitalized patients. This is true of SUD as well. Other addiction consultation service team members may include advanced practice providers (APPs), nurses, social workers or psychologists, drug and alcohol counselors, case managers, trainees, pharmacists, and peer recovery mentors. The availability and scope of care provided by the addiction consultation service will also vary, though having a broad scope of practice, flexibility, and high accessibility can help make the consultation service successful. Chapter 4 provides greater detail about hospital-based SUD models of care and their specific components. Chapter 6 describes ED-based SUD treatment care models.

Building processes to support hospital-to-community SUD treatment linkage is an essential part of the SUD care continuum. A systematic review of care transition programs and practices identified 45 studies with different models of ED or hospital-based SUD transitional programs.[67] The majority of programs (62%) were developed and implemented in the ED and 44% of programs were developed and implemented in the hospital setting.[67] The most common strategy to address transitions of care was scheduling an appointment with a community-based treatment provider prior to discharge.[67] Chapter 20 describes best practices in hospital-to-community care transitions for people with SUD.

Regardless of the model of care and transition of care design, successful integration of hospital-based SUD care can be challenging. Having a dedicated clinical champion who has protected time, passion, and dedication can help the work of integration succeed.[68] See Chapter 2 for more information about implementation and Chapter 3 about essential components of hospital-based SUD care.

Patients' Perspective on Hospitalization

Hospitalization is challenging for all individuals, but particularly for individuals who use alcohol and/or other substances, many of whom may not come to the hospital seeking SUD treatment. Hospitalized patients with SUD may fear that their substance withdrawal and pain may be inadequately treated and that their complaints may be overlooked by their medical team. This can lead to patients considering premature discharge and not completing necessary medical and surgical treatments. A qualitative study by Velez et al, of hospitalized patients with SUD identified themes describing patient-, clinician-, and health-system factors experienced by hospitalized people who use substances (Figure 1.10). Identified

Patient-Related Factors

- Hospitalization is a wake-up call
- Mortality is motivating
- Hospitalization interupts a cycle of drug use
- Cravings and pain complicate medical care

Clinician and Hospital Staff-Related Factors

- Being involved in treatment decisions (patient-centered care)
- Having a clinicial who understands SUD and associated treatments
- Being treated nonjudgmentally and with compassion
- Being offered appropriate and effective withdrawal management

Limitations of the Health Care System

- Hospitalization does not address life stressors and trauma
- Hositalization does not adress basic needs
- Greater need for coordinated and timely SUD care after discharge

Benefits of the Health Care System

- Great value in having peers (people with lived experience) in the hospital
- Low barrier access ot medication treatment

Figure 1.10: Emergent themes related to the experience of hospitalizations among people who use substances.[69]

patient factors included "hospitalization serves as a wake-up call, mortality is motivating, hospitalization interrupts drug use, overpowering compulsion to use [substances], and pain complicates care." Identified clinician-level factors included: "the importance of choice (patient-centered treatment options), clinician understanding of SUD is important, importance of caring and nonjudgmental staff, importance of effective withdrawal management; health system-level factors: hospitalization does not address life stressors and trauma, hospitalization does not address basic needs, value of peers in the hospital setting, access to medication [treatment]; and need for coordinated, timely care after discharge."[69] One specific patient quote from the study states:

> *"I wish I didn't put myself in the predicament of coming to the hospital so much. It's been an experience, a life learning experience. Coming here so much has helped me notice and realize to wake up. It's time to stop doing what I'm doing, to get to the sober and clean path."*[69]

In sum, this study describes the complexity of caring for people with SUD in the hospital setting as well as the importance of addressing pain, substance withdrawal, substance craving, and doing so with compassion and evidence-based treatment. This can be a tall order for clinicians who may not have received dedicated training in addiction medicine in their medical or postgraduate training. Therefore, building this capacity via expert clinical staff or a dedicated team can greatly facilitate the integration of effective hospital-based SUD care.

Communication That Promotes Effective Hospital-Based SUD Care

"Patients emphasized the need for clear, reliable, and frequent communication from health care [clinicians], valuing collaborative dialogue, shared decision making, and empathetic nonstigmatizing interactions that incorporated their prior experiences, full personhood, and current symptoms."[70]

In addition to the SUD care that is provided, communication is also a vital component of hospital-based SUD care. Davis et al, conducted a qualitative study asking hospitalized individuals with SUD about their preferred communication values with their inpatient care teams. The study found three themes: "effectiveness, reciprocity, and empathy."[70] The study reported that "patients emphasized the need for clear, reliable, and frequent communication from health care [clinicians], valuing collaborative dialogue, shared decision making, and empathetic nonstigmatizing interactions that incorporated their prior experiences, full personhood, and current symptoms."[70] On the topic of compassionate care, one participant was quoted saying,

> *"People think they're better than [you]. You're nothing but a drug addict...you're taking up space that other people need. You can see it in the way they deal with you, and the way they handle you, the way they treat you..."*[70]

When compassion was evident from the hospital team, a participant was quoted saying,

> *"Why didn't I leave? You know, they cared. They seemed like they cared. They asked me not to. 'Please give us a chance..." He asked me to stay. And that was important to me-that somebody else gave a shit...[Someone] cared enough to want me to stay here and not go back other there."*[70]

These studies emphasize that although many individuals with SUD may not come to the hospital seeking SUD treatment, when offered to them without judgment and with compassion and respect, they have high interest in it and value having it offered to them. Hospitalization is the "reachable moment" many have described about hospital-based SUD care. Therefore, these qualities of hospital-based SUD care are as important and necessary as any of the other components, like SUD screening and medication treatment. Chapter 15 provides language and communication techniques with prompts to discuss SUD and goals of care with hospitalized patients.

Case Study

The Genesis of Hospital-Based SUD Treatment in a Large Health System: A Case Example From Yale New Haven Hospital

Prior to 2018, Yale New Haven Hospital (YNHH), a premier health institution affiliated with Yale University with 1,500 beds and two hospital campuses in New Haven, Connecticut did not have a coordinated and systematic approach to address SUD for hospitalized individuals. While there were some innovative SUD treatments offered in the ED setting, once a patient was admitted to the hospital, medication treatment for SUD was generally not offered. There was no formal screening process to identify patients with SUD. If a patient was identified to have SUD, a hospital social worker provided them with a list of local SUD treatment resources to engage in care after hospital discharge. There was no formal approach to opioid withdrawal management, though some inpatient teams would offer patients a 3-day taper of methadone. Methadone initiation for OUD treatment was not offered because hospital leadership was unsure of federal and state regulations around methadone use in the hospital and assumed it was not legal. Buprenorphine was also not used for OUD treatment for the same reason and because clinicians did not know where to refer people posthospitalization for continuation of buprenorphine treatment. Alcohol withdrawal was routinely treated, but patients were not offered medications for AUD prior to hospital discharge. Tobacco withdrawal was not regularly treated with nicotine replacement therapy and patients were not offered TUD treatment. These lost opportunities contributed to premature discharge of patients from the hospital, high readmission rates, high ED visits, and long lengths of stay. Surveys of hospitalists at YNHH described SUD identification and management as the "wild west" and identified SUD as a major factor contributing to staff burnout and job dissatisfaction. Hospitalists reported that the care provided to hospitalized patients with SUD neither met accepted standards of care, nor was adequate for their patients. Hospitalists requested YNHH create an addiction consultation team and provide additional hospitalist education to ensure patients received evidence-based medical treatment of SUD.

In response, YNHH leadership committed to starting a pilot consultation team called "The Yale Addiction Medicine Consult Service (YAMCS)." In 2018, YNHH leadership recruited a dually board-certified internal medicine and addiction medicine physician to design, implement, and direct the service. YAMCS was designed to be multidisciplinary with addiction medicine attending physicians, APP, drug and alcohol counselors called health promotion advocates, and addiction medicine fellows.

YAMCS started at one of the YNHH campuses on the general medicine services. With YNHH leadership support, YAMCS expanded over the next 6 years to consult at both YNHH campuses, including the Children's Hospital, for all medical and surgical services. A timeline for the growth of YAMCS is shown in Figure 1.11. Over these 6 years, YAMCS went from seeing no patients to seeing a total 10,000 patients. To meet demand, the YAMCS team grew from a team of one physician, one APP, one health promotion advocate to three physicians, three APPs, three health promotion advocates, two addiction medicine fellows, and one social worker. In addition to providing SUD treatment, YAMCS helped change hospital culture with a reduction of stigma toward the identification and treatment of individuals with SUD, improved standards of care for individuals with SUD, increased medication treatment options for individuals with SUD, and improved connection to ongoing SUD care posthospitalization. From a financial perspective, the clinician billing generated enough relative value units (RVUs) to support the salaries of its physicians and APPs, reduced length of stay for individuals admitted for primary SUD, and decreased hospital 30-day readmissions. At the state level, YAMCS created a new standard by which other Connecticut hospitals were measured for their SUD care and changed the framework by which Connecticut hospitals address SUD.

Evidence for Screening for Unhealthy Substance Use in the ED and Hospital Setting

Screening for unhealthy substance use using validated screening tools is the first step to accurately identify individuals who will likely benefit from additional evaluation and treatment for SUD. In primary care settings, the United States Preventive Services Task Force (USPSTF) gives a "B" grade (ie, recommends the service; there is high certainty that the net benefit is moderate or there is moderate certainty that the net benefit is moderate to substantial) to "screening by asking questions about unhealthy drug use in adults aged 18 and older.[71] Screening should be implemented when services for accurate diagnosis, effective treatment, and appropriate care can be offered or referred. (In this context, screening refers to asking questions about unhealthy drug use, not testing biological specimens.)"[71] The USPSTF concludes that "the current evidence is insufficient to assess the balance of benefits and harms of screening for unhealthy drug use in adolescents."[71] Notably, these recommendations apply to primary care settings because the preponderance of evidence for screening comes from studies completed in this

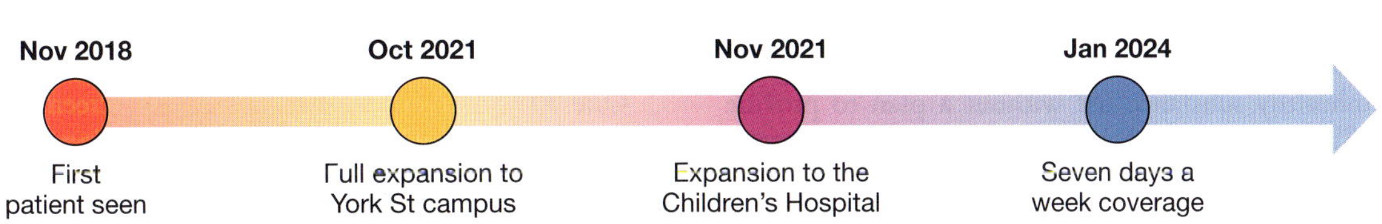

Figure 1.11: Yale New Haven hospital expansion of hospital-based SUD services.

Given how busy the hospital setting is, there may be other effective ways to adequately screen individuals that do not rely on staff time. One study found that an electronic medical record–embedded artificial intelligence (AI) screening tool was effective to identify individuals with unhealthy opioid use and deploy an addiction consultation service to see them in the hospital.[99,100] The use of the AI screening tool was associated with a reduction in 30-day readmissions and cost savings.[99] The study authors noted that the use of AI to identify patients with unhealthy opioid use to direct dedicated SUD treatment services has potential as a generalizable and cost-effective solution for hospital-based OUD care.[99]

One study assessed health care utilization for individuals who received SBIRT delivered by hospital-based mental health counselors.[101] The study found that the receipt of SBIRT reduced hospital readmission, ED visits, and costs for patients with unhealthy alcohol use, but not for other substances.[101]

Like in the ED setting, in the hospital setting, there are clear benefits to universal SBIRT to identify patients at risk for unhealthy alcohol use. If universal screening for unhealthy opioid use is employed in the hospital setting, then screening should be followed by the use of the DSM-5 to diagnose OUD and the initiation of medications for opioid use disorder (MOUD) (eg, buprenorphine, methadone, and extended-release naltrexone). Finally, every patient who is initiated on MOUD in the hospital should be referred to posthospital discharge OUD treatment. Currently, the evidence to support hospital-based universal screening for other substances like stimulants and cannabis use is less clear. In these cases, the benefits of universal SBIRT should be weighed against the time spent in a busy hospital setting.

Evidence for Interventions to Address SUD in the ED and Hospital Setting

As previously mentioned, many individuals who have SUD do not come to the ED or hospital seeking SUD treatment. Generally, these patients have a medical or surgical condition that leads them to seek acute medical care. This makes them a uniquely different population than individuals who seek SUD care in an outpatient SUD clinic, an Opioid Treatment Program for methadone treatment, or an inpatient SUD treatment center (ie, "rehab"). To best support and engage hospitalized patients into SUD treatment, interventions must be targeted to the specific needs of these medically ill patients. In addition, because treatment of SUD with medications or psychosocial interventions are not offered in more than half of US hospitals,[59] individuals who have SUD may have low expectations for dedicated SUD treatment when hospitalized. However, studies report that most hospitalized individuals with SUD express interest in receiving medication or other types of SUD treatments during hospitalization when those treatments are offered to them.[102]

ED-Based SUD Interventions

Hospital-based SUD treatment integration begins in the ED. Chapter 6 will delve into this in depth, but broadly, interventions to address SUD in the ED increase access to medication treatment, encourage linkage to outpatient treatment, promote retention in SUD treatment, reduce the risk of death (particularly for OUD), and reduce subsequent acute care utilization.[103]

For tobacco, interventions in the ED include motivational interviewing–based brief interventions, booster telephone calls, providing nicotine replacement therapy, and other resources like brochures discussing tobacco cessation and resources and referral to tobacco quit support lines.[104] Eleven studies reported in a systematic review identified reductions in tobacco use up to 12 months following receipt of the ED-based tobacco cessation interventions.[104]

For alcohol, ED-based interventions focus on providing brief interventions in the ED to individuals with unhealthy alcohol use (ie, those without an AUD diagnosis) by clinicians, counselors, social workers, or health promotion advocates.[88,103] These interventions often utilize a motivational interviewing framework to help individuals reduce the frequency and quantity of alcohol used and injury prevention.[103] Collectively, these studies have mixed results to help patients sustain reductions in alcohol use, but have shown up to a 41% reduction in the odds of sustaining an alcohol-related injury.[105,106] These interventions are also cost effective with savings as much as $2,100 per patient per year.[103]

Medications for AUD (MAUD) can, and should, be prescribed by ED clinicians. A systematic review of MAUD use in the ED and a small feasibility study reported that naltrexone (oral and extended release) are both feasible to prescribe or administer in the ED setting and promote increased connection to ongoing AUD treatment following ED discharge.[107,108]

ED-based interventions for individuals with nonopioid illicit substances mostly focus on providing brief intervention and referral to treatment with mixed results. OUD-focused interventions that include providing initiation of medication treatment such as buprenorphine have shown great promise. A

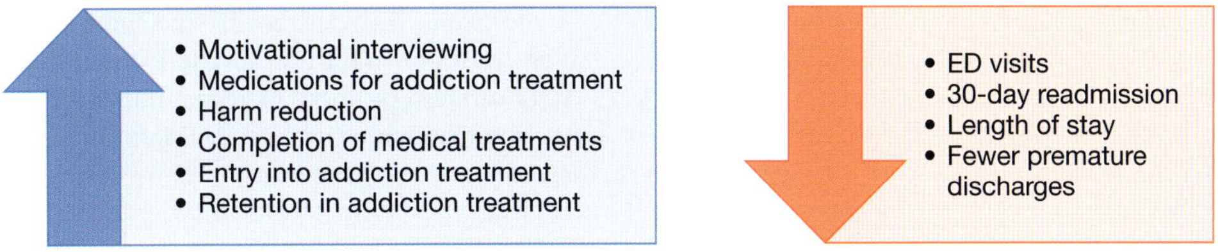

Figure 1.12: Summary of hospital SUD intervention outcomes.*
*Studies supporting these outcomes are described below.

landmark RCT from 2015 demonstrated that 78% of individuals with a urine sample positive for opioids and who met criteria for OUD were provided brief intervention, buprenorphine initiation, and facilitated follow-up in primary care were engaged in OUD treatment at 30 days after the ED visit and had reduced their opioid use.[109] The results of that study led EDs to consider OUD treatment as part of general ED-based care for patients with OUD. Soon thereafter, ACEP published a consensus statement recommending that all patients with OUD are offered effective medication treatment for OUD.[110]

Methadone can also be provided for the treatment of OUD in the ED setting, and some EDs utilize the "72-hour rule" (eg, Code of Federal Regulations, 1306.07c) to facilitate transitions of care to opioid treatment programs after discharge.[111] One observational study found that most individuals who were provided methadone for this purpose successfully connected to care in an OTP after receiving it from the ED.[112]

Additional interventions for opioid overdose prevention recommend providing naloxone freely at discharge from the ED. Some EDs are integrating the use of peer specialists into their workforce for individuals with SUD as well as the use of electronic medical record–best practice guidance for initiation of AUD and OUD treatment.

Hospital-Based SUD Interventions

Over the last 15 years, evidence for hospital-based SUD interventions has greatly evolved. Overall, most of these interventions demonstrate that hospital-based, integrated SUD treatment improves a multitude of outcomes for hospitalized patients (adults and children) including:

- Increased use of evidence-based practices for SUD
- Increased use of medication treatment for SUD
- Increased use of harm reduction counseling
- Lower incidence of patients leaving prior to medical treatment completion
- Lower incidence of 30-day rehospitalizations and ED encounters
- Higher incidence of patient entry into SUD treatment and retention in SUD treatment
- Lower all-cause mortality
- Shorter length of hospital stay
- Improved patient and clinical satisfaction (Figure 1.12)

The next section outlines specific interventions for patients with SUD and the evidence supporting their benefits. Each SUD and associated interventions have a dedicated chapter with greater detail on how to apply these interventions in the hospital setting. Interventions for adolescents and pregnant individuals will be addressed in their own chapters.

Tobacco Use Disorder

Tobacco use is the most prevalent substance used globally and in North America. It is the number one cause of preventable death in most countries and contributes to countless hospitalizations related to lung disease, lung cancer, other types of cancer, and cardiovascular disease, among others. Many hospitals have become "tobacco free" which creates an opportunity to start treatment for TUD early in the hospital course to manage tobacco and nicotine withdrawal. Liberal treatment of acute nicotine withdrawal with short-acting nicotine replacement treatments, with nicotine gum or lozenges and nicotine patches, support ongoing medical care and is the first step to engage individuals in nicotine cessation conversations.[113]

Boston Medical Center has an inpatient tobacco cessation program called Tobacco Treatment Consult (TTC). The TTC consists of a hospital-based respiratory therapist, nurse practitioner and pulmonologist who provide brief counseling, pharmacotherapy, and linkage to outpatient treatment and a smoking cessation quit line. Compared to hospitalized patients who did not receive TCC services, patients who received TCC services had increased receipt of pharmacotherapy and tobacco abstinence at 6 months.[114]

Initiation of medication treatment for tobacco cessation for patients who are hospitalized for related medical conditions, like acute coronary syndrome, is also an effective practice.[115] A multicenter, double-blind RCT of 302 patients hospitalized with acute coronary syndrome were randomized to hospital-based varenicline treatment plus manualized low-intensity counseling or placebo plus manualized low-intensity counseling.[116] The group of individuals in the study smoked an average of 1 pack of cigarettes per day for 36 years.[116] Patients in the varenicline group were significantly more likely to abstain from tobacco use and to reduce their tobacco use at 24 weeks (number needed to treat 6.8).[116]

Other forms of integrated TUD treatment include order sets to facilitate treatment of nicotine withdrawal and to initiate TUD treatment, electronic medical record–based clinical guidance, and health care system–integrated tobacco cessation ambulatory programs provided at discharge.[117]

Alcohol Use Disorder

Unhealthy alcohol use and AUD contribute to a high number of ED visits and hospitalizations each year in North America. Prevalence of unhealthy alcohol use depends on the hospital and the patient population, but has been reported to be as high as 50% in some hospitalized populations and is estimated to be 4 to 5 times higher than the general adult non-hospitalized population.[45,84] Individuals who screen positive for unhealthy alcohol use in the hospital are also more likely to have AUD. Importantly, once a patient is determined to have AUD, screening and brief intervention alone is insufficient, and treatment for AUD is recommended. Despite known effective treatments for AUD, <2% of individuals who are hospitalized related to AUD receive effective medication treatments.[118]

One RCT that compared a 30-minute session of motivational counseling versus usual care reported no increase in linkage to alcohol treatment from the hospital for individuals with AUD who received counseling and concluded that "medical inpatients with unhealthy alcohol use require more extensive, tailored alcohol interventions."[119]

Interventions for AUD should include initiation of MAUD and direct referrals to treatment via primary medical teams or consultation services at hospital discharge. Initiation of hospital-based MAUD is feasible and effective, though it is not done in most hospitals.[118,120] One intervention to increase use of MAUD during hospitalization focused on providing educational interventions to primary medical teams and development of order sets to support MAUD initiation for individuals with AUD before hospital discharge.[121–123] Three studies utilizing this intervention reported an increase in MAUD prescription for patients at discharge, though had conflicting results about reduction in health care utilization at 30 days.[121–123]

Electronic medical record–integrated clinical guidance that supports the use of MAUD for individuals with AUD can also promote increased initiation of MAUD. An observational study of 2,600 hospital admissions across 6 hospitals in one large health system showed that an electronic health record-integrated clinical pathway was used by 18% of hospital-based clinicians.[124] When the pathway was used, the odds of MAUD initiation was 4.3 (Confidence Interval [CI] 3.1 to 5.9, $P < .001$) compared to encounters that did not use the clinical pathway, though MAUD initiation in that study did not improve future acute care utilization.[124]

Hospital-based MAUD initiation has been shown to decrease mortality and acute care utilization in other studies. In a propensity-matched cohort study of Medicare beneficiaries, MAUD prescription within 2 days of hospital discharge reduced the incidence of all-cause mortality and 30-day readmission to the hospital by 42% and reduced all-cause ED visits, and increased 30-day primary care or mental health follow-up.[125] Other interventions for increasing MAUD prescribing focus on addiction consultation services and are described below.[126,127]

Opioid Use Disorder

Unhealthy opioid use and OUD are highly associated with comorbid conditions, including infections and overdose events, which contribute to a high number of annual ED visits and hospitalizations in North America. Individuals who are hospitalized related to OUD can have a 1-year mortality comparable to individuals hospitalized with acute coronary syndrome.[128] Like other treatments for SUD, initiation of OUD treatment during hospitalization can be lifesaving.

When individuals are determined to have OUD either via screening or formal diagnosis, brief intervention and referral to treatment is insufficient to address OUD, and medication treatment initiation cannot be deferred to the outpatient setting. All hospitalized patients experiencing opioid withdrawal symptoms should be offered MOUD, including methadone or buprenorphine, their pain should be assessed and adequately treated, which may involve the use of short-acting opioids, and they should be provided support for transition of ongoing OUD treatment outside of the hospital.[77,128] A systematic review found 17 studies of interventions to address OUD that involved initiation of MOUD during hospitalization and connection to postdischarge OUD treatment.[129] Overall, those studies found that these interventions increased postdischarge connection to OUD treatment, increased initiation of MOUD, increased completion of medical treatments, and reduced premature hospital discharges.[129] Other outcomes that have been described from hospital initiation of MOUD include reduced opioid use, increased retention in OUD treatment, reduced acute care utilization, and reduced mortality.[66,130] Interventions that treat opioid withdrawal alone (ie, "detox") without initiation of MOUD greatly increase the risk of unintentional overdose after hospitalization due to return to opioid use, are not the standard of care, and should universally be avoided. Consensus guidance based on a combination of evidence and expert opinion recommends that every hospitalized patient experiencing objective signs of opioid withdrawal should be offered MOUD.[77] If a patient declines MOUD, then options such as full agonist opioids like oxycodone or hydromorphone can be considered with the goal of supporting the patient to remain in the hospital to receive essential medical or surgical therapies.[131,132]

Other Substance Use Disorders

Cannabis, stimulants, benzodiazepines, hallucinogens, phencyclidine (PCP), and dissociative substances like ketamine can all lead to medical complications that require hospitalization. Cannabis and stimulants have specifically been shown to increase mortality of individuals who require hospitalization.[29] Interventions to address the use of these substances generally involve management of withdrawal syndromes, supportive care, and assessment of SUD treatment need. Chapter 10 covers these substances in detail.

Integrated cardiology and addiction treatment is an intervention that has been studied for individuals with stimulant-associated cardiomyopathy and can begin in the hospital setting. A feasibility study showed that most individuals who were hospitalized for stimulant-associated cardiomyopathy were retained in postdischarge ambulatory treatment with medical management and contingency management.[133] Future interventions to expand hospital-based provision of contingency management for StUD hold promise.[134]

Addiction Consultation Services

A systematic review of addiction consultation services found 41 studies, most of which were observational, but included three RCTs.[135] The most commonly described composition of the addiction consultation teams were physicians, social workers, nurses, and recovery staff.[135] The most common interventions offered to patients by the addiction consultation services included initiation of medications to treat SUD, referral to posthospital SUD care, deployment of behavioral interventions (ie, motivational interviewing), and harm reduction counseling (ie, overdose prevention education and safe injection practice).[135] Not all addiction consultation services have the same focus; in some studies, the consultation services only provided care for OUD. The majority of studies in the systematic review reported increased initiation of medications for SUD and increased linkage of patients to posthospital SUD care.[135] One RCT reported increased odds of patients receiving MOUD (Odds Ratio [OR] 6.26, 95% CI 2.38 to 16.48).[135] Results were mixed regarding postdischarge substance use, but three observational studies reported a reduction in substance use after discharge.[135] Study results were mixed demonstrating decreases in hospital readmission, ED visits, length of stay, and patient-directed discharges.[135] However, focusing on the results of a high-quality RCT that included hospital consultation followed by 3 months of posthospital case management, individuals who received addiction medicine consultation and 3 months of ongoing case management following hospital discharge had a cost-saving of $17,780 per patient.[136] Cost savings were attributed to reduced hospital and ED use compared to the group who received hospital-based addiction medicine consultation without postdischarge case management.[136] These results suggest that having dedicated hospital-based SUD care paired with postdischarge case management supports patients with SUD to succeed both in the hospital, after hospitalization, and reduce overall costs to the health system.

An RCT not included in the aforementioned systematic review examined the impact of an addiction consultation service on receipt of MOUD and postdischarge OUD treatment engagement among hospitalized patients with OUD across 6 public hospitals in New York City.[60] The results showed that, compared to usual care, individuals who received an addiction consultation, had almost eight times higher odds of initiating MOUD and almost seven times higher odds of entering MOUD treatment after hospitalization.[60]

An additional observational study of the impact of an addiction consultation service on AUD outcomes reported that those who received an addiction consultation had an increased odds of receiving MAUD (OR 52.5, 95% CI 12.6 to 218.6).[127] Consultation was not significantly associated with reduced ED visits in that study.

Finally, an addiction medicine consultation service positively impacts the hospital-based clinician and staff who provide direct patient care. A qualitative study of hospital-based clinicians found that having an addiction consultation service increased staff confidence using MOUD.[137] Staff also reported improved patient outcomes and greater job satisfaction.[137,138] Furthermore, hospital-based addiction clinicians describe their work as rewarding because they have an opportunity to advocate for patients who frequently experience stigma in the health care setting.[138]

Together, these findings highlight the positive impact that robust hospital-based SUD interventions, like an addiction consultation service, can have for hospitalized patients with SUD. Given the high prevalence of unhealthy substance use and SUD among patients receiving care in the ED or hospital setting, it is essential to offer SUD treatment in these settings. Providing dedicated treatment, whether that is referral to postdischarge SUD treatment or initiation of medications to treat the SUD, is evidence-based care and should be the standard of care in these settings. Of all the interventions designed to address SUD in the hospital setting, addiction consultation services certainly have significant value and potential to improve outcomes on multiple levels.

Systemic Reform to Increase Hospital-Based SUD Care

National organizations endorse the integration of hospital-based SUD treatment. Professional societies like the SHM and the ASAM also specifically endorse these practices.[64,77,139] The American Heart Association recommends integration of SUD care for treatment of injection drug use–related infective endocarditis.[140] The Joint Commission recognizes how the hospital fits in the larger treatment continuum related to the opioid overdose epidemic with its requirements for pain evaluation and pain treatment. For other forms of substance use, the Joint Commission standards and measures include screening and assessment, care planning, treatment services, discharge and care continuity, education and training, environment of care, and performance improvement.[78] Despite this shared consensus for the value of integrated hospital-based SUD care, most hospitals do not provide this care. The hospitals that do offer hospital-based SUD care are generally doing so based on the work of highly motivated local champions and individual hospital priorities. As described by Englander and Davis in their poignant editorial:

> *"Changing the standard of care requires reforms [beyond] what individual champions or hospitals can accomplish. The path forward [requires] bold actions across multiple agencies and policy domains, including development and dissemination of national clinical guidance, implementation of financing reforms and new quality metrics, provision of implementation support, and workforce education…"*[53]

Systemic reform is essential to facilitate expansion of urgently needed SUD care to all hospital settings. Current state of SUD care in most hospitals falls far below the standard of care. Health care systems, clinicians, and payers must be motivated to make sweeping changes, and this may only happen with concerted and dedicated efforts.

Recommendations for Hospital-Based SUD Care

Many of the following recommendations were discussed in this chapter or will be covered in depth in their respective subsequent chapters.

- Provide education and workforce expansion efforts to support integration of hospital-based SUD care
- Consider starting with small hospital-based SUD screening and treatment pilots and then expand them through iterative processes
- Conduct universal screening for unhealthy substance use among all hospitalized patients
- Develop clinical guidance, hospital policies, and pharmacy formulary changes to support integrated SUD treatment
- Ensure all patients who meet DSM-5 criteria for SUD are offered medication treatment, when indicated
- Offer expert addiction consultation to support and enable the hospital's ability to provide integrated SUD treatment
- Develop patient-centered interventions to support patients while they are hospitalized
- Connect with community partners and/or outpatient resources for ongoing SUD treatment after hospitalization
- Address social determinants of health as essential recovery supports

REFERENCES

1. Serota DP, Kraft CS, Weimer MB. Treating the symptom but not the underlying disease in infective endocarditis: a teachable moment. *JAMA Intern Med.* 2017;177(7):1026–1027.
2. Suen LW, Makam AN, Snyder HR, et al. National prevalence of alcohol and other substance use disorders among emergency department visits and hospitalizations: NHAMCS 2014–2018. *J Gen Intern Med.* 2022;37(10):2420–2428.
3. Agency for Healthcare Research and Quality. *Analysis of Data from the 2020 National Emergency Department Sample.* Healthcare Cost and Utilization Project (HCUP); 2022. https://hcup-us.ahrq.gov/nedsoverview.jsp
4. Ball A, Hadland S, Rodean J, Hall M, Mendoza J, Ahrens K. Trends in substance-related visits among youth to us children's hospitals, 2016–2021: an analysis of the pediatric health

information system database. *J Adolesc Health*. 2024;75(1): 76–84.
5. National Institute on Alcohol Abuse and Alcoholism. *Alcohol's Effects on Health and Deaths in the United States*. Accessed January 31, 2025. https://www.niaaa.nih.gov/alcohols-effects-health/alcohol-topics-z/alcohol-facts-and-statistics/alcohol-related-emergencies-and-deaths-united-states
6. Radhakrishnan L, Leeb RT, Leeb RT, et al. *Key Substance Use and Mental Health Indicators in the United States: Results from the 2023 National Survey on Drug Use and Health*. SAMHSA; 2024.
7. VanFrank B, Malarcher A, Cornelius ME, Schecter A, Jamal A, Tynan M. Adult smoking cessation – United States, 2022. *MMWR Morb Mortal Wkly Rep*. 2024;73:633–641.
8. Roehler DR, Hoots BE, Holland KM, Baldwin GT, Vivolo-Kantor AM. Trends and characteristics of cannabis-associated emergency department visits in the United States, 2006–2018. *Drug Alcohol Depend*. 2022;232:109288.
9. Suen LW, Davy-Mendez T, LeSaint KT, Riley ED, Coffin PO. Emergency department visits and trends related to cocaine, psychostimulants, and opioids in the United States, 2008–2018. *BMC Emerg Med*. 2022;22(1):19.
10. McNeely J, Hamilton L. Screening for unhealthy alcohol and drug use in general medicine settings. *Med Clin North Am*. 2022;106(1):13–28.
11. U.S. Department of Agriculture, U.S. Department of Health and Human Services. *Dietary Guidelines for Americans, 2020–2025*. 9th ed. Accessed February 2, 2026. https://www.dietaryguidelines.gov/about-dietary-guidelines/previous-editions/2020-dietary-guidelines
12. American Psychiatric Association (APA). Substance use disorder. *Diagnostic and Statistical Manual of Mental Disorders*. 5th ed. APA; 2013.
13. Shearer RD, Bart G, Reznikoff C. Rethinking the use of "polysubstance" to describe complex substance use patterns. *J Gen Intern Med*. 2022;37(12):3174–3175.
14. National Institute on Alcohol Abuse and Alcoholism. *NIAAA Recovery Research Definitions*. Accessed March 18, 2025. https://www.niaaa.nih.gov/research/niaaa-recovery-from-alcohol-use-disorder/definitions
15. American Society of Addiction Medicine. *Definition of Addiction*. Updated September 15, 2019. Accessed March 5, 2026. https://www.asam.org/Quality-Science/definition-of-addiction
16. Strang J, Volkow ND, Degenhardt L, et al. Opioid use disorder. *Nat Rev Dis Primers*. 2020;6(1):3.
17. Olsen Y. What is addiction? history, terminology, and core concepts. *Med Clin North Am*. 2022;106(1):1–12
18. Zou Z, Wang H, d'Oleire Uquillas F, Wang X, Ding J, Chen H. Definition of substance and non-substance addiction. *Adv Exp Med Biol*. 2017;1010:21–41.
19. Arias-Carrión O, Stamelou M, Murillo-Rodríguez E, Menéndez-González M, Pöppel E. Dopaminergic reward system: a short integrative review. *Int Arch Med*. 2010;3:24.
20. Volkow ND, Fowler JS, Wang GJ, Swanson JM. Dopamine in drug abuse and addiction: results from imaging studies and treatment implications. *Mol Psychiatry*. 2004;9(6): 557–569.
21. Volkow ND, Chang L, Wang G-J, et al. Loss of dopamine transporters in methamphetamine abusers recovers with protracted abstinence. *J Neurosci*. 2001;21(23):9414–9418.
22. Kaplan GB, Thompson BL. Neuroplasticity of the extended amygdala in opioid withdrawal and prolonged opioid abstinence. *Front Pharmacol*. 2023;14:1253736.
23. McLellan AT, Lewis DC, O'Brien CP, Kleber HD. Drug dependence, a chronic medical illness: implications for treatment, insurance, and outcomes evaluation. *JAMA*. 2000;284(13): 1689–1695.
24. Morales AM, Jones SA, Kliamovich D, Harman G, Nagel BJ. Identifying early risk factors for addiction later in life: a review of prospective longitudinal studies. *Curr Addict Rep*. 2020;7(1):89–98.
25. Volkow ND, Koob GF, McLellan AT. Neurobiologic advances from the brain disease model of addiction. *N Engl J Med*. 2016;374(4):363–371.
26. Nelson LF, Weitzman ER, Levy S. Prevention of substance use disorders. *Med Clin North Am*. 2022;106(1):153–168.
27. Peacock A, Leung J, Larney S, et al. Global statistics on alcohol, tobacco and illicit drug use: 2017 status report. *Addiction*. 2018;113(10):1905–1926.
28. Gale A. Sacklers sacked but purdue still caused opioid epidemic. *Mo Med*. 2022;119(2):109.
29. Myran DT, Pugliese M, McDonald AJ, et al. Cannabis use disorder emergency department visits and hospitalizations and 5-year mortality. *JAMA Netw Open*. 2025;8(2):e2457852.
30. Canadian Institute for Health Information. *Alcohol Harm in Canada: Examining Hospitalizations Entirely Caused by Alcohol and Strategies to Reduce Alcohol Harm*. Accessed February 2, 2026. https://www.cihi.ca/sites/default/files/document/report-alcohol-hospitalizations-en-web.pdf
31. Federal Provincial, and territorial Special Advisory Committee on Toxic Drug Poisonings. *Opioid- and Stimulant-Related Harms in Canada*. Accessed January 31, 2025. https://health-infobase.canada.ca/substance-related-harms/opioids-stimulants/
32. Drug Policy Facts. *Mexico*. Accessed February 2, 2026. https://www.drugpolicyfacts.org/region/mexico
33. Multilateral Evaluation Mechanism, Governmental Expert Group (GEG). *Mexico: Evaluation of Progress in Drug Control 2007–2009*. Accessed January 31, 2025. https://www.oas.org/ext/en/main/oas/our-structure/agencies-and-entities/cicad-commission
34. Strathdee SA, Goodman-Meza D, Rafful CM. Addressing opioid use disorder: Mexico's step backwards. *Lancet Reg Health Am*. 2023;23:100520.
35. Centers for Disease Control and Prevention. *Behavioral Risk Factor Surveillance System*. Accessed February 29, 2024. https://www.cdc.gov/brfss/
36. Garnett MF, Minino AM. *Drug Overdose Deaths in the United States, 2003–2023*. 2024. NCHS Data Brief, No. 522. https://www.cdc.gov/nchs/products/databriefs/db522.htm#Suggested_citation
37. Centers for Disease Control and Prevention, National Center for Health Statistics. *U.S. Overdose Deaths Decrease in 2023, First Time Since 2018*. Accessed March 18, 2025. https://www.cdc.gov/nchs/pressroom/nchs_press_releases/2024/20240515.htm#:~:text=The%20new%20data%20show%20overdose,psychostimulants%20(like%20methamphetamine)%20increased
38. Centre for Addiction and Mental Health. *Mental Illness and Addiction: Facts and Statistics*. Accessed January 31, 2025. https://www.camh.ca/en/driving-change/the-crisis-is-real/mental-health-statistics
39. Peterson C, Xu L, Florence C, Mack KA. Opioid-related US hospital discharges by type, 1993–2016. *J Subst Abuse Treat*. 2019;103:9–13.
40. Ronan MV, Herzig SJ. Hospitalizations related to opioid abuse/dependence and associated serious infections increased sharply, 2002–12. *Health Aff (Millwood)*. 2016;35(5):832–837.
41. Winkelman TN, Admon LK, Jennings L, Shippee ND, Richardson CR, Bart G. Evaluation of amphetamine-related hospitalizations and associated clinical outcomes and costs in the United States. *JAMA Netw Open*. 2018;1(6):e183758.
42. Laswi H, Attar B, Kwei R, Ojemolon P, Ebhohon E, Shaka H. Trends of alcohol withdrawal delirium in the last decade: analysis of the nationwide inpatient sample. *Gastroenterology Res*. 2022;15(4):207–216.
43. Addiction Help. *Canadian Substance Abuse Statistics*. Accessed January 31, 2025. https://www.addictionhelp.com/addiction/canadian-statistics/#:~:text=Canadian%20

Substance%20Abuse%20Statistics,for%20addiction%20in%20their%20lifetime
44. Englander H, Priest KC, Snyder H, Martin M, Calcaterra S, Gregg J. A call to action: hospitalists' role in addressing substance use disorder. *J Hosp Med.* 2020;15(3):184–187.
45. Saitz R, Freedner N, Palfai TP, Horton NJ, Samet JH. The severity of unhealthy alcohol use in hospitalized medical patients. The spectrum is narrow. *J Gen Intern Med.* 2006;21(4):381–385.
46. Walley AY, Paasche-Orlow M, Lee EC, et al. Acute care hospital utilization among medical inpatients discharged with a substance use disorder diagnosis. *J Addict Med.* 2012;6(1):50–56.
47. Kadri AN, Wilner B, Hernandez AV, et al. Geographic trends, patient characteristics, and outcomes of infective endocarditis associated with drug abuse in the United States from 2002–2016. *J Am Heart Assoc.* 2019;8(19):e012969.
48. Chang JE, Cronin CE, Pagán JA, Simon J, Lindenfeld Z, Franz B. Trends in the prioritization and implementation of substance use programs by nonprofit hospitals: 2015–2021. *J Addict Med.* 2023;17(4):e217–e223.
49. Internal Revenue Service. *Community Health Needs Assessment for Charitable Hospital Organizations—Section 501(r)(3).* Accessed March 18, 2025. https://www.irs.gov/charities-non-profits/community-health-needs-assessment-for-charitable-hospital-organizations-section-501r3
50. Peterson C, Li M, Xu L, Mikosz CA, Luo F. Assessment of annual cost of substance use disorder in US hospitals. *JAMA Netw Open.* 2021;4(3):e210242.
51. Chen C, Yoon Y-H. *Trends in Alcohol-Related Morbidity Among Community Hospital Discharges, United States, 2000–2015.* https://www.niaaa.nih.gov/publications/surveillance-reports/surveillance112
52. Healthcare Cost and Utilization Project (HCUP). *Statistical Brief #257.* Accessed February 2, 2026. https://hcup-us.ahrq.gov/reports/statbriefs/sb257-ED-Costs-Mental-Substance-Use-Disorders-2017.pdf
53. Englander H, Davis CS. Hospital standards of care for people with substance use disorder. *N Engl J Med.* 2022;387(8):672–675.
54. South AM, Hawk K, Friedman S, Lofwall MR, Fanucchi LC, Cohen SM. Civil rights laws for people with opioid use disorder in the emergency department. *J Addict Med.* 2025;19(6):643–645.
55. Priest KC, McCarty D. Making the business case for an addiction medicine consult service: a qualitative analysis. *BMC Health Serv Res.* 2019;19(1):822.
56. Englander H, Collins D, Perry SP, Rabinowitz M, Phoutrides E, Nicolaidis C. "We've learned it's a medical illness, not a moral choice": qualitative study of the effects of a multicomponent addiction intervention on hospital providers' attitudes and experiences. *J Hosp Med.* 2018;13(11):752–758.
57. Barocas JA, Savinkina A, Adams J, et al. Clinical impact, costs, and cost-effectiveness of hospital-based strategies for addressing the US opioid epidemic: a modelling study. *Lancet Public Health.* 2022;7(1):e56–e64.
58. Priest KC, Englander H, McCarty D. "Now hospital leaders are paying attention": a qualitative study of internal and external factors influencing addiction consult services. *J Subst Abuse Treat.* 2020;110:59–65.
59. Franz B, Cronin CE, Lindenfeld Z, et al. Rural-urban disparities in the availability of hospital-based screening, medications for opioid use disorder, and addiction consult services. *J Subst Use Addict Treat.* 2024;160:209280.
60. McNeely J, Wang SS, Rostam Abadi Y, et al. Addiction consultation services for opioid use disorder treatment initiation and engagement: a randomized clinical trial. *JAMA Intern Med.* 2024;184(9):1106–1115.
61. Bahji A, Lusty E, Majere R, Newman A, Reshetukha T, Carvalhal A. Piloting an addictions medicine consultation team in Kingston, Ontario, Canada: Results of an inpatient needs assessment. *CJAM.* 2019;10:29–32.
62. Braithwaite V, Ti L, Fairbairn N, et al. Building a hospital-based addiction medicine consultation service in Vancouver, Canada: the path taken and lessons learned. *Addiction.* 2021;116(7):1892–1900.
63. Galanter M, Karasu TB, Wilder JF. Alcohol and drug abuse consultation in the general hospital: a systems approach. *Am J Psychiatry.* 1976;133(8):930–934.
64. American Society of Addiction Medicine. *The ASAM Criteria.* 4th ed. Hazelden Publishing; 2023.
65. U.S. Department of Health and Human Services, Office of Inspector General. *The Emergency Medical Treatment and Labor Act (EMTALA).* Accessed March 18, 2025. https://oig.hhs.gov/reports/featured/emtala/#:~:text=Last%20Updated%3A%2009%2D11%2D,hospitals%20that%20offer%20emergency%20services
66. Englander H, Jones A, Krawczyk N, et al. A taxonomy of hospital-based addiction care models: a scoping review and key informant interviews. *J Gen Intern Med.* 2022;37(11):2821–2833.
67. Krawczyk N, Rivera BD, Chang JE, et al. Strategies to support substance use disorder care transitions from acute-care to community-based settings: a scoping review and typology. *Addict Sci Clin Pract.* 2023;18(1):67.
68. Williams BE, Patten A, Peng L, Englander H. "Just be relentless," lessons learned from in-hospital addiction consult service implementation. *J Gen Intern Med.* 2025;40(12):2916–2925.
69. Velez CM, Nicolaidis C, Korthuis PT, Englander H. "It's been an experience, a life learning experience": a qualitative study of hospitalized patients with substance use disorders. *J Gen Intern Med.* 2017;32(3):296–303.
70. Davis MH, French R, Crowe M, et al. Exploring preferences for communication and care among hospitalized patients with opioid use disorder: a qualitative descriptive study. *J Addict Med.* 2025;19(4):423–429. American Society of Addiction Medicine. https://journals.lww.com/journaladdictionmedicine/abstract/2025/07000/exploring_preferences_for_communication_and_care.14.aspx
71. United States Preventive Services Task Force; Krist KH, Davidson KW, Mangione CM, et al. Screening for unhealthy drug use: US preventive services task force recommendation statement. *JAMA.* 2020;323(22):2301–2309.
72. Patnode CD, Perdue LA, Rushkin M, et al. *Screening for Unhealthy Drug Use in Primary Care in Adolescents and Adults, Including Pregnant Persons: Updated Systematic Review for the U.S. Preventive Services Task Force [Internet].* Agency for Healthcare Research and Quality (US); 2020. Report No: 19-05255-EF-1.
73. American Academy of Pediatrics. *Substance Use Screening and Intervention Implementation Guide.* Accessed February 2, 2026. https://www.aap.org/en/patient-care/substance-use-and-prevention/
74. ACOG Committee Opinion No. 762: Prepregnancy counseling. *Obstet Gynecol.* 2019;133:e78–e89.
75. Obstetric Care Consensus No. 8: Interpregnancy care. *Obstet Gynecol.* 2019;133:e51–e72.
76. American College of Emergency Physicians. Alcohol screening in the emergency department. Accessed February 2, 2026. https://www.acep.org/siteassets/uploads/uploaded-files/acep/clinical-and-practice-management/resources/publichealth/alcohol-screening/alcohol_screening_kit_overview.pdf
77. Calcaterra SL, Martin M, Bottner R, et al. Management of opioid use disorder and associated conditions among hospitalized adults: a Consensus Statement from the

Society of Hospital Medicine. *J Hosp Med.* 2022;17(9): 744–756.
78. Joint Commission. R3 Report: Requirement, Rationale, Reference. Accessed February 2, 2026. https://www.jointcommission.org/en-us/standards/r3-report/r3-report-25
79. Moe J, Koh J, Ma JA, et al. Screening for harmful substance use in emergency departments: a systematic review. *Int J Emerg Med.* 2024;17(1):52.
80. Bush K, Kivlahan DR, McDonell MB, Fihn SD, Bradley KA. The AUDIT alcohol consumption questions (AUDIT-C): an effective brief screening test for problem drinking. Ambulatory Care Quality Improvement Project (ACQUIP). Alcohol Use Disorders Identification Test. *Arch Intern Med.* 1998;158(16):1789–1795.
81. Saunders JB, Aasland OG, Babor TF, de la Fuente JR, Grant M. Development of the Alcohol Use Disorders Identification Test (AUDIT): WHO collaborative project on early detection of persons with harmful alcohol consumption–II. *Addiction.* 1993;88(6):791–804.
82. Cherpitel CJ. Screening for alcohol problems in the emergency room: a rapid alcohol problems screen. *Drug Alcohol Depend.* 1995;40(2):133–137.
83. Smith PC, Schmidt SM, Allensworth-Davies D, Saitz R. A single-question screening test for drug use in primary care. *Arch Intern Med.* 2010;170(13):1155–1160.
84. Roche AM, Freeman T, Skinner N. From data to evidence, to action: findings from a systematic review of hospital screening studies for high risk alcohol consumption. *Drug Alcohol Depend.* 2006;83(1):1–14.
85. Humeniuk R, Ali R, Babor TF, et al. Validation of the alcohol, smoking and substance involvement screening test (ASSIST). *Addiction.* 2008;103(6):1039–1047.
86. Punches BE, Freiermuth CE, Sprague JE, et al. Screening for problematic opioid use in the emergency department: comparison of two screening measures. *J Am Coll Emerg Physicians Open.* 2024;5(1):e13106.
87. Barbosa C, McKnight-Eily LR, Grosse SD, Bray J. Alcohol screening and brief intervention in emergency departments: review of the impact on healthcare costs and utilization. *J Subst Abuse Treat.* 2020;117:108096.
88. D'Onofrio G, Degutis LC. Integrating Project ASSERT: a screening, intervention, and referral to treatment program for unhealthy alcohol and drug use into an urban emergency department. *Acad Emerg Med.* 2010;17(8):903–911.
89. Bogenschutz MP, Donovan DM, Mandler RN, et al. Brief intervention for patients with problematic drug use presenting in emergency departments: a randomized clinical trial. *JAMA Intern Med.* 2014;174(11):1736–1745.
90. Serowik KL, Yonkers KA, Gilstad-Hayden K, Forray A, Zimbrean P, Martino S. Substance use disorder detection rates among providers of general medical inpatients. *J Gen Intern Med.* 2021;36(3):668–675.
91. American College of Surgeons. Resources for optimal care of the injured patient, 2022 standards. 2022.
92. Ewing JA. Detecting alcoholism. The CAGE questionnaire. *JAMA.* 1984;252(14):1905–1907.
93. Pokorny AD, Miller BA, Kaplan HB. The brief MAST: a shortened version of the Michigan alcoholism screening test. *Am J Psychiatry.* 1972;129(3):342–345.
94. Hearne R, Connolly A, Sheehan J. Alcohol abuse: prevalence and detection in a general hospital. *J R Soc Med.* 2002; 95(2):84–87. Copyright © 2002. Reprinted by Permission of Sage Publications.
95. McQueen J, Howe TE, Allan L, Mains D, Hardy V. Brief interventions for heavy alcohol users admitted to general hospital wards. *Cochrane Database Syst Rev.* 2009;(3): CD005191.
96. McNeely J, Strauss SM, Saitz R, et al. A brief patient self-administered substance use screening tool for primary care: two-site validation study of the Substance Use Brief Screen (SUBS). *Am J Med.* 2015;128(7):784.e9–e19.
97. McNeely J, Wu LT, Subramaniam G, et al. Performance of the tobacco, alcohol, prescription medication, and other substance use (TAPS) tool for substance use screening in primary care patients. *Ann Intern Med.* 2016;165(10): 690–699.
98. NIDA Clinical Trials Network. Drug abuse screening test (DAST-10). Accessed February 2, 2026. https://cde.nlm.nih.gov/formView?tinyId=QJPG1TWwl
99. Afshar M, Resnik F, Joyce C, et al. Outcomes and cost-effectiveness of an EHR-Embedded AI screener for identifying hospitalized adults at risk for opioid use disorder. *Res Sq.* 2024:rs.3.rs-5200964.
100. Afshar M, Sharma B, Bhalla S, et al. External validation of an opioid misuse machine learning classifier in hospitalized adult patients. *Addict Sci Clin Pract.* 2021;16(1):19.
101. McCall MH, Wester KL, Bray JW, et al. SBIRT administered by mental health counselors for hospitalized adults with substance misuse or disordered use: evaluating hospital utilization and costs. *J Subst Abuse Treat.* 2022;132:108510.
102. Englander H, Weimer M, Solotaroff R, et al. Planning and designing the Improving Addiction Care Team (IMPACT) for hospitalized adults with substance use disorder. *J Hosp Med.* 2017;12(5):339–342.
103. Hawk K, D'Onofrio G. Emergency department screening and interventions for substance use disorders. *Addict Sci Clin Pract.* 2018;13(1):18.
104. Lemhoefer C, Rabe GL, Wellmann J, et al. Emergency department-initiated tobacco control: update of a systematic review and meta-analysis of randomized controlled trials. *Prev Chronic Dis.* 2017;14:E89.
105. Havard A, Shakeshaft A, Sanson-Fisher R. Systematic review and meta-analyses of strategies targeting alcohol problems in emergency departments: interventions reduce alcohol-related injuries. *Addiction.* 2008;103(3):368–376; discussion 377–378.
106. Barata IA, Shandro JR, Montgomery M, et al. Effectiveness of SBIRT for alcohol use disorders in the emergency department: a systematic review. *West J Emerg Med.* 2017;18(6):1143–1152.
107. Punia K, Scott W, Manuja K, et al. SAEM GRACE: Anti-craving medications for alcohol use disorder treatment in the emergency department: a systematic review of direct evidence. *Acad Emerg Med.* 2024;31(5):504–514.
108. Cowan E, O'Brien-Lambert C, Eiting E, et al. Emergency department-initiated oral naltrexone for patients with moderate to severe alcohol use disorder: a pilot feasibility study. *Acad Emerg Med.* 2025;32(5):488–497.
109. D'Onofrio G, O'Connor PG, Pantalon MV, et al. Emergency department–initiated buprenorphine/naloxone treatment for opioid dependence: a randomized clinical trial. *JAMA.* 2015;313(16):1636–1644.
110. Hawk K, Hoppe J, Ketcham E, et al. Consensus recommendations on the treatment of opioid use disorder in the emergency department. *Ann Emerg Med.* 2021;78(3):434–442.
111. Code of Federal Regulations. *Title 21, Chapter 2, Part 1306.07 Administering or Dispensing Narcotic Drugs.* Accessed March 18, 2025. https://www.ecfr.gov/current/title-21/chapter-II/part-1306/subject-group-ECFR1eb5bb3a23fddd0/section-1306.07
112. Huo S, Heil J, Salzman MS, et al. Emergency department utilization of the methadone "72-hour rule" to bridge or initiate and link to outpatient treatment. *Am J Emerg Med.* 2024;89:209–215.

113. Palmer AM, Rojewski AM, Chen LS, et al. Tobacco treatment program models in us hospitals and outpatient centers on behalf of the SRNT treatment network. *Chest.* 2021; 159(4):1652–1663.
114. Herbst N, Wiener RS, Helm ED, et al. Effectiveness of an opt-out electronic heath record-based tobacco treatment consult service at an urban safety net hospital. *Chest.* 2020;158(4): 1734–1741.
115. Moiz A, Eisenberg MJ. Initiation of varenicline in people hospitalized for acute coronary syndrome who smoke. *Circulation.* 2023;147(25):1869–1871.
116. Eisenberg MJ, Windle SB, Roy N, et al. Varenicline for smoking cessation in hospitalized patients with acute coronary syndrome. *Circulation.* 2016;133(1):21–30.
117. Rigotti NA, Chang Y, Davis EM, et al. Comparative effectiveness of postdischarge smoking cessation interventions for hospital patients: the helping hand 4 randomized clinical trial. *JAMA Intern Med.* 2022;182(8):814–824.
118. Bernstein EY, Baggett TP, Trivedi S, Herzig SJ, Anderson TS. Pharmacologic treatment initiation among medicare beneficiaries hospitalized with alcohol use disorder. *Ann Intern Med.* 2023;176(8):1137–1139.
119. Saitz R, Palfai TP, Cheng DM, et al. Brief intervention for medical inpatients with unhealthy alcohol use: a randomized, controlled trial. *Ann Intern Med.* 2007;146(3):167–176.
120. Busch AC, Denduluri M, Glass J, et al. Predischarge injectable versus oral naltrexone to improve postdischarge treatment engagement among hospitalized veterans with alcohol use disorder: a randomized pilot proof-of-concept study. *Alcohol Clin Exp Res.* 2017;41(7):1352–1360.
121. Wei J, Defries T, Lozada M, Young N, Huen W, Tulsky J. An inpatient treatment and discharge planning protocol for alcohol dependence: efficacy in reducing 30-day readmissions and emergency department visits. *J Gen Intern Med.* 2015;30(3):365–370.
122. Arms L, Johl H, DeMartini J. Improving the utilisation of medication-assisted treatment for alcohol use disorder at discharge. *BMJ Open Qual.* 2022;11(4):e001899.
123. Stephens JR, Moore C, Stepanek KV, et al. Implementation of a process for initiating naltrexone in patients hospitalized for alcohol detoxification or withdrawal. *J Hosp Med.* 2018;13(4):221–228.
124. Cole KO, Weimer MB, Wang K, et al. Impact of an electronically-integrated clinical pathway on hospital initiation of medications for alcohol use disorder and subsequent hospital utilization. *J Hosp Med.* 2025;20(10):1044–1051.
125. Bernstein EY, Baggett TP, Trivedi S, Herzig SJ, Anderson TS. Outcomes after initiation of medications for alcohol use disorder at hospital discharge. *JAMA Netw Open.* 2024; 7(3):e243387.
126. Englander H, King C, Nicolaidis C, et al. Predictors of opioid and alcohol pharmacotherapy initiation at hospital discharge among patients seen by an inpatient addiction consult service. *J Addict Med.* 2020;14(5):415–422.
127. Singh-Tan S, Torres-Lockhart K, Jakubowski A, et al. Addiction consult service and inpatient outcomes among patients with alcohol use disorder. *J Gen Intern Med.* 2023; 38(14):3216–3223.
128. Calcaterra SL, Bottner R, Martin M, et al. Management of opioid use disorder, opioid withdrawal, and opioid overdose prevention in hospitalized adults: a systematic review of existing guidelines. *J Hosp Med.* 2022;17(9):679–692.
129. French R, Aronowitz SV, Brooks Carthon JM, Schmidt HD, Compton P. Interventions for hospitalized medical and surgical patients with opioid use disorder: a systematic review. *Subst Abus.* 2022;43(1):495–507.
130. Englander H, Thakrar AP, Bagley SM, Rolley T, Dong K, Hyshka E. Caring for hospitalized adults with opioid use disorder in the era of fentanyl: a review. *JAMA Intern. Med.* 2024;184(6):691–701.
131. Stern SJ, D'Orazio JL, Work BD, Calcaterra SL, Thakrar AP. Point/counterpoint: should full agonist opioid medications be offered to hospitalized patients for management of opioid withdrawal? *J Hosp Med.* 2024;19(4):339–343.
132. Thakrar AP, Uritsky TJ, Christopher C, et al. Safety and preliminary outcomes of short-acting opioid agonist treatment (sOAT) for hospitalized patients with opioid use disorder. *Addict Sci Clin Pract.* 2023;18(1):13.
133. Leyde S, Abbs E, Suen LW, et al. A mixed-methods evaluation of an addiction/cardiology pilot clinic with contingency management for patients with stimulant-associated cardiomyopathy. *J Addict Med.* 2023;17(3):312–318.
134. Peng L, Titus H, Roellich P, Englander H. Adapting contingency management for hospitalized patients with stimulant use disorder. *J Addict Med.* 2023;17(5):580–586.
135. Danovitch I, Korouri S, Kaur H, et al. The addiction consultation service for hospitalized patients with substance use disorder: an integrative review of the evidence. *J Subst Use Addict Treat.* 2024:163:20937.
136. Orme S, Zarkin GA, Dunlap LJ, et al. Cost and cost savings of navigation services to avoid rehospitalization for a comorbid substance use disorder population. *Med Care.* 2022;60(8):631–635.
137. Callister C, Lockhart S, Holtrop JS, Hoover K, Calcaterra SL. Experiences with an addiction consultation service on care provided to hospitalized patients with opioid use disorder: a qualitative study of hospitalists, nurses, pharmacists, and social workers. *Subst Abus.* 2022;43(1):615–622.
138. Bredenberg E, Tietbohl C, Dafoe A, Thurman L, Calcaterra S. Identifying factors that contribute to burnout and resilience among hospital-based addiction medicine providers: a qualitative study. *J Subst Abuse Treat.* 2023;144:108924.
139. The ASAM Clinical Practice Guideline on alcohol withdrawal management. *J Addict Med.* 2020;14(3S Suppl 1):1–72.
140. Baddour LM, Weimer MB, Wurcel AG, et al. management of infective endocarditis in people who inject drugs: a scientific statement from the American Heart Association. *Circulation.* 2022;146(14):e187–e201.

2

Implementation and Sustainability of Hospital-Based Addiction Treatment

Susan L. Calcaterra, Itai Danovitch

When I began practicing as a hospitalist, black tar heroin dominated the drug supply in my community. Common complications related to injection of black tar heroin included skin and soft tissue infections, abscesses, osteomyelitis, and endocarditis. While skin and soft tissue infections and abscesses were treated with incision and drainage and a short course of antibiotics, osteomyelitis and endocarditis treatment required weeks of intravenous antibiotics, administered during a 6- to 8-week hospitalization. For many patients, a prolonged hospitalization led to boredom, isolation, and depression. My most memorable patient during my early career was a 20-something year-old man, Jake, who worked in food delivery. Jake maintained his job and housing with an active opioid use disorder (OUD) because he used heroin throughout his workday to avoid experiencing withdrawal. After 2 weeks of rigors, night sweats, and exhaustion, Jake went to the emergency department (ED) and was admitted to the hospital with sepsis. Within a few hours, Jake was assigned to my hospital team, and we diagnosed him with tricuspid valve endocarditis complicated by septic pulmonary emboli and opioid withdrawal. At the time, the hospital policy prohibited the use of methadone to manage opioid withdrawal unless patients were enrolled in an opioid treatment program. Buprenorphine, now regularly used to treat OUD, was rarely, if ever used, and only then as an intravenous analgesic.

In an attempt to manage Jake's opioid withdrawal, I prescribed escalating doses of extended-release morphine, oxycodone, and clonidine. My goal was to support Jake to remain in the hospital to receive antibiotic treatment. Unfortunately for Jake, I had no concept of how immense his opioid deficit was or how to best manage it. Ultimately, my treatment of Jake's opioid withdrawal was inadequate. Overwhelmed by his withdrawal symptoms, he ultimately left the hospital before completing antibiotic treatment. Residency trained me to manage endocarditis and other medical complications related to substance use disorder (SUD), but I was wholly unprepared to support Jake in the way he needed.

Despite receiving inadequate OUD treatment, Jake returned to the hospital three more times over the next 6 months, fully knowing he would experience horrific withdrawal each time. During one hospitalization, he received a bioprosthetic tricuspid valve replacement due to new-onset heart failure from inadequately treated endocarditis and valvular destruction. Unfortunately, with each hospitalization, Jake left early due to inadequately controlled opioid withdrawal. Jake later died from an opioid overdose—I received notification of his death in the electronic health record (EHR). During his four hospitalizations, Jake was never offered methadone or buprenorphine to treat his OUD, nor was he prescribed naloxone at hospital discharge. In-hospital initiation of medications for OUD was not standard practice at that time. Naloxone use was limited to paramedics on ambulances, EDs, and hospital settings. This lack of treatment contributed to endless patient suffering, death, and moral distress among clinicians and hospital staff. Personally, I felt complicit in Jake's death.

Jake, and other patients with SUD, led me to pursue addiction medicine training. With the support of colleagues and mentors, I learned that many hospital policies were grounded in stigma, not in federal or state law. According to U.S. Federal Code of Regulations Title 21, Part 1306.07, there are no restrictions on the use of methadone, buprenorphine, or any opioids to manage opioid withdrawal among hospitalized patients. Over time, and with the support of hospital leadership, pharmacy leadership, state grant funding, and the tenacity of dedicated clinicians, we developed and implemented an addiction consultation service (ACS) to better support hospitalized patients with SUD. Our team started out small, but in time the service grew as hospitalizations related to fentanyl and methamphetamine use surged. Today, our ACS is comprised of a group of addiction medicine board certified physicians who are also practicing hospitalists, addiction-trained advance practice professionals, fellows, resident physicians, and importantly, a licensed clinical counselor with addiction expertise, and a person in recovery who supports our patients as they move from the hospital to community setting.

Witnessing and participating in the efforts to transform hospital-based care for patients with SUD has been the most fulfilling part of my career. To date, these efforts are primarily championed by motivated clinicians who recognize the importance of treating SUD in the hospital, with most gains occurring in academic medical centers.[1] Significant disparities in SUD treatment persist. Even after an overdose, most people do not receive OUD treatment, and rates are lowest among racial and ethnic minority individuals.[2] Rural hospitals are 25% less likely to support an ACS, and are 50% less likely to support initiation of medications for OUD.[3] Interventions to promote hospital-based SUD treatment must address local factors reported by hospital-based clinicians and staff as barriers to providing this care. This chapter will outline how to develop and implement hospital-based SUD treatment interventions and programs informed by local needs and by leveraging existing resources.

Today, if Jake were hospitalized with injection-related endocarditis, our ACS would offer him methadone or buprenorphine to manage his opioid withdrawal and short-acting opioids to treat his pain from septic pulmonary emboli. Our team would adjust medication doses to meet his needs informed by both subjective and objective information. Once Jake's bacteremia cleared, we would discuss with our infectious disease colleagues if he would be a candidate for a long-acting injectable lipoglycopeptide to shorten his hospital stay. We would offer Jake infectious disease screening and treatment. We would offer direct linkage to an opioid treatment program for methadone continuation after hospital discharge, or a buprenorphine prescription and a follow-up appointment to ensure treatment continuation. If Jake were interested, we would facilitate direct linkage to a residential addiction treatment program. Finally, Jake would receive harm reduction education, naloxone, wound care supplies, and a list of local syringe service programs at hospital discharge. If we had provided this care to Jake back then, he may still be alive today.

—Susan L. Calcaterra

Key Points

- **Developing and implementing a hospital-based SUD treatment program requires significant time, energy, and resources. Beginning with a well-thought out plan is a major key to future success.**
- **Identify a core team of partners. Ensure that the core team members bring unique skills, ideas, and experiences to the program development and implementation.**
- **Identify key partners who are committed to supporting the program's development, implementation, and sustainment.**
- **Conduct a needs assessment to identify SUD treatment gaps.**
- **Use the results of the needs assessment to create an intervention(s) and determine the most appropriate outcome measures to demonstrate if the intervention has closed existing gaps.**
- **Pilot the intervention, study outcomes, adapt the program, when necessary, and report successes to hospital leadership.**
- **Disseminate the program and identify resources and avenues to ensure program sustainability.**

Historically, substance use disorder (SUD) treatment programs, including the treatment of alcohol and other substances, were separated from general health care and mental health care services.[4] Siloed SUD care reinforces the stigma that SUD is a choice with support limited to social programs, historically located outside of the medical system.[5–8] The separation of traditional medical and SUD treatment has impacted the quality and consistency of care provided to people with SUD.[4,9] Until recently, poor insurance reimbursement for SUD treatment,[10] limited educational opportunities to learn about SUD in health professional training,[11] and a lack of regular substance screening limited SUD treatment accessibility for most people.[12–14] Importantly, the separation of SUD treatment from general health care contributed to stigma and structural racism in every sector of SUD treatment from health care policy, to coverage, to care delivery and research.[9,15] Major disparities exist in SUD treatment access and treatment completion. Black and Hispanic people constitute approximately 40% of the publicly-funded SUD treatment admissions in the US, but are 8% less likely to complete treatment.[16] To address the deep health inequities experienced by minoritized populations related to SUD treatment, it will be necessary to diversify leadership, fund underrepresented groups to support program development and implementation, and dedicate resources to recruit and hire a medical and academic workforce that is reflective, inclusive, and welcoming of people from all backgrounds.[17]

Several research studies over many years have reported on the high prevalence of SUD among people seeking care in emergency departments (EDs), hospitals, and general medical settings; historically, SUD treatment was rarely, if ever, offered in primary care or acute care settings.[4,14] It was the opioid overdose epidemic, one of the deadliest in US history, that spurred SUD treatment into mainstream medical care.[18–20] The steep increase in costly hospitalizations related to opioid, stimulant, and alcohol use[21–24] contributed to the development and implementation of hospital-based addiction care models, including the addiction consultation service (ACS).[18,25] Hospital-based addiction treatment provision is often championed by clinicians who understand that 10% of hospitalized patients have SUD,[23] and if undiagnosed or untreated, SUD often contributes to rehospitalizations and death.[18,26–30]

Rationale for Addressing SUD in the Hospital

As described in Chapter 1, hospitalization provides a critical opportunity to engage patients with SUD into treatment. Hospital-based SUD care with referral to treatment increases outpatient SUD treatment engagement.[31] Hospitals have both an obligation and opportunity to improve the health of their patients and community by supporting the systematic detection and treatment of SUD. Untreated SUD is associated with higher complications, greater utilization of emergency services,[23,32] hospital readmissions,[27,28] workforce turnover and burnout,[33–35] and negative care experiences for people with SUD.[36–38] Many patients who are hospitalized with SUD have difficulty accessing SUD treatment services due to social determinants of health.[39,40] Hospital-based SUD treatment is an important means of overcoming access barriers that exist in other settings.[41] The failure to address SUD exacerbates public health issues, such as the spread of infectious diseases, the rise in overdose deaths, and the broader societal and economic impacts associated with SUD.[21–23,28,42,43] The cost of effective prevention and treatment, both in the hospital setting and in outpatient medical practices, may be substantially offset by a reduction in the high direct medical cost of SUD hospital care.[21]

Models of Hospital-Based Addiction Care

This chapter addresses how to develop, implement, and sustain integrated hospital-based SUD services. Chapter 4 will review various models of hospital-based SUD care.[18] Many of these SUD care models developed organically based on the recognition that there was a site-specific need to provide SUD treatment to hospitalized patients. Successful hospital-based SUD treatment programs share key features including the identification of a project champion, a subject matter expert, and creating a core team who are committing to expanding SUD services. These teams partner with hospital leaders and colleagues across disciplines in the hospital and outpatient setting to obtain buy-in and support of the program for long-term success. Finally, programs leaders leverage existing resources to improve success in implementation and sustainment of hospital-based SUD treatment.

One example of a hospital-based care model that has emerged to improve care for patients with SUD is the ACS.[18,20,31] The ACS includes an interprofessional team that may be comprised of physicians with expertise managing SUD and related complications, advanced practice professionals who provide dedicated SUD services, social workers, licensed therapists, or counselors, and people with lived/living experience with addiction (Figure 2.1).[18,25,44]

Research demonstrates that the ACS model increases SUD treatment initiation and posthospital SUD treatment linkage; it is less clear if the ACS model reduces postdischarge substance use or rehospitalization.[25]

ACS teams have predominantly grown at academic hospitals; the majority of community and rural hospitals do not have the funding to support an ACS.[18,25] In smaller hospitals, an addiction expert may work as a consultant, either in-person or by telephone, to provide support to hospital-based clinicians on challenging cases that are outside of their practice scope.[18]

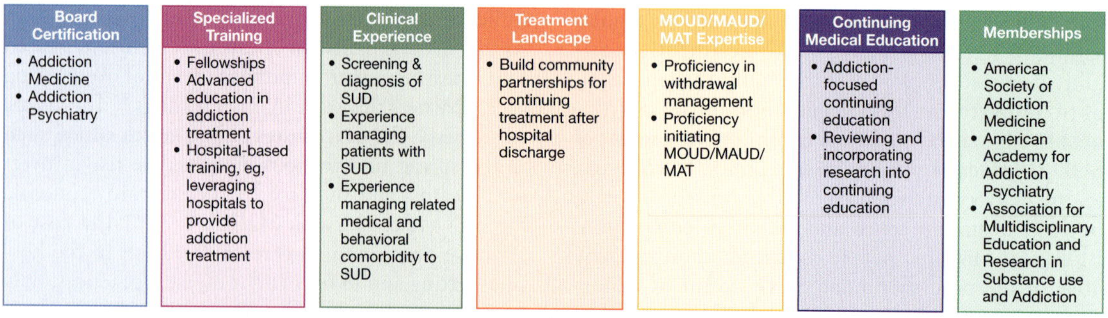

Figure 2.1: Range of medical expertise and skills to support hospital-based SUD treatment. SUD, substance use disorder; MOUD, medications for opioid use disorder; MAUD, medications for alcohol use disorder; MAT, medications for addiction treatment to include tobacco use disorder and stimulant use disorder.

Another model, described as the hospital-based opioid treatment (HBOT) and hospital-based alcohol treatment (HBAT) model, leverages the hospital-based clinician workforce to treat SUD in the hospital. For this model to work effectively, hospital-based clinicians must learn the clinical skills necessary to provide basic SUD care, including diagnosing and treating opioid use disorder (OUD) and AUD, managing withdrawal syndromes, treating common comorbidities, and referring patients to local SUD treatment.[18] Hospital-based guidelines direct best care for opioid withdrawal and OUD management, alcohol withdrawal and AUD management, and stimulant intoxication and withdrawal management should be integrated into all hospital medicine practices.[45–47]

Hospitals and associated health care systems vary greatly in size, location, availability of resources, level of acuity of care provided, patient population, and funding sources. Identifying site-specific SUD needs and implementing targeted evidence-based interventions is the first step to changing hospital-based SUD clinical practice. Sustaining the practice change requires regular assessments with adaptations based on iterative feedback from multidisciplinary collaborators.

This chapter outlines processes to develop and implement hospital-based SUD treatment services that can be adapted to meet the needs of any hospital setting. This chapter begins by distinguishing quality improvement (QI) processes, implementation science frameworks, and examples of each. Next, the chapter provides a step-by-step approach to develop, implement, maintain, and sustain a hospital-based SUD treatment program with example metrics to track progress and to identify areas that need ongoing improvement. Included at the end of the chapter is a detailed case study of an intervention aimed to expand inpatient screening for unhealthy substance use with team members, project activities, and an associated timeline that may be used as a template and adapted by individuals who are interested in building hospital-based SUD treatment processes in their hospital.

Understanding the Difference Between QI and Implementation Science

QI and implementation science are related but distinct fields—both efforts share the goal of improving the quality of health care.

Quality Improvement

QI focuses on enhancing health care services and outcomes through systematic efforts to improve processes, reduce errors, and increase efficiency, usually at a single site or in a health care system.[48] It involves specific interventions aimed at making measurable improvements in health care settings. QI initiatives are informed by data and involve interdisciplinary teams to ensure a broad representation of key partners to maximize the success and impact of the intervention. Successful QI interventions involve specific key strategies: conduct a local needs assessment; engage leadership and staff; adopt evidence-based practices (EBP); monitor progress; and adapt and repeat. Table 2.1 lists key strategies involved in QI initiatives versus key strategies used when implementing and disseminating an intervention using implementation science methods.

Examples of Commonly Used QI Methods

Common QI methods include Plan-Do-Study-Act (PDSA) cycles (Figure 2.2), Root Cause Analysis (RCA), and Lean or Six Sigma methodologies and are listed in Table 2.2.[49–52] These methods share common goals of first clearly identifying, describing, or defining a problem or gap that needs addressing. The next step involves gathering data to better understand the problem or gap. Data should be gathered from multiple

TABLE 2.1

Key Strategies Involved in a Quality Improvement (QI) Initiative Versus Implementation Science

Key strategies involved in a QI initiative	
Conduct a needs assessment	Identify specific areas for improvement based on local data and key partner input
Engage leadership, staff, and other key partners	Involve leadership and frontline staff early in the planning phases, later in the implementation phases, and routinely thereafter to increase buy-in of the QI initiative
Adopt evidence-based practices (EBP)	Utilize proven methodologies like PDSA cycles, Lean, or Six Sigma to guide implementation of the QI initiative
Monitor progress and adapt	Regularly collect and analyze data to measure the effect of the QI intervention, making adjustments informed by data to maximize the effects of the intervention
Key strategies involved in implementation science	
Assessment of needs and context	Conduct a thorough assessment of the specific needs of the target population and the context in which the EBP will be implemented to tailor implementation strategies for improved adoption and uptake
Engage key partners	Actively involve key partners. Key partners are people who will support implementation of the EBP (ie, high-level and mid-level leaders, opinion leaders), people who incorporate the EBP into their clinical practice (ie, frontline clinicians, staff), people who will lead the implementation of the EBP locally (ie, clinical leaders), people who will receive the EBP (ie, patients), policy makers, and others. This will foster buy-in and ensure the EBP meets the needs of the people who will adopt it and who will benefit from it
Use of theories, models, and/or frameworks (TMF) to implement the EBP	Use of TMFs are important to systematically guide the implementation of the EBP for reproducibility, to inform implementation strategies, and to inform needed adaptations to the implementation strategies or EBP
Use tailored implementation strategies to implement the EBP	Identify barriers and facilitators to uptake and impact of the EBP and use targeted implementation strategies to minimize or maximize site-specific barriers and facilitators
Adapt the EBP	Based on qualitative and quantitative data, modify the EBP to fit the local context while maintaining its core components to enhance its relevance and effectiveness
Evaluate the impact of the implementation of the EBP	Using a systematic approach or framework, evaluate implementation outcomes. Commonly assessed outcomes include Reach, Effectiveness, Adoption, Implementation, and Maintenance (REAIM)

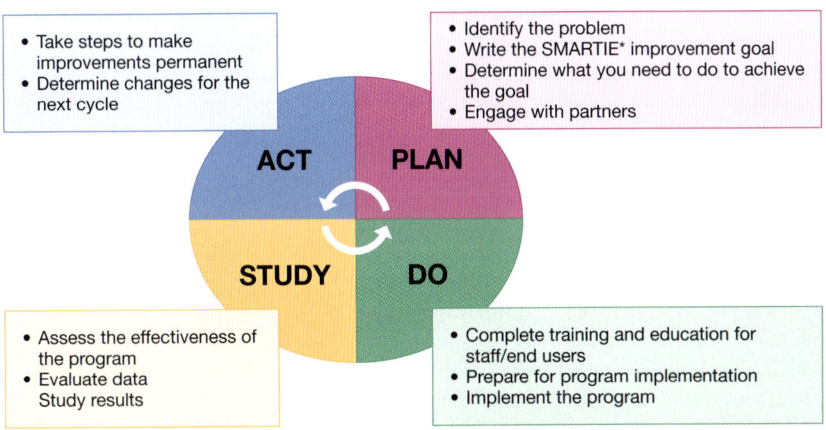

*SMARTIE stands for Strategic, Measurable, Ambitious, Realistic, Time-bound, Inclusive, and Equitable

Figure 2.2: Plan-Do-Study-Act (PDSA) cycle.

TABLE 2.2

Three Commonly Used Quality Improvement Frameworks and Associated Processes

A Plan-Do-Study-Act (PDSA) cycle[53]
Plan: Identify a goal or change that needs to be made locally; develop a plan for how to implement that change and define the objectives, the resources needed, and a timeline for change
Do: Implement the plan on a small scale to test its effectiveness while collecting data on how it performs
Study: Analyze the data collected during the "Do" phase; assess the outcomes against the objectives identified in the planning phase to determine what did and did not work, and why
Act: Based on the information in the "Study" phase, decide whether to adopt, adapt, or reject the change; if the change met the objectives, consider scaling it up or integrate it as local best practices; if not, consider restarting the cycle
Root Cause Analysis (RCA)
Define the problem: Clearly describe the problem, including its symptoms, scope, and impact by gathering relevant data including timeline of events, impact, and observations of the problem by personnel; frame the problem as a "why" to be solved
Gather and organize data: Collect the evidence using existing documents, logs of data, interviews, and observations; with these data, develop a timeline of events to understand what happened and when; then, validate the data to ensure it reflects actual events
Identify possible causes: Brainstorm potential causes using the "5 Whys Analysis"[54] or a "Fishbone Diagram"[55]
Analyze and prioritize causes: Evaluate possible causes to determine its relevance using a "Pareto Analysis"[56] or a "Fault Tree Analysis[57]: validate the findings with a subject matter expert and data
Identify the root cause: Determine the primary reason(s) the problem occurred; ensure the identified root cause is actionable and within the organization's control
Develop solutions: Brainstorm solutions to correct and prevent the root cause, evaluation solutions for feasibility, effectiveness, and potential risks
Implement the solution: Create a detailed action plan by assigning responsibility, deadlines, and resources to team members; communicate the plan to all key partners
Monitor and validate results: Track the implementation of the solution; measure effectives of the correct actions using key performance indicators (KPIs), or follow-up evaluations; make necessary adjustments
Document and share process, outcomes, interventions: Integrate RCA findings into broader process quality improvement initiatives; review and refine RCA practices
Six Sigma Methodologies[51,58]
Define: Identify the problem or opportunity for improvement; define the project scope and goals; develop a project document describing the project aims to align key partners
Measure: Collect data to establish a baseline for current process performance; define KPIs; map the process using tools like flowcharts or value stream mapping
Analyze: Examine the data to identify root causes of problems; use statistical tools such as cause-and-effect diagrams, hypothesis testing, or regression analysis; validate findings with subject matter experts
Improve: Develop and test solutions to address root causes; implement changes using techniques like pilot testing or simulations; optimize the process for efficiency and effectiveness
Control: Establish controls to sustain improvements; develop monitoring plans, control charts, and standard operating procedures (SOPs); conduct periodic reviews to ensure the process remains stable and effective

sources including interviews with key partners, reviewing records or logs, and conducting observations of workflow, work process, and work interactions. Collecting, organizing, and analyzing data from various sources allows for a deeper understanding of the situation before, during, and after a problem with an overview of the current state and practices (or lack of) that may need adjustment. Next, informed by the results of the data analysis, develop solutions to the problem or gap. Involve key partners in developing solutions with iterative refinement. Before implementing the solution, identify key performance indicators (KPIs) to track success and failures of planned solution(s). Finally, implement and study the solution(s) while collecting outcomes data of the KPIs. Use the results of the KPIs to modify the solution to improve its success. Advertise the work to leadership, key partners, and peers. This chapter will provide a detailed map to inform the development and implementation of a hospital-based SUD treatment program. As a reference, Table 2.3 lists examples of SUD-related interventions that can be tailored to individual hospitals with example KPIs to track successes and failures of a hospital-based SUD treatment program.

TABLE 2.3

Examples of Interventions and Programs to Expand Hospital-Based SUD Treatment[59]

Intervention/Program	Intervention description	Who is responsible for completing the task
Develop an interprofessional Addiction Consultative Service (ACS)[18] Resources: Bridge[60,61] Implementation guides[59,62]	▪ Inpatient/hospital setting ▪ Funding to pay for staff, implementation and training, management of team, electronic health record (EHR) tools, data analysis	Person capable to work with leadership to support this endeavor, who can obtain funding and who is (or who can identify) a subject matter expert to provide training, education, advertise the service, and sustain the service **Considerations (applies throughout):** Partnering with key partners, including: ▪ Local opioid treatment programs ▪ Outpatient/inpatient addiction treatment facilities ▪ Bridge clinics ▪ Subacute nursing facilities ▪ Primary care clinics ▪ Behavioral health clinics ▪ Federally qualified health centers Partner with clinical pharmacists to ensure that: ▪ Medications for AUD, OUD, TUD, and nicotine replacement therapy are available on the inpatient formulary ▪ Policies and procedures support use of medications to treat SUD
Hospital-based opioid treatment; alcohol treatment (HBOT/HBAT)[18]	▪ Primary team (eg, hospitalist) or specialist consultant (eg, infectious disease provider) offer MOUD/MAUD as part of their standard practice	Leader and champion who can convince peers to provide this treatment, offer education and training, develop protocols, pathways, or ordersets to support the initiation of these medications, and sustain the efforts
Access to an individual addiction-trained consultant[18]	▪ Provides telephone consults to hospital-based clinicians on difficult cases ▪ Provides remote video consults to hospitalized patients	Person capable to work with leadership to support this endeavor, who can obtain funding and who is (or who can identify) a subject matter expert to provide training, education, advertise the service, and sustain the service
Universal screening for unhealthy substance use[46,63]	▪ Embed validated screening questions in EHR ▪ Examples of validated screening tools: Single-item screeners, DAST-10, AUDIT, CUDIT, TAPS tool	Nurse driven/social work driven
Standardize opioid withdrawal assessments by nursing staff[64]	▪ Embed Clinical Opiate Withdrawal Scale (COWS) in EHR	Nurse driven

(continued)

TABLE 2.3

Examples of Interventions and Programs to Expand Hospital-Based SUD Treatment[59] (*Continued*)

Intervention/Program	Intervention description	Who is responsible for completing the task
Use of DSM-5 to diagnose SUD[65]	■ Embed DSM-5 calculator in EHR	Physician/advance practice professional-driven or social work driven
Standardize documentation of SUD in EHR[65]	■ Embed DSM-5 calculator in EHR	Physician/advance practice professional driven or social work driven
Develop ordersets/protocols for buprenorphine initiation[66]	■ Embed in EHR	Physician/advance practice professional driven **Considerations:** Partner with pharmacist to ensure buprenorphine formulations are available
Develop ordersets/protocols for methadone initiation[66]	■ Embed in EHR	Physician/advance practice professional driven
Develop ordersets/protocols for take-home methadone (72-hour rule)[67]	■ Embed in EHR	Pharmacist and clinical champion driven in a partnership
Develop ordersets/protocols to manage precipitated opioid withdrawal[66]	■ Embed in EHR	Physician/advance practice professional driven
Automate naloxone prescribing for OUD/Stimulant use disorder (StUD) (contamination of drug supply)[68]	■ Embed in EHR	Physician/advance practice professional driven
Develop ordersets/protocols to manage alcohol withdrawal (CIWA, MINDS)[45,69,70]	■ Embed in EHR	Physician/advance practice professional driven **Considerations** Partner with pharmacist, and nursing lead to consider safety, rules, protocols to treat complicated alcohol withdrawal[71]
Develop ordersets/protocols to prescribing medications for AUD[66]	■ Embed in EHR	Physician/advance practice professional driven
Review hospital policies addressing in-hospital substance use; develop patient-centered guidelines to mitigate and address in-hospital substance use[72]	■ Create a multidisciplinary committee responsible for developing, implementing, and periodically reassessing the guidelines	Multidisciplinary committee members may include nurses, clinicians, behavioral health specialists, addiction specialist, legal counsel, patient representatives
Integrate harm reduction services and supplies into hospital care with patient educational materials[73]	■ Identify funding source to pay for supplies; create orders for syringes, in-hand/take-home naloxone, test strips, etc in EHR	Clinical champion driven
Created processes to facilitate postdischarge SUD treatment linkage ■ Buprenorphine prescribers ■ Opioid treatment programs ■ Inpatient and outpatient SUD treatment	■ Identify local SUD treatment resources for post discharge treatment linkage; embed these resources in EHR	Social work driven/case management driven
Address stigma in the workforce, trauma informed care[17,74,75]	■ Provide education to staff and clinicians about person first language; stigma-free documentation in the EHR; how to provide trauma-informed care	Clinical champion driven

Implementation Science

Implementation science is "the scientific study of methods to promote the systematic uptake of research findings and other evidence-based practices (EBP) into routine practice to improve the quality and effectiveness of health services."[76] Implementation science studies how to effectively integrate underutilized EBPs into real world settings with a focus on the context, that is, the hospital, staff, local politics and policies, etc, in which the EBP is being implemented.[48] Implementation science is informed by theories, models, and frameworks (TMF) used in psychology, sociology, public health, and organization studies.[77] The use of TMFs allows for a deeper understanding of the complexities involved with implementation of EBP across various settings. TMFs facilitate the systematic examination of barriers and facilitators to the uptake of EBPs into clinical practice leading to greater success when implementing and disseminating the EPBs across sites with different clinical staff, patient populations, missions, and resources.[78] Key strategies involved in implementation science include assessing the needs and context of the individual site, engaging key partners, using a theory, model, or framework to inform the EPB's implementation, tailoring the implementation strategies to the context, adapting the EBP to facilitate improved uptake and impact, and systematically evaluating the impact of the EBP.

Implementation Strategies

Central to implementation science is use of targeted implementation strategies to increase the uptake and impact of the EBP. Implementation strategies are defined as "methods or techniques used to address barriers and facilitators for uptake of the EBP." Specifically, implementation strategies enhance the adoption, implementation, and sustainability of a clinical program or EBP.[79] Examples include audit and feedback, educational outreach and visits, conducing a local needs assessment, creating a learning collaborative, engaging leadership, identifying and preparing champions, incentivizing or disincentivizing, among many others.[80] Included in this chapter is a case example highlighting various targeted implementation strategies used to enhance SUD treatment uptake in ED settings.[81]

Examples of Commonly Used Implementation Theories, Models, and Frameworks Used in Implementation Science

According to Nilsen,[77] there are three overarching aims of the use of TMF in implementation science: (1) to describe or guide the process of translating research into practice, (2) to understand or explain what influences implementation outcomes; and (3) to evaluate the implementation of an EBP. Nilsen describes five categories of TMF to achieve these aims including: (1) process models, (2) determinant frameworks, (3) classic theories, (4) implementation frameworks, and (5) evaluation frameworks.[77] Table 2.4 lists categories of TMF used in implementation science.

Process models specify steps, stages, or phases in the process of translating research into practice. Process models aim to describe or guide the process of translating research into practice.[82–86] An *action model* is a type of process model that provides practical guidance in the planning and execution of implementation strategies to facilitate implementation of an EBP.

Determinant frameworks describe groups, domains, or classes of factors that may impact an implementation outcome(s).[78,87–94] For example, the experience of burnout may impact whether or not a clinician adopts an EBP, even when they are presented with its evidence of effectiveness. Each group, domain, or class of factors is typically classified as a barrier or facilitator to implementation outcomes related to the EBP including adoption of the EBP in a certain site or community, the effectiveness of the EBP in a certain site or community, whether or not the EBP is sustained in that site or community over time, and how successfully the EBP was implemented in that site or community. Identifying site-specific information about what may influence implementation outcomes is useful when designing and executing implementation strategies that aim to target and reduce identified barriers to EPB uptake.

Classic theories originate from fields outside of implementation science and include psychology, sociology, and organizational theory. These theories are described as "classic change theories." Classic change theories describe mechanisms of change within a context and examine how change occurs organically when there is no active intervention. Change theories can be applied to implementation science to understand or explain aspects of implementation of an EBP.[95–98] Theories exploring group behaviors, that is, health care team, professional groups, communities, and the relationships between and across groups to explore social capital and social networks can be helpful in implementation science. Increasingly, implementation scientists are turning to organizational theory to explore organizational culture, climate, and leaders to better understand organizational influences on implementation processes, especially as it pertains to the learning health system.[99,100] Finally, theories that explore the spread of EBPs have influenced implementation science. This may include particular attributes of the EBP, that is, its compatibility or complexity within a particular site, and also understanding the importance of how key partners, including opinion leaders, change agents, and gate-keepers

TABLE 2.4

Categories of Theories, Models, and Frameworks Used in Implementation Science[77]

TMFs	Examples of TMFs
Process models	■ ACE star model of knowledge transformation[82] ■ Knowledge-to-action model[83] ■ Iowa model[84,85] ■ Ottawa model[86,101]
Determinant frameworks	■ Exploration, preparation, implementation, sustainment (EPIS) framework[78] ■ Consolidated framework for implementation research (CFIR)[87,88] ■ Practical, robust implementation and sustainability model (PRISM)[89–91] ■ Promoting action on research implementation in health services (PARIHS) framework[92,93] ■ Theoretical domains framework[94,102]

Classic theories	■ Change theories:
	  ■ Theory of reasoned action[95]
	  ■ Social cognitive theory[96]
	  ■ Theory of interpersonal behavior[97]
	  ■ Theory of planned behavior[98]
	■ Organizational theories
	  ■ Situated change theory[99]
	  ■ Institutional theory[100]
	■ Theory on the spread of innovations:
	  ■ Theory of diffusion[103]

Implementation theories	■ Implementation climate[104] ■ Absorptive capacity[105] ■ Organizational readiness[106] ■ COM-B[107] ■ Normalization process theory[108]
Evaluation frameworks	■ Reach, effectiveness, adoption, implementation, maintenance (RE-AIM) (a part of PRISM)[89,109] ■ PRECEDE-PROCEED[110,111] ■ Implementation outcomes framework[112,113]
Health equity frameworks	■ PRISM/RE-AIM with a health equity focus[114–116] ■ Health equity implementation framework[117,118] ■ Transcreation framework[119] ■ Behavior change wheel[120]

influence the successful adoption and implementation of an EBP.[103]

Implementation theories are developed or adapted by researchers to provide an understanding or explanation of various aspects of implementation. These theories explore what motivates and directs behaviors,[107] identify capability and opportunity as necessary conditions for change,[106] and examine the relationships between normalizing behaviors, behavioral engagement, collective action, and reflexive monitoring of actions.[108]

Evaluation frameworks provide structure to evaluate aspects of implementation strategies. Commonly measured implementation outcomes include an assessment of:

- The **acceptability** of the EBP in a particular site
- The **adoption** or **uptake** of the EBP in a particular site
- The **appropriateness** of implementing the EBP in a particular site
- The **cost** of implementing the EBP in a particular site
- The **feasibility** of implementing an EBP in a particular site
- If the EBP was implemented with **fidelity** at a particular site
- How well the EBP was **integrated** into a particular site
- Whether or not the EBP **reached** the intended population at a particular site
- The **effectiveness** of the EBP in a particular site
- Whether or not the EBP was **sustained, maintained, or institutionalized** into a particular site.[109,112,121]

Health Equity in Implementation Science

More recently, implementation scientists developed or modified frameworks to explicitly address health equity. Braveman defines health equity as "the principle underlying a commitment to reduce, and ultimately eliminate, disparities in health and in its determinants, including social determinants."[122] The use of determinant frameworks to understand why disparities exist in access, receipt, use, quality, or outcomes of health care are urgently needed.[117] Frameworks that systemically study factors that predict successful and equitable implementation should include an in-depth assessment of the culturally relevant factors of recipients of the EBP.[117,118] These factors may explore how medical mistrust, socioeconomic status, race/ethnicity, language, health literacy, health beliefs, immigrant acculturation, and other factors impact implementation of an EBP.[117,118]

Health Equity Frameworks to Systematically Assess Factors That Contribute to Inequity in Implementation, Dissemination, and Sustainment of EBPs

Health equity frameworks provide a structured approach to examining factors that influence clinical encounters. These frameworks help explore whether EBPs are offered, accepted by the patient, or deemed unacceptable to the patient. They also consider how perceptions or unconscious biases might impact the clinician–patient relationship.

A framework that incorporates health equity will consider the role that societal context plays in implementation of an EBP. Woodward et al, further classifies societal context into three categories (1) economies, (2) physical structures, and (3) sociopolitical forces.[117,118] Before, during, and after implementation of an EPB, it is important to understand how economic structures affect access to resources for implementation. Equity can be impacted by the "built environment" and how people move from one space to another, particularly when accessing health care. One example of this includes systematic rejection of referrals of hospitalized patients with OUD to post–acute medical care facilities.[123] The successful implementation of a hospital to post–acute care facility linkage program must include developing partnerships between hospitals and post–acute care facilities that directly address and resolve reasons for rejection of patients on MOUD.

Finally, sociopolitical forces include political support, laws, and social structures, all of which interact to propagate the status quo including racism, misogyny, ableism, classism, or heterosexism.[117,118] One example of a law that inadvertently propagated stigma toward people with OUD was the X-waiver. In 2000, the Drug Addiction Treatment Act (DATA 2000) required clinicians to obtain a special waiver on their DEA licenses after completing 8 hours (physician) or 24 hours (advanced practice professionals) of training to prescribe buprenorphine for OUD.[124] This created inequities in OUD treatment access where buprenorphine treatment was concentrated among white persons and those with private insurance or among those who paid out of pocket for treatment services.[125] Following calls to remove the X-waiver,[126–128] in 2023, the federal government eliminated the X-waiver.[129]

Implementation scientists have also modified existing frameworks to enhance the focus on health equity by (1) focusing attention on representation in planning, implementation, and evaluation stages of an EBP; (2) engaging participants to cocreate and/or adapt the EBP and implementation strategies to enhance equity; (3) assessing structural drivers of inequity, and capacity and infrastructure needs and resources; and (4) conducting iterative assessment of implementation outcomes to identify equity-enhancing approaches and address unintended consequences.[114]

Case Example of the Use of an Implementation Framework With Targeted Implementation Strategies to Enhance SUD Treatment in ED Settings

Bozinoff et al conducted a scoping review of the literature to systematically identify barriers and facilitators to buprenorphine initiation in the ED setting and associated strategies used to increase treatment uptake.[81] The authors used the Consolidated Framework for Implementation Research (CFIR), an implementation framework, to organize and synthesize their findings into barriers and facilitators identified in the *inner setting*, that is, the hospital and ED setting, and in the *outer setting*, that is, community partnerships and connections.[87,88] Distinguishing the two settings is important to inform resource allocation and direct process changes. Bozinoff et al highlighted facilitators that lead to successful implementation of ED-buprenorphine initiation including a greater days' supply of a buprenorphine prescription from ED clinicians (inner setting), rapid access to an on-site clinic that provides OUD treatment or an addiction medicine clinic (inner setting), that is, low-barrier linkage, care/peer navigators (inner setting), use of extended release buprenorphine in the ED (inner setting), registering patients for public insurance programs while in the ED, programs that support multidisciplinary SUD treatment teams (inner setting), and programs that colocate low-barrier and harm reduction–informed services to support ED to outpatient transitions (outer setting).[81] The authors identified commonly described barriers to successful ED-buprenorphine initiation programs including challenges with communication with outpatient buprenorphine prescribers for linkage (outer setting), both generally, and outside office hours, long wait times to get an outpatient appointment for follow-up (outer setting), difficulty with insurance coverage (both inner and outer setting), lack of care coordination support in the ED for scheduling of outpatient follow-up (inner setting), high rate of no-shows in the outpatient setting (outer setting), unaddressed structural stigma (both inner and outer setting), client complexity (both inner and outer setting), and an increasingly toxic drug supply (both inner and outer setting).[81] The result of this scoping review can inform the development and implementation of hospital-based SUD care because many of these facilitators and barriers are also present during hospital-to-community treatment transitions.

Putting It All Together: A Step-by-Step Guide to Implement a Hospital-Based SUD Treatment Program

Whether or not the intent is to develop hospital-based SUD treatment (ie, a QI-focused local program) or to build an evidence base to inform the development, implementation, and sustainment of hospital-based SUD care more generally (ie, the use of implementation science TMF), many of the concepts are similar. The following section outlines a series of steps, informed by both QI and implementation frameworks, for establishing hospital-based SUD care. While these steps represent an ideal approach based on extensive research of successful program launches, the key to success also lies in having a passionate clinical champion, a solid understanding of EBP, and persistent efforts to improve the health system. It is important to prioritize *progress* over *perfection*. Even if not all steps can be followed, using this framework can help overcome common barriers and increase the likelihood of achieving sustainable success (Figure 2.3).

Initial Steps to Implement a Hospital-Based SUD Treatment Program

When considering hospital-based SUD treatment, it is important to acknowledge and amplify the vast body of literature that demonstrates the effectiveness of SUD treatment interventions. Extensive evidence, for example, demonstrates that MOUD reduces mortality related to OUD.[130–133] Similarly, evidence demonstrates that MAUD reduces any alcohol use and heavy alcohol use.[134] Harm reduction interventions, including the distribution of unused syringes

- **Step 1**. Garner Institutional Support
- **Step 2.** Identify a Core Team
- **Step 3.** Identify a Support Network
- **Step 4.** Conduct a Needs Assessment
    - **Step 4a.** Clarify the Goals of the Needs Assessement
    - **Step 4b.** Determine What Data Are Needed to Describe & Quantify SUD-Treatment Gaps
    - **Step 4c.** Develop Succinct Questions the Assessment Will Answer to Identify the Current State of SUD Delivery & Associated Gaps in Care
    - **Step 4d.** Organize & Analyze the Data to Identify Gaps Based on the Data Query
    - **Step 4e.** Map Out How the Hospital-based SUD Treatment Program Will Address Identified Gaps
        - *Ensure the Solutions are **S**pecific, **M**easurable, **A**ttainable, **R**elevant, **T**ime-bound, **I**nclusive, and **E**quitable (**SMARTIE**)*
- **Step 5.** Write Up a Brief Report of the Above & Present to Leadership
- **Step 6.** Assemble the Implementation Team
- **Step 7.** Develop & Implement a Pilot, Measure Associated Outcome Metrics
- **Step 8.** Consider Necessary Adaptions to the Program Before Widespread Dissemination
- **Step 9.** Dissemination & Sustainability

Figure 2.3: Practical steps to implement a hospital-based SUD treatment program.

and condoms, reduces the spread of infectious diseases.[135,136] Overwhelming evidence demonstrates that community distribution of naloxone prevents fatal opioid overdoses.[137] Many of these interventions have shown benefit when initiated in the hospital or ED setting. Bringing these EBPs into the hospital setting using a systematic approach will reduce morbidity and mortality among people with SUD.[73,138] Identifying how to implement these and other EBPs within a particular hospital requires an in-depth understanding of the hospital's organizational capacities, culture, leadership, existing resources, and community goals.

Step 1: Garner Institutional Support

Obtaining hospital leadership support (eg, "C-suite") will facilitate buy-in and increase the success of the development, implementation, and sustainment of the new programs or services. Which hospital leaders to approach will depend on a variety of factors. For instance, is the hospital academic, private, not-for-profit, for-profit, rural, suburban, or urban? Is the hospital embedded within a larger health care system? Is the hospital a nonprofit community hospital with a mission to address the gaps identified in its annual community health needs assessment? If yes, is there an opportunity to frame hospital-based SUD treatment as aligning with its mission?

Next, develop a broad overview of the problem, and draft a preliminary proposal for how to address it (a detailed needs assessment with identified outcome measures will follow later in the chapter). List potential partners for collaboration, including a request for administrative support and access to SUD-related data and acute care utilization. This may be in the form of monthly tailored reports or a data analyst who can build dashboards linked to the electronic health record (EHR). With this preliminary information, briefly outline potential solutions. Consider reaching out to colleagues across the country who built hospital-based SUD programs to ask for advice and guidance on the proposal draft.[18] Incorporate feedback while revising the proposal and, when ready, request a meeting with the identified hospital leaders. Ideally, these leaders will understand how to build support and garner resources within their system. Keep in mind that it may take a series of meetings to identify a hospital leader who supports the proposal. Finding a leader who agrees to offer administrative support upfront may be challenging. If administrative support is not offered, then consider what can be realistically done with limited time and funds. Be persistent about needing resources to track patient-level and encounter-level data as a marker of productivity and program impact. These data will be necessary when asking for resources for future growth. Once the hospital leader agrees, obtain a signed letter of support acknowledging the proposed project and support as a commitment to the requisite resources over the duration of the program. This is important if there is leadership change during the program's development and implementation. Finally, ask the hospital leader to serve as the executive sponsor who will be the primary contact for the project team.[62]

Step 2: Identify a Core Team

The **core team** is responsible for leading the project to expand hospital-based SUD treatment and will include: a **project leader**, a hospital-based clinician who is familiar with the hospital culture, current practices, and workflow, and a **subject matter expert**, a person with specialized knowledge in SUD treatment provision. It may be that the **project lead** has both of these qualities and can serve in these capacities. The **core team** in a hospital-based SUD program should also ideally include a physician, nurse, pharmacist, and social worker, and, if possible, a data analyst who is familiar with quantitative data sources that may be extracted from the EHR. Enlisting community partners as part of the core team may also be beneficial if the health system relies on community partners as primary referral sources. If it is not possible to include these individuals, consider partnering with individuals with experience building programs in other institutions through national professional organizations like American Society of Addiction Medicine (ASAM),

Step 3: Identify a Support Network

Keep in mind that providing care to hospitalized patients with SUD may require buy-in from a range of people: hospital leadership, an executive sponsor, nursing staff, pharmacists, physicians and advanced practice professionals from various medical (internal medicine, family medicine, cardiology, gastroenterology/hepatology, psychiatry) and surgical specialties (obstetrics and gynecology, general surgery, trauma/burn, orthopedics, transplant), social workers, case management, and data officers. If the program will address interventions to mitigate in-hospital substance use and associated harms, consider involving leaders from psychiatry, risk management, and hospital security.[139] Whenever possible, involve people with lived/living experience with SUD who have engaged in hospital services. Finally, involve nursing educators, clinician educators, and pharmacy educators who will support efforts to acculturate the hospital-based SUD program. Reach out to individuals representing these areas, define their role in the program's development or implementation, and certify their commitment to participating in that capacity. Identify partners representing most, if not all, of these disciplines. The level of involvement of specific individuals in the support network will vary depending on the project and its goals. For example, a nursing educator may agree to develop education and curriculum for nurses once the program is ready for implementation, while a hospital leader may agree to send an email or announcement to hospital staff encouraging them to participate in the program.

Step 4: Conduct a Needs Assessment

The **core team** will conduct a needs assessment, which is a key strategy for any QI or implementation initiative. A needs assessment is a systematic process used to identify and evaluate gaps between the existing state (ie, the current provision of SUD treatment) and the ideal state within a specific context (ie, a hospital, its staff, and hospitalized patients). The information obtained during a needs assessment will be used to prioritize actions, to allocate resources, to gain buy-in from key partners, and to create strategies for improvement. The **core team** will complete the steps listed below when conducting a needs assessment to expand hospital-based SUD treatment. Table 2.5 outlines the steps involved when conducting a needs assessment.

TABLE 2.5

Steps Involved in a Needs Assessment[140]

Part 1. Plan for the needs assessment

- Define the goals of the needs assessment in relation to the program goals
- Describe the gaps by identifying outcomes that are not currently happening; focus on the current situation
- Identify decision makers or partners who will use the needs assessment and how
- Engage with diverse and relevant partners who will use or implement the program; provide them with updates during the needs assessment process
- Develop evaluation questions that will direct the evaluation and reflect the priorities of the program, the key partners, and patients

Part 2. Understand the current state by collecting data and information about gaps

- Identity existing resources to query data that provide answers to the evaluation questions
- Conduct interviews with hospital staff (nurses, clinicians, pharmacists, patients) that answer the evaluation questions

Part 3. Analyze the data; focus on areas with the greatest potential for improvement

- Identify gaps in screening, diagnosis, and treatment
- Identify gaps in knowledge or education to treat SUD
- Identity gaps in medications available to treat SUD
- Identify gaps in linkage to posthospital discharge SUD treatment
- Identify potential causes for the gaps
- Determine the scope of the intended program to address gap
  - Recognize that addressing individual gaps sequentially may be more successful than addressing all the identified gaps at once
- Review the literature to identify possible solutions
- Collaborate with key partners to decide on solutions
- Identify existing resources to leverage to facilitate solutions to close the gap

Part 4. Summarize and develop an action plan/program to close the identified gaps; write up a report to disseminate and discuss with key partners and hospital leadership for transparency

- Provide a high-level description of the goals of the needs assessment with background for context
- A description of the core team and their credentials; this lends credibility that the needs assessment was informed by a diverse group of people with varied skills, expertise, and perspectives
- Summarize the source of data, the methods used to collect, analyze, and interpret the data
- Summarize the findings of the data collected, organize the data based on the evaluation questions
  - Create a gap analysis,[141,142] a logic model,[143] PDSA cycle,[63] or a swim lane diagram[144]
  - Define how you will measure "success" in your gap analysis, logic model, PDSA cycle
- Provide the core group's recommendations—these recommendations should involve actionable steps required to close the identified gaps

Case Study 1

A Preimplementation Needs Assessment

- Using semistructured interviews with hospital administrators, physicians, physician assistants, nurses, and social workers, Evans et al identified reported barriers and facilitators to the implementation of hospital-based OUD treatment program across three hospitals.
- Emergent themes included:
  - A perceived need for hospital-based OUD treatment.
  - An OUD program should be adapted to meet local and cultural needs.
  - An OUD program should include clear hospital-to-community OUD treatment resources.
  - From program start to finish, engage key partners across a variety of departments and with diverse roles to ensure many voices and experiences are considered.
  - By identifying these contextual factors that may impact the success of hospital-based OUD treatment, the program implementors could preemptively incorporate implementation strategies to mitigate future barriers to program success.[145]

Step 4a. The **core team** will clarify the goals of the needs assessment. This is an important step because it will frame every subsequent step in the needs assessment. Be sure to create goals that are realistic when considering the allotted time and resources available to develop and implement a hospital-based SUD treatment program at an individual site. The goals are directly related to the perceived gaps in SUD care that prompted the needs assessment. By clarifying the goals of the needs assessment, the **core team** can then identify the ***current state*** and ***existing gaps*** using data available in the EHR or obtained through interviews with patients and hospital staff or through simple staff and patient surveys described later in greater detail. Once the goals are identified, then the core team will focus on understanding the current state and gaps around the goals. Below are example goals and associated considerations for a needs assessment.

- **Example Goal 1:** To conduct universal screening for unhealthy substance use among all hospitalized patients.
  - **Question 1:** What are the current processes to conduct universal screening for unhealthy substance use for hospitalized patients? Who conducts the screening? What evidence-based screening tools are used? How is this information documented in the EHR?
- **Example Goal 2:** To offer all hospitalized patients with a Diagnostic and Statistical Manual of Mental Disorders 5th Edition (DSM-5)[145] SUD diagnosis medication for addiction treatment, when indicated.
  - **Question 2:** What are the current processes to ensure that medications for opioid, alcohol, stimulant, and tobacco use disorder (TUD) are offered to hospitalized patients with a DSM-5 confirmed SUD? Which medications are available on the hospital formulary?
- **Example Goal 3.** To ensure all hospitalized patients with OUD, an overdose event, or who use multiple substances are offered harm reduction education and naloxone for overdose prevention before, or at the time of, hospital discharge.
  - **Question 3.** What processes are in place to identify patients who meet criteria to receive harm reduction education and supplies? Who provides harm reduction education and supplies? How are harm reduction supplies obtained and paid for?
- **Example Goal 4.** To ensure a patient-centered approach to address and mitigate in-hospital substance use.
  - **Question 4.** What policies and procedures are in place to address and mitigate in-hospital substance use? How are hospital staff informed of hospital policies and procedures? How are the policies and procedures implemented uniformly across hospital units?
- **Example Goal 5.** To ensure all hospitalized patients initiated on medications for SUD are referred to community SUD treatment resources after hospital discharge.
  - **Question 5.** What current community SUD treatment resources are available to support posthospital discharge treatment linkage? Who is responsible for maintaining a current list of community SUD resources? Who is responsible for making follow-up appointments for patients with SUD? How are these follow-up appointments communicated to patients?

The goals of the needs assessment must be realistic within the specific hospital setting, the resources available, and the hospital leadership's support. Goals that are overly ambitious are more likely to be unsuccessful. By tackling individual goals over time, the program's success may gain momentum with greater uptake by hospital staff, leading to ongoing hospital leadership support.

Step 4b. After the **core team** chooses three to five goals, they will determine what data are needed to describe and quantify the perceived gaps. For example, if the core team's long-term goal is to build and implement an ACS, then they should begin by quantifying the annual percentage of hospitalized patients with SUD. If the scope of the long-term goal is smaller, for example, to provide naloxone to people with OUD who are prescribed high-dose opioids, or who have stimulant use disorder (StUD), then the data inquiry may be narrower.

When developing the goals for the needs assessment, identify who will be delivering the program, that is, nurses, clinicians, or social workers, and who are the intended recipients of the program (ie, hospitalized patients with SUD). The program must be designed with these key partners in mind because if it does not fit in their workflow, is too extensive or too superficial, or is not what the patient wants or needs, it will not be successful. To improve the success of the future program, the core team should meet with these key partners to understand their perceived challenges and barriers when caring for hospitalized patients with SUD; what do they need to better support these patients? From the patient perspective—what do people with SUD experience when they are hospitalized? What do they need to improve their hospital experience?

Step 4c. After clarifying the goals of the needs assessment, the **core team** will develop questions that the assessment will answer to identify the current state of SUD care delivery and gap(s). When developing questions, it is important to consider potential data sources to query—are the data available electronically or elsewhere? Where are the data stored? How will the data be accessed and by whom? Or will the data require primary data collection? If yes, in what format? By whom? Both quantitative and qualitative may be needed to answer these questions. Cataloguing and reviewing results from data collection will help identify areas to target for improvement.

Quantitative data sources may include the EHR to query in-hospital medication orders and discharge prescriptions for SUD medication or to identify the frequency of International Classification of Disease (ICD)[146] codes for various SUD diagnoses in billing and encounter data. It will be necessary to partner with an EHR analyst who can query the data and provide the **core team** with reports. A manual chart review is extensive and time consuming, so, whenever possible, use data already available to describe the current state of SUD care. An EHR query may be supplemented with a simple staff survey to investigate how staff perceive the current state and the ideal state to provide hospital-based SUD care.

Obtain patient-level and encounter-level data to quantify the number of hospitalized patients with a SUD. For example, determine what percentage of all hospitalized patients (monthly/quarterly/annually) have an ICD code for OUD, AUD, StUD, TUD, cannabis use disorder listed in their admission or discharge diagnosis. First, consider all hospitalizations during a specific time frame. Within that time frame, identify hospitalizations with a specific SUD-related ICD code. Table 2.6 includes conditions used in health care and death certificate documentation that can be used for substance-related hospitalizations. To do this, first extract all patient encounters from the hospital's EHR or claims database for the designated time period. Once the dataset is compiled, encounters that include a SUD-related diagnosis can be identified by filtering for ICD-10 codes within the F10–F19 category, which encompasses all SUDs. These diagnoses may appear as a primary (the main reason for the encounter) secondary condition contributing to hospitalization. Another useful method to capture hospitalizations related to SUD is through the use of diagnosis-related groups (DRGs), which categorize hospital admissions based on the conditions treated and the complexity of care required. Some DRGs are explicitly tied to SUD and can be used to track admissions where substance use was a primary factor. For example, DRG 894 refers to patients who left prior to treatment completion after an admission related to alcohol or drug use. Beyond these direct SUD-related DRGs, a broader picture can be obtained by analyzing hospitalizations for conditions commonly associated with substance use, such as infectious diseases, liver disease, encephalopathy, and poisoning or overdose. By incorporating these related DRGs into the analysis, hospitals can better capture the indirect impact of substance use on health care utilization.

Once the SUD-related encounters are, the next step is to determine the total number of encounters during the same period. This serves as the denominator, while the count of encounters with a SUD diagnosis serves as the numerator, generating a proportion. Repeat this over time, that is, months, quarterly, or annually, to determine the proportion of SUD-related hospitalizations over a specific time period to assess trends.

Prolonged hospitalizations are costly, and hospital leadership may be interested in reducing length of hospital stay to reduce costs and increase bed availability. Patients with injection-related infections who require prolonged courses of intravenous antibiotics may be an area to intervene with SUD treatment to reduce costs. First, define prolonged hospitalization. Is it one month, 2 months, or longer? Next, identify the monthly/quarterly/annual percentage of hospitalizations with ICD codes related to SUD that meet the predetermined definition of a prolonged hospitalization. Among these hospitalizations, determine the average LOS. Next, compare the average

TABLE 2.6

Conditions Used in Health Care and Death Certificate Documentation

Alcohol-related conditions

Poisoning by ethanol, accidental (unintentional)
Poisoning by ethanol, intentional self-harm
Poisoning by ethanol, assault
Poisoning by ethanol, undetermined
Adverse effect of ethanol
Alcohol substance use disorder, mild
Alcohol substance use disorder, moderate
Alcohol substance use disorder, severe
Sequela due to alcohol use

Amphetamine and methamphetamine-related conditions

Poisoning by, adverse effect of, and underdosing of unspecified psychostimulant
Poisoning by amphetamines, accidental (unintentional)
Poisoning by amphetamines, intentional self-harm
Poisoning by amphetamines, assault
Poisoning by amphetamines, undetermined
Adverse effect of amphetamines, subsequent encounter
Amphetamine-type substance use disorder, mild
Amphetamine-type substance use disorder, moderate
Amphetamine-type substance use disorder, severe
Other or unspecified stimulant use disorder, mild
Other or unspecified stimulant use disorder, moderate
Other or unspecified stimulant use disorder, severe

Cocaine-related conditions

Poisoning by cocaine, accidental, unintentional
Poisoning by cocaine, intentional self-harm
Poisoning by cocaine, assault
Poisoning by cocaine, undetermined
Adverse effect of cocaine
Cocaine use disorder, mild
Cocaine use disorder, moderate
Cocaine use disorder, severe

Opioid-related conditions

Poisoning by opium, accidental (unintentional)
Poisoning by opium, intentional self-harm
Poisoning by opium assault
Poisoning by opium, undetermined
Adverse effect of opium
Poisoning by heroin, accidental (unintentional)
Poisoning by heroin, intentional self-harm
Poisoning by heroin, assault
Poisoning by heroin, undetermined
Adverse effect of heroin
Poisoning by other opioids, accidental (unintentional)
Poisoning by other opioids, intentional self-harm
Poisoning by other opioids, assault
Poisoning by other opioids, undetermined
Adverse effect of other opioids
Poisoning by fentanyl or fentanyl analogs, accidental (unintentional)
Poisoning by fentanyl or fentanyl analogs, intentional self-harm
Poisoning by fentanyl or fentanyl analogs, assault
Poisoning by fentanyl or fentanyl analogs, undetermined
Adverse effect of fentanyl or fentanyl analogs
Poisoning by tramadol, accidental (unintentional)
Poisoning by tramadol, intentional self-harm
Poisoning by tramadol, assault
Poisoning by tramadol, undetermined
Adverse effect of tramadol
Poisoning by other synthetic narcotics, accidental (unintentional)
Poisoning by other synthetic narcotics, intentional self-harm
Poisoning by other synthetic narcotics, assault
Poisoning by other synthetic narcotics, undetermined
Adverse effect of other synthetic narcotics
Poisoning by unspecified narcotics, accidental (unintentional)
Poisoning by unspecified narcotics, intentional self-harm
Poisoning by unspecified narcotics, assault
Poisoning by unspecified narcotics, undetermined
Adverse effect of unspecified narcotics
Poisoning by other narcotics, accidental (unintentional)
Poisoning by other narcotics, intentional self-harm
Poisoning by other narcotics, assault
Poisoning by other narcotics, undetermined
Adverse effect of other narcotics
Opioid abuse, uncomplicated
Opioid abuse with intoxication
Opioid abuse with opioid withdrawal
Opioid abuse with opioid-induced mood disorder
Opioid abuse with opioid-induced psychotic disorder
Opioid abuse with other opioid-induced disorder
Opioid abuse with unspecified opioid-induced disorder
Opioid dependence, uncomplicated
Opioid dependence with intoxication
Opioid dependence with opioid withdrawal
Opioid dependence with opioid-induced mood disorder
Opioid dependence with opioid-induced psychotic disorder
Opioid dependence with other opioid-induced disorder
Opioid dependence with unspecified opioid-induced disorder
Opioid use, unspecified, uncomplicated
Opioid use, unspecified with intoxication
Opioid use, unspecified with opioid withdrawal
Opioid use, unspecified with opioid-induced mood disorder
Opioid use, unspecified with opioid-induced psychotic disorder
Opioid use, unspecified with other opioid-induced disorder
Opioid use, unspecified with unspecified opioid-induced disorder

LOS among these SUD-related hospitalizations to prolonged hospitalizations without an ICD code for SUD. Ensure that hospitalizations are matched by patient age, medical and psychiatric comorbidities, case mix index, and housing status. Finally, determine the cost per day and report to hospital leadership an expected cost saving with introduction of SUD-related services.

> **Case Study 2**
>
> **A Needs Assessment to Inform a Business Case for In-Hospital SUD Treatment**
>
> - Englander et al conducted a thorough needs assessment, which informed a business case and secured funding from Medicaid and hospital payers to support in-hospital SUD treatment services within a large academic hospital.
> - The authors surveyed hospitalized patients with SUD to inquire about their readiness to change their substance use behaviors.
> - The authors conducted in-depth qualitative interviews exploring patient perceptions of substance use treatment needs.
> - The authors convened a group of hospital leaders, frontline hospital staff, and representatives of community organizations to develop strategies to address patient and system needs to better serve hospitalized patients with SUD.
> - The authors used administrative data to describe rates of rehospitalization and length of stay among hospitalized patients with SUD compared to those without documented SUD.
> - The authors presented their findings to hospital leadership and state insurers and secured funding to implement a multicomponent SUD intervention across hospital and post–acute care settings.[147]

Qualitative data sources may include face-to-face interviews or focus groups involving nurses, social workers, physicians, advanced practice professionals, pharmacists, and hospital leaders to inquire about topics related to the current state of SUD treatment. Additional data sources may include guidelines outlining evidence-based SUD treatment[45,46,63,148–150] and publications describing the benefits of in-hospital SUD treatment.[25,28,31,36,44,151] These examples involve primary data collection and will require more time and resources. Primary data collection allows for more nuanced data (ie, perceptions of care provision by staff) collection not available in the EHR. Example questions may include:

Meet with pharmacy staff to determine:

- What policies and procedures facilitate or are barriers to use of medications for SUD?
  - Assess if there are misconceptions about the legality of offering methadone or buprenorphine in the hospital for prevention of opioid withdrawal and OUD treatment.[147]
- What SUD medications are available on the hospital formulary?
  - Clarify available formulations of buprenorphine (sublingual film, sublingual tablet, transdermal patch, and intravenous formulations).
  - Clarify available formulations of methadone (liquid, tablet, intravenous).
  - Clarify if injectable extended release medications, e.g., buprenorphine and naltrexone, are available on formulary.
  - Clarify available formulations of other medications for AUD and TUD.

Meet with nursing staff to determine:

- What is the current practice to screen for unhealthy substance use?
  - If already happening, what questions are used to screen for unhealthy opioid, alcohol, stimulant, cannabis use?
  - Where are the patient's answers documented in the EHR?
  - What happens if a patient screens positive for unhealthy substance use?
  - Describe the workflow in the EHR.
- Do you use the Clinical Opiate Withdrawal Scale (COWS)[64] to assess for opioid withdrawal severity?
  - Describe the workflow in the EHR.
- Do you use a scoring tool to assess for severity of alcohol withdrawal (CIWA-Ar,[69] MINDS,[70] etc)?
- What policies and procedures are in place to address in-hospital substance use?
  - Describe the workflow if a patient uses substances in their hospital room.
  - Describe the workflow if a patient has drug paraphernalia in their room.
  - Describe if/where this is documented in the EHR.
- The Joint Commission has several standards and measures related to SUD. To what extent is the hospital meeting them?
  - Joint Commission standards and measures include: screening and assessment, care planning, treatment services, discharge and care continuity, education and training, environment of care, performance improvement.[152]

Meet with clinician staff to assess:

- Current state of addiction expertise
  - Are there existing addiction-trained clinicians working in the hospital?
  - Are there existing addiction-trained clinicians in the outpatient setting?

   - Are there readily available post discharge SUD treatment resources? If not, what services would need to be built?
- How do clinicians diagnose SUD? Do clinicians regularly use the DSM-5[145] to diagnose SUD?
- Do clinicians document SUD diagnoses, severity of SUD, and the associated plan related to SUD treatment in their notes?
- How comfortable are clinicians in initiating SUD medications?
- What do clinicians need to support them to provide hospital-based SUD treatment?
   - Access to regular educational sessions to treat SUD and harm reduction education
   - Protocols, order sets, embedded pathways in the EHR to direct SUD medication initiation
   - EHR alerts when a patient meets criteria for naloxone at discharge
   - Clear referral pathways to postdischarge treatment linkage
   - Psychiatric services to address common mental health comorbidities
- What SUD services would clinicians like to see in their hospital setting?
   - ACS
   - Access to an addiction specialist on site
   - Telephone consultations between the clinician and addition specialist
   - Virtual consultations with addiction specialists

Meet with social work staff to assess:

- What are existing community referral networks for SUD treatment posthospital discharge?
- What are existing resources for patient transportation for postdischarge appointments?
- What are existing community resources for social determinants of health, for example, food insecurity?
- What are existing community resources and services for patients who are unstably housed or homeless?
- What role do social workers play in providing motivational interviews for patients with SUD, and in assessing and addressing common mental health comorbidities?
- What role do social workers play in linking patients to inpatient or outpatient SUD treatment after hospital discharge?
- Are there syringe service providers, that is, needle exchange programs, and other harm reduction services in the community?

Meet with hospital leadership to assess:

- What are the organization's strategic priorities? How can improving SUD treatment directly address the organization's priorities, that is, reducing rehospitalizations, reducing length of stay, etc.
- Are there opportunities to leverage existing resources and strategic priorities to provide hospital-based SUD services?
- Are there potential philanthropic funders or foundations to support the development of these programs and services?
- Are there opportunities to present ideas to the hospital's board of directors to gain buy-in?

Clarify state-level rules, regulations, and payment models related to medications for OUD/AUD:

- Meet with the state opioid treatment authority (SOTA is a designated entity within each US state that oversees and coordinates the implementation of opioid treatment programs)
   - Are there barriers to link patients to an opioid treatment program for methadone after discharge?
   - Are there barriers to providing take-home methadone doses from the hospital to support hospital to opioid treatment program linkage?[67,147]
- Meet with the Department of Health Care Policy and Financing.
   - Did the state expand Medicaid with the Affordable Care Act?
   - Are there discount health care programs for people who lack insurance coverage?
   - Are there opioid abatement funds/grant opportunities/philanthropic dollars that can be used to pay for services and program development?

Next, using the above-identified information, create questions with discreet outcomes. These questions will be used to measure areas of success and areas for improvement once the hospital-based SUD program has been implemented. Whenever possible, include percentages, proportions, or a discreet number over a specific time frame. Clearly define how data will be obtained, that is, use of ICD codes to identify a SUD-related encounters, use of prescription data from the EHR to identify SUD medications, electronic referrals to SUD treatment post discharge, etc. Examples of succinct questions with measurable outcomes are listed in Table 2.7.

This list of questions is not exhaustive, and all of these questions do not need to be addressed. Rather, the data query should focus on addressing the goals and questions addressed during the needs assessment.

Step 4d. After the data are collected, organize and analyze the data to identify gaps based on the data query (informed by the goals of the needs assessment). The core team will rank the identified gaps to determine which gaps must be addressed first and which gaps will be deferred while recognizing that

TABLE 2.7

Examples of SUD-Related Outcomes[a]

Measure/description/ measure concept	Numerator	Denominator	Desired outcome/ process	Notes
(For an ACS) Number of consultations ordered over X time period	Number of consults completed	Number of hospitalized patients with a documented SUD	**Outcome** 100% completed consults	Tracking this will provide data for future staffing and financial support
(For an ACS) Consultations completed over X time period	NA	NA	**Outcome** Number of amount billed for services provided Number of amount reimbursed for services provided	
Naloxone prescribed for opioid overdoses or high-risk patients	Number of naloxone prescriptions	Number of patients presenting with overdose or high risk for opioid overdose	**Outcome** Increase in naloxone prescriptions	NOTE: This may be challenging to track if a hospital does not have its own retail pharmacy
Urine drug test strips (eg, fentanyl) distributed among patients at high risk for an opioid overdose	Number of test strips distributed	Number of patients with OUD/StUD diagnosis	**Outcome** Increase in distribution of urine test strips	NOTE: This will be challenging to track without associated documentation of number distributed
Screening for unhealthy substance use	Number of percentage of patients screened	Number of hospital admissions	**Process** Increase in number of completed screenings	Merit-based incentive payment system Quality measure
Identification and planning for patients with SUD upon admission	Number of plans documented	Number of patients with SUD diagnosis	**Process** Increase in number of documented plans	Medicaid Adult Core Set
Number of referrals for SUD treatment	Number of referrals ordered	Number of patients identified with untreated SUD	**Outcome** Increase in referrals	Medicaid Adult Core Set, The Joint Commission Quality metric
Completed/successful referrals for SUD treatment	Number of referrals completed	Number of referrals ordered	**Outcome** Increase in number of completed referrals	Medicaid Adult Core Set, The Joint Commission Quality Metric
New medication starts for OUD treatment; AUD treatment	MOUD ordered at hospital discharge; MAUD ordered at hospital discharge	Number of patients identified with OUD/ AUD	**Outcome** Increase in number of prescriptions	Medicaid Adult Core Set
	Methadone ordered and dispensed among patients with documented OUD		**Outcome** Increase in dispensation of methadone in-hospital with an OUD diagnosis	
Screening patients with SUD for infectious diseases (eg, Hepatitis B/C, HIV)	% of patients screened	Number of patients with SUD	**Process** Increase in number of screens	

TABLE 2.7

Examples of SUD-Related Outcomes[a] (*Continued*)

Measure/description/ measure concept	Numerator	Denominator	Desired outcome/ process	Notes
Number of referred patients with SUD in treatment after 30 d	Number of patients still in active SUD treatment program	Number of SUD treatment referrals completed	**Outcome** Increase in number of patients still engaged in SUD treatment	Medicaid Adult Core Set
Engagement in outpatient SUD treatment program for 3, 6, 12 mo or longer	Number of patients engaged in SUD treatment program	Number of SUD treatment referrals	**Outcome** Increase in number of patients engaging in SUD treatment	Merit-based incentive payment system Quality measure
30-d emergency department encounters among patients started on MOUD/ MAUD in previous hospitalization	Number of patients admitted for any cause within 90 d after initial hospital encounter	Number of individuals started on inpatient MOUD and/or MAUD	**Outcome** Decrease in number of emergency department encounters among patients who were started on MOUD/ MAUD	NOTE: Reducing utilization of acute care at large and for conditions related to OUD/AUD aligns with federal incentive programs
30-d rehospitalization among patients started on MOUD/ MAUD in previous hospitalization	Number of patients admitted for any cause within 90 d after initial inpatient encounter	Number of individuals started on inpatient MOUD and/or MAUD	**Outcome** Decrease in number of rehospitalizations among patients who were started on MOUD/MAUD	

[a]Adapted from Colorado Hospital Association. *Colorado MAT: 2020 Key Considerations for Hospitalized Patients with Opioid Use Disorder.* 2020. https://cha.com/wp-content/uploads/2020/10/MAT-Implementation-Guide_final.pdf

some gaps will require greater resources than others. When considering which gaps to address, the **core team** should refer back to the original scope and priorities of the project to expand SUD treatment while also considering organizational capacity for change. Always work to align identified gaps and priorities to treat SUD in the hospital with executive leadership priorities. In some hospitals, hospital leadership may focus on reducing 30-day hospital readmissions, reducing racial/ethnic inequities, developing a skilled work force, or improving the patient experience. In hospitals that predominately serve populations with Medicaid, there may be opportunities to align with health plans on strategic priorities.[62] Table 2.7 lists a number of hospital-based programs that address screening, diagnosis, treatment, and linkage to SUD services for hospitalized patients.

Step 4e. Once the **core team** identifies the program to be implemented, they will use structured methods to map out how the program will address the gaps in hospital-based SUD treatment. There are various strategies that can be used to plan, implement, and evaluate an intervention. A commonly used strategy is to conduct a **gap analysis.** This section will describe three commonly used strategies to evaluate an intervention: a gap analysis, the creation of a logic model, and the use of SMARTIE Goals.

Gap Analysis

A **gap analysis** is a systematic method used to evaluate the difference between the *current state*, that is, routine screening for unhealthy substance use, and the *desired future state* or *goal*, that is, universal screening for unhealthy substance use among hospitalized patients (Figure 2.4). By working through the steps in the gap analysis, the **core team** will describe the current state and identify the strengths and weaknesses in the current state. Next, the **core team** will define desired **goals** and **associated outcome measures**, that is, >80% of hospitalized patients will have completed screening questions documented in the EHR within 48 hours of their admission. The **core team** will then compare the current state and the ideal state, pinpointing differences and identifying specific areas that can be intervened upon to reach the ideal state. Finally, the **core team** will develop a program to address the gap, implement the program, and measure associated outcomes to assess for impact. When creating a gap analysis, make sure to include resource

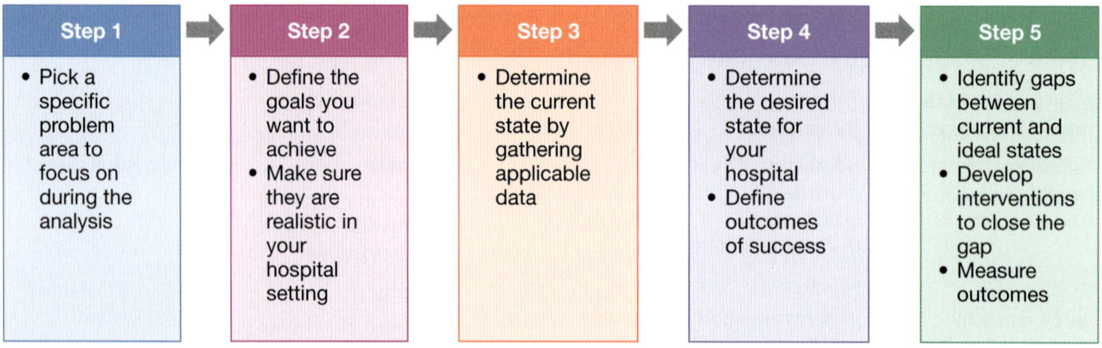

Figure 2.4: Steps in a gap analysis.

allocation, a timeline, and assign responsibilities to core team members and, whenever possible, members of the support network. Check in regularly to ensure team members are meeting their timeline metrics.

Logic Model

Another commonly used strategy to plan, implement, and evaluate a program is the development of a **logic model** (Figure 2.5). A **logic model** involves the creation of a system and visual representation of how a program is intended to work. The logic model illustrates the relationship between the resources invested, "inputs," the "activities" conducted, and the "outcomes" achieved. "Inputs" are the existing resources that can be leveraged or used to develop an intervention/program. For example, if the future intervention/program is to implement universal screening for unhealthy substance use in the hospital, then the "inputs" to leverage are: (1) integrating screening questions into the EHR platform and (2) having nurses complete the screening questions with patients at hospital admission.

Next, describe the "activities" that need to be completed to successfully integrate the "inputs" into workflow. In the example of routine screening for unhealthy substance use, the "inputs" are the integration of screening questions into the EHR to be completed by nursing staff. Necessary "activities" may involve (1) using hospital-employed or contracted EHR analysts to integrate the screening questions into admission workflows, (2) working with nursing leadership to gain buy-in to add this work to nursing workflow, and (3) working with social work leadership to gain buy-in to have social worker complete a full screening, brief intervention, and referral to SUD treatment if a patient is identified as having unhealthy substance use. It should be noted that Medicare will reimburse for Screening, Brief Intervention, and Referral to Treatment (SBIRT) services with appropriate documentation when it completed in the ED setting. To date, Medicare does not reimburse for these services when it is completed in the inpatient setting, though some states may have different reimbursement allowances.[153] Additional "activities" will require gaining buy-in from clinicians to diagnose SUD using DSM-5 criteria and to offer medication treatment, when appropriate, and will providing education to nurses, social workers, and clinicians about the program and its intended purpose.

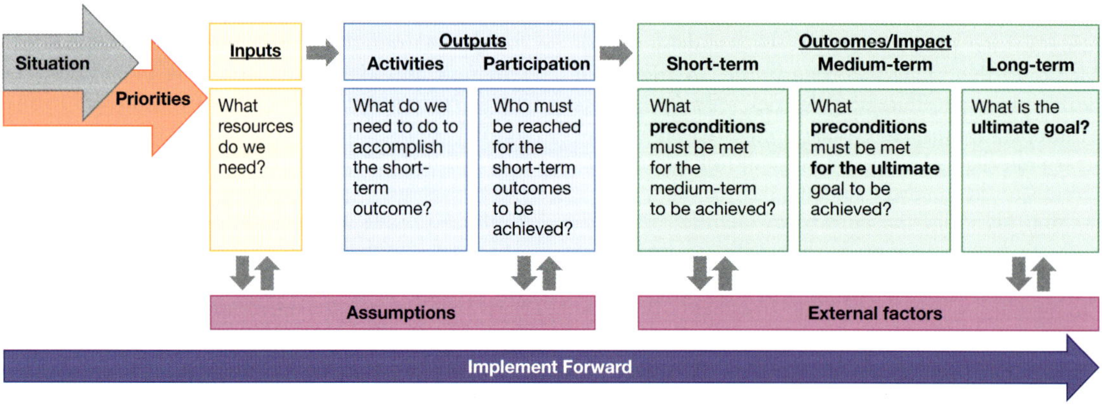

Figure 2.5: Logic model.

After identifying the "activities", develop quantifiable short-term, medium-term, and long-term outcome metrics to assess the impact of the program. For the screening example, a short-term outcome may be to identify what validated screening tools should be included, that is, the Alcohol Use Disorders Identification Test (AUDIT-C),[154] the Drug Abuse Screening Test (DAST)-10,[155] the TAPS tool,[60] and/or the Single-Question Screening Test for Drug Use[156] to identify hospitalized patients with unhealthy substance use. A medium-term outcome may be building the tools into the EHR, providing education to nurses, social workers, and clinicians about the change, and piloting the intervention in one unit of the hospital. The long-term outcome may be implementation of the intervention across one unit in the hospital and, after 3 months, at least 80% of all hospitalized patients will have documented screening questions for unhealthy substance use in their admission assessment. If these goals are met, the final outcome would be to expand the screening intervention to all hospital units.

When developing the logic model, it is important to acknowledge "assumptions" about the intended intervention and "external factors" that may impact the success of the intervention's implementation or outcomes. With universal screening, it must be assumed that if a patient screens positive for unhealthy substance use, then the social worker completes a full SBIRT, that clinicians will be alerted that the patient should be assessed further for SUD, and that the clinician will prescribe medications if the patient meets criteria for SUD.[157] If there is no plan for intervening once a patient screens positive, then the utility of completing universal screening must be reconsidered. External factors that affect the program's success must be consider, that is, competing demands for nurse's time to complete the screening questions, lack of available analysts to incorporate the screening questions into the EHR, or resistance of clinician staff to diagnose SUD and to initiate SUD medications. The **core team** should identify these external factors that may inhibit successful implementation of the intervention/program and develop strategies to address and mitigate these barriers throughout the development, implementation, and sustainment processes.

Specific, Measurable, Attainable, Relevant, Time-Bound, Inclusive, and Equitable (SMARTIE) Goal Framework

Developing specific strategies to target gaps and identifying outcome measures to determine success of the program can be challenging. The SMARTIE Goal Framework will help the **core team** clearly identify what they want to achieve while making sure the goals are objective, reasonable, and that progress can be tracked over time. SMARTIE goals incorporate an equity and inclusion component to ensure that the **core team** is committed to addressing racial equity and inclusion, anchored by tangible and actionable objectives. The SMARTIE statement will guide the steps needed to meet the long-term program objectives, to keep the project moving forward, and to provide specific outcome measures to assess if the future program closes identified treatment gaps.[158] For the example of universal screening, consider these SMARTIE statements:

- **Specific:** Embed screening questions from one or more validated screening tools (AUDIT-C,[154] DAST-10,[155] the TAPS tool,[60] and/or the Single-Question Screening Test for Alcohol and Drug Use[156]) in the EHR to be completed by nursing staff at hospital admission.
- **Measurable:** >80% of hospitalized patients will complete screening questions at the time of hospital admission in the pilot unit.
- **Attainable:** Use existing EHR platforms and analysts to embed screening questions into nursing workflow with alerts to complete the tasks. If the patient screens positive, the EHR will automatically order a social work consult to complete a full SBIRT.
- **Relevant:** This will provide early identification of patients who may develop withdrawal symptoms and who may benefit from medications and referral to SUD treatment after hospital discharge.
- **Time-bound:** Complete EHR integration in 6 months.
- **Inclusive and Equitable:** All hospitalized patients in the pilot unit will universally be screened by nursing staff thereby reducing stigma and bias among who is and is not screened.

Outcome measures will depend on the specific program being implemented and the **core team's** goals. Englander et al[18] and Danovitch et al[25] systematically reviewed hospital-based SUD treatment models and measured how these treatment models affected the SUD treatment provision using specific and measurable outcomes (Table 2.7). The **core team** must consider various factors when choosing the most suitable outcome measures to assess. Some considerations include: What data are available and how/who will access/gather, clean, and analyze the data? If the program is framed as a QI project and process development is informed using a PDSA cycle,[53] an RCA, or Six Sigma methodologies,[51,58] then the outcomes assessed should be directly related to outcomes that are meaningful to the hospital in which the program will be implemented.

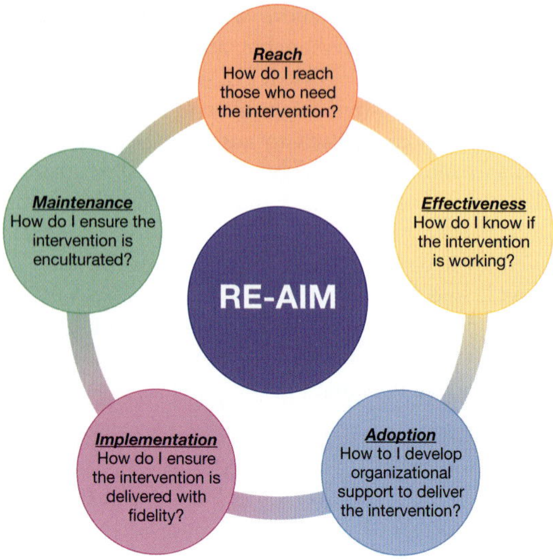

Figure 2.6: RE-AIM. (Figure adapted from Ory MG, Altpeter M, Belza B, Helduser J, Zhang C, Smith ML. Perceived utility of the RE-AIM Framework for health promotion/disease prevention initiatives for older adults: a case study from the U.S. Evidence-based disease prevention initiative. *Front Public Health.* 2014;2:143.)

The Reach, Effectiveness, Adoption, Implementation, and Maintenance (RE-AIM) Framework

If the program being implemented is supported by evidence of efficacy/effectiveness (ie, the use of buprenorphine or methadone to treat OUD), and the **core team** intends to study the impact of the program in multiple dimensions, then outcome metrics should be informed by an implementation model or framework.[89,109,110,112,113] A commonly used implementation evaluation framework is the Reach, Effectiveness, Adoption, Implementation, and Maintenance (RE-AIM) framework (Figure 2.6),[109,159,160] which is integrated into the Practical Robust Implementation and Sustainability Model (PRISM).[89–91,114–116] RE-AIM outcomes are measured at the individual level and multiple ecologic levels, including staff and setting levels in health systems. Its key dimensions are **Reach, Effectiveness** (measured at the individual level), **Adoption, Implementation**, that is, fidelity, feasibility, acceptability, appropriateness (measured at the staff, setting, system, or policy/other levels), and **Maintenance/Sustainability** (measure both at the individual and staff/setting, system, or policy levels).[161] Table 2.8 outlines each RE-AIM dimension, what level the dimension can be measured at, how to report it, and examples of SUD outcomes for each RE-AIM dimension.

Step 5: Write Up a Brief Report to Present to Hospital Leadership and the Executive Sponsor. Include the Signed Letter of Executive Support in the Report

The report should provide a concise background explaining the purpose of the needs assessment, along with a description of the core team members, emphasizing their diverse perspectives and areas of expertise. It should also include a summary of the data sources and detail the methods used for data collection, analysis, and interpretation. Next, summarize three to five key findings that highlight the gap in SUD care in the hospital to emphasize the core team's case for change. The report will include the recommended program and how it will close the treatment gaps, the expected project timeline, and expected outcomes. The report will include a rough estimate of expenses to include staffing costs, data extraction costs and analyst time, and administrative costs of the **core team** to complete the proposed project. If hospital leadership approves the program but does not offer funding or other types of support, consider how the project can be adapted to increase its feasibility. Still, plan to collect data and measure outcomes using iterative cycles (PDSA cycle). Schedule regular meetings with your executive sponsor to update him/her on the progress of the program. Highlight success by including a patient story or staff quotations that demonstrates the program's value. Keep in mind that many programs are not fully funded until the **core team** provides evidence for potential cost savings, improved patient safety, patient satisfaction, mission relevance, or other outcomes that impact the hospital's bottom line or reputation. Over time, and with persistence, the **core team** will gain buy-in for future funding and program expansion.

At the end of **Step 5**, the **core team** should know what program they will implement, which outcome measures will be linked to each intervention, and how they will access outcomes data, and at what frequency (Tables 2.3 and 2.7). These details should be summarized and outlined succinctly in a brief report (Table 2.5; Part 4). If these steps are incomplete, the **core team** should return to **Step 4** "conduct a needs assessment" and work their way through **Steps 4a to 4f** until the program and associated outcomes are clear. Thoroughly and thoughtfully completing these steps will increase the future program's success.

TABLE 2.8

RE-AIM Outcomes[a]

RE-AIM dimension and definition	Reporting classifications	SUD example
Reach (individual level): The absolute number, proportion, and representativeness of individuals who are willing to participate in an intervention, a program, or an initiative, and reason why or why not	Report on both the percentage of individuals who participate based on a valid denominator and characteristics of individual who participate compared to nonparticipants. Use qualitative methods to understand why a person/group of people may accept or decline an intervention	Identify all the patients in the hospital with OUD and/or a COWS score >10 and offer them MOUD (denominator). Determine the number of patients who accepted MOUD (numerator). Reach is the proportion of patients who accepted MOUD. Conduct key informant interviews among people who declined MOUD to understand why—this information can be used to improve reach by adaption how MOUD is offered, for example
Effectiveness (individual level): The impact of the intervention on individual outcomes, including potential negative outcomes or impacts on quality of life, economic outcomes, and how this varies across subgroups	Report on the primary outcome, measures of broader outcomes, ie, quality of life, and short-term outcomes by patient characteristics Use qualitative methods to understand variability in effectiveness across subgroups, ie, lack of transportation, lack of insurance, etc	For patients who accepted MOUD initiation in the hospital, potential short-team outcomes include: 7-d hospital to outpatient appointment linkage; 30-d treatment engagement; 30-d rehospitalization. Longer-term outcomes include 6-mo retention, 1-y retention, and mortality
Adoption (multiple settings or staff levels): The absolute number, proportion, and representativeness of settings and intervention agents (people who deliver the intervention) who are willing to initiate the program, and why	At the staff level, report percentage of staff who were invited to participate, percentage excluded, and characteristics of staff who did and did not participate Qualitatively assess why some staff adopt the program/intervention and others do not	Provide a 5-part educational session to 10 hospital-based physicians on MOUD initiation. After the educational session is complete, identify patients with OUD who received care from one of the 10 physicians. Review the medication orders to see which physicians initiated MOUD after the educational sessions (numerator) divided by the 10 physicians × 100. This is the percentage of staff who adopted MOUD initiation
Implementation (multiple settings and especially devilry staff level): Assess the fidelity to various elements of an intervention's key components or functions including the consistency of delivery as intended, the time and cost of implementing the intervention, and assess adaptations made to the intervention to make its implementation smoother or "fit better" in the site	Report on the costs related to implementing the intervention (time and money), adaptations made to the intervention's implementation, consistency, and adherence of intervention delivery within and across sites	A team develops a clinical decision support (CDS) tool that alerts prescribers to order naloxone for a patient when there is a positive urine drug test for fentanyl, or an ICD-10 code for OUD. Midway through the intervention, the team realized that the CDS tool is missing patients who presented with an overdose who primarily use methamphetamine. The team modifies the alert criteria to also include an ICD code for overdose. This adaptation should be reported with the end goal of increasing **Reach**
Maintenance/Sustainability (individual and setting levels): At the individual level—long-term effects of an intervention once its completed. At the setting level, the extent to which has become institutionalized	At the setting level, report if the intervention is still ongoing at different time points after its initial implementation	An ACS was started with a 2-y grant. During that time, ACS leaders collected data on cost savings related to provision of SUD services with reporting on reduction of rehospitalizations or length of stay. The ACS team leaders approach hospital leadership with these data and they decided to include the ACS team as part of the annual hospital budget. The ACS team is in its 8th year

[a]This table is adapted from Holtrop JS, Estabrooks PA, Gaglio B, et al. Understanding and applying the RE-AIM framework: clarifications and resources. *J Clin Transl Sci*. 2021;5(1):e126.

Step 6: Assemble the Program Implementation Team

The **implementation team** is responsible for completing the implementation activities necessary for program success. The **implementation team** will likely include some or all of the **core team** members and it may also include individuals from the **support network** identified in Step 3. At this stage, it is important to reassess who is on the team, recognizing that people join and leave organizations and their priorities and ability to participate in the program's development may change over time.

Similar to the **core team**, one person will serve as the **project leader** who is responsible for leading the program development and implementation. Also, similar to the **core team**, and because this is a hospital-based program, it is recommended that the **implementation team** includes people familiar with the inpatient workflow, patient flow, and hospital system. Ideally the **implementation team** will include a hospital-based physician or advanced practice professional, a subject matter expert (who might be the hospital-based clinician), a nurse, a social worker, and a pharmacist. The team composition will depend on the intervention or program. Once the **implementation team** members are solidified, the **project leader** should clearly define their role in the program and certify their commitment to participating in that capacity. The project leader should make it clear to **implementation team** members that their commitment is time limited and will end upon completion of the program goals. A team charter is a useful tool to articulate the implementation team member's roles, responsibilities, and is matched with a timeline listing key prespecified goals to be completed over the implementation period.

Once the **implementation team** members' roles are solidified, update members of the **support network** that the program is forthcoming and provide them with regular updates as the program completes milestones or KPIs. Depending on the program, consider engaging a broader group of hospital-based employees, including nursing leaders and nursing educators, pharmacist leaders, patient safety officers, social work team leaders, case managers, regulatory team members, and frontline staff. If the hospital has a patient and family advisory committee or patient experience office, the **implementation team** should present the program to them and incorporate early feedback from those stakeholders. Early and regular involvement of these people will improve the success of the program and will help it to become a part of the hospital's culture.

Step 7: Develop and Implement a Pilot, Then Assess Outcome Metrics

If the success of the program requires that nurses, social workers, or clinicians adopt practice change, and to do so will require significant education and training, it is optimal to pilot the program in one to two hospital units before widespread dissemination. The pilot period will allow for adaptations to be made to the program to increase its success and to determine opportunities for greater uptake and expansion. Considerations for selecting the pilot location in the hospital include the ability to identify available staff who are willing to implement the program, the typical patient population in that unit, the unit's workflow and patient volume, and the unit's leadership buy-in and potential for partnership and collaboration. For a SUD intervention, the **implementation team** should consider piloting the program in units or departments with the highest volume of patients with SUD. For example, the leader of the cardiac unit may be motivated to participate as a pilot unit because many of their patients have infective endocarditis from injection drug use and current clinical care does not address the underlying SUD, leading to difficult patient/staff interactions and high rates of premature discharge.

Steps involved in developing and implementing the pilot include:

- Identify select services or areas to pilot the program
- Create a timeline for the pilot project, that is, to start in 1 month and to be completed in 6 months
- Set the pilot up for success by obtaining buy-in from each key team member *before* deploying the pilot
  - Provide education to the unit staff and promote the pilot project for increased awareness
    - Implementation team members will commit to presenting at team meetings across various staff groups (social workers, clinicians, pharmacists, nurses, care management)
      - Present at monthly meetings, grand rounds, noon conference, divisional meetings
        - The focus of these sessions is to review current best practice
        - Discuss the gaps that have been identified
        - Present the logic model of how the program will address the gaps
          - Include the essential components necessary for success
          - Present anticipated outcomes that will define success

    - Create a nurse campaign with education on their specific role
    - Hang posters, signs, project boards to remind the unit staff of the pilot project and its timeline
- Collect outcomes data
- Use *audit and feedback* as an evidence-based strategy for improving adherence to best practice
  - Create reports detailing changes in care processes and outcomes: these can be unit or provider specific
    - Consider potential adaptations based on outcome assessment
    - Incorporate adaptations into the EHR and test adaptations in workflow
- Present to leadership/individuals listed above, obtain leadership approval to expand to all inpatient units
- Identify steps for dissemination and sustainability

Step 8: Considerations Before Widespread Dissemination

Congratulations! As a result of the thorough groundwork completed by the **core team** and the **implementation team**, hospital leadership recognizes the value of the intervention/program and its benefit to patients and staff. The **implementation team** is now permitted to expand the intervention/program across the entire hospital. Before jumping in and fully committing, consider the following:

Fatigue

Is the **project leader** or are the **implementation team** members interested in working on the next steps required for the program's expansion? At this point, the **project leader** and **implementation team** members should regroup and reassess whether any of the team members would prefer to step back and encourage others to step forward. It is important for all team members to be committed to the project's success. Reaffirming the team's commitment is *essential* before proceeding with the program's expansion. Once the **implementation team** has reassessed and reorganized, the newly created **dissemination team** and its **project leader** are responsible for all activities related to successful dissemination of the program.

Administrative Resources

With expansion of the program, it is important to consider what additional resources are required for success. For example, will the hospital leadership support the **dissemination team** members with administrative time to lead the program expansion across the hospital? How many hours per week do **dissemination team** members anticipate dedicating to this project, and over what time period? If program expansion will be time consuming and require resources, the **dissemination team** should create a budget and negotiate with hospital leaders for financial and administrative support. If hospital leaders will not provide support for expansion, consider alternative funding sources, including state or federal grants, foundational grants, philanthropy, or in-kind support. The **dissemination team** should consider how the goals of the project align with the goals of the hospital.

Data Analytics Support

With the program expanding, there will be more data to gather, report, and interpret. The **dissemination team** should consider if more analytics support is needed to assess outcomes reliably, accurately, and in a timely manner. Talk to data analytics experts to determine how many hours per week they would need to meet the program's needs and deadlines. This should be included in the budget.

Inpatient Formulary Resources

If the program involves use of medications for OUD, AUD, TUD, or StUD, pharmacy involvement is necessary to ensure that medications are available in all hospital units. If new medications are needed, a pharmacist would likely champion the request through the hospital's pharmacy and therapeutic's committee (P&T) (see Chapter 3).[162] Including injectable buprenorphine and naltrexone on the inpatient formulary will likely require additional work due to potential insurance reimbursement challenges.[163–165]

Staffing Positions

Depending on the program, the **dissemination team** should consider if new/additional staff will need to be hired. If yes, who will be responsible for paying their salaries? Is it the hospital? If the hospital is affiliated with an academic institution, then will a certain department or division be responsible for paying the salaries of new hires? If the **dissemination team** intends to create an ACS, they need to consider which team members will work on the ACS? Will an addiction-certified physician be hired? Will the team include an advanced practice professional with addiction skills? Will a social worker, a care coordinator, and/or a person in recovery as a patient navigator be hired to work on the ACS? How many days a week will an ACS operate? Who will post the positions for hire? Who will manage the staff? The **dissemination team** should consider all of this when creating their budget.

Medical Staff Education/Training

How will the intervention be socialized across the hospital units? Will nursing interventions be taught by nurse educators? Will social work interventions, that is, linkage to outpatient treatment, be taught by social work team leaders? Who will provide the physician/advance practice professional education? Who will develop or decide on SUD education? Who will decide where education will occur (online/in-person/both), when (during work hours/after-hours/early morning/during business meetings), and with what frequency and repetitiveness? Who will designate and train nurses? Will online training modules be developed for nursing education? Developing educational materials and providing education is time consuming. The **dissemination team** should ensure that the time needed to complete these administrative tasks are reflected in the budget.

Medical Education for House Staff (If Applicable)

If the program involves the development of an ACS and the hospital supports residency programs, then the **dissemination team** should consider if and how residents will rotate on the service as part of their residency training. Who will be responsible for scheduling resident rotations? Who will be responsible for developing and delivering a SUD curriculum for residents? Highlighting this education benefit as a service to the residency training programs will reflect well on the hospital and should be highlighted to residency program and hospital leadership to increase the change for administrative and staffing support.

Discharge Planning and Care Coordination

The **dissemination team** should consider who will be responsible for establishing protocols to support hospital-to-SUD treatment linkage at hospital discharge? Who will develop relationships with community partners to link patients from the hospital to the SUD treatment care continuum? Who will update and maintain these relationships as community treatment organizations close and new ones open? Who will be responsible for ensuring patients have access to transportation to get to follow-up appointments after hospital discharge? Who will develop relationships with subacute nursing facilities that are open to accepting patients on MOUD? Who will be responsible for ensuring that local pharmacies stock buprenorphine? These responsibilities may be best suited for the ACS social worker and/or ACS care coordinator.

Billing and Revenue Generation

Whenever possible, bill for services rendered. The **dissemination team** should meet with their hospital's billing department to create charge capture tools that accurately reflect the addiction care provided. Billing for addiction services provided by physicians and advanced practice professionals in the hospital setting can be based on time spent providing medical services or on the complexity of medical care provided, per usual evaluation and management (E/M) current procedural terminology (CPT) codes.[166] The physician and advanced practice professionals will bill for either an initial consultation encounter, a subsequent encounter, and whenever applicable, prolonged services.[166] Depending on hospital bylaws and state scope of practice, advance practice professionals may bill on their own or via shared billing under the supervision of a physician. To maximize billing on an ACS, the physician may prioritize seeing and billing for new encounters and the advanced practice professionals would see and bill for subsequent encounters. ACS workflow and billing will depend on patient volume the ACS team composition. The **dissemination team** should keep in mind that rules around billing change frequently, and that collections from billing vary widely across different insurers and often do not cover the total costs of an ACS. They should stay in touch with the hospital's billing department and update billing practices based on these changes.

Cost Savings

The **dissemination team** should estimate cost savings (ie, return on investment) related to in-hospital SUD treatment provision. There may be great potential for reducing hospital readmissions, hospital length of stay LOS, and improving patient satisfaction metrics and should be reported to hospital leadership. Many studies have estimated cost savings with the implementation of hospital-based SUD care.[27,167–169] While downstream costs savings may not be captured by a hospital, it is important to highlight robust cost-effectiveness data for the interventions (ie, MOUD) that ACS models seek to deliver.

Step 9: Dissemination and Sustainability

The process of disseminating the program across all hospital units is similar to the dissemination of the pilot, however, it is on a larger scale. If, during the pilot study, it became clear that some of the original data sources were not useful to assess program outcome, then the **dissemination team** should revise the data source, consider alternative data sources, or revise the outcome measure.

If the **dissemination** team intends to rigorously study the implementation of the program and associated outcomes, then the team should use an implementation framework like PRISM/RE-AIM, EPIS, or CFIR during the planning, implementation, and evaluation phases. If the intent is to publish the results for greater dissemination, the **dissemination team** should obtain institutional review board (IRB) approval early because the IRB may have recommendations or requirements related to data collection and reporting of identifiable or deidentifiable data.

If the **dissemination team** identified barriers or facilitators to the program's adoption or reach identified during the pilot study, these should be addressed and resolved before its widespread dissemination. This may require obtaining feedback from hospital staff and individuals in the **support network** who could recommend ideas or suggestions to adapt the program to make it more user-friendly without reducing its effectiveness.

Once the **dissemination team** implements the program across all hospital units, they should assess outcomes data on a prespecified schedule with the goal to regularly identify areas for improvement. As the program becomes part of the hospital's culture and its funding source is solidified, the frequency of outcome assessment can be reassessed and adjusted to the needs of the patients, hospital staff, and hospital leaders. Periodic assessments will identify a need for ongoing adaptations—checking for drifts or changes in the intervention/program, with continued modifications.

Finally, the **dissemination team** should identify a person who will lead the program over the long term. This person should receive administrative support for taking on this role. Potential candidates include members of the **core team**, the **implementation team**, or the **dissemination team**. If the program is large or if there is demand/interest to expand the program, the **dissemination team** may conduct a local, state, or national search to identify the best candidate for this position. In the case of an ACS, the ACS director is responsible for leading the team. This may include hiring and training staff and clinicians, ensuring cohesiveness and collaboration between ACS team members, ensuring continued support from hospital leadership, engaging in ongoing implementation and expansion efforts, and maintaining community partners. Other responsibilities may include developing innovative programs within the ACS to improve the care provided to hospitalized patients with SUD, publishing on ACS-related treatment outcomes and successes, and becoming a leader in the addiction community.

Case Study 3

The Use of a SMARTIE Statement and Gap Analysis to Develop and Implement Universal Screening for Unhealthy Substance Use

Example: *Intervention to Expand Inpatient Screening for Unhealthy Substance Use*

Project lead: Dr Julie Smith, MD, Hospital Medicine

Subject matter expert: Dr Julie Smith, MD

Project partner: Mary Carter, MSN, Nursing Supervisor and Nursing Educator

Project partner: Jennifer Adams, MS, Epic Analyst

Project partner: Joe Ford, MSW, Social Work Lead, Inpatient Unit

Project activities:

May 1st: Project team meets with chief nursing officer and head of inpatient social work to present the planned intervention to incorporate universal screening for unhealthy substance use at hospital admission (nurses) with completion of a full SBIRT by social workers if the nursing screen is positive. During this meeting, the team will present why this intervention is needed and the intended outcomes.

May 20th: the chief nursing officer and head of inpatient social work agree to support the project.

June 1st to August 30th: Dr Smith will review information about screening, brief intervention, and referral to treatment (SBIRT) including validated screening tools[170] and reimbursement for providing these services by the Substance Abuse and Mental Health Services Administration (SAMHSA) describing coding for screening and brief intervention reimbursement.[171]

September 1st to October 1st: Dr Smith will decide which screening tools to use and which questions in the screening tools to include in initial prescreening assessment to be completed by nurses at admission, that is, AUDIT-C,[154] DAST-10,[155] CUDIT,[172] a single-question screen,[156] or the TAPS tool,[60] etc.

October 15th: Team meeting (Dr Smith, MD; Mary Carter, MSN; Jennifer Adams, MS; and Joe Ford, MSW) discuss Dr Smith's findings and an opportunity for the team to offer feedback.

October 16th to October 30th: Dr Smith incorporates the team's feedback and provides finalized screening questions for unhealthy substance use.

November 1st to November 15th: Dr Smith, Ms Carter, and Mr Ford provide updates to the chief nursing officer and head of inpatient social work to solicit (and incorporate) their feedback. They decide on a unit to pilot the screening tool.

November 30th to January 1st: Ms Adams (Epic analyst) builds the new workflow into the Epic admission navigator to incorporate one question from the

AUDIT-C and the Single Item Screener for drug use.[156] The nurses will be prompted to complete the screening questions at the time of hospital admission. If the patient answers "yes" to either question, then an automatic order will be placed to the inpatient social worker assigned to the patient's floor to complete a full SBIRT and to provide resources for treatment. The clinical team (physician) will receive a "best practice alert" that their patient had a full SBIRT completed by the social worker, and the clinician should assess for alcohol or opioid withdrawal symptoms and provide medical treatment, as indicated.

November 30th to January 1st: Dr Smith provides education to her physician and advanced practice professional peers who work in the pilot unit during a monthly team meeting. She will outline the gaps in care, describe the intervention and its intent, discuss outcomes that will be measured, and describe how the change will (or will not) impact current workflow. Dr Smith sends out three waves of email communication to nursing leaders, social work leaders, and physician leaders and asks them to send out her email on their behalf. She then asks her direct leadership to support the intervention by announcing it in meetings and via email to increase action by physicians and advance practice providers to provide interventions for opioid or alcohol withdraw.

November 30th to January 1st: Ms Carter and a nursing educator provide education at team meetings and additional education to nurses who work in the pilot unit. Ms Carter and the nursing educator will outline the gaps in care, describe the intervention and its intent, discuss outcomes that will be measured, and describe who the change will (or will not) impact. They will describe the upcoming change in workflow. She provides email communication and asks her direct leadership to support the intervention by announcing it in meetings and via email to increase adoption of the intervention.

November 30th to January 1st: Mr Ford provides education to his social work colleagues who work in the pilot unit at team meetings to outline the gaps in care, describe the intervention and its intent, discuss outcomes that will be measured, and describe who the change will (or will not) impact, and any change in workflow. He provides email communication and asks his direct leadership to support the intervention by announcing it in meetings and via email to increase adoption of the intervention.

January 10th: The workflow is "turned on" in Epic but is limited to the pilot unit.

April 1st: Completion of screening questions are accessed in Epic: (number of completed screening questions documented in each encounter per month)/(denominator: number of monthly encounters) during February, March, and April. Outcomes are reported as rates.

Additional outcomes:

- Number of patients who screened positive by nurses who had a completed full SBIRT by social workers
- Number of patients who screened positive by social workers with full SBIRT who received a new diagnosis of AUD or OUD
- Number of patients who screened positive by nurses who had completed full SBIRT by social workers
- Number of patients who screened positive for OUD by social workers with full SBIRT who were also prescribed methadone or buprenorphine for opioid withdrawal/OUD
- Number of patients who screened positive for AUD by social workers with full SBIRT who were also prescribed naltrexone or acamprosate at hospital discharge

May 1st: Review outcomes—how do they compare to the original goals? If the intervention/program underperformed, the team will regroup, revise, and reinvent. If the intervention/program met the project goals, the team will celebrate and advertise the program's success to hospital leadership, to the support network, and to frontline staff by presenting the data, posting fliers in work areas, and sending emails to team leaders.

May 15th: Gain leadership support to expand the screening questions to all hospital units.

May 20th to June 20th: Provide education across the inpatient units (repeat of education provided during the pilot).

June 25th: The workflow is "turned on" in Epic across all hospital units.

July 1st to Sept 30th: Gather data and repeated outcome assessments.

- Completion of screening questions are accessed in Epic: (number of completed screening questions documented in each encounter per month)/(denominator: number of monthly encounters) during February, March, and April. Outcomes are reported as rates.

Additional outcomes:

- Number of patients who screened positive by nurses who had completed full SBIRT by social workers
- Number of patients who screened positive by social workers with full SBIRT who received a new diagnosis of AUD or OUD
- Number of patients who screened positive by nurses who had completed full SBIRT by social workers
- Number of patients who screened positive for OUD by social workers with full SBIRT who were also prescribed methadone or buprenorphine for opioid withdrawal/OUD

- Number of patients who screened positive for AUD by social workers with full SBIRT who were also prescribed naltrexone or acamprosate at hospital discharge

November 15th: Compare outcomes to original goals and to the outcomes from the pilot. If the intervention underperformed, the team will regroup, revise, and reinvent. If the intervention met the project goals, the team will celebrate and advertise the program's success to hospital leadership, to the support network, and to frontline staff by presenting the data, posting fliers in work areas, and sending emails to team leaders.

December 1st and thereafter: Develop a sustainability plan

Conclusion

Hospitalization is an important opportunity to engage and initiate treatment among out-of-treatment adults with SUD. To reduce the morbidity and mortality associated with untreated SUD, and to save health care dollars, hospital leaders would be well served to support and invest in innovative programs championed by well-informed subject matter experts that incorporate EBP to screen, diagnosis, and treat SUD among hospitalized patients. Hospital leaders should recognize that developing a successful in-hospital SUD treatment program requires participation and buy-in from a diverse group of people with various skills and experiences. Hospital leaders who support these efforts will be remembered as trailblazers to improve the care of all hospitalized patients with SUD.

REFERENCES

1. Azoulay P, Heggeness ML, Kao JL. Medical research and health care finance: evidence from academic medical centers. *Res Policy*. 2025;54(2):105163.
2. Kilaru AS, Xiong A, Lowenstein M, et al. Incidence of treatment for opioid use disorder following nonfatal overdose in commercially insured patients. *JAMA Netw Open*. 2020;3(5):e205852.
3. Franz B, Cronin CE, Lindenfeld Z, et al. Rural-urban disparities in the availability of hospital-based screening, medications for opioid use disorder, and addiction consult services. *J Subst Use Addict Treat*. 2024;160:209280.
4. Substance Abuse and Mental Health Services Administration (SAMHSA), Office of the Surgeon General (OSG). *Reports of the Surgeon General. Facing Addiction in America: The Surgeon General's Report on Alcohol, Drugs, and Health*. US Department of Health and Human Services; 2016.
5. Leshner AI. Addiction is a brain disease, and it matters. *Science*. 1997;278(5335):45–47.
6. Daley DC. Family and social aspects of substance use disorders and treatment. *J Food Drug Anal*. 2013;21(4):S73–S76.
7. Henden E, Melberg HO, Røgeberg OJ. Addiction: choice or compulsion? *Front Psychiatry*. 2013;4:77.
8. Schaler JA. *Addiction Is a Choice*. Open Court; 2011.
9. Richter L, Vuolo L, Salmassi MS. Stigma and addiction treatment. In: Avery JD, Avery JJ, eds. *The Stigma of Addiction: An Essential Guide*. Springer; 2019:93–130.
10. Barry CL, Huskamp HA. Moving beyond parity–mental health and addiction care under the ACA. *N Engl J Med*. 2011;365(11):973–975.
11. Richardson C, Daniels K, Confer A, et al. Internal medicine resident addiction training at the veteran's health administration: a qualitative evaluation of site directors' response to the 2022 ACGME requirements. *J Gen Intern Med*. 2024;39(8):1393–1399.
12. Atkins J, Dopp AL, Temaner EB. Combatting the stigma of addiction—the need for a comprehensive health system approach. *NAM Perspect*. 2020;2020:10.
13. McKnight-Eily LR, Liu Y, Brewer RD, et al. Vital signs: communication between health professionals and their patients about alcohol use—44 states and the District of Columbia, 2011. *MMWR Morb Mortal Wkly Rep*. 2014;63(1):16–22.
14. Institute of Medicine Committee on Crossing the Quality Chasm: Adaptation to Mental Health and Addictive Disorders; The National Academies Collection: Reports funded by National Institutes of Health. *Improving the Quality of Health Care for Mental and Substance-Use Conditions: Quality Chasm Series*. National Academies Press; 2006.
15. Jackson DS, Nguemeni Tiako MJ, Jordan A. Disparities in addiction treatment: learning from the past to forge an equitable future. *Med Clin North Am*. 2022;106(1):29–41.
16. Saloner B, Lê Cook B. Blacks and Hispanics are less likely than whites to complete addiction treatment, largely due to socioeconomic factors. *Health Aff (Millwood)*. 2013;32(1):135–145.
17. Calcaterra SL, Peterkin AF. Antiracist strategies to combat racial disparities in the delivery of hospital-based addiction care. *J Gen Intern Med*. 2024;39(2):165–167.
18. Englander H, Jones A, Krawczyk N, et al. A taxonomy of hospital-based addiction care models: a scoping review and key informant interviews. *J Gen Intern Med*. 2022;37(11):2821–2833.
19. Gottschalk M. The opioid crisis: the war on drugs is over. long live the war on drugs. *Annu Rev Criminol*. 2023;6(1):363–398.
20. Priest KC, McCarty D. Role of the hospital in the 21st century opioid overdose epidemic: the addiction medicine consult service. *J Addict Med*. 2019;13(2):104–112.
21. Peterson C, Li M, Xu L, Mikosz CA, Luo F. Assessment of annual cost of substance use disorder in US hospitals. *JAMA Netw Open*. 2021;4(3):e210242.
22. Singh JA, Cleveland JD. National US time-trends in opioid use disorder hospitalizations and associated healthcare utilization and mortality. *PLoS One*. 2020;15(2):e0229174.
23. Suen LW, Makam AN, Snyder HR, et al. National prevalence of alcohol and other substance use disorders among emergency department visits and hospitalizations: NHAMCS 2014–2018. *J Gen Intern Med*. 2022;37(10):2420–2428.
24. Ronan MV, Herzig SJ. Hospitalizations related to opioid abuse/dependence and associated serious infections increased sharply, 2002–12. *Health Aff (Millwood)*. 2016;35(5):832–837.
25. Danovitch I, Korouri S, Kaur H, et al. The addiction consultation service for hospitalized patients with substance use disorder: an integrative review of the evidence. *J Subst Use Addict Treat*. 2024;163:209377.

26. Englander H, Davis CS. Hospital standards of care for people with substance use disorder. *N Engl J Med.* 2022; 387(8):672–675.
27. Gryczynski J, Nordeck CD, Welsh C, Mitchell SG, O'Grady KE, Schwartz RP. Preventing hospital readmission for patients with comorbid substance use disorder: a randomized trial. *Ann Intern Med.* 2021;174(7):899–909.
28. Nordeck CD, Welsh C, Schwartz RP, et al. Rehospitalization and substance use disorder (SUD) treatment entry among patients seen by a hospital SUD consultation-liaison service. *Drug Alcohol Depend.* 2018;186:23–28.
29. Hser Y-I, Mooney LJ, Saxon AJ, et al. High mortality among patients with opioid use disorder in a large healthcare system. *J Addict Med.* 2017;11(4):315–319.
30. Hjemsæter AJ, Bramness JG, Drake R, et al. Mortality, cause of death and risk factors in patients with alcohol use disorder alone or poly-substance use disorders: a 19-year prospective cohort study. *BMC Psychiatry.* 2019;19:101.
31. McNeely J, Wang SS, Rostam Abadi Y, et al. Addiction consultation services for opioid use disorder treatment initiation and engagement: a randomized clinical trial. *JAMA Intern Med.* 2024;184(9):1106–1115.
32. Lewer D, Freer J, King E, et al. Frequency of health-care utilization by adults who use illicit drugs: a systematic review and meta-analysis. *Addiction.* 2020;115(6):1011–1023.
33. Bredenberg E, Tietbohl C, Dafoe A, Thurman L, Calcaterra S. Identifying factors that contribute to burnout and resilience among hospital-based addiction medicine providers: a qualitative study. *J Subst Abuse Treat.* 2023;144:108924.
34. Stelson EA, Sabbath-Clayton LL, Sorensen G, Kubzansky LD, Berkman LF, Sabbath EL. Residential addiction treatment providers: identifying the role of social context in worker health and turnover. *Soc Sci Med.* 2022;314:115462.
35. Murphy J. Improving the recruitment and retention of counselors in rural substance use disorder treatment programs. *J Drug Issues.* 2022;52(3):434–456.
36. Hoover K, Lockhart S, Callister C, Holtrop JS, Calcaterra SL. Experiences of stigma in hospitals with addiction consultation services: a qualitative analysis of patients' and hospital-based providers' perspectives. *J Subst Abuse Treat.* 2022;138: 108708.
37. Muncan B, Walters SM, Ezell J, Ompad DC. "They look at us like junkies": influences of drug use stigma on the healthcare engagement of people who inject drugs in New York City. *Harm Reduct J.* 2020;17:53.
38. Simon R, Snow R, Wakeman S. Understanding why patients with substance use disorders leave the hospital against medical advice: a qualitative study. *Subst Abus.* 2020;41(4):519–525.
39. Dasgupta N, Beletsky L, Ciccarone D. Opioid crisis: no easy fix to its social and economic determinants. *Am J Public Health.* 2018;108(2):182–186.
40. Lee CA, Bonar EE, Ilgen MA. Impact of social determinants of health and individual characteristics on substance use disorder treatment utilization among emerging adults aged 18–25. *Addict Res Theory.* 2025;33(1):65–71.
41. Roberts K, Smith E, Sousa C, et al. Centering persons who use drugs: addressing social determinants of health among patients hospitalized with substance use disorders. Social Work in Health *Care.* 2024;63(1):19–34.
42. Rehm J, Gmel G, Sempos CT, Trevisan M. Alcohol-related morbidity and mortality. *Alcohol Res Health.* 2003; 27(1):39–51.
43. Kimmel SD, Kim J-H, Kalesan B, Samet JH, Walley AY, Larochelle MR. Against medical advice discharges in injection and non-injection drug use-associated infective endocarditis: a nationwide cohort study. *Clin Infect Dis.* 2021;73(9): e2484–e2492.
44. Institute for Community Health. *Inpatient Addiction Consult Services in Massachusetts: Insights and Recommendations from Six Model Programs.* 2024. Accessed January 7, 2026. https://www.rizema.org/wp-content/uploads/2024/03/Inpatient-addiction-consult-services-in-MA-final-for-distribution.pdf#:~:text=An%20inpatient%20ACS%20program%20can,with%20expertise%20in%20addiction%20medicine
45. Lindsay DL, Freedman K, Jarvis M, et al. Executive summary of the American Society of Addiction Medicine (ASAM) clinical practice guideline on alcohol withdrawal management. *J Addict Med.* 2020;14(5):376–392.
46. Calcaterra SL, Martin M, Bottner R, et al. Management of opioid use disorder and associated conditions among hospitalized adults: a Consensus Statement from the Society of Hospital Medicine. *J Hosp Med.* 2022;17(9):744–756.
47. Logan AA, Haber LA, Martín M. Clinical progress note: management of the hospitalized patient who uses methamphetamine. *J Hosp Med.* 2025;20(4):380–384.
48. Bauer MS, Damschroder L, Hagedorn H, Smith J, Kilbourne AM. An introduction to implementation science for the non-specialist. *BMC Psychol.* 2015;3(1):32.
49. Centers for Medicare & Medicaid Services. *Quality Improvement Organizations.* Accessed December 5, 2024. https://www.cms.gov/medicare/quality/quality-improvement-organizations
50. Agency for Healthcare Research and Quality. *Research Tools, Data, and Funding.* Updated January 2024. Accessed December 5, 2024. https://www.ahrq.gov/health-literacy/research/index.html
51. Montgomery DC, Woodall WH. An overview of six sigma. *Int Stat Rev.* 2008;76(3):329–346.
52. What is lean healthcare? *NEJM Catalyst.* 2018;4(2). doi: 10.1056/CAT.18.0193
53. Services CfMaM. *PDSA Cycle Template.* Accessed December 16, 2024. https://www.cms.gov/medicare/provider-enrollment-and-certification/qapi/downloads/pdsacycledebedits.pdf
54. Serrat O. The five whys technique. Knowledge solutions: Tools, methods, and approaches to drive organizational performance. 2017:307–310.
55. Ilie G, Ciocoiu CN. Application of fishbone diagram to determine the risk of an event with multiple causes. *Knowl Manag Res Pract.* 2010;2(1):1–20.
56. Karuppusami G, Gandhinathan R. Pareto analysis of critical success factors of total quality management: a literature review and analysis. *Total Qual Manag.* 2006;18(4):372–385.
57. Lee W-S, Grosh DL, Tillman FA, Lie CH. Fault tree analysis, methods, and applications: a review. *IEEE Trans Reliab.* 1985;34(3):1–17.
58. Zimmermann GDS, Siqueira LD, Bohomol E. Lean six sigma methodology application in health care settings: an integrative review. *Rev Bras Enferm.* 2020;73(suppl 5): e20190861.
59. Association CH. *ColoradoMAT: 2020 Key Considerations for Hospitalized Patients with Opioid Use Disorder.* 2020. https://cha.com/wp-content/uploads/2020/10/MAT-Implementation-Guide_final.pdf
60. McNeely J, Wu L-T, Subramaniam G, et al. Performance of the tobacco, alcohol, prescription medication, and other substance use (TAPS) tool for substance use screening in primary care patients. *Ann Intern Med.* 2016;165(10):690–699.
61. Bridge. *Rapid Implementation of OUD Treatment in the Hospital Nationwide. CA Bridge.* Accessed December 18, 2024. https://bridgetotreatment.org/resource/rapid-implementation-of-opioid-use-disorder-treatment-in-the-hospital-nationwide/

62. Martin MCSL. *Improving Care for Hospitalized Patients with Opioid Use Disorder: Implementation Guide.* 2023. https://www.hospitalmedicine.org/globalassets/clinical-topics/clinical-pdf/oud-implementation-guide.pdf
63. Calcaterra SL, Bottner R, Martin M, et al. Management of opioid use disorder, opioid withdrawal, and opioid overdose prevention in hospitalized adults: a systematic review of existing guidelines. *J Hosp Med.* 2022;17(9):679–692.
64. Wesson DR, Ling W. The clinical opiate withdrawal scale (COWS). *J Psychoactive Drugs.* 2003;35(2):253–259.
65. Shearer RD, Bart G, Reznikoff C. Rethinking the use of “polysubstance” to describe complex substance use patterns. *J Gen Intern Med.* 2022;37(12):3174–3175.
66. Bridge C. *CA Bridge Treatment Protocols.* CA Bridge. Accessed December 18, 2024. https://bridgetotreatment.org/wp-content/uploads/protocol-packet.pdf
67. Skogrand E, Sharpe J, Englander H. Dispensing methadone at hospital discharge: one hospital’s approach to implementing the “72-hour rule” change. *J Addict Med.* 2024;18(1):71–74.
68. Sommers SW, Tolle HJ, Trinkley KE, et al. Clinical decision support to increase emergency department naloxone coprescribing: implementation report. *JMIR Med Inform.* 2024;12(1):e58276.
69. Sullivan JT, Sykora K, Schneiderman J, Naranjo CA, Sellers EM. Assessment of alcohol withdrawal: the revised clinical institute withdrawal assessment for alcohol scale (CIWA-Ar). *Br J Addict.* 1989;84(11):1353–1357.
70. Smith RM, Benzio B, Hendrickson AL, Telford ED, Franck AJ. Implementation of the Modified Minnesota Detoxification Scale (mMINDS) for alcohol withdrawal syndrome in critically ill patients. *Jt Comm J Qual Patient Saf.* 2020;46(11):656–658.
71. Langlois H, Cormier M, Villeneuve E, Hoffman RS, Longo C, Gosselin S. Benzodiazepine resistant alcohol withdrawal: what is the clinician’s preferred definition? *CJEM.* 2020;22(2):165–169.
72. Martin M, Snyder HR, Otway G, Holpit L, Day LW, Seidman D. In-hospital substance use policies: an opportunity to advance equity, reduce stigma, and offer evidence-based addiction care. *J Addict Med.* 2023;17(1):10–12.
73. Perera R, Stephan L, Appa A, et al. Meeting people where they are: implementing hospital-based substance use harm reduction. *Harm Reduct J.* 2022;19(1):14.
74. Calcaterra SL, Buresh M, Weimer MB. Better care at the bedside for hospitalized patients with opioid use disorder. *J Hosp Med.* 2023;18(12):1134–1138.
75. Hagle HN, Martin M, Winograd R, et al. Dismantling racism against black, indigenous, and people of color across the substance use continuum: a position statement of the association for multidisciplinary education and research in substance use and addiction. *Subst Abus.* 2021;42(1):5–12.
76. Eccles M, Mittman B. Welcome to implementation science [Internet]. Vol. 1 *Implement Sci BioMed Central.* 2006:1.
77. Nilsen P. Making sense of implementation theories, models and frameworks. *Implement Sci.* 2015;10(1):53.
78. Moullin JC, Dickson KS, Stadnick NA, et al. Ten recommendations for using implementation frameworks in research and practice. *Implement Sci Commun.* 2020;1(1):42.
79. Curran GM, Bauer M, Mittman B, Pyne JM, Stetler C. Effectiveness-implementation hybrid designs: combining elements of clinical effectiveness and implementation research to enhance public health impact. *Med Care.* 2012;50(3):217–226.
80. Powell BJ, Waltz TJ, Chinman MJ, et al. A refined compilation of implementation strategies: results from the Expert Recommendations for Implementing Change (ERIC) project. *Implement Sci.* 2015;10(1):21.
81. Bozinoff N, Grennell E, Soobiah C, et al. Facilitators of and barriers to buprenorphine initiation in the emergency department: a scoping review. *Lancet Reg Health Am.* 2024;38:100899.
82. Stevens K. *ACE Star Model of EBP: Knowledge Transformation.* Academic Center for Evidence-Based Practice, The University of Texas Health Science Center; 2004;30:2009.
83. Wilson KM, Brady TJ, Lesesne C; NCCDPHP Work Group on Translation. An organizing framework for translation in public health: the Knowledge to Action Framework. *Prev Chronic Dis.* 2011;8(2):A46.
84. Titler MG, Kleiber C, Steelman V, et al. Infusing research into practice to promote quality care. *Nurs Res.* 1994;43(5):307–313.
85. Titler MG, Kleiber C, Steelman VJ, et al. The Iowa model of evidence-based practice to promote quality care. *Crit Care Nurs Clin North Am.* 2001;13(4):497–509.
86. Logan J, Graham ID. The Ottawa model of research use. *Models and Frameworks for Implementing Evidence-Based Practice: Linking Evidence to Action.* Wiley-Blackwell; 2010:83–108.
87. Damschroder LJ, Reardon CM, Widerquist MAO, Lowery J. The updated consolidated framework for implementation research based on user feedback. *Implement Sci.* 2022;17(1):75.
88. Damschroder LJ, Aron DC, Keith RE, Kirsh SR, Alexander JA, Lowery JC. Fostering implementation of health services research findings into practice: a consolidated framework for advancing implementation science. *Implement Sci.* 2009;4:50.
89. Feldstein AC, Glasgow RE. A practical, robust implementation and sustainability model (PRISM) for integrating research findings into practice. *Jt Comm J Qual Patient Saf.* 2008;34(4):228–243.
90. McCreight MS, Rabin BA, Glasgow RE, et al. Using the Practical, Robust Implementation and Sustainability Model (PRISM) to qualitatively assess multilevel contextual factors to help plan, implement, evaluate, and disseminate health services programs. *Transl Behav Med.* 2019;9(6):1002–1011.
91. Rabin BA, Cakici J, Golden CA, Estabrooks PA, Glasgow RE, Gaglio B. A citation analysis and scoping systematic review of the operationalization of the Practical, Robust Implementation and Sustainability Model (PRISM). *Implement Sci.* 2022;17(1):62.
92. Rycroft-Malone J. Promoting Action on Research Implementation in Health Services (PARIHS). *Models and frameworks for implementing evidence-based practice: linking evidence to action.* 2010;109:135. https://books.google.com/books?hl=en&lr=&id=EpDbQSI1390C&oi=fnd&pg=PA109&dq=Promoting+action+on+research+implementation+in+health+services+(PARIHS)&ots=efhJxWVALK&sig=6_Foc0O7WmMUwr8pscUoTOmxPb8#v=onepage&q=Promoting%20action%20on%20research%20implementation%20in%20health%20services%20(PARIHS)&f=false
93. Helfrich CD, Damschroder LJ, Hagedorn HJ, et al. A critical synthesis of literature on the promoting action on research implementation in health services (PARIHS) framework. *Implement Sci.* 2010;5:82.
94. Cane J, O’Connor D, Michie S. Validation of the theoretical domains framework for use in behaviour change and implementation research. *Implement Sci.* 2012;7:37.
95. Fishbein M, Ajzen I.Belief, attitude, intention, and behavior: an introduction to theory and research. 1975.
96. Bandura A. *Social Foundations of Thought and Action: A Social Cognitive Theory.* Prentice-Hall, Inc.; 1986.
97. Triandis HC. *Values, Attitudes, and Interpersonal Behavior.* University of Nebraska Press; 1979.

3

Health System Optimizations to Support Treatment of Substance Use Disorders

Alia Bodnar, Lindsay A. Bowman, Olivia Berger, Megan E. Buresh

In 2018, I was medical director of a successful hospital-based addiction consultation service. We were starting more and more patients on evidence-based addiction treatment, including initiating methadone and buprenorphine for opioid use disorder (OUD). We had lots of success, particularly with patients we could directly connect to our outpatient primary care clinic on discharge. I continue to see many patients I met in the hospital for primary care and buprenorphine, and many are doing well in long-term recovery.

However, it was a struggle to find quality, patient-centered options for patients with more complex medical needs, particularly those requiring post–acute care (usually intravenous [IV] antibiotics or wound care). Ironically, skilled nursing facilities (SNFs) were less likely to accept patients on methadone and buprenorphine than if they were on short-acting full agonists like oxycodone alone. Our consult team social worker, generally an advocate for medications for OUD, started asking me not to start buprenorphine in patients going to SNF because of the difficulty of finding a facility, or worse, being accepted to a sub-par facility. A patient who desired OUD treatment described one SNF as an "open air drug market" and begged us not to send him there. Patients often languished in the hospital and lacked an option where they could receive both evidence-based OUD treatment and their other medical care.

One such patient is Lisa (pseudonym) with severe OUD from injection heroin and fentanyl use, alcohol use disorder, benzodiazepine use disorder driven by an underlying anxiety disorder, and unstable housing. I first met her in 2019 when she was 31 years old. Between 2019 and 2022, she had over 20 hospital admissions to our health system alone for complications of her OUD, including cellulitis, chronic wounds, osteomyelitis, and deep vein thrombosis. She had a strong desire to get her infections treated, but struggled with anxiety, ongoing desire to use substances, and finding a place where her goals could be met. She benefitted from methadone initiated in the hospital, but struggled to find a methadone clinic outside of the hospital that met her goals. She used alprazolam obtained from the street to self-treat her severe anxiety. Over her many hospitalizations, our team was able to build trust with Lisa. We often continued a low dose of benzodiazepines to help treat her anxiety. She did well with methadone initiation.

Despite these "wins," we couldn't find a place outside of the hospital for her to continue antibiotics. She was rejected by many facilities due to "behavioral issues," and often required prolonged stays in the hospital to complete antibiotics. When we did find a facility, she often left by self-directed discharge and re-presented to the hospital with untreated infection. She ultimately died of a fentanyl overdose—had reportedly used fentanyl on top of her methadone to self-treat chronic pain due to leg wounds.

Lisa's case, and others like hers, led me to partner with local outpatient treatment program (OTPs) and SNFs in 2019 to develop pathways for patients to initiate medications for OUD and continue them at SNF posthospital, which developed into the OUD Medical Patient Engagement, Enrollment in treatment and Transitional

Supports (MEETS) partnership.[1] It took a lot of work, strong support from hospital leadership, and complex care coordination, including determining how to enroll patients in OTP so that they could continue to receive methadone at SNF. I recognize that as a physician at an academic center with an addiction consultation service, I am in a privileged position with more support than many have. My goal is to continue to share and disseminate practical ways to improve substance use disorder (SUD) care for hospitalized patients so that all patients receive life-saving treatment.

Like many institutions, we are getting much better at initiating SUD treatment in the hospital, but there are still large system gaps in continuity of care and integration of SUD treatment with the rest of medical treatment. I continue to advocate for patients with SUD and complex medical needs to have options posthospital, where they can have all of their medical needs addressed. This includes advocating for change in home care policies so that patients with stable housing can be discharged home on IV antibiotics and working to find residential SUD treatment facilities and SNFs who are willing to accept patients. It has also involved implementing policies to dispense up to 3 days of methadone at discharge to facilitate transitions of care. Recently, this allowed one of my primary care continuity patients to be discharged home on Thanksgiving and spend the holiday with his family. These partnerships speak to what is possible, even within our current regulatory framework. Ongoing creative work, both at the health-system level and through advocating for policy changes, is needed to increase patient-centered care options for patients with SUD and complex medical needs.

—Megan E. Buresh

Key Points

- **Addressing substance use disorder (SUD)-related stigma is key to health system and hospital culture change.**
- **Billing guidelines and current procedural terminology (CPT) codes used on inpatient addition medicine consultation services are consistent with guidelines and CPT codes used for other inpatient consultation services.**
- **Embedding universal SUD screening and order sets for substance withdrawal treatment into the electronic medical record (EMR) can help improve guideline-concordant practice.**
- **Key procedures and policies, including initiation of medication treatment for SUD, are key to implementing patient-centered SUD care in hospitals.**
- **EMR-based templates can support hospital-based SUD treatment.**
- **Medications for opioid use disorder (OUD) can and should be initiated and continued for most hospitalized patients with OUD.**
- **Recent changes in regulations allow hospital pharmacies to dispense up to 3 days of methadone at hospital discharge, helping with transitions of care.**

Historically, substance use disorder (SUD) has been treated as a moral failing rather than a medical disease, and much of SUD treatment had a nonmedical focus (eg, abstinence only recovery houses, emphasis on mutual help meetings). In the United States, treatments like methadone have been segregated to highly federally regulated opioid treatment programs (OTP) in the outpatient setting, which are siloed from the rest of health care (including medical notes and clinical information made inaccessible due to privacy regulations under 42 CFR, Part 2). Despite caring for patients admitted with medical complications of SUD, historically hospitals have not viewed treating SUD as within their scope of care. Prior to the past decade, most medical staff received little to no training in the treatment of SUD. Given this historic segregation between SUD treatment and other medical treatment in the United States, a systems-level approach is key to integrating SUD treatment services into hospitals.

Key components to a sustainable, systems-level approach includes education and training of existing hospital staff, so that all care team members view treating SUD within their scope of practice. This is particularly important in resource-limited settings where having dedicated addiction consultation services may not be feasible. Existing clinicians (hospitalists, surgeons, etc) can be educated in basic substance withdrawal management and initiation of pharmacotherapy, with decision support from embedded hospital-based guidelines and order sets. Pharmacists can be educated in how regulations apply to hospitals and become key advocates for adding essential medications to the hospital formulary. Social workers and case managers can help with referral and linkage to ongoing SUD treatment. Other clinicians, such as infectious disease specialists can become champions of increasing access to postdischarge intravenous antibiotics in SUD treatment settings. There are multiple other care optimizations that are possible when health systems and hospitals embrace SUD care as part of medical care.

The hopeful news is that this systems-level work can be done, and much of it can be accomplished within existing staffing and infrastructure. In addition, if one is strategic about identifying and tracking impact on critical metrics that matter to hospital leaderships and staff (ie, 30-day readmissions, length of stay, staff wellness), it can help with generating commitment for further change and garnering hospital resources to help hire staff, including peer recovery specialists and dedicated addiction medicine clinicians. This chapter outlines real-world, practical examples of how to implement these changes at your institution, from culture change to billing to electronic medical record (EMR) integration and sample order sets.

Creating a Culture of SUD Care

The optimal treatment environment for people with SUD is one in which evidence-based care is delivered in a low-barrier, destigmatized, and patient-centered way. Treatment of SUD during hospitalization improves engagement in other aspects of medical care and increases the likelihood that patients will continue treatment for SUD after hospital discharge.[2,3] Despite this, an insufficient proportion of hospitalized patients with SUDs receive disease specific treatment.[4] It is imperative that medical clinicians caring for people with SUDs have a basic understanding of evidence-based care for the most common SUDs affecting their patients, as well as an understanding of the rationale for minimizing stigma and other barriers to care.

While there is a growing understanding of the value of education regarding management of SUDs early and throughout medical education,[5] medical clinicians already in practice often have limited formal education or teaching, which may hinder comfort and readiness to provide evidence-based care of SUDs.[6] Formal didactic sessions during onboarding or at intervals can be tailored to clinician's scope of practice, and offer opportunities to share the evidence supporting treatment of SUD during hospitalization, as well as diagnosis and management of SUDs most frequently encountered during hospitalization. In addition, clinical decision-making tools, as described later in this chapter, support evidence-based treatment while actively providing care.

In addition to education supporting diagnosis and management of SUDs, measures to provide destigmatized care are also crucial to maintaining a therapeutic environment and supporting recovery for hospitalized patients with SUD. Stigma and misconceptions about people with and treatment of SUD affect both individual care and the policies and resources available to address SUD, and it has been well characterized that this negatively impacts both the quality of care delivered and outcomes[7] and limits patient's ability to engage in treatment.[8] Studies of interventions to minimize stigma regarding SUD amongst health care professionals have evaluated a range of interventions, from online education only to combined training and direct contact with individuals in recovery. While interventions that include contact with those in recovery show the most meaningful effect on clinician attitudes and enthusiasm for treating SUD, education alone offers at least short-term changes in attitudes.[9]

Notably, specific terminology, for example, the word "abuser," has been shown to negatively affect care and perceptions of patients with SUD, even amongst experienced clinicians,[8] and "antistigma" campaigns have included initiatives to promote use of destigmatized language. In addition, for those working at institutions without existing antistigma campaigns, there are tool kits and resources available to support development of interventions to prevent or reduce the impact of stigma. For example, the Providers Clinical Support System (PCSS) for Medications for Opioid Use Disorder (MOUD) offers a free toolkit as well as online learning modules that guide a multipronged approach to reducing stigma targeting people with SUD.[10] This including both measures that can be adopted by individuals as well as broader, community or system level interventions.[11,12] Boston Medical Center also created a pledge called, "Words Matter: My Pledge" that members of the medical center sign as their commitment to promoting dignity and respect in their language related to SUD.[13]

Person-first language demonstrating diagnostic accuracy and a scientific understanding of disease is recommended when speaking with patients, speaking with clinicians, and when documenting in the medical record. The National Institute for Drug Abuse (NIDA) published preferred terminology including rational for use,[14] and individual institutions have promoted similar language as part of a strategy to dispel misconceptions regarding SUD while advancing the understanding of SUD as a chronic disease with evidence-based treatments to support recovery.[15] While to date, there is not specific data validating this approach, these resources do offer high-yield access to information needed to promote a culture of comprehensive and patient-centered SUD care. Examples of nonstigmatizing language to use, and the stigmatizing language that it replaces, are provided in Table 3.1.

While it is important to promote an understanding of SUD as a chronic but treatable disease, it is

TABLE 3.1

SUD Terminology

Nonstigmatizing language	Stigmatizing language
Person with a substance use disorder	Substance abuser or drug abuser Alcoholic Addict User Abuser Drunk Junkie
Babies born with an opioid dependency	Addicted babies/Born addicted
Substance use disorder or addiction Use, misuse Risky, unhealthy, or heavy use	Drug habit Abuse Problem
Person in recovery Abstinent Not drinking or taking drugs	Clean
Treatment or medication for addiction	Substitution or replacement therapy
Medication for opioid use disorder/alcohol use disorder	Medication-assisted treatment
Positive, negative (toxicology screen results)	Clean, dirty

Adapted from Boston Medical Center. *Words Matter Pledge.* Grayken Center for Addiction Medicine.[16]

also important to support an understanding of the role of harm reduction, or a focus on mitigating the harms of substance use rather than cessation of use itself, to support patients who may not yet be ready to engage in treatment with recovery as a goal.[17] In addition, it must be recognized that individuals who use substances experience trauma at a higher rate than the general population, whether as a trigger for or associated with substance use. This can also limit engagement with the health care system, use of a trauma-informed approach is imperative to support a safe, therapeutic treatment environment and avoid inflicting additional harm. See Chapter 16 for more information on this topic.

Establishing Addiction Specialty Credentials and Billing for Services

As discussed throughout this book, there are multiple models to provide hospital-based SUD care. The simplest model that does not rely on specialty care involves integrating SUD care into existing hospital teams' general medical or surgical care. In this model, credentialing and billing utilize existing structures.

If the hospital wants to provide specialty addiction consultative services provided by physicians, there are several steps they should consider. The first step is to establish hospital-specific experience and board certification requirements. Clinicians acting in a consultative role to provide SUD-specific care to hospitalized patients can come from addiction medicine or addiction psychiatry. Addiction medicine has been recognized as a subspecialty by the American Board of Medical Specialties (ABMS) since 2016, and physicians can become board certified by the American Board of Preventive Medicine (ABPM) from any of the 24 primary ABMS. Since the ABPM addiction medicine certifying exam's first cycle in 2017 until 2025, physicians with sufficient practice experience as well as those who completed an addiction medicine fellowship could apply to sit for the ABPM addiction medicine certification exam; starting in 2026 completion of an accredited addiction medicine fellowship is required to certify. Despite its relatively new designation, accredited fellowships in addiction medicine are growing, offering comprehensive training in management of SUDs in a variety of inpatient and outpatient settings.[18]

There is significant overlap in the principles and goals of addiction medicine and addiction psychiatry, though certification in addiction psychiatry has been available through the American Board of Psychiatry and Neurology since 1993. As its name suggests, addiction psychiatry fellowships are available to psychiatrists only, and completion is necessary to take the addiction psychiatry certifying exam.[19]

Once board certification is confirmed, hospital credentialing staff can apply the physician's primary and secondary billing taxonomy codes. If the physician is primarily working in addiction medicine or addiction psychiatry, their primary taxonomy should be addiction medicine or addiction psychiatry, respectively. Unfortunately, board eligibility alone does not allow the additional taxonomy assignment and could lead to payment delays.

The essential tasks of the addiction medicine or addiction psychiatrist include diagnosis and characterization of SUD identified in the DSM-5, as well as identification and management of associated toxidromes and withdrawal. The bulk of this work is done through direct history taking, examination of the patient, and assessment of diagnostic testing (laboratory results, electrocardiograms, etc), and there is rarely a role for procedural interventions. Advanced practice providers (APPs) may also provide these services under the supervision of a physician certified in addiction medicine or addiction psychiatry. See Chapter 5 for more information about the training available to APPs.

Addiction medicine or addiction psychiatry board-certified physicians seeing patients with SUDs in a consultative capacity should bill under their respective Addiction Medicine or Addiction Psychiatry taxonomy using standard CPT codes for inpatient consultation. For initial hospital consultation, CPT codes 99252–99255 may be used, with CPT codes 99231–99233 used for hospital follow-up visits, or subsequent hospital care. The parameters guiding use of medical decision making or time to identify the correct code are consistent with other specialty consultations like cardiology and neurology.[20] Notably, ICD-10 includes codes referring to "abuse" and "dependence" that correlate with severity of disease but are inconsistent with current DSM-5 definitions of SUDs. As ICD-10 also includes codes that are consistent with DSM-5 classifications, those less familiar with the coding definitions may use these preferentially. In general, use codes that are consistent with DSM-5 diagnoses.

Inpatient addiction medicine consultation services are often multidisciplinary and may include medical clinicians, pharmacists, social workers, behavioral health therapists, peer recovery coaches, and more. Though a range of services are provided, only physicians and APPs can bill for their hospital work. Though the information here reflects The Centers for Medicare & Medicaid Services (CMS) guidance at the time of this writing, readers should consult billing and coding experts at their own institutions to ensure compliance with any institutional-specific policies and any CMS updates or changes.

Billing With APPs

Though both physicians and APPs may bill for visits using the CPT codes above, if patients are seen by multiple billing clinicians from the same practice or group (also called a shared or split visit), only one clinician may bill. Consistent with CMS guidelines for shared visits in any specialty, the billing clinician is the person who performs a "substantive" portion of the visit, either defined by independent qualifying time spent or medical decision making. Documentation from both clinicians should reflect individual contributions to the visit (each should note time spent independently and/or fully describe their own medical decision making), and an "FS" modifier should be used to identify a shared visit.[21] Physicians can place the primary bill for a shared visit if they perform a substantive portion of the visit and document to support their involvement, otherwise they can attest a shared visit note and the APP would place the primary bill. Some hospitals may preferentially require physicians to see all new consultations. Clinicians are encouraged to check their local hospital bylaws to ensure compliance.

Billing With Residents and Fellows

Attending, teaching physicians may also bill for care provided with trainees and can addend and sign documentation to support billing. When providing care with an intern or resident physician, the attending physician must actively participate in management, and either be present for or independently perform all key portions of the service. This must be documented in the medical record, and a "GC" modifier used to indicate that care was provided by a resident and supervised by a teaching physician. When providing care with a student, the teaching physician must verify all portions of the visit (witness or confirm history, re-perform physical exam, verify medical decision making), though may addend a student's documentation if correctly documented. In both cases, billing reflects medical decision making or the teaching physician's time, and must not include the trainee's time.[22] As above, this is not specific to care of patients with SUD and rather reflects general CMS guidance.

Universal Screening for SUD in Hospital Systems

How to Integrate Universal Screening in Hospital Practice

In order to identify unhealthy substance use and SUDs in hospitalized patients, it is important to have standardized and universal screening, both to identify all cases and to avoid bias in who receives screening. Chapter 1 covers screening for SUD in detail, including characteristics of validated screening measures. Screening for unhealthy alcohol use was adopted in 2006 as a quality care measure by the Joint Commission, which is the major accrediting body for US hospitals.[23]

Most of the literature on universal screening comes from primary care and emergency departments (EDs), which have shown that embedding screening into the EMR is feasible and increases screening rates.[23] One option is to integrate screening into nursing workflows during ED triage or as part of hospital admission assessments.[24,25] For hospitalized patients first seen in ED, there should be a standardized way that

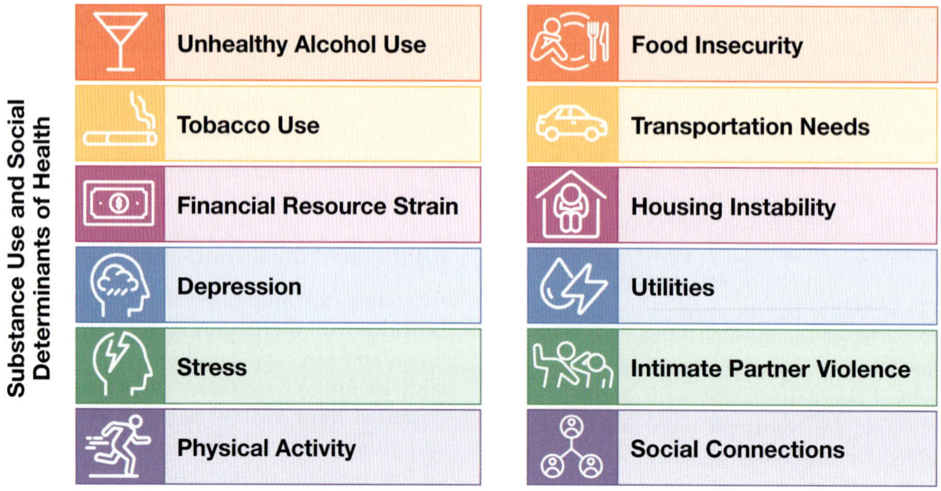

Figure 3.1: Example of EMR-integrated social determinants of health.

ED screening appears for hospital teams (eg, on flowsheets), both to avoid duplication of screening and to ensure that positive screening results receive follow-up.

In order to ensure that hospital teams see positive results, some EMR systems integrate screening for other specific social determinants of health information as well, such as housing security, food security, and transportation (Figure 3.1).

What Screening Tests to Use

In hospital settings, a feasible screening protocol is to use the three-item Alcohol Use Disorders Identification Test-Consumption (AUDIT-C) for alcohol[26] plus Single Item Screening Questions (SISQs) for tobacco and other substance use. All positive screens should trigger further assessment (eg, full 10-item AUDIT for positive AUDIT-C and best practice advisory (BPA) to order alcohol withdrawal assessments). In a study of screening, brief intervention and referral to treatment (SBIRT) in 23 EDs across Maryland, ED nurses completed screening using AUDIT-C plus a single screening question for substance use, with positive screens triggering an automatic referral to peer recovery coach for further assessment.[27] An alternative tool to screen for substances, alcohol and tobacco is the eight-item Alcohol, Smoking, and Substance Involvement Screening Test (ASSIST), but this is lengthier. A third proposed strategy is to use three SISQs (one for tobacco, one for alcohol, and one for other substances).[28] Sample screenings protocols are shown in Table 3.2.

Emerging research points to the potential additional utility of artificial intelligence (AI)[29] and natural language processing (NLP)[30,31] to further identify patients with SUD based on clinical notes. One study validated unhealthy alcohol use with a NLP classifier in hospitalized trauma patients that may better identify patients with unhealthy alcohol use rather than solely identifying based on billing and diagnostic codes.[32] There is also potential for Embodied Conversational Agents (ECAs), virtual agents that display on computer screens, to conduct unhealthy substance use screening using a smartphone app.[33,34] Further work is needed to determine practical ways to implement these tools in clinical practice.

Diagnosis of SUDs

In the authors' experience, SUDs are generally underdocumented in medical records, even for patients who are receiving appropriate clinical care (eg, withdrawal treatment, referral to SUD treatment). DSM-5 criteria[35] is the gold standard for diagnosing the type and severity of SUD. Each substance should have its own associated diagnosis and severity. For example, if a patient uses opioids, cocaine, cannabis, and tobacco, the patient would have four separate SUD diagnoses: severe opioid use disorder (OUD), moderate cocaine use disorder, severe cannabis use disorder, and tobacco use disorder. "Polysubstance use" is not an accurate diagnosis and does not assist with treatment decisions.

DSM-5 can be added to templated EMR notes and manually completed. Alternatively, decision support can be embedded into the EMR to help with linking to DSM-5 criteria for SUD.

TABLE 3.2

Options for Universal Unhealthy Substance Use Screening

Screening methods	Initial screening questions	Number of items, time	Additional screening questions in response to positive initial screen
Single Item Screening Questions (SISQ)	SISQ for tobacco	One item, 1 min	"Would you be interested in quitting tobacco use within the next few weeks?"
	SISQ for alcohol	One item, 1 min	AUDIT-C (three-item)
	SISQ for other drugs	One item, 1 min	10-item Drug Abuse Screening Test (DAST10)[36]
Alcohol Use Disorder Identification Test-Consumption (AUDIT-C)[37] plus SISQs for tobacco and alcohol	Alcohol: AUDIT-C	Three items, 1–2 min	Full eight-item AUDIT[38,39]
	SISQ for tobacco	One item, 1 min	"Would you be interested in quitting tobacco use within the next few weeks?"
	SISQ for other substances	One item, 1 min	DAST10[36]
Alcohol, Smoking, and Substance Involvement Screening Test (ASSIST)[40]	Eight-item assessment for alcohol, tobacco, and other substances	Eight items, 5–10 min	—
Tobacco, **A**lcohol, **P**rescription medication, and other **S**ubstance use (TAPS)	Four-item screening for tobacco, alcohol, prescription medication, and other substance use	Four items, 3–5 min	TAPS-2[41]
Severity of Dependence Scale (SDS)[42]	Five-item screening for risky cannabis use	Five-items, 2–3 min	—

Placing SUD Diagnosis in the Problem List

Any SUD diagnoses should be placed on the patient's problem list so that they are visible to all care team members. SUD information should be coded in standardized places (eg, clinical flowsheets). It should not be documented in social history fields, as this is inappropriate for a chronic medical condition with available treatments and makes information more difficult for care team members to find.

Toxicology Testing

Toxicology is frequently used in acute care settings, and can be useful, but should be done with care. There is no evidence that toxicology improves clinical care, so it should be used with caution. Toxicology can detect exposure to substances, both intentional and unintentional, and help with clinical treatment (particularly toxidromes or risk for withdrawal), but cannot be used to diagnose a SUD. Clinicians should not wait for toxicology results to treat withdrawal syndromes or toxidromes—often initial management relies on patient history of substance use and clinical assessment.

The most common form of hospital-based toxicology testing is urine toxicology, but serum testing can also be used for patients who are anuric. Usually, testing starts with immunoassay, which has faster processing time and is highly sensitive but less specific and can lead to false positives. Positive results that are inconsistent with patient report and/or known in-hospital exposures should receive confirmatory testing through gas chromatography-mass spectrometry (GC-MS) or liquid chromatography-mass spectrometry (LC-MS) to confirm that it is a true positive.

It is important to understand what standard toxicology testing can and cannot detect, which substances within a structurally similar family of medications may trigger a positive result (eg, codeine, morphine, hydromorphone, and heroin may all trigger a positive screen for a codeine/morphine antigen), and the window of detection for various substances following last use. For example, given protracted renal clearance of fentanyl (mean of 2 weeks in persons with OUD),[43] repeat fentanyl testing is not useful for assessing for in-hospital illicit fentanyl use if a patient already had a fentanyl-positive test. When interpreting toxicology results, it is also critical to note the specimen collection time relative to the administration time of medications given during the course of medical care (either en route or after arrival to the institution).

Toxicology testing can be helpful to counsel patients about unknown exposures to substances. For example, with increasing fentanyl contamination of the illicit stimulant supply, patients using stimulants may be unknowingly exposed to fentanyl, and thus at risk of unintentional opioid overdose. A positive fentanyl test on toxicology can lead to patient counseling on harm reduction, including prescribing naloxone on discharge.

Hospitals are encouraged to work with their laboratory medicine colleagues to determine appropriate toxicology testing. It is also helpful to work with laboratory medicine to increase ability to test for new and emerging drugs of concern, such as xylazine.

Hospital Policies and Procedures

Hospital policies standardize an approach to management of an issue or use of a hospital resource to improve patient safety, staff efficiency, and patient outcomes. Through clear delineation of staff roles and responsibilities as well as relevant processes, policies serve as a common guideline so that all staff members are working from the same set of rules, expectations, and foundational knowledge. Policies and procedures come in many forms, including administrative policies, clinical practice policies, and medication policies, to name a few.

In the care of patients with SUD specifically, policies are helpful tools to establish a standard of care within an institution or health system, fill knowledge gaps in areas where expert treatment is not readily accessible, and dispel myths or misconceptions related to SUD care. For example, a policy about management of OUD in hospitalized patients can clearly state that all patients with OUD shall be offered a medication for OUD (ie, methadone, buprenorphine) followed by clinical guidance for how to safely initiate these medications. The policy can then elaborate that federal law does not prohibit the use of methadone in the hospital, thus dispelling this myth and serving as a helpful reference should this question arise. In this way, the policy can help to reduce stigma surrounding MOUD, establish a culture in which evidence-based SUD care is expected and prioritized, and reduce staff discomfort by offering reassurance about pertinent regulations and providing clinical guidance. Components of key policies such as in-hospital drug use and management of OUD, are described in more detail in Table 3.3.

Dispensing Medications for OUD During Hospitalization

Misconceptions surrounding MOUD still abound, creating unnecessary barriers to accessing these critical therapies during hospitalization. One particularly disruptive misconception is the belief that federal regulations pertaining to outpatient methadone use also govern use of methadone in the hospital. However, the code of federal regulations (CFR) 1306.07(c) specifically states that this regulation "is not intended to impose any limitations on a physician or authorized hospital staff to administer or dispense narcotic drugs in a hospital to maintain or detoxify a person as an incidental adjunct to medical or surgical treatment of conditions other than addiction."[44]

While this clearly delineates that federal limitations around methadone (and other scheduled drugs, including buprenorphine) do not apply to patients admitted to the hospital for issues besides opioid dependence or withdrawal, some institutions ban the use of methadone and/or buprenorphine in the hospital or limit their use to continuation of outpatient treatment only, erroneously citing federal regulations as the limitation. As a result, patients who are not actively treated with methadone are often unnecessarily limited to buprenorphine as their only agonist medication option for management of OUD, or in more severe cases, left without access to either of the most evidence-based therapies for OUD. A careful reading of the federal regulations and developing policy and procedure with hospital leadership is recommended in order to offer these life-saving treatments.

Hospital Formulary Management

It is common practice for health systems and hospitals to have committees that assess and regulate the hospital medication formulary. Most hospitals may refer to this as a Pharmacy and Therapeutics (P&T) Committee, but it is possible another name is used to describe a similar concept. A formulary is a list of medications that are purchased, stocked, and available for use at the hospital.[45] Many factors are considered when a new medication is reviewed by a P&T committee, such as cost, appropriate care setting, similar medications already on formulary, therapeutic evidence, and patient outcomes. Medications may be restricted for use by indication, clinical setting, or patient population, amongst other possible restrictions. P&T committees often also oversee any medication-related policies and procedures as well. Ultimately, a P&T committee will decide whether to add a medication to formulary based on the previously mentioned factors.

When thinking about hospital-based SUD care, there are essential medications to have available for use for the treatment of SUD (Table 3.4). For OUD, methadone and buprenorphine are necessary to have on the hospital formulary. Methadone tends to be

TABLE 3.3

Example Hospital Policies Related to SUD Care

Issue	Key highlights

Inpatient management of opioid use disorder (OUD)	▪ Standardize an assessment process to identify and evaluate OUD and/or opioid withdrawal
	▪ Establish offering of medications for OUD (MOUD) as a standard of care
	▪ Address misconceptions related to treatment of individuals with OUD, including:
	  ▪ Federal law does not prohibit use of buprenorphine or methadone in the hospital
	  ▪ OUD and/or treatment with methadone or buprenorphine do not preclude the use of opioid analgesics when clinically appropriate for moderate–severe acute pain
	  ▪ An X-waiver is no longer required to prescribe buprenorphine at hospital discharge
	  ▪ Methadone or buprenorphine dispensed via an opioid treatment program is generally not included in the Prescription Drug Monitoring Program
	▪ Provide clinical guidance for key issues:
	  ▪ Initiation and titration of MOUD
	  ▪ Discharge planning, including referral to treatment
	  ▪ Provision of naloxone

In-hospital substance use[46]	▪ Highlight the link between in-hospital substance use and insufficient treatment of SUD, withdrawal syndromes, pain, and other related symptoms to promote evidence-based treatment ▪ Promote therapeutic rather than punitive responses to in-hospital substance use with a focus on patient safety ▪ Delineate a process for how substances, if found on hospital premises, should be handled or disposed of ▪ Identify who should be notified of in-hospital substance use when suspected and what circumstances may prompt a property search ▪ Discuss the role for toxicology testing in the case of in-hospital substance use and offer guidance on interpretation of results ▪ Provide a range of medical or psychosocial interventions to optimize patient and staff safety in the event of in-hospital substance use, including differentiation between first and repeated in-hospital substance use events
Alcohol withdrawal management	▪ Establish a standard screening process and/or screening tool(s) that will be used to identify at-risk patients ▪ Select a validated symptom-assessment tool for us in symptom-triggered treatment pathways (eg, CIWA, BAWS, etc) ▪ Highlight risk factors that may indicate a higher risk for severe or complicated withdrawal ▪ Provide clinical guidance for management of alcohol withdrawal syndrome

straightforward because there are only three formulations to consider (oral tablet, oral liquid, and intravenous); however, different concentrations may be available and may need to be considered for different populations and uses. For example, the hospital may choose to have one concentration of methadone liquid that is 5 mg/1 mL which might be used for analgesic purposes and another concentration 10 mg/1 mL for the treatment of OUD. Buprenorphine can be more complicated because there are multiple different formulations and products available for different therapeutic purposes. Buprenorphine has many important considerations, such as indication (products for chronic pain vs OUD), route of administration (sublingual, buccal, intravenous/intramuscular, subcutaneous, transdermal), and formulation (tablet, film, short-acting injection, extended-release subcutaneous injection). As such, it is common for hospitals to carefully select which product/formulations will be on the formulary, and it is possible that all formulations will not be available for use. It is important to have access to these evidence-based medication treatments in order to most effectively treat patients with SUD.

Long-Acting Injectable Formulations

The long-acting injectable (LAI) formulations of buprenorphine (Sublocade, Brixadi) and naltrexone (Vivitrol) are essential medications, however, due to their cost, it can be challenging to obtain hospital approval to add them to hospital formularies.

Some institutions have successfully obtained LAI for hospitalized patients using outpatient prescription coverage and administering medication to patient directly after discharge in outpatient care (eg,

TABLE 3.4

Hospital Formulary Recommendations for Medications for SUD

Medication	Formulation	Essential or aspirational
Alcohol use disorder		
Acamprosate	Oral	Essential
Disulfiram	Oral	Essential
Gabapentin	Oral	Essential
Naltrexone	Oral	Essential
Naltrexone	Extended-release intramuscular	Aspirational[a]
Topiramate	Oral	Essential
Opioid use disorder[b]		
Buprenorphine	Sublingual	Essential
Buprenorphine/naloxone	Sublingual	Essential
Buprenorphine	Extended-release subcutaneous	Aspirational
Methadone	Oral tablet	Essential
Methadone	Oral liquid	Essential
Methadone	Intravenous/intramuscular	Essential
Naltrexone	Extended-release intramuscular	Aspirational[a]
Opioid overdose reversal		
Naloxone	Intravenous/intramuscular	Essential
Naloxone	Intranasal	Aspirational
Tobacco use disorder		
Bupropion	Oral	Essential
Nicotine replacement	Transdermal patch	Essential
Nicotine replacement	Gum	Essential
Nicotine replacement	Lozenge	Essential
Nicotine replacement	Inhaler	Aspirational
Varenicline	Oral	Essential

[a]Lower cost options for ER Naltrexone may be available to nonprofit hospitals.

[b]Buccal buprenorphine, IV/IM buprenorphine, and transdermal buprenorphine, indicated for the treatment of pain, may also be considered. Buccal and IV/IM buprenorphine can assist with low-dose buprenorphine transitions as discussed in Chapter 7.

infusion suite, outpatient pharmacy). Other hospitals have approved these treatments with specific restrictions for their use. For instance, for patients with high risk for rehospitalization, homelessness, history of medication nonadherence, or patients going to settings where medications are not available (carceral setting or SNF), the cost of the medication is less than the cost of ongoing care in the hospital or hospital readmission. Hospitals may also be able to apply for reduced costs of the medications from the manufacturer for some treatments.

Practice Optimizations

SUD Assessment Templates

Note templates and EMR smart phrases can help with standardizing SUD assessments. An example initial SUD evaluation template is shown here.

The following clinical information related to substance use is CONFIDENTIAL and protected by Federal Law. ACCESS TO THIS INFORMATION IS ON A NEED-TO-KNOW BASIS ONLY AND IS PROVIDED FOR THE PURPOSE OF ASSURING APPROPRIATE MEDICAL CARE. Federal regulations (42 CFR, Part 2) prohibit the release of this information without specific written consent of the patient. A general authorization for the release of medical information is NOT sufficient for the purpose of releasing the following information.

INPATIENT INITIAL ADDICTION MEDICINE CONSULT NOTE

Author: @ME@

PCP: @PCP@

Date of Admission: @ADMITDTY@

Hospital Day: @LOS@

Reason for admission: @ADMITDX@

Consult requested by: @ATTENDINGNAMENUMBER@

REASON FOR CONSULTATION: ***

IMPRESSION:

@NAME@ is a @AGE@ @SEX@ with PMH of *** who presents with ***

Diagnosis:

#*** Use Disorder

#***

RECOMMENDATIONS:

____

CONSULT HISTORY/OBJECTIVE

HPI:

@NAME@ is a @AGE@ @SEX@ with PMH of ***

Signs of * use disorder in the last 12 months:**

(1) Recurrent use resulting in failure to fulfill major role obligations {YES:25828}

(2) Recurrent use in physically hazardous situations {YES:25828}

(3) Continued use despite recurrent social or interpersonal problems exacerbated by substance {YES:25828}

(4) Tolerance: {YES:25828}

(5) Withdrawal: {YES:25828}

(6) Taking substance in larger amounts and longer than intended: {YES:25828}

(7) Having a persistent desire or unsuccessful effort to cut down or control use: {YES:25828}

(8) Spending a great deal of time to obtain substance or recover from its effects: {YES:25828}

(9) Giving up important social, occupational, or recreational activities: {YES:25828}

(10) Using the substance despite knowledge of having a persistent physical or psychological problem that has been caused by the substance: {YES:25828}

(11) Craving {YES:25828}

TOTAL = ***

2–3 = mild, 4–5 = moderate, >6 severe

OTHER SUBSTANCE USE HISTORY:

Injection Substance use: {YES:28767}

Opioid Overdose in the last year: {YES:28767}

Past Tobacco or vaping use: {YES:25828} Current Tobacco or vaping use: {YES:25828}

Interested in nicotine replacement? {YES:25828} Interested in quitting? {YES:25828}

Past EtOH use: {YES:25828} Current EtOH use: {YES:25828}

Past substance use: {YES:25828}; Current substance use: {YES:25828}

Other notable substance or behavioral use: ***

Family Hx of substance use disorder: {YES:25828} Active substance use in household: {YES:25828}

History of substance use disorder treatment: {YES:25828} Where and when? ***

Hx of incarceration/probation? {YES:25828}

Prescription drug monitoring checked: {YES:25828}, Appropriate? {YES:25828}

ROS:

Withdrawal symptoms currently: {sx; tobacco withdrawal lower case:22640}

Concern for abscess or induration: {YES:25828}

Concern for STI or s/s of STI: {YES:25828}

Consents to HIV testing: {YES:25828}

Hx of Mental Illness or trauma: ***

PMH: @PMHP@

INPATIENT MEDS:

@CMEDS@ @ALGP@

SOCIAL Hx:

Address: @ADDCAP@

Homeless: {YES:25828}

Has *** child(ren) who live with ***.

Current DHS involvement: {YES:25828}

Current Legal issues: {YES:25828}

PHYSICAL EXAM:

@VS@

DATA:

Signed: @ME@

Dispensing MOUD at Hospital Discharge

Health care teams are able to initiate or continue medications for OUD (ie, methadone or buprenorphine) in acute care settings, such as EDs or hospitals. In December 2022, the Mainstreaming Addiction Treatment (MAT) and Medication Access and Training Expansion (MATE) Acts were passed as part of the Consolidated Appropriations Act (the Omnibus Bill). Prior to this time, clinicians who intended to prescribe buprenorphine for treatment of OUD were required to submit a "Notice of Intent" to Substance Abuse and Mental Health Services Administration (SAMHSA), and to be granted an "X-waiver" allowing prescription of buprenorphine outside of an Outpatient Treatment Program (OTP). Those intending to treat more than 30 patients at a time were required to participate in a specific training program (8 hours for physicians, 24 hours for advance practice providers). The MAT Act eliminated the X-waiver, allowing any clinician with DEA registration that includes schedule III controlled substances to prescribe buprenorphine for treatment of OUD.[47] Concurrently, the MATE Act implemented a one-time requirement indicating that clinicians applying for or renewing their DEA registration on or after June 27, 2023

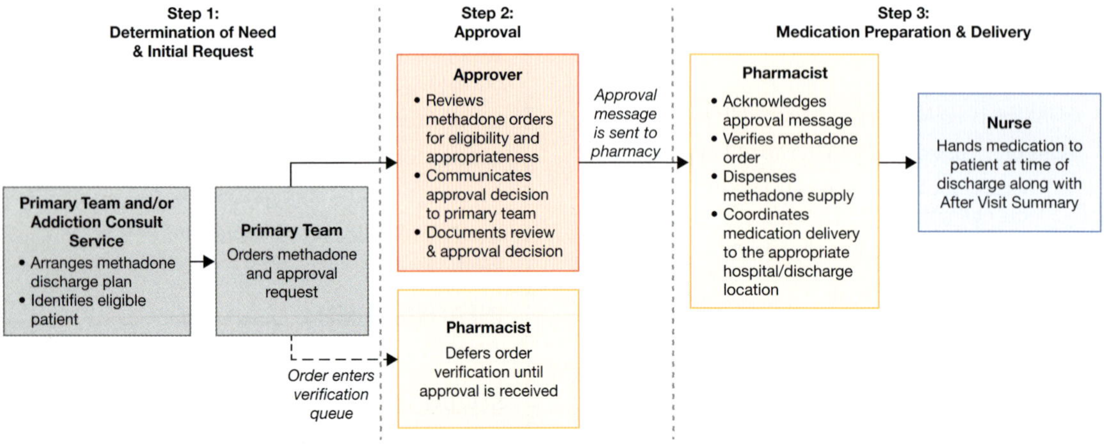

Figure 3.2: Example of workflow for ordering and dispensing methadone at discharge.

must complete 8 hours of training on management of OUD or other SUD.[48] Graduates within 5 years from U.S. health professional schools may also use training completed in their curriculum to fulfill the requirement. Clinicians already board certified in addiction medicine or addiction psychiatry are assumed to have fulfilled the requirement. Thus, all clinicians with an active DEA registration are able to prescribe up to 30 days of buprenorphine at hospital discharge, assisting with linkage to ongoing treatment.

Methadone, however, cannot be prescribed for OUD treatment upon ED or hospital discharge due to regulations that only allow methadone to be dispensed at an OTP in the outpatient setting. This historically has led to challenging transitions of care. In addition, for patients who are newly initiating treatment with methadone, an in-person medical history and physical exam is also required. Because of this, next-day appointments must be arranged at the time of ED or hospital discharge, which can be difficult for a number of reasons including limited OTP hours of operation (particularly on weekends or holidays), functional or medical limitations that limit ability to present to an OTP the following day, or potential challenges in rural or underserved areas (distance, lack of available intake appointments, or simply fewer OTPs). Consequently, treatment initiation during acute hospitalization is often deferred, or hospital length of stay is unnecessarily prolonged until next-day dosing with an OTP can be arranged. In response, the DEA has amended associated regulations (21 CFR 1306.07(b)) to allow for an entity to dispense to the patient up to a 3-day supply of methadone while ongoing outpatient treatment is being arranged.[44] While this new exception addresses a gap in care, no guidance was provided on how to successfully implement this service within health systems. Table 3.5 outlines how different addiction programs throughout the United States have implemented hospital-based methadone dispensing.

One approach to implementation is a workflow within the EMR that guides primary teams, with approval by select approvers (addiction medicine team or selected ED provider), on how to provide patients with up to a 3-day supply of methadone at time of discharge for patients who are discharging to community settings or skilled nursing facilities (Figure 3.2).[49] Involvement of addiction medicine may be preferred by your institution, but is not required by federal regulations. Collaboration with the hospital pharmacy is essential because that is where the methadone is dispensed from. Because methadone cannot be prescribed, it cannot be filled by a traditional outpatient or community pharmacy. Developing a workflow of this complexity may require support and input from several key stakeholders, such as pharmacy, relevant physician groups (including addiction medicine physicians), nursing, clinical informatics, legal/regulatory representatives, and relevant hospital committees. Sample workflow is illustrated in Figure 3.1.

Other Regulatory Changes and Updates

In addition to the exception to 21 CFR 1306.07(b) as described above, other changes have been made to expand access to MOUD and to better support clinicians and hospitals to deliver evidence-based care of SUDs.

As of April 2, 2024, multiple changes were made to 42 CFR, Part 8, the section of the federal code of regulating OTPs. These changes were also intended to improve access to MOUD while removing barriers to care, improve retention, eliminate stigmatizing language from the regulations, and support clinician

TABLE 3.5

Implementation of Hospital-based Methadone Dispensing at Discharge[50]

State of implementation	Maryland	Oregon	Washington	Connecticut	Colorado
How ordered	Order set in Epic	Order set in Epic	Order set in Epic	Order set in Epic	Order set in Epic
Who can order	Any ED or hospital clinician can order; requires review and approval by hospital addiction consult service or group of designated ED clinician/PharmDs	Any ED or inpatient clinician	Any inpatient clinician	Restricted to inpatient addiction medicine consult team	Any inpatient clinician (requires attestation that addiction medicine was involved if not ordered by addiction medicine)
Formulation of methadone	Liquid	Liquid	Liquid	Oral tablets	Liquid
Chain of custody	Pharmacy → Inpatient nurse → patient (delivered to patient bedside)	Pharmacist → patient	Pharmacist → prescriber → patient. All three are together at the pharmacy window	Inpatient pharmacy → prescriber → patient (delivered at patient bedside)	Pharmacy → inpatient nurse → patient (delivered to patient bedside)

autonomy in treatment decisions. Among these are the use of telehealth when assessing patients for treatment with MOUD, liberalization of the timing and number of "take-home" doses of methadone from the first week of treatment, and prioritization of treatment for vulnerable groups, such as pregnant people.[51] While this does not directly affect how MOUD may be administered in the hospital setting, hospital-based clinicians should be aware of these changes as they may improve access to MOUD and affect transitions of care at discharge. Continued attention to regulatory changes is necessary to ensure treatment patterns are consistent and offer the greatest access to care within current regulations.

Electronic Medical Record Optimizations

Order Sets

Order sets are another invaluable tool in the hospital to promote evidence-based care and improve efficiency, accuracy and safety of ordering medications and related interventions.[52] Order sets are a form of clinical decision support in which common orders related to management of a particular condition are grouped into a single template where they can be ordered at once. Orders within an order set may include medications, nursing interventions, labs, imaging, or even consult requests. Medication orders within an order set can specify appropriate starting dosing, titration or taper strategies, and/or as-needed indications, thus offering an opportunity to educate on and standardize the use of best practices for a particular disease state. By clearly delineating the intended indication for contained orders and using a dosing strategy that has been vetted and approved by hospital committees, order sets improve efficiency and safety of downstream processes as well, like pharmacist order verification or nursing administration. In some cases, order sets have even been shown to reduce hospital mortality.[53] Order sets that may be integrated within the EMR as traditional order sets or clinical guidance prove particularly helpful in the hospital management of SUD and related syndromes include methadone initiation (Figure 3.3A), methadone initiation for pregnant patients (Figure 3.3B), buprenorphine initiation (Figure 3.4A), buprenorphine initiation for pregnant patients (Figure 3.4B), supportive medications for opioid withdrawal (Figure 3.5), medications for alcohol use disorder (Figure 3.6), and management of alcohol withdrawal (Figure 3.7).

Upkeep is an important consideration when introducing a new order set, as order sets can be an equally powerful force in perpetuating outdated practices. For example, old opioid withdrawal order sets may contain tapers to abstinence that can be particularly harmful for patients if implemented. An inventory of existing order panels may be a helpful initial step in reducing harmful practices, and regular review cycles should be established for remaining order sets to ensure they stay current and consistent with best medical practice.

Best Practice Advisories and Embedded Decision Support Tools

Many EMRs contain other useful tools to offer clinical guidance, improve efficiency, and shape the standard of care. BPAs are one such example in which an alert fires in the EMR to prompt a specific action based on patient characteristics or conditions. The alert may contain direct links to the suggested action to simplify the ordering process and increase likelihood of follow-through. For example, a BPA may be used to alert clinicians to order naloxone at discharge for patients meeting criteria to suggest a high risk for opioid overdose (example shown in Figure 3.8). This alert type has been associated with significant increases in prescribing patterns, particularly when paired directly with order entry support.[54,55]

Many EMRs have functionality to embed more complex, noninterruptive clinical decision support

Initiating long-term methadone ✕

Order: COWS q4h for 36 hours

Day 1:

1. If COWS Is >8, **order:** methadone 30 mg once daily
2. If 6 hours after initial dose COWS is >8, **order an additional:** methadone 10 mg once
3. Do not give more than 40 mg on day 1
4. Use clonidine and other adjuvant treatments for ongoing symptoms

If vomits after dose: re-dose only, if emesis is witnessed and occurs <15 minutes after dose administration

Day 2:

1. If COWS is >8 in the AM, **order:** methadone 50 mg once daily
2. If COWS is <8 in the AM, administer total dose from day 1
3. Use clonidine and other adjuvant treatments for orgoing symptoms

Day 3:

- Adjust methadone dose by no greater than 10 mg/d every 3–4 days
- Methadone dose should be adjusted for objective signs of withdrawal (eg, sweating, pupillary dilation, piloerection, restlessness) and subjective opioid cravirg
- If patients is sedated, do not give methadone ard seek consultation
- At discharge, arrange for next day transition to an Opioid Treatment Program
- Do not prescribe methadone at discharge

Decrease initial dose if low opioid tolerance, risk of oversedation with other substances/medications, decompensated cirrhosis, or prolonged QTc

Figure 3.3: **A:** Methadone initiation in nonpregnant patients. (Care Signature Program at Yale New Haven Hospital, Kelsey Cole, PA-C, and AgileMD.)

Methadone initiation guidance
Day 1

<u>DAY 1</u> (midnight is switch over to new day—establish regimen for morning start): **maximum daily dose 50 mg**

- Evaluate for signs/symptoms of active opioid withdrawal

1. **Order:** COWS q2h for 48 hours—click here for educaton on COWS administration
   a. **With 1st** COWS that is ≥8, dose with methadone 20 mg once
   b. **2nd** COWS assessment at 2 hours: if COWS ≥8, dose one time PRN once oxycodone IR PO
   c. **3rd** COWS assessment 4 hours after first dose: if COWS is ≥8, give an additional 20 mg of methadone once
   d. **4th** COWS assessment 2 hours later: if COWS ≥8, dose one time PRN once oxycodone IR PO
   e. **5th** COWS assessment 4 hours after 3rd COWS: if COWS ≥8, can dose with methadone 10 mg PO once—must be at least 4 hours after last methadone dose
   f. Continue COWS every 2 hours
      - **If 50 mg total dose reached and COWS remains ≥8:** treat breakthrough symptoms with PRN medications for symptomatic management

- **If vomits after dose:** re-dose <u>only</u> if emesis is witnessed and occurs <15 minutes after dose administration. Any emesis outside this timeframe please contact provider—if unable to tolerate liquid, consider crushed tablets

↓

Methadone initiation guidance
Day 2

<u>DAY 2</u>: **maximum daily dose 60 mg**

1. Give total dose from day 1 as either a single dose or split dose (q12h) depending upon patient preference
   a. Discuss with patient that if splitting dose in 2, that this is an inpatient option and may not be continued outpatient
2. Continue COWS every 2 hours assessment
3. **4 hours after initial dose:** If COWS is ≥8, give an additional 10 mg of methadone
4. Treat breakthrough symptoms with PRN medications for symptomatic management

↓

Methadone initiation guidance
Day 3

<u>DAY 3</u>: **maximum daily dose 70 mg**

1. Give total dose from day 2 as either a single dose or split dose (q12h) depending upon patient preference
   a. **Order:** methadone daily or methadone q12h
2. Continue COWS assessment—space to every 4 hours: **Order:** COWS q4h
3. **4 hours after initial dose:** if COWS is ≥8, give an additional 10 mg of methadone
4. Continue COWS assessment every 4 hours
5. Treat breakthrough symptoms with PRN medications for symptomatic management

↓

Methadone initiation guidance
After Day 3

<u>After Day 3</u>:

- There should be at least 3 days at day 3 total dose before continued uptitration
- Methadone dose should be adjusted for objective signs of withdrawal (eg, sweating, pupillary dilation, piloerection, restlessness) and subjective opioid craving
- Treat breakthrough symptoms with PRN medications for symptomatic management
- If patient is continuing to have ongoing withdrawal symptoms/craving, contact Addiction Medicine for guidance

Figure 3.3: (*Continued*) **B:** Methadone initiation in pregnant patients. (Care Signature Program at Yale New Haven Hospital, Kelsey Cole, PA-C, and AgileMD.)

platforms seamlessly into the EMR. These tools require specific software such as AgileMD and may be referred to by different names such as Clinical Care Pathways. They offer an opportunity to support higher-level clinical decision making at the point of care. They may be targeted to a specific medication (eg, buprenorphine initiation)[56] or address a disease state more globally (eg, management of OUD—see Figures 3.3, 3.4, 3.6, and 3.9). Clinical care pathways have been shown to increase initiation of medications for alcohol use disorder when integrated into one large health system.[57]

Addressing Privacy

42 CFR, Part 2, or "the Confidentiality of Substance Use Disorders Records" addresses federal regulations specific to treatment records from federally assisted SUD programs (Part 2 programs). Part 2 programs are individuals or entities that specifically provide diagnosis and management of SUD, and though federally assisted programs may be programs conducted by a federal agency, those operating under a federal license to dispense MOUD or those participating in Medicare. The goal of the regulations is to protect the

Initiating long-term buprenorphine-naloxone ×

To avoid precipitating acute opioid withdrawal, *do not begin treatment until >12 hours since last opioid use, COWS is 8–12, and patient has objective signs of opioid withdrawal (eg, dilated pupils, vomiting, gooseflesh)*

Patients with higher opioid tolerance (eg, fentanyl use) may need higher doses of buprenorphine

Order: COWS q4h for 36 hours

Day 1:

1. **Order: buprenorphine-naloxone 4 mg SL once** *(if fentanyl use can start with 8 mg SL once)*
2. May repeat up to 4–8 mg every 1–2 hours as needed up to a maximum of 32 mg on day 1 (patients who experience precipitated opioid withdrawal or with tolerance to fentanyl may require a higher dose on first day of treatment)
   a. **Order: buprenorphine-naloxone SL**
3. If precipitated withdrawal occurs, consider specialty consultation
   a. **Order: Addiction Medicine consult** or **Psychiatry consult**

Day 2:

1. Administer 8–16 mg (select dose based on prior total dose from previous day, severity of opioid use disorder, and level of physical dependence)
   a. **Order: buprenorphine-naloxone SL**

Day 3:

1. Administer 16–24 mg (select dose based on prior total dose from previous day, severity of opioid use disorder, and level of physical dependence)
   a. **Order: buprenorphine-naloxone SL once**

Day 4:

1. Continue dose from day 3 and connect to treatment

If emesis occurs: check mouth for whether film is still in place

- **If film is no longer present within 10 minutes of administration due to emesis:** give buprenorphine 2 mg SL or half of current dose
- **If film is still in place or ≥10 minutes since dose administration:** fully absorbed, no repeat dosing required but COWS should be reassessed 1 hour postemesis to guide further treatment

Figure 3.4: A: Buprenorphine initiation guidance for nonpregnant patients. (Care Signature Program at Yale New Haven Hospital, Kelsey Cole, PA-C, and AgileMD.)

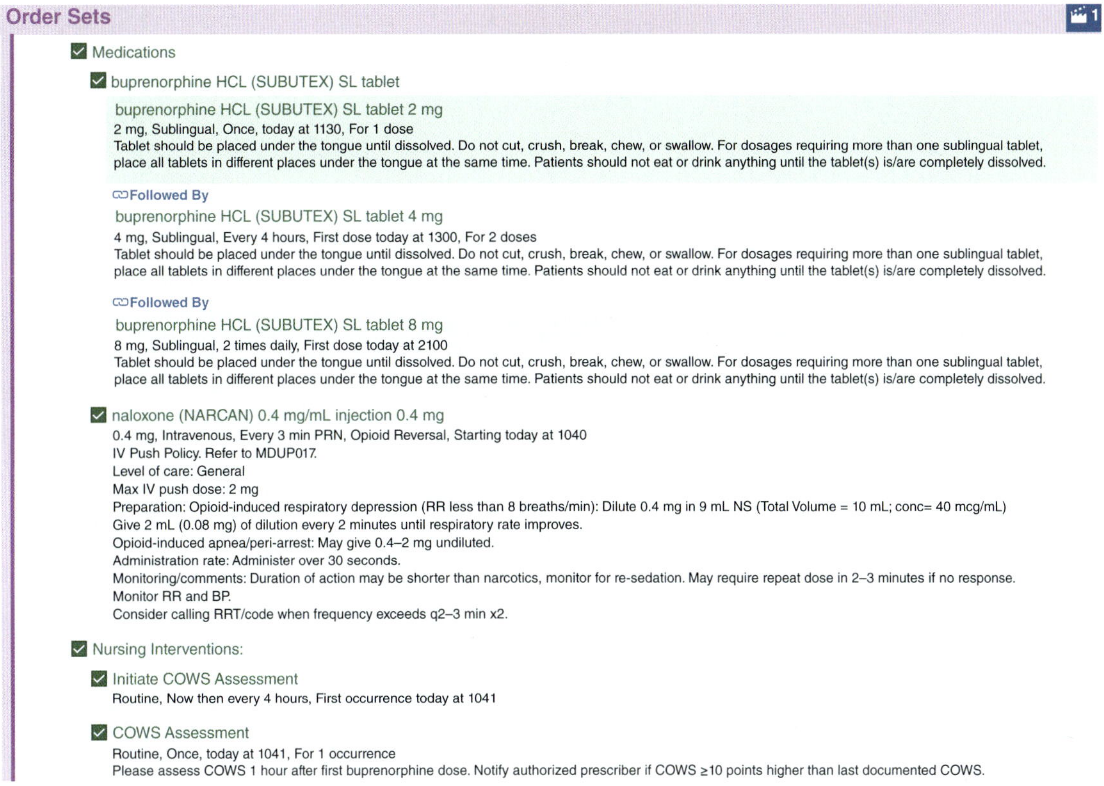
Order Sets

Medications

buprenorphine HCL (SUBUTEX) SL tablet

buprenorphine HCL (SUBUTEX) SL tablet 2 mg
2 mg, Sublingual, Once, today at 1130, For 1 dose
Tablet should be placed under the tongue until dissolved. Do not cut, crush, break, chew, or swallow. For dosages requiring more than one sublingual tablet, place all tablets in different places under the tongue at the same time. Patients should not eat or drink anything until the tablet(s) is/are completely dissolved.

Followed By
buprenorphine HCL (SUBUTEX) SL tablet 4 mg
4 mg, Sublingual, Every 4 hours, First dose today at 1300, For 2 doses
Tablet should be placed under the tongue until dissolved. Do not cut, crush, break, chew, or swallow. For dosages requiring more than one sublingual tablet, place all tablets in different places under the tongue at the same time. Patients should not eat or drink anything until the tablet(s) is/are completely dissolved.

Followed By
buprenorphine HCL (SUBUTEX) SL tablet 8 mg
8 mg, Sublingual, 2 times daily, First dose today at 2100
Tablet should be placed under the tongue until dissolved. Do not cut, crush, break, chew, or swallow. For dosages requiring more than one sublingual tablet, place all tablets in different places under the tongue at the same time. Patients should not eat or drink anything until the tablet(s) is/are completely dissolved.

naloxone (NARCAN) 0.4 mg/mL injection 0.4 mg
0.4 mg, Intravenous, Every 3 min PRN, Opioid Reversal, Starting today at 1040
IV Push Policy. Refer to MDUP017.
Level of care: General
Max IV push dose: 2 mg
Preparation: Opioid-induced respiratory depression (RR less than 8 breaths/min): Dilute 0.4 mg in 9 mL NS (Total Volume = 10 mL; conc= 40 mcg/mL)
Give 2 mL (0.08 mg) of dilution every 2 minutes until respiratory rate improves.
Opioid-induced apnea/peri-arrest: May give 0.4–2 mg undiluted.
Administration rate: Administer over 30 seconds.
Monitoring/comments: Duration of action may be shorter than narcotics, monitor for re-sedation. May require repeat dose in 2–3 minutes if no response.
Monitor RR and BP.
Consider calling RRT/code when frequency exceeds q2–3 min x2.

Nursing Interventions:

Initiate COWS Assessment
Routine, Now then every 4 hours, First occurrence today at 1041

COWS Assessment
Routine, Once, today at 1041, For 1 occurrence
Please assess COWS 1 hour after first buprenorphine dose. Notify authorized prescriber if COWS ≥10 points higher than last documented COWS.

Figure 3.4: (*Continued*) **B:** Buprenorphine initiation order set for pregnant patients.

privacy of people accessing treatment for SUDs, and to answer concerns regarding risk of discrimination and prosecution associated with disclosure of SUDs diagnosis or treatment. In practice, this has meant that SUD treatment is behind a firewall (even within a health-system EMR), and non-Part 2 clinicians cannot access this information without written consent. The regulations do not apply to documentation of SUDs by non-Part 2 clinicians. It is important to note that some health systems may interpret the 42 CFR Part 2 differently and may consider clinicians providing hospital-based SUD care as Part 2. Each health system should review the law and determine their best course to address and follow the law. Onerous processes around confidentiality are not recommended because they may discourage the exact access that hospital-based SUD care programs intend to provide. If hospital-based SUD services are deemed to be Part 2 programs (as some programs have determined in 2026), it is important to streamline and integrate consent processes as much as possible to preserve access to care and care coordination in the hospital.

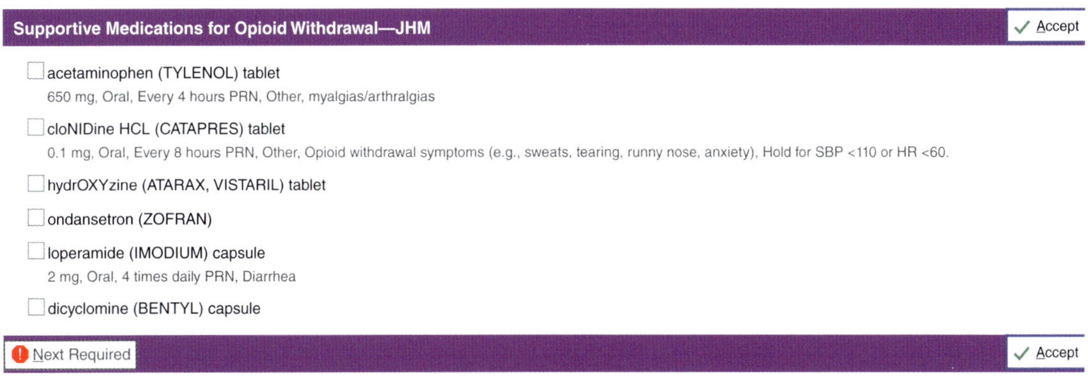
Supportive Medications for Opioid Withdrawal—JHM
Accept

acetaminophen (TYLENOL) tablet
650 mg, Oral, Every 4 hours PRN, Other, myalgias/arthralgias

cloNIDine HCL (CATAPRES) tablet
0.1 mg, Oral, Every 8 hours PRN, Other, Opioid withdrawal symptoms (e.g., sweats, tearing, runny nose, anxiety), Hold for SBP <110 or HR <60.

hydrOXYzine (ATARAX, VISTARIL) tablet

ondansetron (ZOFRAN)

loperamide (IMODIUM) capsule
2 mg, Oral, 4 times daily PRN, Diarrhea

dicyclomine (BENTYL) capsule

Next Required
Accept

Figure 3.5: Supportive medications for opioid withdrawal order set. (© 2025 Epic Systems Corporation.)

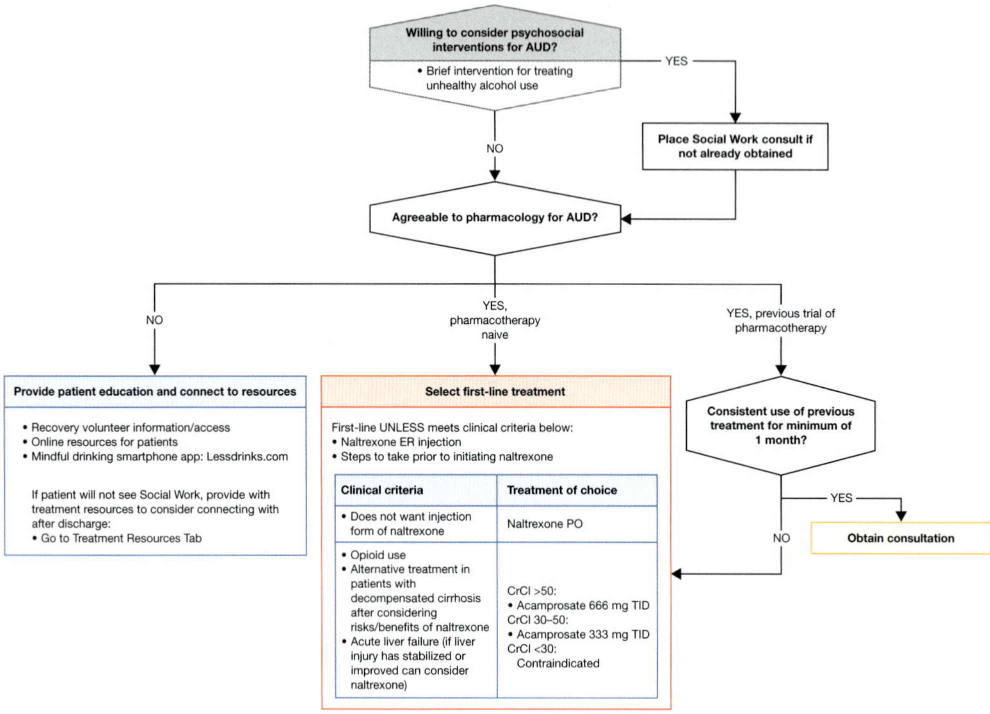

Figure 3.6: Medications for alcohol use disorder clinical guidance. (Care Signature Program at Yale New Haven Hospital, Kelsey Cole, PA-C, and AgileMD.)

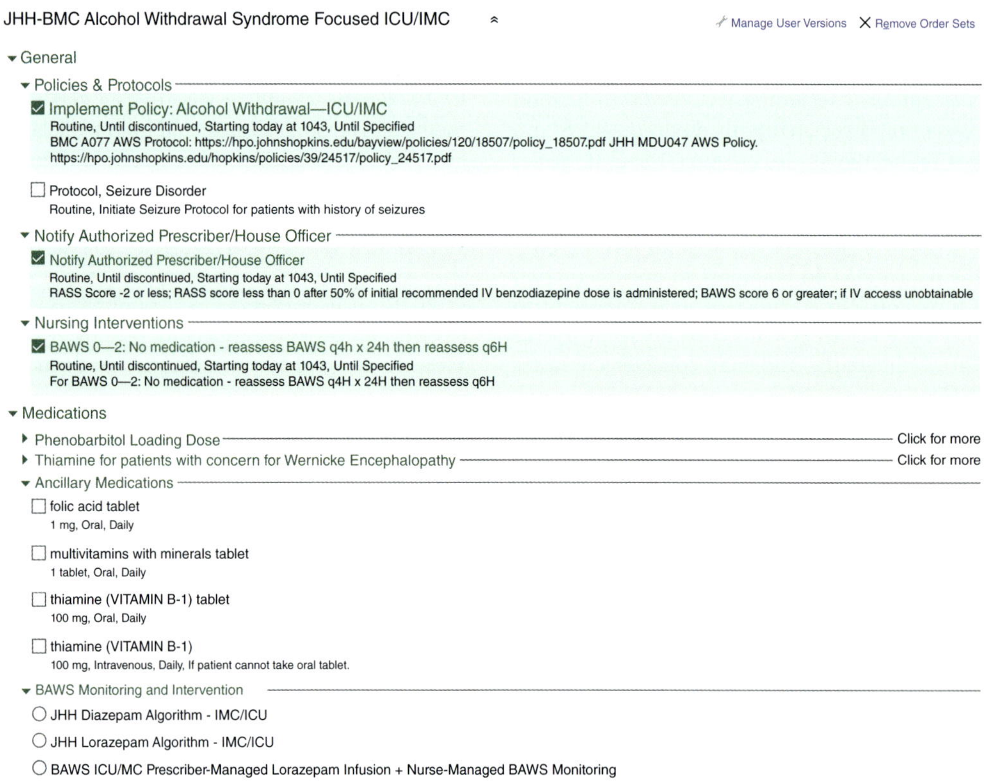

Figure 3.7: Sample alcohol withdrawal order set. (© 2025 Epic Systems Corporation.)

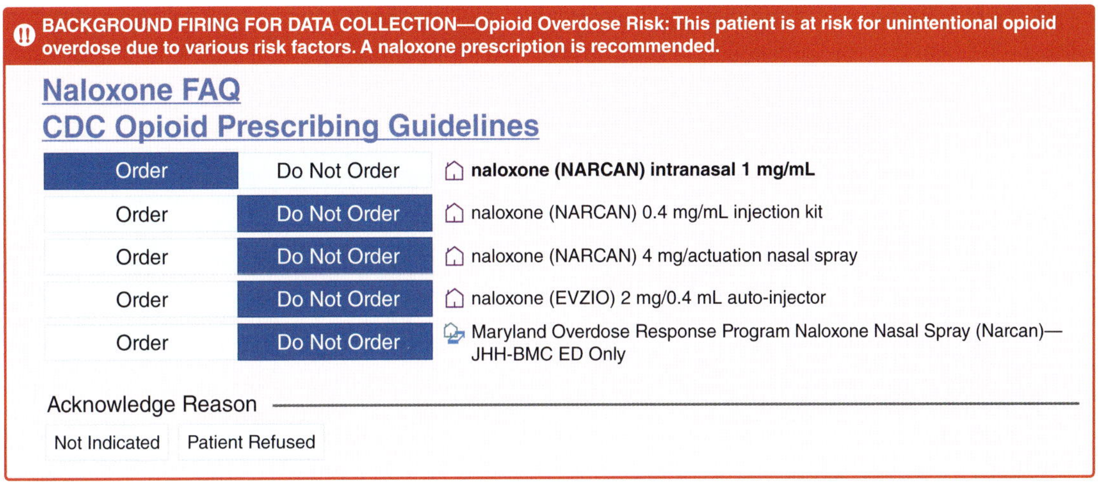

Figure 3.8: Example best practice advisory for naloxone prescribing. (© 2025 Epic Systems Corporation.)

As of April 16, 2024 changes were made to the regulations implementing elements of the Coronavirus Aid, Relief, and Economic Security (CARES) act addressing confidentiality, and aligning certain aspect of privacy of Part 2 records with Health Insurance Portability and Accountability Act (HIPAA) and HITECH.[58] Specifically, a single consent can now be used for Treatment, Payment, and Operations (TPO) (consistent with other health care records), and notes that segregation of Part 2 data is not required. Notably, SUD counseling notes are not covered by TPO consent and require specific permission to disclose, similar to HIPAA protections for psychotherapy notes. Updates to the regulations do not affect protections limiting disclosure for legal purposes (other than mandatory reporting), which still requires express written consent or a court order.[58]

In order to transmit information about hospital-based SUD care to community SUD treatment providers, a 42-CFR and institution-compliant release of information should be signed by the patient and can be sent by fax or secure email to community treatment providers (eg, OTP or residential addiction treatment program where patient will transition after discharge).

Conclusion

In summary, existing health system resources can be effectively leveraged to implement SUD care into health systems. Embedding screening and diagnosis into the EMR, antistigma education, expansion of hospital formularies, developing SUD-related order sets and clinical guidance, and policies and procedures can help put evidence-based SUD care into practice using existing hospital teams. Addiction medicine or addiction psychiatry specialists can also help advance SUD care.

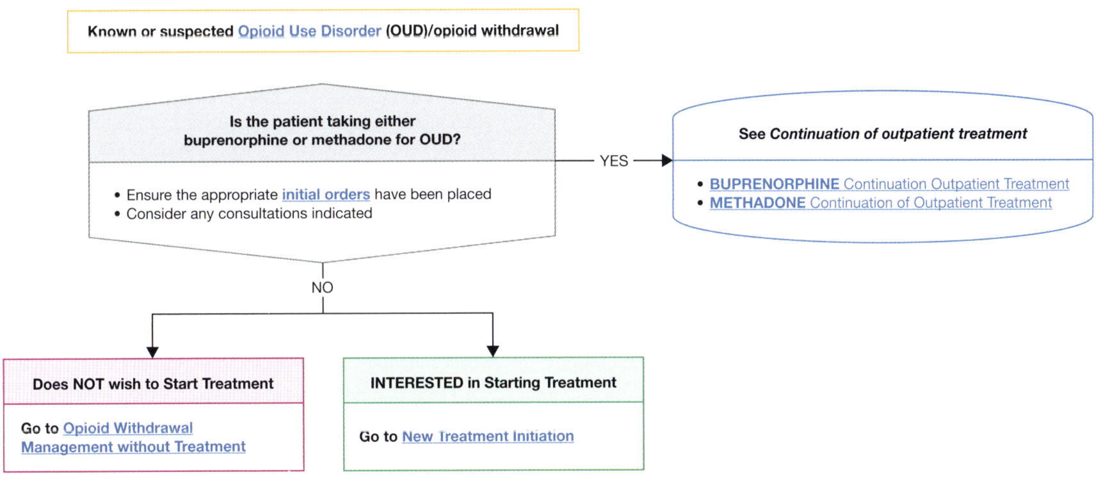

Figure 3.9: Embedded clinical guideline for management of opioid use disorder.

REFERENCES

1. Tassey TE, Ott GE, Alvanzo AAH, Peirce JM, Antoine D, Buresh ME. OUD MEETS: a novel program to increase initiation of medications for opioid use disorder and improve outcomes for hospitalized patients being discharged to skilled nursing facilities. *J Subst Abuse Treat.* 2022;143:108895.
2. Ober AJ, Murray-Krezan C, Page K, et al. Hospital addiction consultation service and opioid use disorder treatment. *JAMA Intern Med.* 2025;185(6):624–633.
3. Englander H, Dobbertin K, Lind BK, et al. Inpatient addiction medicine consultation and post-hospital substance use disorder treatment engagement: a propensity-matched analysis. *J Gen Intern Med.* 2019;34(12):2796–2803.
4. Danovitch I, Korouri S, Kaur H, et al. The addiction consultation service for hospitalized patients with substance use disorder: an integrative review of the evidence. *J Subst Use Addict Treat.* 2024;163:209377.
5. Klimas J, McCracken R, Robertson R, Cullen W. Towards a framework for implementing physician education in substance use disorders. *Drug Alcohol Depend Reports.* 2021;1:100001.
6. Von Klimo MC, Nolan L, Corbin M, et al. Physician reluctance to intervene in addiction: a systematic review. *JAMA Netw Open.* 2024;7(7):e2420837.
7. Van Boekel LC, Brouwers EPM, Van Weeghel J, Garretsen HFL. Stigma among health professionals towards patients with substance use disorders and its consequences for healthcare delivery: systematic review. *Drug Alcohol Depend.* 2013; 131(1–3):23–35.
8. Kelly JF, Westerhoff CM. Does it matter how we refer to individuals with substance-related conditions? A randomized study of two commonly used terms. *Int J Drug Policy.* 2010; 21(3):202–207.
9. Bielenberg J, Swisher G, Lembke A, Haug NA. A systematic review of stigma interventions for providers who treat patients with substance use disorders. *J Subst Abuse Treat.* 2021;131: 108486.
10. Providers Clinical Support Network. Accessed June 19, 2025. https://pcssnow.org/
11. ATTC—Anti-Stigma Toolkit: A Guide to Reducing Addiction-Related Stigma—Providers Clinical Support System-Medications for Opioid Use Disorders. Accessed June 9, 2025. https://pcssnow.org/courses/attc-anti-stigma-toolkit-a-guide-to-reducing-addiction-related-stigma-2/
12. Reducing Stigma Education Tools (ReSET)—Dell-Medical-School—Providers Clinical Support System-Medications for Opioid Use Disorders. Accessed June 9, 2025. https://pcssnow.org/courses/reducing-stigma-education-tools-reset-dell-medical-school/
13. What We Say and How We Say It Makes a Difference to Our Patients with Substance Use Disorder. Accessed June 19, 2025. https://www.bmc.org/sites/default/files/Patient_Care/Specialty_Care/Addiction-Medicine/LANDING/files/Words-Matter-Pledge.pdf
14. Words Matter: Preferred Language for Talking About Addiction | National Institute on Drug Abuse (NIDA). Accessed May 9, 2025. https://nida.nih.gov/research-topics/addiction-science/words-matter-preferred-language-talking-about-addiction
15. Join the "Words Matter" campaign! | Public Health Institute at Denver Health | Public Health Institute at Denver Health. Accessed May 9, 2025. https://www.phidenverhealth.org/blog/2024/05/join-the-words-matter-campaign
16. Boston Medical Center Grayken Center for Addiction. *Words Matter Pledge.* Accessed February 24, 2026. https://www.addictiontraining.org/documents/resources/355_Words_Matter_Pledge.pdf
17. Progress Over Perfection: Redefining Success—Providers Clinical Support System-Medications for Opioid Use Disorders. Accessed June 9, 2025. https://pcssnow.org/courses/progress-over-perfection-redefining-success/
18. Finding and Applying to Fellowships. Accessed June 9, 2025. https://www.acaam.org/finding-and-applying-to-fellowships
19. Fellowship and Programs – AAAP. Accessed June 9, 2025. https://www.aaap.org/fellowship/
20. American Medical Association. *CPT Evaluation and Management Code and Guideline Changes. JAMA.* Published 2022. Accessed May 13, 2025. https://www.ama-assn.org/system/files/2023-e-m-descriptors-guidelines.pdf
21. Updates for Split or Shared Evaluation & Management Visits. 2023. Accessed June 9, 2025. https://www.cms.gov/files/document/mm13592-updates-split-or-shared-evaluation-management-visits.pdf
22. Guidelines for Teaching Physicians, Interns, and Residents.; 2024. https://www.cms.gov/files/document/guidelines-teaching-physicians-interns-residents.pdf
23. Barclay C, Viswanathan M, Ratner S, Tompkins J, Jonas DE. Implementing evidence-based screening and counseling for unhealthy alcohol use with epic-based electronic health record tools. *Jt Comm J Qual Patient Saf.* 2019;45(8):566–574.
24. Keen A, Thoele K, Oruche U, Newhouse R. Perceptions of the barriers, facilitators, outcomes, and helpfulness of strategies to implement screening, brief intervention, and referral to treatment in acute care. *Implement Sci.* 2021;16(1):44.
25. Thoele K, Draucker CB, Newhouse R. Implementation of screening, brief intervention, and referral to treatment (SBIRT) by nurses on acute care units: a qualitative descriptive study. *Subst Abus.* 2021;42(4):662–671.
26. Haroon S, Wooldridge D, Hoogewerf J, et al. Information standards for recording alcohol use in electronic health records: Findings from a national consultation. *BMC Med Inform Decis Mak.* 2018;18(1):36.
27. Monico LB, Oros M, Smith S, Mitchell SG, Gryczynski J, Schwartz R. One million screened: Scaling up SBIRT and buprenorphine treatment in hospital emergency departments across Maryland. *Am J Emerg Med.* 2020;38(7):1466–1469.
28. Tai B, McLellan AT. Integrating information on substance use disorders into electronic health record systems. *J Subst Abuse Treat.* 2012;43(1):12–19.
29. Afshar M, Sharma B, Dligach D, et al. Development and multimodal validation of a substance misuse algorithm for referral to treatment using artificial intelligence (SMART-AI): a retrospective deep learning study. *Lancet Digit Health.* 2022;4(6):e426–e435.
30. Afshar M, Phillips A, Karnik N, et al. Natural language processing and machine learning to identify alcohol misuse from the electronic health record in trauma patients: development and internal validation. *J Am Med Inform Assoc.* 2019;26(3):254–261.
31. Riddick TA, Choo EK. Natural language processing to identify substance misuse in the electronic health record. *Lancet Digit Heal.* 2022;4(6):e401–e402.
32. To D, Sharma B, Karnik N, Joyce C, Dligach D, Afshar M. Validation of an alcohol misuse classifier in hospitalized patients. *Alcohol.* 2020;84:49–55.
33. Auriacombe M, Fournet L, Dupuy L, et al. Effectiveness and acceptance of a smartphone-based virtual agent screening for alcohol and tobacco problems and associated risk factors during COVID-19 pandemic in the general population. *Front Psychiatry.* 2021;12:693687.
34. Auriacombe M, Moriceau S, Serre F, et al. Development and validation of a virtual agent to screen tobacco and alcohol use disorders. *Drug Alcohol Depend.* 2018;193:1–6.

35. American Psychiatric Association. *Diagnostic and Statistical Manual of Mental Disorders*. 5th ed, text rev (DSM-5-TR). American Psychiatric Association Publishing; 2022.
36. Skinner HA. The drug abuse screening test. *Addict Behav*. 1982; 7(4):363–371.
37. Bush K, Kivlahan DR, McDonell MB, Fihn SD, Bradley KA. The AUDIT alcohol consumption questions (AUDIT-C): an effective brief screening test for problem drinking. *Arch Intern Med*. 1998;158(16):1789–1795.
38. Saunders JB, Aasland OG, Babor TF, de la Fuente JR, Grant M. Development of the Alcohol Use Disorders Identification Test (AUDIT): WHO collaborative project on early detection of persons with harmful alcohol consumption-II. *Addiction*. 1993;88(6):791–804.
39. Alcohol Use Disorders Identification Test (AUDIT). Accessed June 9, 2025. https://auditscreen.org/
40. Humeniuk R, Henry-Edwards S, Ali R, et al. *The Alcohol, Smoking and Substance Involvement Screening Test (ASSIST) : Manual for Use in Primary Care*. 2nd ed. World Health Organization; 2010.
41. Tobacco, Alcohol, Prescription medication, and other Substance use (TAPS) Tool. Accessed June 9, 2025. https://nida.nih.gov/taps2/
42. Van der Pol P, Liebregts N, de Graaf R, Korf DJ, van den Brink W, "van Laar M. Reliability and validity of the severity of dependence scale for detecting cannabis dependence in frequent cannabis users. *Int J Methods Psychiatr Res*. 2013;22(2):138–143.
43. Huhn AS, Hobelmann JG, Oyler GA, Strain EC. Protracted renal clearance of fentanyl in persons with opioid use disorder. *Drug Alcohol Depend*. 2020;214:108147.
44. eCFR :: 21 CFR 1306.07—Administering or dispensing of narcotic drugs. Accessed May 9, 2025. https://www.ecfr.gov/current/title-21/part-1306/section-1306.07#p-1306.07(c)
45. Ciccarello C, Leber MB, Leonard MC, et al. ASHP guidelines on the pharmacy and therapeutics committee and the formulary system. *Am J Health Syst Pharm*. 2021;78(10):907–918.
46. Huxley-Reicher Z, Puglisi LB, Tetrault JM, et al. Response to substance use during hospitalization: a survey study of current and ideal policies and practices. *J Hosp Med*. 2023;18(9):829–834.
47. Waiver Elimination (MAT Act) | SAMHSA. Accessed May 9, 2025. https://www.samhsa.gov/substance-use/treatment/statutes-regulations-guidelines/mat-act
48. Training Requirements (MATE Act) Resources | SAMHSA. Accessed May 9, 2025. https://www.samhsa.gov/substance-use/treatment/resources/mat-act/training-requirements
49. Bowman LA, Berger O, Nesbit S, Stoller KB, Buresh M, Stewart R. Operationalizing the new DEA exception: a novel process for dispensing of methadone for opioid use disorder at discharge from acute care settings. *Am J Health Syst Pharm*. 2024;81(6):204–218.
50. Calcaterra SL, Weimer MB, Grimm E, et al. Leveraging the 72-hour rule change to support transition from hospital to opioid treatment program. *JAMA Netw Open*. 2025;8(11): e2544996.
51. The 42 CFR Part 8 Final Rule Table of Changes | SAMHSA. Accessed May 9, 2025. https://www.samhsa.gov/substance-use/treatment/opioid-treatment-program/42-cfr-part-8/changes
52. Cohen SM, Kashyap N, Steel TL, Edelman EJ, Fiellin DA, Joudrey PJ. Guideline concordance of electronic health record order sets for hospital-based treatment of alcohol withdrawal syndrome. *J Hosp Med*. 2025;20(6):550–561.
53. Ballard DJ, Ogola G, Fleming NS, et al. The impact of standardized order sets on quality and financial outcomes. In: Henriksen K, Battles JB, Keyes MA, Grady ML, eds. *Advances in Patient Safety: New Directions and Alternative Approaches*. Agency for Healthcare Research and Quality (US); 2008. Accessed May 13, 2025. http://www.ncbi.nlm.nih.gov/pubmed/21249907
54. Funke M, Kaplan MC, Glover H, et al. Increasing naloxone prescribing in the emergency department through education and electronic medical record work-aids. *Jt Comm J Qual Patient Saf*. 2021;47(6):364–375.
55. Hussain S, Lehmann H, Buresh ME, et al. Academic detailing to enhance adoption of clinical decision support for patients at risk of opioid overdose. *Appl Clin Inform*. 2025; 16(02):393–401.
56. Melnick ER, Nath B, Dziura JD, et al. User centered clinical decision support to implement initiation of buprenorphine for opioid use disorder in the emergency department: EMBED pragmatic cluster randomized controlled trial. *BMJ*. 2022;377:e069271.
57. Cole KO, Weimer MB, Wang K, et al. Impact of an electronically-integrated clinical pathway on hospital initiation of medications for alcohol use disorder and subsequent hospital utilization. *J Hosp Med*. 2025;20(10):1044–1051.
58. Fact Sheet 42 CFR Part 2 Final Rule | HHS.gov. Accessed May 13, 2025. https://www.hhs.gov/hipaa/for-professionals/regulatory-initiatives/fact-sheet-42-cfr-part-2-final-rule/index.html#ftn1

4

Hospital-Based Substance Use Disorder Care Delivery Models

Honora Englander, Beth Williams, Linda Peng

Tim* eyed me skeptically as I entered his hospital room. A young man hospitalized for complications of diabetes; he had been referred to our team after his urine drug test came back positive for opioids. He greeted me with clipped, one-word answers and then, clearly uncomfortable, asked me to leave because he wasn't feeling well. Later that day, I returned with Traci, our hospital peer who brings her own lived experience with addiction to her work. Traci began by sharing her story, explaining that she was there to advocate for him and provide nonjudgmental support. As she spoke, I saw Tim's* skepticism evolve into disbelief.

He was cautious at first but shared that although he'd been hospitalized many times before, no one had ever addressed his addiction. He described feeling stigmatized by hospital staff, who he felt judged his choices and dismissed his complaints of pain. The lack of trust and support had made his hospital stays unbearable, often causing him to leave against medical advice. For the first time in the hospital, Tim* felt heard. He opened up as we validated his experiences and treated him with respect. When I offered medications for opioid use disorder (MOUD), his eyes lit up with relief. He confided in us that he had hidden fentanyl in his socks, fearing the discomfort of opioid withdrawal. With a newfound sense of hope, he chose to start methadone, taking a significant step toward managing his health and addiction.

After speaking with Tim*, Traci and I sought out his bedside nurse, who was visibly frustrated, remarking that Tim* was refusing all care. We took a moment to explain that Tim* was feeling unwell due to opioid withdrawal and shared his story of struggling to have his addiction addressed during previous hospitalizations. Traci added her personal perspective, recounting the challenges she faced when hospitalized with addiction and highlighting how empathetic care from a nurse made a huge difference. While the nurse initially seemed unimpressed, she listened to us and ultimately ensured that Tim* received his ordered methadone doses.

The next day, Tim* was feeling significantly better. Throughout the rest of his hospitalization, we worked closely with him to adjust his methadone dose and support his goals. Our social worker referred him to an opioid treatment program, set him up with primary care follow-up, and provided him with transportation resources.

On the day of his discharge, Tim's* initial nurse approached us, clearly moved by his transformation. She admitted she was astonished by the change in his demeanor once his opioid withdrawal was addressed. She shared that she was rooting for him and his substance use disorder (SUD) recovery journey as he prepared to leave the hospital and thanked us for providing education around his care.

The interprofessional addiction consultation service at our hospital has not only transformed patient care but has also driven a palpable shift in the hospital's culture. As Traci put it for a recent hospital newsletter highlighting our team, "Over the past three years, I've watched the culture shift and change in reducing stigma in the hospital. It's a huge honor to be a part of that and get to support patients here and see people transform their lives."

By bringing together professionals from various health disciplines, our team provides comprehensive support for hospitalized patients as they work toward their SUD and health goals. Traci refers to herself as the "Hope Dealer," who works in partnership with the social worker (who she sometimes refers to as the "Resource

*Name changed to protect patient's identity.

Dealer") and the addiction medicine clinician and others on the health care team. Traci's description summarizes team members' core role–each vital in addressing SUD. Yet the whole is greater than the sum of the parts, not only for improving patient care but for transforming hospital systems. Together, these disciplines create a holistic approach that empowers patients on their journey to improving their health and their lives.

—Linda Peng, Beth Williams, and Honora Englander

Key Points

- **Over the last decade, there has been a proliferation of hospital-based substance use disorder (SUD) care models in the United States (US).**
- **A recent taxonomy of US hospital models defined three main categories of models: 1) consultation models, wherein addiction specialists deliver care, sometimes as part of an interprofessional team (ACS), psychiatry consult liaison service, or as an individual consultant; 2) practice-based models, wherein generalists such as hospitalists deliver medications for OUD and other elements of hospital-based SUD care; and 3) in-reach models, wherein community clinicians may offer some recommendations and serve as a post-hospital care linkage.**
- **Interprofessional addiction consultation services (ACS) are the most rigorously studied care models, and have potential to deliver direct patient care, educate and train a workforce, and transform hospital systems to improve care for people with SUD.**
- **Regardless of care model or approach, diverse medical professionals (eg, physicians, nurses, pharmacists, social workers) have a critical role in caring for hospitalized people with SUD.**
- **Future research should use standard model definitions and explore core questions related to outcomes, population health and innovation, implementation, and dissemination of hospital-based SUD care.**

In the US, at least one in nine hospitalized adults has a SUD,[1] and in many hospitals, rates are much higher.[2] Hospitalized people with SUD are at high risk for overdose and death.[3,4] Many are not engaged in medical care before hospitalization, and many avoid or delay necessary hospital care for fear of stigma, discrimination, and other harms, such as experiencing acute withdrawal.[5,6] However, hospitalization is a critical opportunity to engage patients with SUD in care, initiate medications and other SUD treatments, and facilitate connection to longitudinal care.[4,7–10] While interprofessional ACS are the most rigorously studied, various approaches or care models exist to deliver hospital-based SUD care.[11] Hospitals may select different models based on local needs and resources. We discuss various care models in this chapter.

Initial steps to implement hospital-based SUD care—regardless of the care model—include understanding local community and health system needs; convening key interdisciplinary stakeholders across hospital and community settings; identifying starting target patient populations; defining initial goals and metrics; and securing funding, executive leadership support, and resources.[12–14] These steps are foundational to implementing innovation in hospital-based SUD care. Steps can help build buy-in and engagement from various stakeholders, and they are likely to be iterative. For example, hospitals may start with an individual consultant (IC) or team of highly motivated hospitalists,[15] and over time, expand to include additional roles such as peers, dedicated social workers, and addiction-trained physicians.[11] Moreover, teams may start serving a specific subset of patients—for example, patients admitted to general medical services—and later expand to include obstetric, surgical, and pediatric patients.

Strong clinical champions are key to successful implementation of hospital-based SUD care.[11,16–19] Beyond foundational understanding of SUD and hospital systems, characteristics of effective champions are that they understand hospital systems; can communicate the importance of change to diverse stakeholders including administrators and frontline clinical staff; can challenge the status quo while bringing others along; and that they be organized and persistent.[18,20] Building teams takes time, and teams often evolve as improvement efforts gain momentum or face unanticipated obstacles, for example, adding new roles such as pharmacists or nurses. As one of our colleagues says, changing hospital SUD systems is a "yellow-brick road, so welcome aboard" (2024 personal conversation from E. Brender with H. Englander). Chapter 2 discusses these early stages of securing buy-in and building teams in greater detail.

The emerging national standard is that all US hospitals should be able to identify and diagnose unhealthy substance use and SUD, offer evidence-based treatments, including appropriate withdrawal management and medications for SUD treatment, and provide linkage to outpatient SUD care.[9,21,22] However, approaches to implementing such care will differ based on local needs and resources, and there is no one-size-fits-all approach.[11] For example, large hospitals serving high proportion of people with SUD may deploy interprofessional ACS, whereas smaller hospitals caring for fewer patients with SUD may leverage general inpatient teams to deliver the essential components of care—for example, treating acute withdrawal and pain and initiating methadone or buprenorphine with linkage to outpatient care for ongoing opioid use disorder (OUD) care.

When considering what services to prioritize, hospitals should focus on interventions that are most likely to improve patient outcomes and experience.[7] Hospital teams should recognize that screening for substance use alone is insufficient and must be accompanied by appropriate clinical management of acute SUD care needs, including withdrawal management, medication initiation, and linkage to ongoing care.[7,23] Moreover, despite its widespread adoption in many hospitals, evidence supports that SBIRT alone (screening, brief intervention, referral to treatment) is not associated with improved clinical outcomes in hospitalized patients[24] and prioritizing SBIRT alone has potential to distract resources and staff energy to more important interventions such as offering medications for SUD.[21,25] If hospitals do screen, screening should be implemented as part of an effort to engage and support patients with evidence-based treatment (eg, MAUD and/or MOUD). Identifying and diagnosing SUD can include recognizing substance-related health conditions—for example, alcohol-related liver disease or drug-related serious bacterial infections,[26] and offering care or linking service delivery with existing approaches to screening.

While they differ in their approaches and resources, all models of hospital-based SUD care can and should incorporate principles of harm reduction and patient-centered care as well. A harm reduction approach does not require abstinence as a precondition of care. It integrates harm reduction and treatment as complementary strategies, supporting people to achieve positive change without judgment, coercion, or discrimination.[27] Moreover, evidence shows implementing hospital-based SUD care can shift clinicians' views of SUD and reduce stigma, alleviate clinicians' moral distress commonly associated with caring for patients with SUD without needed supports, and educate the workforce, making hospital systems more trauma informed and responsive to care of people with SUD.[11,28–30]

Models of Hospital-Based SUD Care Delivery

A recent taxonomy defines current US models of hospital-based SUD care.[11] Included care models had to address SUD (excluding tobacco use disorder alone), serve adults in a US hospital setting (eg, excluded emergency department [ED] only settings), and have a medical component (eg, excluded models that included only peers or counselors). Care models were classified as **consult models** wherein addiction specialists deliver care; **practice-based models** where generalist physicians or clinicians provide SUD care as part of routine hospital practice; and **in-reach models** wherein community clinicians offer SUD guidance to hospital teams and provide post–hospital SUD follow-up. Standard model definitions provide a framework to guide the adoption, implementation, expansion, and evaluation of hospital-based SUD care across diverse hospital settings.[11] Figure 4.1 compares three common care models, including brief model descriptions and core services that the models deliver. **Here, we describe unique model types, summarizing their key characteristics and implementation considerations.**

Consultation Models of Care

Consultation models include interprofessional ACS, psychiatry consultation liaison (PCL) services, and ICs.

Interprofessional Addiction Consultation Services

Interprofessional ACS are the most rigorously studied and comprehensive of all the hospital-based SUD care models. ACS provide comprehensive care through expert addiction clinicians (eg, board-certified physicians or advanced practice providers), dedicated coordinators (eg, social workers or case managers), and patient engagement staff (eg, peers), along with other roles such as nurses and pharmacists. ACS teams care for patients with any SUD and at all stages of change. They address complex patient needs, including polysubstance use, serious medical conditions (eg, pain management, end-of-life care), challenging medical decisions (eg, valve surgery, transplant), and often address policies and work to support resolution of conflicts between patients and staff (eg, active substance use during hospitalization). ACS teams focus explicitly on patient engagement, including for those not seeking SUD treatment, and may deliver tailored harm reduction services based on patient priorities and risks.[31,32] They also prioritize care transformation through staff and trainee education[11,28,33] and hospital-wide improvement efforts such as local policy and protocol development[34] and responding to emerging needs such as changes in the drug supply or in adapting care during public health emergencies such as the SARS-CoV-2 pandemic.[30,35] ACS teams

<table>
<tr><th></th><th>Interprofesional addiction consult service (ACS)</th><th>Practice-based model (HBOT)</th><th>In-reach model</th></tr>
<tr><td>Model descriptions</td><td>ACS provide comprehensive care through expert addiction clinicians (eg, MD), dedicated coordinators (eg, social workers or case managers), and patient engagement staff (eg, peers). Teams may also include other roles such as nurses and pharmacists.</td><td>General hospital clinicians (eg, hospitalist, ED clinicians) offers medication for opioid use disorder as part of their standard practice.</td><td>Community-based clinician provides remote support to initiate or sustain SUD medications during admission.</td></tr>
<tr><td rowspan="13">Services delivered</td><td colspan="3">Clinicians start and continue SUD medications</td></tr>
<tr><td colspan="3">FDA-approved SUD medications are available on hospital formulary</td></tr>
<tr><td colspan="3">Care pathways support linkage to ongoing SUD care after discharge</td></tr>
<tr><td>Clinicians conduct comprehensive SUD assessments</td><td>Clinicians conduct basic SUD assessments</td><td></td></tr>
<tr><td colspan="2">Provide post-overdose care and distribute naloxone</td><td></td></tr>
<tr><td>Provide complex withdrawal management</td><td>Provide basic withdrawal management</td><td></td></tr>
<tr><td colspan="2">Review hospital policies with a lens of assessing whether they are causing unintended harms</td><td></td></tr>
<tr><td>Support management of co-occuring medical (eg, endocarditis, transplant) and psychiatric conditions (eg, suicidality, psychosis)</td><td></td><td></td></tr>
<tr><td>Provide complex pain management</td><td></td><td></td></tr>
<tr><td>Provide dedicated patient engagement support (eg, peers)</td><td></td><td></td></tr>
<tr><td>Provide advanced SUD medication management (eg, low-dose buprenorphine)</td><td></td><td></td></tr>
<tr><td>Serve as platform for change for transformational SUD improvements and innovation (eg, methadone dispensation via 72-hour rule, developing bridge clinics)</td><td></td><td></td></tr>
<tr><td>Lead interprofessional staff-wide SUD education activities</td><td></td><td></td></tr>
</table>

Figure 4.1: Figure comparing three common care models. (American Society of Addiction Medicine. *Implementation Guide for Hospital and Emergency Department Substance Use Disorder Care*. Accessed March 30, 2026. https://www.asam.org/quality-care/implementation-guidance/implementation-guide-hospital)

partner across hospital and community settings, often developing new treatment pathways or collaborating to expand access through initiatives like outpatient low-barrier (aka, "bridge") clinics. ACS implementation depends on strong clinical champions, as well as addiction medicine expertise and adequate resources and funding.[18] ACS have demonstrated improvements in rates of MOUD and medications for alcohol use disorder (MAUD) initiation,[36,37] post–hospital SUD treatment engagement,[38–41] and mortality,[42,43] and in transforming hospital care for people who use drugs (PWUD).[11,44] ACS often have dedicated partnerships with outpatient SUD or primary care clinics that can strengthen post–hospital care linkages and promote care.[11,16] ACS provide expert SUD care to hospitalized patients just as cardiology consult services provide specialty care for people with advanced heart failure or acute myocarditis. However, unlike cardiology services treating heart disease, ACS face unique challenges, which can both hinder implementation and increase their importance as levers for change within hospitals. Specifically, many hospitals are largely unprepared to deliver SUD care (eg, lacking key medications on formulary)[45] or hospital staff may not view addressing SUD as part of hospital care.[28,46] Moreover, building interprofessional teams,

Interprofessional Addiction Consult Services Function as a Platform for Change

Redesign Care
- Develop and implement medication protocols
- Implement patient-centered approaches to common population health needs (eg, endocarditis care)
- Support post–acute care transitions, including bridge clinics or skilled nursing facilities

Transform Culture
- Promote trauma-informed policies (eg, management of in-hospital substance use, off-unit/visitor policies, child protective services reporting)
- Provide workforce education
- Address individual and structural stigma

Build Responsive Systems
- Develop and sustain pathways to community SUD and other care
- Address emerging population needs (eg, COVID-19, fentanyl)

Figure 4.2: Describes how interprofessional ACS serve as a platform for change through multiple mechanisms.

including incorporating peers with lived or living experience, requires unique considerations, time, and resources.[47] Figure 4.2 demonstrates the ways in which interprofessional ACS can serve as a platform for change across hospital systems.

Psychiatry Consultation Liaison Services

PCL services are another type of consultation model for hospital-based SUD care. PCLs specialize in managing patients with complex psychiatric conditions, which often co-occur with SUD.[11,48] PCL services are staffed by psychiatrists and sometimes include social workers or psychologists with expertise in community mental health resources.[11,49–54] PCL teams commonly focus on diagnosis and provide acute psychiatric medication management (eg, for psychosis or depression), and behavioral interventions such as motivational interviewing and cognitive-behavioral therapy.[54,55] In academic settings, medical students, residents, and PCL fellows are integral team members.[11]

Historically, many PCLs have not prioritized SUD within their primary scope and not all provide medications for SUD treatment,[49,50,54] likely due to high consultation volumes, limited staffing, and gaps in addiction training for psychiatrists.[11] However, this can and may be changing.[44] Compared to ACS, PCLs often focus less on acute medical and surgical needs related to SUD (eg, pain, infections) and hospital policies[56]; though, with their focus on integrated mental health and SUD, they have an opportunity to connect with community mental health resources that provide co-occurring treatment.[11] It is important to recognize that not all community mental health treatment provides co-occurring SUD treatment, such as buprenorphine for OUD or medication for AUD. As such, PCLs—as with all models—must consider the capacity and services of their community referral partners to assure seamless transitions of care after hospitalization.

Individual Consultant Model

In the IC model, a single addiction medicine-trained clinician (eg, MD/DO, PA, NP) provides consultations for acute medical needs, including withdrawal management, MOUD, and MAUD initiation. The IC then partners with usual care hospital staff (eg, medical social workers and discharge planners) to support post–hospital treatment referrals. This model is less resource-intensive than ACS and hence may be more feasible to finance or staff in areas with a limited SUD workforce. Moreover, it can also serve as a precursor to developing a full ACS. Limitations include reduced capacity to engage non–treatment-seeking patients, address complex discharge needs, and fully tackle social determinants of health and engage interprofessional hospital staff due to the lack of dedicated interdisciplinary team members. It may be important for IC to identify interdisciplinary champions within the hospital (eg, a nurse, social worker, and pharmacy champion) to implement and lead change. In addition, compared to an ACS or PCL, the IC model typically places less emphasis on behavioral health unless the consultant has a psychiatry background.

Practice-Based Models of Care

Practice-based models are distinct in that they rely on general hospital staff (eg, hospitalists) and do not rely on expert addiction medicine consultants.

The Hospital-Based Opioid Treatment (HBOT)

The HBOT model, as one example, relies on generalists (eg, hospitalists) or nonaddiction specialists (eg, infectious disease clinicians) who integrate MOUD care into routine practice. HBOT clinicians typically utilize protocols and order sets to spread best practices among clinicians, and they may also draw on local expertise, such as a clinical champion, to lead local improvement efforts, provide staff education, and assure system-level preparedness (eg, having methadone and buprenorphine on inpatient formularies). Practice models are best described in ED settings, where clinical protocols and point-of-care decision aids, embedded in the electronic health record, can lead to broader adoption of buprenorphine initiation and other SUD care.[57] HBOT typically only targets motivated patients who want MOUD, despite our understanding that MOUD should be offered to all patients. Moreover, HBOT teams may struggle to engage and support patients who are more psychosocially complex. An HBOT model has many strengths, including mainstreaming and normalizing MOUD as standard of care, being scalable for hospitals without addiction medicine specialists, and not requiring additional staffing. Technical support for HBOT champions is available through local, regional, and national outlets, with notable programs like California Bridge offering structured training, technical assistance, system infrastructure, and navigator funding to expand HBOT statewide[58,59] or telementoring programs such as ECHOs (which stands for Extension for Community Healthcare Outcomes).[60–62] However, HBOT has limitations, including challenges with complex SUD management (eg, polysubstance use, complex withdrawal syndromes, acute pain, limited experience coordinating with specialty addiction community programs), risks of dosing errors, and limited capacity for formal OUD assessments or advocacy. Similarly, while HBOT can include protocol-driven naloxone prescribing, typically it does not include the broader range of harm reduction approaches that are more common in ACS. While most HBOT models are physician driven, it is a flexible model, and examples exist of pharmacist-led HBOT.[63] Despite these limitations, HBOT is often a steppingstone toward a full ACS and can evolve to include broader supports by partnering with pharmacy, palliative care, and other services, expanding its scope and impact.

Other Hospital-Based Treatment Teams

While most practice-based models focused on care of people with OUD, there are examples of integrated hospital-based alcohol treatment (HBAT) that integrate MAUD as a routine part of hospital care,[64] and most hospitals staffed by generalists are prepared to identify and treat acute alcohol withdrawal, though may have less knowledge about MAUD. Models exist for tobacco use disorder treatment as well.[65]

Community-Based In-Reach Models of Care

Community-based in-reach involves clinicians from primary or specialty SUD care "reaching in" to hospitals to deliver SUD care—most typically MOUD—and establish post–hospital treatment pathways. This approach can include MOUD initiation or continuation, bridging prescriptions, and follow-up appointment coordination, supporting hospital staff who lack training to prescribe MOUD.[11,66] In-reach requires minimal hospital investment, as community clinicians often volunteer their time without billing. The model is flexible, and may include in-person, telephonic, or video visits. Further, in-reach can be a starting point to support patients and provide staff education in hospitals that lack SUD expertise. However, in-reach generally focuses on highly motivated patients with OUD, with limited capacity to address polysubstance use or patients' complex medical and behavioral needs. Implementation challenges include reliance on hospital staff to identify OUD and contact in-reach clinicians, potential credentialing hurdles for community clinicians, and insurance barriers that may hinder treatment linkage. Moreover, in-reach generally does not create systemic change within hospitals and depends on outpatient clinicians willing to work for little or no reimbursement. In one study that included interviews with staff working in in-reach model, informants cautioned that hospital leaders might view in-reach as a sufficient solution, despite its limitations, rather than investing in more comprehensive SUD care systems. While valuable as a stopgap measure, in-reach may underscore the need for broader structural solutions to meet the full scope of hospital-based SUD care.

Models in Context

In practice, various hospital-based SUD care models can coexist or build on each other. For example, a large health system might deploy hospitalists to initiate MOUD (using an HBOT model) in patients with fewer psychosocial needs or with shorter hospitalizations, while simultaneously offering an ACS for patients with complex withdrawal, polysubstance use, co-occurring pain, or serious conditions like infectious endocarditis requiring cardiac valve replacement. Similarly, a rural hospital with limited local SUD expertise can implement HBOT/HBAT and collaborate with telehealth addiction specialists to provide in-reach services. This approach ensures patients receive MOUD/MAUD during and after hospitalization, enhances community treatment options, and increases hospital staff's access to SUD expertise. Approaching service delivery this way can help allocate scarce resources (eg, ACS) and assure that all patients receive necessary care. This approach is similar to other services, for example, palliative care, where any clinician can discuss patient goals of care and code status, and palliative consultation services may be best suited to addressing complex symptom management or end-of-life decision making.

Moreover, various care models may deploy additional technology and community resources that are not part of the specific model but can improve care. For example, embedded electronic health record tools can screen patients for unhealthy substance use[67] and promote best practices through clinician decision support.[68] Clinicians across a range of care models can also tap into resources such as tele-mentoring and training supports and community warmlines that can provide clinicians with guidance, coaching, and a community of practice to drive practice change.[57,59–61,69,70]

A quickly growing body of emerging evidence supports the value of hospital-based SUD care (Table 4.1), including outcomes related to rates of

TABLE 4.1

Categories of Value-Add Associated With Hospital-Based SUD Care and Representative Citations

Value-add categories	Key findings, with representative citations
Improved rates of medically necessary services	ACS improves rates of MOUD and MAUD, and linkage to aftercare.[11,36–38,71–75]
Reduced mortality	ACS associated with reduced all-cause mortality.[3,42]
Improved patient experience	ACS improves patient experience and trust in hospital physicians.[76,77]
Improving treatment engagement and reducing addiction severity postdischarge	ACS increases post–hospitalization SUD treatment engagement and reduces addiction severity and days of alcohol and drug use.[38,41]
Reducing readmissions and acute care utilization	ACS associated with reduced 30-day readmission.[72,78]
Providing cost-effective care	Hospital-based SUD care can reduce costs by increasing adoption of cost-effective treatments which reduce downstream medical expenses by preventing complications of untreated addiction.[79]
	Hospital-based SUD care can reduce costly hospital days by supporting patients to receive necessary medical care in lower-acuity ambulatory settings.[80]
Supporting institutional priorities	Addressing SUD during hospitalizations contributes to broader institutional objectives, such as value-based care, patient satisfaction, and reduced disparities, which can justify investments to hospital administrators.[81]
Reducing staff moral distress and burnout	ACS can reduce staff "moral distress," and limit staff fears about workplace harms. This is particularly important given workforce shortages across US hospitals.[28,82]
Reducing stigma and educating the workforce, including trainees, in SUD care	ACS and other models of hospital addiction care can reduce provider stigma toward patients with SUD and improve staff knowledge and preparedness to provide SUD care.[11,29,33,83,84]
Hospital policy change	ACS can facilitate hospital policy change around in hospital drug use.[14,85]
	ACS may address some risk factors for "against medical advice" discharge.[86,87]
	ACS may play a role in guiding change in mandatory reporting policies.[88]
	ACS may provide input on hospital policies around leaving the hospital floor.[85,89]
Driving systems' change	ACS can develop protocols for rapid methadone initiation among hospitalized patients.[90–92]
	ACS and hospital-based SUD care can facilitate improvements in postacute linkage.[93]
	ACS may facilitate outpatient parenteral antibiotic therapy for people with a history of injection substance use.[80,94,95]
	ACS involvement may elevate other policy arenas where ethical issues related to hospitalized people with SUD exist, such as transplantation and SUD.[96]

American Society of Addiction Medicine. *Implementation Guide for Hospital and Emergency Department Substance Use Disorder Care.* Accessed March 30, 2026. https://www.asam.org/quality-care/ implementation-guidance/implementation-guide-hospital medically necessary services, patient experience, engagement in post–hospital SUD care, health care utilization and cost, and mortality.

Interprofessional Roles

Integrating diverse health professions as part of hospital SUD care provides patients with comprehensive care needed to address SUD, including medical, psychosocial, and post–discharge community support.[7] Collaboration across disciplines can promote evidence-based interventions, allow clinicians to work at the top of their licensure, promote resilience and professional satisfaction among addiction clinicians,[97] and promote positive change in hospital culture and care systems.[11]

The interventions and roles of each health professional may vary depending on patient's needs. For example, a patient experiencing acute substance withdrawal may need immediate medical intervention, whereas a patient struggling with boredom during a prolonged hospital stay may benefit from peer support. Every role in the interdisciplinary team can play a part in integrating harm reduction principles and practices as part of hospital care, ensuring that care is compassionate, nonjudgmental, and focused on partnering with the patient to achieve their individual goals. This approach acknowledges the complexity of SUD and that some patients will not be seeking abstinence from substance use.[98] Here, we describe diverse roles of various health professions and how they can contribute to meeting the complex needs of hospitalized adults with SUD.

Table 4.2 describes the various roles within an interprofessional addiction consultation service (ACS) team and highlights additional ways in which the team may function collectively to advance hospital-based SUD care.

Physicians

Physicians are responsible for assessing and diagnosing SUD (eg, DSM-5), including engaging patients, assessing patient goals around their hospitalization and their substance use, and promoting shared decision making. Physicians identify and treat substance withdrawal; initiate evidence-based medication treatments; address pain and mental health needs; and contextualize SUD care as it relates to other medical and surgical comorbidities.[1,2] For example, hospitalized patients with endocarditis may face key decisions related to eligibility and appropriateness for cardiac surgery or home antibiotic infusion; addiction-informed clinicians can help lead these discussions to overcome stigma, prioritize patients' values and needs, and ensure patients have access to the highest-quality care.[80,99,100] Physicians with many backgrounds can play critical roles in adopting, developing, and spreading best practices in hospital-based SUD care, including physicians with training in addiction medicine, addiction psychiatry, general medicine, emergency medicine, obstetrics, pediatrics, infectious diseases, trauma and cardiac surgery, and numerous other backgrounds.[11,39,57,101–104] Patients with SUD have wide range of health care conditions, and this should be reflected in the range of physicians and clinicians seeking to support their care.

Clinical Champions

Beyond clinical care, physicians frequently serve as leaders and clinical champions, spearheading efforts to improve hospital-based SUD care. This often involves leading multidisciplinary teams or driving efforts to implement hospital-based SUD treatment. Effective clinical champions are change leaders who are respected in their organization, are skilled communicators, and know how to leverage power within their institution.[3] In the face of barriers, including pervasive stigma and lack of clear financial incentives to implement hospital-based SUD care, clinical champions are persistent and creative while lobbying for change.[18] To support this work, champions find that access to external support—including informal coaching or peer networks and formal online tools and tele-mentoring programs—is critical.[18] While physicians are often seen in the role of champion, other health professionals can also serve as impactful leaders and clinical champions in improving hospital SUD care.[4]

Hospital executive champions can also help lay the foundation for systems of SUD care. This includes support for funding and advocacy within the "C Suite," incorporating SUD care into the strategic plan, and supporting changes in hospital policy to facilitate SUD treatment. Executive-level support results in resources for SUD care and also sets a precedent to prioritize the work throughout the hospital. An executive champion may also drive policy change at the state level, for example, through advocacy for SUD-specific funding or Medicaid reimbursement rates.

Within the hospital, nursing and pharmacy champions are crucial to the integration of SUD treatment into routine care. A nursing champion partners with hospital addiction teams to implement SUD care at the bedside, including nursing withdrawal management protocols or naloxone education and distribution. Nurse champions also provide essential input on training of RNs in SUD-related care, including management of co-occurring SUD and

TABLE 4.2

Description of Interprofessional ACS Roles

Role	Description	Hospital SUD care–related activities
Core Interprofessional Addiction Consultation Service (ACS) Team Members[11]		
Addiction clinician[a]	Board-certified addiction medicine/addiction psychiatry physician and/or APP with training and expertise in SUD care	■ Diagnose SUD (DSM-5) ■ Identify and treat withdrawal, including complex withdrawal from multiple substances ■ Address pain and mental health needs ■ Contextualize SUD care in relation to other comorbidities
Social worker, counselor, or navigator[a]	Social workers are trained professionals who assess patient needs and provide resources. Counselors or navigators focus on more limited evaluation and help with transitions of care	■ Social workers can conduct psychosocial and ASAM assessments ■ Provide therapeutic interventions during hospitalization (eg, brief intervention, counseling) ■ Coordinate and facilitate referrals to posthospital care (eg, SUD services, skilled nursing facility, etc) ■ Arrange recovery supports to address social determinants of health (eg, housing, social services)
Peer recovery support specialist[a,47]	Individuals with lived or living experience in addiction and recovery who are certified to support patient's SUD goals	■ Draw on personal experience to connect with patients ■ Serve as "cultural brokers" helping bridge communication between patients and health care teams ■ Offer emotional and social support ■ Discuss harm reduction strategies
Other possible roles		
Nurse[31]	Nurses who bring understanding of SUD, harm reduction, and hospital systems and culture	■ Provides direct patient care (eg, harm reduction education) ■ Provides coaching and other staff support around conflict de-escalation, in-hospital substance use, and patient-centered approaches to care
Pharmacist[105]	Experts in medication management and hospital systems that deliver medications	■ Develop and implement medication protocols and order sets ■ Inform hospital policies around medications for SUD ■ Advance hospital formularies to include novel forms of medications for SUD ■ Provide education around medication indications and dosing
Team		
Team-based care	■ ACS members collaborate in an integrated, team-based care model. Teams may structure daily huddles to review patient cases and often designate regular time for focused population health, quality improvement efforts (eg, through weekly operations and/or quality improvement meetings)	
Team-led transformation	■ Develop workflows and protocols to support evidence-based SUD care (eg, buprenorphine order sets, naloxone dispensation workflows) ■ Review, revise, develop, and implement policies that commonly affect hospitalized people who use substances (eg, off-unit policies, substance possession policies, room search policies) ■ Lead education and training to other hospital staff to deliver evidence-based, patient-centered SUD care (eg, targeted efforts to support nurses, hospitalists, others) ■ Transform hospital systems to deliver patient-centered, trauma-informed care ■ Develop and sustain pathway from hospital to community SUD care ■ Respond to emerging population health needs, for example, during COVID-19 pandemic	

[a]By definition, interprofessional ACS includes clinician, coordinator, and patient engagement roles. Addiction physician, social worker, and peers are one such way of meeting these core elements.

pain, recognizing and treating withdrawal, and harm reduction education. Meanwhile, hospital pharmacist champions establish pharmacy and EHR workflows to improve access to SUD medication, including for patients transitioning out of the hospital. They make important contributions to hospital policies around MOUD and pain management, for example, leading implementation of methadone dispensation at hospital discharge utilizing the "72-hour rule."[34] or developing order sets and protocols to facilitate low-dose buprenorphine initiations.[106,107]

Advanced Practice Professionals

Bringing a range of backgrounds, perspectives, and strengths, advanced practice professionals (APPs) are critical to the addiction workforce.[108] APPs include nurse practitioners (NPs), physician associates/assistants (PAs), and psychiatric-mental health nurse practitioners (PMHNPs). Depending on experience and the state of practice, APPs require varying levels of supervision and training. With appropriate training, guidance, and experience, APPs can deliver expert SUD care and play a similar role to those of physicians as described above. Importantly, APPs can help address addiction physician workforce shortages by expanding access to high-quality care for patients with SUD.[82] NPs can gain formal certification as Certified Addictions Registered Nurses—Advanced Practice (CARN-AP) through the Addictions Nursing Certification Board (ANCB). This credential certifies knowledge of the essential clinical competencies for an NP providing SUD care, but remains underutilized; only 57 new CARN-NPs became certified between 2020 and 2023.[109] Currently, there is no path for PAs to receive specialty certification in addiction medicine. Several APP fellowships in addiction medicine in the US provide the opportunity for APPs to gain advanced training in SUD care.[110,111]

Social Workers

Social workers are essential partners in hospital SUD care, particularly because psychosocial factors are deeply intertwined with SUD.[112] Socials workers conduct psychosocial and ASAM level of care assessments[113] that guide and facilitate referrals to post–hospital care and recovery support services. These referrals include SUD treatment as well as connection to essential recovery support services, such as housing and other social services.[114] Beyond resource referrals, social workers provide evidence-based behavioral treatments, such as motivational interviewing, brief treatment, and cognitive-behavioral therapy.[112] They can also offer crisis intervention, de-escalation, and emotional support, which can support patients with the challenges of hospitalization. In the hospital setting, medical social workers also work closely with other health care professionals and support patients with medical illnesses. Chapter 15 further describes hospital-based behavioral treatments for SUD.

Just as SUD training gaps exist in other professions and disciplines, social workers often lack training in SUD, including evidence-based medication and behavioral treatments.[115] They may not have the training to perform standard SUD assessments (such as ASAM assessments) and may not understand differences across community treatment settings and levels of care. As such, teams looking to hire social workers with SUD expertise should inquire about clinical experience and skills and offer supplemental training to build these skills when necessary.

Pharmacists

Pharmacists are uniquely positioned to integrate SUD care in hospitals[105]—both through providing direct patient care and in building prepared and responsive systems—given their expertise in medication management, hospital systems, and patient safety. They can provide guidance on appropriate dosing, drug interactions, and appropriate treatment of patients with SUD during hospitalization. For hospital clinicians less familiar with these medications, pharmacists can often help close a knowledge gap to support treatment decisions. Pharmacists can also develop and implement medication protocols and embedded electronic health record order sets,[107] develop care pathways, and inform hospital policies. For example, pharmacists can help advance hospital formularies to include novel forms of medication such as long-acting injectable buprenorphine. Pharmacists can also play a role in developing and disseminating innovation. For example, pharmacists are critical to implementing methadone dispensing at hospital discharge via the "72-hour rule,"[34] anticipating pharmacy shortages and prior authorization requirements for post–hospital buprenorphine access,[116] and can play a key role in developing naloxone distribution processes.

Pharmacists can also support staff, patient, and community education about SUD, particularly in settings such as hospitals and EDs, where high clinician turnover and the fast pace of care can predispose to error where clinicians may need support to navigate complex prescribing decisions and nuances of medication management.

Regulatory pathways in some states allow pharmacists to dispense naloxone[117] to patients before hospital discharge, and pharmacists can be key leaders in implementing naloxone distribution and adoption of other evidence-based practices.[118–120]

Nurses

Nurses are the health care team members who interact with patients the most during hospitalization. As such, their role in caring for patients with SUD is expansive and includes both physical and psychosocial aspects of care. Nurses are also crucial in shaping hospital culture and are instrumental in deconstructing existing stigma faced by hospitalized patients with SUD.[120]

Nurses play an important role in substance withdrawal management, including performing ongoing symptomatic assessment that may trigger medication administration (eg, benzodiazepines for acute alcohol withdrawal, opioid administration for acute pain management).

Nurses also play an important role in facilitating communication between patients and other health care clinicians, communicating acute care needs (eg, advocating for multimodal pain management) and anticipating post–hospital transitional care needs. Notably, most nurses receive minimal education on SUD and addiction at the undergraduate or graduate level training.[121–123] Research suggests nurses are eager to gain this foundational knowledge, particularly given the growing prevalence of SUD in hospitalized populations. This is an important opportunity for nursing programs to expand curricula to include content on addiction, harm reduction, and patient-centered communication strategies. However, research also supports that nurses need more than education to shape attitudes and improve skills in caring for patients with SUDs.[124] Research supports the benefit that nurses gain from leadership support and a workplace culture that encourages their important work with this population.[124] Mentorship from an "SUD nurse liaison," clear delineation of roles, and training in motivational interviewing and harm reduction have been highlighted as ways to increase nurses' feelings of efficacy and reduce burnout when working with patients with SUD.[120,125]

Nurse care managers can play a key role in helping overcome barriers to discharge for patients needing skilled nursing facility (SNF) or long-term care after hospitalization. Patients with SUD frequently experience explicit discrimination when rejected from SNF care despite federal and state protections.[126–128] Nurses can help address these challenges by using nonstigmatizing language and advocating for patients with SNF partners.[129,130]

Finally, nurses have been recognized for their potential as powerful harm reduction proponents in their care of hospitalized patients with SUD.[131] Nurses can support harm reduction by educating patients on safe use and overdose prevention and connecting patients to resources to address the underlying drivers of substance use while in the hospital (eg, mental health or social work assessment, specialty SUD care when).

Peers

Peers are individuals with lived and living experience of addiction who support people with SUD. Common titles for peers include peer recovery support specialists, recovery mentors, peer providers, and certified peer specialists. Unlike "sponsors" or mentors involved in mutual aid programs such as Alcoholics Anonymous (eg, 12-step fellowships), most states require peers to obtain certification and complete peer-specific training.[12] Certification and training requirements vary across states, which leads to variation in the scope of work and may impact their general acceptance as part of a hospital care team.[132]

Through lived experience, peers use personal experiences to connect with people in a way that may be difficult for traditional health care professionals.[76] For example, peers may serve as "cultural brokers,"[76] helping bridge communication between patients and health care teams,[76] thereby increasing patients' trust in the care they receive.[10] Peers can offer emotional and social support during challenging or prolonged hospitalizations through actions like accompanying patients on walks or braiding hair.[133] Their support may also include conflict de-escalation. Finally, peers often provide harm reduction services, including distributing supplies (eg, safe injection kits) and teaching harm reduction strategies to patients and their families. One important function of many hospital-based peers is to serve as a bridge to community treatment by connecting patients with resources and ongoing support after discharge. Findings are mixed, however,[134–136] on what model of peer intervention best supports retention in SUD care, and further research is needed in this area. Specific challenges that contribute to this evidence gap include the difficulty of tracking care transitions postdischarge and lack of information sharing between hospitals and community providers.[136]

Peers working in hospitals may encounter challenges performing their duties and becoming fully integrated members of care teams.[47,76] Peers sometimes experience a lack of role definition and sense of place within the traditional hospital medical hierarchy. They may hold different boundaries with patients around information sharing and privacy compared with other medical staff. They may also be disproportionately affected by the emotionally taxing nature of caring for hospitalized patients with SUD[47,132] compared to other team members. These challenges can be helped by clearly defining peer roles and publicizing the peer model widely across the hospital, ensuring peers feel they have a "home" within the hospital setting (eg, with an established office space and welcoming team), and offering opportunities for professional development.[47]

Studies on peer interventions are heterogeneous with few controlled trials focusing on peer work in hospital settings.[137,138] Peer interventions may lead to decreases in substance use, increased engagement in treatment, and lower hospital readmission rates, but systematic reviews to date emphasize the need to overcome methodological limitations through better standardization of peer roles and interventions.[137–139]

Counselors

Addiction counselors, such as Certified Alcohol and Drug Counselors (CADCs), Licensed Alcohol and Drug Counselors (LADCs), and Certified Substance Abuse Counselors (CSACs), receive certification and licensure after meeting state-level standards. These include completing a minimum amount of clinical experience, passing an exam, and participating in continuing education. Addiction counselors work in diverse clinical settings and are specifically trained to evaluate SUD, support treatment planning, and coordinate referrals and services, including conducting ASAM assessements.[8,11] They also provide individual and group counseling, utilizing approaches such as motivational interviewing and recovery skill building to help patients achieve their SUD goals.[11] In the hospital, addiction counselors can play an important role in supporting patients in goal setting and referral to treatment or other SUD services. While their responsibilities in the hospital may overlap with those of social workers, addiction counselors do not generally have advanced secondary education, have less training in managing medical illnesses, and may not be equipped to provide more complex mental health counseling.

Navigators

SUD navigators support patients to navigate healthcare systems—including SUD treatment—during and after hospitalization. Some other commonly used terms include behavioral health navigator, health promotion advocate, community health worker (CHW), and patient navigator.[132,140] Navigators can help identify patients, conduct brief assessments, provide education, and facilitate referrals to various SUD treatment and recovery support resources.[20] Navigators are a key component of SUD care for many hospitals, especially in ED settings. The California Bridge Navigator Program utilizes trained behavioral health navigators to facilitate MOUD referrals and has been implemented in over 100 California hospitals.[141] Implementing SUD navigators in the ED has been associated with higher engagement rates in SUD treatment after discharge[142,143] and cost savings. Future trials on navigation services will evaluate whether these services improve hospital utilization metrics.[144]

Team-Based Care Versus Individual Clinicians

As described, diverse disciplines can contribute to hospital-based SUD care in unique and important ways. However, as clinicians, hospital leaders, and payors consider the role of individuals, it is important to underscore the role of the team—working together, with dedicated time—to advance hospital care quality and population health for people with SUD and serious illness. This is most evident in experience and the literature describing interprofessional ACS (Table 4.2), where activities extend beyond the role of direct patient care, and can advance key needs, including staff education, hospital policies, and health system preparedness to treat SUD.[11] Commonly, the ACS team—with dedicated time, effort, and leadership—is transformative. In these instances, the whole is often more than the sum of its parts.

Moreover, ACS can respond to emerging population health needs in a way that hospitals are not typically prepared to do. For example, during the SARS-CoV-2 (COVID-19) pandemic—when closing of community resources threatened patients' basic survival outside of the hospital, changes in outpatient care increased patients' reliance on hospitals, and hospital policies made hospitalization more difficult to tolerate—ACS were often the sole structures within hospitals focused on meeting needs of highly marginalized people with SUD.[30] In times of crisis and in general, an ACS team can make hospitals more prepared and more responsive to needs of people with SUD.[35]

Partnerships Within the Hospital

Population-based approaches to conditions such as infectious endocarditis, care for patients needing prolonged intravenous antibiotics, and managing SUD in pregnancy are emerging. These approaches span various approaches to SUD care (eg, for example, interprofessional ACS or practice-based models). Figure 4.3 shows a range of hospital and community partnerships that can support implementation for hospital-based SUD care.

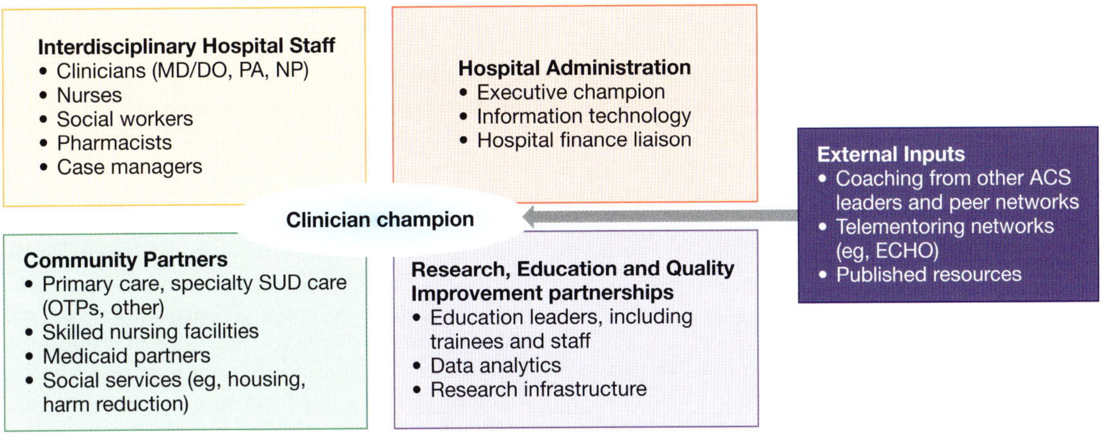

Figure 4.3: Key partnerships to consider when implementing hospital-based SUD care.

Multidisciplinary care conferences involving infectious disease and addiction consultation teams can facilitate patient-centered discharge planning by exploring and supporting options such as outpatient parenteral antibiotic therapy (OPAT). This collaborative approach ensures that care plans are tailored to the patient's preferences, reducing the risk of premature discharge and adverse outcomes.[80,145,146] Such teams can support patient-level clinical decision making, and may also work to reform hospital policies (eg, those governing time on- and off-the-unit) and care pathways (eg, building relationships with skilled nursing facilities [SNFs] and home infusion companies) to support patients to receive antibiotics in settings outside of the hospital.

Similar collaborative approaches have been used to improve surgical management of drug use–associated infective endocarditis.[99,147] Patients may not be offered necessary cardiac surgeries due to concerns among surgical teams about the potential risk of subsequent prosthetic infection from ongoing drug use. While older guidelines presented conflicting guidance on this topic, newer guidance supports a collaborative approach, including initiation of SUD treatment for patients with drug use–associated endocarditis.[145,148,149] Interdisciplinary collaboration can address stigma, ensure equitable care, and assist in developing individualized treatment plans for this complex patient population. Other partnerships that may be particularly important to include are those that bridge SUD care with obstetrical and pediatric care,[101] acute pain services, palliative care, and SNFs.[127]

Partnering With Hospital Stakeholders to Change Policies

Collaborations with social workers and other hospital departments are also crucial in addressing and changing stigmatizing hospital policies.[150] For instance, hospital policies may prohibit patients with SUD from leaving their rooms or require that all patients with a SUD diagnosis have visitors and personal belongings searched.[85] Such policies are typically implemented with the goal of reducing in-hospital substance use or improving staff safety, but can quickly lead to patients not disclosing SUD, mistrust between patients and staff, patient-directed discharge, and widespread discrimination. More trauma-informed approaches are possible.[14] Other examples include hospital policies on child protective services (CPS) reporting, which may be overly strict compared with federal or state mandatory reporting requirements, leading to excessive reporting. This can contribute to stigmatizing care practices and impose significant stress on parents, underscoring the need for a more nuanced, multidisciplinary approach to hospital policy reform.[151]

While clinical partnerships are crucial, nonclinical hospital roles also significantly influence patient care. Building relationships with these departments is essential for driving meaningful improvements in patient care. For example, off-unit (eg, allowing patients to go outside to smoke a cigarette) and in-hospital substance use policies are often stigmatizing, frequently causing patients to leave the hospital prematurely. To create more equitable, patient-centered policies, public safety/security, legal, nursing, and leadership support and buy-in is essential. The University of California at San Francisco ACS describes their process of convening an interprofessional group of key stakeholders to help create more patient-centered, trauma-informed policies while balancing hospital system concerns around patient safety and legal concerns.[14] Other institutions are taking similar approaches.

Forming effective and impactful partnerships starts with establishing shared goals of improving patient care and developing an understanding of diverse perspectives. Given how deeply stigma is embedded within hospital systems, these internal partnerships are critical to driving meaningful and necessary changes in patient care, hospital practice, and hospital policy. By intentionally fostering collaborative relationships across hospital departments and disciplines, addiction medicine teams and champions can more effectively identify opportunities and engage diverse stakeholders in improving care for patients with SUD.

Community Partnerships

Hospital-based SUD care represents just one part of the broader continuum of SUD care. To effectively address the many barriers to SUD care, working in a silo is not sufficient. Within hospitals and EDs, there may already be ecosystems and initiatives focused on improving SUD care. Proactively identifying and engaging champions and community partners who can support and extend hospital-based efforts is essential for building a more integrated and effective approach to SUD care.

Community partners play a critical role in supporting hospital-based SUD care, ensuring continuity of care and effective transitions for patients after discharge. These partners include specialty SUD clinics, such as opioid treatment programs (OTPs), residential SUD treatment facilities, withdrawal management programs, harm reduction agencies, street medicine programs, and primary care clinics. Building strong partnerships with these organizations is essential for enabling seamless care transitions (discussed in more detail in Chapter 20). For example, ensuring that a local OTP will continue hospital-initiated methadone dosing and understanding when they complete new patient intakes can prevent gaps in care. Similarly, certain residential SUD programs may be able to coordinate with hospital staff to facilitate direct transitions from hospitalization into their programs upon discharge. Several examples exist describing innovative approaches and partnerships, some successful and others unsuccessful. For example, the University of Colorado deploys a physician who is dually affiliated with the hospital ACS and a community OTP. In the hospital, the ACS physician can then complete a face-to-face medical assessment and provide linkage to post–hospital SUD care, and an OTP-affiliated nurse with hospital privileges completes a psychosocial evaluation and provides case management by arranging transportation and providing weekly telephone check-ins.[152] Such a program streamlines care coordination and has led to high rates of methadone initiation and engagement in care after discharge. The interprofessional ACS at Oregon Health & Science University (OHSU) has developed and adapted a series of approaches to post–hospital SUD care linkages, including developing prioritized rapid-access linkages to care, which were foundational to initial ACS implementation,[2] bridge clinic implementation, and trial of medically enhanced residential treatment model wherein patients could receive intravenous antibiotics in residential SUD care.[153] While the rapid-access pathways and bridge clinic proved essential to supporting patients' needs, the medically enhanced residential model was unsuccessful and unable to support patient care needs, and did not warrant significant time and attention from ACS leadership to justify its continuation.[153] Facing the need to find alternatives to in-hospital antibiotics for patients with SUD, the OHSU team subsequently developed an interdisciplinary structured case conference that includes partnerships within and across hospital and community settings. Simpler and more broadly applicable, this approach delivers more patient-centered care and has led to significant savings in hospital length of stay.[80] Other novel approaches to IV antibiotics and partnerships with SNFs exist, for example, a novel partnership with a Johns Hopkins Bayview hospital, two SNFs and two OTPs, to improve recovery supports and access to MOUD for patients discharged to SNF.[93]

Effective partnerships are essential for facilitating timely referrals that can reduce barriers to care. Building strong community partnerships requires developing meaningful relationships and aligning on shared goals. Site visits and in-person meetings can support relationship building by demonstrating commitment, fostering open communication, and building trust. Community partners may also have valuable expertise that will inform the needs of hospitalized patients with SUD. Building strong partnerships is a continuous process that requires regular communication about challenges and successes, along with a willingness to adapt and make improvements.

Developing and sustaining strong community partnerships is critical to bridging gaps in SUD care, reducing barriers, and ensuring that patients receive comprehensive, continuous support during and after hospitalization.

Future Research

Advancing science related to hospital-based SUD care models relies on research studies that use standard model definitions to describe interventions and outcomes.[11] Key questions for future research center in four main domains, including outcomes of hospital-based SUD care, population health and innovation, questions of implementation, and dissemination (see Table 4.3).

TABLE 4.3

Future Research Directions

Knowledge gap	Key questions	Research strategy
Outcomes	■ What are the effects of hospital-based SUD care?	■ Observational and experimental studies describing outcomes using standard model definitions
Population health and innovation	■ How do we improve care models?	■ Studies that explore and address racial disparities; transitional care gaps; population-specific needs and opportunities (eg, end of life, rural, tribal, pregnant populations); specific health conditions (eg, endocarditis, transplant)
Implementation	■ How do we implement hospital-based SUD care across diverse settings?	■ Mixed-methods studies that explore integration of specific team members (such as peers); compare different model types and combinations; explore role for telehealth/tele-ACS; and other aspects of implementation (eg, supports for clinician champions) ■ Studies exploring alternative payment models and value-based care
Dissemination	■ How do we promote broad adoption and diffusion of innovation?	■ Mixed-methods studies that explore clinician, hospital, health system, and policy-factors, including metrics and incentives ■ Studies that assess policies influencing adoption of hospital-based SUD services

American Society of Addiction Medicine. *Implementation Guide for Hospital and Emergency Department Substance Use Disorder Care.* Accessed March 30, 2026. https://www.asam.org/quality-care/ implementation-guidance/implementation-guide-hospital

REFERENCES

1. Suen LW, Makam AN, Snyder HR, et al. National prevalence of alcohol and other substance use disorders among emergency department visits and hospitalizations: NHAMCS 2014–2018. *J Gen Intern Med.* 2022;37(10):2420–2428.
2. Englander H, Weimer M, Solotaroff R, et al. Planning and designing the Improving Addiction Care Team (IMPACT) for hospitalized adults with substance use disorder. *J Hosp Med.* 2017;12(5):339–342.
3. King C, Cook R, Korthuis PT, Morris CD, Englander H. Causes of death in the 12 months after hospital discharge among patients with opioid use disorder. *J Addict Med.* 2022; 16(4):466–469.
4. Larochelle MR, Bernstein R, Bernson D, et al. Touchpoints opportunities to predict and prevent opioid overdose: a cohort study. *Drug Alcohol Depend.* 2019;204:107537.
5. McNeil R, Small W, Wood E, Kerr T. Hospitals as a 'risk environment': an ethno-epidemiological study of voluntary and involuntary discharge from hospital against medical advice among people who inject drugs. *Soc Sci Med.* 2014; 105:59–66.
6. Biancarelli DL, Biello KB, Childs E, et al. Strategies used by people who inject drugs to avoid stigma in healthcare settings. *Drug Alcohol Depend.* 2019;198:80–86.
7. Englander H, Thakrar AP, Bagley SM, Rolley T, Dong K, Hyshka E. Caring for hospitalized adults with opioid use disorder in the era of fentanyl: a review. *JAMA Intern Med.* 2024;184(6):691–701.
8. Incze MA, Kelley AT, James H, et al. Post-hospitalization care transition strategies for patients with substance use disorders: a narrative review and taxonomy. *J Gen Intern Med.* 2024;39(5):837–846.
9. Krawczyk N, Miller M, Englander H, et al. Toward a consensus on strategies to support opioid use disorder care transitions following hospitalization: a modified Delphi process. *J Gen Intern Med.* 2025;40(5):1048–1058.
10. Velez CM, Nicolaidis C, Korthuis PT, Englander H. "It's been an experience, a life learning experience": a qualitative study of hospitalized patients with substance use disorders. *J Gen Intern Med.* 2017;32(3):296–303.
11. Englander H, Jones A, Krawczyk N, et al. A taxonomy of hospital-based addiction care models: a scoping review and key informant interviews. *J Gen Intern Med.* 2022;37(11):2821–2833.
12. Englander H, Kansagara D. Planning and designing the care transitions innovation (C-Train) for uninsured and Medicaid patients. *J Hosp Med.* 2012;7(7):524–529.
13. Fielman S, McNeely J, Fitzpatrick A, et al. A clinical guide to support the implementation of addiction consult services and the value of teaching and technical assistance. *J Addict Med.* 2024;18(3):215–217.
14. Martin M, Snyder HR, Otway G, Holpit L, Day LW, Seid man D. In-hospital substance use policies: an opportunity to advance equity, reduce stigma, and offer evidence-based addiction care. *J Addict Med.* 2023;17(1):10–12.
15. Bottner R, Moriates C, Tirado C. The role of hospitalists in treating opioid use disorder. *J Addict Med.* 2020;14(2):178.
16. Incze MA, Kelley AT, Gordon AJ. Champions among us: leading primary care to the forefront of opioid use disorder treatment. *J Gen Intern Med.* 2022;37(7):1771–1773.
17. Wood K, Giannopoulos V, Louie E, et al. The role of clinical champions in facilitating the use of evidence-based practice in drug and alcohol and mental health settings: a systematic review. *Implement Res Pract.* 2020;1:2633489520959072.
18. Williams B, Patten A, Peng L, Englander H. "Just be relentless," lessons learned from in-hospital addiction consult service implementation. *J Gen Intern Med.* 2025;40(12):2916–2925.
19. Gordon AJ, Kavanagh G, Krumm M, et al. Facilitators and barriers in implementing buprenorphine in the Veterans Health Administration. *Psychol Addict Behav.* 2011; 25(2):215–224.
20. The Network for the Improvement of Addiction Treatment. *Workbook: An Introduction to the NIATx Model of Process Improvement.* University of Wisconsin-Madison. Accessed December 11, 2024. https://niatx.wisc.edu/wp-content/uploads/sites/1871/2023/02/NIATxWorkbook_2.pdf

21. Calcaterra SL, Martin M, Bottner R, et al. Management of opioid use disorder and associated conditions among hospitalized adults: a consensus statement from the society of hospital medicine. *J Hosp Med.* 2022;17(9):744–756.
22. Englander H, Davis CS. Hospital standards of care for people with substance use disorder. *N Engl J Med.* 2022; 387(8):672–675.
23. McNeely J, Hamilton L. Screening for unhealthy alcohol and drug use in general medicine settings. *Med Clin North Am.* 2022;106(1):13–28.
24. Tanner-Smith EE, Parr NJ, Schweer-Collins M, Saitz R. Effects of brief substance use interventions delivered in general medical settings: a systematic review and meta-analysis. *Addiction.* 2022;117(4):877–889.
25. Saitz R. Candidate performance measures for screening for, assessing, and treating unhealthy substance use in hospitals: advocacy or evidence-based practice? *Ann Intern Med.* 2010;153(1):40–43.
26. Capizzi J, Leahy J, Wheelock H, et al. Population-based trends in hospitalizations due to injection drug use-related serious bacterial infections, Oregon, 2008 to 2018. *PLoS One.* 2020;15(11):e0242165.
27. Harm Reduction International. *What is Harm Reduction?* Accessed December 9, 2024. https://hri.global/what-is-harm-reduction/
28. Englander H, Collins D, Perry SP, Rabinowitz M, Phoutrides E, Nicolaidis C. "We've learned it's a medical illness, not a moral choice": qualitative study of the effects of a multicomponent addiction intervention on hospital providers' attitudes and experiences. *J Hosp Med.* 2018;13(11):752–758.
29. Hoover K, Lockhart S, Callister C, Holtrop JS, Calcaterra SL. Experiences of stigma in hospitals with addiction consultation services: a qualitative analysis of patients' and hospital-based providers' perspectives. *J Subst Abuse Treat.* 2022;138: 108708.
30. King C, Vega T, Button D, Nicolaidis C, Gregg J, Englander H. Understanding the impact of the SARS-COV-2 pandemic on hospitalized patients with substance use disorder. *PLoS One.* 2021;16(2):e0247951.
31. Goff A, Lujan-Bear S, Titus H, Englander H. Integrating hospital-based harm reduction care-harnessing the nursing model. *Subst Use Addctn J.* 2024;45(2):307–313.
32. Perera R, Stephan L, Appa A, et al. Meeting people where they are: implementing hospital-based substance use harm reduction. *Harm Reduct J.* 2022;19(1):14.
33. Wakeman SE, Kanter GP, Donelan K. Institutional substance use disorder intervention improves general internist preparedness, attitudes, and clinical practice. *J Addict Med.* 2017;11(4):308–314.
34. Skogrand E, Sharpe J, Englander H. Dispensing methadone at hospital discharge: one hospital's approach to implementing the "72-hour rule" change. *J Addict Med.* 2024;18(1):71–74.
35. Harris MTH, Peterkin A, Bach P, et al. Adapting inpatient addiction medicine consult services during the COVID-19 pandemic. *Addict Sci Clin Pract.* 2021;16(1):13.
36. Englander H, King C, Nicolaidis C, et al. Predictors of opioid and alcohol pharmacotherapy initiation at hospital discharge among patients seen by an inpatient addiction consult service. *J Addict Med.* 2020;14(5):415–422.
37. Nordeck CD, Welsh C, Schwartz RP, Mitchell SG, O'Grady KE, Gryczynski J. Opioid agonist treatment initiation and linkage for hospitalized patients seen by a substance use disorder consultation service. *Drug Alcohol Depend Rep.* 2022;2:100031.
38. Englander H, Dobbertin K, Lind BK, et al. Inpatient addiction medicine consultation and post-hospital substance use disorder treatment engagement: a propensity-matched analysis. *J Gen Intern Med.* 2019;34(12):2796–2803.
39. Bhatraju EP, Ludwig-Barron N, Takagi-Stewart J, Sandhu HK, Klein JW, Tsui JI. Successful engagement in buprenorphine treatment among hospitalized patients with opioid use disorder and trauma. *Drug Alcohol Depend.* 2020;215: 108253.
40. Liebschutz JM, Crooks D, Herman D, et al. Buprenorphine treatment for hospitalized, opioid-dependent patients: a randomized clinical trial. *JAMA Intern Med.* 2014;174(8): 1369–1376.
41. Wakeman SE, Metlay JP, Chang Y, Herman GE, Rigotti NA. Inpatient addiction consultation for hospitalized patients increases post-discharge abstinence and reduces addiction severity. *J Gen Intern Med.* 2017;32(8):909–916.
42. Wilson JD, Altieri Dunn SC, Roy P, Joseph E, Klipp S, Liebschutz J. Inpatient addiction medicine consultation service impact on post-discharge patient mortality: a propensity-matched analysis. *J Gen Intern Med.* 2022;37(10): 2521–2525.
43. King CA, Cook R, Wheelock H, et al. Simulating the impact of addiction consult services in the context of drug supply contamination, hospitalizations, and drug-related mortality. *Int J Drug Policy.* 2022;100:103525.
44. Danovitch I, Korouri S, Kaur H, et al. The addiction consultation service for hospitalized patients with substance use disorder: an integrative review of the evidence. *J Subst Use Addict Treat.* 2024;163:209377.
45. Pham S, Haigh A, Barrett E. Statewide availability of buprenorphine/naloxone in acute care hospitals. *J Addict Med.* 2022;16(1):e48–e51.
46. Shearer R, Englander H, Hagedorn H, Hospital provider's perspectives on MOUD initiation and continuation ater inpatient discharge. *J Gen Intern Med.* 2024;40(12):2926–2933.
47. Englander H, Gregg J, Gullickson J, et al. Recommendations for integrating peer mentors in hospital-based addiction care. *Subst Abus.* 2020;41(4):419–424.
48. Greenfield SF, Hennessy G, Sugarman DE, Weiss RD. What general psychiatrists ask addiction psychiatrists: a review of 381 substance abuse consultations in a psychiatric hospital. *Am J Addict.* 2003;12(1):18–28.
49. Suzuki J, DeVido J, Kalra I, et al. Initiating buprenorphine treatment for hospitalized patients with opioid dependence: a case series. *Am J Addict.* 2015;24(1):10–14.
50. Murphy MK, Chabon B, Delgado A, Newville H, Nicolson SE. Development of a substance abuse consultation and referral service in an academic medical center: challenges, achievements and dissemination. *J Clin Psychol Med Settings.* 2009;16(1):77–86.
51. Bourgeois JA, Wegelin JA, Servis ME, Hales RE. Psychiatric diagnoses of 901 inpatients seen by consultation-liaison psychiatrists at an academic medical center in a managed care environment. *J Acad Consult Liaison Psychiatry.* 2005;46(1):47–57.
52. Hassamal S, Goldenberg M, Ishak W, Haglund M, Miotto K, Danovitch I. Overcoming barriers to initiating medication-assisted treatment for heroin use disorder in a general medical hospital: a case report and narrative literature review. *J Psychiatr Pract.* 2017;23(3):221–229.
53. Grant JE, Meller W, Urevig B. Changes in psychiatric consultations over ten years. *Gen Hosp Psychiatry.* 2001; 23(5):261–265.
54. Kathol RG, Kunkel EJ, Weiner JS, et al. Psychiatrists for medically complex patients: bringing value at the physical health and mental health/substance-use disorder interface. *Psychosomatics.* 2009;50(2):93–107.
55. Martino S, Zimbrean P, Forray A, et al. Implementing motivational interviewing for substance misuse on medical inpatient units: a randomized controlled trial. *J Gen Intern Med.* 2019;34(11):2520–2529.

56. Marcovitz D, Nisavic M, Bearnot B. Staffing an addiction consult service: psychiatrists, internists, or both? *Gen Hosp Psychiatry.* 2019;57:41–43.
57. Englander H, Priest KC, Snyder H, Martin M, Calcaterra S, Gregg J. A call to action: hospitalists' role in addressing substance use disorder. *J Hosp Med.* 2019;14(3):E1–E4.
58. Snyder H, Kalmin MM, Moulin A, et al. Rapid adoption of low-threshold buprenorphine treatment at California Emergency Departments participating in the CA bridge program. *Ann Emerg Med.* 2021;78(6):759–772.
59. CA Bridge. *Bridge to Treatment. [Internet].* California Department of Health Care Services. 2024. Accessed November 6, 2024. https://bridgetotreatment.org/addiction-treatment/ca-bridge/
60. Englander H, Patten A, Lockard R, Muller M, Gregg J. Spreading addictions care across Oregon's rural and community hospitals: mixed-methods evaluation of an interprofessional telementoring ECHO program. *J Gen Intern Med.* 2021;36(1):100–107.
61. Englander H, Patten A, Gregg J. Collaboration in a time of crisis: adapting a telementoring ECHO for addiction leaders during COVID-19. *Subst Abus.* 2022;43(1):547–550.
62. Project ECHO. *A Revolution in Medical Education and Care Delivery [Internet].* The University of New Mexico. Accessed November 15, 2024. https://echo.unm.edu/
63. Andrews LB, Bridgeman MB, Dalal KS, et al. Implementation of a pharmacist-driven pain management consultation service for hospitalised adults with a history of substance abuse. *Int J Clin Pract.* 2013;67(12):1342–1349.
64. Wei J, Defries T, Lozada M, Young N, Huen W, Tulsky J. An inpatient treatment and discharge planning protocol for alcohol dependence: efficacy in reducing 30-day readmissions and emergency department visits. *J Gen Intern Med.* 2015;30(3):365–370.
65. Herbst N, Wiener RS, Helm ED, et al. Effectiveness of an opt-out electronic heath record-based tobacco treatment consult service at an urban safety net hospital. *Chest.* 2020; 158(4):1734–1741.
66. Shanahan CW, Beers D, Alford DP, Brigandi E, Samet JH. A transitional opioid program to engage hospitalized drug users. *J Gen Intern Med.* 2010;25(8):803–808.
67. Afshar M, Sharma B, Dligach D, et al. Development and multimodal validation of a substance misuse algorithm for referral to treatment using artificial intelligence (SMART-AI): a retrospective deep learning study. *Lancet Digit Health.* 2022;4(6): e426–e435.
68. Forrest GN, Van Schooneveld TC, Kullar R, Schulz LT, Duong P, Postelnick M. Use of electronic health records and clinical decision support systems for antimicrobial stewardship. *Clin Infect Dis.* 2014;59(suppl_3):S122–S133.
69. Providers Clinical Support System. *Discover the Rewards of Treating Patients with Opioid Use Disorders* [Internet]. Accessed May 21, 2019. https://pcssnow.org/
70. Clinical Consultation Center. *Substance Use Resources.* 2019. Accessed November 21, 2024. https://nccc.ucsf.edu/clinical-resources/substance-use-resources/
71. McNeely J, Wang SS, Abadi RY, et al. Addiction consultation services for opioid use disorder treatment initiation and engagement: a randomized clinical trial. *JAMA Intern Med.* 2024;184(9):1106–1115.
72. Lambert E, Regan S, Wakeman SE. The impact of addiction consultation and medication for opioid or alcohol use disorder on hospital readmission. *J Gen Intern Med.* 2025; 40(12):2989–2996.
73. Jakubowski A, Singh-Tan S, Torres-Lockhart K, et al. Addiction consult service and inpatient outcomes among patients with OUD. *J Gen Intern Med.* 2024;39(15):2961–2969.
74. Singh-Tan S, Torres-Lockhart K, Jakubowski A, et al. Addiction consult service and inpatient outcomes among patients with alcohol use disorder. *J Gen Intern Med.* 2023; 38(14):3216–3223.
75. Ober AJ, Murray-Krezan C, Page K, et al. Hospital addiction consultation service and opioid use disorder treatment: the START randomized clinical trial. *JAMA Intern Med.* 2025;185(6):624–633.
76. Collins D, Alla J, Nicolaidis C, et al. "If it wasn't for him, I wouldn't have talked to them": qualitative study of addiction peer mentorship in the hospital. *J Gen Intern Med.* 2019.
77. King C, Collins D, Patten A, Nicolaidis C, Englander H. Trust in hospital physicians among patients with substance use disorder referred to an addiction consult service: a mixed-methods study. *J Addict Med.* 2022;16(1):41–48.
78. Wakeman SE, Kane M, Powell E, Howard S, Shaw C, Regan S. Impact of inpatient addiction consultation on hospital readmission. *J Gen Intern Med.* 2021;36(7):2161–2163.
79. Barocas JA, Savinkina A, Adams J, et al. Clinical impact, costs, and cost-effectiveness of hospital-based strategies for addressing the US opioid epidemic: a modelling study. *Lancet Public Health.* 2022;7(1):e56–e64.
80. Sikka MK, Gore S, Vega T, Strnad L, Gregg J, Englander H. "OPTIONS-DC", a feasible discharge planning conference to expand infection treatment options for people with substance use disorder. *BMC Infect Dis.* 2021;21(1):772.
81. Priest KC, Englander H, McCarty D. "Now hospital leaders are paying attention": a qualitative study of internal and external factors influencing addiction consult services. *J Subst Abuse Treat.* 2020;110:59–65.
82. McNeely J, Schatz D, Olfson M, Appleton N, Williams AR. How physician workforce shortages are hampering the response to the opioid crisis. *Psychiatr Serv.* 2022;73(5):547–554.
83. Heil JM, Lassiter JM, Salzman MS, et al. A qualitative assessment of emergency physicians' experiences with robust emergency department buprenorphine bridge programs. *Acad Emerg Med.* 2024;31(6):576–583.
84. Callister C, Lockhart S, Holtrop JS, Hoover K, Calcaterra SL. Experiences with an addiction consultation service on care provided to hospitalized patients with opioid use disorder: a qualitative study of hospitalists, nurses, pharmacists, and social workers. *Subst Abus.* 2022;43(1):615–622.
85. Nessen SJ, Thakrar A, Perrone J, Xu L, McFadden R, Lowenstein M. Hospital security searches among patients with substance-related encounters. *JAMA Network Open.* 2025;8(3):e251068.
86. Lail P, Fairbairn N. Patients with substance use disorders leaving against medical advice: strategies for improvement. *J Addict Med.* 2018;12(6):421–423.
87. Reed MK, Sarpoulaki N, Murali V, et al. A Qualitative analysis of hospitalist perceptions of self-directed discharge among inpatients with opioid use disorder. *Subst Use Misuse.* 2023;58(7):881–888.
88. Khazanchi R, Wachman EM, Schiff DM, Modest A, Saia KA, Hsu HE. Mandatory child protective services reporting for substance-exposed newborns and peripartum outcomes: a difference-in-differences analysis. *JAMA Pediatr.* 2024;178(7):719–722.
89. Simon R, Snow R, Wakeman S. Understanding why patients with substance use disorders leave the hospital against medical advice: a qualitative study. *Subst Abus.* 2020;41(4):519–525.
90. Liu P, Chan B, Sokolski E, Patten A, Englander H. Piloting a hospital-based rapid methadone initiation protocol for fentanyl. *J Addict Med.* 2024;18(4):458–462.
91. Casey S, Regan S, Gale E, et al. Rapid methadone induction in a general hospital setting: a retrospective, observational analysis. *Subst Abus.* 2023;44(3):177–183.

92. Nacev EC, Prewitt KC, Yang WT, et al. Feasibility of an inpatient split-dose rapid methadone induction protocol for pregnant individuals. *J Addict Med.* 2025. doi:10.1097/ADM.0000000000001548. Online ahead of print.
93. Tassey TE, Ott GE, Alvanzo AAH, Peirce JM, Antoine D, Buresh ME. OUD MEETS: a novel program to increase initiation of medications for opioid use disorder and improve outcomes for hospitalized patients being discharged to skilled nursing facilities. *J Subst Abuse Treat.* 2022;143:108895.
94. Price CN, Solomon DA, Johnson JA, Montgomery MW, Martin B, Suzuki J. Feasibility and safety of outpatient parenteral antimicrobial therapy in conjunction with addiction treatment for people who inject drugs. *J Infect Dis.* 2020;222(Suppl 5):S494–S498.
95. Cortes-Penfield N, Cawcutt K, Alexander BT, Karre VMM, Balasanova AA. A proposal for addiction and infectious diseases specialist collaboration to improve care for patients with opioid use disorder and injection drug use-associated infective endocarditis. *J Addict Med.* 2022;16(4):392–395.
96. Greenberg R, Goldberg A, Anthony S, et al. Canadian society of transplantation white paper: ethical and legal considerations for alcohol and cannabis use in solid organ listing and allocation. *Transplantation.* 2021;105(9):1957–1964.
97. Bredenberg E, Tietbohl C, Dafoe A, Thurman L, Calcaterra S. Identifying factors that contribute to burnout and resilience among hospital-based addiction medicine providers: a qualitative study. *J Subst Abuse Treat.* 2023;144:108924.
98. Krawczyk N, Fawole A, Yang J, Tofighi B. Early innovations in opioid use disorder treatment and harm reduction during the COVID-19 pandemic: a scoping review. *Addict Sci Clin Pract.* 2021;16(1):68.
99. O'Donnell M, Englander H, Strnad L, Bhamidipati CM, Shalen E, Riquelme PA. Expanding the team: optimizing the multidisciplinary management of drug use-associated infective endocarditis. *J Gen Intern Med.* 2022;37(4):935–939.
100. Vyas DA, Marinacci L, Bearnot B, et al. Creation of a multidisciplinary drug use endocarditis treatment (DUET) team: initial patient characteristics, outcomes, and future directions. *Open Forum Infect Dis.* 2022;9(3):ofac047.
101. Schiff DM, Walt G, Kane M, et al. Development of a clinical decision-making framework to address parental substance use and child safety. *Parent Sci Pract.* 2024.
102. Rapoport AB, Rowley CF. Stretching the scope—becoming frontline addiction-medicine providers. *N Engl J Med.* 2017;377(8):705–707.
103. Englander H. Addiction physician specialty training: how does the USA compare with Europe? *Eur Addict Res.* 2024; 30(3):153–155.
104. Nunes EV, Kunz K, Galanter M, O'Connor PG. Addiction psychiatry and addiction medicine: the evolution of addiction physician specialists. *Am J Addict.* 2020;29(5): 390–400.
105. Englander H, Sharpe J, Skogrand E. Leveraging a clinical pharmacist as part of an interprofessional addiction medicine consult service: supporting and spreading best practices. *J Hosp Med.* 2025. doi:10.1002/jhm.70197. Online ahead of print.
106. Button D, Hartley J, Robbins J, Levander XA, Smith NJ, Englander H. Low-dose buprenorphine initiation in hospitalized adults with opioid use disorder: a retrospective cohort analysis. *J Addict Med.* 2021;17:17.
107. Sokolski E, Skogrand E, Goff A, Englander H. Rapid low-dose buprenorphine initiation for hospitalized patients with opioid use disorder. *J Addict Med.* 2023;17(4):e278–e280.
108. Hass V. Physician assistants and nurse practitioners are not interchangeable. *JAAPA.* 2016;29(4):9–12.
109. Addictions Nursing Certification Board. *Statistics & Studies: Role Delineation, Annual Reports, Exam Data & Recertification Totals.* Accessed September 5, 2025. https://ancbonline.org/Stats-&-Studies_subpage_newdies
110. Fox JM, Wason K, Beers D, et al. The creation of an addiction nursing fellowship program for registered nurses: a unique approach to enhancing the addiction-treatment workforce. *Subst Abus.* 2023;44(1):24–31.
111. Yale School of Medicine. *Addiction Medicine APP Fellowship (SUSTAIN).* Accessed September 5, 2025. https://medicine.yale.edu/internal-medicine/genmed/addictionmedicine/education/sustain/
112. Wells EA, Kristman-Valente AN, Peavy KM, Jackson TR. Social workers and delivery of evidence-based psychosocial treatments for substance use disorders. *Soc Work Public Health.* 2013;28(3–4):279–301.
113. ASAM Criteria Intake Assessment Guide. Default. Accessed November 19, 2024. https://www.asam.org/asam-criteria/implementation-tools/criteria-intake-assessment-form
114. Daley DC, Feit MD. The many roles of social workers in the prevention and treatment of alcohol and drug addiction: a major health and social problem affecting individuals, families, and society. Introduction. *Soc Work Public Health.* 2013;28(3–4):159–64.
115. Castillo J, Hendrix E, Tobar K. Examining the inclusion of substance use content in the curriculum of undergraduate social work education. *JBSW.* 2024;27–28(1):102–112.
116. Peckham AM, Ball J, Colvard MD, et al. Leveraging pharmacists to maintain and extend buprenorphine supply for opioid use disorder amid COVID-19 pandemic. *Am J Health Syst Pharm.* 2021;78(7):613–618.
117. Weiner J MS, Behrends C. Expanding access to naloxone: a review of distribution strategies. *Penn LDI.* May 29, 2019. Accessed September 15, 2024. https://ldi.upenn.edu/our-work/research-updates/expanding-access-to-naloxone-a-review-of-distribution-strategies/
118. Vadiei N, Axon DR, Eckert B. Naloxone distribution models in the united states: a scoping review. *Subst Use Addctn J.* 2025;46(2):391–404.
119. Sindhwani MK, Friedman A, O'Donnell M, Stader D, Weiner SG. Naloxone distribution programs in the emergency department: a scoping review of the literature. *J Am Coll Emerg Physicians Open.* 2024;5(3):e13180.
120. Horner G, Daddona J, Burke DJ, Cullinane J, Skeer M, Wurcel AG. "You're kind of at war with yourself as a nurse": perspectives of inpatient nurses on treating people who present with a comorbid opioid use disorder. *PLoS One.* 2019;14(10):e0224335.
121. Compton P, Blacher S. Nursing education in the midst of the opioid crisis. *Pain Manag Nurs.* 2020;21(1):35–42.
122. Kelleher S, Cotter P. A descriptive study on emergency department doctors' and nurses' knowledge and attitudes concerning substance use and substance users. *Int Emerg Nurs.* 2009;17(1):3–14.
123. Knopf-Amelung S, Gotham H, Kuofie A, et al. Comparison of instructional methods for screening, brief intervention, and referral to treatment for substance use in nursing education. *Nurse Educ.* 2018;43(3):123–127.
124. Ford R, Bammer G, Becker N. Improving nurses' therapeutic attitude to patients who use illicit drugs: workplace drug and alcohol education is not enough. *Int J Nurs Pract.* 2009;15(2):112–118.
125. Ford R. Interpersonal challenges as a constraint on care: the experience of nurses' care of patients who use illicit drugs. *Contemp Nurse.* 2011;37(2):241–252.
126. Wakeman SE, Rich JD. Barriers to post-acute care for patients on opioid agonist therapy; an example of systematic stigmatization of addiction. *J Gen Intern Med.* 2017;32(1):17–19.
127. Kimmel SD, Rosenmoss S, Bearnot B, et al. Northeast post-acute medical facilities disproportionately reject referrals for

patients with opioid use disorder. *Health Aff (Millwood).* 2022;41(3):434–444.
128. Kimmel SD, Rosenmoss S, Bearnot B, Larochelle M, Walley AY. Rejection of patients with opioid use disorder referred for post-acute medical care before and after an anti-discrimination settlement in Massachusetts. *J Addict Med.* 2021;15(1): 20–26.
129. Saitz R, Miller SC, Fiellin DA, Rosenthal RN. Recommended use of terminology in addiction medicine. *J Addict Med.* 2021;15(1):3–7.
130. National Institute of Drug Abuse. *Words Matter: Preferred Language for Talking About Addiction.* National Institutes of Health. Updated January 20, 2021. Accessed December 16, 2024. https://nida.nih.gov/research-topics/addiction-science/words-matter-preferred-language-talking-about-addiction
131. American Nurses Association Issue Brief. *The Opioid Epidemic—The Evolving Role of the Nurse.* 2018. Accessed December 11, 2024. https://www.ncsbn.org/public-files/2018_ANA_Opioid_Epidemic.pdf
132. Stack E, Hildebran C, Leichtling G, et al. Peer recovery support services across the continuum: in community, hospital, corrections, and treatment and recovery agency settings—a narrative review. *J Addict Med.* 2022;16(1):93–100.
133. Englander H, Mahoney S, Brandt K, et al. Tools to support hospital-based addiction care: core components, values, and activities of the improving addiction care team. *J Addict Med.* 2019;13(2):85–89.
134. Jack HE, Denisiuk ED, Collins BA, et al. Peer providers and linkage with buprenorphine care after hospitalization: a retrospective cohort study. *Subst Abus.* 2022;43(1): 1308–1316.
135. Suzuki J, Martin B, Loguidice F, et al. A peer recovery coach intervention for hospitalized patients with opioid use disorder: a pilot randomized controlled trial. *J Addict Med.* 2023;17(5):604–607.
136. Gormley MA, Pericot-Valverde I, Diaz L, et al. Effectiveness of peer recovery support services on stages of the opioid use disorder treatment cascade: a systematic review. *Drug Alcohol Depend.* 2021;229(Pt B):109123.
137. Eddie D, Hoffman L, Vilsaint C, et al. Lived experience in new models of care for substance use disorder: a systematic review of peer recovery support services and recovery coaching. *Front Psychol.* 2019;10:1052.
138. Bassuk EL, Hanson J, Greene RN, Richard M, Laudet A. Peer-delivered recovery support services for addictions in the United States: a systematic review. *J Subst Abuse Treat.* 2016;63:1–9.
139. O'Connell MJ, Flanagan EH, Delphin-Rittmon ME, Davidson L. Enhancing outcomes for persons with co-occurring disorders through skills training and peer recovery support. *J Ment Health.* 2020;29(1):6–11.
140. D'Onofrio G, Degutis LC. Integrating Project ASSERT: a screening, intervention, and referral to treatment program for unhealthy alcohol and drug use into an urban emergency department. *Acad Emerg Med.* 2010;17(8):903–911.
141. Bridge. Public Health Institute. CalBridge Navigator Program. California Department of Health Care Services. Updated September 20, 2024. Accessed September 5, 2025. https://bridgetotreatment.org/addiction-treatment/ca-bridge/calbridge-navigator-program/
142. Anderson ES, Rusoja E, Luftig J, et al. Effectiveness of substance use navigation for emergency department patients with substance use disorders: an implementation study. *Ann Emerg Med.* 2023;81(3):297–308.
143. Orme S, Zarkin GA, Dunlap LJ, et al. Cost and cost savings of navigation services to avoid rehospitalization for a comorbid substance use disorder population. *Med Care.* 2022;60(8): 631–635.
144. Nordeck CD, Welsh C, Schwartz RP, et al. Navigation services to avoid rehospitalization among medical/surgical patients with comorbid substance use disorder: rationale and design of a randomized controlled trial. *J Psychiatr Brain Sci.* 2020;5(3):e200013.
145. Yucel E, Bearnot B, Paras Molly L, et al. Diagnosis and management of infective endocarditis in people who inject drugs. *JACC.* 2022;79(20):2037–2057.
146. Appa A, Barocas JA. Can I safely discharge a patient with a substance use disorder home with a peripherally inserted central catheter? *NEJM Evidence.* 2022;1(2):EVIDccon2100012.
147. Weimer MB, Falker CG, Seval N, et al. The need for multidisciplinary hospital teams for injection drug use-related infective endocarditis. *J Addict Med.* 2022;16(4): 375–378.
148. Baddour LM, Wilson WR, Bayer AS, et al. Infective endocarditis in adults: diagnosis, antimicrobial therapy, and management of complications: a scientific statement for healthcare professionals from the American Heart Association. *Circulation.* 2015;132(15):1435–1486.
149. Baddour LM, Weimer MB, Wurcel AG, et al. Management of infective endocarditis in people who inject drugs: a scientific statement from the American Heart Association. *Circulation.* 2022;146(14):e187–e201.
150. Lennox R, Martin L, Brimner C, O'Shea T. Hospital policy as a harm reduction intervention for people who use drugs. *Int J Drug Policy.* 2021;97:103324.
151. Work EC, Muftu S, MacMillan KDL, et al. Prescribed and penalized: the detrimental impact of mandated reporting for prenatal utilization of medication for opioid use disorder. *Matern Child Health J.* 2023;27(Suppl 1):104–112.
152. Calcaterra SL, Saunders S, Grimm E, et al. In-hospital methadone enrollment: a novel program to facilitate linkage from the hospital to the opioid treatment program for vulnerable patients with opioid use disorder. *J Gen Intern Med.* 2024;39(3):385–392.
153. Englander H, Wilson T, Collins D, et al. Lessons learned from the implementation of a medically enhanced residential treatment (MERT) model integrating intravenous antibiotics and residential addiction treatment. *Subst Abus.* 2018; 39(2):225–232.

5

Substance Use Disorder Training in the Hospital Setting

Carolyn A. Chan, Eleasa Sokolski, Kento Sonoda, Kenneth L. Morford

When entering his hospital room, I first noticed the three bags of belongings sitting on the hospital windowsill, two bags near the closet, and framed family photos, including two kids sitting on his side table. Along the windowsill, I saw snack bags of Doritos and handmade children's art lovingly taped along the wall. The room had all the hallmarks of a patient with a prolonged hospital stay. At the time, I was the senior internal medicine resident coming to assess Mr H, who had been transferred from the cardiac intensive care unit to the general internal medicine floor. Mr H was in his 40s and had just completed a prosthetic valve surgery for injection drug use–related infective endocarditis. I had reviewed the plan for his post-op pain management, antibiotics, and bacteremia before entering his room. His clinical care had succeeded by all accounts in the medical record. He had a lifesaving surgery to manage his infection, responded well to the antibiotics, and had a strong social support system. At first glance, it appeared to be a straightforward case of a patient pending care coordination for hospital discharge care.

As I walked into the room, Mr H was sitting on the side of his hospital bed, hovering over the framed images of his kids with silent tears on his face. I introduced myself and my role and asked how I could support him. He responded with, "Start me on buprenorphine." For the next 30 minutes, Mr H taught me more about opioid use disorder (OUD) than any lecture I had received during my medical training. Approximately 10 years prior, he had started taking opioids for back pain after a car accident. When his pain management clinic stopped prescribing him opioids, he quickly turned to heroin to avoid feeling sick from withdrawal and to care for his family.

He explained how he started buprenorphine in an outpatient substance use disorder (SUD) clinic and that it had made him feel normal after nearly a decade of struggling with heroin use. He had no heroin use when he was on buprenorphine, and he was able to stay on the medication for an entire year. At the one-year mark of receiving buprenorphine, a first-line medication for opioid use disorder (MOUD), his doctor informed him that MOUD was only needed for 1 year and tapered him off. About 6 months after tapering off the medication, Mr H had intense cravings that led him to return to heroin use. Mr H informed me that he had asked every doctor he met in the hospital the same question, "Can I please restart buprenorphine in the hospital?" After hearing about his journey, it became clear that starting buprenorphine treatment in the hospital was the key intervention to promote his long-term recovery.

The year was 2013, and inspired by Mr H's story, I began reading about how to start buprenorphine. At the time, additional training called the X-waiver was needed to prescribe buprenorphine upon discharge from the hospital. Neither I nor my attending had any training on the use of this medication. We tried to order it, but the pharmacy informed us that we did not have the credentials to prescribe the medication per the hospital policy. I reached out to the psychiatry consultation service and other individuals with an X-waiver who could have prescribed it. Yet, each time, I was informed that it was not an option to start buprenorphine in the hospital without having already been established as an outpatient. After 3 days, numerous phone calls, and following every potential lead, I had run out of options for accessing this medication for Mr H. I informed him it was not possible due to the barriers I encountered. He graciously thanked me for my efforts, and tears streamed down his face. He told me he was not sure he would make it through a prolonged stay for intravenous antibiotics at the nursing home without the medication, but was going to try for his family. The multiple barriers this patient faced in accessing evidence-based SUD treatment in the hospital deeply impacted my views and approach to caring for patients with SUD.

Shortly after his hospital encounter, I completed X-waiver training through a local course, knowing that I wanted to have the knowledge and ability to prescribe buprenorphine in my next career step as a hospitalist. Once I graduated, I started prescribing buprenorphine in the hospital. The experience affirmed everything Mr H had informed me—that the medication was lifesaving and made patients feel like themselves again. I thought of Mr H and how, if hospital-based MOUD had been accessible, our interaction could have been different. I continue to hope he found a way to start buprenorphine in the outpatient setting. Based on how fulfilling it was to provide hospital-based SUD treatment, I decided to pursue an addiction medicine fellowship to develop further expertise and be able to provide better care for patients like Mr H.

Now, I spend my clinical time as an attending on a hospital-based addiction consultation service where I can spread the knowledge, skills, and joy of providing hospital-based SUD care. Starting SUD treatment in the hospital can be a reachable moment for many patients. Furthermore, it can offer rich educational opportunities to train and inspire the next generation of health professionals to provide effective and compassionate SUD care so that no other patients like Mr H are denied lifesaving treatment.

—Carolyn A. Chan

Key Points

- **Significant gaps exist in substance use disorder (SUD) knowledge, attitudes, and skills among health professionals.**
- **The hospital setting can provide numerous educational opportunities on evidence-based SUD care for learners from various professions and at different training levels.**
- **Hospital-based SUD education should align learner goals and learning objectives with clinical teaching activities and didactics that are evaluated with competency-based assessments to ensure the education is achieving its goals.**
- **Faculty should be prepared to navigate challenges unique to hospital-based SUD care and provide emotional debriefing with learners when needed.**
- **Faculty lacking expertise in hospital-based SUD education can benefit from continuing medical education programs designed to fill gaps in knowledge, skills, and attitudes related to SUD care.**

SUDs are prevalent worldwide, and it is crucial for health professionals to provide evidence-based SUD treatment and care. Overdose remains a leading cause of death, and SUD is associated with significant morbidity. Hospitals, serving as primary clinical teaching sites, provide a unique and rich learning environment for SUD education. Most SUD care has historically been concentrated in outpatient settings; however, implementing evidence-based practices to screen, diagnose, and treat SUD within hospital settings is essential. Hospitals offer a critical opportunity to engage patients in discussions about their substance use goals and to provide evidence-based treatment, harm reduction services, and other resources.

Hospitals expose health professional learners to a wide spectrum of SUD severity and related comorbidities. This diverse exposure is vital for learning clinical SUD care. Furthermore, the emergence of hospital-based addiction consultation services enables dedicated clinical rotations to enhance the training experience. As hospital-based addiction consultation services expand, ensuring a well-trained specialty workforce to meet the unique needs of hospital-based SUD care is essential.

This chapter will discuss hospital-based SUD education for health professionals, including physicians (DO, MD), physician associates (PAs), advanced practice registered nurses (APRNs), registered nurses (RNs), pharmacists, and social workers (SWs). The focus will primarily be centered on the education of clinicians who prescribe, progressing from the student level such as medical, APRN, and PA students, to postgraduate medical education (ie, residency and fellowship), and finally faculty continuing education efforts. Although focused on disciplines who prescribe, many teaching methods and assessments can be adapted to other health professionals.

SUD Education Requirements

To increase the uptake of evidence-based SUD care to address the opioid epidemic, various health professional accrediting bodies have opted to require

SUD education. There is wide variability in educational requirements related to SUD across different health professions and training levels. As such, there are knowledge and skills gaps among health professionals caring for patients with SUD in the hospital setting. Requirements specific to hospital-based SUD only exist for specialty addiction training programs like addiction medicine and addiction psychiatry fellowships and are further described in the section on fellowship education.

At the level of health professional students, medical and APRN schools do not currently have a formal SUD education requirement from their accrediting bodies. However, the Accreditation Review Commission on Education for the Physician Assistant (ARC-PA) requires SUD education within the curriculum.[1]

For postgraduate physician trainees, the Accreditation Council for Graduate Medical Education (ACGME) sets educational standards for US allopathic and osteopathic medical residents and fellows. In 2018, the ACGME published common program requirements for all residency programs to "provide instruction and experience in pain management if applicable for the specialty including recognition of the signs of addiction."[2] While this ACGME core program requirement does not require specific curricular elements, the Graduate Medical Education (GME) Stakeholders Congress on preparing residents and fellows to manage pain and SUD convened in March 2021 and developed recommendations for all GME trainees related to pain management, communication, and treatment for SUD.[3] The Congress also proposed specialty-specific recommendations for family medicine, internal medicine, emergency medicine, obstetrics & gynecology, pediatrics, and psychiatry programs.[3] Sokolski et al proposed examples of curricular experiences for various GME programs along with relevant resources for residency SUD education.[4]

In addition to the ACGME common program requirements, some GME specialties have specific program requirements on SUD education. Notably, the educational requirements vary for each specialty. For example, family medicine residents must recognize the intersection of social and governmental contexts, including SUD and health.[5] Internal medicine residents must demonstrate knowledge and have clinical experience in addiction medicine.[6] Psychiatry residents must complete a 1-month clinical experience caring for individuals with SUD and dual diagnosis.[7] Furthermore, the ACGME specifies that psychiatry residents must have experience with treatment modalities that include pharmacotherapy for SUD, medically supervised withdrawal, overdose management, and therapeutic techniques such as cognitive-behavioral therapy.[7]

For practicing prescribers, the US Congress passed the Medication Access and Training Expansion (MATE) included in the Consolidated Appropriations Act of 2023.[8] As of June 2023, all practitioners applying for or renewing their Drug Enforcement Agency (DEA) registration to prescribe controlled substances must complete a one-time 8-hour training on the treatment and management of patients with SUD.

Gaps and Barriers in SUD Training

Despite increased efforts to improve SUD education, significant gaps exist in the knowledge, attitudes, and skills needed to care for this population among health professionals. Historically, SUD educational content has focused on outpatient settings. While significant overlap exists in the knowledge, attitudes, and skills needed to provide outpatient and hospital-based SUD care, special attention must be given to the unique clinical environment of the hospital setting.

Hospital-based clinicians should be experienced in screening, diagnosis, withdrawal management, pharmacotherapy initiation, motivational interviewing, harm reduction counseling, interprofessional teamwork, and care coordination for complex linkage for SUD treatment plans. Yet, in practice, hospital-based screening for unhealthy substance use is often suboptimal.[9] General medicine physicians and PAs have reported barriers to starting medications for opioid use disorder (OUD) in the hospital, including lack of experience, inadequate training, and the need for more addiction specialist support.[10] In a systematic review, nearly 74% of physicians reported that they did not intervene in SUD due to a lack of skill, and 72% did not intervene due to a lack of knowledge.[11] Physicians commonly report institutional and structural barriers as reasons to not intervene in SUD treatment.[12]

Low levels of physicians' comfort in SUD knowledge and clinical skills have reverberating effects on SUD training among medical students and residents. At the medical student level, a survey of medical school deans found that most schools taught some domains of SUD treatment, which was often integrated throughout the students' preclerkship and clerkship years.[13] However, respondents described challenges teaching students about the topic of SUD, including a lack of curricular time and faculty expertise.[13] At the resident level, residency programs have reported low levels of SUD content and educational effectiveness. In a survey study of family medicine program directors, only 29% reported offering a formal SUD curriculum.[14] In a survey of internal medicine residency program directors, only 15% reported that their programs are very effective in teaching the treatment of SUD.[15] Barriers to education among residency programs include a need for more trained faculty.[15] In addition, residents interested in hospital-based SUD clinical rotations may have limited opportunities. Among internal medicine residency programs, only 4.6% reported clinical rotation opportunities with hospital-based addiction consultation services.[15]

Many allied health professionals, such as pharmacists, RNs, and SWs, face similar gaps and barriers in SUD education. While most pharmacy graduate programs teach SUD content, an average of only 2.7 hours are dedicated to this content.[16] Among a sample of practicing pharmacists, nearly 29% reported receiving no SUD education, less than half said they had much or very much knowledge on counseling patients about potentially addictive medications, and 54% had never referred a patient to SUD treatment in their careers.[17] Nursing professions have described similar low levels of curriculum time dedicated to teaching SUD and a lack of faculty as a common barrier to addressing this gap.[18] RNs play an essential role in the care for hospitalized patients with SUD, but many do not receive formal SUD education during training.[19] Addiction RNs in Australia, have reported stigma toward the addiction nursing specialty itself, lack of awareness, and stigma toward patients, as having made the field of addiction nursing less attractive to new nurses.[20] In addition, a survey of SWs reported that more than 25% of their clients have SUD, though few respondents had addiction and SUD as their area of practice.[21] Similar to nursing education, there exists a large training gap in SUD education for those completing Masters of Social Work (MSW) programs, and most students acquire these skills through field internships and work experience rather than formal classroom settings.[22,23] Specific SUD training has been shown to increase SWs' likelihood of assessing and intervening with SUD.[24] Among MSW degree programs, few offer addiction specializations, and only 4.7% require at least one addiction course.[22] Gaps remain in bridging SW knowledge, skills and attitudes to caring for this population. Clinical SW faculty have reported barriers including only superficially covering the content, a lack of integration of SUD content into SW programs, limited curricular time, and a lack of faculty knowledge.[25] Efforts are needed to decrease these knowledge gaps to improve the consistency of hospital-based SUD education within various health professional disciplines.

Uniqueness of Hospital Setting for SUD Education

The hospital is a rich training environment for health professionals to learn about evidence-based SUD care. Educators arranging required or elective clinical rotations should consider the benefits and limitations of hospital-based experiences in the context of learner level, discipline, and treatment delivery model. Insight into these factors can help faculty develop SUD rotations with appropriate learning objectives and assessments. Hospital-based SUD care can be delivered in consult models (eg, through addiction medicine or psychiatry consult services) or practice-based models where generalists integrate SUD care into their core specialties.[26] For educators who lack access to a consultation service for their learners, they can consider collaborative training opportunities with other specialties who may offer SUD care such as through psychiatry, toxicology, or emergency medicine. Furthermore, hospital-based SUD treatment often provides opportunities for interprofessional learning. Unique considerations for educators in charge of developing clinical rotations that provide hospital-based SUD care are discussed in this section.

There are numerous benefits of using the hospital as a training site for SUD education. From a practical standpoint, hospitals are already a primary training environment for health professional learners. This environment provides a rich array of acute and complex cases to learn from, including severe cases of SUD that are unsafe to manage in outpatient settings. Patients in the hospital are often admitted for a co-occurring medical or psychiatric disorder related to their SUD diagnosis, providing learners with a critical understanding of the most acute manifestations and adverse consequences of SUD. In addition, hospital-based care can include managing SUD in the perioperative context. This experience helps learners develop skills in complex pain management; preventing, assessing and managing substance withdrawal symptoms; and collaborating effectively with surgical teams.

The hospital setting can provide opportunities for direct observation of skills such as taking a SUD history, using nonjudgmental language, and practicing motivational interviewing and shared decision making. It allows learners to see the results of their care plans in real time (eg, managing opioid withdrawal with buprenorphine). In addition, patients in the hospital are not necessarily seeking treatment for SUD, but rather seeking treatment for an acute medical condition (eg, cellulitis). This can provide opportunities for learners to practice motivational interviewing skills as well as harm reduction counseling for individuals who are not ready to engage in SUD treatment.

Learners in the hospital setting often gain exposure to SUD care with high levels of social complexity. Some patients in the hospital are unable to receive

TABLE 5.1

Examples of Hospital-Based SUD Cases and Associated Educational Domains for Health Professional Learners

Hospital-based addiction case	Potential learning domains
A patient with opioid use disorder, unstable housing, and a history of infective endocarditis status post two bioprosthetic valve replacements presented to the emergency department with a fever. The patient was found to have recurrent infective endocarditis requiring a third valve replacement during this admission. However, the cardiothoracic team informed him that this would be the last surgery they could perform due to ongoing injection opioid use. When he was admitted to the general internal medicine team, infectious disease, cardiology, cardiothoracic surgery, addiction medicine, and palliative care were consulted to optimize his care plan. Methadone was started for opioid use disorder by the addiction medicine consultation team. Social work and case management were closely involved to address social determinants of health for the patient.	Patient care Medical knowledge of SUD pharmacotherapy Care coordination management of multiple consultants Ethical principles Interprofessional collaboration Professionalism and well-being Communication—patient shared decision making
A patient with alcohol use disorder and alcohol-associated cirrhosis was brought to the emergency department by a family member due to altered mental status with suspected ingestion of a nonbeverage alcohol. In the emergency department, she developed a seizure and was admitted to the intensive care unit. Toxicology, neurology, and hepatology teams were consulted. Medications for alcohol use disorder were initiated by the general medicine team while case management linked the patient to outpatient SUD care.	Patient care—management of withdrawal in the hospital setting Medical knowledge of AUD pharmacotherapy Communication—motivational interviewing Care coordination management of multiple consultants Interprofessional collaboration

These scenarios highlight the complexity of managing substance use and its complications and the critical role of interprofessional collaboration in patient care and addiction education. Learning experiences include navigating the interplay between acute management, specialty care, transitions of care, and addressing the underlying SUD.

treatment in outpatient settings due to social barriers, including financial concerns, transportation insecurity, and lack of housing. In addition, care in the hospital often requires a multidisciplinary approach to manage SUD-related complications and presents unique opportunities for health professionals and trainees to engage in collaborative learning. Table 5.1 provides two examples of multidisciplinary, hospital-based SUD cases and associated learning domains.

There are some limitations to hospital settings for SUD education that are important to note. One drawback is the short-term nature of hospital-based SUD care, though some patients are admitted for extended stays. Trainees are often unable to observe the chronic nature or the full course of SUD recovery, as the focus is primarily on addressing acute conditions. As trainees rotating in the hospital are commonly exposed to severe SUD conditions and return to use episodes of SUD, they may miss opportunities to see mild and moderate SUD. This focus may leave knowledge gaps in long-term SUD management, such as adjusting medication doses during the maintenance phase of treatment, tailoring return to use prevention strategies over time, integrating behavioral therapies into care, and managing SUD in sustained remission. These aspects are essential for comprehensive SUD education but are less commonly addressed in hospital settings.

Clinical Learning Environment

At the beginning of a hospital-based addiction rotation, orienting learners to provide SUD care in the hospital is an important step. Educators should formalize an orientation process that includes identifying learner goals, setting expectations, reviewing schedules, introducing members of the care team, navigating the clinical environment including locations of patients and workplaces, and ensuring access to the electronic medical record and other relevant clinical information. The orientation should also address unique aspects of providing SUD care in the hospital, which are discussed in this section. Importantly, learner orientations should be tailored to each institution as there can be variable institutional and state policies.

TABLE 5.2

A Three-Pronged Approach to Using Nonstigmatizing Language When Describing SUD and Related Conditions

Approach to using nonstigmatizing language	Example language to avoid	Example language to utilize
Updated clinical terminology	Substance abuse	Substance use disorder
Person-first language	Alcoholic cirrhosis	Person with alcohol-associated liver disease
	Addict	Patient with substance use disorder
Nonstigmatizing language	Dirty and clean urine drug test	Positive or negative urine drug test

Nonstigmatizing Language

The use of stigmatizing language related to substance use and SUD is widespread in health care both in verbal communication and clinical documentation. Furthermore, learners may encounter and adopt behaviors that stigmatize patients with SUD within the hidden curriculum, as many health professionals have negative attitudes toward individuals with SUD.[27] Learners on a hospital-based addiction rotation may be the first health care contact for a patient with SUD. Using patient-centered, nonstigmatizing, clinically accurate, and up-to-date medical language in verbal and written communication can help reduce stigma and help patients feel more empowered to engage in care (Table 5.2).[28] When working with new learners in the hospital setting, it is important to address this concept early and role-model appropriate language in observed interactions with patients and colleagues.

Educators can consider using a three-pronged approach to ensuring learners utilize nonstigmatizing language when describing substance-related conditions, individuals with SUD, and SUD treatments (Table 5.2). First, it is important for clinical terminology related to substance use and SUD to be both accurate and current. Educators should consider providing historical context on the evolution of relevant terms. For instance, the shift from "alcohol abuse" in the DSM-IV to "alcohol use disorder" in the DSM-5 reflects a broader transition from a moral model of addiction to a biopsychosocial, medical model. This updated terminology underscores the complexity of SUD and helps reduce stigma by framing it as a medical condition rather than a moral failing. Second, educators should emphasize the importance of using person-first language. This approach highlights the individual rather than defining them by their disease. For example, replacing terms like "alcoholic cirrhosis" with "person with alcohol-associated liver disease" serves as a reminder that individuals are not solely defined by their SUD. Such language fosters respect and empathy, which are crucial for effective patient care. In addition, common stigmatizing terms pervasive in health care should be identified and replaced with preferred terms in both clinical documentation and interpersonal communications. For instance, when discussing toxicology results, terms like "clean" or "dirty" urine drug screens can be replaced with "positive" or "negative" results for a particular substance.

It can be helpful to let learners know in advance that faculty will correct stigmatizing language identified in case presentations and documentation with appropriate terminology. When a learner uses stigmatizing language, educators should provide clear feedback in the moment and explain why using medically based language is important. Feedback in clinical settings should be viewed as an opportunity for growth and development rather than a final assessment of a learner's skills.[29]

Ensuring the use of clinically accurate, person-first, and respectful language during case presentations, in clinical notes, and in consultation with care teams is essential for maintaining a supportive and nonjudgmental health care environment. By embedding these practices into the curriculum, educators can help reshape perceptions and improve the overall care provided to individuals with SUD.

Taking a SUD History

Historically, asking about substance use is often relegated to the social history of a clinical note. Learners often narrowly focus on questions about the type of substance being used and the quantity and frequency of use. Educators should provide a framework on how to take a comprehensive substance use history during learner orientation, as well as how to apply the DSM-5 criteria to make a SUD diagnosis. One framework that has been described is the use of the mnemonic RIP-TEAR, which represents risks (eg, withdrawal seizures, overdose), initiation of substance use, pattern of use, treatment history, effects (positive and negative), abstinence, and return to use prevention (see Table 5.3).[30] If applicable, educators can consider developing a note template designed to

TABLE 5.3

The RIP-TEAR Framework for Teaching the Substance Use History

Framework component	Item	Sample questions
Risks of current use	Are there immediate risks to address (eg, recent overdose, acute withdrawal, injection-related infections)?	Have you ever had a seizure or needed to be in the ICU for alcohol withdrawal treatment?
Initiation	When and how did the substance use start?	Tell me about how you started using cocaine.
Pattern	What is the quantity and frequency of substance use?	How many beers do you drink per day, how many ounces, what brand? How many grams of fentanyl do you use a day? Do you snort, inject, or smoke it?
Treatment	Have there been prior treatment episodes? With what? Were they effective?	Have you ever received medications, counseling, or gone to any programs for opioid use?
Effects	What are the positive and negative effects of substance use?	How has the substance helped you? For example, some people have told me using fentanyl helps treat their physical pain or depression.
Abstinence	Have there been periods of not using the substance? What were the circumstances? How long did they last?	What was your longest period of not using? What was occurring then that was helping you achieve this goal?
Return to use prevention	What triggers for substance use have been identified? Are there factors to help prevent returning to use?	After you leave the hospital in the first week, what is going to be your biggest trigger to start drinking again?

walk the learner through key components of taking a SUD history.

The use of slang terms to describe certain substances and routes of substance use can vary geographically. Providing learners with common terminology that they may be unfamiliar with is recommended. In addition, it is recommended to normalize the process of learning from patients with SUD who often have a wealth of information about local substance–related terminology and use patterns. Learners should be prepared to expect that patients may use unfamiliar terms and to ask for clarification when such terms arise.

In the hospital setting, patients with SUD may be experiencing acute withdrawal, intoxication, or uncontrolled pain during the initial encounter. In these scenarios, a learner may be unable to complete a comprehensive assessment. It is recommended that educators normalize with the learner that iterative patient visits may be required to obtain a comprehensive history, which may differ from expectations on prior rotations.

Confidentiality Considerations

It is always important to abide by standards of confidentiality, and special attention must be paid to the risk of unintentional disclosure of a SUD to a family member, friend, or associate of a patient in the hospital environment. Learners should be briefed on how this diagnosis could potentially harm patients' relationships with family, employers, Child Protective Services, or aspects of the legal systems. Unintentional disclosure could have profound consequences for patients. To encourage patients to seek treatment without fear of stigma, retaliation, or legal prosecution, additional safeguards should be considered in the hospital setting. Depending on what setting the learner is rotating, their services may fall under 42 CFR Part 2 regulations, which requires additional privacy protection (see Chapter 3 in book for additional discussion). If 42 CFR part 2 does apply, it is recommended that educators include a discussion of this requirement during learner orientation.

Along these lines, learners should be taught to always ask individuals accompanying patients to step out before introducing themselves and their role on a SUD care team to prevent unintentional disclosure of substance use or a SUD diagnosis. During the visit, it is recommended that learners ask the patient which individuals are aware of their substance use and how the team should approach any visitors who may be at the bedside. Notably, with the implementation of the 21st Century Cures Act, many patients have access to their medical records in real-time patient portals.[31] Some patients may share their access with family members. Learners can prevent notes from being released to patient portals based on the preference of the patient if there is a risk of unintentional disclosure. Educators are encouraged to verify a patient's expectations and concerns regarding privacy to decrease the risk of an unintentional SUD disclosure.

Regulatory Considerations

Advanced learners, such as residents and fellows, may provide clinical services under indirect supervision. As such, educators should ensure that these learners have foundational knowledge necessary to provide safe patient care within regulatory constraints. While it is outside of the scope of this chapter to discuss all regulatory considerations for hospital-based SUD treatment, supervising faculty should clarify any key federal, state, and institutional-level regulations that the learner must abide by during orientation. For example, incoming first-year residents may be unaware that a prescription for methadone cannot be sent to a pharmacy upon discharge for the treatment of OUD. Furthermore, hospitals may have their own policies on medication for opioid use disorder (MOUD) initiation, in-hospital substance use, and opioid prescribing, among others, that a learner may need to be familiar with to provide care under indirect supervision.

Curriculum Design Best Practices

Educators should use a structured approach to develop a hospital SUD curriculum to ensure that essential content is covered effectively. It is recommended that educators use a structured framework to design hospital-based SUD curricula, which include learning objectives and goals, teaching method, and curricular evaluation. When designing a curriculum, educators should take the following factors into their consideration: learner types and levels, specialty, duration of topics, prior and current SUD education, and local resources. Barriers to implementing effective SUD curricula may include time constraints, lack of trained faculty, state-level or institutional regulations, and limited local resources. Educators can address these barriers through creative solutions and collaboration with institutional and community partners.

Educators can utilize tools such as Bloom's taxonomy to design measurable learning objectives to guide the curriculum. Existing frameworks can aid in designing a curriculum, such as Kern's 6-Step Approach and the Backward Design Model.[16,32] Table 5.4 provides an example of learning objectives, and the clinical duties, didactics, and assessments that could be utilized to

TABLE 5.4

Example of Components of a 2-Week Addiction Medicine Rotation for a Medical Resident

Rotation component	Examples
Learning Objectives	1. Utilize person-first and nonstigmatizing terminology when discussing substance use disorders (SUD) 2. Take a comprehensive SUD history 3. Diagnose an individual with SUD using DSM-5 criteria 4. Interpret a urine drug test 5. Elicit patient goals regardless of readiness to engage in SUD treatment 6. Manage opioid withdrawal 7. Manage alcohol withdrawal 8. Develop a patient-centered treatment plan incorporating evidence-based medication for SUD 9. Describe psychosocial interventions for SUD 10. Apply motivational interviewing strategies during patient encounters 11. Counsel a patient on harm reduction strategies related to SUD 12. Coordinate linkage to care plans upon discharge
Clinical Duties	▪ Monday–Friday, 8 AM–5 PM: Perform comprehensive SUD assessments, develop treatment and linkage to care plans on the hospital-based addiction consultation service as assigned and precepted by clinical supervisor ▪ Participate in multidisciplinary huddle from 9 AM–9:30 AM ▪ Document a note in the electronic medical system and discuss recommendations with the primary medical team
Didactics	▪ Attend monthly addiction medicine grand rounds and journal club ▪ Faculty to present 6 chalk talks on the following topics: Completing a SUD assessment, interpreting urine drug testing, alcohol use disorder pharmacotherapy, opioid use disorder pharmacotherapy, principles of substance withdrawal management, harm reduction principles and practice ▪ Learner to present a 10-min chalk talk to the addiction team on SUD-related topic
Assessments	▪ In-person learner feedback midway through rotation ▪ End of rotation faculty evaluation of learner competency of learning objectives

design a curriculum and clinical rotation on an addiction consultation service. To ensure that the curriculum is effective, it is encouraged that educators develop an evaluation method, seek feedback from learners, and then regularly adjust their curriculum as needed. The Kirkpatrick Model is a recognized method of evaluating the effectiveness of a curriculum through four different levels of evaluation, including reaction (eg, learner satisfaction with the course), learning (eg, passing a multiple-choice test), behavior (eg, resident prescribing naloxone for patients with OUD), and results (eg, tracking patient premature discharges).[33]

Training Across the Continuum of Education

A coordinated training strategy across the continuum of education is essential for preparing health professionals to provide effective, compassionate, and competent care to individuals with SUD in the hospital setting. As learners progress from students to residents to fellows, the complexity of their roles and educational needs evolve. In this section, a framework for hospital-based SUD training (Figure 5.1, Table 5.5) is proposed where core SUD content and skills are introduced and practiced in health professions schools (basic level), implemented and reinforced under supervision in hospital settings during residency (intermediate level), and then applied at the level of an expert consultant for select learners during fellowship (advanced level). In addition, trained faculty require continuing education and ongoing support to teach up-to-date SUD content, supervise clinical encounters, and develop hospital-based SUD curricula for learners at different training levels. While residency and fellowship are typically focused on physician training, this structured framework can be applied and adapted to meet the unique needs of diverse learners from various health professions. It is also recommended to adapt this framework to leverage existing strengths of teaching hospitals based on the SUD resources and services they offer.

Health Professions Students

All health professions students (eg, medical, PA, APRN, RN, pharmacy, social work) should develop a strong foundation of knowledge in basic SUD content and skills (Figure 5.1, Table 5.5). Curricula should include content such as using person-centered and nonstigmatizing language, the biopsychosocial model of SUD; prevention, screening, diagnosis, assessment, treatment of SUD; basic motivational interviewing skills; and harm reduction. Topics tailored to the hospital setting may include safer opioid prescribing for acute pain (prevention), initiation of MOUD in the hospital (treatment), and overdose prevention with naloxone education (harm reduction). The Substance Abuse and Mental Health Services Administration (SAMHSA) has developed a resource guide on core curricular elements of SUD education, designed for early health professions learners.[1] The resource guide provides additional details on core content, discipline-specific recommendations, models of integration of content into the curriculum, and ways to promote institutional-level integration of the SUD curriculum. Notably, early SUD education may decrease stigma by improving student attitudes toward patients with SUD.[34,35] Implementing longitudinal SUD education has been described as feasible and encouraged as it may enhance knowledge and skill retention.[36] After learning foundational SUD

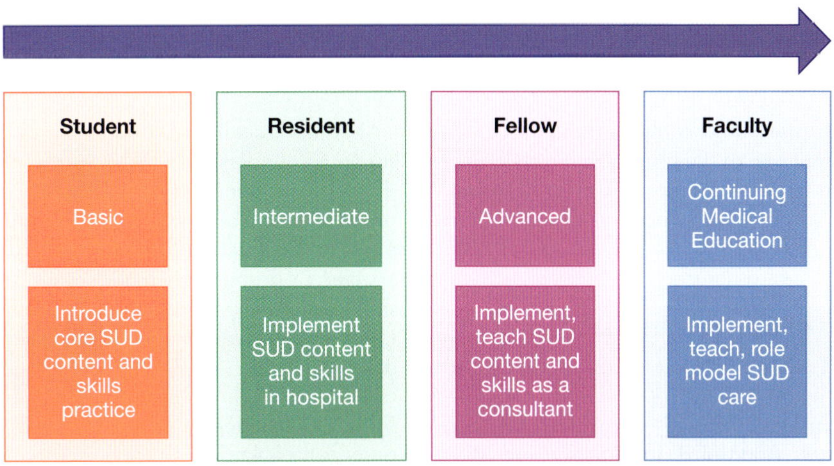

Figure 5.1: Overview of framework for hospital-based SUD education across the continuum of medical education in the hospital setting including learner type, skill level, and training goals.

TABLE 5.5

Detailed Framework for Hospital-Based SUD Education Including Content and Skills, Assessments, and Examples of Activities by Learner Level

Learner level	Content and skills	Assessment	Examples of activities[a]
Health Professions Students (MD, DO, RN, PA, APRN)	■ Stigma reduction ■ Prevention ■ Screening ■ Diagnosis ■ Treatment ■ Harm reduction ■ Core motivational interviewing skills	■ Knowledge assessment ■ Direct observation ■ Simulation ■ Standardized patients	■ Perform a SUD history ■ Demonstrate use of nonstigmatizing language ■ Apply SBIRT ■ Explain how to respond to an opioid overdose ■ Discuss service learning
Residents (MD/DO)	■ Withdrawal and intoxication management ■ Initiation of pharmacotherapy ■ Harm reduction counseling ■ Intermediate motivational interviewing skills	■ Direct observation ■ OSCEs ■ Milestones ■ Entrustable professional activities	■ Manage inpatient alcohol withdrawal ■ Initiate medications for OUD in the hospital
Fellows	■ Inpatient consultation ■ Complicated withdrawal and intoxication management ■ Initiation of pharmacotherapy in patients with complex comorbidities ■ SUD and pain management ■ Competency in motivational interviewing ■ Return to use prevention counseling	■ Direct observation ■ Milestones ■ Entrustable professional activities ■ Board certification	■ Initiate buprenorphine for OUD via low-dose or high-dose protocol ■ Develop a return-to-use prevention plan for a patient with AUD discharging from the hospital ■ Teach students opioid overdose response
Faculty	■ SUD curriculum development ■ Clinical supervision ■ Quality improvement ■ Career advising and mentorship ■ Role modeling ■ Leadership and teaching skills	■ CME activities ■ Maintenance of certification	■ Develop a hospital-based SUD curriculum ■ Supervise and debrief learners in challenging cases ■ Develop a SUD journal club ■ Implement inpatient buprenorphine order sets

[a]Activities written as measurable learning objectives.

SUD, substance use disorders; SBIRT, screening, brief intervention and referral to treatment; OSCE, objective structured clinical exam; CME, continuing medical education.

content, health professions students should focus on skills practice, tailored to their profession, which may occur through clinical rotations, service learning, simulations, and objective structured clinical exams (OSCEs).

Teaching Methods and Strategies

This section describes SUD teaching methods and strategies, with an emphasis on clinical rotations for student education focused on medical, PA, and APRN students. Additional information on RN, pharmacist, and social work training is described in the section on allied health professionals.

Various teaching strategies may be used to teach students foundational SUD content. Medical school deans have reported using case-based learning, problem-based learning, role-play, simulation, and other pedagogical methods to teach SUD content.[13] Specific to hospital-based SUD care, simulation sessions and movie-based education focusing on alcohol withdrawal management for students have been described.[37,38] In addition, opioid overdose prevention training with naloxone can engage preclinical students in SUD education as an early clinical skill.[39] At this time, little is known about how the medical knowledge content is targeted to hospital-based versus outpatient SUD care for health professions students.

Building on the foundational knowledge throughout the curriculum, implementing skills practice for key items such as Screening, Brief Intervention, and Referral to Treatment (SBIRT), and taking a SUD history are important.[40,41] Numerous interprofessional SBIRT curricula have been described, and can serve as unique opportunities for interprofessional education.[42] It is recommended that educators align knowledge, skills, and attitudes of preclinical content with clinical experiences during clerkship years. Notably, one study found that nursing students who received SBIRT training followed by skills practice during hospital-based clinical rotations had improved confidence in their ability to perform SBIRT.[43]

Clinical Experiences

Students should have opportunities for meaningful clinical experiences to care for patients with SUD during clinical years through required and/or elective rotations. For applicable students, these experiences may be integrated within core rotations such as psychiatry, internal medicine, family medicine, or emergency medicine, where they actively manage acute intoxication, withdrawal syndromes, and initiate evidence-based SUD pharmacotherapy. If a hospital has an addiction consultation service, it is an opportunity to develop a required or elective rotation on the specialty service. Hospital-based addiction rotations are thought to decrease SUD stigma by teaching learners patient-shared decision models, harm reduction, person-centered language, and skills such as motivational interviewing.[44,45] For institutions with no immediate clinical opportunity, simulation activities may be considered to ensure students have skills practice. In addition, institutions can partner with local SUD outpatient or inpatient programs (eg, medically supervised withdrawal units) or coordinate rotations at outside institutions to provide these experiences.

Currently, many students are exposed to hospital-based SUD within core specialty rotations rather than addiction consultation service experiences or on medically supervised withdrawal units. However, there may be additional benefits in having learners rotate on specialty addiction services. In one study, medical students who completed an elective on a hospital-based addiction consultation service demonstrated improved SUD knowledge and were more likely to report career aspirations to practice addiction medicine.[46,47] Additional research is needed to better understand how hospital-based SUD experiences in core specialty rotations versus addiction-specific rotations impact learners' knowledge, attitudes, skills, and career aspirations.

Beyond traditional teaching methods, service learning may provide opportunities for early exposure to SUD care, such as working in a syringe service program, shadowing at a medically supervised withdrawal unit, or attending a mutual support meeting (eg, 12-step Alcoholics Anonymous) and reflecting on their experience.[48] Several hospital-based SUD service learning experiences have been described. Medical student programs have been developed to support bedside tobacco cessation counseling in the hospital setting.[49–51] In addition, a service learning program that enrolled medical students to cuddle infants experiencing neonatal opioid withdrawal found that students were more likely to feel comfortable with patient-centered language and talking to patients about substance use or recovery.[52] Ensuring students are aware of and can apply for service learning opportunities outside of their institution is also important. The Hazelden Betty Ford Foundation's Summer Institute for Medical Students is a week-long program that provides didactics and experiential sessions in groups and residential treatment.[53] Service learning can occur at any time during their education and provides unique opportunities for students to better understand SUD, biopsychosocial aspects of the disease, and how they impact their community.

Assessments, using tools such as exams, direct observation, and standardized patients, should be utilized to ensure that students learn key knowledge, skills, and attitudes during their preclinical and clinical years. Educators can consider brief assessments, such as 1-minute papers, in-class polls, and short feedback surveys, to continuously improve the content and learning environment.

Residents

Resident physicians have completed medical school and have distinct educational specialties within the continuum of medical training. While medical students primarily concentrate on acquiring clinical knowledge and practicing skills, resident physicians are expected to apply that knowledge in clinical practice. As described previously, the ACGME requires that all residency programs teach SUD content and certain specialties have additional core program requirements on the topic. Hospital-based SUD education at the residency level should emphasize implementation of skills in the clinical environment, such as making a SUD diagnosis, management of acute intoxication and withdrawal, harm reduction counseling, intermediate motivational interviewing skills, and initiation of evidence-based pharmacotherapy.

It is recommended that all residency programs develop longitudinal curricula and clinical rotations in hospital-based SUD care to build on foundational knowledge and develop the skills necessary to care for individuals with SUD. Curricula should be tailored to the needs of a specialty, and required rotations may occur within the core specialty, addiction consultation services, or other subspecialty services and institutional structures. For example, internal medicine residents may benefit from working with a general medicine attending who also has addiction medicine specialization to better understand SUD treatment in patients admitted to a general medical floor (eg, providing comprehensive alcohol use disorder [AUD] care for a patient admitted with alcohol withdrawal by managing acute withdrawal, initiating a medication for AUD, and linking to outpatient follow-up). A surgical resident may benefit from rotating with an acute pain service to understand how to best treat pain with nonopioid regimens to prevent potential opioid-related harms.

Teaching Methods and Strategies

Most residency education occurs through experiential learning with clinical supervision, though all programs must provide protected time for education. Residency programs can offer SUD education through various strategies to augment clinical learning and provide an educational structure for SUD clinical experiences. These include didactic lectures, workshops, simulation, role-playing, journal clubs, and mentorship.[54–57] Novel strategies such as improvisational theater and virtual avatars have been described to teach residents motivational interviewing.[58,59] Longitudinal SUD curricula have been described and can equip resident physicians with progressively advanced skills throughout their education.[60,61] In addition, grand rounds and morbidity and mortality conferences can provide opportunities to teach SUD content. Educators should tailor teaching methods and strategies to the resident's unique needs, institutional resources, and be intentionally designed to address gaps in resident knowledge and skills.

Clinical Experiences

It is recommended that residents have meaningful clinical experiences with hospital-based SUD care that may occur through a variety of mechanisms. Residents commonly care for patients with SUD during required core specialty hospital rotations, such as managing alcohol withdrawal on a hospital medicine rotation. Depending on the institution, some residents may have more or less exposure to specific clinical scenarios, such as starting MOUD in the hospital or managing acute stimulant intoxication.

Hospital-based addiction consultation rotations for residents offer a valuable opportunity to learn SUD topics and leverage the unique aspects of hospital-based training. Rotations with addiction consultation services allow residents to learn how to care for patients with acute complications related to SUD, manage underlying SUD, and work in multidisciplinary teams that may include peer support specialists and SWs. A mixed-methods study in Canada examined the educational impact of a 4-week addiction medicine elective curriculum, including clinical experiences with an addiction consultation service, didactic lectures, journal clubs, mortality and morbidity rounds, and grand rounds presentations.[46] This study demonstrated that residents reported self-perceived improvement in clinical knowledge related to substance use screening, history taking, treating withdrawal, return to use prevention, OUD, nicotine use disorder, safer opioid prescribing, and the neurobiology of SUD.[46] Furthermore, addiction consultation services may contribute to combating the stigma surrounding SUD by observing patient-centered and destigmatizing approaches role modeled by addiction specialists.[44]

For programs that do not have access to addiction consultation services, clinical opportunities may be available through collaboration with other disciplines providing SUD care and taking advantage of SUD services unique to their hospital system. For example, residents may rotate in the following settings if they exist at their institution: hospitalist-led buprenorphine teams, toxicology services that care for patients with SUD, psychiatry consult-liaison teams that treat co-occurring mental health and SUD, medically supervised withdrawal units, and emergency departments that initiate MOUD.[62–64] Developing away rotations at institutions with addiction consultation service rotations may also be explored.

Addiction Concentrations and Tracks

For resident physicians interested in SUD care, several programs have developed addiction medicine tracks or concentrations to provide enhanced SUD training and support for residents interested in pursuing specialty training.[65–67] These tracks/concentrations typically include additional elective rotations, a longitudinal ambulatory clinic, hospital-based addiction consultation service rotations, scholarly activities, and mentorship.[67] While the specifics of each track/concentration vary, they offer residents with a particular interest in SUD to gain enhanced clinical knowledge and skills in SUD care. It is encouraged that residents who participate in addiction tracks have a required clinical experience in hospital-based SUD treatment. This could occur through a rotation on a hospital addiction consultation service or through a community partner that provides subacute withdrawal management services (American Society of Addiction Medicine level of care 3.7).

Example of an Addiction Medicine Residency Training Track: Yale Primary Care CHAMP Track

In 2019, the Yale Primary Care Internal Medicine Residency Program launched an addiction medicine training track as part of the *Collaborative Behavioral Health and Addiction Medicine in Primary Care (CHAMP)* program funded by the Health Resources and Services Administration (HRSA). The goals of the CHAMP track are to improve knowledge, skills, and readiness of participating residents to care for patients with SUD. Two interns are recruited each year for a total of six residents participating in the 3-year track annually. Each resident is assigned a faculty advisor board-certified in addiction medicine. CHAMP residents complete clinical rotations on the hospital-based Yale Addiction Medicine Consult Service and longitudinal outpatient experiences at a community-based opioid treatment program, an academic addiction medicine clinic embedded in a federally qualified health center, and elective experiences on a street medicine team and at a transitions clinic for patients who were recently incarcerated.[68,69] Didactic activities include weekly training with a licensed psychologist to practice motivational interviewing and cognitive-behavioral therapy, as well as attendance at monthly addiction medicine grand rounds, journal clubs, and case conferences. CHAMP residents also participate in addiction-related teaching activities for medical, APRN, and PA students.

Fellowship

During addiction medicine or addiction psychiatry fellowship training, trainees should continue to advance their knowledge, skills, and attitudes necessary to be an addiction specialist. Fellowship is a time to focus on advanced skills such as developing competency in advanced medication initiation for OUD, medication treatment for AUD or other SUD, treatment of patients with co-occurring mental illness and SUD, management of polysubstance or complicated substance withdrawal syndromes, motivational interviewing, return to substance use prevention, harm reduction, and cognitive-behavioral therapy, among others. They should know and be able to critically appraise landmark studies and emerging research in the field of SUD, as well as the impact of federal, state, and local regulations on SUD practice. In addition, they should develop skills to serve as expert consultants in the hospital setting, as well as gain leadership and education skills as they prepare to step into faculty positions and independent practice. Here is an overview of addiction fellowships with a focus on hospital-based training for physicians and allied health professionals who prescribe medications.

History of Physician Addiction Fellowships

Addiction fellowship training and its first recognition as a subspecialty occurred within the field of psychiatry.[70] The American Academy of Addiction Psychiatry (AAAP) was established in 1985 and played a significant role in advocating that addiction psychiatry become a subspecialty. In 1991, the American Board of Psychiatry and Neurology granted addiction psychiatry as a subspecialty.[70] Currently, there are a total of 54 ACGME-accredited addiction psychiatry fellowships.[71] Over time, the importance of SUD treatment expanded beyond psychiatry and the American Board of Medical Specialties officially recognized addiction medicine as a multispecialty subspecialty in 2015. Prior to this, in 2007, the American Board of Addiction Medicine became a nonprofit and began to develop and accredit non-ACGME addiction medicine fellowships.[70] This eventually led to the ACGME accreditation of addiction medicine fellowships in 2018. As of 2024, there are 105 ACGME-accredited addiction medicine fellowships across the US.[71]

While addiction psychiatry fellowships require completion of psychiatry residency training, physicians from any medical specialty are eligible to pursue an addiction medicine fellowship. Qualified candidates can sit for the addiction medicine board certification exam through the American Board of Preventive Medicine (ABPM) or the American Osteopathic Association (AOA) if they meet requirements for the ACGME-accredited fellowship pathway or the clinical practice pathway.[72] Notably, the clinical practice pathway through the AOA will close for new applicants in December 2026, and the ABPM closes in June 2025.[72,73]

Fellowship Hospital-based Training Requirements

Per ACGME, all addiction fellows must have clinical experience evaluating and treating patients in a hospital setting. Within addiction medicine fellowships, trainees must complete a minimum of 3 months of structured inpatient rotations that may include hospital-based addiction consultation services, residential SUD treatment, medically managed residential SUD programs, or hospital-based rehabilitation programs.[74] The ACGME does not provide specific guidance on the minimum number of inpatient rotations for addiction psychiatry fellows, but requires that they should have clinical experience providing consultation to acute and chronically ill patients with SUD being treated in settings that can include a general hospital and emergency room.[75] Addiction fellowships are heterogeneous, and a fellow's inpatient experience can vary depending on the program.

Only some fellowship sites have a hospital-based addiction consultation service. The current number of fellowships with addiction consultation rotations is unclear, as the implementation of these services across hospital systems is rapidly evolving. Little is known about the impact of hospital-based addiction consultation services on fellow education compared to other inpatient learning opportunities. One study examining fellows' experiences on a 4-week addiction consultation elective demonstrated improved medical knowledge on a pre-post test.[46] While graduates of addiction fellowships should have the knowledge, skills, and behaviors to lead a hospital-based addiction consultation service, additional research is needed to clarify educational outcomes of hospital-based experiences.

Additional Health Professional Postgraduate Training

Beyond physician fellowships, there is a growing number of postgraduate training programs for various health care specialties aimed at developing expertise in caring for individuals with SUD. Postgraduate addiction programs ranging from 6 to 12 months have been described for APRNs and PAs.[76,77] The goal is to provide specialty training to APRNs and PAs interested in providing specialty SUD care within their practice. For example, in 2023, the Yale School of Medicine implemented a 1-year addiction medicine fellowship program for APRNs and PAs. This Health Resources and Services Administration (HRSA)-funded program, called *Substance Use Skills Training to Advance Integrated Care (SUSTAIN)*, trains one APRN or PA fellow each year alongside addiction medicine physician fellows. Clinical rotations alternate between 6-week blocks on a hospital-based addiction medicine consult service and 2-week outpatient blocks at a community-based opioid treatment program, primary care-based addiction medicine clinic, adolescent addiction clinic, and street medicine service.[68] SUSTAIN fellows attend weekly didactics with addiction medicine and addiction psychiatry fellows, complete a scholarly project, and participate in teaching activities for medical, APRN, and PA students. SUSTAIN fellows are supervised by addiction medicine physicians, APRNs, and PAs. To support APRN and PA faculty, the SUSTAIN fellowship additionally offers a faculty development program for two APRN or PA faculty each year to improve clinical teaching skills and provide mentorship on career development and educational projects.

Addiction Fellowship Assessment and Competencies

To ensure addiction fellows are equipped with the skills necessary for independent practice, they must be deemed ready for independent practice based on their competency. The ACGME looks at six domains of competence, including medical knowledge, patient care, professionalism, communication and interpersonal skills, practice-based learning and improvement, and systems-based practice.[78] In addition, the International Society of Addiction Medicine has identified core addiction competencies for undergraduate, graduate, and continuing medical education (CME).[79] Faculty must assess fellows to help them improve their skills, provide a direction for future learning, and protect the public by training individuals who can safely practice independently.[78] This is particularly important for hospital-based SUD care, which often involves management of acute medical conditions, such as complicated withdrawal syndromes and SUD-related systemic infections, associated with significant morbidity and mortality.

Two common frameworks used for assessment in competency-based education are milestones and entrustable professional activities (EPA). Milestones refer to a point along the competency continuum and are often clearly described with specialty-specific accreditation.[80] An EPA is a discrete clinical task or responsibility (eg, managing alcohol withdrawal) that can be measured and observed by faculty to assess the level of supervision required by a trainee.[81] EPAs serve as a tool to translate competencies into clinical practice and can be mapped to align with milestones. The ACGME has developed milestones for fellows in addiction medicine and addiction psychiatry that include key competencies for addiction specialists to practice independently in the hospital setting.[82,83] While the ACGME milestones are designed for physicians, adapting and applying them to APRN and PA postgraduate addiction programs is an area for future study.

Fellowship programs should use a combination of methods to provide formative and summative feedback to fellows throughout their training. These may include rotation evaluations, patient feedback, narrative feedback, in-person feedback to fellows, simulation, direct observation, 360-degree evaluations, and data reviewed at clinical competency committees. At the end of the fellowship, individuals should be deemed competent for every ACGME milestone, and medical knowledge can be formally assessed by encouraging addiction fellows to sit and pass a board certification exam.

Faculty

With the rapid expansion of addiction fellowships, hospital systems have a growing opportunity to recruit board-certified physicians in addiction medicine, addiction psychiatry, or other allied health professionals with addiction specialty training. Faculty play a crucial role in hospital-based addiction care as they develop SUD curricula, provide clinical supervision, lead quality improvement projects, serve as role models, assess learners, and provide mentorship. Learners may become interested in a career in addiction medicine or addiction psychiatry after working with faculty who inspire them. Furthermore, faculty shape the attitudes and values of the hidden curriculum of health professions education. They can help decrease the stigma toward patients with SUD by utilizing patient-centered language, using shared decision making, and demonstrating what harm reduction looks like in clinical practice. Board-certified faculty can enhance and assess their knowledge base by participating in CME programs and utilizing longitudinal assessments, such as those provided by the ABPM.[84] There is also a need to gain knowledge and skills in SUD care among faculty who have not received sufficient training. While faculty do not need to be board-certified to teach SUD content, many will need to pursue advanced education through CME to gain competence teaching this subject matter. Here, opportunities are discussed for faculty to use CME to address this gap and develop expertise outside of formal addiction fellowship training.

Continuing Medical Education Opportunities for Faculty

Studies have shown that CME experiences that include interactive components, such as small group learning, role-play, and skills practice, are more effective in changing practice.[85] There are many high-quality and interactive SUD educational opportunities, several of which are detailed below (Table 5.6). These programs can effectively increase the faculty contributing to trainee SUD education. For example, junior faculty who participated in the Alcohol Medical Scholars Program (AMSP), which is an individual mentoring program developed to improve SUD education in US medical schools, increased SUD lecture hours fourfold, increased clinical rotations for trainees, and designed new SUD-related electives.[86]

Chief residents are the newest faculty members at academic institutions and provide a vital role in resident medical education. The Chief Resident Immersion Training (CRIT) program through Boston University provides a 4-day immersive training in diagnosing and managing SUD for incoming chief residents.[87] After completing the on-site training, chief residents work with their faculty mentors to develop and implement a teaching project at their

TABLE 5.6

Continuing Medical Education Resources for Faculty Interested in Increasing Their SUD Knowledge

Category of resource	Resource	Website
Professional Organizations	American Society of Addiction Medicine[88]	https://www.asam.org/
	American Academy of Addiction Psychiatry (AAAP)[89]	https://www.aaap.org/
	Association for Multidisciplinary Education and Research in Substance Use and Addiction (AMERSA)[90]	https://amersa.org/
	Society of Hospital Medicine[91]	https://www.hospitalmedicine.org
Podcasts	ASAM's Practice Pearls[92]	https://asampracticepearls.podbean.com/
	AMERSA's Podcast Series[90]	https://amersa.org/amersa-podcast/
	Curbsiders Addiction Medicine[93]	https://thecurbsiders.com/addiction
	Behind the Evidence: An Addiction Medicine Podcast[94]	https://www.bu.edu/aodhealth/2023/02/14/out-now-behind-the-evidence-podcast/
Other	Providers Clinical Support System (PCSS)—Opioid Use Disorder[95]	https://pcssnow.org/
	Providers Clinical Support System (PCSS)—Alcohol Use Disorder[96]	https://www.pcss-maud.org/
	Alcohol, Other Drugs, and Health Newsletter[97]	https://www.bu.edu/aodhealth/
	Opioid Response Network[98]	https://opioidresponsenetwork.org
Immersive Programs	Chief Resident Immersion Training (CRIT)[99]	https://www.bumc.bu.edu/care/education-and-training-programs/training-programs/crit/
	Clinical Addiction Research Faculty Scholars (CARE)[100]	

population with a high prevalence of SUD.[25] SWs who have completed their bachelor's degree may consider pursuing an advanced degree such as an MSW or a Doctorate in Social Work. They may choose a degree program that provides addiction certificates or specialization.[115,116] Among SWs who qualify through an MSW, those with 3,000 hours of post-MSW supervision and 180 hours of professional education can apply to be a Certified Clinical Alcohol, Tobacco, and other Drugs Social Worker through the National Association of Social Workers (NASW).[117]

In addition, core competencies for SWs addressing SUD have been developed through the Association for Multidisciplinary Education and Research in Substance Use and Addiction (AMERSA).[23] These competencies are divided into recommended knowledge, attitudes, and skills for SWs across a continuum of care settings and align with the NASW code of ethics, and NASW Standards for Social Work Practice with Clients with Substance Use Disorders.[118] The NASW has also developed credential standards to become a Certified Clinical Alcohol and Other Drugs Social Worker (CATODSW).[117] In addition, the Canadian Center on Substance Abuse has developed 18 core competencies for SWs working with clients with SUD.[111] While not specific to the hospital, many of these principles may be adapted for the hospital setting.

Pharmacists

Hospital pharmacists frequently check medication orders for dosage safety reviews, alert prescribers of drug-to-drug interactions to ensure the safe administration of SUD pharmacotherapy, and lead hospital pharmacy and therapeutics committees that determine hospital formularies, making them key stakeholders in providing SUD care for hospitalized patients. While most pharmacy students receive some education in evaluating and managing SUD, significant knowledge gaps persist, as detailed earlier in this chapter. Institutions have described training pharmacy students to educate patients admitted to the hospital on overdose education and naloxone distribution to patients (OEND).[119] Pharmacy school graduates may go on to complete 1-year general practice residencies followed by a second year of a specialty residency, some of which offer additional training in SUD. The most robust training is found in psychiatric pharmacy residencies. There are currently 1540 pharmacists with a Psychiatric Pharmacy Specialty Certification (BCPP) in the US. Pharmacists who pass this specialized board certification are tested on comprehensive SUD content, including treatment of SUD, motivational interviewing, reducing barriers to care, and harm reduction.[120] AMERSA has called for expanded education efforts and developed a list of core competencies pertaining to SUD for all practicing pharmacists.[113]

Interprofessional Education

Hospital care is delivered in interprofessional settings, collaborating with clinicians, nurses, pharmacists, SWs, and other hospital staff. Hospital-based SUD care has unique learning opportunities for interprofessional collaboration, as many hospitals are already teaching sites for multiple professions. Hospital-based addiction consultation services provide opportunities to place learners from different disciplines, such as pharmacy, physicians, and social work, in a shared clinical learning environment. Educators interested in this work should consider developing new or utilizing existing educational structures and using a competency framework to assess their educational sessions as described below.

A scoping review of 14 studies on interprofessional SUD education in health professions students found that SUD educational interventions enhanced students' knowledge, skills, and attitudes toward SUD care and improved interprofessional collaboration.[121] Many of the interventions included either a simulation with standardized patients or supervised counseling of patients with SUD, allowing students to apply learned skills in real-life scenarios.[37,122–125]

Using existing conference structures can be one modality of encouraging interprofessional learning. For example, a morbidity–mortality conference on a recently discharged patient with SUD who had an adverse outcome or left the hospital prematurely could provide opportunities for interprofessional learning. Shared formal didactics, interprofessional team huddles, and interactive workshops all provide opportunities for interprofessional SUD learning.

It is recommended that educators using the hospital learning environment for interprofessional learning select a competency framework for their educational work. Interprofessional competency frameworks have been developed and can be summarized into themes of (1) roles and responsibilities, (2) ethical practice, (3) conflict resolution, (4) communication, and (5) collaboration and teamwork.[126] While not specific to the hospital setting, this framework can be adapted when developing interprofessional education experiences for learners at all levels.

Tips on Navigating Challenging Situations as an Educator

Challenging clinical and ethical scenarios may arise when caring for hospitalized patients with SUD. These situations can lead to significant distress for

TABLE 5.8

A Challenging Hospital Scenario and Specific Components of an Emotional Debriefing That Uses the Mnemonic WATER

Example Scenario: A resident on an addiction consultation service has returned after seeing a new consult for a patient with opioid use disorder currently on methadone who has been admitted 4 times this month, now admitted with infective endocarditis. They cared for the patient on 3 out of 4 of these admissions. The resident appears frustrated during multidisciplinary rounds when describing the patient's continued substance use and hospital stay. The addiction consultation team includes a social worker, an addiction fellow, a resident, and an attending physician.

Debrief component	Goal	Example debriefing
Welfare check	Brief check-in to gauge their state of mind and if they are able to continue providing care	The attending checks in on the resident's emotional state. The resident reports they feel frustrated and that they have failed the patient because the patient keeps using substances and returning to the hospital.
Acute/short-term corrections	Review active medical issues and any matters to be addressed, caring for the next clinical case	Ask if the patient is describing any new pain, withdrawal, cravings, or anxiety that may be new to this admission. The resident reports that the patient has been feeling more withdrawal symptoms since starting a new antibiotic, rifampin.
Team reactions and reflections	Summarize the case and listen to learner and/or team member reactions	The attending summarizes that this is a patient with OUD and frequent hospital admissions due to continued substance use and acknowledges that the consult team has invested a lot of time caring for this patient on multiple admissions. The social worker notes that this month is tough for the patient as their friend passed away from an overdose, which could be contributing. The addiction fellow remembers the patient from earlier that month who stated a goal of reducing rather than abstaining from opioid use.
Education from a professional and resources	Provide teaching pearls, discuss lessons learned, and share resources	The attending reframes the case through a harm reduction lens of "any positive change" as a measure of success and reinforces that continued opioid use does not mean the resident is failing. The attending shares learning pearls that rifampin increases the clearance rate of methadone putting the patient at risk of opioid withdrawal and suggests offering an increased methadone dose.

both patients and clinicians. Educators should be prepared to help learners navigate complex situations, such as in-hospital substance use, severe agitation, reporting mandates to child protective services, and legal system involvement. In addition, learners at all levels and disciplines who work with this population may experience burnout and moral distress. Educators should anticipate and be prepared to support learners through emotional debriefing and supervision tailored to different training levels when these challenging scenarios occur. A framework for emotional debriefing, called WATER, can be found in Table 5.8, and practical tips for faculty navigating a selection of common challenging situations in hospital-based SUD care are discussed here (see Table 5.9).[127]

In-hospital Substance Use

In-hospital substance use is a frequent occurrence among patients with SUD.[128,129] Hospitals often lack a unified policy addressing this issue, leading to conflicts between medical staff and patients.[130] Learners may interpret in-hospital substance use as a personal failure to address patients' care needs. In some cases, more advanced learners such as residents or fellows may be asked to discharge patients from the hospital to "punish" them for in-hospital use of substances. Preceptors can support learners facing this scenario on multiple levels. First, modeling how to talk with patients about in-hospital substance use can help normalize this phenomenon and create a plan for how to address it when it occurs. This includes having a plan to address overdoses that occur in the hospital. In addition, when learners perceive in-hospital substance use as a personal failure to address patients' pain or withdrawal symptoms, educators should reframe this occurrence as a symptom of the SUD itself (eg, strong cravings, withdrawal) that is part of the patients' medical illness. Finally, preceptors can support learners by role modeling or being present for difficult discussions with other hospital staff and providing space to debrief after these interactions occur. For those working in hospitals without a clear policy around in-hospital substance use, this also provides an opportunity for quality improvement.

TABLE 5.9

Challenging Hospital Scenarios and Discussion Points for Learner Debriefing

Scenarios	Suggested reflections and teaching points during a debrief
In-hospital substance use	■ Prepare the learner before the encounter to ask, "are you having withdrawal, cravings, or pain?" ■ Ask the learner how they feel about the case ■ Review biopsychosocial model of addiction to reframe use as a moral failing
Acutely agitated patient	■ Prepare the learner before the encounter to step away at any time during the assessment to maintain individual safety first and foremost ■ Reflect on the targeted assessment and triage of the patient
A patient is using substances and is also a parent of a young child. Child Protective Services is called by a hospital social worker to report concern of neglect	■ Review requirements of mandatory reporting and avoiding punitive Child Protective Service calls ■ Reflect on the complexity of the case holistically ■ Review strategies to avoid snap judgments to prevent conflating poverty with abuse ■ Ask the learner about what aspects of the case were emotionally challenging
The patient has to go to jail as a result of substance use–related activity	■ Review inequality in the criminal-legal system ■ Provide a toolkit to be an effective advocate at the individual, state, and federal level ■ Ask the learner about their emotions and how they managed them during the case
Patient dies of overdose	■ Reflect with the learner on self-care and coping with grief ■ Reflect on ways to improve patient care moving forward ■ Consider having morbidity/mortality case conferences
Learner burnout and moral distress	■ Reflect on ways to provide self-care ■ Review and refer individuals to local resources such as counseling services ■ Ask what aspects of the rotation have been emotionally challenging

Severe Agitation

Hospital-based addiction clinicians and the learners they supervise play an important role in supporting the medical management of substance withdrawal and intoxication, which may result in acute agitation. Agitation can progress from mild physical or emotional symptoms, such as fidgeting and anxiousness, to severe symptoms, resulting in combative behavior. Often, acute agitation can be effectively managed with behavioral interventions and de-escalation techniques. If these are unsuccessful, pharmacologic management and restraint may be required in severe situations. When working with learners, preceptors must remain keenly aware that acute agitation can place the patient at risk of harming themselves and others, including health care staff.

To promote safety, educators should consider the learner level and their prior clinical experiences to determine the level of faculty supervision needed when learners are managing acutely agitated patients. Faculty may consider direct observation for early learners or those without experience managing acute agitation. In a review of curricula on managing acute agitation among health professionals, less than 20% of the studies focused on acute agitation in the general medical setting.[131] Preceptors should check in with a learner before having them see a patient with acute agitation and discuss their management approach, as well as systems-level considerations such as the patient, staff, health care team, unit environment/logistics, health system (eg, policies on restraints) to ensure the learner has appropriate supervision and support to navigate the encounter safely.[132] Safety must be prioritized, and learners should know to step away and end the encounter early to maintain individual safety first and foremost.

Child Protective Services

Another difficult scenario is mandatory reporting to child protective services, either for patients with children at home or those presenting for obstetrical care. It is important to be aware of state-specific laws around mandated reporting, as well as federal laws that govern policy related to substance use and families that can be found in the Child Abuse Prevention and Treatment (CAPTA) and Comprehensive Addiction Recovery Act (CARA)[133,134] Learners should be encouraged to discuss situations where reporting may be required and avoid snap judgments that can result in unnecessary reporting. Depending on the learner's level of education (ie, student vs resident or fellow), it may be more appropriate for the educator to complete reporting requirements. In hospitals where SWs typically make these reports, encourage open communication between the SWs and medical teams. Maintaining transparent communication with patients around reporting is essential and allows educators to model trauma-informed care. Learners may have strong feelings or responses to reporting. Provide time and space to debrief. In states with laws that punish and criminalize substance use during pregnancy, consider using these events as an opportunity to teach learners about advocacy and opportunities for change.

Criminal-Legal Involvement

Some patients with SUD hospitalized for acute care needs may be incarcerated. This poses specific challenges, including additional layers of stigma, patient privacy during clinical encounters (eg, an officer in the room), and uncertainty about continued care after discharge when starting medications for SUD. Learners may struggle with both conscious and unconscious bias toward those who are incarcerated, particularly if they have not received training in working with this population.[135] Preceptors can utilize these experiences as an opportunity for education and advocacy to reduce inequities in the criminal legal system. For example, a preceptor can use such an encounter to model a nonjudgmental interview style, provide education on overdose risk upon release from incarceration, review the privacy rights of incarcerated patients who are hospitalized and coordinate with medical units of local jails and prisons to determine which medications can be continued after hospitalization.[136]

Maintaining Wellness and Navigating Moral Distress

Health professionals, such as physicians, SWs, and advanced practice providers, have found working on a hospital-based addiction consultation service intrinsically satisfying.[137] Despite this, addiction clinicians are at risk of experiencing burnout and moral distress as they care for patients with complex social determinants of health and behavioral health needs. Furthermore, clinicians may experience secondary trauma through working with individuals who may have suffered from traumatic events. Clinicians working on an addiction consultation service have described system barriers, such as limited resources contributing to provider burnout, and team dynamics that can influence perceptions of burnout and resilience.[137] In addition, a staggering number of drug overdose deaths continue each year, and many addiction clinicians may experience grief from the loss of patients to overdose or other causes of premature death.[138] If left unaddressed, these disturbances may negatively impact the clinician's well-being. Educators should be aware of how this work may impact individual learners. Strategies to help mitigate intense emotions, maintain wellness, and support individual learners are described here.

Depending on the length of the clinical experience, educators may consider asking learners to complete formal self-assessment tools, such as the Maslach Burnout Inventory, or Measure of Moral Distress for Health professionals.[139,140] Using validated tools may be helpful to trend learner wellness over time, such as for learners completing a fellowship. For shorter rotations, it is recommended that educators create a safe environment to discuss topics such as moral distress and inform learners at the start of the rotation that they can be a resource to support emotional processing and well-being.[141]

If learners experience an acutely distressing clinical scenario, expressing signs of burnout, moral distress, or secondary trauma, educators should proactively check in with the learner and offer support. Emotional debriefing can be one way that supervisors can support learners in navigating challenging scenarios and intense emotions that may occur within hospital-based SUD care.[142] Several models for psychological debriefing have been described within health care.[142] One debriefing model utilizes a mnemonic WATER, which was developed to debrief the clinical care of a patient and the clinician's well-being described in Table 5.8.[127] Debriefing components of WATER include the following: welfare check, acute/short-term corrections, team reactions and reflections, education from a professional, and resource awareness.[127] It is recommended that preceptors select an emotional debriefing model that fits the context of the scenario, learner, and institution when utilizing this strategy. Table 5.9 provides some sample reflections and teaching points preceptors may consider using during common hospital-based SUD scenarios that may involve learner emotional debriefing.

Beyond emotional debriefing, strategies to decrease health care burnout may include small group discussions, mindfulness, stress management, and structural interventions.[143] Additional research is needed to determine the context in which specific interventions may be the most effective. Among addiction clinicians, a qualitative study found that engaging in meaningful work, such as supporting underserved patients, advocacy, and education, helped increase their resilience.[137]

Educators can consider supporting and developing opportunities to promote patient advocacy for learners. In addition, strategies to address grief associated with patient deaths may include memorial services, support groups, retreats, and emotional debriefing.[138,144] Some learners may benefit from formalized counseling services. It is important to be familiar with institutional resources, such as employee assistance programs (EAP) that offer counseling and university resources.

Conclusion

Expanding SUD treatment within hospitals is crucial for addressing morbidity and mortality associated with SUD. Hospitals are well suited to provide training environments where health professionals can learn evidence-based practices to address SUD prevention, screening, diagnosis, treatment, and learn harm reduction principles. Clinical rotations in the hospital setting give health professional learners the opportunity to practice skills such as managing substance withdrawal, starting pharmacotherapy, providing overdose education, and treating co-occurring medical and psychiatric conditions.

Conducting needs assessments can guide the development of curricula and clinical rotations to create impactful hospital-based SUD clinical experiences. Curricula and rotations should be tailored to the needs of various learner level, discipline, and when possible, include interprofessional collaborations. Several resources are available and described in this chapter that educators may utilize to support their efforts in curriculum design, and evaluation. Clinical rotations may occur through addiction consultation services or general practice models offer rich learning opportunities across a spectrum of SUD severity. Faculty who routinely supervise learners providing SUD care should be prepared to support them in navigating challenging scenarios unique to hospital-based SUD care. Limited literature exists on the impact of hospital-based addiction rotations on learners' attitudes, knowledge, skills, and future careers in the field. Although the impact of an addiction consultation services rotation has been described, additional research is needed to evaluate learner outcomes and identify best practices for effective hospital-based SUD educational interventions.[46,47]

The hospital environment can be a robust clinical learning environment for health professional trainees to learn how to care for individuals with SUD. Hospital systems should ensure they have well-trained faculty and allied health professionals to educate the next generation of health professionals to provide evidence-based SUD care. Many freely available educational resources exist to support faculty. Ultimately, a well-trained hospital workforce will expand access to evidence-based SUD care, reduce structural stigma in health systems, and better address the health needs of patients with SUD.

REFERENCES

1. Substance Abuse and Mental Health Services Administration. Core curriculum elements on substance use disorder for early academic career: medical and health professions education programs. Updated March 12, 2024. Accessed October 12, 2024.
2. Accreditation Council for Graduate Medical Education. *Common Program Requirements*. Updated February 9, 2025. https://www.acgme.org/programs-and-institutions/programs/common-program-requirements
3. Schleiter K, Johnson L, Combes JR. GME stakeholders congress on preparing residents and fellows to manage pain and substance use disorder. *J Grad Med Educ*. 2021;13(5):739–742.
4. Sokolski E, Buchheit BM, Desai S, Englander H. It's time to train residents in addiction medicine. *J Grad Med Educ*. 2023;15(6):632–637.
5. Accreditation Council for Graduate Medical Education program requirements for graduate medical education in family medicine. Accessed January 16, 2026. https://www.acgme.org/globalassets/pfassets/programrequirements/2026-prs/120_familymedicine_2026.pdf
6. Accreditation Council for Graduate Medical Education program requirements for graduate medical education in internal medicine. Accessed January 16, 2026. https://www.acgme.org/globalassets/pfassets/programrequirements/2026-prs/140_internalmedicine_2026.pdf
7. Accreditation Council for Graduate Medical Education program requirements for graduate medical education in psychiatry. Accessed January 16, 2026. https://www.acgme.org/globalassets/pfassets/programrequirements/2026-prs/400_psychiatry_2026.pdf
8. Consolidated Appropriations Act, 2023, Pub L No. 117-328, § 1263, 136 Stat 4459 (2022) (Medication Access and Training Expansion Act).
9. Holt SR, Ramos J, Harma M, et al. Physician detection of unhealthy substance use on inpatient teaching and hospitalist medical services. *Am J Drug Alcohol Abuse*. 2013;39(2):121–129.
10. Jakubowski A, Singh-Tan S, Torres-Lockhart K, et al. Hospital-based clinicians lack knowledge and comfort in initiating medications for opioid use disorder: opportunities for training innovation. *Addict Sci Clin Pract*. 2023;18(1):31.
11. Campopiano von Klimo M, Nolan L, Corbin M, et al. Physician reluctance to intervene in addiction: a systematic review. *JAMA Netw Open*. 2024;7(7):e2420837.
12. Farhoudian A, Razaghi E, Hooshyari Z, et al. Barriers and facilitators to substance use disorder treatment: an overview of systematic reviews. *Subst Abuse*. 2022;16:11782218221118462.
13. Howley L, Whelan A, Rasouli T. Addressing the opioid epidemic: U.S. medical school curricular approaches. *AAMC Analysis in Brief*. 2018;18(1).

14. Tong S, Sabo R, Aycock R, et al. Assessment of addiction medicine training in family medicine residency programs: a CERA study. *Fam Med.* 2017;49(7):537–543.
15. Windish DM, Catalanotti JS, Zaas A, Kisielewski M, Moriarty JP. Training in safe opioid prescribing and treatment of opioid use disorder in internal medicine residencies: a national survey of program directors. *J Gen Intern Med.* 2022;37(11):2650–2660.
16. Thomas K, Muzyk AJ. Surveys of substance use disorders education in US pharmacy programs. *Ment Health Clin.* 2018;8(1):14–17.
17. Lafferty L, Hunter TS, Marsh WA. Knowledge, attitudes and practices of pharmacists concerning prescription drug abuse. *J Psychoactive Drugs.* 2006;38(3):229–232.
18. Farrell ML. Substance use disorders: a curriculum response. *Online J Issues Nurs.* 2020;25(1).
19. Knopf-Amelung S, Gotham H, Kuofie A, et al. Comparison of instructional methods for screening, brief intervention, and referral to treatment for substance use in nursing education. *Nurse Educ.* 2018;43(3):123–127.
20. Searby A, Burr D, Abram MD. Stigma towards a nursing specialty: a qualitative analysis of the perceptions of the addiction nursing workforce. *Int J Ment Health Nurs.* 2024;33(5):1460–1470.
21. Smith MJ, Whitaker T, Weismiller T. Social workers in the substance abuse treatment field: a snapshot of service activities. *Health Soc Work.* 2006;31(2):109–115.
22. Wilkey C, Lundgren L, Amodeo M. Addiction training in social work schools: a nationwide analysis. *J Soc Work Pract Addict.* 2013;13(2):192–210.
23. Osborne-Leute V, Pugatch M, Hruschak V. Social work: addressing substance use in the 21st century. *Subst Abus.* 2019;40(4):435–440.
24. Amodeo M. The therapeutic attitudes and behavior of social work clinicians with and without substance abuse training. *Subst Use Misuse.* 2000;35(11):1507–1536.
25. Krull I, Salas-Wright CP, Amodeo M, Hall T, Alford DP, Lundgren L. Integrating alcohol and other drug content in the social work curriculum: practices and perceived barriers. *J Soc Work Pract Addict.* 2018;18(1):30–48.
26. Englander H, Jones A, Krawczyk N, et al. A taxonomy of hospital-based addiction care models: a scoping review and key informant interviews. *J Gen Intern Med.* 2022;37(11):2821–2833.
27. Van Boekel LC, Brouwers EP, Van Weeghel J, Garretsen HFL. Stigma among health professionals towards patients with substance use disorders and its consequences for healthcare delivery: systematic review. *Drug Alcohol Depend.* 2013;131(1–2):23–35.
28. Zgierska AE, Miller MM, Rabago DP, et al. Language matters: it is time we change how we talk about addiction and its treatment. *J Addict Med.* 2021;15(1):10–12.
29. Brand PL, Jaarsma ADC, van der Vleuten CPM. Driving lesson or driving test? A metaphor to help faculty separate feedback from assessment. *Perspect Med Educ.* 2021;10(1):50–56.
30. Tetrault JM, Krause R, Roessler E, et al; Coursera. *Addiction Treatment: Clinical Skills for Healthcare Providers.* Accessed February 9, 2025. https://www.coursera.org/learn/addiction-treatment
31. Chan CA, Tetrault JM, Fiellin DA, Weimer MB. SOAPs and SUDs: patients with substance use disorders and what clinicians should know about the Cures act. *J Addict Med.* 2022;16(2):141–142.
32. Daugherty KK. Backward course design: making the end the beginning. *Am J Pharm Educ.* 2006;70(6):135
33. Smidt A, Balandin S, Sigafoos J, Reed VA. The Kirkpatrick model: a useful tool for evaluating training outcomes. *J Intellect Dev Disabil.* 2009;34(3):266–274.
34. Ayu AP, van der Ven M, Suryani E, et al. Improving medical students' attitude toward patients with substance use problems through addiction medicine education. *Subst Abuse.* 2022;43(1):47–55.
35. Avra T, Cowan A, Friedman J, et al. Decreasing stigma toward people who inject drugs: harm reduction training for first-year medical students. *Acad Med.* 2024;99(6):613–617.
36. Muvvala SB, Schwartz ML, Petrakis I, O'Connor PG, Tetrault JM. Stitching a solution to the addiction epidemic: a longitudinal addiction curricular thread across four years of medical training. *Subst Abuse.* 2020;41(4):475–479.
37. Gates SA, Brown JR. Preparing nursing and social work students to care for patients in acute alcohol withdrawal. *J Addict Nurs.* 2017;28(3):143–147.
38. Welsh CJ. OD's and DT's: using movies to teach intoxication and withdrawal syndromes to medical students. *Acad Psychiatry.* 2003;27(3):182–186.
39. Berland N, Fox A, Tofighi B, Hanley K. Opioid overdose prevention training with naloxone, an adjunct to basic life support training for first-year medical students. *Subst Abuse.* 2017;38(2):123–128.
40. Reynolds MD, Santa H, Hoffman J, et al. Training health professional students to conduct SBIRT: a step forward to interprofessional collaboration to address substance use. *J Interprof Educ Pract.* 2024;35:100701.
41. Clauser J, Richardson BB, Odom-Maryon T, et al. Standardized patient simulation using SBIRT (screening, brief intervention, and referral for treatment) as a tool for interprofessional learning. *MedEdPORTAL.* 2020;16:10955.
42. McAfee NW, Schumacher JA, Madson MB, Villarosa-Hurlocker MC, Williams DC. The status of SBIRT training in health professions education: a cross-discipline review and evaluation of SBIRT Curricula and Educational Research. *Acad Med.* 2022;97(8):1236–1246.
43. Braxter BJ, Puskar K, Mitchell AM, Hagle H, Gotham H, Terry MA. Nursing students' experiences with screening, brief intervention, and referral to treatment for substance use in the clinical/hospital setting. *J Addict Nurs.* 2014;25(3):122–129.
44. Balasanova AA, Eagen K, Marcovitz D. Rewriting the hidden curriculum via addiction consult services: meeting patients where they are at. *J Gen Intern Med.* 2023;38(9):2194–2197.
45. Marcovitz DE, Sidelnik SA, Smith MP, Suzuki J. Motivational interviewing on an addiction consult service: pearls, perils, and educational opportunities. *Acad Psychiatry.* 2020;44:352–355.
46. Gorfinkel L, Klimas J, Reel B, et al. In-hospital training in addiction medicine: a mixed methods study of health care provider benefits and differences. *Subst Abus.* 2019;40(2):207–213.
47. Gooding L, Hamilton M-A, Dong H, et al. Educational studies examining knowledge of substance use disorders and career aspirations among medical trainees in an inner-city hospital. *J Addict Med.* 2022;16(1):72–76.
48. Rose AJ, Stein MR, Arnsten JH, Saitz R. Teaching internal medicine resident physicians about Alcoholics Anonymous: a pilot study of an educational intervention. *Subst Abus.* 2006;27(3):5–11.
49. Grable JC, Shan K, Wang M, et al. training medical student counselors for the Rochester model, a hospital tobacco treatment program. *J Multidiscip Healthc.* 2024;17:601–607.
50. Stack NM, Zillich AJ. Implementation of inpatient and outpatient tobacco-cessation programs. *Am J Health Syst Pharm.* 2007;64(19):2074–2079.
51. Kumar A, Ward KD, Mellon L, et al. Medical student INtervention to promote effective nicotine dependence and tobacco HEalthcare (MIND-THE-GAP): single-centre

feasibility randomised trial results. *BMC Med Educ.* 2017;17:1–13.
52. Gummadi NH, D'Amico M, Chandra P, et al. Impact of cuddler service-learning program in medical student education of opioid use disorder in pregnancy and neonatal opioid withdrawal syndrome. *Subst Abuse.* 2021;42(4):951–956.
53. Barron R, Frank E, Gitlow S. Evaluation of an experiential curriculum for addiction education among medical students. *J Addict Med.* 2012;6(2):131–136.
54. Karam-Hage M, Nerenberg L, Brower KJ. Modifying residents' professional attitudes about substance abuse treatment and training. *Am J Addict.* 2001;10(1):40–47.
55. Meltzer EC, Suppes A, Burns S, et al. Stigmatization of substance use disorders among internal medicine residents. *Subst Abuse.* 2013;34(4):356–362.
56. Graddy R, Accurso AJ, Nandiwada DR, Shalaby M, Holt SR. Models of resident physician training in opioid use disorders. *Curr Addict Rep.* 2019;6:355–364.
57. Rastegar DA, Bertram A, Sisson SD. Use of an internet-based curriculum to teach internal medicine residents about addiction. *J Addict Med.* 2010;4(4):233–235.
58. Shershneva M, Kim JH, Kear C, et al. Motivational interviewing workshop in a virtual world: learning as avatars. *Fam Med.* 2014;46(4):251–258.
59. Chan CA, Cabaniss P, Morford KL, Martino S, Martin A, Windish DM. Medical improvisation-based motivational interviewing for internal medicine residents: mixed-methods evaluation of a novel course. *Med Teach.* 2023;45(12):1411–1418.
60. Iannucci R, Sanders K, Greenfield SF. A 4-year curriculum on substance use disorders for psychiatry residents. *Acad Psychiatry.* 2009;33:60–66.
61. Canver B, Liptak A, Clark K, Tetrault JM, Holt SR. Preparing physicians to treat addiction: inclusion of dedicated addiction training during internal medicine residency. *Subst Use Addctn J.* 2024;45(3):408–414.
62. Bottner R, Harvey JB, Baysinger AN, et al. The development and implementation of a "B-Team" (buprenorphine team) to treat hospitalized patients with opioid use disorder. *Healthc (Amst).* 2021;9(4):100579.
63. Laes JR. The integration of medical toxicology and addiction medicine: a new era in patient care. *J Med Toxicol.* 2016;12(1):79–81.
64. Whiteside LK, D'Onofrio G, Fiellin DA, et al. Models for implementing emergency department–initiated buprenorphine with referral for ongoing medication treatment at emergency department discharge in diverse academic centers. *Ann Emerg Med.* 2022;80(5):410–419.
65. *St. Louis Family Medicine Residency Curriculum: Addiction Medicine Concentration.* Accessed January 3, 2024. https://www.slu.edu/medicine/family-medicine/residency/curriculum.php
66. University of Kentucky Internal Medicine Residency. *Addiction Medicine Track.* Accessed January 3, 2024. https://medicine.uky.edu/departments/internalmedicine/addiction-medicine-track
67. Morford KL. Yale primary care's CHAMP: the case for addiction medicine training tracks. *Gen Intern Med.* 2025;48(2):14.
68. Holt SR, Segar N, Cavallo DA, Tetrault JM. The addiction recovery clinic: a novel, primary-care-based approach to teaching addiction medicine. *Acad Med.* 2017;92(5):680–683.
69. Howell BA, Puglisi L, Clark K, et al. The Transitions Clinic Network: Post Incarceration Addiction Treatment, Healthcare, and Social Support (TCN-PATHS): a hybrid type-1 effectiveness trial of enhanced primary care to improve opioid use disorder treatment outcomes following release from jail. *J Subst Abuse Treat.* 2021;128:108315.
70. Kunz K, Adger H, White WL, Brennan T, Lévesque A, Wilson DA. Chapter 35: Addiction medicine in America: its birth, early history, and current status (1750–2022). In: Miller SC, Rosenthal RN, Levy S, Saxon AJ, Tetrault JM, Wakeman SE, eds. *The ASAM Principles of Addiction Medicine.* 7th ed. Wolters Kluwer; 2024.
71. Accreditation Council for Graduate Medical Education (ACGME) – Public. Accessed December 15, 2024. https://apps.acgme.org/ads/Public/Programs/Search
72. Medicine TABoP. *Addiction Medicine Eligibility Requirements.* Accessed February 11, 2024. https://www.theabpm.org/become-certified/subspecialties/addiction-medicine/table/
73. AOA. *Addiction Medicine Subspecialty Certification.* Accessed February 11, 2025. https://certification.osteopathic.org/addiction-medicine/certification-process/
74. Accreditation Council for Graduate Medical Education Program. *Requirements for Graduate Medical Education in Addiction Medicine.* Accessed January 11, 2025. https://www.acgme.org/globalassets/pfassets/programrequirements/2026-prs/404_addictionmedicine_2026.pdf
75. Accreditation Council for Graduate Medical Education Program. *Requirements for Graduate Medical Education in Addiction Psychiatry.* Accessed January 11, 2025. https://www.acgme.org/globalassets/pfassets/programrequirements/2024-prs/401_addictionpsychiatry_2024.pdf
76. Yale School of Medicine. *Addiction Medicine APP Fellowship (SUSTAIN).* Accessed January 11, 2025. https://medicine.yale.edu/internal-medicine/genmed/addictionmedicine/education/sustain/
77. MetroHealth Addiction Medicine APP Fellowship. Accessed January 11, 2025. https://gme.metrohealth.org/en/programs/advanced-practice-provider-fellowships/addiction-medicine-app-fellowship/application-process/
78. Epstein RM. Assessment in medical education. *N Engl J Med.* 2007;356(4):387–396.
79. Ayu AP, El-Guebaly N, Schellekens A, et al. Core addiction medicine competencies for doctors: an international consultation on training. *Subst Abuse.* 2017;38(4):483–487.
80. Sklar DP. Competencies, milestones, and entrustable professional activities: what they are, what they could be. *Acad Med.* 2015;90(4):395–397.
81. Cate OT. Nuts and bolts of entrustable professional activities. *J Grad Med Educ.* 2013;5(1):157–158.
82. The Accreditation Council for Graduate Medical Education. *The Addiction Medicine Milestone Project.* Accessed January 11, 2025. https://www.acgme.org/globalassets/pdfs/milestones/addictionmedicinemilestones.pdf
83. The Accreditation Council for Graduate Medical Education. *Addiction Psychiatry Milestones.* Accessed January 11, 2025. https://www.acgme.org/globalassets/pdfs/milestones/addictionpsychiatrymilestones.pdf
84. Medicine ABoP. *Addiction Medicine Longitudinal Assessment Program (LAP).* Accessed February 11, 2025. https://www.theabpm.org/continuing-certification-program-ccp/addiction-medicine-longitudinal-assessment-program-lap
85. Davis D, O'Brien MAT, Freemantle N, Wolf FM, Mazmanian P, Taylor-Vaisey A. Impact of formal continuing medical education: do conferences, workshops, rounds, and other traditional continuing education activities change physician behavior or health care outcomes? *JAMA.* 1999;282(9):867–874.
86. Neufeld KJ, Schuckit MA, Hernandez-Avila CA. Alcohol medical scholars program—a mentorship program for improving medical education regarding substance use disorders. *Subst Abuse.* 2011;32(3):121–127.
87. Chief Resident Immersion Training (CRIT) Program in Addiction Medicine. Accessed January 11, 2025. https://

www.bumc.bu.edu/care/education-and-training-programs/training-programs/crit/
88. American Society of Academic Addiction Medicine. Accessed March 13, 2025. https://www.asam.org/
89. American Academy of Academic Addiction Psychiatry. Accessed March 13, 2025. https://www.aaap.org/
90. AMERSA's Podcast Series. Accessed March 13, 2025. https://amersa.org/amersa-podcast/
91. Society of Hospital Medicine. Accessed March 13, 2025. https://www.hospitalmedicine.org/
92. ASAM's Practice Pearls. Accessed March 13, 2025. https://asampracticepearls.podbean.com/
93. Curbsiders. *Addiction Medicine Season 1–3*. Accessed March 13, 2025. https://thecurbsiders.com/category/curbsiders-podcast/addictionmed
94. Alcohol, Other Drugs, and Health: Current Evidence. Behind the evidence: an addiction medicine podcast. Accessed March 13, 2025. https://www.bu.edu/aodhealth/podcast/
95. Providers Clinical Support System. *Medications for Opioid Use Disorder*. Accessed March 26, 2025. https://pcssnow.org/medications-for-opioid-use-disorder/
96. PCSS. *Providers Clinical Support System Medications for Alcohol Use Disorder*. Accessed March 26, 2025. https://www.pcss-maud.org/
97. Alcohol, Other Drugs, and Health Newsletter. Accessed March 26, 2025. https://www.bu.edu/aodhealth/
98. Opioid Response Network. Accessed March 12, 2025. https://opioidresponsenetwork.org
99. Alford DP, Bridden C, Jackson AH, et al. Promoting substance use education among generalist physicians: an evaluation of the Chief Resident Immersion Training (CRIT) program. *J Gen Intern Med*. 2009;24:40–47.
100. Boston University Chobanian & Avedisian School of Medicine: Clinical Addiction Research & Education (CARE) Unit. *CARE Faculty Scholars (CFS) Program in Addiction Medicine*. Accessed January 11, 2025. https://www.bumc.bu.edu/care/education-and-training-programs/training-programs/cfs/
101. Providers Clinical Support System. Accessed January 11, 2025. https://pcssnow.org/
102. Englander H, Patten A, Lockard R, Muller M, Gregg J. Spreading addictions care across Oregon's rural and community hospitals: mixed-methods evaluation of an interprofessional telementoring ECHO program. *J Gen Intern Med*. 2021;36:100–107.
103. Lindsey AC, Deem-Bolton C, Finley E, Potter JS, Lanham H, Fleming S. Leveraging Project ECHO to implement a suite of substance use learning communities for statewide impact. *Subst Use Addctn J*. 2024;45(4):690–697.
104. El-Dalati S, Cronin D, Riddell IV J, et al. The clinical impact of implementation of a multidisciplinary endocarditis team. *Ann Thorac Surg*. 2022;113(1):118–124.
105. Van Camp J, Chappy S. The effectiveness of nurse residency programs on retention: a systematic review. *AORN J*. 2017;106(2):128–144.
106. Fox JM, Wason K, Beers D, et al. The creation of an addiction nursing fellowship program for registered nurses: a unique approach to enhancing the addiction-treatment workforce. *Subst Abuse*. 2023;44(1-2):24–31.
107. Wason K, Potter A, Alves J, et al. Addiction nursing competencies: a comprehensive toolkit for the addictions nurse. *J Nurs Adm*. 2021;51(9):424–429.
108. Kane C, Brackley M. Psychiatric mental health substance abuse essential competencies taskforce of the American academy of nursing psychiatric mental health substance abuse expert panel. Essential psychiatric, mental health and substance use competencies for the registered nurse. *Arch Psychiatr Nurs*. 2012;26(2):80–110.
109. Finnell DS, Tierney M, Mitchell AM. Nursing: Addressing substance use in the 21st century. *Subst Abus*. 2019;40(4):412–420.
110. Education CoSW. *Specialized practice curricular guide for substance use social work practice*. CSWE. Accessed February 11, 2025. https://www.cswe.org/products/specialized-practice-curricular-guide-for-substance-use-social-work-practice/
111. Graves G, Csiernik R, Foy J, Cesar J. An examination of Canadian social work program curriculum and the addiction core competencies. *J Soc Work Pract Addict*. 2009;9(4):400–413.
112. Tran T, Ball J, Bratberg JP, et al. Report of the 2020 special committee on substance use and pharmacy education. *Am J Pharm Educ*. 2020;84(11):8421.
113. Bratberg J. Article commentary: pharmacy: addressing substance use in the 21st century. *Subst Abuse*. 2019;40(4):421–434.
114. Addictions Nursing Certification Board. Accessed January 11, 2025. https://ancbonline.org/
115. USC. *Social Work Practice in Addiction*. Accessed January 11, 2025. https://dworakpeck.usc.edu/academic-programs/graduate-certificates/social-work-practice-addiction-graduate-certificate
116. Indianna Wesleyan University Online B.S. Social Work Degree. *Addictions Specialization*. Accessed February 11, 2015. https://www.indwes.edu/program/bs-social-work/addictions/
117. National Association of Social Workers. *Certified Clinical Alcohol, Tobacco & Other Drugs Social Worker (C-CATODSW)*. Accessed January 11, 2025. https://www.socialworkers.org/Careers/Credentials-Certifications/Apply-for-NASW-Social-Work-Credentials/Certified-Clinical-Alcohol-Tobacco-Other-Drugs-Social-Worker
118. National Association of Social Workers. *Standards for Social Work Practice with Clients with Substance Use Disorders*. Accessed February /12, 2025. https://www.socialworkers.org/LinkClick.aspx?fileticket=ICxAggMy9CU%3D&portalid=0
119. Nguyen TT, Applewhite D, Cheung F, Jacob S, Mitchell E. Implementation of a multidisciplinary inpatient opioid overdose education and naloxone distribution program at a large academic medical center. *Am J Health Syst Pharm*. 2022;79(24):2253–2260.
120. BoP Specialties. *Psychiatric Pharmacy Specialty Certification (BCPP®)*. Accessed January 11, 2025. https://bpsweb.org/psychiatric-pharmacy/
121. Muzyk A, Smothers ZPW, Andolsek KM, et al. Interprofessional substance use disorder education in health professions education programs: a scoping review. *Acad Med*. 2020;95(3):470–480.
122. Monteiro K, Dumenco L, Collins S, et al. An interprofessional education workshop to develop health professional student opioid misuse knowledge, attitudes, and skills. *J Am Pharm Assoc (2003)*. 2017;57(2):S113–S117.
123. Mitchell AM, Riccelli A, Boucek L, Puskar KR, Hagle H, Lindsay D. Effect on dental hygiene students of a substance use simulation conducted with nursing students. *J Dent Educ*. 2018;82(5):469–474.
124. Tsu L, Buckley K, Early N, Jackowski R. Evaluation of multidisciplinary and pharmacy-only student-run clinics on student's perceptions of interprofessional roles. *Curr Pharm Teach Learn*. 2018;10(6):785–794.
125. Myers Virtue S, Rotz ME, Boyd M, Lykon JL, Waldron EM, Theodorou J. Impact of a novel interprofessional dental and pharmacy student tobacco cessation education programme on dental patient outcomes. *J Interprof Care*. 2018;32(1):52–62.
126. van Diggele C, Roberts C, Burgess A, Mellis C. Interprofessional education: tips for design and implementation. *BMC Med Educ*. 2020;20(Suppl 2):455.

127. Chen Y-YK, Szyld D, Clapp JT, et al. Crisis checklist for critical event debriefings: findings from a mixed-methods study. *JCA Advances.* 2024;1(3–4):100057.
128. Martin M, Snyder HR, Otway G, Holpit L, Day LW, Seidman D. In-hospital substance use policies: an opportunity to advance equity, reduce stigma, and offer evidence-based addiction care. *J Addict Med.* 2023;17(1):10–12.
129. Parmar GS, Hayashi K, Nolan S, et al. Non-medical prescription opioid use and in-hospital illicit drug use among people who use drugs. *Drug Alcohol Rev.* 2021;40(6): 959–963.
130. Strike C, Robinson S, Guta A, et al. Illicit drug use while admitted to hospital: patient and health care provider perspectives. *PLoS One.* 2020;15(3):e0229713.
131. Leppla I, Tobolowsky W, Patel S, et al. Scoping review on educational programs for medical professionals on the management of acute agitation. *J Acad Consult Liaison Psychiatry.* 2023;64(5):457–467.
132. Wong AH, Ray JM, Iennaco JD. Workplace violence in health care and agitation management: safety for patients and health care professionals are two sides of the same coin. *Jt Comm J Qual Patient Saf.* 2019;45(2):71–73.
133. Comprehensive Addiction and Recovery Act of 2016, Pub L No. 114-198, 130 Stat 695 (2016).
134. Child Abuse Prevention and Treatment Act, Pub L No. 93-247, 88 Stat 4 (1974) (codified as amended at 42 U.S.C. § 5101 et seq.).
135. Suh MI, Robinson MD. Vulnerable yet unprotected: the hidden curriculum of the care of the incarcerated patient. *J Grad Med Educ.* 2022;14(6):655–658.
136. Victor G, Zettner C, Huynh P, Ray B, Sightes E. Jail and overdose: assessing the community impact of incarceration on overdose. *Addiction.* 2022;117(2):433–441.
137. Bredenberg E, Tietbohl C, Dafoe A, Thurman L, Calcaterra S. Identifying factors that contribute to burnout and resilience among hospital-based addiction medicine providers: a qualitative study. *J Subst Abuse Treat.* 2023;144:108924.
138. Morford KL, Batchelor HM, Tetrault JM. Grief at the heart of the opioid overdose crisis: past lessons and present implications. *J Addict Med.* 2022;16(6):613–615.
139. Maslach C, Jackson SE, Leiter MP. *Maslach Burnout Inventory.* Scarecrow Education; 1997.
140. Epstein EG, Whitehead PB, Prompahakul C, Thacker LR, Hamric AB. Enhancing understanding of moral distress: the measure of moral distress for health care professionals. *AJOB Empir Bioeth.* 2019;10(2):113–124.
141. Beck J, O'Hara KL, Falco CN, et al. How attendings can help residents navigate moral distress: a qualitative study. *Acad Pediatr.* 2021;21(8):1458–1466.
142. Baum S, Lee P, Awan MU, et al. Assessment of psychological debriefing models' components & effective implementation, and its impact on healthcare professionals stress management skills, mental wellbeing, and clinical performance. *Am J Surg.* 2025;240:116118.
143. West CP, Dyrbye LN, Erwin PJ, Shanafelt TD. Interventions to prevent and reduce physician burnout: a systematic review and meta-analysis. *Lancet.* 2016;388(10057):2272–2281.
144. Yazdan R, Corey K, Messer SJ, et al. Hospital-based interventions to address provider grief: a narrative review. *J Pain Symptom Manage.* 2023;66(1):e85–e107.

6

Emergency Department Management of Substance Use Disorders

Sarah Follman, Arianna Campbell, Josh Luftig, Andrew Herring, Gail D'Onofrio

When Marcus was 20 years old, he underwent knee surgery and was prescribed oxycodone for severe postoperative pain. After the initial recovery period, his orthopedist transitioned him to nonopioid analgesics and stopped prescribing oxycodone. Marcus still had pain and had developed a craving for opioids, so began seeking oxycodone from friends and family and then turned to buying pills online. For the next 10 years he suffered with a worsening opioid use disorder (OUD), until finding hope and a new path forward through buprenorphine treatment offered through a telehealth clinic.

Then came a setback—Marcus reinjured his knee and was again prescribed oxycodone and continued buprenorphine as part of the plan developed with his orthopedist and addiction medicine provider. However, once again, he returned to opioid use, and after repeated positive urine drug toxicology screens, both his orthopedist and telemedicine addiction medicine physicians terminated his care. Frustrated and desperate, Marcus was out of oxycodone and buprenorphine and got into his car, intending to buy street pills he knew were assuredly fentanyl. On his way to the spot where he knew he could find pills on the street, he spotted a hospital sign and had second thoughts about his plan. Though he initially checked into the ED complaining of knee pain, after seeing signs about offerings for opioid treatment services, he opened up about his true reason for coming in.

With this information, the treatment was clear. Marcus was prescribed buprenorphine in the fast-track area, and he was connected to ongoing OUD care at the low-barrier bridge clinic. Today, Marcus receives monthly buprenorphine injections and is grateful he was able to get immediate treatment at a moment of vulnerability, and when he felt abandoned by health care. He has since earned a promotion at work and is enjoying life with his young children and partner. He often reflects on that pivotal moment—with his tolerance down, seeking street pills could have ended in a fatal overdose. Instead, having an accessible way to restart treatment saved his life.

—Sarah Follman

Key Points

- **Emergency departments (EDs) are critical entry points for individuals with substance use disorder (SUD).**
- **Medications for opioid use disorder (OUD) can be safely and effectively started in the ED and can save lives.**
- **Alcohol withdrawal syndrome management and medications for alcohol use disorder (MAUD) can safely and effectively be started in the ED.**
- **Other substance use disorders, such as stimulant use disorder, need a structured ED response including referral to treatment.**

- **Patients and ED clinicians benefit from a substance use navigator (SUN) to assist with patient ED and follow-up care in the community.**
- **Core components of successful ED-based SUD programs include physician champion, SUNs, access to medications, and easily accessible care pathways to ensure adoption.**
- **Feedback and monitoring metrics drive improvement of ED-based SUD programs.**

Emergency departments (EDs) play a pivotal role in caring for individuals presenting with a wide spectrum of substance use and substance use disorders (SUDs). Beyond treating acute conditions such as substance intoxication, overdose, and withdrawal, EDs are uniquely positioned to reach complex, stigmatized populations that often face prejudice, overt discrimination, and structural exclusion from other settings in the health care system such as people struggling with SUD.[1,2] The combined infrastructure of emergency care in the US is massive and well distributed with over 155 million ED visits annually; this 24/7 open access infrastructure provides an opportunity for ED interventions to have a population-level impact on public health challenges.[3] Thus, the ED encounter is an important touchpoint for initiation of medications for SUDs including alcohol use disorder (AUD) and OUDs,[2,4] and studies show that when medications are offered in ED settings, people often accept treatment.[5] The ED visit also offers an opportunity to introduce and provide harm reduction strategies, and facilitate community connections and referrals to ongoing SUD care.[3]

Epidemiology of SUD in the ED Setting

In 2023, SAMHSA estimated that almost 49 million people in the US have a SUD and more than 11% of ED patients have a SUD.[1,6] With almost half of all hospital-associated medical care in the US delivered in EDs, and with an almost 39% increase in ED visits for SUD between 2018 and 2021,[1,7] it is crucial that EDs have updated and evidence-based policies and procedures in place to treat people with SUD.[8] The most recent data from the Drug Abuse Warning Network (DAWN) that reports data on national estimates of substance-related ED visits from 53 participating hospitals estimated that there were 7,590,202 substance-related ED visits in 2023, or 2,266 per 100,000 visits, and increase by 5.8% compared to 2022, with similar rates across regions.[9] Alcohol was the most prevalent substance reported in substance-related ED visits (41%), followed by cannabis (11.8%), and opioids (11.6%). Of note, 21.6% of substance-related ED visits involved more than one substance.[9] The rate of ED visits related to substances was noted to be higher for males (2,778/100,000), Black individuals (4,053/100,000), and those aged 26 to 44 (3,245/10,000).[9]

While opioid overdose deaths overall have started to decelerate, there are regions such as the western US that may be accelerating and in certain populations.[10] Racial, ethnic, and sex disparities exist in the receipt of buprenorphine in EDs with patients who experience overdose or withdrawal.[11] Thirty years into the opioid epidemic, overdose deaths remain at levels never imagined possible in the US with more than 1 million deaths since the 1990s.[12,13]

Alcohol is the most prevalent substance reported in ED visits related to substance use at twice the rate of other substances,[14] and the third-leading preventable cause of cancer-related death in the US.[15] Though EDs routinely provide care for alcohol withdrawal, few provide medications for alcohol use disorder (MAUD), or medications to treat craving and decrease heavy drinking days.[16] Alcohol has been estimated to be a contributor to more than 178,000 deaths annually, making it one of the highest rates of preventable deaths in the US.[17] It is estimated that alcohol plays a role in more than 7% of all ED visits annually,[18] and alcohol preventable deaths and years of potential life lost due to alcohol have been increasing.[19]

With known evidence-based treatments for stimulant use disorder, discussed below, the ED visit is a prime opportunity to engage patients in treatment and harm reduction.[20] Stimulant-related overdose deaths and stimulant-related ED visits have also increased sharply.[13,21,22] Many of the complications arising from stimulant use and stimulant use disorder can be addressed in ED settings. Improving access to care with connections to cognitive behavioral therapy and treatments such as contingency management holds an opportunity to improve outcomes.[23] Recognition of different toxicities associated with stimulant use and pairing with treatment opportunities holds promise to improve care in ED settings.[20] Unfortunately, many patients present with polysubstance use, intoxications, and withdrawal states, making clinical care even more complicated.[24]

Evidence for ED-Based SUD Interventions

This section of the chapter will review each SUD with a focus on OUD, AUD, and methamphetamine use disorder (MUD) and summarize specific evidence regarding ED-based interventions for addressing different SUDs.

Screening, Brief Intervention, and Referral to Treatment

Screening, brief intervention, and referral to treatment (SBIRT) represents a comprehensive, integrated approach for identifying and addressing unhealthy substance use and SUD in ED settings. While SBIRT can be implemented at relatively modest costs, evidence regarding its clinical and economic benefits in ED settings have shown mixed results, most likely due to inclusion of different populations and wide variety of specific substances.[25–27]

SBIRT that includes specific psychosocial and pharmacotherapeutic interventions have been shown to be effective. Brief interventions, specifically the brief negotiation interview, for AUD and OUD have been documented in robust randomized clinical trials to decrease alcohol use in harmful and hazardous drinkers[28,29] and improve engagement in treatment for OUD.[30] Overall, brief interventions and referral for more severe AUD and SUD have improved engagement in community treatment programs.[29,31] In addition, integrating staff such as certified alcohol and drug counselors (CADCs) in the ED significantly improves the identification of patients with unhealthy substance use and SUD and increases successful referrals to treatment.[32–34] In one study examining CADC integration, EDs showed a 67% reduction in visits among patients who had high utilization of services in the 6 months following SBIRT intervention compared to baseline.[35] Substance use navigators (SUNs), such as in California Bridge programs or Health Promotion Advocates in the Project ASSERT model in Connecticut provide evidence that interventions provided by counselors embedded in the ED itself with fidelity to interventions and local champions can improve engagement in treatment.[5,29,33,36]

SBIRT typically begins with standardized screening using validated tools such as the Alcohol Use Disorders Identification Test (AUDIT) or Drug Abuse Screening Test (DAST-10).[35] In the ED setting, these are long and may not be as useful. Brief adaptations of screening questions, such as the National Institute on Drug Abuse (NIDA) and National Institute on Alcohol Abuse and Alcoholism (NIAAA) brief two-question screens are most effective.[37] The important goal is detection by any means, whether from screens, patient requests, presentation with complications of alcohol and substance use, or identified as part of the history, physical exam and ED stay. Brief intervention employs motivational interviewing techniques to engage patients in discussing their substance use and exploring readiness for change.[37] Evidence shows these interventions can be effectively administered by clinicians, nurses, social workers, dedicated counselors, and automatic digital health tool for Latino patients.[27,33,37,38]

Opioid Use Disorder

Large-scale engagement of people living with OUD with evidence-based treatment and harm reduction practices at critical touch points such as EDs hold the potential to change the course of the opioid epidemic and decrease overdose deaths by more than 50%.[4] While some communities are experiencing a deceleration in overdose deaths from a peak during the COVID-19 pandemic,[10] excess mortality remains alarmingly high, and in many particularly vulnerable communities, overdose rates continue to rise.[13] According to the Centers for Disease Control and Prevention (CDC), opioid overdose rates in Black and Indigenous/Native American individuals have grown while the death rates for White individuals declined.[13] This elevates the need to continue to expand access to medications through all entry points, importantly EDs.[8]

The consequences of untreated OUD are well described. The overall mortality risk in the 12 months following an ED visit for a nonfatal overdose approaches 5%.[35] If medications for opioid use disorder (MOUD), specifically buprenorphine or methadone is initiated, mortality decreased by more than 50%.[39] This mortality risk within the first year resembles that of other high-risk conditions like myocardial infarction.[40] This risk is mitigated by provision of opioid agonist such as buprenorphine or methadone in these settings.[5,30,41,42]

In a landmark randomized clinical trial published in the Journal of American Medical Association (JAMA) in 2015, D'Onofrio and colleagues demonstrated that initiating buprenorphine treatment in the ED significantly outperformed brief intervention and referral in several key outcomes.[30] At 30 days, 78% of patients in the buprenorphine group were engaged in OUD treatment, compared to 45% in the brief intervention group and 37% in the referral-only group.[30] Buprenorphine treatment also led to a substantial reduction in illicit opioid use, with patients decreasing use from 5.4 days per week to 0.9 days, compared to reductions of 2.3 days in the referral group and 2.4 days in the brief intervention group.[30] Furthermore, the use of hospital-based OUD treatment was notably lower among the buprenorphine group, with only 11% of patients requiring hospital care, compared to 35% in the brief intervention group and 37% in the referral group.[29] This important trial expanded the role of the ED to reach high-risk individuals with evidence-based OUD treatments.[29,36,41]

The California Bridge program has accelerated emergency physician administration and prescribing of buprenorphine with accessible follow-up bridge clinics.[5] CA Bridge found that providing buprenorphine treatment to ED patients with OUD was associated with significantly higher rates of engagement in OUD treatment 1 month later.[5] Among patients treated with buprenorphine in the ED, nearly 50% were still in treatment at 30 days, compared to only 23% of those not given buprenorphine initially.[5] Buprenorphine can be effectively implemented in a variety of ED settings. Over 14 months, CA Bridge established a buprenorphine treatment program in 52 diverse hospitals across California, emphasizing low-barrier initiation, patient navigation, and harm reduction strategies.[36] The program was successfully adopted by a range of facilities, including rural and teaching hospitals. Together, the hospitals identified more than 12,000 ED patients with OUD; 60% received buprenorphine, and 40% were connected to follow-up OUD care.[36] Notably, all participating hospitals continued offering buprenorphine 9 months after the funding ended, demonstrating the program's sustainability.[36] To incentivize system change, the California Department of Health Care Services offered financial support to hospitals to hire a SUN on-site in the ED and participate in a statewide CA Bridge training and technical assistance program. This program successfully reached 92% (291/316) of all the EDs in California to implement ED-initiated buprenorphine with patient navigation.[43] Prescribing of buprenorphine by ED clinicians increased from 2% to 16%, and buprenorphine initiation increased from 0.1% to 5%.[41] Of note, when buprenorphine is prescribed from the ED setting, one in nine patients who fill the prescription achieve 6 months of continuous treatment engagement, underscoring the essential role of EDs in providing access to lifesaving medication.[8,41]

In addition, a systematic review of studies examining emergency medical services (EMS) and ED-initiated buprenorphine found that buprenorphine significantly improved OUD treatment engagement at 30 days in both randomized (OR 5.97) and observational (OR 4.28) studies. Retention rates varied, ranging from 77% within 24 hours to 35% at 12 months, with a low incidence of precipitated withdrawal (0.00%).[44]

Safety and efficacy of buprenorphine appears consistent regardless of initiation dosing. A case series examined high-dose buprenorphine induction (>12 mg).[45] Data from 579 encounters involving 391 unique patients revealed that 63.2% received high-dose buprenorphine, including 23.8% with doses ≥28 mg.[45] No cases of respiratory depression or sedation were reported, and precipitated withdrawal (0.8%) was rare and unrelated to dose. Adverse events were minimal.[45] These findings suggest that high-dose buprenorphine initiation is safe, well tolerated, and feasible in the ED setting.[45,46]

Injectable, extended-release buprenorphine formulations (ie, lasting 7 days or 28 days) represent a newer treatment option for patients and offer the advantage of reducing the burden of taking daily medication. A nonrandomized control trial assessed the feasibility of administering a 7-day injectable extended-release buprenorphine in the ED.[47] This trial consisted of 100 adults with OUD and Clinical Opiate Withdrawal Scale (COWS) scores less than 8.[47] In this trial, 10% of patients experienced a significant increase in COWS scores, 7% transitioned to moderate or greater withdrawal, and 2% experienced precipitated withdrawal within 1 hour.[47] A majority of patients reported no cravings or opioid use during the study period, and injection site pain was reportedly minimal.[47] A majority of patients (73%) were engaged in OUD treatment by day 7.[47] The authors concluded that the 7-day injectable, extended-release buprenorphine formulation is acceptable, well tolerated, and safe for patients with minimal to mild opioid withdrawal.[47] This innovation in practice demonstrates the opportunity to offer "direct to inject" options for those individuals that present with lower COWS scores (4 or greater) while improving engagement in the cascade of care.

Methadone initiation is also feasible in the ED setting.[48] Newer regulations are making it easier to initiate and dispense methadone from the ED.[49,50] In 2022 Drug Enforcement Agency (DEA) implemented and update to the "72-hour rule" that allows clinicians to administer or *dispense* up to 72 hours of opioids for withdrawal treatment as a bridge to ongoing treatment. Each state is implementing this rule differently, and a first step to planning local implementation is to assure alignment with State Pharmacy and Medical Board regulations. Every patient who receives dispensed methadone should have an expected intake at opioid treatment program (OTP) for ongoing methadone maintenance treatment.

Guidelines can be interpreted differently regarding the appropriateness of repeat methadone dispensing for patients who do not succeed with initial engagement. To assure consistency, it is important that any health care setting that implements 3-day dispensing of methadone or buprenorphine establishes a clear governance and oversight of the program with multidisciplinary participation and clear documentation in the form of health system guidelines or protocols.

Alcohol Use Disorder

The ED provides unique opportunities to address AUD, as individuals with AUD utilize EDs at disproportionately high rates.[51,52] Clinical management guidance from the American Academy of Emergency Medicine outlines the emergency physicians' role in AUD treatment encompassing "withdrawal management, comorbid medical, social, substance, or psychiatric conditions, referral for ongoing medical and community-based wrap around care, and prescribing anticraving and withdrawal medications."[53] Evidence suggests that MAUD is both feasible[54,55] and associated with improved patient outcomes, such as reduced alcohol use and improved quality of life.[55] In addition, ED clinicians have also been optimistic about the opportunity to provide treatment to decrease heavy drinking days and improve outcomes for people with AUD.[3] However, adoption of initiation of MAUD from the ED has lagged.

Murphy et al, conducted a 12-week prospective open-label single-arm study of a multimodal treatment for AUD.[55] Patients were enrolled in the ED, received extended-release naltrexone, and referred for monthly injections with the help of case management services. Of the 32 enrolled patients, 25 (78%) completed all visits. This study underscored the feasibility of initiating extended-release naltrexone and case management in the ED. The authors found significant reductions in daily alcohol use and improvements in quality of life at 12 weeks. Sixty-nine percent of study participants continued naltrexone after the trial, demonstrating retention and adherence to ongoing naltrexone treatment.[55]

A protocol that combined medications with either oral naltrexone or extended-release intramuscular (IM) naltrexone for patients with AUD, along with substance use navigation to promote bridge clinic adherence, similarly demonstrated the feasibility of using MAUD in the ED setting.[54] This study further demonstrated that those who received extended-release IM naltrexone had better follow-up in formal SUD treatment at 30 days than those who received oral naltrexone (27.8% and 9.8%, respectively), which suggests a potential benefit to using extended-release IM naltrexone.[54]

A systematic review published by the Society for Academic Emergency Medicine identified studies that showed both oral and extended-release naltrexone provided in the ED setting resulted in decreased alcohol consumption up to 3 months after index visit.[56] In addition, monthly extended-release naltrexone injections resulted in significant improvements in drinking and quality of life.[56] However, the authors note that more direct evidence is needed with respect to using anticraving medications for AUD in the ED, and they acknowledge that it is challenging to connect patients with AUD to follow-up care after MAUD initiation.[56]

Gabapentin is another medication that is increasingly considered for treatment of AUD from the ED, particularly for the treatment of low-risk acute alcohol withdrawal. Gabapentin can be used instead of benzodiazepines for certain patients without risk for complicated alcohol withdrawal.[57] More studies are needed to look specifically at ED-initiated gabapentin, but there is increasing potential for its use at ED discharge. Hawk and colleagues are currently conducting an NIAAA study investigating the initiation of naltrexone and gabapentin in moderate–severe AUD compared with usual care.[58]

Stimulant Use Disorder

Presentations for stimulant-related ED visits differ from opioid-related ED visits. When compared to opioids, ED presentations related to methamphetamine, cocaine, and other psychostimulants are less often identified as related to substance toxicity or withdrawal. In addition, stimulant presentations more often require interventions to address acute cardiopulmonary and psychiatric complications.[59] Currently, ED-based interventions aimed at stimulant-focused harm reduction are less common and less well defined. CA Bridge has proposed a framework for management of MUD that combines pharmacologic treatment targeted to the phases of methamphetamine use with harm reduction and behavioral health interventions[31] (Figure 6.6). Future efforts could benefit from focusing on developing more robust support for patients with stimulant use disorders in the ED.

Cannabis Use Disorder

Rates of cannabis-associated ED visits are on the rise, and potential explanations for this include increased use, availability, and diversity of cannabis products.[60] ED visits for cannabis use often present as cannabinoid hyperemesis syndrome or psychiatric symptoms such as anxiety, paranoia, suicidal ideation, or cognitive impairment.[61] The treatment of cannabis use in the ED focuses on managing manifestations of acute toxicity and associated conditions such as cannabinoid hyperemesis syndrome. The latter is primarily managed in the ED with a combination of dopamine agonists and capsaicin cream and some patients require hospital admission for ongoing care.[62,63]

Substance Use Navigators

There is evidence that utilization of SUNs—health care professionals who connect patients with SUD to appropriate treatment and support services—is an important component of ED-based interventions to address SUD. Anderson et al demonstrated that whole person care-informed interventions delivered by SUNs for ED patients with SUD was strongly associated with higher engagement rates in SUD treatment after discharge.[33] A randomized controlled trial conducted by Gryczynski et al showed that substance use navigation services reduced hospital readmissions and ED visits for patients with comorbid SUD.[64] Their intervention, which featured proactive case management, advocacy, service linkage, and motivational support, led to a 36% reduction in ED visits and a 26% reduction in hospital readmissions over 12 months.[64]

Implementation Strategies to Improve Adoption

Implementation barriers for initiation of SUD treatment commonly cited by ED clinicians include time constraints, competing clinical demands, limited privacy, stigma, and insufficient referral resources.[65–67] However, these barriers can be mitigated through:

- Integration into existing ED workflows to minimize disruption
- Strategic staffing models aligned with peak substance use presentation times
- Comprehensive staff training with ongoing supervision
- Strong partnerships with community treatment providers
- Regular monitoring of both clinical and economic outcomes

Successful implementation has been shown to require more than education alone, but attention to both clinical processes and operations. Implementation facilitation strategies, including identifying local champions, developing community partnerships, employing ED navigators, having formal feedback and monitoring systems and availability of real time experts all make a difference.[65,67] Having dedicated SUD counselors or case managers appears particularly impactful. One study found that homeless patients were more than twice as likely to enter SUD treatment when working with a SUD counselor or case manager (OR = 2.34).[27] However, system-level challenges persist, including proper documentation. Research indicates that up to 45% of patients who screen positive for unhealthy substance use and SUD may not receive appropriate diagnostic coding at discharge.[68]

Future research should focus on identifying optimal program models, improving multilingual access, and determining which patient populations benefit most from ED-based interventions. While current evidence shows promises for reducing ED utilization,[69,70] more work is needed to establish the most cost-effective approaches to implementation.[69]

Integrating SUD Treatment in the ED Setting

This section delivers concise, evidence-based guidance to transform ED encounters into life-saving interventions, bridging acute care to lasting SUD recovery. It focuses on practical, actionable steps—program setup, patient assessment, treatment initiation, care navigation, and quality metrics—tailored to the high-stakes, fast-paced ED environment.

Building SUD Services in the ED

Effective ED management of SUD hinges on a lean, adaptable infrastructure. This setup empowers EDs to initiate evidence-based treatment and bridge patients to SUD recovery, even in resource-strapped settings. Start with essentials, then scale as capacity grows—evidence shows this approach doubles treatment engagement[30] and sustains programs long term.[36,41]

- **Clinical Champion:** An ED physician or advanced practice provider (APP), ideally with addiction medicine interest, leads program initiation and development. This person crafts protocols, develops electronic health record (EHR) pathways, trains staff, directs navigators, and troubleshoots resistance. Champions should have administrative support for this work, as their efforts will reduce unnecessary repeat ED visits and hospitalizations.
- **Substance Use Navigators (SUNs):** SUNs play a crucial role in ED settings, enhancing early SUD detection, treatment protocol adherence, care referrals, and community partnerships. By guiding patients through complex ED, hospital, and postdischarge treatment system, these professionals ensure continuity of care, with one navigator per shift recommended for optimal coverage. Evidence demonstrates SUNs increase treatment engagement by 34.5%,[33] and entry by 15%, while reducing hospital readmissions.[64] To maximize impact across diverse patient needs, navigators require training in SUD and medication treatment basics, local treatment ecosystems, and harm reduction strategies, such as naloxone distribution.[33,64] Comprehensive training materials are available at bridgetotreatment.org. EDs can staff navigators through direct hiring, harm reduction-focused staffing agencies, or partnerships with external clinics and community organizations. Success factors include thorough training, immediate ED availability, accountability to designated SUD program leaders (eg, a clinical champion), and access to expert consultation—all ensuring intervention quality and effective SUD care support.[65]
- **Medication Access:** The pharmacy must stock key medications and make them accessible within

TABLE 6.1

Risk Factors Amplifying Mortality and Morbidity From SUD in the ED

Risk factor	Clinical implications	Evidence-based intervention	Expected outcome
History of opioid overdose	High risk of recurrence and increased mortality risk	Immediate OUD medication initiation (buprenorphine or methadone); Naloxone distribution	Reduces subsequent fatal events
Use of multiple substances	Increased overdose risk, complex withdrawal, organ damage	Stabilization with medications targeting each substance (eg, buprenorphine + phenobarbital for opioid withdrawal + alcohol withdrawal)	Reduces synergistic risks; prevents withdrawal complications
Injection drug use	Elevated overdose risk, infection risk (HCV, HIV, abscess, endocarditis)	Immediate OUD treatment, infectious disease screening, harm reduction resources	Reduces risk for overdose; prevents complications; decreases in injection-related harms
Recent overdose/binge	Acute vulnerability period; cognitive impairment affecting decision making	Treatment initiation before discharge; warm handoff to treatment; peer recovery support	Addresses immediate mortality risks; capitalizes on "reachable moment" for intervention

30 minutes via automated dispensing (eg, Pyxis). For OUD, sublingual (SL) buprenorphine (8 mg doses) is essential, and long-acting injectables (24 mg weekly–300 mg monthly) are emerging as another crucial formulation.[31,47] Managing AUD necessitates availability of benzodiazepines (lorazepam and diazepam), phenobarbital (10 mg/kg) and naltrexone (50 mg PO and extended release 380 mg IM); MUD requires olanzapine (5 to 10 mg) and mirtazapine (30 mg). Prenegotiate with the hospital pharmacy to avoid delays—rural EDs in CA Bridge adapted this rapidly.[5]

- **Protocols and EHR Pathways:** Standardize care with clear guidelines: withdrawal management for OUD and AUD, buprenorphine initiation, treatment of worsening or precipitated withdrawal for OUD, and crisis deescalation. It is important to keep protocols and pathways simple and update annually with evidence.[46] Pathways embedded in the EHR with ordering and note writing are the gold standard and can be accomplished in many EHRs. Other workflows can be developed while pathways are automated.
- **Partnerships:** Forge ties with community providers—buprenorphine prescribers, SUD clinics, mutual support programs—for rapid referrals. Add harm reduction groups (eg, syringe services) and social services for housing or transport. Formal memorandum of understanding beat casual handshakes; CA Bridge sustained 100% hospital participation postfunding via these links.[36] ED clinicians often do not know that these services exist, nor the exact admission criteria or clinic times for specific programs, often leading to frustration on the part of the patient and clinician. The SUN will assist with making sure that most referrals are seamless.

Start with essentials: a single clinician champion, a navigator, core medications, and protocols. Research has demonstrated the effectiveness of multicomponent implementation involving local champions and protocol use while engaging in learning collaboratives with performance feedback compared to more passive educational offerings alone.[65] The local ED SUD team can work with the ED administrators to embed their work into the EHR and flow of the ED.[71] This framework provides critical support for patients and clinicians and will improve the care of those with SUD.

Developing Assessments

Rapid, targeted assessment in the ED is key for managing SUD. Universal screening for unhealthy substance use may not meet the needs of ED patients or staff. In the ED environment, there are over 50 potential screenings that could be of value to individuals, thus making them often irrelevant in this chaotic environment, and leading staff to rush through questions.[72] An alternative approach would be to use case finding to identify patients via clinical cues (eg, overdose, withdrawal, infections) or self-disclosure. Bold signage in waiting rooms, bathrooms, and treatment areas—"Want help with Fentanyl, Heroin or Pain Pills? Ask about trying Buprenorphine HERE in the Emergency Department TODAY!"—encourages patients with SUD to seek SUD treatment.[36]

- **Withdrawal Severity:** Gauge substance withdrawal with a mix of objective signs and patient reports—speed matters more than perfection. For OUD, an evidence-based scale such as the COWS can be helpful. It is important to focus on objective signs such as pupillary dilation, yawning, diaphoresis, tremor, diarrhea, vomiting, or tachycardia when assessing readiness for buprenorphine, as an example. AUD demands vigilance: tachycardia, hypertension, and tremors flag severity, with Clinical Institute Withdrawal Assessment-revised (CIWA-Ar) ≥15 marking high risk for seizures or delirium.[73] MUD lacks a formal withdrawal scale—focus on postbinge exhaustion, depression, or psychosis (eg, paranoia, hallucinations).[20] Experienced clinicians may skip formal assessment measures for gestalt, but tools standardize care in busy shifts and can be done by trained registered nurses.[74]

- **Risk Stratification:** Table 6.1 outlines key risk factors amplifying fatality and morbidity, guiding urgent intervention.[30,35] Identify these rapidly—each escalates mortality odds if unaddressed.
- **Documentation:** Briefly capture essential components of the patient's history: last use of substances (time, amount), withdrawal symptoms, risks (eg, overdose history), and patient goals ("I want to quit"). Example: "32 y/o M, smoking 1–2 g fentanyl daily, last use 10 hours ago, prior overdose ×2, presents experiencing severe withdrawal—hot/cold sensation, body aches, abdominal cramping, nausea, diarrhea—seeks treatment." While clinicians focus on medical decisions, support staff (SUNs, social workers) can obtain social history (housing, prior treatment history). This baseline documentation justifies intervention decisions, enable monitoring of treatment response, and facilitates effective care transitions.

ED Management of OUD

EDs serve as critical intervention points for OUD, where initiation of medications for OUD reduces mortality by over 50% and doubles treatment engagement at 30 days.[30] This section delineates evidence-based protocols for treatment initiation, management of complications, and coordination of ongoing care, aligning with the urgent needs of patients presenting with signs of OUD.

Buprenorphine Initiation

Implementation studies, such as the CA Bridge program, demonstrate feasibility of buprenorphine initiation for OUD across diverse ED settings.[36] Engaging patients through collaboration and shared decision making—eg, confirming readiness for initiation—enhances adherence. Importantly, patients do not need to commit to long-term treatment when they agree to ED-based buprenorphine initiation—they only need to express a willingness to try buprenorphine to manage their acute withdrawal symptoms. Further assessment of treatment goals and duration of treatment can be conducted at follow-up as an outpatient.

Web applications such as the "BUP Initiation" app can facilitate opioid withdrawal assessment and buprenorphine initiation.[71] Upon confirmation of opioid withdrawal, evidenced by objective signs of opioid withdrawal (eg, tachycardia, yawning, pupil dilation, diaphoresis, piloerection) and a COWS score ≥8, administer buprenorphine 8 to 16 mg SL[31,75,76] (Figure 6.1).

Given the prevalence of fentanyl in illicit opioid supplies—approximately 80% per recent analyses[77]—opioid withdrawal may present with heightened severity, necessitating titration to buprenorphine 24 to 32 mg SL in 8 to 16 mg increments every 30 to 60 minutes on the first day of initiation if symptoms (eg, nausea, myalgias) persist.[45,46]

High-dose buprenorphine initiation (starting with a single buprenorphine dose >8 mg) can be safely provided; a case series of 579 ED encounters reported no instances of respiratory depression or sedation.[45] Postadministration reassessment at 30 to 60 minutes should confirm withdrawal amelioration (COWS reduction >5), stable vital signs (heart rate <100 bpm), and ability to tolerate oral intake.

For patients who present to the ED with COWS scores less than 8, buprenorphine can be prescribed for unwitnessed, home initiation (Figure 6.2).[78,79] Another, more novel option is giving a 7-day extended-release buprenorphine injection at 24 mg (equivalent to buprenorphine SL 16 mg daily) for patients with COWS 4 or more with objective signs of withdrawal. This has been described as the "Direct to Inject" option.[47]

Risk Factors Amplifying Mortality and Morbidity From SUD in the ED

Patient: 32 y/o female, G2P1, 14 weeks pregnant
Chief Complaint: Fentanyl withdrawal, desire to quit

History of Present Illness

32 y/o female, G2P1, 14 weeks pregnant by LMP, past medical history chronic back pain s/p motor vehicle collision (MVC) 10 years ago, presents for evaluation of fentanyl withdrawal and wanting to quit using fentanyl. Smokes approximately 1–2 g fentanyl daily, has overdosed × 2 in the past, last use 12 hours ago. Feels "bad" from withdrawal, estimates 8/10 withdrawal severity. +Nausea, abdominal cramping, diarrhea, body aches, hot/cold sensation, nasal congestion, anxiety, and irritation. Occasionally smokes meth, last use 1 week ago. No other street drugs or ethanol. Previously on buprenorphine for ~6 months

when incarcerated 2 years ago, was on 24 mg daily and cravings were well controlled at that dose, but was frequently having breakthrough back pain in afternoons/evenings. No history of methadone use. No history of injection drug use. No chest pain, no SOB, no pelvic pain, no vaginal bleeding. Not receiving prenatal care. No other complaints.

Physical Exam

Vitals: BP 134/88, HR 102, RR 20, SpO_2 96%, Temp 37 °C
General: Anxious-appearing, uncomfortable, diaphoretic, occasionally yawning
HEENT: Nasal congestion, pupils mildly dilated, no rhinorrhea
CV: Tachycardic, regular rhythm, no murmurs
Lungs: Clear bilaterally, no wheezing or rales
Abdomen: Soft, no tenderness, no guarding, mildly hyperactive bowel sounds
Extremities: No edema, mild tremor noted
Neuro: Alert, oriented ×3, restless, no focal deficits
Psych: Anxious, irritable, no suicidal ideation

Medical Decision Making

32 y/o female, 14 weeks pregnant, with OUD, presenting with opioid withdrawal (last use 12 hours ago). Symptoms consistent with opioid withdrawal (nausea, diarrhea, cramps, myalgias, anxiety, autonomic instability) with COWS score likely elevated based on severity (not formally calculated) with ≥2 objective signs (yawning, tremor, tachycardia, dilated pupils). Patient is interested in buprenorphine treatment for her OUD. No evidence of acute overdose, infection, or other emergent pathology (eg, no chest pain, SOB, or vaginal bleeding). Differential includes withdrawal vs early pregnancy–related symptoms, though history strongly favors opioid withdrawal.

Plan

1. Lorazepam 2 mg PO × 1 for intense anxiety.
2. SUN engaging patient since their arrival at ED intake, providing motivational interviewing, discussing treatment options, and is supporting at bedside.
3. Buprenorphine start: 16 mg SL now, reevaluate in 30–60 minutes, titrate as needed (target 16–32 mg total).
4. PO hydration (initiate 20 minutes after sublingual [SL] dose to allow for full SL dose absorption).
5. Reassess symptoms and withdrawal severity postdose.
6. Ondansetron 4 mg PRN nausea.
7. Consult OB for outpatient prenatal care coordination.
8. SUN providing outpatient OUD treatment planning.
9. Discharge with buprenorphine prescription 8 mg TID (TID split dosing for optimal chronic pain management), take-home naloxone kit, prenatal vitamins, and follow-up if stable.

ED Course

- 1320: Patient received lorazepam 2 mg and buprenorphine 16 mg SL. PO hydration subsequently started.
- 1400: Reevaluation post-buprenorphine: Patient reports feeling "much better," withdrawal severity now 3/10. Vitals improved (BP 128/82, HR 88, RR 18, SpO_2 97%). Tolerating PO, declined ondansetron, eating a sandwich. Shared decision making regarding second dose—agreed upon an additional 8 mg SL buprenorphine, which was administered (total 24 mg).
- 1420: Patient stable, symptoms controlled, vitals normal. OB consulted; outpatient follow-up arranged. SUN provided harm reduction supplies, arranged a Bridge Clinic appointment tomorrow at 9 AM, and will give an appointment reminder call tomorrow at 8 AM. Discharged with buprenorphine 8 mg SL TID prescription (14-day supply with 1 refill), take-home naloxone (4 mg nasal spray), prenatal vitamins, and strict return precautions.

Complications

Precipitated withdrawal, occurring in less than 1% of cases,[45,46] generally manifests within 1 hour of buprenorphine initiation as an acute exacerbation of withdrawal symptoms (eg, agitation, vomiting, diffuse pain). This uncommon event, more likely with recent full-agonist use (eg, fentanyl within 6 hours), requires immediate intervention per (Figure 6.3). After precipitated withdrawal related to buprenorphine initiation is recognized, administer an additional buprenorphine 16 mg SL combined with lorazepam 2 mg PO to address autonomic instability and anxiety. Reassess every 30 minutes. Further buprenorphine 16 mg SL doses may be provided, with total doses reaching 48 mg safely due to buprenorphine's respiratory ceiling effect. In severe refractory cases, consider ketamine 0.3 mg/kg IV q 15 min PRN and fentanyl 200 mcg IV q10min PRN with close monitoring and continuous cardiac, pulse oximetry, and end-tidal CO_2 monitoring. Adjunctive therapies—eg, clonidine 0.1 to 0.3 mg PO for sympathetic symptoms and pramipexole 0.25 to 0.5 mg PO for restlessness—may supplement care. Avoid frequent repeat doses of benzodiazepines given risk of respiratory depression. Stabilization typically occurs within 2 to 3 hours; and patients can be discharged. Severe refractory cases requiring ongoing ketamine and fentanyl dosing require admission.

Special Cases

Pregnancy: Buprenorphine monoproduct (without naloxone) at 16 to 32 mg SL daily is the preferred agent, mitigating risks of maternal overdose and fetal

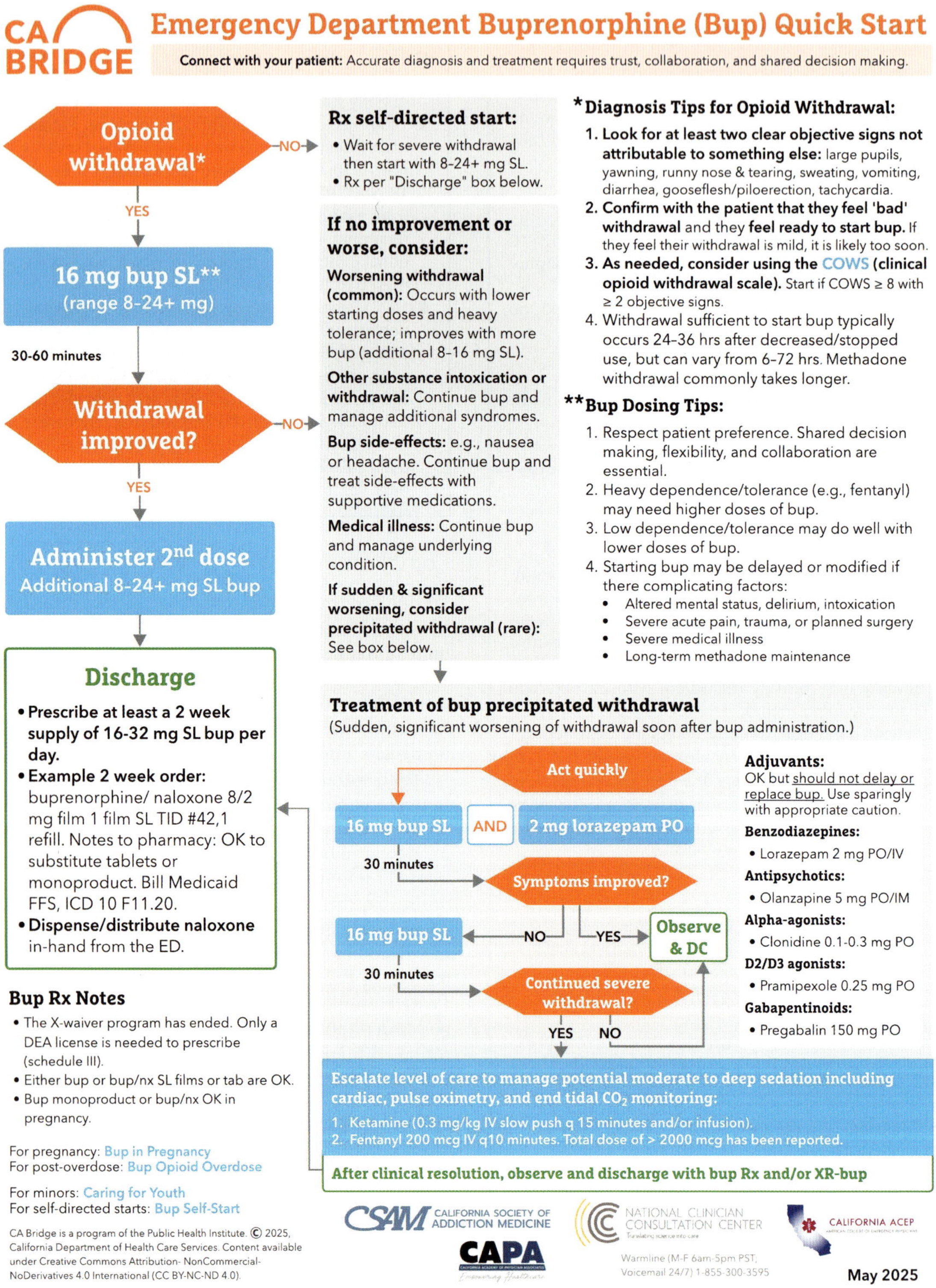

Figure 6.1: Emergency department buprenorphine quick start. (The California Department of Health Care Services funds this work through CA Bridge, a program of the Public Health Institute, via State Opioid Response (SOR) grants.)

A Guide to Begin Buprenorphine Treatment on Your Own

Before you being you want to feel **very sick** from your withdrawal symptoms

It should be at about...

- 12 hours or longer since you used fentanyl
- 12 hours since you snorted pain pills (oxycodone)
- 16 hours since you swallowed pain pills
- 48–72 hours since you used methadone

You should feel at least three of these symptoms...

- Restlessness
- Heavy yawning
- Enlarged pupils
- Runny nose
- Body aches
- Tremors/twitching
- Chills or sweating
- Goose pimples
- Stomach cramps, nausea, vomiting or diarrhea

Once you are withdrawing, follow these instructions to start the

DAY 1:
8–16mg of buprenorphine
Most people feel better the first day after 8–12mg
(dosing depends on: how early on the 1st day you started and severity of use)

Step 1

Take the first dose	Wait 60 minutes
8mg	60 minutes

- Put the tablet or strip under your tongue
- Keep it there until fully dissolved (about 15 min)
- Do NOT eat or drink at this time
- Do NOT swallow the medicine

Step 2

Still feel sick? Take next dose	Wait
4–8mg	1–2 hours

Most people feel better after 8mg, but some may need additional dosing

Step 3 (Ongoing symptoms)

Still uncomfortable? Take more	Stop
4mg	Stop

People with heavy use may need more buprenorphine. Most will do well with 8–16mg

DAY 2:
16mg of buprenorphine

Take one 16 mg dose

Most people feel better with a 16mg dose

16mg

Repeat this dose until your next follow-up appointment

If you develop worsening symptoms while starting buprenorphine before outpatient appointment return to the emergency department

A

CA BRIDGE

Buprenorphine Self-Start

Guidance for patients starting buprenorphine outside of hospitals or clinics

1. Plan to take a day off and have a place to rest.
2. Stop using and wait until you feel very sick from withdrawals (at least 12 hours is best, if using fentanyl it may take a few days).
3. Dose one or two 8mg tablets or strips UNDER your tongue (total dose of 8-16mg).
4. Repeat dose (another 8mg-16mg) in an hour to feel well.
5. The next day, take 16-32mg (2-4 tablets or films) at one time.

If you have started bup before:

- If it went well, that's great! Just do that again.
- If it was difficult, talk with your care team to figure out what happened and find ways to make it better this time. You may need a different dosing plan than what is listed here.

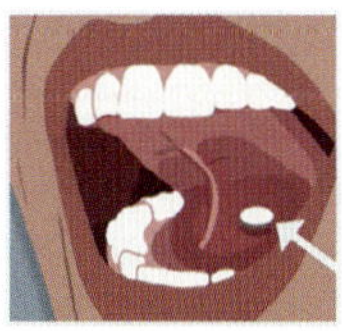

Place dose under your tongue (sublingual).

If you have never started bup before:

- Gather your support team and if possible take a "day off."
- You are going to want space to rest. Don't drive.
- Using cocaine, meth, alcohol or pills makes starting bup harder, and mixing in alcohol or benzos can be dangerous.

If you have a light habit: *(For example, 5 "Norco 10's" a day)*

- Consider a low dose: start with 4mg and stop at 8mg total.
- **WARNING:** Withdrawal will continue if you don't take enough bup.

If you have a heavy habit: *(For example, injecting 2g heroin a day or smoking 1g fentanyl a day)*

- Consider a high dose: start with a first dose of 16mg.
- For most people, the effects of bup max out at around 24-32mg.
- **WARNING:** Too much bup can make you feel sick and sleepy.

Not going well? Have questions? Contact your Navigator for help!

B

Figure 6.2: Buprenorphine home initiation instructions. **A:** Buprenorphine initiation protocol. **B:** California bridge self-start buprenorphine guidance. (The California Department of Health Care Services funds this work through CA Bridge, a program of the Public Health Institute, via State Opioid Response (SOR) grants.)

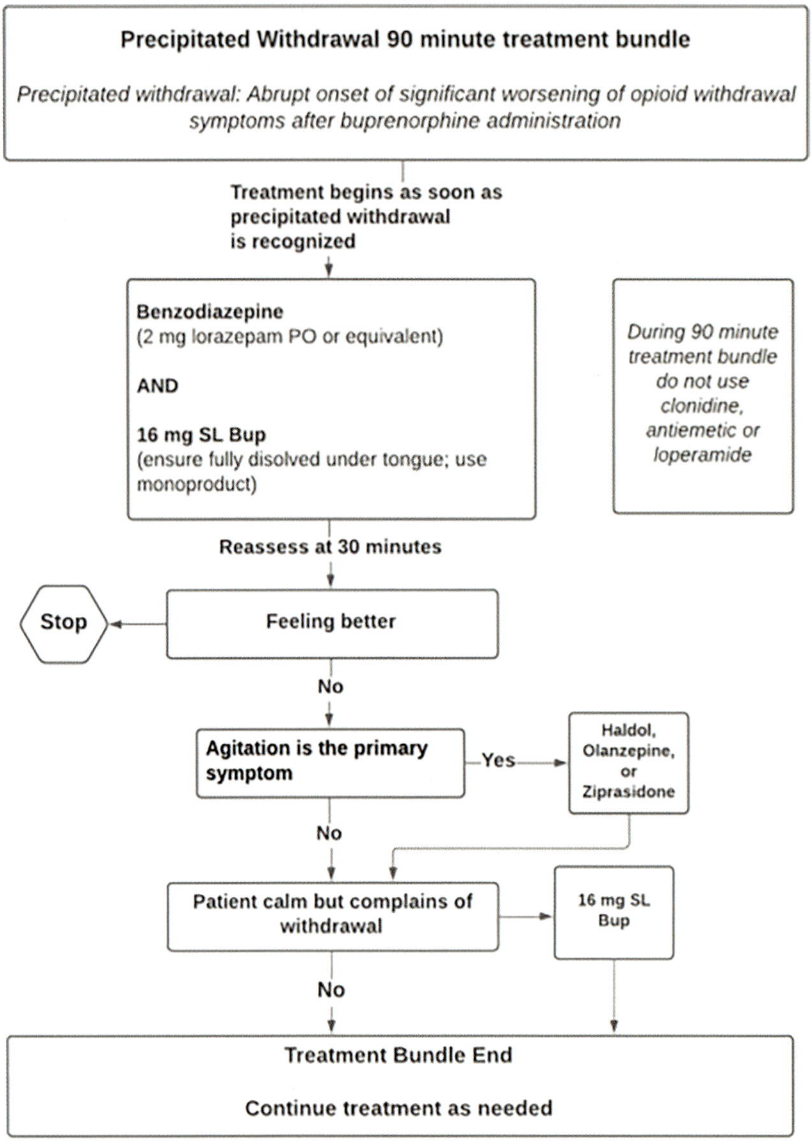

Figure 6.3: Buprenorphine precipitated opioid withdrawal management. (The California Department of Health Care Services funds this work through CA Bridge, a program of the Public Health Institute, via State Opioid Response (SOR) grants.)

harm.[80] Combination product (buprenorphine with naloxone) is also acceptable. Fetal monitoring is not required in the ED; obstetrical consultation should be arranged postdischarge.

Postopioid Overdose: For patients with a heroin, fentanyl, or short-acting opioid overdose reversed by naloxone, clinicians can initiate SL buprenorphine for stabilization.[81] Screen for exclusion criteria: benzodiazepine/sedative use, altered mental status, severe illness, methadone use, or inability to consent. If absent, confirm opioid withdrawal (COWS >4) and patient agreement for buprenorphine initiation. Can also consider buprenorphine home initiation. Use motivational interviewing to support ongoing care. Tailor to clinical judgment.

Methadone Use: Prolonged receptor occupancy increases precipitation risk; outpatient transition under the current prescriber is optimal.

Acute Pain, Already on Buprenorphine: Buprenorphine's high receptor affinity complicates full-agonist opioid analgesia (Figure 6.4). Leverage buprenorphine's potent analgesic properties with

CA BRIDGE

Acute Pain Management in Patients on Buprenorphine (Bup) Treatment for Opioid Use Disorder

Emergency Department / Critical Care

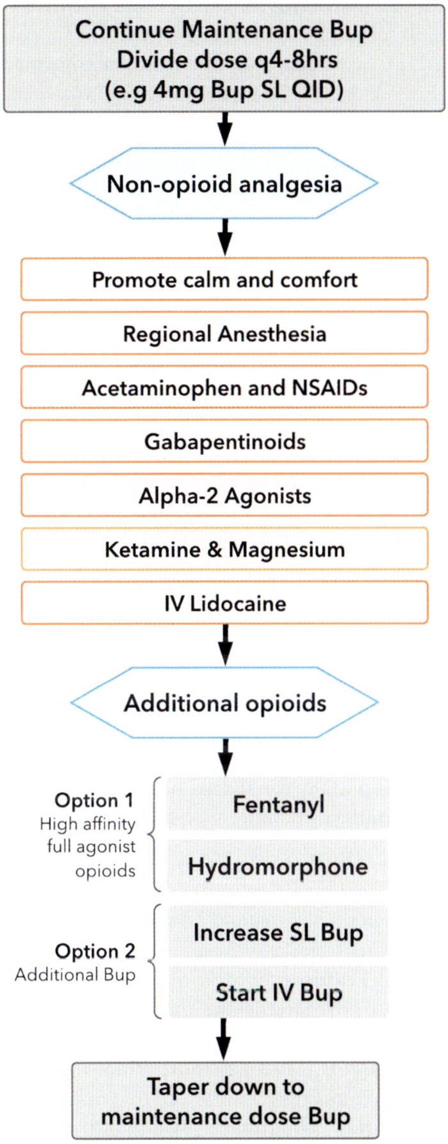

Promote calm and comfort

Anxiety, fear, depression are common: Instill sense of control, provide education on self-management techniques such as mindfulness or meditation. Reduce noise, uncertainty, confusion.
Positioning, splinting, and physical comfort should be maximized.
Minimize unnecessary NPO status.

TREAT UNPLEASANT SYMPTOMS:
Diphenhydramine 25-50mg PO q8h prn insomnia/anxiety
Tizanidine 2-4mg q6h prn muscle spasms
Ondansetron 4mg PO q6h prn nausea
Trazadone 50mg PO qhs prn insomnia
Melatonin 3mg PO qhs prn insomnia
Lorazepam 0.5-1mg PO prn anxiety
Antipsychotics prn psychotic disorder symptom control
Nicotine replacement prn tobacco dependence

Regional Anesthesia

Peripheral nerve blocks: superficial cervical plexus, brachial plexus, radial/median/ulnar, PECS, erratus plane, TAP, femoral, sciatic, posterior tibial.
Spinal and Epidural anesthesia

Acetaminophen and NSAIDs

Acetaminophen and **NSAIDs,** when not contraindicated, are the foundation of a multimodal analgesic strategy.

Gabapentinoids

In opioid depenent patients, the calcium channel inhibitors, gabapentin and pregabalin reduce postoperative pain and reduce opioid consumption. Gabapentin 300-600mg PO TID.

Alpha-2 agonists

Clonidine and Dexmedetomidine are anxiolytic and analgesic with significant opioid sparing affects. e.g. **Clonidine** 0.1-0.3mg PO q6-8h prn pain or anxiety (NTE 1.2mg/day, hold if BP <100/70).

Ketamine & Magnesium (NMDAR antagonists)

Ketamine is the most potent non-opioid analgesic for opioid tolerant patients. A brief infusion of 0.3mg/kg IV over 15min is followed by 0.3-1mg/kg/hr as needed.
Magnesium is also an NMDAR with analgesic and opioid sparing effect. eg. 30-50mg/kg bolus followed by 10-mg/kg/hr.

IV Lidocaine (Na channel antagonist)

Opioid sparing analgesic. A bolus of 1-1.5mg/kg is followed by 1.5-3 mg/kg/h. Contraindications include cardiac dysrthymias. Must monitor serum levels after 24hrs.

High Affinity Full agonist Opioids

Hydromorphone, fentanyl, and sufentanil can be added to maintenance Bup to provide synergistic analgesia. Titrate to analgesia and side effects. This will NOT cause withdrawal.

Additional Bup

There is no clinical ceiling on Bup analgesia. SL Bup can be given as frequently as q2h. IV Bup is a potent analgesic start at 0.3mg IV and titrate as needed. At higher doses respiratory depression does occur.

Guidelines are options for multimodal analgesic therapy. Use clinical judgement and avoid use if contraindicated.

November 2025

Provider Resources

California Poison Control
Available 24 hours a day, 365 days a year
1-800-411-8080

National Clinician Consultation Center
Warmline (M-F 6am-5pm PST; Voicemail 24/7)
1-855-300-3595

Figure 6.4: Acute pain management in patients treated with buprenorphine. (The California Department of Health Care Services funds this work through CA Bridge, a program of the Public Health Institute, via State Opioid Response (SOR) grants.)

higher, more frequent doses (eg, 8 mg SL QID, rather than 16 mg daily). Employ multimodal analgesia strategies (eg, NSAIDs, acetaminophen, ketamine) and regional anesthesia. High receptor affinity opioids (eg, hydromorphone, fentanyl) in elevated doses with appropriate monitoring can also be beneficial.

Concurrent Alcohol Withdrawal or Other Substance Use/Withdrawal: Start with alcohol withdrawal treatment before starting buprenorphine. If unsure whether it is opioid withdrawal versus a mixed substance withdrawal picture, start with adjunctive treatments.

Transition to Ongoing OUD Care

Prescribe a 14-day supply of buprenorphine (16 to 32 mg/d), 1 refill to address cravings or pain,[82] alongside take-home naloxone (4 mg intranasal) with administration instructions. Follow-up within 72 hours is ideal—telehealth options suit remote settings. One in nine patients sustains treatment at 6 months with this approach.[36] Discharge documentation should include: dosing regimen (eg, "8 mg SL TID"), naloxone instructions, follow-up appointment details (date, time, location), indications for ED return (eg, severe withdrawal). Hospital admission is warranted for severe complications (eg, endocarditis) or unstable comorbidities, though most patients are managed outpatient.

Methadone Initiation

Patients have a choice in evidence-based medications for OUD, which includes methadone, a synthetic full mu-receptor agonist that can be initiated in the ED or hospital setting with connection to ongoing care in an OTP. Methadone is ideal for those who are unable to be stabilized on a high enough dose of buprenorphine given it is a partial agonist with ceiling effects, or who prefer to have more frequent interactions with staff at OTP. However, barriers exist, in that one must travel to an OTP daily for often long periods of time before being eligible for take-home dosing. In addition, there are deserts of available OTP programs throughout the US.[83]

Initiation of methadone in the ED is feasible with similar follow-up rates to buprenorphine initiation in the ED.[84] The "72-hour rule" can be utilized for methadone initiation with a typical initial starting dose of 30 to 40 mg.[49,85,86] Federal regulation 1306.07b allows DEA-registered prescribers to dispense from the ED or hospital up to 3 days of methadone to initiate or continue treatment for OUD.[86–88] This 3-day supply provides a critical bridge for patients to connect with their local OTP for continued OUD care, with case studies demonstrating successful implementation of ED-dispensed methadone supplies.[89]

ED Management of AUD

AUD accounts for over 7% of annual ED visits in the US[18] presenting opportunities for withdrawal management and initiation of MAUD to reduce heavy alcohol use and mortality. This section outlines evidence-based protocols for acute care and care transitions for patients with AUD. See Chapter 8 for additional information.

Withdrawal Management

When patients present to the ED with alcohol withdrawal symptoms, rapid assessment is essential to determine the need for hospital-based withdrawal management versus ambulatory care. The Prediction of Alcohol Withdrawal Severity Scale (PAWSS) can help identify patients at risk for severe withdrawal.[90] Hospital admission is warranted for patients with severe symptoms, high-risk features, or inadequate social support. Other individuals without a history of delirium tremens, complex comorbidities (ie, cirrhosis, severe kidney disease, heart failure, COPD), unstable psychosocial factors, pregnancy, and mild alcohol withdrawal symptoms may be safely treated in the ambulatory setting (Figure 6.5).

Diagnosis and Evaluation

Accurate diagnosis of alcohol withdrawal syndrome (AWS) relies on a detailed alcohol history, including the amount, pattern (daily vs binge), and timing of the last drink, as well as prior withdrawal episodes.[91] Collateral information from family or friends may be necessary, especially for altered patients. Key diagnostic considerations include:

- **Timing of Symptoms:** Withdrawal symptoms can begin as early as 6 hours after alcohol cessation, with seizures occurring 12 to 48 hours and delirium tremens typically 2 to 4 days postcessation.
- **Clinical Features:** Symptoms include autonomic activation (hypertension, tachycardia, diaphoresis), neurologic signs (tremors, anxiety, seizures, hallucinations), and gastrointestinal disturbances (nausea, vomiting).
- **Differential Diagnosis:** Rule out alternative causes of delirium (eg, hypoglycemia, infection, hepatic encephalopathy) and other alcohol-related neurologic disorders (eg, Wernicke encephalopathy, subacute encephalopathy with seizures in alcoholics syndrome).[91]
- **Initial Evaluation:**
  - **Labs:** ethanol level, STAT fingerstick glucose, electrolytes (Ca/Mg/Phos), CBC, INR, PTT, and liver function tests
  - **Imaging:** Chest x-ray and consider a head CT to exclude subdural hematoma, especially in patients with trauma history

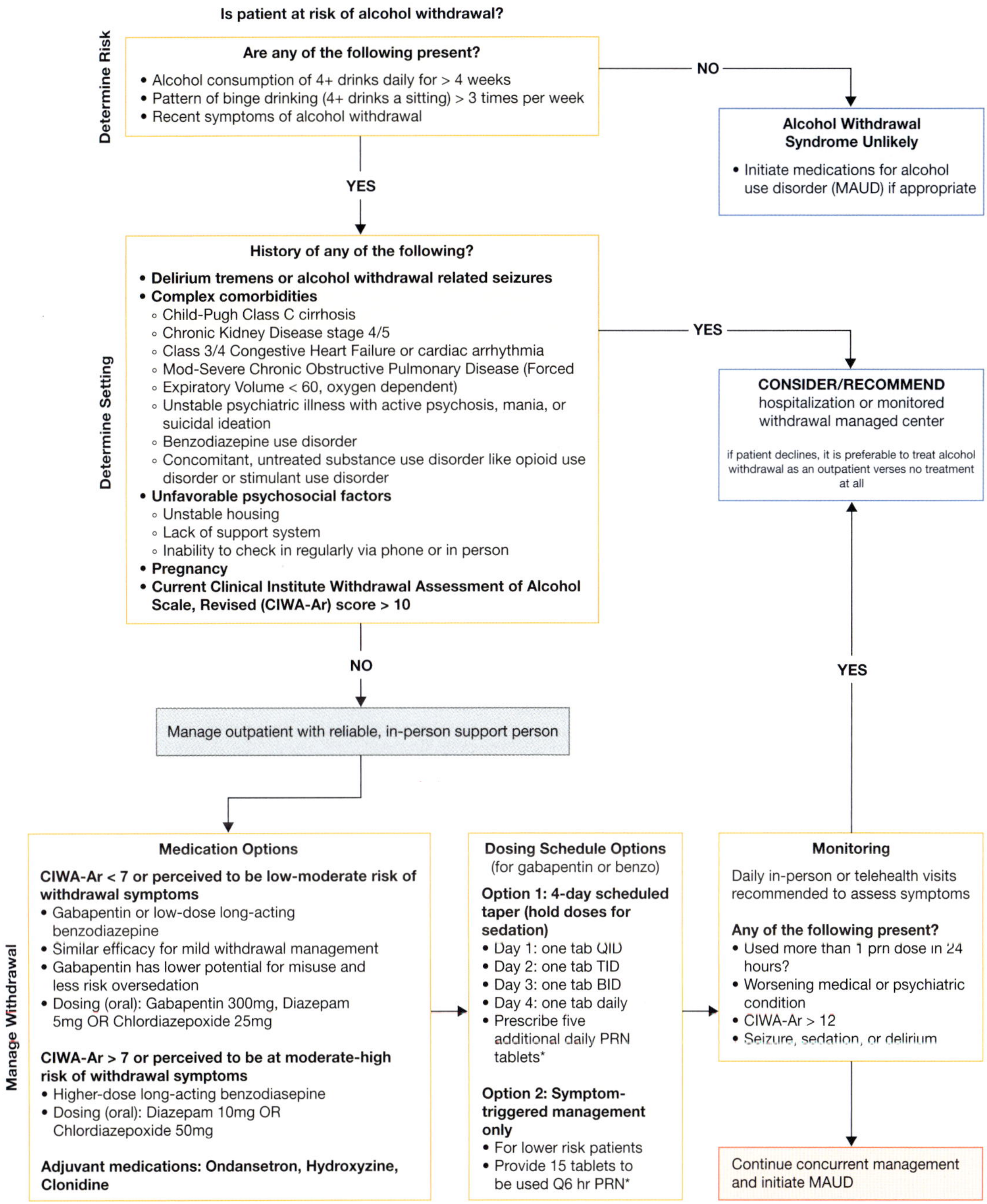

*For PRN assessment, use score > 12 on Short Alcohol Withdrawal Scale (SAWS).

Figure 6.5: Assessing patients for ambulatory alcohol withdrawal. (Providers Clinical Support System—Medications for Alcohol Use Disorder. *Outpatient Management of Alcohol Withdrawal.* Accessed September 12, 2025. https://learning.pcss-maud.org/resources Created by PCSS-MAUD with funding from SAMSHA.)

Early in the evaluation process, consider thiamine administration, management of dehydration, nutritional deficits and electrolyte abnormalities. If a patient has suspected Wernicke encephalopathy, administer thiamine 500 mg IV q8h. If the patient has normal mental status, administer thiamine 100 mg IV daily to prevent Wernicke encephalopathy. After thiamine, administer 5% dextrose/normal saline 1 L IV to correct fluid, glucose, and electrolyte abnormalities such as magnesium, calcium, and phosphorus.

Therapeutic Targets

The Richmond Agitation and Sedation Scale (RASS) is gaining favor over the CIWA-Ar for guiding therapy in critical care settings due to its simplicity, reproducibility, and ability to be administered for individuals who have delirium.[92] CIWA is labor intensive and less reliable in critically ill patients with confounding factors (eg, tachycardia from other causes, delirium). The target RASS score is typically 0 to −1, indicating a calm and alert state.

The vast number of patients stabilizes within 2 to 4 hours, facilitating discharge in socially supported cases for community withdrawal management units or outpatient management with appropriate medication regimens and follow-up. Admission is indicated for persistent severe withdrawal (RASS >0, CIWA >10 posttreatment), hepatic complications, or inadequate social support.

Treatment Protocols

Benzodiazepines

Traditional practice is to stabilize AWS with benzodiazepines based on the CIWA-Ar scale. Standard CIWA protocols are based around benzodiazepine administration, typically using either symptom-triggered or fixed dosing.[93] Guidelines recommend dosing based on objectively measured symptoms (known as symptom-triggered therapy) rather than fixed-dose regimens. However, concerns have been raised about its inappropriate use and safety. Moderate strength evidence suggests that symptom-triggered therapy improves duration of therapy and total benzodiazepine dose in low-risk patients.[93] Higher-risk patients, such as those with a history of severe withdrawal in the past, may benefit from fixed-dosing regimens.

For symptom-triggered dosing, it is recommended to give either diazepam or lorazepam. Diazepam is longer lasting, but absorption and painful IM or IV, and should be used in caution with liver failure patients. A dose of 5 to 10 mg IV, which can be repeated every 5 to 10 min for severe withdrawal with increases up to a maximum dose of 200 mg. For lorazepam, it is recommended to give 1 to 4 mg IV, which can be repeated every 15 to 20 minutes for severe withdrawal.[94] For both options, dosing is typically based on severity of symptoms as measured by CIWA-Ar scores.

Phenobarbital Monotherapy

Phenobarbital is increasingly favored as a first-line agent for AWS due to its predictable pharmacokinetics, efficacy, and broader neurochemical action compared to benzodiazepines.[91,95–97,98] It enhances GABA activity and inhibits glutamate signaling, addressing both components of withdrawal pathophysiology.[91,96–102]

Consider phenobarbital in individuals with a definite diagnosis of alcohol withdrawal and who do not have contraindications (eg, hepatic encephalopathy, acute intermittent porphyria, chronic phenobarbital use, significant drug interactions). Its advantages are that it has uniform efficacy (even in benzodiazepine refractory cases), it has a long half-life that allows autotapering and may reduce rebound symptoms that cause return visits to the ED,[103] it has minimal risk of paradoxical agitation, and it is effective for seizure prevention and treatment.

Phenobarbital is generally started with a loading dose, which is given as a single dose or several doses over several hours. Each health system is encouraged to establish their own protocol for the management of phenobarbital. See Chapter 8 for a sample phenobarbital protocol.[104] It is important to track cumulative doses to avoid toxicity and check phenobarbital levels if uncertainty arises about dosing or response.

AUD Maintenance Treatment

Medications for AUD can be safely and effectively initiated in the ED. Options are naltrexone, acamprosate, disulfiram, topiramate, and gabapentin. Naltrexone is 50 mg orally once daily or 380 mg IM once every 28 days and can be given prior to discharge. Naltrexone is contraindicated for individuals who have physical dependence on opioids from long-term use of short-acting opioids within 5 to 7 days or use of long-acting opioids within 7 to 10 days. If the history is unclear, then one can administer a small test dose of naloxone (2 to 4 mg) to ensure that withdrawal symptoms do not occur or obtain urine testing to check for opiates, methadone, or other opioids.

Acamprosate (666 mg TID) can be prescribed as an alternative MAUD for individuals who use opioids, however, dosing 3 times a day is very difficult. Topiramate can be started at 25 mg PO QHS but will need to be titrated in the outpatient setting. Gabapentin can be started at 300 mg PO TID and titrated in the outpatient setting. Disulfiram 250 mg once daily is another option but should not be started until the individual has abstained from alcohol for at least 72 hours. See Chapter 8 for more information.

Transition to Ongoing Care

Provide a 14-day prescription with follow-up ideally arranged within 72 hours via a navigator. Include thiamine (100 mg PO daily) and harm reduction guidance (eg, pacing alcohol consumption). Discharge materials should comprise medication instructions, follow-up appointment specifics, and criteria for ED return (eg, seizures, altered mentation). Additional resources are available at https://learning.pcss-maud.org/resources.

TABLE 6.2

Stabilization Protocol for Stimulant Use Disorder in the ED

Condition	Initial intervention	Pharmacotherapy	Goal
Agitation/psychosis	Verbal deescalation	Olanzapine 5–10 mg PO/IM or Lorazepam 2 mg PO/IM	HR <120 bpm, calm behavior
Hyperthermia (>39 °C)	Cooling (ice packs), IV fluids	N/A	Temp <38 °C, CK <1,000 U/L
Persistent psychosis	Olanzapine 5–10 mg	As needed, max 20 mg/24 h	Behavioral stabilization

ED Management of Methamphetamine Use Disorder

MUD significantly drives stimulant-related ED visits and overdose deaths, with hospitalizations showing rising clinical severity and costs.[105] Stimulants often present regionally with cocaine being much more prevalent on the East Coast of the US. The ED serves as a critical hub for managing acute neuropsychiatric crises and facilitating care linkage, despite fewer pharmacotherapeutic options for MUD compared to OUD or AUD.[20] This section describes evaluation, management, and treatment for the acute effects of stimulant use disorders.

Acute Stabilization

Acute MUD presentations often involve agitation, psychosis, or mania, requiring rapid stabilization (See Table 6.2). Begin with verbal deescalation—calm dialogue, reduced stimuli, and a private setting—to ease patient distress. If unresolved, administer olanzapine (5 to 10 mg PO or IM) or lorazepam (2 mg PO or IM); approximately 70% of patients stabilize within 30 minutes.[20] For severe agitation, olanzapine may be repeated every 30 minutes (max 20 mg/24 h).[31] Treat hyperthermia (>39 °C) with external cooling (eg, ice packs) and IV fluids, monitoring for rhabdomyolysis (creatine kinase >5 to 10 times normal). Avoid physical restraints to prevent worsening hyperthermia or agitation. Check vital signs every 15 to 30 minutes, aiming for heart rate <120 bpm, temperature <38 °C, and behavioral control, with stabilization typically resolving within 1 to 2 hours. Assess differential diagnoses (eg, delirium) and screen for suicidal/homicidal ideation, initiating a psychiatric hold if indicated[106] (See Figure 6.6).

Withdrawal Support

The postbinge "crash" brings profound exhaustion, depression, and heightened suicide risk. Offer a quiet bed, encourage sleep (often absent for over 7 days), and provide nutrition (eg, double portions for severe hunger). Screen for suicidal intent with direct questions (eg, "Are you feeling hopeless?") and monitor mood/behavior every 1 to 2 hours. Start mirtazapine (30 mg PO nightly) after psychosis resolves to improve sleep and reduce cravings, with 60% reporting relief within 24 hours.[107–110] Use hydration (oral or IV) and high-calorie meals to address depletion. Withdrawal peaks within 48 hours, making the ED a key stabilization and referral point. Consult psychiatry for suicidal ideation with a plan (See Table 6.3).[111]

Special Cases

- **Cardiovascular Complications:** Manage arrhythmias or hypertensive crises (systolic BP >180 mm Hg) with labetalol (10 mg IV) and ECG evaluation to reduce risks like stroke or heart failure, which increase with chronic methamphetamine use.[106]
- **Infectious Sequelae:** Treat injection-related infections (eg, endocarditis) with antibiotics and admission. Screen for HIV, hepatitis C, and STIs due to prevalent high-risk behaviors.[106]
- **Polysubstance Use:** For concurrent alcohol or opioid use, consider gabapentin (600 mg TID), monitoring for sedation. Avoid naltrexone if opioids are present due to contraindications.

Transition to Ongoing Care

Prescribe olanzapine (5 mg PO PRN every 4 hours, #30, max 20 mg/24 h) for persistent racing thoughts or "overamping," and mirtazapine (30 mg PO nightly, #30) for sleep and mood support, offering a first dose in the ED. For stimulant use disorder treatment refer to outpatient treatment, which is noted to be difficult to find. Provide harm reduction resources—naloxone (in-hand preferred), fentanyl test strips, and safer-use supplies—with overdose prevention education (eg, "start low, go slow, never use alone") as stimulants can often be contaminated with fentanyl and other opioids. Screen for STIs and offer ED pre-exposure prophylaxis (PrEP)/postexposure prophylaxis (PEP)/emergency contraception (EC) if indicated (see Chapter 11). Discharge documentation should detail medications, appointments, and return indications (eg, chest pain, suicidal intent). Admit patients with refractory psychosis, acute decompensation (eg, stroke), or no social support. Connections to contingency management programs enhance outpatient efficacy, despite limited ED-initiated pharmacotherapy options.[23,112]

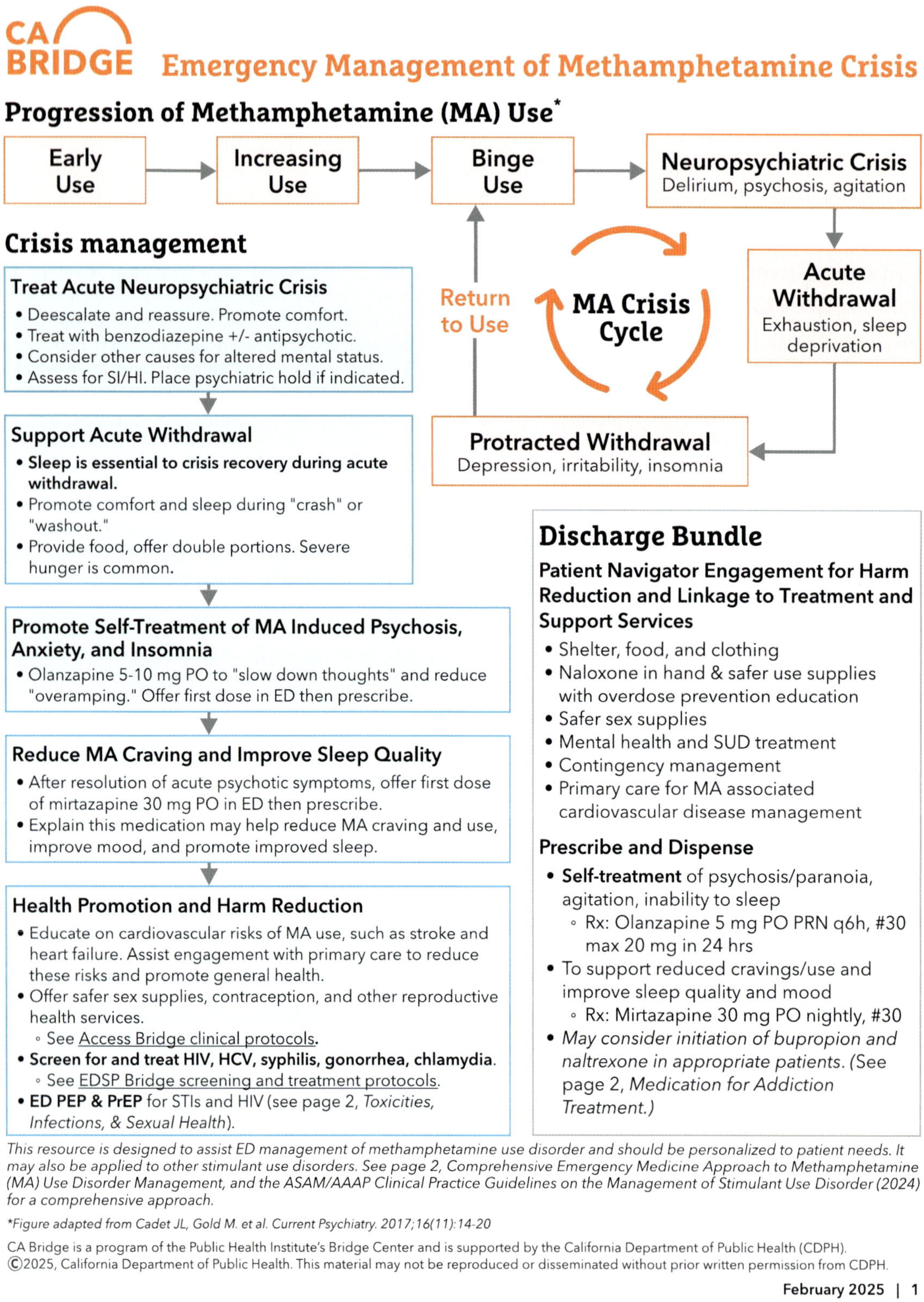

CA BRIDGE **Emergency Management of Methamphetamine Crisis**

Progression of Methamphetamine (MA) Use*

Crisis management

Treat Acute Neuropsychiatric Crisis

- Deescalate and reassure. Promote comfort.
- Treat with benzodiazepine +/- antipsychotic.
- Consider other causes for altered mental status.
- Assess for SI/HI. Place psychiatric hold if indicated.

Support Acute Withdrawal

- **Sleep is essential to crisis recovery during acute withdrawal.**
- Promote comfort and sleep during "crash" or "washout."
- Provide food, offer double portions. Severe hunger is common.

Promote Self-Treatment of MA Induced Psychosis, Anxiety, and Insomnia

- Olanzapine 5-10 mg PO to "slow down thoughts" and reduce "overamping." Offer first dose in ED then prescribe.

Reduce MA Craving and Improve Sleep Quality

- After resolution of acute psychotic symptoms, offer first dose of mirtazapine 30 mg PO in ED then prescribe.
- Explain this medication may help reduce MA craving and use, improve mood, and promote improved sleep.

Health Promotion and Harm Reduction

- Educate on cardiovascular risks of MA use, such as stroke and heart failure. Assist engagement with primary care to reduce these risks and promote general health.
- Offer safer sex supplies, contraception, and other reproductive health services.
  - See Access Bridge clinical protocols.
- **Screen for and treat HIV, HCV, syphilis, gonorrhea, chlamydia.**
  - See EDSP Bridge screening and treatment protocols.
- **ED PEP & PrEP** for STIs and HIV (see page 2, *Toxicities, Infections, & Sexual Health*).

Discharge Bundle

Patient Navigator Engagement for Harm Reduction and Linkage to Treatment and Support Services

- Shelter, food, and clothing
- Naloxone in hand & safer use supplies with overdose prevention education
- Safer sex supplies
- Mental health and SUD treatment
- Contingency management
- Primary care for MA associated cardiovascular disease management

Prescribe and Dispense

- **Self-treatment** of psychosis/paranoia, agitation, inability to sleep
  - Rx: Olanzapine 5 mg PO PRN q6h, #30 max 20 mg in 24 hrs
- To support reduced cravings/use and improve sleep quality and mood
  - Rx: Mirtazapine 30 mg PO nightly, #30
- *May consider initiation of bupropion and naltrexone in appropriate patients. (See page 2, Medication for Addiction Treatment.)*

This resource is designed to assist ED management of methamphetamine use disorder and should be personalized to patient needs. It may also be applied to other stimulant use disorders. See page 2, Comprehensive Emergency Medicine Approach to Methamphetamine (MA) Use Disorder Management, and the ASAM/AAAP Clinical Practice Guidelines on the Management of Stimulant Use Disorder (2024) for a comprehensive approach.

**Figure adapted from Cadet JL, Gold M. et al. Current Psychiatry. 2017;16(11):14-20*

CA Bridge is a program of the Public Health Institute's Bridge Center and is supported by the California Department of Public Health (CDPH).

February 2025 | 1

Figure 6.6: ED management of methamphetamine crisis. (The California Department of Health Care Services funds this work through CA Bridge, a program of the Public Health Institute, via State Opioid Response (SOR) grants.)

TABLE 6.3

Interventions for Methamphetamine and Cocaine Use Disorder Management

Intervention	Dosing	Use	Comments
Labetalol	10 mg IV	Treats arrhythmias or hypertensive crises (systolic BP >180 mm Hg) in cardiovascular complications	Used with ECG evaluation; reduces risks like stroke or heart failure from chronic methamphetamine use
Mirtazapine	30 mg PO nightly #30	Improves sleep and reduces cravings during withdrawal; supports mood in ongoing care	60% of patients report relief within 24 h; prescribed for outpatient use after psychosis resolves
Olanzapine	5–10 mg PO/IM, repeatable up to 20 mg/24 h; #30 (5 mg PRN every 4 h)	Stabilizes agitation, psychosis, or mania; manages persistent racing thoughts	Initial dose stabilizes 70% of patients within 30 min; outpatient prescription for symptom control
Naloxone	Not specified (in-hand delivery)	Reverses opioid overdose in polysubstance use scenarios	Provided as a harm reduction tool; not for methamphetamine itself, but addresses co-occurring opioid risks
Naltrexone	Extended-release injectable (dose per outpatient protocol)	Part of combination therapy with bupropion to reduce methamphetamine use long term	Contraindicated with opioid use; typically, outpatient initiation, not ED administered; paired with bupropion
Bupropion	Extended-release oral (dose per outpatient protocol)	Part of combination therapy with naltrexone to reduce methamphetamine use long-term	Paired with naltrexone, increased negative urine tests by 27% vs 11% placebo in trials; outpatient use
Contingency management	N/A (behavioral therapy)	Provide referral for this behavioral therapy that rewards abstinence to reinforce sobriety in outpatient settings	Uses incentives (eg, vouchers, prizes); evidence based for reducing methamphetamine use long term

Harm Reduction in the ED Setting

Harm reduction in the ED represents a pragmatic approach to public health that aims to minimize negative consequences associated with high-risk behaviors like substance use.[113] The ED serves as a crucial setting for harm reduction interventions, as it often represents a primary point of health care contact for marginalized populations engaged in substance use or other high-risk behaviors.[113–115]

Harm reduction philosophy acknowledges that while certain behaviors carry risks, a nonjudgmental, evidence-based approach focused on reducing negative outcomes is more effective than punitive or abstinence-only models.[113] This approach is particularly vital in emergency settings where clinicians encounter patients experiencing acute consequences of various high-risk behaviors, including SUD, unprotected sexual encounters, and complications related to unplanned pregnancies.

Key Interventions

Key harm reduction interventions commonly implemented in EDs include naloxone distribution programs, which provide overdose-reversal medication to patients at risk.[116,117] Additional strategies include sterile syringe distribution, referrals to syringe service programs, education on safer substance injection practices, opioid agonist treatment (OAT), and testing for HIV, hepatitis, and other infectious diseases[114,115,118] (Table 6.4). See www.bridgetotreatment.org for naloxone and harm reduction resources.

HIV Prevention: PEP and PrEP in the ED Setting

PEP for HIV represents a critical time-sensitive intervention that can be initiated in the ED. PEP involves administering antiretroviral medications within 72 hours of potential HIV exposure to prevent infection. EDs are ideally positioned to identify candidates for PEP, including individuals presenting after sexual assault, occupational exposures, known substance use exposure, or high-risk sexual encounters.[119,120]

PrEP referral programs in the ED connect high-risk individuals with preventive medication regimens that can significantly reduce HIV transmission risk.[121–123] While the ED typically cannot provide ongoing PrEP prescriptions, it serves as an essential identification and linkage point, particularly for individuals who may not access routine preventive care.[121–123] ED-based PrEP navigation programs can facilitate connections with community providers for continued care.

TABLE 6.4

ED-Based Harm Reduction Interventions

Intervention	Dosing	Use	Comments
Naloxone	4 mg nasal spray	Reverses opioid overdose	Critical harm reduction tool addressing opioid overdose risk. Now over-the-counter (OTC) allowing ED-based low-barrier, high-volume distribution. Methods: take-home in-hand (active distribution) or distribution stand, vending machine (passive distribution)
Sterile syringes	Provided as needed, variable supply	Prevents transmission of bloodborne infections (eg, HIV, HCV) through injection substance use	Distributed via ED-based harm reduction initiatives often in partnership with community-based syringe service programs (SSPs). Paired with education on safe injection practices and disposal to reduce community health risks
Emtricitabine and tenofovir disoproxil fumarate	200 mg/300 mg PO daily	Pre-exposure prophylaxis (PrEP) for HIV prevention	Can be initiated in ED for ongoing HIV prevention in injection substance use/needle-sharing risk, high-risk sexual activity. Supports long-term HIV risk reduction with regular STI screening and adherence support
Doxycycline	200 mg PO single dose	Postexposure prophylaxis ("Doxy PEP") for bacterial STIs after sexual risk (≤72 h)	Complements HIV PrEP in ED for comprehensive STI risk management
Ulipristal Acetate	30 mg PO single dose	Emergency contraception after unprotected sex (≤5 d)	Consistent effectiveness across all 5 days. Wait at least 5 days before starting or resuming hormonal birth control to avoid interaction
Levonorgestrel	1.5 mg PO single dose	Emergency contraception after unprotected sex. Most effective within 72 h (3 d) but can work up to 5 d (effectiveness declines)	OTC: Available without a prescription or ID (*state dependent*)

Pregnancy Prevention and Reproductive Health

Emergency contraception (EC) provision represents another cornerstone of ED-based harm reduction. EDs routinely provide levonorgestrel or ulipristal acetate for pregnancy prevention to patients presenting after unprotected intercourse, contraceptive failures, or sexual assault.[124] Education about correct EC usage and timing maximizes effectiveness.[124]

Comprehensive reproductive health counseling in the ED setting can include discussion of longer-term contraceptive options with appropriate referrals. Some EDs have implemented rapid-start contraception programs that initiate hormonal methods immediately and connect patients with resources for long-acting reversible contraception (LARC).[125]

Challenges and Implementation Considerations

Despite proven efficacy, harm reduction programs in emergency settings face numerous barriers, including resource constraints, stigma among health care clinicians, and regulatory challenges.[114,125] Successful implementation requires institutional commitment, interdisciplinary collaboration, and ongoing education to address biases and misconceptions about harm reduction approaches.[113,115] For opioid-specific interventions, limited access to SUD specialists can hinder 24/7 service delivery, compounded by concerns about safety and regulatory restrictions.[114,115]

Effective harm reduction programs also acknowledge the social determinants of health that contribute to high-risk behaviors, incorporating trauma-informed care principles and culturally responsive practices.[113,126] EDs implementing these approaches have demonstrated improvements in patient outcomes, reduction in repeat ED visits, and cost-effectiveness.[116] Physicians' willingness to adopt harm reduction is often high, but barriers such as lack of confidence, time, training, and institutional support limit translation into practice, necessitating leadership endorsement and evidence dissemination.[114]

Conclusion

Harm reduction represents an essential component of comprehensive emergency care that bridges immediate crisis management with longer-term public health goals. By meeting patients "where they are" while simultaneously creating pathways to improved health, ED harm reduction initiatives embody the ethical principles of beneficence and respect for patient autonomy while addressing critical public health challenges.[113]

Substance Use Navigators (Care Coordination)

Effective management of SUD in EDs extends beyond acute intervention to encompass seamless transitions to ongoing SUD care. Care coordination, facilitated by dedicated personnel and strategic partnerships, is essential to sustain treatment engagement, reduce ED revisits, and address disparities in outcomes, such as elevated overdose rates among Black and Native populations.[127] This section delineates the infrastructure and processes required to bridge ED-initiated care to longitudinal recovery.

As previously described, the SUN, a specialized coordinator (eg, social worker, addiction counselor, health promotion advocate), serves as the cornerstone of ED-based SUD care transitions. Their responsibilities include conducting comprehensive patient assessments—encompassing substance use patterns, social determinants (eg, housing instability), and treatment preferences—followed by linkage to appropriate community resources and SUD treatment. Navigators provide motivational interviewing to enhance patient commitment and perform follow-up contact within 24 to 48 hours post discharge to address barriers (eg, prescription access, transportation). Evidence demonstrates that navigator-led interventions increase treatment retention by 26% to 34% at 1 year and reduce ED visits by 26%.[64] Training should emphasize cultural competence and knowledge of local treatment ecosystems to ensure equitable access, particularly for underserved groups. They must be integrated into the ED staff structure and responsible to ED management/champion for ensuring fidelity to their interventions and success.

- **Community Partnerships:**
  Successful care coordination necessitates robust alliances with external, community-based entities. Formal memoranda of understanding with office-based buprenorphine clinicians or clinics, federally qualified health centers, and specialty SUD treatment programs ensure rapid referral pathways.[55] Partnerships with harm reduction organizations provide naloxone and safer-use education, while social service agencies address structural barriers like housing or insurance gaps. These relationships require regular updates on capacity, insurance requirements, and wait times to optimize patient placement.
- **After-Hours Management:**
  EDs must accommodate care transitions during off-hours when navigator availability may be limited. Protocols should include extended prescriptions—eg, 2-week supplies of medications—to bridge to navigator contact and follow-up care. Relationships with 24/7 treatment access points, such as crisis stabilization units or telehealth services, provide interim support; 75% of patients accept telehealth follow-up postoverdose.[5] Standardized handoff procedures—eg, electronic referrals flagged for navigator review—ensure continuity. These strategies mitigate disruptions, sustaining the care continuum established during the ED encounter.

Care coordination transforms ED visits into sustained recovery opportunities, aligning with evidence that structured linkage reduces hospital readmissions and improves outcomes.[128] By integrating navigators and partnerships, EDs can operationalize a safety net that addresses both clinical and social complexities of SUD, enhancing access for vulnerable populations and supporting program scalability.

Quality Metrics

Systematic evaluation of ED-based SUD treatment programs is imperative to ensure quality, demonstrate efficacy, and guide resource allocation. Quality metrics provide an evidence-based framework to assess clinical processes, patient outcomes, and program sustainability, aligning with the broader imperative to reduce overdose mortality and address disparities.[127] This section delineates key performance indicators and operational strategies for their implementation, supporting continuous improvement and institutional justification. Programs require mechanisms to track basic metrics, including numbers of patients treated, follow-up rates, and clinical outcomes.[5,36,129–133] While sophisticated databases may support mature programs, initial monitoring can utilize simple spreadsheets or EHR reports. These data support continuous program improvement while demonstrating value to institutional stakeholders.

Regular reassessment of infrastructure needs allows programs to scale appropriately as volume increases. Many successful programs begin with minimal infrastructure and add elements as experience demonstrates specific needs. This approach allows rapid implementation while ensuring sustainable growth.

TABLE 6.5

Quality Metrics for ED-Based SUD Programs

Metric	Domain	Target/benchmark	Source
Treatment initiations (eg, buprenorphine, naltrexone) Or discussion with patient (they may decline)	Process	>90% of eligible patients	Snyder et al, 2021[36]
Naloxone distribution	Process	Offered to 100% of patients with OUD	N/A
Follow-up rate (within 30 d)	Outcome	>50%	Snyder et al, 2021[36] D'Onofrio et al, 2010[29]
ED return visits (30 d)	Outcome	<20%	Gryczynski et al, 2021[64]
Prescription fill rate	Outcome	>75%	N/A
Patient satisfaction (Likert)	Outcome	>4/5 average	N/A
Initiation rate by race/ethnicity	Equity	Parity across groups	Herring et al, 2024[5] Chhabra et al, 2025[11]

Key Measures

Table 6.5 outlines essential metrics across process and outcome domains, with benchmarks informed by evidence.[36,64] Disparity-focused metrics enable targeted interventions to mitigate inequitable outcomes.[5]

- **Data Collection and Analysis:**
  Data collection should integrate seamlessly with ED workflows to minimize burden. EHR systems, where available, facilitate automated extraction of initiation and follow-up data via standardized order sets and discharge codes; alternatively, simple spreadsheets suffice for initial tracking, capturing core variables (eg, patient ID, treatment date, navigator contact). SUNs play a pivotal role in logging encounter-specific outcomes, such as appointment adherence, during routine follow-ups. Monthly multidisciplinary reviews—engaging physicians, navigators, and administrators—analyze trends, identify barriers (eg, prolonged time to buprenorphine administration), and refine protocols. Statistical benchmarks guide performance targets.
- **Program Improvement:**
  Regular metric assessment informs iterative enhancements—eg, increasing navigator hours if follow-up rates lag or strengthening pharmacy partnerships if fill rates falter. Reporting to hospital leadership, emphasizing outcomes like reduced readmissions (aligned with CMS priorities), secures sustained support.[134,135] External collaboration with research networks or state agencies amplifies impact through benchmark comparisons and funding opportunities. This rigorous approach ensures ED SUD programs evolve as dynamic, evidence-driven systems, optimizing patient care and public health benefits.

REFERENCES

1. Zhang X, Wang N, Hou F, et al. Emergency department visits by patients with substance use disorder in the United States. *West J Emerg Med.* 2021;22(5):1076–1085.
2. Medications for Substance Use Disorders. April 11, 2024. Accessed January 6, 2025. https://www.samhsa.gov/substance-use/treatment/options
3. Philippine T, Forsgren E, DeWitt C, Carter I, McCollough M, Taira BR. Provider perspectives on emergency department initiation of medication assisted treatment for alcohol use disorder. *BMC Health Serv Res.* 2022;22(1):456.
4. Larochelle MR, Bernstein R, Bernson D, et al. Touchpoints—opportunities to predict and prevent opioid overdose: a cohort study. *Drug Alcohol Depend.* 2019;204:107537.
5. Herring AA, Rosen AD, Samuels EA, et al. Emergency department access to buprenorphine for opioid use disorder. *JAMA Netw Open.* 2024;7(1):e2353771.
6. 2023 National Survey on Drug Use and Health (NSDUH) Releases | CBHSQ Data. Accessed April 28, 2025. https://www.samhsa.gov/data/data-we-collect/nsduh-national-survey-drug-use-and-health/national-releases/2023
7. Marcozzi D, Carr B, Liferidge A, Baehr N, Browne B. Trends in the contribution of emergency departments to the provision of hospital-associated health care in the USA. *Int J Health Serv.* 2018;48(2):267–288.
8. D'Onofrio G, Cole JB, Perrone J. State investment in emergency department buprenorphine pays off. *JAMA.* 2025;333(14):1209–1211.
9. DAWN National Annual Estimates | CBHSQ Data. Accessed April 23, 2025. https://www.samhsa.gov/data/data-we-collect/dawn-drug-abuse-warning-network/annual-releases
10. Kiang MV, Humphreys K. Recent drug overdose mortality decline compared with pre–COVID-19 trend. *JAMA Netw Open.* 2025;8(2):e2458090.
11. Chhabra N, Smith D, Parde N, et al. Racial, ethnic, and sex disparities in buprenorphine treatment from emergency

departments by discharge diagnosis. *Acad Emerg Med.* 2025; 32(9):985–993.
12. Ahmed FB, Cisewski JA, Rossen LM, Sutton P. County-level provisional drug overdose death counts. National Center for Health Statistics; 2025. doi:10.15620/cdc/20250305008
13. Spencer M, Miniño A, Warner M. Drug overdose deaths in the United States, 2001–2021. *NCHS Data Brief*; 2022; (457):1–8. doi:10.15620/cdc:122556
14. Drug Abuse Warning Network (DAWN) Short Report | Alcohol-related ED visits. https://library.samhsa.gov/product/dawn-alcohol-related-short-report/pep24-07-019
15. Islami F, Marlow EC, Thomson B, et al. Proportion and number of cancer cases and deaths attributable to potentially modifiable risk factors in the United States, 2019. *CA Cancer J Clin.* 2024;74(5):405–432.
16. Han B, Jones CM, Einstein EB, Powell PA, Compton WM. Use of medications for alcohol use disorder in the US: Results from the 2019 National Survey on drug use and health. *JAMA Psychiatry.* 2021;78(8):922–924.
17. Alcohol-Related Disease Impact | CDC. Accessed April 28, 2025. https://nccd.cdc.gov/DPH_ARDI/default/default.aspx
18. Suen LW, Makam AN, Snyder HR, et al. National prevalence of alcohol and other substance use disorders among emergency department visits and hospitalizations: NHAMCS 2014–2018. *J Gen Intern Med.* 2022;37(10):2420–2428.
19. Esser MB, Sherk A, Liu Y, et al. Deaths and years of potential life lost from excessive alcohol use—United States, 2011–2015. *MMWR Morb Mortal Wkly Rep.* 2020;69(30):981–987.
20. Coffin PO, Suen LW. Methamphetamine toxicities and clinical management. *NEJM Evid.* 2023;2(12):EVIDra2300160. doi:10.1056/EVIDra2300160
21. Beckerleg W, Hudgins J. Substance use-related emergency department visits and resource utilization. *West J Emerg Med.* 2022;23(2):166–173.
22. CDC. Stimulants. November 7, 2024. Accessed April 28, 2025. https://www.cdc.gov/overdose-prevention/about/stimulant-overdose.html
23. Rash CJ. Implementing an evidence-based prize contingency management protocol for stimulant use. *J Subst Use Addict Treat.* 2023;151:209079.
24. Pickens CM, Hoots BE, Casillas SM, Scholl L. Prevalences of and characteristics associated with single- and polydrug-involved U.S. emergency department visits in 2018. *Addict Behav.* 2022;125:107158.
25. Horn BP, Crandall C, Forcehimes A, French MT, Bogenschutz M. Benefit-cost analysis of SBIRT interventions for substance using patients in emergency departments. *J Subst Abuse Treat.* 2017;79:6–11.
26. Bernstein E, Bernstein J, Feldman J, et al. An evidence-based alcohol screening, brief intervention and referral to treatment (SBIRT) curriculum for emergency department (ED) providers improves skills and utilization. *Subst Abuse.* 2007;28(4):79–92.
27. Moulin AK, Wu EF, Trevino TG, Richards JR. The impact of SBIRT and dedicated alcohol and drug counseling for domiciled and homeless patients in the emergency department. *J Subst Use.* 2021;26(2):156–159.
28. D'Onofrio G, Fiellin DA, Pantalon MV, et al. A brief intervention reduces hazardous and harmful drinking in emergency department patients. *Ann Emerg Med.* 2012;60(2):181–192.
29. D'Onofrio G, Degutis LC. Integrating project ASSERT: a screening, intervention, and referral to treatment program for unhealthy alcohol and drug use into an urban emergency department. *Acad Emerg Med.* 2010;17(8):903–911.
30. D'Onofrio G, O'Connor PG, Pantalon MV, et al. Emergency department–initiated buprenorphine/naloxone treatment for opioid dependence: a randomized clinical trial. *JAMA.* 2015;313(16):1636.
31. CA Bridge. Resources. CA Bridge. Accessed August 31, 2024. https://cabridge.org/tools/resources/
32. Giraldo A, Shah P, Zerbo E, Nyaku AN. The role of recovery peer navigators in retention in outpatient buprenorphine treatment: a retrospective cohort study. *Ann Med.* 2024;56(1): 2355566.
33. Anderson ES, Rusoja E, Luftig J, Nyaku AN. Effectiveness of substance use navigation for emergency department patients with substance use disorders: an implementation study. *Ann Emerg Med.* 2023;81(3):297–308.
34. Samuels EA, Bernstein SL, Marshall BDL, Krieger M, Baird J, Mello MJ. Peer navigation and take-home naloxone for opioid overdose emergency department patients: preliminary patient outcomes. *J Subst Abuse Treat.* 2018;94:29–34.
35. Weiner SG, Baker O, Bernson D, Schuur JD. One-year mortality of patients after emergency department treatment for nonfatal opioid overdose. *Ann Emerg Med.* 2020;75(1):13–17.
36. Snyder H, Kalmin MM, Moulin A, et al. Rapid adoption of low-threshold buprenorphine treatment at California emergency departments participating in the CA Bridge program. *Ann Emerg Med.* 2021;78(6):759–772.
37. Hawk K, D'Onofrio G. Emergency department screening and interventions for substance use disorders. *Addict Sci Clin Pract.* 2018;13(1):18.
38. Vaca FE, Dziura J, Abujarad F, et al. Use of an automated bilingual digital health tool to reduce unhealthy alcohol use among Latino Emergency department patients: a randomized clinical trial. *JAMA Netw Open.* 2023;6(5):e2314848.
39. Larochelle MR, Bernson D, Land T, et al. Medication for opioid use disorder after nonfatal opioid overdose and association with mortality: a cohort study. *Ann Intern Med.* 2018;169(3):137.
40. Bouisset F, Ruidavets JB, Dallongeville J, et al. Comparison of short- and long-term prognosis between ST-elevation and non-ST-elevation myocardial infarction. *J Clin Med.* 2021; 10(2):180.
41. Dekker AM, Schriger DL, Herring AA, Samuels EA. Emergency clinician buprenorphine initiation, subsequent prescriptions, and continuous prescriptions. *JAMA.* 2025;333(14): 1232–1241.
42. Hawk K, Hoppe J, Ketcham E, et al. Consensus Recommendations on the treatment of opioid use disorder in the emergency department. *Ann Emerg Med.* 2021;78(3):434–442.
43. Samuels EA, Rosen AD, Speener M, et al. Scaling emergency department opioid use disorder treatment across California to reduce overdose deaths, 2019–2023. *Am J Public Health.* 2024;114(9):874–878.
44. Armour R, Nielsen S, Buxton JA, Bolster J, Han MX, Ross L. Initiation of buprenorphine in the emergency department or emergency out-of-hospital setting: a mixed-methods systematic review. *Am J Emerg Med.* 2025;88:12–22.
45. Herring AA, Vosooghi AA, Luftig J, et al. High-dose buprenorphine induction in the emergency department for treatment of opioid use disorder. *JAMA Netw Open.* 2021;4(7):e2117128.
46. Snyder H, Chau B, Kalmin MM, et al. High-dose buprenorphine initiation in the emergency department among patients using fentanyl and other opioids. *JAMA Netw Open.* 2023; 6(3):e231572.
47. D'Onofrio G, Herring AA, Perrone J, et al. Extended-release 7-day injectable buprenorphine for patients with minimal to mild opioid withdrawal. *JAMA Netw Open.* 2024; 7(7):e2420702.
48. Huo S, Heil J, Salzman MS, Carroll G, Haroz R. Methadone initiation in the emergency department for opioid use disorder: a case series. *J Emerg Med.* 2023;64(3):391–396.
49. Skogrand E, Sharpe J, Englander H. Dispensing methadone at hospital discharge: one hospital's approach to

implementing the "72-hour rule" change. *J Addict Med.* 2024; 18(1):71–74.
50. Request for Exception to Limitations on Dispensing for Opioid Use Disorder. Accessed May 1, 2025. https://lsbme.la.gov/in-the-news/request-for-exception-to-limitations-on-dispensing-for-opioid-use-disorder
51. Mintz CM, Hartz SM, Fisher SL, et al. A cascade of care for alcohol use disorder: using 2015–2019 National Survey on Drug Use and Health data to identify gaps in past 12-month care. *Alcohol Clin Exp Res.* 2021;45(6):1276–1286.
52. Yin X, O'Jiaku-Okorie A, Lucas CA. Rate of emergency department visits for alcohol-specific diagnoses, by sex: United States, 2003–2004 to 2021–2022. *NCHS Health E-Stat.* 2026;(109):1–5. https://dx.doi.org/10.15620/cdc/174637
53. Strayer RJ, Friedman BW, Haroz R, et al. Emergency department management of patients with alcohol intoxication, alcohol withdrawal, and alcohol use disorder: a white paper prepared for the American Academy of Emergency Medicine. *J Emerg Med.* 2023;64(4):517–540.
54. Anderson ES, Chamberlin M, Zuluaga M, et al. Implementation of oral and extended-release naltrexone for the treatment of emergency department patients with moderate to severe alcohol use disorder: feasibility and initial outcomes. *Ann Emerg Med.* 2021;78(6):752–758.
55. Murphy CE IV, Coralic Z, Wang RC, Montoy JCC, Ramirez B, Raven MC. Extended-release naltrexone and case management for treatment of alcohol use disorder in the emergency department. *Ann Emerg Med.* 2023;81(4): 440–449.
56. Punia K, Scott W, Manuja K, et al. SAEM GRACE: Anti-craving medications for alcohol use disorder treatment in the emergency department: a systematic review of direct evidence. *Acad Emerg Med.* 2024;31(5):504–514.
57. PCSS-MAUD Learning: Resources. Accessed April 23, 2025. https://learning.pcss-maud.org/resources
58. Hawk KF, D'Onofrio G. Time to treat alcohol use disorder in the emergency department. *Ann Emerg Med.* 2023; 81(4):450–452.
59. Suen LW, Davy-Mendez T, LeSaint KT, Riley ED, Coffin PO. Emergency department visits and trends related to cocaine, psychostimulants, and opioids in the United States, 2008–2018. *BMC Emerg Med.* 2022;22(1):19.
60. Roehler DR, Hoots BE, Holland KM, Baldwin GT, Vivolo-Kantor AM. Trends and characteristics of cannabis-associated emergency department visits in the United States, 2006–2018. *Drug Alcohol Depend.* 2022;232:109288.
61. Kim C, Chum A, Nielsen A, et al. Associations between recreational cannabis legalization and cannabis-related emergency department visits by age, gender, and geographic status in Ontario, Canada: an interrupted time series study. *PLOS ONE.* 2022;17(10):e0268718.
62. Sabbineni M, Scott W, Punia K, et al. SAEM GRACE: Dopamine antagonists and topical capsaicin for cannabis hyperemesis syndrome in the emergency department: a systematic review of direct evidence. *Acad Emerg Med.* 2024; 31(5):493–503.
63. Borgundvaag B, Bellolio F, Miles I, et al. Guidelines for Reasonable and Appropriate Care in the Emergency Department (GRACE-4): alcohol use disorder and cannabinoid hyperemesis syndrome management in the emergency department. *Acad Emerg Med.* 2024;31(5):425–455.
64. Gryczynski J, Nordeck CD, Welsh C, Mitchell SG, O'Grady KE, Schwartz RP. Preventing hospital readmission for patients with comorbid substance use disorder: a randomized trial. *Ann Intern Med.* 2021;174(7):899–909.
65. D'Onofrio G, Edelman EJ, Hawk KF, et al. Implementation facilitation to promote emergency department-initiated buprenorphine for opioid use disorder. *JAMA Netw Open.* 2023;6(4):e235439.
66. Hawk KF, D'Onofrio G, Chawarski MC, et al. Barriers and facilitators to clinician readiness to provide emergency department–initiated buprenorphine. *JAMA Netw Open.* 2020;3(5):e204561.
67. Strout T, Dziura J, Barrett TW, et al. Implementation facilitation improves readiness for emergency department-initiated buprenorphine to treat opioid use disorder. *J Subst Use Addict Treat.* 2025:209845.
68. Kirchner JE, Owen RR, Nordquist C, Fischer EP. Diagnosis and management of substance use disorders among inpatients with schizophrenia. *Psychiatr Serv.* 1998;49(1): 82–85.
69. Busch SH, Fiellin DA, Chawarski MC, et al. Cost-effectiveness of emergency department-initiated treatment for opioid dependence. *Addict Abingdon Engl.* 2017;112(11): 2002–2010.
70. Lu T, Ryan D, Cadet T, et al. Cost-effectiveness of implementation facilitation to promote emergency department-initiated buprenorphine for opioid use disorder. *Ann Emerg Med.* 2025;85(3):205–213.
71. Melnick ER, Nath B, Dziura JD, et al. User centered clinical decision support to implement initiation of buprenorphine for opioid use disorder in the emergency department: EMBED pragmatic cluster randomized controlled trial. *BMJ.* 2022:377:e069271.
72. Donley E. Supports and barriers to implementing screening tools in public hospital emergency departments. *J Emerg Crit Care Med.* 2024;8:19–19.
73. Saitz R, Mayo-Smith MF, Roberts MS, Redmond HA, Bernard DR, Calkins DR. Individualized treatment for alcohol withdrawal: a randomized double-blind controlled trial. *JAMA.* 1994;272(7):519–523.
74. Tomaszewski CA, Quenzer F, Corbett B, et al. Interobserver agreement between emergency clinicians and nurses for Clinical Opiate Withdrawal Scale. *J Am Coll Emerg Physicians Open.* 2021;2(3):e12462.
75. Wesson DR, Ling W. The clinical opiate withdrawal scale (COWS). *J Psychoactive Drugs.* 2003;35(2):253–259.
76. Guo CZ, D'Onofrio G, Fiellin DA, et al. Emergency department-initiated buprenorphine protocols: a national evaluation. *J Am Coll Emerg Physicians Open.* 2021;2(6):e12606.
77. Ciccarone D. The triple wave epidemic: supply and demand drivers of the US opioid overdose crisis. *Int J Drug Policy.* 2019;71:183–188.
78. D'Onofrio G, Hawk KF, Herring AA, et al. The design and conduct of a randomized clinical trial comparing emergency department initiation of sublingual versus a 7-day extended-release injection formulation of buprenorphine for opioid use disorder: project ED innovation. *Contemp Clin Trials.* 2021;104:106359.
79. B. CA Bridge of the Public Health Institute, California Department of Health Care Services. *Site Example: Enhanced Care Practice: Precipitated Withdrawal 90-Minute Bundle.* Accessed September 12, 2025. https://bridgetotreatment.org/wp-content/uploads/CA_BRIDGE_SITE-EXAMPLE_Enhanced-Care-Practice-Precipitated-Withdrawal-90-Minute-Bundle_June_2025.pdf
80. Jones HE, Kaltenbach K, Heil SH, et al. Neonatal abstinence syndrome after methadone or buprenorphine exposure. *N Engl J Med.* 2010;363(24):2320–2331.
81. Herring AA, Schultz CW, Yang E, Greenwald MK. Rapid induction onto sublingual buprenorphine after opioid

overdose and successful linkage to treatment for opioid use disorder. *Am J Emerg Med.* 2019;37(12):2259–2262.
82. Alford DP, Compton P, Samet JH. Acute pain management for patients receiving maintenance methadone or buprenorphine therapy. *Ann Intern Med.* 2006;144(2):127–134.
83. Joudrey PJ, Kolak M, Lin Q, Paykin S, Anguiano V, Wang EA. Assessment of community-level vulnerability and access to medications for opioid use disorder. *JAMA Netw Open.* 2022;5(4):e227028.
84. Wolfson D, King R, Lamberson M, et al. Methadone initiation in the emergency department for opioid use disorder. *West J Emerg Med.* 2024;25(5):668–674.
85. Methadone Hospital Quick Start. *Bridge to Treatment.* Accessed April 29, 2025. https://bridgetotreatment.org/resource/methadone-hospital-quick-start/
86. *Dispensing of Narcotic Drugs to Relieve Acute Withdrawal Symptoms of Opioid Use Disorder. Federal Register.* August 8, 2023. Accessed April 29, 2025. https://www.federalregister.gov/documents/2023/08/08/2023-16892/dispensing-of-narcotic-drugs-to-relieve-acute-withdrawal-symptoms-of-opioid-use-disorder
87. *21 CFR 1306.07—Administering or dispensing of narcotic drugs.* Accessed April 29, 2025. https://www.ecfr.gov/current/title-21/part-1306/section-1306.07
88. *DEA's Commitment to Expanding Access to Medication-Assisted Treatment.* Accessed April 29, 2025. https://www.dea.gov/press-releases/2022/03/23/deas-commitment-expanding-access-medication-assisted-treatment
89. Huo S, Heil J, Salzman MS, Carroll G, Haroz R. Methadone initiation in the emergency department for opioid use disorder: a case series. *J Emerg Med.* 2023;64(3):391–396.
90. Maldonado J, Sher Y, Das S, et al. Prospective validation study of the prediction of alcohol withdrawal severity scale (PAWSS): a new scale for the prediction of moderate to severe alcohol withdrawal. *Alcohol Alcohol. 2015*;50(5):509–518.
91. Farkas J. *Alcohol Withdrawal & Alcohol Use Disorder.* The Internet Book of Critical Care. 2023. Accessed May 1, 2025. https://emcrit.org/ibcc/etoh/
92. Oks M, Cleven KL, Healy L, et al. The safety and utility of phenobarbital use for the treatment of severe alcohol withdrawal syndrome in the medical intensive care unit. *J Intensive Care Med.* 2020;35(9):844–850.
93. Holleck JL, Merchant N, Gunderson CG. Symptom-triggered therapy for alcohol withdrawal syndrome: a systematic review and meta-analysis of randomized controlled trials. *J Gen Intern Med.* 2019;34(6):1018–1024.
94. The ASAM clinical practice guideline on alcohol withdrawal management. *J Addict Med.* 2020;14(3S):1–72.
95. Nisavic M, Nejad SH, Isenberg BM, et al. Use of phenobarbital in alcohol withdrawal management—a retrospective comparison study of phenobarbital and benzodiazepines for acute alcohol withdrawal management in general medical patients. *Psychosomatics.* 2019;60(5):458–467.
96. Umar Z, Haseeb Ul Rasool M, Muhammad S, et al. Phenobarbital and alcohol withdrawal syndrome: a systematic review and meta-analysis. *Cureus.* 2023;15(1):e33695.
97. Rogers TA, Cambron JD. *Phenobarbital as First-Line Medication for Alcohol Withdrawal: Have You Switched From Benzodiazepines Yet?* Academic Life in Emergency Medicine (ALiEM). 2023. Accessed May 1, 2025. https://www.aliem.com/phenobarbital-first-line-medication-alcohol-withdrawal/
98. Rosenson J, Clements C, Simon B, et al. Phenobarbital for acute alcohol withdrawal: a prospective randomized double-blind placebo-controlled study. *J Emerg Med.* 2013;44(3):592–598.e2.
99. Gold JA, Rimal B, Nolan A, Nelson LS. A strategy of escalating doses of benzodiazepines and phenobarbital administration reduces the need for mechanical ventilation in delirium tremens. *Crit Care Med.* 2007;35(3):724–730.
100. Hammond DA, Rowe JM, Wong A, Wiley TL, Lee KC, Kane-Gill SL. Patient outcomes associated with phenobarbital use with or without benzodiazepines for alcohol withdrawal syndrome: a systematic review. *Hosp Pharm.* 2017;52(9):607–616.
101. Holleck JL, Merchant N, Gunderson CG. Symptom-triggered therapy for alcohol withdrawal syndrome: a systematic review and meta-analysis of randomized controlled trials. *J Gen Intern Med.* 2019;34(6):1018–1024.
102. Kattimani S, Bharadwaj B. Clinical management of alcohol withdrawal: a systematic review. *Ind Psychiatry J.* 2013;22(2):100–108.
103. Lebin JA, Mudan A, Murphy CE, Wang RC, Smollin CG. Return encounters in emergency department patients treated with phenobarbital versus benzodiazepines for alcohol withdrawal. *J Med Toxicol.* 2022;18(1):4–10.
104. Centanni N, Mezoian T, Gilboy J, et al. Effect of phenobarbital-based alcohol withdrawal protocol on provider practice and patient outcomes—a quality improvement study. *Hosp Pharm.* 2024;59(5):562–567.
105. Winkelman TNA, Admon LK, Jennings L, Shippee ND, Richardson CR, Bart G. Evaluation of amphetamine-related hospitalizations and associated clinical outcomes and costs in the United States. *JAMA Netw Open.* 2018;1(6):e183758.
106. Cadet JL. Methamphetamine-induced psychosis: who says all drug use is reversible? *Curr Psychiatr.* 2017;16(11):14–20.
107. Coffin PO, Santos GM, Hern J, et al. Effects of mirtazapine for methamphetamine use disorder among cisgender men and transgender women who have sex with men: a placebo-controlled randomized clinical trial. *JAMA Psychiatry.* 2020;77(3):246.
108. Colfax GN. Mirtazapine to reduce methamphetamine use: a randomized controlled trial. *Arch Gen Psychiatry.* 2011;68(11):1168–1175.
109. Acheson LS, Clay S, McKetin R, et al. Participant experiences in a pilot study for methamphetamine withdrawal treatment: implications for retention. *Int J Drug Policy.* 2024;126:104383.
110. Hassanein EHM, Althagafy HS, Baraka MA, Abd-alhameed EK, Ibrahim IM. Pharmacological update of mirtazapine: a narrative literature review. *Naunyn Schmiedebergs Arch Pharmacol.* 2024;397(5):2603–2619.
111. Naji L, Dennis B, Rosic T, et al. Mirtazapine for the treatment of amphetamine and methamphetamine use disorder: a systematic review and meta-analysis. *Drug Alcohol Depend.* 2022;232:109295.
112. Rash CJ, Alessi SM, Petry NM. Cocaine abusers with and without alcohol dependence respond equally well to contingency management treatments. *Exp Clin Psychopharmacol.* 2008;16(4):275–281.
113. Hawk M, Coulter RWS, Egan JE, et al. Harm reduction principles for healthcare settings. *Harm Reduct J.* 2017;14(1):70.
114. Samuels EA, Dwyer K, Mello MJ, Baird J, Kellogg AR, Bernstein E. Emergency department-based opioid harm reduction: moving physicians from willing to doing. *Acad Emerg Med.* 2016;23(4):455–465.
115. Jiao S, Bungay V, Jenkins E, Gagnon M. How an emergency department is organized to provide opioid-specific harm reduction and facilitators and barriers to harm reduction implementation: a systems perspective. *Harm Reduct J.* 2023;20(1):139.

116. Gunn A, Smothers Z, Schramm-Sapyta N, Freiermuth C, MacEachern M, Muzyk A. The emergency department as an opportunity for naloxone distribution. *West J Emerg Med.* 2018;19(6):1036–1042.
117. Samuels EA, Hoppe J, Papp J, Whiteside L, Raja AS, Bernstein E. Emergency department naloxone distribution. *Ann Emerg Med.* 2022;80(4):371–379.
118. Centers for Disease Control and Prevention. *Syringe Services Programs (SSPs).* 2019. https://archive.cdc.gov/#/details?q=Syringe%20Services%20Programs%20(SSPs)&start=0&rows=10&url=https://www.cdc.gov/hepatitis/policy/FO-CDC-RFA-PS22-2208.htm?
119. Heck J, Höner Zu Siederdissen C, Krause O, et al. Concordance of emergency department physicians' decisions on HIV post-exposure prophylaxis with national guidelines: results from a retrospective cohort study. *Int Health.* 2024;16(2):219–226.
120. White DAE, Jewett M, Burns M, et al. A quality improvement initiative to increase HIV post-exposure prophylaxis treatment for emergency department patients after sexual assault: a pre-post study. *PLoS ONE.* 2025;20(3):e0320690.
121. Bisom-Rapp E, Patel K, Jaradeh K, Hayirli TC, Peabody CR. Feasibility of emergency department-initiated HIV pre-exposure prophylaxis. *West J Emerg Med.* 2024;25(6):985–992.
122. Gormley MA, Nagy TR, Moschella P, Lu Z, Rodriguez J, Roth P. HIV pre-exposure prophylaxis in the emergency department: a systematic review. *Ann Emerg Med.* 2023;81(4):468–481.
123. Shull JA, Attys JM, Amutah-Onukagha NN, Hill MJ. Utilizing emergency departments for pre-exposure prophylaxis (PrEP). *J Am Coll Emerg Physicians Open.* 2020;1(6):1427–1435.
124. Rosenberg KD, DeMunter JK, Liu J. Emergency contraception in emergency departments in Oregon, 2003. *Am J Public Health.* 2005;95(8):1453–1457.
125. American College of Obstetricians and Gynecologists. Access to emergency contraception. Committee Opinion No. 707: Improving awareness of and screening for health risks among sex workers. *Obstet Gynecol.* 2017;130(1):e53–e57.
126. Israel BS, Belcher AM, Ford JD. A harm reduction framework for integrated treatment of co-occurring opioid use disorder and trauma-related disorders. *J Dual Diagn.* 2024;20(1):52–85.
127. CDC. *SUDORS Dashboard: Fatal Drug Overdose Data. Overdose Prevention.* February 13, 2025. Accessed February 22, 2025. https://www.cdc.gov/overdose-prevention/data-research/facts-stats/sudors-dashboard-fatal-overdose-data.html
128. Orme S, Zarkin GA, Dunlap LJ, et al. Cost and cost savings of navigation services to avoid rehospitalization for a comorbid substance use disorder population. *Med Care.* 2022;60(8):631–635.
129. LaPietra A, Simon B, Maybloom R, et al. 106 emergency physician quality improvement metric increases utilization of medication for opioid use disorder. *Ann Emerg Med.* 2024;84(4):S47.
130. Samuels EA, D'Onofrio G, Huntley K, et al. A quality framework for emergency department treatment of opioid use disorder. *Ann Emerg Med.* 2019;73(3):237–247.
131. Williams AR, Mauro CM, Huber B, et al. Defining discontinuation for buprenorphine treatment: implications for quality measurement. *Am J Psychiatry.* 2024;181(5):457–459.
132. Anderson KE, Saloner B, Eckstein J, et al. Quality of buprenorphine care for insured adults with opioid use disorder. *Med Care.* 2021;59(5):393–401.
133. Gordon A, Lo-Ciganic WH, Cochran G, Gellad WF, Cathers T, Donohue JM. Treatment quality for buprenorphine care: the pot at the end of the rainbow. *J Addict Med.* 2016;10(3):210–211.
134. CMS Office of Minority Health. Impact of hospital readmissions reduction initiatives on vulnerable populations. *Baltim MD Cent Medicare Medicaid Serv.* Published online September, 2020. https://www.cms.gov/files/document/impact-readmissions-reduction-initiatives-report.pdf
135. CMS. *Hospital Readmission Reduction Program.* Accessed April 28, 2025. https://www.cms.gov/medicare/quality/value-based-programs/hospital-readmissions

7

Opioid Use Disorder Evaluation and Management

Ashish P. Thakrar, Kristine E. Torres-Lockhart, Leslie Suen

Jonathan (a pseudonym) was an unhoused man in his 30s admitted to our safety-net hospital for an infection he developed as a complication of smoking and injecting fentanyl. During his hospitalization, Jonathan developed sepsis and necrotizing fasciitis of both lower limbs that required bilateral amputations. He required an extended stay in the intensive care unit (ICU) and his hospital course was complicated by end-stage renal failure requiring dialysis. Our addiction medicine consult service was consulted for treatment of opioid use disorder (OUD).

Initial Treatment Plan: Consideration of Methadone

Jonathan initially wanted to start methadone treatment for OUD because methadone offered him the best control of opioid withdrawal and craving based on his prior experience. However, after starting methadone in the setting of progressive kidney failure and, ultimately, uremia, Jonathan had repeated episodes of oversedation. In addition, our consult service was concerned about his ability to access an opioid treatment program (OTP) for daily methadone dosing given leg infections that ultimately required amputation. He would need a wheelchair, and OTPs can be hard to access for people with mobility and transportation challenges.

Transition to Buprenorphine

In light of his oversedation, ongoing critical illness, and access concerns, Jonathan and the addiction consult team agreed to transition to buprenorphine for OUD treatment. After a few days on buprenorphine, however, Jonathan reported that buprenorphine did not adequately address his severe opioid cravings. Jonathan had feelings of isolation during his extended hospitalization, and despite his determination to manage his OUD, he had a few episodes of substance use in the hospital that he felt could have been mitigated by methadone rather than buprenorphine. These incidents of in-hospital substance use additionally strained his relationships with some ICU nurses, leaving him feeling ashamed and stigmatized.

Adjustment of Care: Back to Methadone

As Jonathan's renal function improved, the addiction consult team worked with him to reconsider his OUD treatment plan in context of his long-term goals. Together, they decided to switch him back to methadone. He responded well to this adjustment and had significant relief from opioid cravings with improved mood and without episodes of sedation. He also secured a place in supportive housing. After hospital discharge, Jonathan continued methadone treatment at a local OTP through support from his case management teams, and he remained engaged with outpatient wound care. Jonathan's medical and social stabilization demonstrates the importance of tailoring OUD treatment to individual needs, addressing stigma, and leveraging community resources to support recovery.

Lessons Learned

Jonathan's case underscores the opportunities to partner with hospitalized patients with OUD, even in light of a severe OUD and significant medical comorbidities. Key takeaways include:

1. **Flexible, Patient-Centered Treatment Approaches**: Methadone and buprenorphine are effective and should be offered to all hospitalized patients with OUD, but individualized treatment plans are essential, particularly in patients with complex medical and social circumstances.
2. **Stigma and Relationships**: Substance use during hospitalization can strain clinician–patient relationships, but maintaining a nonjudgmental and supportive approach is critical to fostering trust and engagement.
3. **Continuity of Care**: Discharge planning should prioritize ensuring access to OUD treatment and medical follow-up, especially for patients in underserved areas.

Jonathan's journey reflects the resilience of patients facing significant medical and psychosocial challenges and highlights the role of compassionate, individualized care in fostering recovery and hope.

—Leslie Suen

Key Points

- **All hospitalized patients with OUD should be offered long-term OUD treatment with methadone, buprenorphine, or, for those who decline these options, extended-release (XR) naltrexone.**
- **Opioid withdrawal should be treated promptly with an evidence-based approach that involves methadone or buprenorphine, other nonopioid medications, and, when necessary, short-acting opioids.**
- **There are novel approaches to starting methadone and buprenorphine that respond to the unique pharmacology of fentanyl and other high-potency synthetic opioids; these approaches are increasingly common and supported by emerging evidence.**
- **Clinical care for OUD should prioritize patients' goals, stigma-free communication, harm reduction, and management of OUD-related complications in addition to OUD treatment.**

Introduction and Epidemiology of OUD in the Hospital Setting

Opioids are the broad class of natural, semisynthetic, or synthetic compounds that bind to opioid receptors and cause morphine-like pharmacologic effects. The term *opiate* refers to the specific group of naturally occurring opioids derived from poppy plants, for example, opium, morphine, codeine, and heroin. In contrast, synthetic opioids are derived solely from precursor chemicals. Since 2014, illicitly manufactured fentanyl and other high-potency synthetic opioids have adulterated and then replaced heroin in the unregulated drug supply in the United States (US).

The spread of fentanyl and other high-potency synthetic opioids has made opioid use more unpredictable and dangerous. Overdose deaths in the US reached a peak of 111,029 deaths in 2022[1]; based on the most recently available data, approximately 87,000 overdose deaths occurred in the US from October 2023 to September 2024.[2] Approximately 75% to 80% of overdose deaths in the US every year are due to opioids, and the vast majority of these deaths are now caused by fentanyl and other high-potency synthetic opioids.[2] Opioid-related hospitalizations rose by 64% between 2004 and 2015[3]; as of 2020, they accounted for about 2% of all hospital admissions.[4] Hospitalization can serve as an important opportunity to offer persons with OUD withdrawal management, OUD treatment, harm-reduction services, and linkage to ongoing care for OUD and related complications.[5] For more details on the epidemiology of OUD, please see Chapter 1.

Summary of Evidence

Meta-analyses and systematic reviews of clinical trials have established a very strong evidence base for the treatment of opioid withdrawal and OUD. The studies included in these reviews enrolled patients across a range of settings including outpatient clinics, medically managed withdrawal (previously known as "detox") units, and human laboratory units, and thus have high relevance to patients who are hospitalized (Table 7.1). Most patients in these studies were using opioids such as heroin or oxycodone that are less potent and less lipophilic than high-potency synthetic opioids like fentanyl. Thus, dosing approaches might have to be adapted for patients using opioids

TABLE 7.1

Level of Evidence and Key Studies for Treatment of Opioid Withdrawal and OUD

Key practice	Level of evidence	Key studies or reviews
Treating opioid withdrawal with methadone, buprenorphine, and/or the $alpha_2$-agonists lofexidine or clonidine	Systematic reviews with meta-analyses of randomized controlled trials	Gowing et al (2017)[6] Gowing et al (2016)[7] Calcaterra et al (2022)[8]
Treating opioid withdrawal with short-acting opioids as an adjuvant or bridge to methadone or buprenorphine	Retrospective cohort studies without comparator group	Steiner et al (2025)[9] Thakrar et al (2023)[10]
Treating OUD with methadone, buprenorphine, or extended-release naltrexone	Systematic reviews with meta-analyses of randomized controlled trials	Santo et al (2021)[11] Sordo et al (2017)[12]
Starting medications for OUD while patients are hospitalized	Randomized controlled trials	Liebschutz et al (2014)[8,13] Calcaterra et al (2022) Englander et al (2024)[5]
Buprenorphine low-dose initiation with opioid continuation	Retrospective cohort studies	Button et al (2022)[14] Jablonski et al (2022)[15] Cohen et al (2021)[16]
Buprenorphine high-dose initiation	Retrospective cohort studies	Herring et al (2021)[17]
Rapid methadone titration for hospitalized patients	Retrospective cohort studies without comparator group	Casey et al (2023)[18] Klaire et al (2023)[19] Martin et al (2023)[20] Bosshardt et al (2025)[34]

in our current era of fentanyl or other high-potency synthetic opioids.

Summary of Evidence: Opioid Withdrawal Treatment

Opioid withdrawal is a syndrome of physical and psychological symptoms that arises after sudden reduction or cessation of opioid use. Opioid withdrawal is uncomfortable and distressing and, in severe cases without treatment, can be fatal.[21] Historically, opioid withdrawal has been undertreated in general medical settings like the hospital,[22,23] contributing to distrust,[24] delayed presentations for care,[25] before medically advised discharges,[4,26] and in-hospital substance use.[27] However, evidence-based treatment of opioid withdrawal is well described with robust evidence and should be offered to all hospitalized patients with opioid withdrawal.

A 2017 meta-analysis[6] of 27 randomized controlled trials (RCTs) with a total of 3,048 participants determined that individuals who had opioid withdrawal treated with buprenorphine had less severe opioid withdrawal and were more likely to complete opioid withdrawal treatment compared to individuals treated with the $alpha_2$-agonists like clonidine or lofexidine. This meta-analysis also found evidence suggesting that buprenorphine and methadone have similar efficacy for opioid withdrawal treatment, although buprenorphine may relieve opioid withdrawal faster. Participants from 17 of these 27 studies were experiencing withdrawal from heroin alone or heroin and methadone; others were withdrawing from oxycodone, opium, buprenorphine, or methadone.

Compared to withdrawal from heroin, oxycodone, or morphine, withdrawal from fentanyl or other high-potency opioids appears to have different severity and time course. One quasi-experimental study found that fentanyl withdrawal, compared to heroin withdrawal, took longer to peak (2 to 3 days for fentanyl vs <1 day for heroin) and involved more severe symptoms (peak clinical opioid withdrawal scale [COWS] about 4 to 5 points higher during days 2 to 4) even while participants were treated with 30 mg subcutaneous morphine four times daily.[28] These findings align with clinical experience, suggesting that patients who chronically use fentanyl have higher opioid tolerance than patients who use other less potent opioids.

Evidence is emerging on how to adapt opioid withdrawal treatment for individuals using fentanyl.[29] Retrospective cohort studies without comparator groups have described the feasibility and safety of methadone and buprenorphine dosing approaches for patients using fentanyl. These approaches, which include rapid methadone titration, buprenorphine low-dose initiation with opioid continuation (LDI-OC), and high-dose buprenorphine initiation, respond to the higher opioid tolerance and lipophilicity of fentanyl (see *OUD Treatment* below for details). In addition, short-acting opioids (most often immediate-release oxycodone, hydromorphone, or morphine) can be used to treat opioid withdrawal in the hospital, usually used as adjuvants to methadone or as a bridge to buprenorphine. Two single-arm retrospective cohort studies with a total of 147 patients found this practice to be feasible with few adverse events.[9,10] In these studies, most patients were using fentanyl prior to hospitalization, an addiction consultation team or expert pharmacist selected patients and guided dosing, patients received an average of 200 to 300 oral morphine milligram equivalents daily (most often in addition to methadone), adverse events were rare, higher doses of short-acting opioids were correlated with less severe withdrawal, and patients had lower risk of discharge before medically advised compared to historical controls.

Summary of Evidence: OUD Treatment

In addition to receiving opioid withdrawal treatment, hospitalized patients should be offered long-term treatment for OUD. In the US, there are three FDA-approved medication treatments for OUD: methadone, buprenorphine, and XR naltrexone. Two systematic reviews with meta-analyses of RCTs and observational studies[11,12] (combined 15 RCTs with 3,852 participants and 36 cohort studies with 872,518 participants) found that individuals in, compared to out of, OUD treatment with methadone or buprenorphine have substantially lower all-cause mortality (relative risk in vs out of treatment 0.47; 95% CI 0.41–0.54[11]). Two single-site RCTs, one in an emergency department (ED)[30] (n = 320) and one among admitted patients[13] (n = 145), found that initiating buprenorphine treatment for OUD in the hospital leads to increased engagement in OUD care and decreased opioid use after hospital discharge. XR naltrexone is also FDA approved for OUD treatment, but has not demonstrated the same reduction in mortality in real-world studies, potentially because it is more difficult to initiate.[31] Based on this evidence, methadone, buprenorphine, and, for those who decline these medications, XR naltrexone should be offered to every hospitalized patient with OUD.

There has been almost no prospective, clinical research on the best way to start methadone treatment of OUD.[32] Methadone has a long half-life of about 24 hours, thus once-daily dosing leads to dose stacking during the first 5 to 7 days. The traditional opioid treatment program (OTP) approach is to start at 10 to 30 mg daily and increase the dose by 5 to 10 mg only after patients reach steady state, after approximately 5 to 7 days. This approach emerged through clinical practice and expert consensus to minimize the risks of opioid overdose in outpatient, unmonitored settings.[33]

At least ten retrospective cohort studies with a total of 649 methadone initiations have described[34] the feasibility, safety, and clinical outcomes of more rapid methadone titrations in hospital settings guided by addiction consultation services.[18,19,35–38] Dosing approaches varied and adverse events related to methadone occurred infrequently, typically only with the most aggressive approaches.[18,35] Further research is needed to understand which dosing approach best balances the benefit of early opioid withdrawal treatment with the risk of methadone dose stacking, which may occur after hospital discharge. For now, expert guidance suggests that for individuals with high opioid tolerance (eg, use of illicit fentanyl), an initial dose of 30 to 40 mg with dose titrations for ongoing withdrawal in 10-mg increments up to 40 mg total on day 1, 50 mg total on day 2, and 60 mg total on day 3 is likely safe with adequate monitoring, and likely improves outcomes for hospitalized patients using fentanyl.[5,20] Supplemental opioids, either short-acting opioids or additional methadone via faster titrations, may be safe and necessary to treat withdrawal in some settings.[35,39]

The standard approach to initiating buprenorphine (wait 8 to 12 hours from last use of a short-acting opioid until objective signs of opioid withdrawal, then give 2 to 4 mg sublingual (SL) buprenorphine followed by additional buprenorphine if no precipitated withdrawal[40]) is associated with only rare instances of precipitated withdrawal for individuals using heroin or oxycodone based on a systematic review,[41] RCTs in observed settings[42] and observational studies of home buprenorphine initiations.[43] There is controversy about whether and to what extent fentanyl use increases the risk of buprenorphine precipitated withdrawal.[44] A secondary analysis of a multisite RCT[45] with 1,200 patients in EDs (75% exposed to fentanyl) found 1% incidence of precipitated withdrawal, while a retrospective cohort study of 226 initiations found an overall incidence of 12% and 16% incidence among patients with confirmed fentanyl use.[45,46] When there is concern for buprenorphine-precipitated withdrawal, LDI-OC[44] or bridging with short-acting opioids can be used as alternative buprenorphine initiation approaches.

LDI-OC has been described in more than two dozen case series or retrospective cohort studies of more than 250 patients in total.[44] A systematic review of buprenorphine initiation strategies for OUD and pain management found 96% success rate of LDI-OC,[47] however, studies of LDI-OC specifically among hospitalized patients with OUD demonstrated lower success rates ranging from 68% to 92%.[14,15,48] Various dosing approaches and buprenorphine formulations have been used and there is insufficient evidence to recommend any one approach over others. Another practice that has emerged is to treat opioid withdrawal with short-acting opioids for 24 to 48 hours while allowing bioaccumulated fentanyl to clear prior to initiating buprenorphine with a standard initiation. This approach has only been described anecdotally.

High-dose initiation, wherein initial doses of 8 to 24 mg SL buprenorphine are given in the same setting as traditional initiation (ie, after a sufficient period of opioid abstinence and once patients demonstrate objective signs of opioid withdrawal), has been described in one prospective study[45] and in two retrospective case series,[17,49] all in EDs, with low rates of sedation and precipitated withdrawal.[17]

Federal Legal and Regulatory Restrictions

Clinicians and staff may have concerns about legal or regulatory barriers to using medications for opioid withdrawal and OUD in the hospital. This section reviews federal regulations. State or local jurisdictions may impose additional restrictions, though the authors are not aware of any that specifically pertain to hospitalized patients.

In federal regulations (most notably Title 21, Chapter II, Part 1300 of the Code of Federal Regulations), there is a distinction drawn between *prescribing*, *dispensing*, and *administering* controlled substances. Based on current interpretation, outpatient clinicians and hospital clinicians on discharge *prescribe* medications to be filled by the patient from a pharmacy, sometimes at a later date. Alternatively, medications may be *dispensed* directly to patients by a hospital pharmacy or an OTP to be taken on-site or at a later time. Last, medications are *administered* to hospitalized patients when they are directly given, often by nurses, during hospitalization (Table 7.2).

Legal and Regulatory Restrictions: Buprenorphine

In the hospital setting, buprenorphine may be administered or dispensed for OUD. In addition, any drug enforcement administration (DEA)-registered physician or advanced-practice clinician may prescribe buprenorphine on hospital discharge. Special buprenorphine training and DEA registration (commonly known as the "X-waiver") is no longer required to prescribe buprenorphine as of January 2023.[50]

Legal and Regulatory Restrictions: Methadone

In the outpatient setting, methadone for OUD can only be dispensed from licensed OTPs. OTPs are

TABLE 7.2

Regulatory Considerations for Opioid Withdrawal and OUD Treatment in Emergency Department and Hospital Settings

Key permitted practices	Relevant federal law, regulations, and citations
▪ Administering or dispensing buprenorphine during hospitalization ▪ Prescribing buprenorphine at hospital discharge	▪ Drug Addiction Treatment Act of 2000 ▪ Consolidated Appropriations Act of 2023[50]
▪ Administering methadone (for withdrawal or OUD treatment) during medical or surgical hospital treatment of conditions other than addiction	▪ 21 CFR 1306.07 (c)[51] ▪ Martin et al (2023)[20]
▪ Administering hydromorphone, oxycodone, morphine, or other short-acting opioids for opioid withdrawal, treatment, or intractable pain during hospitalization	▪ 21 CFR 1306.07 (c)[51] ▪ Thakrar et al (2023)[10] ▪ Steiner et al (2025)[9]
▪ Dispensing up to 3 d of methadone for OUD to bridge patients from hospital or ED discharge to linkage at an OTP	▪ 21 CFR 1306.07 (b)[51] ▪ Skogrand et al (2023)[52] ▪ Bowman et al (2024)[53] ▪ Huo et al (2025)[54]
▪ Buprenorphine treatment at SNF prescribed by SNF clinicians ▪ Methadone treatment at SNF with methadone dispensed by an OTP	▪ Pytell et al (2019)[55] ▪ Cohen et al (2023)[56]

sometimes referred to as "methadone clinics" or, in older federal regulations, "narcotic treatment programs." Methadone cannot be prescribed for OUD treatment in the outpatient setting. Thus, hospital clinicians may not prescribe methadone for OUD on discharge, for example, to bridge a patient from discharge to intake at an OTP. Practically, this means hospital clinicians must ensure a patient can access methadone for OUD starting the day following discharge. Most often, this is accomplished through enrollment at an OTP, but some hospitals have established pathways to directly dispense up to a 3-day supply of methadone for patients to take home on discharge (see exception 3 below).[52,53]

Three federal regulatory exceptions allow methadone to be administered or dispensed, but not prescribed, to hospitalized patients with OUD:

1. First, methadone (or any "narcotic drug") may be administered or dispensed "to maintain or detoxify a person as an incidental adjunct to medical or surgical treatment of conditions other than addiction" (see *21 CFR 1306.07 (c)*). Under this exception, patients hospitalized for medical or surgical conditions may be administered methadone without dose or time limitations.[20,57]
2. Second, methadone (or any "narcotic drug") may be administered or dispensed to persons with OUD and "intractable pain in which no relief or cure is possible, or none has been found after reasonable efforts" (see *21 CFR 1306.07 (c)*).
3. Third, methadone (or any "narcotic drug") can be dispensed "for the purpose of initiating maintenance treatment or detoxification" for up to 3 days (with up to a 3-day supply dispensed) "while arrangements are being made for referral for treatment" (see *21 CFR 1306.07 (b)*). Under this exception, patients hospitalized specifically for addiction (eg, in medically managed withdrawal units) and patients being discharged from the hospital or ED can be dispensed methadone for up to 3 days at a time.[52,53] This is sometimes referred to as the "3-day" or "72-hour" rule. Note, methadone must be dispensed specifically from the hospital-based pharmacy and cannot be prescribed for OUD treatment to an external pharmacy. This is described further in Chapter 3.

Legal and Regulatory Restrictions: Other Opioids

As with methadone, other opioids besides buprenorphine cannot be prescribed for OUD treatment in the outpatient setting.[58] However, "narcotic drugs" such as the short-acting opioids hydromorphone, oxycodone, or morphine can be administered to hospitalized patients in the specific situations described in the exceptions above.[22,23]

Legal and Regulatory Restrictions: Skilled Nursing Facilities

Hospital clinicians must ensure OUD care can continue if patients are discharged directly to a skilled nursing facility (SNF). Any DEA-registered physician or advanced-practice clinician at an SNF may prescribe buprenorphine for OUD treatment. As noted above, there is no longer a requirement for documented training or a dedicated "X-waiver."

The provision of methadone for OUD at SNFs is more complicated. SNF admissions are not considered hospitalizations, thus the exceptions noted above for administering or dispensing methadone in the hospital do not apply to SNFs. As a result, SNF clinicians may not prescribe methadone to treat OUD.[55] Instead, SNF patients receiving methadone treatment for OUD must have methadone dispensed from an OTP while at an SNF. Approaches to enrolling patients in an OTP while hospitalized for ongoing OUD care at an SNF are described below. See Chapters 3 and 20 for more information as well.

Of note, it is a violation of the Americans with Disabilities Act (ADA), the Rehabilitation Act of 1973, and the Patient Protection and Affordable Care Act for an SNF to refuse to admit a patient because they are treated with medications for OUD.[56]

Clinical Evaluation and Management of OUD

Diagnosis of OUD and Related Conditions

This section defines the related conditions of OUD, opioid dependence, and opioid misuse (Table 7.3). While there may be overlap between these diagnoses, it is important to understand their unique aspects to ensure hospitalized patients are offered appropriate, evidence-based, and legally permissible treatments and services.

Opioid Use Disorder

OUD is the ongoing, compulsive use of opioids despite significant impairment, distress, and/or negative consequences. Key characteristics of OUD are sometimes described by the "3 Cs" of "craving, compulsive use, and negative consequences."[3] Formally, OUD is defined and diagnosed using the *Diagnostic and Statistical Manual of the Mental Disorders*, 5th edition (DSM-5).[3,59] DSM-5 describes 11 criteria for OUD: opioid tolerance, opioid withdrawal, using

TABLE 7.3

Summary of Distinguishing Characteristics between OUD, Opioid Dependence, and Opioid Misuse

Clinical characteristics	OUD	Opioid dependence	Opioid misuse
Opioid tolerance	Yes	Yes[a]	No
Opioid withdrawal	Yes	Yes[a]	Maybe[b]
Compulsive use of opioids	Yes	No	Maybe[b]
Opioid use despite negative consequences	Yes	No	Maybe[b]
Opioid craving	Yes	No	Maybe[b]

[a]Individuals are taking prescribed opioids as directed by their prescriber.

[b]Individuals with opioid misuse should undergo a full evaluation for possible OUD. They may be a high risk for opioid overdose and may benefit from medications for opioid use disorder, particularly buprenorphine.

more opioids than intended, inability to cut down on opioid use, opioid craving, increased time spent using or recovering from opioid use, physically hazardous use (eg, driving while impaired), opioid use despite negative health consequences, opioid use despite social/interpersonal problems, inability to carry out roles or obligations, and important activities have been given up or reduced due to opioid use. OUD severity is defined based on the number of criteria, with mild OUD defined as 2 to 3 criteria, moderate OUD as 4 to 5 criteria, and severe OUD as 6 or more criteria.[3,59] Note that opioid dependence and opioid withdrawal are not considered diagnostic of OUD for individuals using only opioids prescribed to them for chronic pain.

Opioid Dependence

Opioid dependence is defined as physical dependence resulting from long-term opioid use. Patients with opioid dependence develop opioid withdrawal symptoms (eg, rhinorrhea, lacrimation, mydriasis, anxiety, restlessness) after abrupt cessation or decrease in opioid use.[60,61] All patients treated with long-term prescription opioid therapy are likely to develop physical dependence and should be counseled accordingly. For example, a patient presenting to the hospital prescribed long-term opioids for years for chronic pain without compulsive use and without associated negative consequences likely has opioid dependence and would develop opioid withdrawal without continued administration of opioids. In the absence of DSM-5 criteria for OUD, this patient would not meet criteria for OUD.

Opioid Misuse

Misuse of opioids is defined as opioid use in any way other than what is prescribed, often for rewarding effects. Opioids, especially at high doses and when used intranasally or intravenously, increase dopamine activity reward and motivation neuropathways (including the ventral tegmental area and nucleus accumbens).[60]

For a patient prescribed long-term opioid therapy for pain, the use of prescribed opioids more often or in higher doses than prescribed (or used for a reason other than its intended use, eg, for sleep or to enhance mood) would be considered opioid misuse. While opioid misuse is not synonymous with OUD, patients misusing prescribed opioids should have a thorough history and assessment for OUD and may meet criteria for OUD.[60]

Role of Toxicology Testing in Diagnosing OUD

OUD, opioid dependence, and opioid misuse are clinical diagnoses that require a thorough patient history. Urine or serum toxicology testing can inform or prompt assessments for these conditions, but toxicology testing is not required or sufficient to make the diagnosis.[62] In addition, it is important to consider that inappropriate use or misinterpretation of toxicology tests can contribute to poor outcomes (eg, family separation for pregnant and parenting patients) or fractured therapeutic relationships.[63,64]

Point-of-care (POC) immunoassay urine toxicology tests can provide rapid results, but they have poor specificity and sensitivity for some opioids and must be interpreted carefully. For example, POC urine tests for opiates assess for the presence of organic opioids derived from poppy such as heroin, morphine, and codeine; these tests do not assess for the presence of fentanyl and other synthetic opioids. In addition, POC urine tests are sometimes used to assess if a substance has been used in a certain window of time, however, this interpretation has to be informed by the unique pharmacology of each substance. For example, among patients with OUD using fentanyl, fentanyl is detectable in urine for an average of 5 to 7 days after last use.[65,66] Given the prolonged clearance of fentanyl during early abstinence, even confirmatory testing using mass spectrometry must be interpreted cautiously.[67]

Several studies and published cases have demonstrated a gap between clinician confidence and clinician knowledge in toxicology interpretation. Improved knowledge around toxicology testing is critical to determining if testing is: (1) indicated and likely to change the course of clinical care, and (2) to ensure accurate interpretation of any testing performed.[62,63,67] In these settings, consulting addiction medicine or toxicology experts can be beneficial.

Opioid Withdrawal Diagnosis and Treatment

Diagnosing and Assessing Opioid Withdrawal

Opioid withdrawal syndrome is a constellation of physical and psychological symptoms that arise with sudden reduction or cessation of opioid use in persons who have used opioids repeatedly over time.[61,68] The most common signs and symptoms are anxiety or irritability, restlessness, insomnia, hot or cold flashes, nausea, vomiting, diarrhea, abdominal cramping, pupil dilation, lacrimation, rhinorrhea, yawning, diaphoresis, piloerection, tachycardia, and hypertension.[61,68] Opioid withdrawal can be very distressing for patients with OUD and fear of withdrawal may be a primary motivation for ongoing use. Although opioid withdrawal itself is infrequently life threatening, untreated opioid withdrawal can cause life-threatening hypovolemia from fluid losses and can prompt patients to leave the hospital before medically advised.[4,26]

Opioid withdrawal typically starts within 12 hours after the last use of a short-acting opioid such as heroin or oxycodone and peaks in severity within 24 hours of cessation. For patients using long-acting opioids such as XR oxycodone, methadone, or buprenorphine, opioid withdrawal symptoms start within 24 to 72 hours after last use and may peak a few days after onset. For individuals with OUD using illicit fentanyl, opioid withdrawal typically arises within 8 to 24 hours of cessation and peaks 2 to 3 days after last use.[28] Although prescribed fentanyl is considered a short-acting opioid when used for analgesia, opioid withdrawal after long-term use of illicitly manufactured fentanyl may take longer to manifest and peak for individuals with OUD because fentanyl exposure over weeks leads to peripheral accumulation in adipose and skeletal muscle.[65,69]

For patients taking prescribed long-term opioids (or any opioid of consistent amount and potency), dose reductions of more than 10% to 20% per week can also lead to opioid withdrawal.[70]

Opioid withdrawal should be diagnosed clinically by assessing for both physical and psychological symptoms. Formal assessment with a validated scale can help guide treatment and dosing, but should not be required to initiate opioid withdrawal care.[5] The most commonly used validated clinical scale is the Clinical Opiate Withdrawal Scale (COWS), which grades withdrawal as mild (5 to 12), moderate (13 to 24), or severe (25 to 36) based on 11 signs and symptoms.[71] Other validated scales include the Short Opioid Withdrawal Scale,[72] the Subjective Opioid Withdrawal Scale,[73] and the Objective Opioid Withdrawal Scale.[73]

Many of the signs and symptoms of opioid withdrawal can occur due to other conditions that are common among hospitalized patients, including acute infection (eg, upper respiratory infections or gastroenteritis), other withdrawal syndromes (eg, alcohol or benzodiazepines), or anxiety (including fear of withdrawal itself).[61,74] Thus, in the hospital, it is particularly important to use a patient-centered, non-judgment approach to obtaining an accurate history of recent opioid use and to integrate this information with objective findings on exam and laboratory testing. Some physical manifestations such as pupil dilation and yawning are more specific to opioid withdrawal compared to other conditions.[61] In addition, patients should be reassured that adequate treatment of opioid withdrawal treatment is a shared priority for the care team.[5]

Management of Acute Opioid Withdrawal

Table 7.4 provides an overview of a recommended approach for management of acute opioid withdrawal in the hospital.

Opioid withdrawal should be managed with a combination of (1) methadone or buprenorphine (or, in Canada, slow-release oral morphine [SROM]); (2) the alpha$_2$-agonists clonidine or lofexidine; (3) other nonopioid medications; and, if necessary, (4) other short-acting opioids. Patients who are ambivalent about or who decline long-term OUD treatment with methadone, buprenorphine, and SROM should still receive one of these for withdrawal treatment while hospitalized based on a large body of evidence on their safety and efficacy in treating opioid withdrawal. Initial opioid withdrawal treatment with one of these medications also gives patients the opportunity to be discharged on OUD treatment if they

TABLE 7.4

Treatment of Acute Opioid Withdrawal

Long-acting opioid		Alpha$_2$-agonist		Other nonopioid medications		Other opioids (if necessary)
▪ Buprenorphine (2–8 mg SL initial dose, titrate in 2–8 mg SL increments every 60–90 min to max 24–32 mg SL daily) *or* ▪ Methadone (20–40 mg PO initial dose, titrate in 5–10 mg increments every 4–6 h to max 40–60 mg PO day 1) *or* ▪ Slow-release oral morphine (in Canada, not available in the US) 30–200 mg PO once daily using the 24 h extended-release formulation, titrate to response	*and*	▪ Lofexidine (0.54 mg PO every 5–6 h) *or* ▪ Clonidine (0.1–0.3 mg PO every 6–8 h)	*and*	▪ Loperamide for diarrhea (4 mg PO, then 2 mg for ongoing loose stools) ▪ Ondansetron for nausea (4–8 mg PO every 4–8 h) ▪ Dicyclomine for intestinal cramping (20 mg PO every 4 h) ▪ Trazodone for insomnia (25–100 PO mg nightly) ▪ Ibuprofen for muscle aches or joint pain (400–600 PO every 6 h) ▪ Hydroxyzine for anxiety and restlessness (25–50 PO mg every 6 h)	*and*	▪ Hydromorphone (4–6 mg PO every 3 h initial dose, titrate to effect) *or* ▪ Morphine (20–30 mg PO every 3–4 h initial dose, titrate to effect) *or* ▪ Oxycodone (15–20 mg PO every 4 h initial dose, titrate to effect)

During the first 1–3 days of opioid withdrawal treatment, monitor patients every 6–8 hours with standardized scales for ongoing withdrawal (eg, with COWS) and for oversedation (eg, with RASS or POSS), especially if using multiple opioids or other sedating medications.

change their mind. If patients wish to be discharged without medications for OUD, these long-acting opioids can be tapered or abruptly discontinued prior to discharge.

In the US, the choice of whether to use methadone or buprenorphine as the long-acting opioid for initial opioid withdrawal management depends on patient preference and clinical context. Patients who wish, at the outset of withdrawal treatment, to start medication treatment for OUD should start with whichever long-acting opioid they plan to use for ongoing OUD treatment outside the hospital. For patients who are unsure about medication treatment for OUD (and in settings where the perceived risk of buprenorphine-precipitated withdrawal is low), buprenorphine might be preferred because of its faster onset of action, its safety, and the ease of transitioning to methadone if patients decide later to use methadone for OUD. For patients with acute pain, patients who will need multiple surgical procedures, or when concern for buprenorphine-precipitated withdrawal is high, methadone might be preferred for opioid withdrawal.

Methadone and buprenorphine are also the foundation of long-term OUD treatment and should be offered to all hospitalized patients with OUD. Given this overlap between medication approaches for acute opioid withdrawal and long-term OUD treatment, the following section provides details on each medication and pharmacologic approach. Conversations about long-term OUD treatment goals should begin when opioid withdrawal treatment is started so that opioid withdrawal can be treated with the same long-term OUD treatment patients want to continue. Patients may be ambivalent about treatment or unable to discuss the nuances of long-term OUD treatment during active opioid withdrawal. In these settings, these conversations can be revisited once opioid withdrawal is stabilized.

Methadone

Methadone is a synthetic long-acting mu-opioid agonist and NMDA-receptor antagonist that is available in oral, intravenous, and intramuscular formulations. The onset of action for oral methadone is typically 30 to 60 minutes with peak effects in about 3 to 4 hours. Methadone is hepatically metabolized and has a long half-life (average 24 hours, range 8 to 59 hours for nonpregnant individuals). For this reason, clinicians need to be aware that once-daily dosing will lead to dose stacking over the first 4 to 7 days of methadone treatment. In addition, methadone prolongs the QT interval, likely in a dose-dependent manner.[74] More details on QT prolongation are provided below. Intravenous and intramuscular methadone is typically given with a 50% dose reduction (ie, 40 mg oral methadone is 20 mg of IV/IM methadone) from the oral formulation and may possess a higher risk for QTc prolongation.

Methadone for Acute Opioid Withdrawal

In the hospital, methadone for opioid withdrawal is typically dosed as 20 to 30 mg initially followed by additional doses of 5 to 10 mg every 4 to 6 hours for ongoing withdrawal, up to 40 mg on the first day. Over days 2 to 3, methadone for opioid withdrawal can be titrated up in 10-mg doses for ongoing withdrawal symptoms. Typically, 40 to 60 mg daily is sufficient to treat opioid withdrawal. Some rapid methadone titrations for individuals using fentanyl reach up to 60 mg on day 1 and up to 80 mg by day 3, though these higher doses require careful clinical assessment (see *Starting Methadone for OUD Treatment*, below). During the first few days of methadone dosing, some patients report the recurrence of withdrawal about 8 to 12 hours after a morning methadone dose; these patients may benefit from receiving an additional 5 to 10 mg of methadone in the evening.

After initial methadone treatment for acute opioid withdrawal, patients who wish to continue long-term methadone treatment for OUD can have methadone titrated up per below (see *Methadone for OUD Treatment*, below). For patients who wish to start buprenorphine after receiving methadone for opioid withdrawal, clinicians can use LDI-OC or bridge patients with short-acting opioids. Details on these approaches can be found below (see *Buprenorphine for OUD Treatment*, below). Patients who wish to be discharged off medications for OUD despite counseling can be continued on methadone during hospitalization, then abruptly discontinued at discharge or tapered off in about 3 days; the decision to abruptly discontinue or taper should be made in conjunction with patients. Note, however, that medically managed withdrawal without ongoing medications for OUD after hospital discharge is associated with poor outcomes like high risk of opioid overdose and death.[75]

Considerations Before Starting Methadone for OUD Treatment

Clinicians treating patients with OUD should discuss the benefits, risks, and requirements of methadone treatment with patients. There are no special requirements for patients who wish to receive methadone for OUD while hospitalized, but patients who wish to continue methadone for OUD after hospital discharge must enroll in an OTP and be willing to go to the OTP multiple times a week (and potentially daily). OTPs provide counseling, case management and peer support services in addition to methadone treatment. Goal doses generally range from 60 to 180 mg but can be higher or lower depending on the individual. Methadone for OUD treatment is titrated until patients report suppression of opioid withdrawal and cessation of opioid craving without side effects like sedation.

Prior to initiation, hospital clinicians should:

- Document history of prior and current opioid use.
- Confirm diagnosis of OUD.
- Assess concurrent SUD, such as benzodiazepine or alcohol use disorders. The presence of these conditions does not preclude methadone initiation but does warrant careful management and consideration of co-occurring withdrawal syndromes.
- Query for use of other controlled substances through the state's prescription drug monitoring program and document findings
- Evaluate comorbid medical conditions which may affect methadone treatment, such as chronic obstructive pulmonary disease, liver disease, renal disease, sleep apnea, etc
- Perform toxicology testing (encouraged and will be needed for OTP admission)
- Perform urine pregnancy test, if relevant
- Assess for QT-interval prolongation (recommended, but not required)

Table 20.2 in Chapter 20 outlines more specific requirements and criteria for methadone treatment from an OTP. It is helpful to be familiar with these criteria, though clinicians do not need to satisfy all of these criteria before making the decision to start methadone treatment. Components of care such as identification and transportation can be arranged by other hospital team members before hospital discharge.

Dosing Methadone to Initiate OUD Treatment

Historically, methadone dose titration in the hospital followed the same approach used in OTPs. In these outpatient settings, methadone initiation typically starts with 10 to 30 mg oral methadone. Most healthy adults start at 30 mg, while those with older age (>65 years old), comorbid end-organ dysfunction, or lower opioid tolerance may start at 10 to 20 mg. Patients are clinically assessed at peak effect after their first methadone dose, or 3 to 4 hours after administration. If patients are not sedated and have ongoing withdrawal symptoms, they can receive an additional 10-mg dose, for a total max dose of 40 mg on day 1. The daily methadone dose is then increased by 5 to 10 mg every 3 to 7 days, only after patients reach a steady state without side effects. This approach minimizes the risks of iatrogenic overdose but exposes patients to ongoing opioid withdrawal and requires at least 1 to 2 weeks, and often longer, to achieve a therapeutic dose for OUD treatment.

In contrast, most hospitalized patients, particularly those using fentanyl or other high-potency opioids, will benefit from more rapid methadone titration to effectively treat opioid withdrawal and craving.[35,36] It is particularly important to prioritize early opioid withdrawal treatment because of the rising rate of before medically advised hospital discharges for patients with OUD in the fentanyl era.[4] As noted above (*Summary of Evidence for OUD Treatment*), evidence is still emerging about what rapid titration approach best balances early withdrawal treatment with the risks of methadone dose stacking later in treatment, potentially after patients are discharged. Based on available evidence and published expert opinion, this section provides recommendations for a more rapid methadone titration for hospitalized patients (Table 7.5).

Most patients hospitalized patients with active OUD tolerate methadone initiation with maximum doses of 40 mg on day 1, 50 mg on day 2, and 60 mg on day 3. Some patients with significant risk factors for methadone-induced sedation (eg, decompensated cirrhosis, renal impairment with eGFR <30) or for ventricular arrhythmias (eg, long-QT syndrome) should be dosed more cautiously and require closer monitoring. Alternatively, some patients with heavy fentanyl use tolerate and may benefit from even more rapid titrations; these patients should be selected carefully, and these cases are generally guided by addiction consultation services. Clinicians should discuss the risks and benefits of these more rapid methadone titration with patients and document these discussions prior to starting treatment. The general guidance that a clinician "can always give more methadone, not less" is a safe guideline to keep in mind when considering any methadone initiation approach. In addition, short-acting opioids can greatly support patients while they are awaiting the full effects of methadone.

Clinical staff should assess for ongoing opioid withdrawal using a standardized assessment such as COWS. This should be reassessed every 4 to 8 hours during titration, particularly early in a patient's hospitalization when withdrawal is dynamic and can escalate quickly. COWS assessments can be discontinued after 3 to 5 days, as withdrawal stabilizes. Ongoing opioid withdrawal symptoms and opioid craving during methadone titration can be treated with short-acting opioids, $alpha_2$-agonists, and other nonopioid medications. Since oral methadone takes 3 to 4 hours to reach peak effects and can lead to dose stacking, patients initiating methadone for OUD should be monitored for sedation during the first 3 to 5 days of inpatient titration. Hospital teams can use the Richmond Agitation-Sedation Scale (RASS) or Pasero Opioid-induced Sedation Scale (POSS) to assess sedation.

Continuing Methadone for OUD Treatment

For patients already receiving methadone from an OTP at the time of hospital admission, it is crucial to ensure continuity of methadone treatment to prevent withdrawal and to maintain stability. When continuing methadone for a hospitalized patient, the admitting team should promptly contact the patient's OTP to verify the patient's methadone dose, confirm the date and time of the last administered dose, and document this information in the medical record. When the dose cannot be confirmed, such as hours when the OTP is closed, clinicians should discuss with their hospital pharmacists regarding hospital policies on what methadone doses to administer. In some hospitals, all patients are assumed to be methadone naïve until proven otherwise with an OTP dose confirmation; in other hospitals, addiction consultation services have the latitude to administer higher methadone doses based on clinical context. To prevent delays in maintaining methadone treatment, the admitting team should prioritize methadone dose confirmation as soon as possible to resume the patient's usual dose.

Methadone withdrawal typically emerges 24 to 36 hours after the last methadone dose. To avoid withdrawal, clinicians should avoid delaying or holding methadone doses unless clinically necessary. However, some clinical situations may warrant temporarily reducing or holding the patient's methadone dose for safety, such as patients presenting with altered mental status or encephalopathy, acute intoxication or ingestion, or new or significantly worsening organ dysfunction (eg, severe respiratory failure, new or worsening renal or hepatic function).

Dose reductions of 10% or higher may also be considered in patients starting new medications during hospitalization that fall into any of three categories:

- New chronic medications that inhibit or slow methadone metabolism
- Medications causing QTc prolongation in patients already with prolonged QTc (>500 ms) prior to hospitalization
- Medications with side effects of sedation or respiratory depression, compounding methadone's sedating effects

TABLE 7.5

Methadone Initiation for OUD Treatment in the Hospital

Titration day	Methadone dosing	Maximum total daily dose[a]	Monitoring
Traditional outpatient titration			
1–3	■ 10–30 mg once ■ Additional doses of 10 mg given at least 3–4 h after the last dose for ongoing withdrawal or craving, if no sedation	40 mg	■ Assess for opioid withdrawal (eg, COWS every 4–8 h × 3 d) ■ Check ECG for QT-interval prolongation
4–7+	■ Increase dose by up to 10 mg once for ongoing withdrawal or opioid craving, if no sedation ■ Increase by 5–10 mg every 3–5 d	Variable	■ Continue withdrawal assessments only if patient has ongoing withdrawal ■ QT interval can be reassessed again if/when patients reach ≥90 mg daily
Inpatient titration (recommended for most hospitalized patients using fentanyl)			
Titration day	**Methadone dosing**	**Range of maximum total daily dose[a]**	**Monitoring**
1	■ 30–40 mg initial dose ■ Additional doses of 10 mg given at least 3–4 h after the last dose for ongoing withdrawal or craving, if no sedation	40 mg–50 mg	■ Assess for sedation (eg, RASS or POSS every 4–8 h) ■ Assess for opioid withdrawal (eg, COWS every 4–8 h) ■ Check ECG for QT-interval prolongation (recommended but not required if no other risk factors)
2	■ Total methadone dose received day 1 as a single dose ■ Additional doses of 10 mg given at least 3–4 h after the last dose for ongoing withdrawal or craving, if no sedation	50 mg–60 mg	■ Assess for sedation (eg, RASS or POSS every 4–8 h) ■ Assess for opioid withdrawal (eg, COWS every 4–8 h) ■ Assess for sedation (eg, RASS or POSS every 4–8 h)
3	■ Total methadone dose received day 2 as a single dose ■ Additional doses of 10 mg given at least 3–4 h after the last dose for ongoing withdrawal or craving, if no sedation	50–70 mg	■ Assess for sedation (eg, RASS or POSS every 4–8 h) ■ Assess for opioid withdrawal (eg, COWS every 4–8 h) ■ Assess for sedation (eg, RASS or POSS every 4–8 h)
4+	■ Total methadone dose received day 3 as a single dose ■ Hold for 2–3 d to assess symptoms ■ Once a patient gets to 70–80 mg of daily methadone, subsequent dose increases titrated to patient-reported cravings and should not exceed 10 mg increase every 3–5 d	Variable	■ Assess for sedation 3–4 h after a dose increase ■ Continue withdrawal assessments only if patient has ongoing withdrawal ■ QT-interval can be assessed again if/when patients reach ≥90 mg daily

[a]Note: Short-acting opioids, $alpha_2$-agonists, other nonopioid medications should be used to treat ongoing withdrawal once the maximum daily dose is reached.

COWS, clinical opiate withdrawal scale; RASS, Richmond Agitation-Sedation Scale; POSS, Pasero Opioid-induced Sedation Scale.

Clinicians should always discuss methadone dose changes with patients and should prioritize resuming the patient's full dose of methadone as soon as clinically safe to do so. Ensuring timely resumption of methadone reflects best practices in managing OUD and supports positive patient outcomes.

If patients have missed multiple consecutive days of methadone dosing from their outpatient OTP clinic prior to hospitalization, patients may have lost their methadone tolerance and warrant retitration back to their usual dose.

Restarting Methadone After Missed Doses

Patients who miss 1 to 2 days of methadone should receive their usual methadone dose as soon as possible without dose reduction, barring any clinical concerns for resuming their usual methadone dose. However, patients who have missed 3 days or more of methadone require dose reduction to reduce the risk of iatrogenic overdose.

There is very little evidence to guide practice on how much to reduce methadone for missed doses. Historically, guidelines based on clinical experience recommended dose reductions of 25% to 50% for patients who have missed 3 to 4 days of methadone and restarting from scratch for patients who miss at least 5 to 7 days. These guidelines generally assume patients are not using other opioids during this time (since other opioids can maintain some cross tolerance for methadone). However, for patients using other opioids, especially high-potency opioids like fentanyl (which can maintain higher opioid tolerance), clinicians may consider resuming methadone doses at faster rates. Sample guidance for reinitiation of methadone is provided in Table 7.6.

Methadone and QT Prolongation

Methadone carries a risk of QT-interval prolongation in a dose-dependent manner. Methadone binds to the cardiac ion channel KCNH2 and prolongs the action potential.[76] It inhibits voltage-gated potassium channels, leading to prolonged repolarization and long QTc. QT-interval prolongation, in general, predisposes patients to ventricular arrhythmias such as torsades de pointes (TdP). However, the clinical relevance of methadone's impact on the QT-interval has not been firmly established.[77] For this reason, ECG screening solely for the purpose of initiating methadone is typically unnecessary in outpatient settings unless patients have predisposing cardiac risk factors (such as underlying heart conditions such as heart failure, prior arrhythmia, or a strong family history of cardiac risk factors) or reach doses of ≥90 mg daily.

Most hospitalized patients will have already had an ECG for other clinical indications prior to starting methadone. In addition, critical illness is an independent risk factor for QT prolongation and many hospitalized patients are treated with new medications that could also prolong the QT interval. For these reasons, it is prudent to assess for QT prolongation before starting methadone treatment in the hospital, but opioid withdrawal treatment with methadone should not be delayed solely to obtain a screening ECG in a patient without other risk factors.

For patients undergoing ongoing methadone dose increases in the hospital, weekly ECG monitoring may be considered, although little evidence supports this approach. This approach minimizes unnecessary testing (compared to daily ECG) while still monitoring for QTc prolongation in patients most at risk. Clinical judgment remains key, and a baseline ECG and subsequent monitoring, including cardiac telemetry, should be considered if the patient develops risk factors for QT prolongation, such as electrolyte disturbances, cardiac illness, or starts other QT-prolonging medications (including CYP 3A4 inhibitors such as ritonavir, diltiazem, ketoconazole).

Although prolonged QTc is formally defined as an interval greater than 450 ms for men and 460 ms for women,[78] clinical action is generally recommended only when the QTc is longer than 500 ms in men or 520 ms in women. For patients with prolonged QTc that is shorter than 500 ms in men or 520 ms in women, clinicians should discuss the risks and benefits of continuing methadone through patient-centered counseling and document outcomes of such discussions.

For QTc greater than 500 ms in men or 520 ms in women, one approach is to reduce the methadone dose by 10% to 25% to see if QTc improves, however close attention should be paid to patient withdrawal symptoms with each dose reduction; residual opioid withdrawal can be treated with short-acting opioids, alpha$_2$-agonists, or other nonopioid medications. Clinicians should also complete a thorough workup for other reasons for prolonged QTc (such as electrolyte imbalance from critical illness, malnutrition, dehydration, transient kidney injury, or diuretic use), or concomitant medications commonly used during hospitalization that prolong QTc, such as antiemetics, antibiotics, or antipsychotic medications.

TABLE 7.6

Restarting Methadone After Missed Doses[a]

Dosing days missed	Restart day 1 dose	Day 2	Day 3
1–2 d	100%	100%	100%
3–4 d	70–90%	80–100%	90–100%
5–7 d	50%	Increase by 10 mg every 2–3 d	Increase by 10 mg every 2–3 d
8+ d	Restart methadone initiation as new methadone start, typically at 40–50 mg depending on their dose		

[a]Percentages are of the patient's last confirmed methadone dose at their OTP.

In many cases, prolonged QTc is temporary and reversible, and methadone dose can respond to these changes in clinical status.

For patients with ongoing prolonged QTc, the risk of TdP must be balanced with the risk of stopping methadone, such opioid withdrawal, opioid craving, and increased rates of discharges before medically advised. For patients without other risk factors or a history of ventricular arrhythmias, TdP is rare, while the risk of overdose death among patients who do not receive medication treatment for OUD and return to nonprescribed opioid use, especially in the fentanyl era, is high. Clinicians should balance these risks with patients, being mindful of patient goals, and document discussions accordingly. Patients with severe or persistent QT prolongation may also consider switching to buprenorphine, which carries minimal risk of QT prolongation.

Buprenorphine

Buprenorphine is a long-acting, partial-agonist opioid most often administered in SL formulation, either as a monoproduct or coformulated with naloxone for the treatment of OUD. SL buprenorphine reaches peak effects in 60 to 90 minutes and has a terminal half-life of approximately 37 hours. Buprenorphine is hepatically metabolized via CYP3A4 enzymes. Buprenorphine is also available in buccal and patch formulations indicated for the treatment of pain. There are also two versions of XR subcutaneous injectable buprenorphine available for OUD treatment.

Buprenorphine-Precipitated Opioid Withdrawal

Buprenorphine has high binding affinity for the mu-opioid receptor. When taken while other, full-agonist opioids are active, buprenorphine can displace the other opioids and cause the sudden onset of opioid withdrawal. This phenomenon is called buprenorphine-precipitated withdrawal. To avoid precipitated withdrawal, clinicians should wait until other opioids have metabolized or cleared and wait for patients to demonstrate objective signs of opioid withdrawal (eg, COWS >8) before giving buprenorphine. For heroin or oxycodone withdrawal, it is sufficient to wait 8 to 12 hours from last use. For methadone at doses of 40 mg or lower taken for 3 days or less, it is typically sufficient to wait 72 hours; higher doses of methadone given for longer periods require 5 to 7 days of washout.

It is unclear how long patients, in general, should remain abstinent from fentanyl before starting buprenorphine to minimize the risk of precipitated withdrawal. Patients and clinicians have described instances of precipitated withdrawal despite fentanyl abstinence for 12 to 48 hours in monitored settings, sometimes with COWS of 13 or higher, however the incidence of buprenorphine-precipitated withdrawal with traditional or high-dose initiation in published studies is low, ranging from 1% to 16%. These complicated buprenorphine initiations may be due to fentanyl's pharmacology. Fentanyl is highly lipophilic with a large volume of distribution leading to peripheral sequestration in fat and skeletal muscle with repeat dosing. This accumulation means it takes longer periods of time for the body to clear fentanyl completely. Fentanyl can be detected for the first 5 to 7 days of abstinence, on average, for people with OUD.

Due to this phenomenon, experts believe some patients using fentanyl must wait longer periods of time before starting buprenorphine to reduce the risk of precipitated withdrawal. The exact amount of time likely depends on patient-specific factors like route of fentanyl administration, frequency of use, and BMI, in addition to geographic factors like the purity of fentanyl in the local substance supply.[46] Based on clinical experience, we recommend at least 12 hours of fentanyl abstinence before buprenorphine initiation in regions with low concern for precipitated withdrawal and at least 24 (ideally 48) hours of fentanyl abstinence in regions with high concern for precipitated withdrawal. During this fentanyl wash-out period, alpha$_2$-agonists, short-acting opioids, and nonopioid adjuvants can be used to treat withdrawal; short-acting opioids should then be held for the last 8 to 12 hours of the wash-out period, after which buprenorphine can be started with traditional or high-dose initiation. If there is concern for buprenorphine-precipitated withdrawal, a lower initial dose of buprenorphine (eg, 2 mg SL) with additional doses given every 1 to 2 hours may lead to precipitated withdrawal less often than a single large dose, although this has not been studied extensively.[79]

Buprenorphine for Opioid Withdrawal

Buprenorphine for opioid withdrawal is traditionally dosed as 2 to 4 mg SL initially, with additional doses given every 1 to 2 hours for ongoing symptoms. A total of 4 to 8 mg SL buprenorphine is typically sufficient to treat heroin withdrawal.[6,42] Some experts have suggested higher doses are required to treat fentanyl withdrawal, but limited data exist. Retrospective data suggests it is safe to reach 16 to 24 mg on the first day of treatment and some hospital systems have started using initial doses of 8 to 16 mg or higher to treat withdrawal and quickly reach OUD treatment doses, an approach called "high-dose" initiation.[17]

Patients starting buprenorphine treatment for OUD after initial withdrawal management should continue buprenorphine (typically dosed 16 to 24 mg daily using 8 or 12 mg SL products). Patients who wish to switch to methadone can abruptly stop buprenorphine and start methadone, typically via rapid initiation. Patients who decline medications for OUD despite counseling can continue buprenorphine for withdrawal treatment while hospitalized, then abruptly discontinue on discharge (or, alternatively, can receive a 3-day buprenorphine taper, eg, 8 mg day 1, 4 mg day 2, 2 mg day 3).

Traditional Buprenorphine Initiation and Titration

Traditional initiation of buprenorphine has been used for more than 25 years with only rare instances of precipitated withdrawal or other adverse effects before the spread of fentanyl in the unregulated opioid supply. This traditional initiation approach continues to work well for individuals using short-acting opioids such as heroin or oxycodone or for individuals using fentanyl or opioids with longer half-life after a longer period of abstinence. Traditional buprenorphine initiation involves:

- **A Period of Opioid Abstinence Prior to Starting Buprenorphine:** For heroin or oxycodone, 8 to 12 hours is sufficient. For long-acting opioids like XR oxycodone, 16 to 24 hours is required; methadone generally requires 48 to 72 hours at a dose <50 mg. Fentanyl may require 24 to 48 hours for some patients. During this period of abstinence, opioid withdrawal is treated with nonopioid adjuvants (and, if a longer period is required, short-acting opioids).
- **Confirmation of Opioid Withdrawal:** Patients should have at least two objective manifestations (eg, gooseflesh, dilated pupils, vomiting, or diarrhea) of opioid withdrawal (often assessed with COWS scores of ≥8).
- **Start Buprenorphine:** Initial doses are typically 2 to 4 mg SL with additional doses given every 60 to 120 minutes if there is no precipitated withdrawal, up to a goal dose of 16 to 24 mg daily. Total daily buprenorphine doses of 16 to 24 mg are associated with improved acute care outcomes and should be reached in the first day.[24]
- **Ongoing Monitoring:** Thereafter, clinicians should continue to assess and titrate buprenorphine doses daily throughout hospitalization based on evolving clinical status and patient reports of ongoing opioid cravings and withdrawal. COWS monitoring every 4 to 8 hours can help monitor withdrawal symptoms until patients receive 16 mg total daily dose. Continuous telemetry or pulse oximetry monitoring is not required for patients with opioid tolerance prior to starting buprenorphine.

Alternative Initiation Approaches

Two alternative initiation strategies can address concern for buprenorphine-precipitated withdrawal with traditional initiation: (1) LDI-OC, which uses small initial doses of buprenorphine (0.5 mg SL or lower) that are increased over days as individuals continue full-agonist opioids, and (2) treating opioid withdrawal ("bridging") with short-acting opioids while fentanyl clears. LDI-OC is also used to start buprenorphine among patients who cannot tolerate even a brief period of withdrawal or who require ongoing opioids for analgesia, for example, after trauma or in the perioperative period. A third alternative, (3) high-dose initiation, involves initial doses of 8 to 32 mg SL buprenorphine after patients demonstrate moderate to severe opioid withdrawal with a validated scale after a sufficient period of abstinence. It is sometimes used in ED settings when there is low concern for buprenorphine-precipitated withdrawal based on higher withdrawal severity, longer time of abstinence, and/or the local drug supply and drug use patterns.

Low-Dose Buprenorphine Initiation With Opioid Continuation

LDI-OC allows for the gradual uptitration of buprenorphine with ongoing full-agonist opioid use, avoiding a period of prerequisite opioid withdrawal.[14,44,47] When successful, this approach allows for the gradual introduction of buprenorphine to slowly replace full-agonist opioids at the mu-opioid receptor, avoiding the sudden displacement of full-agonists that is experienced as precipitated withdrawal.[80] Since buprenorphine doses are too small to prevent the emergence of opioid withdrawal, full-agonist opioids are continued throughout the process and stopped only once the patient reaches a therapeutic buprenorphine dose (8 mg SL or higher). This method has gained particular popularity in hospital settings since there is no regulatory restriction to administering full-agonist opioids to patients during most hospitalizations (for details, see *Regulatory Concerns* above). Clinicians should note that evidence supporting LDI-OC is nascent and mostly limited to small, uncontrolled, retrospective cohort studies.[14] See Table 7.7 for four examples of LDI-OC approaches.

There are many dosing strategies and formulations used for LDI-OC, however a few principles are consistent between approaches[16]:

TABLE 7.7

Buprenorphine Low-Dose Initiation With Opioid Continuation (LDI-OC) Strategies for Hospitalized Patients

Day	Full-agonist opioid continuation strategy	2-d low-dose approach (SL, buccal)[15]	4-d low-dose approach (SL, buccal)[81]	7-d low-dose approach (SL, buccal)[16]	7-day low-dose approach (TD patch)[82]
1	Initiate *before* starting buprenorphine low-dose approach, titrate to resolution of opioid withdrawal, and continue based on low-dose strategy	0.5 mg SL q6h × 2 doses, followed 6 h later by 1 mg q6h × 2 doses	0.5 mg SL BID	0.5 mg SL once	Apply one 20 mcg transdermal patch and leave on for 7 d
2	For 2-d approach, taper by 50% per day or stop after the first dose of 8 mg if there is no other indication For 4- or 7-d approach, continue consistent opioid dose	2 mg SL q6h × 2 doses, followed 6 h later by 4 mg × 1 dose, followed 6 h later by 8 mg	1 mg SL BID	0.5 mg SL BID	Apply second 20 mcg transdermal patch and leave on for 7 d
3	For 2-d approach, discontinue or continue taper For 4- or 7-d approach, continue consistent opioid dose	Continue 16–24 mg SL daily	2 mg SL BID	1 mg SL BID	2 mg SL once (while continuing two patches)
4	For 2-d approach, discontinued For 4-d approach, taper by 50% per day or stop after the first dose of 8 mg if there is no other indication For 7-d approach, continue consistent opioid dose	Continue 16–24 mg SL daily	4 mg once, then 8 mg SL BID–TID	2 mg SL BID	2 mg SL BID (while continuing two patches)
5	For 2-d or 4-d approach, discontinued or continue taper For 7-d approach, continue consistent opioid dose	Continue 16–24 mg SL daily	Continue 16–24 mg SL daily	3 mg SL BID	4 mg SL BID (while continuing two patches)
6	For 2-d or 4-d approach, discontinued For 7-d approach, continue consistent opioid dose	Continue 16–24 mg SL daily	Continue 16–24 mg SL daily	4 mg SL BID	8 mg SL BID–TID (while continuing two patches)
7	For 2-d or 4-d approach, discontinued For 7-d approach, taper by 50% per day or stop after the first dose of 8 mg if there is no other indication	Continue 16–24 mg SL daily	Continue 16–24 mg SL daily	8 mg SL BID-TID	Remove patches Continue 16–24 mg SL daily

[a]Buccal formulations can be used for buprenorphine doses <2 mg SL; 0.5 mg SL buprenorphine is approximately equivalent to 225-mcg buccal buprenorphine and 450 mcg of buccal buprenorphine is equivalent to 1 mg of buprenorphine.

TD, transdermal.

- **Start and Continue a Full-Agonist Opioid:** Since administered buprenorphine doses are too small to stave off withdrawal symptoms, full-agonist opioids should be started before buprenorphine, titrated to clinical response with no opioid withdrawal, and maintained during LDI. Full-agonist opioids are tapered or discontinued after reaching at least 8 mg SL buprenorphine.
- **Start Buprenorphine at a Low Dose:** The typical initial dose is 0.5 mg SL (or equivalent in patch or buccal formulation, based on local availability and regulations), but it can range from 0.25 to 1 mg.

- **Gradually Increase Buprenorphine Dose:** Dose escalation generally occurs over 1 to 10 days until patients reach treatment doses (usually 16 to 24 mg SL daily). Longer periods with more gradual dose increases might reduce the risk of precipitated withdrawal, particularly when transitioning from methadone.
- **Clear Communication and Frequent Monitoring:** Patients should be well informed about the process, and frequent check-ins are essential with regular monitoring for withdrawal. If withdrawal occurs, dose increases should be paused to allow for stabilization. Adjunctive medications like clonidine, ondansetron, and short-term use of benzodiazepines can be used for symptom relief.
- **Care Coordination:** Effective communication among health care professionals, including OTPs, outpatient pharmacies, primary care clinicians, and hospital teams, ensures smooth transitions and mitigates barriers during treatment.

Quicker approaches (eg, completing LDI-OC in 1 to 3 days) allow LDI-OC to be completed prior to discharge without prolonging hospitalization and were found to have high success rates in at least one setting (about 92% completion without moderate to severe opioid withdrawal).[15] Longer approaches (eg, completion in 7 days) may be preferred for transitions from methadone and might allow more time to respond to emergent withdrawal symptoms during LDI-OC. Dosing frequency and time to completion should be tailored to the clinical situation, patient preference, and anticipated discharge date; intermediate approaches of about 3 to 4 days are probably the most common.

Various buprenorphine formulations have been used for LDI-OC. Buprenorphine/naloxone SL films, SL tablets, or buprenorphine monoproduct tablets can be used if splitting films or tablets is allowed by hospital pharmacy leadership. The buprenorphine monoproduct may have a lower risk of precipitated withdrawal given recent evidence of naloxone absorption with combination SL product.[83] Some hospital pharmacies do not allow 2 mg SL buprenorphine to be split into quarters because of Centers for Medicare and Medicaid Services (CMS) regulation interpretation, unpredictable stability concerns, and inexact dosing of the split product. To respond to this challenge, published protocols have used transdermal,[84] intravenous,[81] and buccal[85] formulations instead. There is no available evidence to recommend one formulation over another and we recommend using whatever is already on-formulary.

Patients who have been maintained on methadone may desire transition to buprenorphine for various reasons, including due to experiencing adverse effects from methadone (eg, QTc prolongation) or having longer medication prescriptions with fewer clinic visits that are more common with buprenorphine than methadone outpatient treatment.

There is no standardized, universally accepted protocol for transitioning from methadone to buprenorphine. Historically, patients were counseled to decrease their methadone dose to 50 mg, abstain from methadone use for 72 hours, and start buprenorphine using traditional initiation, though this often led to experiences of withdrawal, increased risk of return to opioid use, and thus has now fallen out of favor.

For patients maintained on >80 mg methadone daily for more than a week, experts now recommend a slow LDI-OC protocol to account for methadone's long half-life, generally taking at least 7 days to complete. As with other full-agonists, methadone can be continued through LDI-OC until patients reach a single dose of 8 to 12 mg SL; alternatively, some published protocols decrease the methadone dose by 50% on the day prior to completing LDI-OC or discontinuing on the last day of LDI-OC. For patients ready to be discharged before completing this transition, it is important to communicate and partner with an outpatient OTP to continue LDI-OC in the outpatient setting.

Bridging With Short-Acting Opioids as Fentanyl Clears

Based on clinical experience, patients in settings with high concern for buprenorphine-precipitated withdrawal may require 24 to 48 hours of abstinence from fentanyl prior to starting buprenorphine. Rather than start a 2- to 7-day LDI-OC initiation, clinicians can treat opioid withdrawal using a combination of short-acting opioids, alpha$_2$-agonists, and nonopioid medications until patients have 24 to 48 hours without fentanyl use. The last short-acting opioid should be administered at least 8 to 12 hours before buprenorphine is initiated. Buprenorphine can then be initiated using a standard or high-dose buprenorphine initiation.

High-Dose Buprenorphine Initiation

High-dose initiation involves administering initial doses of 8 to 24 mg SL buprenorphine to individuals in moderate to severe opioid withdrawal after a sufficient period of opioid abstinence. This approach should only be used for individuals already in acute moderate or severe opioid withdrawal in time-constrained settings where it is infeasible to reassess and redose the patient multiple times and where it is crucial to achieve therapeutic doses for OUD as quickly as possible (eg, in EDs). Three studies have shown that this approach is acceptable and tolerable in ED settings, including among patients using fentanyl.[17,45,49] It is important to note that these were settings with a low baseline rate of buprenorphine-precipitated withdrawal; it remains unclear whether high-dose (compared to standard) initiation increases, reduces, or does not change the rate of precipitated withdrawal in settings where this is a major concern. There are four general principles for high-dose initiation:

- **Ensure a Sufficient Period of Opioid Abstinence:** Ensure that the patient has sufficiently abstained from full opioid agonists to avoid precipitated withdrawal. This typically means at least 12 to 24 hours since last opioid use; waiting at least 24 to 36 hours from last fentanyl use may be required in some settings.
- **Assess for Opioid Withdrawal Severity:** High-dose initiation is most appropriate for patients in moderate to severe withdrawal with at least two objective signs of opioid withdrawal (eg, COWS score ≥13).
- **Achieve Therapeutic Levels Quickly:** Administer an initial dose of 8 to 24 mg SL, with reassessment for additional dosing within hours if symptoms persist. The total dose on the first day may reach 24 to 32 mg depending on the clinical situation and patient needs.
- **Monitoring and Support:** Closely monitor patients during and after initiation for signs of oversedation, withdrawal symptoms, or other adverse effects. Provide adjunctive medications (eg, clonidine, antiemetics) as needed to manage residual withdrawal symptoms.

Continuing Buprenorphine Treatment for OUD

Patients receiving buprenorphine for OUD treatment prior to admission should be continued on buprenorphine during hospitalization. Buprenorphine serves as both a treatment for OUD and an analgesic, providing dual benefits. Patients who have buprenorphine discontinued will experience iatrogenic opioid withdrawal, potentially contributing to before medically advised discharge, and are less likely to have buprenorphine continued after hospital discharge.[86]

It was previously recommended that buprenorphine be discontinued perioperatively or for patients with acute pain to allow for adequate opioid analgesia.[1] This practice was based on buprenorphine's pharmacology as a partial-opioid agonist with high-binding affinity for the mu-opioid receptor and experimental evidence demonstrating that even high doses short-acting opioids (up to 16 mg IV hydromorphone) are indistinguishable from placebo for acute pain among patients receiving buprenorphine for OUD.[87]

However, expert guidelines and evidence have now shifted towards recommending buprenorphine continuation during the preoperative period, sometimes at a reduced dose, due to the risks of OUD destabilization, return to use, and overdose.[3,4] Patients on buprenorphine and undergoing surgery may require higher amounts of short-acting opioids to achieve sufficient analgesia but have similar lengths of stay and long-term surgical outcomes compared to controls, underscoring that the benefits of buprenorphine continuation during surgery often outweigh the risks.[5,21–23] Clinicians may consider splitting buprenorphine doses into twice or thrice daily dosing, as more frequent buprenorphine dosing has shown to have more analgesic benefits.[3] In addition, they can consider titrating buprenorphine up to 32 mg/d in divided doses if using buprenorphine as the only opioid for acute pain management. Any adjustment of the buprenorphine dose would need to be weighed against the risk of patients going into opioid withdrawal from a dose reduction. A recent systematic review did not find evidence supporting a need for buprenorphine dose reductions in the perioperative period.[88]

Cases where patients have not used buprenorphine in more than 3 to 5 days should be treated as new buprenorphine initiations.

Continuing Buprenorphine on Discharge

Buprenorphine treatment for OUD reduces all-cause mortality and morbidity across a host of outcomes and should be continued after hospital discharge. Clinicians should establish an appointment for outpatient buprenorphine follow up and should prescribe sufficient buprenorphine for patients to take until that appointment (typically up to 1 to 2 weeks of buprenorphine). When looking for an outpatient buprenorphine clinician, it is important to note that a buprenorphine X-waiver is no longer required; any clinician with a DEA license can prescribe buprenorphine treatment for OUD in the outpatient setting.

Long-Acting Injectable Buprenorphine

Buprenorphine for OUD treatment is available as long-acting injectable buprenorphine (LAIB, sometimes referred to as XR buprenorphine). LAIB use has increased due to the convenience of weekly or monthly dosing and the extended overdose protection provided by the long-acting formulation.

First-generation LAIB, brand name Sublocade, is a monthly buprenorphine injection first FDA approved in 2017 initially indicated for patients who had taken daily SL doses of 8 to 24 mg for at least a week. A recent update to the product information allows patients to receive Sublocade after tolerating just a single 4 mg SL dose of buprenorphine. The medication comes as 300 mg or 100 mg monthly doses and is administered into subcutaneous tissue of the abdomen, thigh, buttocks, or underside of the arm by a health care professional. Sublocade creates a nodule that releases buprenorphine over 4 weeks. Patients are typically administered 300 mg for the first dose, then given 300 mg for the second dose 7 to 28 days after the first dose. After two 300-mg doses, buprenorphine serum levels approach steady state and patients are typically switched to once-monthly injections of 100 mg, with the third dose given at least 26 days after the second dose. In some cases, patients are maintained on monthly 300-mg injections.

Second-generation LAIB, brand name Brixadi, was FDA approved in 2023. As with Sublocade, it can be initiated for any patient who has tolerated at least a single dose of SL buprenorphine 4 mg. Brixadi comes in both weekly and monthly versions with multiple dosing options (see Table 7.8). It can also be administered in other subcutaneous sites, including the buttocks, thighs, abdomen, or upper arms, which may reduce injection-related pain (however, the upper arm should not be used for initial doses of weekly Brixadi). Brixadi may be appropriate for individuals who wish to try LAIB for a week before committing to a full month, individuals who do not tolerate first-generation LAIB (eg, due to injection-related pain), or those desiring a lower dose than Sublocade.

It should be noted that it takes at least two doses of Sublocade to reach a steady state for trough buprenorphine serum levels to remain at goal levels. This means that patients might experience withdrawal symptoms in the days or weeks leading up to the second or third injection. Supplemental SL doses of buprenorphine can be given to improve patient comfort and reduce the risk of returning to opioid use, generally in the form of SL buprenorphine 8 mg one to three times daily.

Recently, there has been growing interest in "direct to inject" initiation strategies where LAIB is administered without an initial dose of SL buprenorphine.[89] LAIB pharmacology mimics the most rapid versions of LDI-OC, with peak effects in about 24 hours (for the weekly version of second-generation LAI buprenorphine). The strategy has been described in one prospective study from four diverse ED settings.[90] In the study, 100 patients with OUD who had minimal to no withdrawal (COWS 0 to 7) received a 24-mg dose of the weekly second-generation buprenorphine LAI. Seven (7%) of patients had precipitated withdrawal, and those who had baseline COWS of 0 to 3 had higher incidence of precipitated withdrawal than those with baseline COWS 4 to 7.

Comparatively, second-generation Brixadi formulations are less expensive than the Sublocade, so hospitals may consider use of Brixadi for this reason. LAIB may be considered for patients who are discharging to settings with limited access to buprenorphine such as SNF or jail. LAIB may also be considered for highly vulnerable unhoused individuals who may not be able to safely store their buprenorphine.

TABLE 7.8

Approximate Equivalent Dosing Between Formulations of Buprenorphine at Steady State

Daily sublingual	Weekly Brixadi	Monthly Brixadi	Monthly Sublocade
≤6 mg	8 mg	—	—
8–10 mg	16 mg	64 mg	300 mg, 300 mg, then 100 mg monthly
12–16 mg	24 mg	94 mg	
18–24 mg	32 mg	128 mg	

Slow-Release Oral Morphine

SROM can be used as an alternative long-acting opioid agonist or as an adjuvant alongside methadone for treatment of opioid withdrawal or treatment of OUD. SROM is available in Canada for the treatment of OUD in the outpatient setting due to different federal and provincial laws that allow for its use. Typical initial dosing of SROM is 30 to 200 mg once daily with the 24-hour XR formulation. Dosing is typically guided by an addiction specialist and should be titrated to patient response.

Alpha$_2$-Agonists and Other Nonopioid Medications

Clonidine and lofexidine are centrally acting alpha$_2$-adrenergic agonists that have been shown to be safe and effective at reducing the severity of opioid withdrawal syndrome. They have demonstrated strong efficacy in reducing a host of opioid withdrawal symptoms.[7]

Oral clonidine for opioid withdrawal is dosed at 0.1 to 0.3 mg every 6 to 8 hours with a maximum dose of 1 mg in a 24-hour period. Clonidine's most common side effects are bradycardia, orthostatic hypotension, dry mouth, and sedation. After 3 to 5 days of daily dosing, clonidine should be tapered because abrupt withdrawal may cause rebound hypertension, sweating, headache, or agitation. Of note, clonidine is used nonmedically to potentiate opioid effects and, in general, should not be prescribed on discharge unless there is a specific indication.

Lofexidine is the only FDA-approved, nonopioid treatment for opioid withdrawal. The starting dose is 0.54 mg four times daily. The most common side effects are bradycardia, hypotension, and dry mouth. Lofexidine's impact on blood pressure and heart rate is less pronounced than clonidine, especially at higher doses. However, lofexidine is much more expensive than clonidine in the US.

Table 7.4 lists other nonopioid medications commonly used to treat specific symptoms of opioid withdrawal. Since opioid withdrawal has different manifestations for different patients, clinicians should tailor treatment and use of these medications to each individual patient.

Other Opioids for Opioid Withdrawal or OUD Treatment

Hospitalized patients with ongoing opioid withdrawal despite the approaches above may benefit from opioids such as short-acting oral hydromorphone, morphine, or oxycodone to treat opioid withdrawal.[9,10,91] As a separate indication, these opioids are often required to treat acute pain. See Chapter 17 for guidance on acute pain management in patients with OUD. A few important considerations should guide their use for withdrawal.

First, the evidence base for these alternative opioids is limited, especially compared to methadone and buprenorphine, and dosing is largely based on clinical experience by addiction specialists. Second, these agents can increase the risk of sedation and iatrogenic overdose; all patients should be closely monitored for sedation, and some patients with severe respiratory depression, hepatic impairment, critical illness, or altered mental status are poor candidates for this approach. Third, the initial doses of these opioids may be insufficient and should be titrated to clinical effect; we recommend titrating until patients no longer manifest objective signs of opioid withdrawal. Fourth, it is critical to have a plan for discontinuing these opioids and to discuss this plan with patients early; based on federal regulations, they cannot be prescribed on discharge for the treatment of OUD, and in the vast majority of cases, they should be used for a few days to help patients transition to methadone or buprenorphine treatment.

With these considerations in mind, opioids such as short-acting oral hydromorphone, oxycodone, or morphine can be used for opioid withdrawal in three, sometimes overlapping, scenarios.

First, they can be used as adjuvants to methadone initiation for opioid withdrawal. Some patients, especially those using fentanyl, have ongoing opioid withdrawal despite the maximum dose of methadone considered safe based on concerns for methadone dose stacking. While methadone is titrated during the first few days of hospitalization, other opioid agonists can treat residual opioid withdrawal. These other opioids can be titrated off over a few days while the methadone dose is increased using a more rapid methadone titration approach compared to OTP settings.

Second, other opioids can be used to bridge patients to buprenorphine while other opioids such as fentanyl or methadone metabolize and clear. For hospitalized patients using fentanyl who wish to start buprenorphine treatment for OUD in regions with high concern for buprenorphine-precipitated withdrawal, opioid withdrawal can be initially managed using a combination of short-acting opioids, alpha$_2$-agonists, and other nonopioid adjuvants to allow for 24 to 48 hours of fentanyl washout. The last short-acting opioid should be administered 8 hours before starting buprenorphine (ie, 16 to 40 hours after last fentanyl use), all subsequent opioids should be held, then buprenorphine can be initiated using a standard or high-dose initiation. For patients transitioning from methadone to buprenorphine, short-acting opioids can be used to bridge patients for 5 to 7 days as an alternative to LDI.

Third, other opioids (eg, XR oxycodone) can be used as alternative long-acting opioids when buprenorphine, methadone, and SROM are all contraindicated or unavailable.[92] However, optimal dosing has not been well established and use of other long-acting opioids misses an opportunity to stabilize patients on medications that can be used for long-term OUD treatment.

For patients using fentanyl, typical dosing starts are 4 to 6 mg oral hydromorphone every 3 hours, 20 to 30 mg oral morphine every 3 to 4 hours, or 15 to 20 mg immediate-release oxycodone every 4 hours. Based on experience, the authors recommend scheduling short-acting opioids so that they do not dose stack (eg, oxycodone every 4 hours) with instructions to hold for sedation, rather than ordering them as needed for withdrawal; this approach pre-empts confusion over their indication, ensures patients receive needed withdrawal treatment, and reduces the chance that patients will feel stigmatized for requesting medications for withdrawal. Doses should be titrated to clinical effect in the first 12 to 24 hours, usually until patients no longer have objective signs of opioid withdrawal. For patients who are already injecting opioids, intravenous formulations can be used by experienced clinicians to titrate doses more quickly, then transitioned to oral formulations with longer opioid effect.

Once opioid withdrawal is stabilized, ideally in the first 12 to 24 hours, a plan should be implemented to discontinue these agents for opioid withdrawal. For patients receiving methadone for withdrawal, short-acting opioids should be titrated down over a few days and then discontinued once patients reach a total daily dose of 60 to 80 mg oral methadone. Patients transitioning to buprenorphine should at least start (and ideally complete) this transition to buprenorphine within 48 to 72 hours.

Patients with acute pain may require ongoing use of these opioids and other medications for analgesia, but should not require indefinite short-acting opioids for opioid withdrawal.

In the outpatient setting in Canada, injectable opioid agonist therapy (iOAT) is an alternative treatment for OUD, particularly for patients who have not responded to traditional therapies like methadone or buprenorphine. iOAT involves the supervised administration of pharmaceutical-grade opioids, such as diacetylmorphine (heroin) or hydromorphone, and has been shown in international studies to improve treatment retention, reduce illicit opioid use, and decrease related harms.[93–97] iOAT is not currently legal or available in the US, however, it is recognized as a valuable treatment strategy for refractory OUD in Canada and parts of Europe.

Critical Care Management of Opioid Withdrawal

Patients with opioid withdrawal in critical care units face additional challenges. Some are sedated and unable to provide a history of opioid use or a subjective account of ongoing opioid withdrawal symptoms. Many have severe organ dysfunction that limits absorption of medications (eg, upper GI bleeding), alters drug metabolism (eg, liver or renal failure) or increases the risks of under and overtreatment of opioid withdrawal (eg, respiratory failure or altered mental status with inability to protect an airway). In addition, many of these other conditions cause symptoms that overlap with opioid withdrawal, confounding clinical assessments.

To assess for opioid withdrawal in patients unable to provide a history, prior documentation in the electronic health record can provide important context. If clinicians believe it is crucial to obtain a collateral history from family or friends, they should ask open-ended questions and should not disclose patients' history of substance use, substance use disorder treatment, or results of toxicology testing without patient consent. The physical exam assessing for objective manifestations of opioid withdrawal can be particularly helpful in critical care settings. The Objective Opioid Withdrawal Scale is one validated scale that can be used.[73] Careful interpretation of urine or serum toxicology testing can provide additional data to guide assessments of opioid withdrawal.

Treatment of opioid withdrawal for critically ill patients should follow the same approach outlined above that prioritizes methadone or buprenorphine alongside alpha$_2$-agonists (when not contraindicated), other nonopioid medications, and, as necessary, short-acting opioids. When it is not possible to ask about a patient's interest in buprenorphine after exposure to long-acting opioids (or after chronic exposure to fentanyl, in areas with high concern for buprenorphine-precipitated withdrawal), scheduled doses of short-acting opioids can be used for the first 24 to 48 hours of withdrawal treatment. Based on clinical experience, 15 to 20 mg of oxycodone scheduled every 4 hours (or 1.5 to 2 mg IV hydromorphone every 3 hours, if there is no enteral access) is typically sufficient to prevent the development of severe opioid withdrawal for patients using fentanyl. After 24 to 48 hours (or once the patient is awake), opioid withdrawal treatment can be transitioned to methadone or buprenorphine based on the patient's OUD treatment goals.

For patients who were previously treated with buprenorphine prior to hospitalization, buprenorphine can be continued on their home dose or adjusted based on clinical scenario. Importantly, buprenorphine can still be safely and effectively given sublingually even to individuals who are intubated or do not have enteral access. Similarly, individuals who were treated with methadone prior to hospitalization, can be continued on their home dose or adjusted based on clinical scenario. If patients lose enteral access, methadone can be transitioned to IV formulation at half the dose (eg, 100 mg of oral methadone is equivalent to 50 mg of IV methadone).

Responding to Opioid Overdose

In the US, there are epidemic levels of fatal and nonfatal overdose deaths related to opioids. Overdoses that occur in the community often present to the ED. Overdoses may also occur in the hospital when patients use their own substances or have iatrogenic overdose. The opioid antagonist naloxone should be given to reverse opioid overdose. Naloxone is available in intramuscular (IM), intravenous (IV), subcutaneous (SQ), intranasal (IN), or nebulized formulations.[98] The traditional dose to reverse opioid overdose is 0.4 mg IM/IV. However, naloxone, particularly this or higher doses, can cause severe opioid withdrawal symptoms or noncardiogenic pulmonary edema for patients with opioid dependence. To prevent these complications, the American Heart Association updated its guidance in 2021 to use "the lowest effective dose" of naloxone to reverse respiratory depression, while avoiding opioid withdrawal.[99] We recommend an initial naloxone dose of 0.04 to 0.4 mg IM/IV during overdose response with doses repeated every 2 to 3 minutes until the patient achieves adequate ventilation.

When repeated doses are needed, for example, from overdose of a long-acting opioid or after concomitant use of benzodiazepines and opioids, a naloxone infusion may be needed. These are patients whose end-tidal CO_2 remains elevated and respiratory rate low. If severe cases, patients may need to be intubated to protect their airways. Naloxone infusions can be stopped once the patient's respiratory status stabilizes (respiratory rate >12). Patients should not be maintained on naloxone infusions until they experience opioid withdrawal. Medications for OUD can and should be offered to patients once they fully stabilize to prevent repeat opioid overdose.

Co-occurring Withdrawal Syndromes

Many patients using opioids also use other substances that lead to withdrawal syndromes, such as alcohol, stimulants, and benzodiazepines. In addition, the unregulated "street" supply of opioids is increasingly adulterated by nonopioids such as nonpharmaceutical benzodiazepines, xylazine, or medetomidine. Patients using opioids may be knowingly or unknowingly exposed to these adulterants.

Clinicians managing co-occurring withdrawal from opioids and other substances should use best practices for each withdrawal syndrome.[5] Many signs and symptoms of alcohol and benzodiazepine withdrawal overlap with opioid withdrawal, however, some physical exam findings (eg, yawning, lacrimation, and pupil dilation) are more specific to opioid withdrawal, and others (eg, disorientation, tactile disturbances, and visual hallucinations) are more specific to alcohol and benzodiazepine withdrawal. Nevertheless, symptom-triggered approaches to both syndromes can be challenging to implement at the same time. In this context, it is even more important to use evidence-based medications and dosing strategies for opioid withdrawal.

For patients co-using opioids and stimulants, clinicians should be aware that acute stimulant withdrawal often leads to a profound desire to sleep paired with depressed moods, dysphoria, anxiety, and irritability. This sleepiness can sometimes be conflated with iatrogenic opioid overdose during opioid withdrawal treatment. Again, using evidence-based opioid agonists and dosing strategies for opioid withdrawal can help clinicians distinguish between these conditions.

Xylazine and medetomidine are veterinary sedative alpha$_2$-agonists that are not FDA approved for use in humans but that are increasingly detected as adulterants of illicitly manufactured fentanyl. People who use substances report increased anxiety and restlessness from xylazine and fentanyl (compared to fentanyl in isolation),[100,101] however, objective manifestations of xylazine withdrawal have not been identified in early studies.[102] In contrast, early studies from Philadelphia and Pittsburgh suggest that medetomidine withdrawal can involve severe and refractory hypertension, tachycardia, nausea, and vomiting, in addition to a high-amplitude tremor, all unresponsive to high doses of opioids.[54,103] Most patients in these early studies required intensive care unit care with dexmedetomidine infusions.

While further evidence develops, the authors' recommendation is to prioritize evidence-based and early treatment of opioid withdrawal and to maintain a broad differential before anchoring on xylazine or medetomidine withdrawal as an explanation for unexplained symptoms.

XR Naltrexone

XR naltrexone is a long-acting opioid antagonist FDA approved for OUD treatment. Administered as a once-monthly injection, it provides consistent blockade of opioid receptors and modulates dopaminergic pathways, thereby preventing the euphoric effects of opioids and reducing cue-induced cravings. Only the intramuscular, XR form of naltrexone is FDA approved for OUD treatment; oral naltrexone has not been shown to be effective for OUD. Although XR naltrexone has shown promise in clinical trials, real-world evidence has not demonstrated the same mortality-reducing benefits as methadone and buprenorphine, likely because of challenges initiating XR naltrexone and reduced retention in care. However, it remains an important treatment modality for patients who strongly desire OUD treatment without opioid agonists.

Naltrexone can precipitate withdrawal in patients with recent opioid use. Thus, the traditional approach to starting XR naltrexone is for patients to abstain from opioid use for at least 7 to 10 days. Patients must be carefully selected and counseled prior to initiation. Patients are suitable candidates for XR naltrexone if they:

- Can tolerate opioid abstinence for at least 7 days (or >14 days if previously on methadone)
- Do not have any acute pain conditions or upcoming procedures or surgeries that may require opioid treatment
- Prefer a nonopioid treatment
- Are at low risk of treatment dropout (missing doses increases overdose risk)

Patients who meet the above criteria and have comorbid alcohol or methamphetamine use disorder may also benefit because XR naltrexone is known to have benefits in both alcohol use disorder and methamphetamine disorder.

XR naltrexone is hepatically cleared, so patients with decompensated liver disease (Child Pugh Class C) should be carefully evaluated for risks versus benefits of starting naltrexone; however, liver disease itself is not a contraindication to naltrexone use.

When starting XR naltrexone for patients with OUD, it is recommended to obtain a urine toxicology test to assess for opioids. If there is concern for opioid exposure, patients may receive a naloxone (0.4 mg IV, IM, or SQ) or naltrexone (one 50 oral dose) challenge. Patients are observed for signs of withdrawal for 30 to 60 minutes after either administration. Absence of withdrawal confirms readiness for XR naltrexone initiation. An alternative, rapid initiation approach was recently described and found to be noninferior to standard initiation. In this approach, patients are administered 1 day of SL buprenorphine for withdrawal, followed by 1 day opioid free and then 3 to 4 days of oral naltrexone titration (with adjunctive withdrawal medications) before XR naltrexone.[104]

The standard XR naltrexone dose is 380 mg admin istered via deep intramuscular injection in the gluteal muscle every 4 weeks. Strict adherence to monthly injections is critical for efficacy, and patients should be counseled about the loss of opioid tolerance while on XR naltrexone and the heightened risk of overdose if returning to their prior levels of opioid use.

Psychosocial Interventions and Other Behavioral Treatments

Many patients with OUD benefit from psychosocial interventions and other behavioral treatments after hospital discharge. These treatment approaches include cognitive-behavioral therapy (CBT), contingency management, motivational interviewing, and peer support groups (eg, Alcoholics Anonymous, Narcotics Anonymous, or SMART recovery). These psychosocial interventions can be helpful for patients by supporting their development of coping skills, addressing underlying psychological factors, and enhancing motivation for substance use disorder recovery. These therapies can also improve adherence to medications for OUD and reduce the risk of returning to opioid use. Referrals to these outpatient resources should be offered to all patients but should not be a prerequisite to start medications for OUD. For more information, see Chapter 15 for details.

Patients Who Decline OUD Treatment

Patients entering the hospital are typically seeking care for an acute medical issue and may not be seeking OUD treatment. While hospitalization can be a point of reflection and an opportunity to stabilize patients on long-term medications for OUD, it is not realistic to expect all patients to start OUD treatment or achieve abstinence after hospitalization. Patients may be in a precontemplative stage of change and opioids or other drugs may serve an ongoing role in patients' lives despite negative consequences, for example, as a coping approach for prior trauma, mental illness, or chronic pain. These patients may continue using opioids despite harms, clinician counseling, and motivational interviewing to harness ambivalence about ongoing opioid use.

Regardless of a patient's interest in treatment after hospitalization, it is still essential to address withdrawal symptoms with evidence-based approaches and to provide comprehensive support during hospitalization. In addition, clinicians should apply a harm-reduction framework for all patients using substances to allow for more patient-centered care.[105] This is especially true for patients who do not plan to stop using opioids after discharge. Harm-reduction principles, including nonjudgmental counseling and tailored interventions, should be incorporated to build a therapeutic relationship and to reduce the risks associated with ongoing drug use. Providing naloxone, education on safer use practices, and addressing barriers to care can help foster trust and promote health, even for patients who decline formal OUD treatment after discharge. See Chapter 15 for more information.

Harm Reduction

Harm-reduction resources are essential for hospitalized patients with OUD, particularly for those who plan to resume substance use after discharge. Providing harm-reduction counseling in a nonjudgmental and patient-centered manner helps build trust and focuses on the patient's goals, such as reducing risks associated with substance use. Patients should be offered supplies like naloxone for overdose prevention, sterile syringes for patients who inject their substance, education on safer substance use practices to minimize harm, and other harm-reduction supplies to reduce their risk of overdose and spread of infectious diseases (eg, tourniquets, sterile saline, cotton, etc).[106] This approach empowers patients to make informed choices, reduces stigma, and enhances their safety and well-being, as well as improves trusting relationships with health care clinicians and systems. For more information, see Chapter 19 for details.

REFERENCES

1. U.S. Overdose Deaths Decrease in 2023, First Time Since 2018. May 14, 2024. Accessed May 12, 2025. https://www.cdc.gov/media/releases/2025/2025-cdc-reports-decline-in-us-drug-overdose-deaths.html
2. CDC. *CDC Reports Nearly 24% Decline in U.S. Drug Overdose Deaths*. CDC Newsroom. February 25, 2025. Accessed May 12, 2025. https://www.cdc.gov/media/releases/2025/2025-cdc-reports-decline-in-us-drug-overdose-deaths.html
3. Wakeman SE. Opioid use disorder diagnosis and management. *NEJM Evid*. 2022;1(4):EVIDra2200038.
4. Thakrar AP, Lowenstein M, Greysen SR, Delgado MK. Trends in before medically advised discharges for patients with opioid use disorder, 2016–2020. *JAMA*. 2023;330(23):2302–2304.
5. Englander H, Thakrar AP, Bagley SM, Rolley T, Dong K, Hyshka E. Caring for hospitalized adults with opioid use disorder in the era of fentanyl: a review. *JAMA Intern Med*. 2024;184(6):691–701.
6. Gowing L, Ali R, White JM, Mbewe D. Buprenorphine for managing opioid withdrawal. *Cochrane Database Syst Rev*. 2017;2(2):CD002025.
7. Gowing L, Farrell M, Ali R, White JM. Alpha$_2$-adrenergic agonists for the management of opioid withdrawal. *Cochrane Database Syst Rev*. 2016;2016(5):CD002024.
8. Calcaterra SL, Bottner R, Martin M, et al. Management of opioid use disorder, opioid withdrawal, and opioid overdose prevention in hospitalized adults: a systematic review of existing guidelines. *J Hosp Med*. 2022;17(9):679–692.
9. Steiner G, Suen LW, Martin M, et al. Treatment of Inpatient opioid withdrawal with short-acting full agonist opioids at a safety-net hospital. *J Gen Intern Med*. 2025;40(12):2890–2895.
10. Thakrar AP, Uritsky UJ, Christopher C, et al. Safety and preliminary outcomes of short-acting opioid agonist treatment (sOAT) for hospitalized patients with opioid use disorder. *Addict Sci Clin Pract*. 2023;18(1):13.
11. Santo T, Clark B, Hickman M, et al. Association of opioid agonist treatment with all-cause mortality and specific causes of death among people with opioid dependence: a systematic review and meta-analysis. *JAMA Psychiatry*. 2021;78(9):979.
12. Sordo L, Barrio G, Bravo MJ, et al. Mortality risk during and after opioid substitution treatment: systematic review and meta-analysis of cohort studies. *BMJ*. 2017;357:j1550.
13. Liebschutz JM, Crooks D, Herman D, et al. Buprenorphine treatment for hospitalized, opioid-dependent patients: a randomized clinical trial. *JAMA Intern Med*. 2014;174(8):1369–1376.
14. Button D, Hartley J, Robbins J, Levander XA, Smith NJ, Englander H. Low-dose buprenorphine initiation in hospitalized adults with opioid use disorder: a retrospective cohort analysis. *J Addict Med*. 2022;16(2):e105–e111.
15. Jablonski LA, Bodnar AR, Stewart RW. Development of an intravenous low-dose buprenorphine initiation protocol. *Drug Alcohol Depend*. 2022;237:109541.
16. Cohen SM, Weimer MB, Levander XA, Peckham AM, Tetrault JM, Morford KL. Low dose initiation of buprenorphine: a narrative review and practical approach. *J Addict Med*. 2021;16(4):399–406.
17. Herring AA, Vosooghi AA, Luftig J, et al. High-dose buprenorphine induction in the emergency department for treatment of opioid use disorder. *JAMA Netw Open*. 2021; 4(7):e2117128.
18. Casey S, Regan S, Gale E, et al. Rapid methadone induction in a general hospital setting: a retrospective, observational analysis. *Subst Abus*. 2023;44(3):177–183.
19. Klaire S, Fairbairn N, Ryan A, Nolan S, McLean M, Bach P. Safety and efficacy of rapid methadone titration for opioid use disorder in an inpatient setting: a retrospective cohort study. *J Addict Med*. 2023;17(6):711–713.
20. Martin M, Englander H, Calcaterra SL. Things We Do for No Reason™: avoiding methadone for opioid withdrawal. *J Hosp Med*. 2023;18(11):1034–1037:jhm.13138.
21. Darke S, Larney S, Farrell M. Yes, people can die from opiate withdrawal. *Addiction*. 2017;112(2):199–200.
22. Kleinman RA, Wakeman SE. Treating opioid withdrawal in the hospital: a role for short-acting opioids. *Ann Intern Med*. 2021;175(2):283–284.
23. Thakrar AP. Short-acting opioids for hospitalized patients with opioid use disorder. *JAMA Intern Med*. 2022;182(3):247–248.
24. Mayer S, Langheimer V, Nolan S, Boyd J, Small W, McNeil R. Emergency department experiences of people who use drugs who left or were discharged from hospital against medical advice. *PLoS ONE*. 2023;18(2):e0282215.
25. Harris M. Normalised pain and severe health care delay among people who inject drugs in London: adapting cultural safety principles to promote care. *Soc Sci Med*. 2020;260:113183.
26. Simon R, Snow R, Wakeman S. Understanding why patients with substance use disorders leave the hospital against medical advice: a qualitative study. *Substance Abuse*. 2020;41(4):519–525.
27. McNeil R, Small W, Wood E, Kerr T. Hospitals as a 'risk environment': an ethno-epidemiological study of voluntary and involuntary discharge from hospital against medical advice among people who inject drugs. *Soc Sci Med*. 2014; 105:59–66.
28. Sharma A, Dunn KE, Schmid-Doyle K, et al. Examining the severity and progression of illicitly manufactured fentanyl withdrawal: a quasi-experimental comparison. *J Addict Med*. 2024;19(2):172–178.
29. Thakrar AP, Kleinman RA. Opioid withdrawal management in the fentanyl era. *Addiction*. 2022;117(9):2560–2561.

30. D'Onofrio G, O'Connor PG, Pantalon MV, et al. Emergency department–initiated buprenorphine/naloxone treatment for opioid dependence: a randomized clinical trial. *JAMA*. 2015; 313(16):1636–1644.
31. Lee JD, Nunes EV, Novo P, et al. Comparative effectiveness of extended-release naltrexone versus buprenorphine-naloxone for opioid relapse prevention (X:BOT): a multicentre, open-label, randomised controlled trial. *Lancet*. 2018;391(10118): 309–318.
32. Strain EC, Stitzer ML. *Methadone Treatment for Opioid Dependence*. Johns Hopkins University Press; 1999.
33. Baxter LE, Campbell A, DeShields M, et al. Safe methadone induction and stabilization: report of an expert panel. *J Addict Med*. 2013;7(6):377–386.
34. Bosshardt Z, Ortega Perez M, Casarella J, Buresh M, Tang Yi-Lang. Dosing and safety of methadone initiation in the setting of fentanyl: a systematic review. *J Addict Med*. 2025. doi: 10.1097/ADM.0000000000001629
35. Martin M, Baisey T, Skinner S, et al. Early results of implementing rapid methadone titration for hospitalized patients: a case series. *J Gen Intern Med*. 2025;40(13):3104–3110.
36. Liu P, Chan B, Sokolski E, Patten A, Englander H. Piloting a hospital-based rapid methadone initiation protocol for fentanyl. *J Addict Med*. 2024;18(4):458–462.
37. Iyer NS, Ferguson EB, Yan VZ, Hand DJ, Abatemarco DJ, Boelig RC. Standard versus rapid inpatient methadone titration for pregnant patients with opioid use disorder: a retrospective cohort study. *J Addict Med*. 2024;18(6): 670–674.
38. Racha S, Buresh ME, Patel B, Harfouch LT, Berger O. Safety of rapid inpatient methadone initiation protocol: a retrospective cohort study. *J Subst Use Addict Treat*. 2023;148: 209004.
39. Steiger S, McCuistian C, Suen LW, Shapiro B, Tompkins DA, Bazazi AR. Induction to methadone 80 mg in the first week of treatment of patients who use fentanyl: a case series from an outpatient opioid treatment program. *J Addict Med*. 2024; 18(5):580–585.
40. American Society of Addiction Medicine. The ASAM National Practice Guideline for the treatment of opioid use disorder: 2020 focused update. *J Addict Med*. 2020;14(2S): 1–91.
41. Gregory C, Yadav K, Linders J, Sikora L, Eagles D. Incidence of buprenorphine-precipitated opioid withdrawal in adults with opioid use disorder: a systematic review. *Addiction*. 2025; 120(1):7–20.
42. Johnson R, Strain EC, Amass L. Buprenorphine: how to use it right. *Drug Alcohol Depend*. 2003;70(2):S59–S77.
43. Lee JD, Grossman E, DiRocco D, Gourevitch MN. Home buprenorphine/naloxone induction in primary care. *J Gen Intern Med*. 2009;24(2):226–232.
44. Weimer MB, Herring AA, Kawasaki SS, Meyer M, Kleykamp BA, Ramsey KS. ASAM clinical considerations: buprenorphine treatment of opioid use disorder for individuals using high-potency synthetic opioids. *J Addict Med*. 2023; 17(6):632–639.
45. D'Onofrio G, Hawk KF, Perrone J, et al. Incidence of precipitated withdrawal during a multisite emergency department–initiated buprenorphine clinical trial in the era of fentanyl. *JAMA Netw Open*. 2023;6(3):e236108.
46. Thakrar AP, Christine PJ, Siaw-Asamoah A, et al. Buprenorphine-precipitated withdrawal among hospitalized patients using fentanyl. *JAMA Network Open*. 2024;7(9):e2435895.
47. Spreen LA, Dittmar EN, Quirk KC, Smith MA. Buprenorphine initiation strategies for opioid use disorder and pain management: a systematic review. *Pharmacotherapy*. 2022; 42(5):411–427.
48. Bhatraju EP, Klein JW, Hall AN, et al. Low dose buprenorphine induction with full agonist overlap in hospitalized patients with opioid use disorder: a retrospective cohort study. *J Addict Med*. 2021;16(4):461–465.
49. Snyder H, Chau B, Kalmin MM, et al. High-dose buprenorphine initiation in the emergency department among patients using fentanyl and other opioids. *JAMA Netw Open*. 2023; 6(3):e231572.
50. *H.R.2617—117th Congress (2021–2022): Consolidated Appropriations Act, 2023*. Accessed May 12, 2025. https://www.congress.gov/bill/117th-congress/house-bill/2617
51. *Title 21 Code of Federal Regulations—Section 1306.07 Administering or Dispensing of Narcotic Drugs*. Accessed November 10, 2021. https://www.deadiversion.usdoj.gov/21cfr/cfr/1306/1306_07.htm
52. Skogrand E, Sharpe J, Englander H. Dispensing methadone at hospital discharge: one hospital's approach to implementing the "72-hour rule" change. *J Addict Med*. 2023;18(1):71–74.
53. Bowman LA, Berger O, Nesbit S, Stoller KB, Buresh M, Stewart R. Operationalizing the new DEA exception: a novel process for dispensing of methadone for opioid use disorder at discharge from acute care settings. *Am J Health Syst Pharm*. 2024;81(6):204–218.
54. Huo S, Heil J, Salzman MS, et al. Emergency department utilization of the methadone "72-hour rule" to bridge or initiate and link to outpatient treatment. *Am J Emerg Med*. 2025;89:209–215.
55. Pytell JD, Sharfstein JM, Olsen Y. Facilitating methadone use in hospitals and skilled nursing facilities. *JAMA Intern Med*. 2019;180(1):7–8.
56. Cohen SM, Joab R, Bolles KM, Friedman S, Kimmel SD. Ending medical complicity with skilled-nursing facility discrimination against people with opioid use disorder. *Ann Intern Med*. 2023;176(3):410–412.
57. Noska A, Mohan A, Wakeman S, Rich J, Boutwell A. Managing opioid use disorder during and after acute hospitalization: a case-based review clarifying methadone regulation for acute care settings. *J Addict Behav Ther Rehabil*. 2015;4(2):1000138.
58. Jackson DS, Nguemeni Tiako MJ, Jordan A. Disparities in addiction treatment: learning from the past to forge an equitable future. *Med Clin North Am*. 2022;106(1):29–41.
59. American Psychiatric Association. Opioid use disorder. *Diagnostic and Statistical Manual of Mental Disorders (DSM-5)*. 5th ed. American Psychiatric Association; 2013.
60. Volkow ND, Jones EB, Einstein EB, Wargo EM. Prevention and treatment of opioid misuse and addiction: a review. *JAMA Psychiatry*. 2019;76(2):208–216.
61. Torres-Lockhart KE, Lu TY, Weimer MB, Stein MR, Cunningham CO. Clinical management of opioid withdrawal. *Addiction*. 2022;117(9):2540–2550.
62. Jarvis M, Williams J, Hurford M, et al. Appropriate use of drug testing in clinical addiction medicine. *J Addict Med*. 2017;11(3):163–173.
63. Khatri UG, Aronowitz SV. Considering the harms of our habits: the reflexive urine drug screen in opioid use disorder treatment. *J Subst Abuse Treat*. 2021;123:108258.
64. Pytell JD, Rastegar DA. Down the drain: reconsidering routine urine drug testing during the COVID-19 pandemic. *J Subst Abuse Treat*. 2021;120:108155.
65. Huhn AS, Hobelmann JG, Oyler GA, Strain EC. Protracted renal clearance of fentanyl in persons with opioid use disorder. *Drug Alcohol Depend*. 2020;214:108147.
66. Luba R, Jones J, Choi CJ, Comer S. Fentanyl withdrawal: understanding symptom severity and exploring the role of body mass index on withdrawal symptoms and clearance. *Addiction*. 2022;118(4):719–726.

67. Weiss ST, Chinn M, Veach L. Reconsidering reliance on confirmatory drug testing in a patient with repeated positive urine drug screen results: a teachable moment. *JAMA Intern Med.* 2021;181(12):1637.
68. Dunn KE, Strain EC. Establishing a research agenda for the study and assessment of opioid withdrawal. *Lancet Psychiatry.* 2024;11(7):566–572.
69. Martinez S, Ellis JD, Bergeria CL, Huhn AS, Dunn KE. Treating opioid use disorder and opioid withdrawal in the context of fentanyl. *Annu Rev Clin Psychol.* 2025;21(1):221–249.
70. Pergolizzi JV, Varrassi G, Paladini A, LeQuang J. Stopping or decreasing opioid therapy in patients on chronic opioid therapy. *Pain Ther.* 2019;8(2):163–176.
71. Wesson DR, Ling W. The clinical opiate withdrawal scale (COWS). *J Psychoactive Drugs.* 2003;35(2):253–259.
72. Gossop M. The development of a short opiate withdrawal scale (SOWS). *Addict Behav.* 1990;15(5):487–490.
73. Handelsman L, Cochrane KJ, Aronson MJ, Ness R, Rubinstein KJ, Kanof PD. Two new rating scales for opiate withdrawal. *Am J Drug Alcohol Abuse.* 1987;13(3):293–308.
74. Hall OT, Vilensky M, Teater JE, et al. Withdrawal catastrophizing scale: initial psychometric properties and implications for the study of opioid use disorder and hyperkatifeia. *Am J Drug Alcohol Abuse.* 2024;51(1):31–43.
75. Wakeman SE, Larochelle MR, Ameli O, et al. Comparative effectiveness of different treatment pathways for opioid use disorder. *JAMA Netw Open.* 2020;3(2):e1920622–e1920622.
76. Ehret GB, Voide C, Gex-Fabry M, et al. Drug-induced long QT syndrome in injection drug users receiving methadone: high frequency in hospitalized patients and risk factors. *Arch Intern Med.* 2006;166(12):1280–1287.
77. Bart G, Wyman Z, Wang Q, Hodges JS, Karim R, Bart BA. Methadone and the QTc interval: paucity of clinically significant factors in a retrospective cohort. *J Addict Med.* 2017;11(6):489–493.
78. Rautaharju PM, Surawicz B, Gettes LS. AHA/ACCF/HRS recommendations for the standardization and interpretation of the electrocardiogram: part IV: the ST segment, T and U waves, and the QT interval: a scientific statement from the American Heart Association Electrocardiography and Arrhythmias Committee, Council on Clinical Cardiology; the American College of Cardiology Foundation; and the Heart Rhythm Society: endorsed by the International Society for Computerized Electrocardiology. *Circulation.* 2009;119(10): e241–e250.
79. Rosado J, Walsh SL, Bigelow GE, Strain EC. Sublingual buprenorphine/naloxone precipitated withdrawal in subjects maintained on 100 mg of daily methadone. *Drug Alcohol Depend.* 2007;90(2–3):261–269.
80. De Aquino JP, Parida S, Sofuoglu M. The pharmacology of buprenorphine microinduction for opioid use disorder. *Clin Drug Investig.* 2021;41(5):425–436.
81. Thakrar AP, Jablonski L, Ratner J, Rastegar DA. Micro-dosing intravenous buprenorphine to rapidly transition from full opioid agonists. *J Addict Med.* 2022;16(1):122–124.
82. Saal D, Lee F. Rapid induction therapy for opioid-use disorder using buprenorphine transdermal patch: a case series. *Perm J.* 2020;24(19):124.
83. Michel I, Ochal D, Paharia A, Jannetto P, Breitinger S, Oesterle T. Absorption of naloxone in patients prescribed buprenorphine-naloxone. *Am J Addict.* 2025;34(3): 350–354.
84. Karavolis ZA, Roy PJ. Adapting low-dose buprenorphine induction to meet patient needs: a pilot study. *Drug Alcohol Depend Rep.* 2022;5:100104.
85. Weimer MB, Guerra M, Morrow G, Adams K. Hospital-based buprenorphine micro-dose initiation. *J Addict Med.* 2020;15(3):255–257.
86. Mosher HJ, Hadlandsmyth K, Alexander B, Lund BC. Continuation of buprenorphine during hospitalization and subsequent retention in therapy: an observational study in veterans administration hospitals. *J Gen Intern Med.* 2024;39(2):207–213.
87. Huhn AS, Strain EC, Bigelow GE, Smith MT, Edwards RR, Tompkins DA. Analgesic effects of hydromorphone versus buprenorphine in buprenorphine-maintained individuals. *Anesthesiology.* 2019;130(1):131–141.
88. Buonora MJ, Mackey K, Khalid L, et al. Acute pain management in people with opioid use disorder: a systematic review. *Ann Intern Med.* 2025;178(4):558–570.
89. Björnsson M, Acharya C, Strandgården K, Tiberg F. Population pharmacokinetic analysis supports initiation treatment and bridging from sublingual buprenorphine to subcutaneous administration of a buprenorphine depot (CAM2038) in the treatment of opioid use disorder. *Clin Pharmacokinet.* 2023;62(10):1427–1443.
90. D'Onofrio G, Herring AA, Perrone J, et al. Extended-release 7-day injectable buprenorphine for patients with minimal to mild opioid withdrawal. *JAMA Network Open.* 2024;7(7):e2420702.
91. Kleinman RA, Thakrar AP. Using short-acting opioids to relieve opioid withdrawal in hospital. *CMAJ.* 2023;195(49): E1718–E1720.
92. Stern SJ, D'Orazio JL, Work BD, Calcaterra SL, Thakrar AP. Point/counterpoint: should full agonist opioid medications be offered to hospitalized patients for management of opioid withdrawal? *J Hosp Med.* 2023;19(4):339–343.
93. Demaret I, Quertemont E, Litran G, et al. Efficacy of heroin-assisted treatment in Belgium: a randomised controlled trial. *Eur Addict Res.* 2015;21(4):179–187.
94. Haasen C, Verthein U, Degkwitz P, Berger J, Krausz M, Naber D. Heroin-assisted treatment for opioid dependence: randomised controlled trial. *Br J Psychiatry.* 2007;191:55–62.
95. Oviedo-Joekes E, Brissette S, Marsh DC, et al. Diacetylmorphine versus methadone for the treatment of opioid addiction. *N Engl J Med.* 2009;361(8):777–786.
96. Oviedo-Joekes E, Guh D, Brissette S, et al. Hydromorphone compared with diacetylmorphine for long-term opioid dependence: a randomized clinical trial. *JAMA Psychiatry.* 2016;73(5):447.
97. Strang J, Groshkova T, Uchtenhagen A, et al. Heroin on trial: systematic review and meta-analysis of randomised trials of diamorphine-prescribing as treatment for refractory heroin addiction. *Br J Psychiatry.* 2015;207(1):5–14.
98. Rzasa Lynn R, Galinkin JL. Naloxone dosage for opioid reversal: current evidence and clinical implications. *Ther Adv Drug Saf.* 2018;9(1):63–88.
99. Dezfulian C, Orkin AM, Maron BA, et al. Opioid-associated out-of-hospital cardiac arrest: distinctive clinical features and implications for health care and public responses: a scientific statement from the American Heart Association. *Circulation.* 2021;143(16):e836–e870.
100. Reed MK, Imperato NS, Bowles JM, Salcedo VJ, Guth A, Rising KL. Perspectives of people in Philadelphia who use fentanyl/heroin adulterated with the animal tranquilizer xylazine; Making a case for xylazine test strips. *Drug Alcohol Depend Rep.* 2022;4:100074.
101. Spadaro A, O'Connor K, Lakamana S, et al. Self-reported xylazine experiences: a mixed-methods study of Reddit subscribers. *J Addict Med.* 2023;17(6):691–694.
102. Thakrar AP, Zwiebel SJ, Christine PJ, et al. Manifestations of potential xylazine withdrawal: a retrospective cohort study

with nested case series. *Drug Alcohol Depend.* 2025;272: 112681.

103. Ostrowski SJ. Notes from the field: severe medetomidine withdrawal syndrome in patients using illegally manufactured opioids—Pittsburgh, Pennsylvania, October 2024–March 2025. *MMWR Morb Mortal Wkly Rep.* 2025;74(15):269–271.
104. Shulman M, Greiner MG, Tafessu HM, et al. Rapid initiation of injection naltrexone for opioid use disorder: a stepped-wedge cluster randomized clinical trial. *JAMA Network Open.* 2024;7(5):e249744.
105. Abuse S. *Mental Health Services Administration. Harm Reduction Framework.* Center for Substance Abuse Prevention, Substance Abuse and Mental Health Services Administration; 2023.
106. Perera R, Stephan L, Appa A, et al. Meeting people where they are: implementing hospital-based substance use harm reduction. *Harm Reduct J.* 2022;19(1):14.

8

Alcohol Withdrawal and Alcohol Use Disorder Evaluation and Management

Shawn M. Cohen, Stephen Holt, Alyssa F. Peterkin

On my desk at work, there is a weathered, silver-dollar–sized, bronze coin with the words "Unity, Service, Recovery" embossed on a triangle on one side. Within the triangle is the numeral "3" and the word "months" beneath it. For anyone who has attended an Alcoholics Anonymous (AA) meeting, and for seasoned Addiction Medicine clinicians, you know this is a treasured coin given to an active AA member who reached 90 days of abstinence. I received this coin from Juan, a young man I met more than 15 years ago. I encountered Juan, then a 32-year-old army veteran with a history of combat-related posttraumatic stress disorder, when he was admitted to my team on the general medicine service for alcohol withdrawal and alcohol-related pancreatitis. This was his sixth admission for alcohol-related complications that year, each time being admitted to a different attending in the hospital. In the emergency department (ED), once determined to be in moderate alcohol withdrawal, he was loaded with chlordiazepoxide before being sent up to the floor, as he had several times before. When I met with Juan to get additional history, his wife Marta arrived—she was distraught, flushed, and tearful. She sat beside him, holding his hand tightly, obviously full of a mix of anguish and frustration. Marta was 5 months pregnant. Thirteen months prior, Juan returned from a traumatic tour in Afghanistan. Since then, he struggled with anxiety and countless cycles of self-medicating with alcohol, intoxication, and regret. Ironically, he found the Veterans Administration (VA) hospital to be triggering and preferred our non-VA hospital. He had trouble looking in his wife's eyes. The shame was palpable. It was clear to me that she loved him, wanted him to get better, and felt powerless to do so.

Over the next several days, we managed his alcohol withdrawal and pancreatitis pain. As the tempest of alcohol, benzodiazepines, opioids, and pain cleared away, I was able to see the disciplined, sincere, resilient, and selfless husband, veteran, and would-be father underneath. He expressed a vehement desire to abstain from alcohol, and I believed him. He knew he was hurting himself and his wife, and he wished to end his enslavement to alcohol. After a 5-day hospitalization, with abstinence as his unequivocal goal, he committed to starting disulfiram and took his first dose before leaving the hospital.

When he arrived home, however, panic set in. He felt guilty over his inability to hold down a job, anxiety over the reality of his wife's pregnancy, and an overwhelming temptation of the liquor store across the street from their apartment. He quickly resumed drinking, consuming a half pint of vodka in the stairwell of their apartment. Within less than an hour, predictably, he began to experience severe nausea, intractable vomiting, headache, and palpitations, consistent with the "alcohol-disulfiram reaction." Seeing Juan unable to keep anything down, Marta brought him back to the hospital. It had been just 12 hours since his last discharge. In the ED, he was given benzodiazepines for presumed alcohol withdrawal despite having only consumed a half-pint of vodka since his last hospital stay. He was admitted again for "alcohol withdrawal." But unlike so many prior admissions, he was serendipitously admitted to the same general medical team that cared for him the day before—my service. Having this spark of continuity proved consequential. I already knew his story—I knew his goals, his anxieties, his unfulfilled commitment to his family. I certainly knew he wasn't here for alcohol withdrawal; he was here because of the alcohol-disulfiram reaction. After 24 hours of supportive care with antiemetics, fluids, and some benzodiazepines, he was ready for discharge again. He thanked me for caring, for not judging him, for sitting beside him—for believing in him. Remarkably, he resumed the disulfiram.

Many months went by. I periodically took a quick look in his chart to see if he had been readmitted. He hadn't. Finally, I came to work one day and the unit clerk on our floor told me someone had dropped off a letter for me. It was from Juan! In a short note, he told me he had made it to "90 meetings in 90 days" as the old AA mantra goes. He found seasonal work doing landscaping. Marta was now 36 weeks pregnant, and he was excited about soon becoming a father. He faithfully took his disulfiram, which was prescribed by his primary care doctor, and he was immensely grateful. Enclosed in the note was the bronze coin stamped with "3 months." I was pleased as punch.

I didn't hear from Juan again for a long time. It wasn't until 4 years later that I received a letter from his wife, Marta. How she found me is anyone's guess. She was writing to inform me that Juan had relapsed to drinking about 18 months prior, and that he had passed away. It was not clear to me from the letter *how* he died, just that he had. Much to my surprise, Marta was writing to express her gratitude. Gratitude that Juan was there for the birth of their son, and that he had been completely sober for the first 2 years of their son's life, watching him learn to crawl and then walk. She still loved Juan very much, and was grateful for those few years they had together before alcohol took ahold of him once more.

His death served as a reminder to me that alcohol use disorder is indeed a relapsing, remitting disease. It reminded me that behind every "frequent flier" in the ED, there is a story, a person who loves them, and the potential for a welcome respite from the tumult that often accompanies severe alcohol use disorder.

—Stephen Holt

Key Points

- **Alcohol withdrawal symptoms are due to neurobiologic adaptations to chronic alcohol use, particularly in gamma-aminobutyric acid (GABA) and glutamate systems.**
- **Delirium tremens and alcohol withdrawal seizures are hallmarks of complicated alcohol withdrawal.**
- **Hospital-based treatment of alcohol withdrawal should begin with risk assessment for development of complicated alcohol withdrawal.**
- **For patients at high risk of complicated alcohol withdrawal, front loading with benzodiazepines is the recommended treatment strategy.**
- **For patients deemed lower risk for complicated alcohol withdrawal, symptom-triggered therapy with benzodiazepines is appropriate.**
- **Medications for alcohol use disorder (MAUD) are associated with reduced hospital readmissions, reduced risk of developing alcohol-related liver disease, lower risk of hepatic decompensation, and should be offered to all hospitalized patients with alcohol use disorder (AUD).**

Alcohol use disorder (AUD), the most prevalent substance use disorder (SUD) in the United States (US), impacts 1 in 10 people over the age of 12, with a disproportionate impact on racially and ethnically minoritized communities.[1] The Centers for Disease Control and Prevention (CDC) estimates that 178,000 persons died from alcohol attributable deaths between 2020 and 2021, roughly 1 person every 3 minutes.[2] Beyond increasing risk of death, alcohol use negatively impacts every organ system as well as increases the risk of several types of cancer; most commonly, breast and colorectal cancers.[3] Given these risks, in 2025 the US Surgeon General issued an advisory raising awareness of direct links between alcohol consumption and cancer.[4] The COVID-19 pandemic further increased alcohol use and its health impacts,[5] an effect which has continued post pandemic.[6]

It is estimated that 17 to 30% of hospitalized patients have AUD depending on geographic location and community.[7,8] Alcohol withdrawal, one of the most common complications of AUD, is estimated to be involved in 2% of all hospitalizations in the US.[9] While hospitalization can be a time of crisis, it also represents a crucial opportunity to engage a population that may be less connected to medical care.[10] It is estimated that only 2% of patients with AUD receive medications for alcohol use disorder (MAUD) on hospital discharge.[11] This is despite compelling evidence that MAUD is associated with decreased hospital readmissions[11] and decreased mortality among those with alcohol-associated liver disease.[12] Black and Latino adults experience disproportionately more alcohol-related health concerns (ie, liver disease and accidents/injuries) and social impacts (ie, legal consequences) but are even less likely to engage in AUD treatment services.[13–15]

As a guide to hospital-based clinicians treating people with AUD, this chapter reviews the spectrum of AUD care among hospitalized patients, with a focus on effective evidence-based treatments for alcohol withdrawal and AUD at the time of discharge.

Pathophysiology of Alcohol Use

Neurobiology of Acute Alcohol Use

Alcohol exerts numerous acute effects via multiple pathways within the central nervous system (CNS). Alcohol acts as a CNS depressant, impacting gamma-aminobutyric acid (GABA) and glutamate activity in the brain. GABA is an inhibitory neurotransmitter that reduces the electrical activity of neurons, and glutamate is an excitatory neurotransmitter which increases the electrical activity of neurons. In a natural state, there exists a balance between CNS excitation and inhibition. Acutely, alcohol enhances the effect of GABA by promoting increased GABA release and facilitating activity at the $GABA_A$ receptor; this contributes to the anxiolytic effects of alcohol.[16,17] Simultaneously, alcohol suppresses extracellular glutamate levels in the striatum,[16] thereby inhibiting glutamatergic activity at N-methyl-D-aspartate (NMDA) glutamate receptors. In addition, entry of calcium ions into neurons is reduced which further decreases CNS excitability. While interventions to address alcohol withdrawal typically focus on the GABA and glutamatergic effects described above, alcohol consumption also acutely increases norepinephrine levels[18] and the release of endogenous opioids which facilitate alcohol's reinforcing effects.[19]

Neurobiology of Chronic Alcohol Use

GABA and Glutamate

Chronic alcohol exposure—episodic or continuous alcohol use over weeks to months—leads to maladaptive neurochemical changes that preserve homeostasis between the GABA and glutamate systems to counterbalance the effects of chronic alcohol use. Chronic alcohol consumption creates a feedback mechanism compensating for the constant depressant effect of alcohol. The inhibitory $GABA_A$ receptors are downregulated in the brain, by way of the alpha-1 subunit (α_1); the excitatory glutamate NMDA receptors[17] are upregulated in the brain through increased gene expression leading to increased glutamate production. The decreased number of α_1 on the $GABA_A$ receptors leads to reduced neuronal responsiveness to alcohol use, manifesting clinically as "tolerance," whereby more alcohol is needed to achieve the same level of inhibition.

Norepinephrine

In people with physiologic tolerance to alcohol, peripheral and central noradrenergic activity is elevated, evidenced by higher plasma levels of norepinephrine and its metabolites compared to those who do not exhibit tolerance.[18] Increased noradrenergic activity plays a role in ongoing alcohol use and anxiety as well as physiologic changes like hypertension. To compensate for alcohol-induced reductions in electrical activity, voltage-operated calcium channels increase which contributes to tolerance and primes the neuron for increased excitation and withdrawal when an individual abstains from alcohol.[17]

Endogenous Opioids, Serotonin, and Dopamine

Chronic alcohol use also leads to reductions in mu-opioid receptor expression in the nucleus accumbens as a compensatory response to the increased release of endogenous opioid with chronic alcohol use.[20] Reductions in serotonin levels[20,21] and concomitant increases in kappa-opioid receptor activity related to chronic alcohol use are linked to impulsivity, alcohol use, and dysphoria.[19,21] After months to years of heavy alcohol use, the anticipation of alcohol consumption leads to dopamine release within the mesocorticolimbic system, manifesting subjectively as intense cravings.[16]

Alcohol Withdrawal

Defining Alcohol Withdrawal

Acute alcohol withdrawal syndrome (AWS) is defined by the Diagnostic and Statistical Manual of Mental Disorders, 5th edition (DSM-5)[22] as the presence of at least two of the following:

- Autonomic hyperactivity
- Increased hand tremor
- Insomnia, nausea, or vomiting
- Transient visual, tactile, or auditory hallucinations or illusions
- Psychomotor agitation
- Anxiety or generalized tonic–clonic seizures

Symptoms must occur within several hours to days after cessation or reduction in heavy and prolonged alcohol use.[22] These signs or symptoms must cause clinically significant distress, social, occupational and/or

TABLE 8.1

Summary of Neuroadaptations Related to Alcohol Use and Alcohol Withdrawal

	GABA	Glutamate	Calcium	Dopamine	Norepinephrine	Serotonin	Endogenous opioids
Alcohol use (acute)	↑	↓	↓	↑	↑	↑	↑
Compensation to chronic alcohol use	↓↓	↑↑	↑↑	↑	↑↑	↓	↓↑
Alcohol withdrawal	↓	↑↑↑	↑↑	↓	↑↑↑	↓	↑

functional impairment, and cannot be attributed to another medical condition or mental disorder.[22] About 50% of people with heavy alcohol use and AUD will experience alcohol withdrawal symptoms following the reduction or cessation of alcohol.[23]

Neurobiology of Alcohol Withdrawal

AWS is characterized by CNS excitation due to the disruption of the neurochemical equilibrium of the GABA and glutamate systems following the cessation or reduction of alcohol use after a period of chronic exposure. Cessation or reduction of alcohol leads to decreased GABA inhibition, resulting in unopposed neuronal excitation from the upregulation of glutamate receptors (hyperglutaminergic state)[17] and calcium channels within the glutamate NMDA receptors.

Alterations in $GABA_A$ receptors, which are potentially related to decreased sensitivity of GABA at the $GABA_A$ receptors, have been linked to the clinical manifestations of alcohol withdrawal including agitation, anxiety, tremors, and seizures. The combination of unopposed glutamate excess and the increased glutamate NMDA receptors play a role in alcohol withdrawal-associated hallucinations and seizures. Glutamate NMDA receptors, which include receptor-operated calcium channels,[17] allow for the entry of more calcium ions into the neuron and consequently increase voltage-operated calcium channels leading to the excitatory state associated with AWS. Finally, the dysphoria of alcohol withdrawal and delirium tremens (DTs) are related to serotonin and dopamine depletion and concomitant increases in dynorphin and kappa-opioid receptor activity (Table 8.1, Figure 8.1).[19]

Timing of Alcohol Withdrawal Symptoms

Acute alcohol withdrawal symptoms only occur in individuals with some degree of physiologic tolerance to alcohol. Alcohol withdrawal symptoms range in severity and present as early as 6 hours after one's last drink, peaking within 48 hours and diminishing after 5 to 7 days.[16] More protracted withdrawal symptoms, also known as "post–acute withdrawal syndrome," including mood dysregulation, (ie, anxiety and depression, insomnia, and alcohol cravings), may persist for several weeks to months after alcohol cessation and often contribute to a return to alcohol use.[19] Alcohol withdrawal can occur with any relative decrease in serum alcohol levels. Undetectable serum alcohol levels are not required for symptom manifestation. Figure 8.2 presents a timeline of alcohol

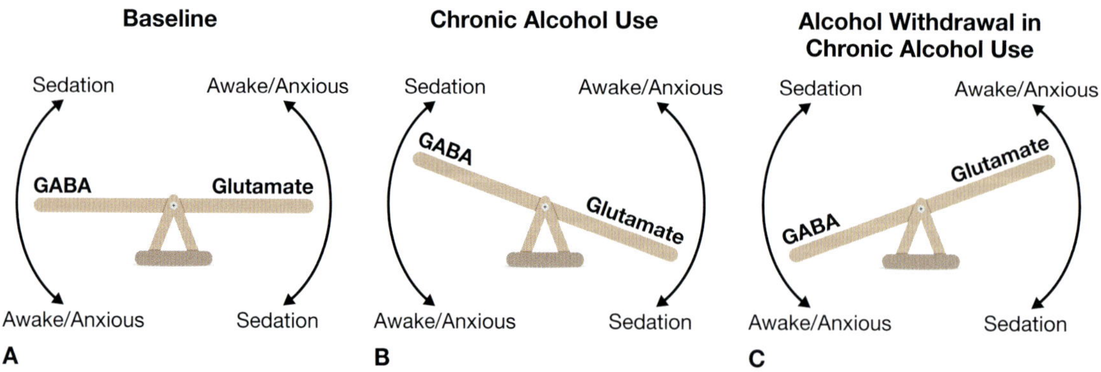

Figure 8.1: Neurobiology of alcohol intoxication and withdrawal. (Part A redrawn from Eickelberg SJ, Gordon AJ. Management of sedative-hypnotic intoxication and withdrawal. In: Miller SC, eds. *The ASAM Principles of Addiction Medicine*. 7th ed. 2024: 888–907.)

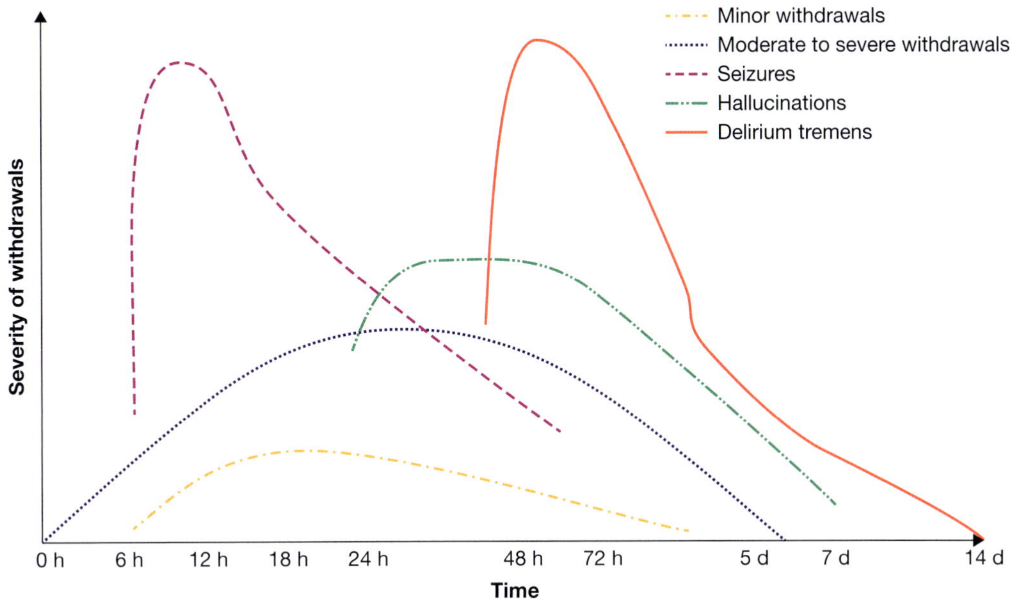

Figure 8.2: Timeline of alcohol withdrawal syndrome. (Kattimani S, Bharadwaj B. Clinical management of alcohol withdrawal: a systematic review. *Ind Psychiatry J.* 2013;22(2):100–108. https://journals.lww.com/inpj/fulltext/2013/22020/clinical_management_of_alcohol_withdrawal__a.2.aspx)

withdrawal symptom presentation from the time of last alcohol use.

Physical Manifestations of Alcohol Withdrawal

Mild to Moderate Alcohol Withdrawal Symptoms

Physical alcohol withdrawal signs include tachycardia, hypertension, hyperthermia, hyperreflexia, tremor, agitation, and diaphoresis, all of which are related to increased sympathetic nervous system activity. Gastrointestinal symptoms such as nausea and vomiting are often present during the acute phase of alcohol withdrawal and are also attributed to increased autonomic activity. Sleep disturbances may manifest as greater rapid eye movement, lengthened sleep latency, increased awakenings, and overall reductions in total sleep.[19]

Alcohol hallucinosis is characterized by perceptual disturbances, which can be auditory, visual, tactile, gustatory, or olfactory, beginning approximately 12 to 48 hours after one's last drink. Hallucinations can occur in the absence of autonomic changes.[24] The majority of hallucinations are short lived and resolve within 24 hours of onset; however in a minority of individuals, they may last for several days.[25] Visual and auditory hallucinations are most common, for example, seeing an animal in the room or hearing voices. In some cases, patients will experience photo- or phonosensitivity or describe a sensation of "pins and needles." Patients experiencing alcohol hallucinosis are alert and oriented and display insight. The presence of normal vital signs and intact orientation distinguishes alcohol hallucinosis from DTs, described below.

Alcohol Withdrawal Seizures

Alcohol withdrawal seizures typically occur within 8 to 24 hours after alcohol cessation. They are grand mal—major generalized convulsions with loss of consciousness—and may present as the first sign of alcohol withdrawal. Most studies demonstrate rates of alcohol withdrawal seizure in people with AUD ranging from 5% to 10%[26] with higher seizure rates in people drinking larger quantities of alcohol over long periods of time. Seizures related to alcohol withdrawal are typically singular but can also appear in clusters. A second convulsion may present within 6 hours of the first.[25] Prompt treatment can prevent seizure recurrence and worsening of alcohol withdrawal symptoms.[27] A third of individuals experiencing a seizure will develop alcohol withdrawal delirium or DTs.[28] In addition, occult traumatic brain injury (ie, subdural hematomas) can also be a source of seizure foci and should be ruled out among patients with a reported or witnessed seizure.

Delirium Tremens

Alcohol withdrawal delirium—more commonly known as DTs—is a rare but serious complication of alcohol withdrawal that appears approximately 72 to 96 hours after alcohol cessation.[29] It is characterized

TABLE 8.2

Risk Factors Associated With Complicated Alcohol Withdrawal

Historical	At presentation
■ History of alcohol withdrawal delirium tremens or alcohol withdrawal seizure ■ Numerous prior alcohol withdrawal episodes ■ Long duration of heavy and regular alcohol use	■ Marked autonomic hyperactivity (heart rate >120) ■ Acute medical illness or surgical condition (eg, traumatic brain injury) ■ Seizure ■ Physiological dependence on other GABAergic agents (ie, benzodiazepines or barbiturates) ■ Age >65 ■ Emergence of alcohol withdrawal symptoms despite detectable blood alcohol level (BAL)

by worsening of alcohol withdrawal symptoms, delirium and autonomic instability manifested as fever, diaphoresis, tremor, and tachycardia.[29] In contrast to alcohol hallucinosis, patients experiencing DTs are disoriented, globally confused, and demonstrate impaired attention. Prior studies identified that 5% of hospitalized patients with alcohol withdrawal experience DTs,[28] though rates as low as 1.25% and as high as 33% have been reported.[30] In some cases, alcohol withdrawal DTs resolves within 24 hours, while in others it may persist for 3 to 4 days. Historically, DTs had a high mortality rate between 5% and 20%[31]; more recently, the mortality rate has decreased to approximately 1% due to medical advancements and increased knowledge of complicated alcohol withdrawal management.[26]

Common causes of death among people experiencing DTs are related to metabolic, cardiovascular, and infectious complications. Prevention of DTs begins with close monitoring and prompt treatment of alcohol withdrawal manifestations, described later in this chapter.

Severe and Complicated Alcohol Withdrawal

The terms "severe" and "complicated" alcohol withdrawal are often used interchangeably with varied definitions in the literature. About 10% of people with physiologic alcohol dependence will experience severe or complicated alcohol withdrawal during their lifetime. Individual variation in alcohol withdrawal symptom manifestation is likely related to several factors including patterns of alcohol use, co-occurring psychiatric and somatic conditions, and genetic variations in neurochemical brain alterations.[24,32]

The American Thoracic Society conceptually defines *severe* alcohol withdrawal as "a progressive state of central nervous system hyperexcitation due to reduction or cessation of alcohol use resulting in severe signs and symptoms of hyperautonomia and hyperactive delirium."[33] In the American Society of Addiction Medicine (ASAM) Clinical Practice Guidelines, a Clinical Institute Withdrawal Assessment for Alcohol, Revised (CIWA-Ar) score of greater than or equal to 19 classifies alcohol withdrawal as *severe*.[34]

Complicated alcohol withdrawal includes the development of alcohol withdrawal seizures or DTs.[34,35] There are several factors that are associated with *complicated* alcohol withdrawal and their use for risk stratification is discussed below in "Principles of Hospital-Based Treatment of Alcohol Withdrawal: *Principle 2 Risk Stratification for Complicated Alcohol Withdrawal.*" The presence of multiple risk factors is additive, increasing the risk of *complicated* alcohol withdrawal (Table 8.2).

Outpatient Alcohol Withdrawal Management

While this chapter primarily focuses on hospital-based management, alcohol withdrawal can be treated in the outpatient setting for individuals experiencing mild to moderate withdrawal symptoms.[34,36,37] While moderate to severe alcohol withdrawal symptoms have been associated with treatment failure in the outpatient setting,[38] outpatient alcohol withdrawal management is less disruptive for patients. Outpatient alcohol withdrawal treatment offers an opportunity to involve family, friends, and the home environments in the treatment and recovery plan. With outpatient alcohol withdrawal management, patients can engage in recovery supports, such as mutual support groups and intensive outpatient programming, while also maintaining employment.

Compared to hospital-based alcohol withdrawal management, outpatient alcohol withdrawal management is less expensive and requires a shorter treatment duration. When discussing the decision to undergo outpatient versus hospital-based alcohol withdrawal management with patients, it is important to emphasize that people who undergo hospital-based withdrawal management are more likely to complete the treatment course than individuals engaging in outpatient withdrawal management.[39] Patients who may safely undergo alcohol withdrawal at home do not

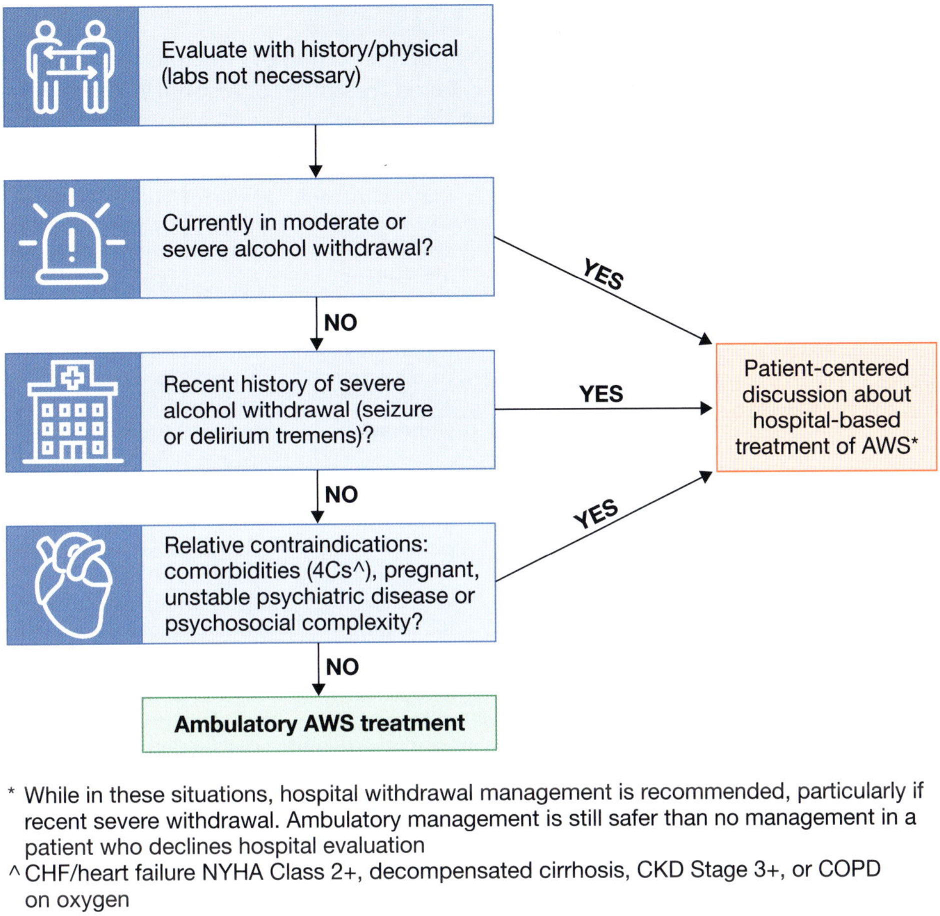

Figure 8.3: Triaging people appropriate for ambulatory management of alcohol withdrawal syndrome (AWS). (Adapted from Cohen SM, Holt S, Williams PN, Chan CA. #2 Get in the spirit of ambulatory alcohol withdrawal. *The Curbsiders Addiction Medicine Podcast.* July 14, 2022. http://thecurbsiders.com/addiction.)

have a history of severe alcohol withdrawal, will have a support system who can monitor them and help administer medications, do not have severe medical comorbidities such as heart failure, chronic obstructive pulmonary disease, decompensated cirrhosis, will be able to check in with a clinician, and do not have active moderate to severe alcohol withdrawal symptoms on presentation (Figure 8.3).

Although its use is not validated in the outpatient setting, some guidelines[40] recommend the Prediction of Alcohol Withdrawal Severity Scale (PAWSS)[41] to determine a patient's candidacy for outpatient alcohol withdrawal management. In addition to using the PAWSS, assessing current alcohol withdrawal symptoms, mental state, status of chronic conditions and any anticipated associated medical complications, for example, gastrointestinal bleeding, acute pancreatitis, related to alcohol use can help with triaging patients to the appropriate care setting.[24] Gabapentin, benzodiazepines, and carbamazepine are evidence-based treatment options and can be used as monotherapy for outpatient alcohol withdrawal management (see Figure 8.4).

Principles of Hospital-Based Treatment of Alcohol Withdrawal

Despite the prevalence of alcohol withdrawal among hospitalized patients, evidence guiding its treatment is predominantly observational. Across research studies, there is wide heterogeneity in treatment protocols with significant variation in alcohol withdrawal management strategies, classes of medications used, medication dosages and frequencies, as well as symptom severity scales, complicating efforts to recommend a particular protocol or strategy. The resultant wide treatment variation seen across institutions[42,43] served as a primary motivation for the creation of the 2020 ASAM Clinical Practice Guideline on Alcohol Withdrawal Management.[34] As in other areas of medical

Best Practices

1. Start in the morning and don't taper alcohol before
2. Check in every other day, can use telehealth (video preferred) to make more accessible
3. Recommend hospitalization if: seizures, altered mental status, using more PRNs than prescribed
4. Don't forget to address and treat AUD

Medication Regimens

	Diazepam based^	Gabapentin based
Day 1	10 mg q6hrs*	300 mg q6hrs*
Day 2	10 mg TID	300 mg TID
Day 3	10 mg BID	300 mg BID
Day 4	10 mg once	300 mg once
Additional PRNs	5 × 10 mg pills	5 × 300 mg pills

^ Can substitute chlordiazepoxide 50 mg for diazepam 10 mg
* If >10 drinks per day double on first day

Figure 8.4: Ambulatory alcohol withdrawal treatment. (Adapted from Cohen SM, Holt S, Williams PN, Chan CA: #2 Get in the spirit of ambulatory alcohol withdrawal. *The Curbsiders Addiction Medicine Podcast.* July 14, 2022. http://thecurbsiders.com/addiction)

TABLE 8.3

Implementation of Principles of Hospital-Based Treatment of Alcohol Withdrawal

Principle	Example of elements using an electronic health record order set
Protocolize care with regular symptom assessment	Order for regular assessment (every 1–4 h) using a validated symptom scale (ie, CIWA-Ar) Vital signs assessment frequency increases if symptoms escalate
Risk stratify for complicated alcohol withdrawal	Guidance for risk assessment for complication using known risk factors (history of delirium tremens, history of seizure) or a risk assessment tool (ie, PAWSS) to guide treatment
In low-risk patients, treat symptomatically with close monitoring	Order for treatment option for low-risk patient, including symptom-triggered therapy using a long-acting benzodiazepine (ie, diazepam) linked to elevated CIWA-Ar
In high-risk patients, treatment should be proactive	Order(s) for treatment option(s) including benzodiazepine front-loading followed by symptom-triggered therapy and/or barbiturate (ie, phenobarbital) loading
When symptoms escalate, escalate care	Orders for transfer to higher level of care in case of seizure, delirium tremens, or nonresponse to current treatment regimen Additional medication options including transition to barbiturate loading, propofol if intubated, adjunctive medications (ie, dexmedetomidine)
Address associated comorbidities	Baseline laboratory tests including electrolytes, liver function, transaminases, and coagulation testing Orders for thiamine for prophylaxis and treatment of Wernicke encephalopathy Orders for medications for alcohol use disorder and referrals to behavioral treatment

practice that lack a clearly superior and specific treatment regimen, principles derived from both the pathophysiology and the literature help guide hospital-based treatment of alcohol withdrawal (Table 8.3). The following section lists six principles recommended for best practices in hospital-based alcohol management. Of note, for this section, the term "complicated alcohol withdrawal" refers to alcohol withdrawal delirium/DTs and alcohol withdrawal seizures, similar to the ASAM Clinical Practice Guideline.[34]

Principle 1: Protocolize Care With Regular Symptom Assessment

Given the wide variation in alcohol withdrawal care, establishing an institutional treatment protocol to ensure treatment consistency is critical. Protocolizing care for alcohol withdrawal, through the use of standard orders guiding medication treatment, is associated with adoption of evidence-based care practices, including the use of symptom-triggered medication therapy[44–47] and the treatment of nutritional deficiencies,[48] often associated with chronic alcohol use. Furthermore, studies assessing the impact of protocolization on alcohol withdrawal treatment outcomes demonstrate shorter intensive care unit (ICU) length

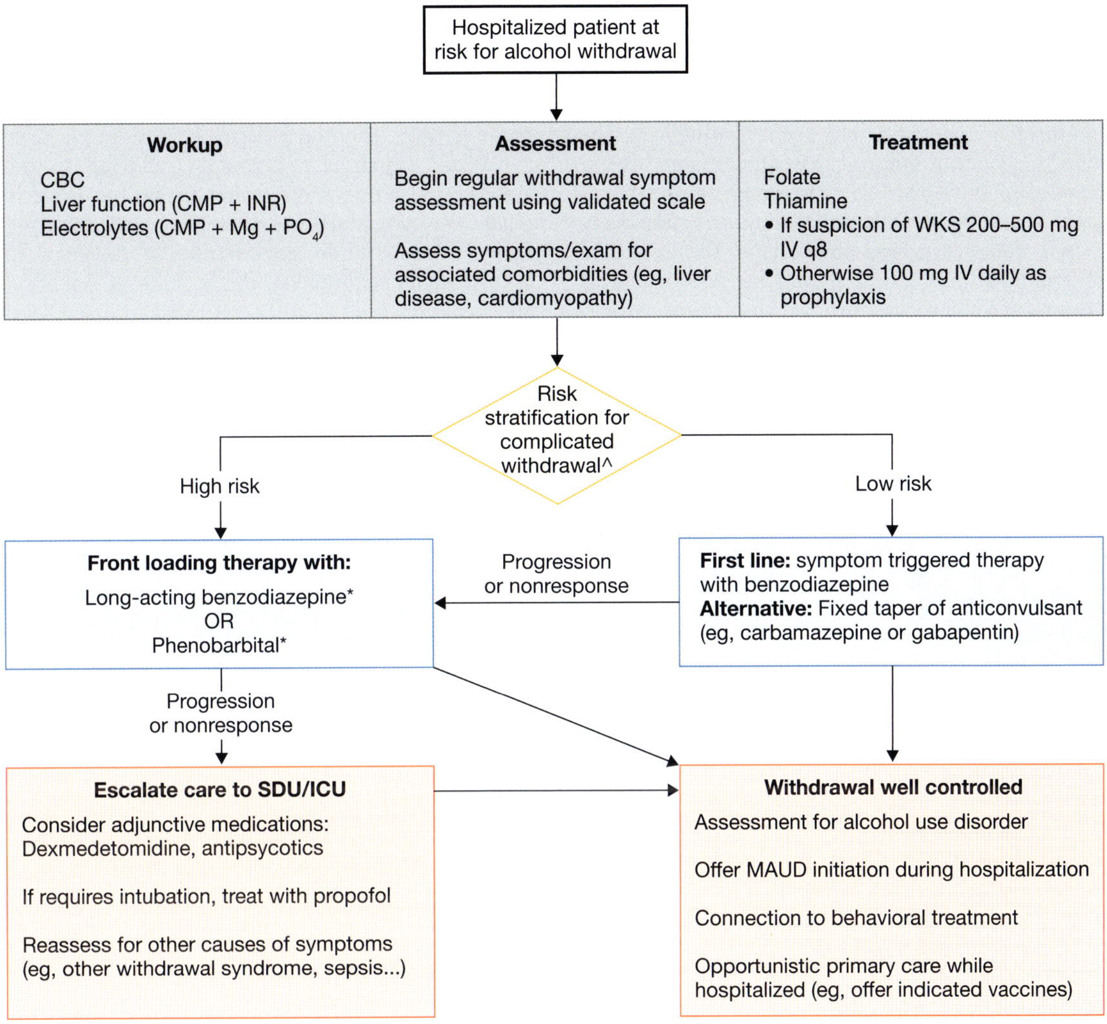

Key:
CBC, complete blood count; **CMP**, comprehensive metabolic panel; **ICU**, intensive care unit; **INR**, international normalized ratio; **IV**, intravenous; **MAUD**, medication for alcohol use disorder; **Mg**, magnesium; **PO_4**, phosphate; **SDU**, step-down unit; **WKS**, Wernicke-Korsakoff syndrome

^Patients in whom significant symptoms of alcohol withdrawal could precipitate further medical decompensation should be treated as high risk

*Loading therapy should be followed by serial reassessment with a validated symptom score with additional as-needed doses of medications

Figure 8.5: Flowchart of hospital care for person with alcohol use disorder.

of stay,[45,46] fewer intubations,[44,46] and a reduction in the composite outcome of severe complications of alcohol withdrawal (defined as hallucinations, use of restraints, admission to the ICU, seizure, request for behavioral emergency team, delirium, cardiovascular event, or death related to alcohol withdrawal).[47] Protocolization of alcohol withdrawal care and implementation of guideline-based care within protocols can be adopted through the use of order sets embedded within the electronic health record, a strategy endorsed by the Institute of Medicine.[49] Figure 8.5 outlines an example of a protocol used for hospital-based alcohol withdrawal management.

Alcohol Withdrawal Severity of Symptom Assessments

The use of a validated symptom scale is a critical component of an institutional protocol to manage alcohol withdrawal. The symptoms and severity of alcohol withdrawal may progress over the course of several days and, in some cases, in an unpredictable manner. Without effective medication treatment, early alcohol withdrawal symptoms may progress to potentially life-threatening complicated alcohol withdrawal. The ideal frequency of symptom assessment is not clearly established, but ASAM guidelines suggest monitoring every 1 to 4 hours with closer monitoring (ie, every 1 to 2 hours) if symptoms escalate. The frequency of symptom monitoring should be de-escalated as symptoms stabilize and improve with treatment and time.[34]

Symptom assessment should be completed using a validated symptom scale in conjunction with monitoring of vital signs for autonomic hyperactivity (ie, tachycardia and hypertension). Validated scales allow for consistent objective and subjective assessments of alcohol withdrawal signs and symptoms across care teams and locations. Their use facilitates trending of symptom severity to guide the patient's level of care and hospital course. Although some symptom scales, such as the Clinical Institute Withdrawal for Alcohol revised (CIWA-Ar), require training to administer validly, they can be properly administered by bedside nurses, allowing for more frequent evaluation. There are clear limitations to all symptom scales that are worth noting:

- No single symptom scale has been shown to be superior to another
- Symptom scales are not diagnostic for alcohol withdrawal and may be elevated due to other acute medical comorbidities (ie, other withdrawal syndromes, infections, delirium from other causes)
- Many symptom scales rely heavily on a patient's *subjective* report of symptoms rather than *objective* data (ie, pulse, blood pressure, temperature, etc)

Given these limitations, symptom scales should be used as an adjunct to clinical judgment.

The most widely used assessment tool across research and clinical practice is the CIWA-Ar.[50] The CIWA-Ar scale has the advantage of decades of prior research and countless readily available protocols for its use. The CIWA-Ar can be more cumbersome than other scales, it does not include objective data, including heart rate or blood pressure, which, when elevated, may be a harbinger of impending or worsening delirium, and it relies heavily on patient-reported symptoms, which are prone to subjectivity. Due to its reliance on patient-reported symptoms, the CIWA-Ar should not be used when a patient is intubated, has loss of or limited consciousness, or is unable to engage in an interview.

Alternative alcohol withdrawal symptom scales include the Brief Alcohol Withdrawal Scale (BAWS),[51] which is shorter and does not rely on patient-reported symptoms, the Minnesota Detoxification Scale (MINDS),[52] which has been validated in the ICU, the acute care unit, and the emergency department settings, the Short Alcohol Withdrawal Scale (SAWS),[53] which is additionally validated in the ambulatory setting and hospital setting but is solely reliant on patient self-assessment of symptoms, and many others. While not specifically designed to assess alcohol withdrawal, the Richmond Agitation and Sedation Scale (RASS),[54] created to assess level of sedation in the intensive care setting, has also been used to assess and guide treatment of alcohol withdrawal.[46]

As no clear symptom scale is superior, choice of scale used should be determined at the institutional level and ideally include a scale that has familiarity at the institution and can be used consistently across care locations and treatment teams (Table 8.4).

Principle 2: Risk Stratify for Complicated Alcohol Withdrawal

Most people who undergo alcohol withdrawal have mild or moderate symptoms without significant risk of complication. Although uncommon, complicated alcohol withdrawal is associated with significant morbidity and risk of mortality. Effectively managing alcohol withdrawal in hospitalized patients necessitates early determination of the risk of complication and initiating treatment accordingly.

Incidence of Complicated Alcohol Withdrawal

The incidence of complicated/severe alcohol withdrawal depends on the patient population, the care setting, and the reason for admission. Wood et al[55] describe this phenomenon well in their systematic review and meta-analysis of studies involving patients with AWS across various care settings noting incidence of severe withdrawal at withdrawal management facilities to be 23% while incidence of alcohol withdrawal in hospitals ranged from 1.9% for those with AUDIT C>8 and 6.7% for those with either a blood alcohol level (BAL) >200 on admission or any reported alcohol use in the past 30 days.

While most alcohol withdrawal is usually limited to mild to moderate withdrawal symptoms and incidence of complicated withdrawal remains hard to pinpoint, roughly 10% of patients will develop complicated alcohol withdrawal, which requires prompt medical management.[27,56] Early recognition of risk factors associated with the development of complicated alcohol withdrawal is essential to

TABLE 8.4

Alcohol Withdrawal Symptom Scales

Symptom scale	Total components	Patient-reported components	Physical exam components	Vital signs	Additional notes
Brief Alcohol Withdrawal Scale (BAWS)[57]	5	0	5 (tremor, diaphoresis, RASS, orientation, hallucinations)	None	Includes RASS in assessment
Clinical Institute Withdrawal for Alcohol Revised (CIWA-Ar)[58]	10	6 (nausea, anxiety, tactile disturbances, auditory disturbances, visual disturbances, headache)	4 (tremor, sweats, agitation, orientation)	None	Most commonly used scale for alcohol withdrawal symptoms
Minnesota Detoxification Scale (MINDS)[59]	9	None	7 (tremor, sweats, hallucination, agitation, orientation, delusions, seizure)	2 (pulse, diastolic blood pressure)	Validation study completed in ICU
Richmond Agitation and Sedation Scale (RASS)[60]	1	None	1 (level of agitation/ sedation)	None	Validated as a scale for agitation/ sedation common in the ICU and subsequently used in studies to guide alcohol withdrawal treatment
Short Alcohol Withdrawal Scale (SAWS)[61]	10	5 (anxious, confused, restless, miserable, memory problems)	5 (tremor, nausea, heart pounding, sleep disturbance, sweating)	None	Able to be self-administered (including physical exam findings)

reduce the morbidity and mortality related to seizures and DTs.

Risk Factors and Signs of Complicated Alcohol Withdrawal

The literature examining risk factors associated with progression to complicated alcohol withdrawal primarily includes observational data. These studies are summarized in two meta-analyses published in 2014[62] and 2018.[55] Both meta-analyses evaluated historical factors, demographics, and laboratory findings associated with the development of complicated alcohol withdrawal and both were limited insofar as many of the findings in the analyses were derived from a single or very few studies.

The 2014 meta-analysis[62] found that a history of DTs was associated with subsequent DTs, a history of alcohol withdrawal seizures and higher blood concentrations of gamma-glutamyl transferase (GGT) was associated with subsequent seizures, lower potassium on admission was associated with both DTs and seizures, and lower platelets and higher alanine aminotransferase (ALT) were associated with DTs, seizures, and complicated alcohol withdrawal.

The 2018 meta-analysis[55] was unique in that it assessed factors both predictive of the development of complicated alcohol withdrawal and factors not predictive of developing complicated alcohol withdrawal. In this study, a history of DTs, a presentation with hypertension, low platelets, elevated GGT, elevated aspartate aminotransferase (AST), and positive BAL were associated with the development of complicated (severe) alcohol withdrawal.

Tools to Stratify Patients at Risk for Complicated Alcohol Withdrawal

Individual risk factors are relatively insensitive and nonspecific to predict which patients are more likely to develop complicated alcohol withdrawal. To account for this, several composite measures of high-risk features (eg, history of DTs, seizures) have been evaluated and validated in various patient populations to identify patients at risk for developing complicated AWS.

Prediction of Alcohol Withdrawal Severity Scale

The PAWSS[41] is a 10-item tool which includes 8 patient interview questions (including a history of alcohol withdrawal seizure and a history of DTs), a single laboratory assessment (BAL), and physical exam for signs of autonomic hyperactivity. Scores ≥4 were shown to correlate with the authors' definition of "complicated/severe alcohol withdrawal" but the definition used was CIWA ≥15 or receiving any medication to treat alcohol withdrawal, rather than emergence of complicated withdrawal symptoms like DTs or seizure. PAWSS has not been validated in youth and pregnant patients (Table 8.5).

Luebeck Alcohol Risk Scale

The Luebeck Alcohol Risk Scale (LARS)[63] is a 10- or 11-item tool including 2 historical components (history of DTs or seizure), patient interview questions (nightmares, sleep disturbances), 5 physical exam findings (3 of which are required to be in the context of elevated BAL), and 2 additional laboratory findings. The LARS has limited utility in hospitalized patients because it was not validated in that population and the definition for complicated withdrawal used in its development was based on a symptom scale cutoff, not the emergence of DTs or seizure (Table 8.5).

The aforementioned 2018 meta-analysis reviewed the PAWSS and LARS risk scoring tools and found that both the PAWSS and LARS were highly sensitivity and specific to identify patients at increased risk to develop complicated/severe alcohol withdrawal (PAWSS sensitivity was 0.93 and specificity was 0.99; LARS-10 sensitivity was 0.95 and specificity was 0.93). Both scoring tools also exhibited high positive and negative predictive values based on their validation studies.

Each scale has a particular limitation, or set of limitations, that must be considered. Neither scoring tool perfectly predicts every patient's risk for developing DTs or alcohol withdrawal seizures. The use of scoring tools should be seen as an additional tool to inform clinical decision making that can be used in combination with the patient's clinical presentation

TABLE 8.5

Prediction of Alcohol Withdrawal Severity Scale (PAWSS) and Luebeck Alcohol Withdrawal Risk Scale (LARS)

Name of risk stratification tool	Prediction of Alcohol Withdrawal Severity Scale (PAWSS)	Luebeck Alcohol Withdrawal Risk Scale (LARS 10)
Screening/threshold question (if no, tool is inappropriate)	Any alcohol consumption in the past 30 d or positive blood alcohol level on admission	None
Components (points per component present)	Ever experienced previous episodes of alcohol withdrawal (1 point) Ever experienced alcohol withdrawal seizure (1 point) Ever experienced delirium tremens (1 point) Ever undergone alcohol treatment (1 point) Ever experienced blackouts (1 point) Combined alcohol and other "downers" like benzodiazepines or barbiturates during the last 90 d (1 point) Combined alcohol with any other substance of abuse during the last 90 d (1 point) Blood alcohol level (BAL) on presentation >200 mg/dL (1 point) Evidence of increased autonomic activity (eg, HR >120, tremor, sweating, agitation, nausea) (1 point)	≥3 episodes of previous withdrawal delirium (3 points) ≥3 episodes of previous withdrawal seizures (3 points) Frequent sleep disturbances during the last week (1 point) Nightmares during the last week (1 point) BAL ≥100 mg/dL (1) Tremor despite BAL ≥100 mg/dL (1 point) Sweating despite BAL ≥100 mg/dL (1 point) Pulse rate ≥100 despite BAL ≥100 mg/dL (1 point) Polyneuropathy (1 point) Ataxia (1 point)
Scoring	≥4 denotes high risk	≥9 denotes high risk

PAWSS score adapted from Maldonado et al.[41]

LARS score adapted from Westerling et al.[63]

and physical examination, laboratory values, the level of care being provided, and the medications available to the clinician to manage complicated alcohol withdrawal.

Practical Implementation of Risk Stratification Tools

Given the limitations of both the risk scoring tools and individual risk factors discussed above, the implementation of risk stratification tools in clinical care should complement, not replace, clinical judgment. For example, electrolyte abnormalities and elevated liver inflammatory markers likely reflect longer-term, heavier alcohol use leading to malnutrition, electrolyte deficiencies, and liver injury, and thus theoretically are consistent with a higher risk of complicated alcohol withdrawal. An elevated BAL on admission, particularly with symptoms of alcohol withdrawal, as presented in the LARS, is likely reflective of higher alcohol tolerance and is likely consistent with a higher risk of complicated alcohol withdrawal. Most notably included in both scoring tools, as well as the meta-analyses, is a finding supported by the kindling phenomenon—a history of withdrawal complications, namely seizures and/or DTs, reflects significant risk for future seizures and/or DTs.[64] As seizures peak early within the course of alcohol withdrawal, presentation with an alcohol withdrawal seizure should be seen as a significant predictor of worsening and complicated alcohol withdrawal. Patients with recent alcohol withdrawal seizure, DTs, those presenting with an alcohol withdrawal seizure, or those with a combination of the above findings should be considered high risk for complication and treated accordingly.

In addition, patients in whom significant symptoms of alcohol withdrawal could precipitate further medical decompensation should be treated similarly to patients who meet high-risk criteria to develop complicated alcohol withdrawal. This includes patients with a seizure disorder, known arrhythmia, unstable psychiatric disease, or active acute severe medical illness (eg, sepsis, shock, myocardial infarction, any illness requiring ICU level of care).

In patients unable to be assessed with symptom scales (eg, CIWA-Ar), or those unable to participate in interviews to allow for risk stratification (ie, intubated trauma patient), fixed-dosing protocols, such as a fixed benzodiazepine taper[34] or phenobarbital loading,[65] can be used.

Principle 3: In Low-Risk Patients, Treat Symptomatically With Close Monitoring

Symptom-Triggered Therapy

Symptom-triggered therapy is recommended in the ASAM guidelines for patients stratified to be at lower risk for the development of complicated alcohol withdrawal.[34] Symptom-triggered therapy is the administration of "as-needed" medications based on the severity of alcohol withdrawal symptoms as assessed by a validated symptom scale.

Prior to the 1990s, the predominant strategy for treating alcohol withdrawal and avoiding complications was prespecified fixed doses of medications, usually benzodiazepines, often administered regardless of symptoms. A landmark paper by Saitz et al published in 1994 identified that symptom-triggered therapy reduced the total medication dose administered during the encounter and the length of stay without an increase in severity of symptoms or complications of alcohol withdrawal, as compared with a fixed-dose regimen.[66] Although this study occurred in a medically managed withdrawal nonhospital unit and may not be reflective of the severity of illness or medical comorbidity seen among patients in the hospital setting, further hospital-based studies also reported improved outcomes related to length of stay and amount of medication administered with symptom-triggered therapy.[44–47] Table 8.6 includes examples of hospital-based alcohol withdrawal management strategies.

TABLE 8.6

Hospital-Based Alcohol Withdrawal Treatment Regimens

Symptom-triggered therapy with benzodiazepines	■ Diazepam 10 mg[a] every 4 h as needed for CIWA-Ar ≥8 ■ Symptom reassessment interval becomes more frequent with elevated scores
Front-loading therapy with benzodiazepines	■ Diazepam 10–20 mg[a] every 1 h as needed for CIWA-Ar ≥8 (IV/IM preferred due to faster onset) ■ Followed by symptom-triggered regimen above
Front-loading therapy with barbiturates	■ Phenobarbital 10–15 mg/kg followed by regular symptom assessment and additional as-needed doses (65–130 mg) (IV/IM preferred due to faster onset) ■ Consider monitoring phenobarbital blood levels during treatment

[a]Can use equipotent doses of other benzodiazepines as well (ie, diazepam 10 mg = chlordiazepoxide 25 mg = lorazepam 2 mg).

Benzodiazepines

Benzodiazepine Mechanism of Action

Benzodiazepines reduce alcohol withdrawal symptoms by potentiating the effect of GABA on the $GABA_A$ receptor. It is important to note that benzodiazepines do not directly bind to the $GABA_A$ receptor. In the presence of benzodiazepines, when GABA binds to the $GABA_A$ receptor, the chloride ion channel opens more frequently, allowing chloride ions to flow across the chloride ion channel, hyperpolarizing the cell, and increasing its inhibition. This leads to the reduction of alcohol withdrawal symptoms exhibited by the patient. Importantly, benzodiazepines' effect on the $GABA_A$ receptors is dependent of the presence of GABA neurotransmitters in the brain. There must be sufficient GABA available in the brain to activate the $GABA_A$ receptor and to facilitate the chloride ion channel's opening.[64] If the brain is depleted of GABA, benzodiazepines will have minimal impact on reducing alcohol withdrawal symptoms. This phenomenon has been described as "benzodiazepine-resistant alcohol withdrawal"[67–69] discussed in more detail below.

Benzodiazepine Are First-Line Treatment of Alcohol Withdrawal

Benzodiazepines are the first-line medication treatment for alcohol withdrawal as endorsed in the ASAM guidelines,[34,70] the Department of Veterans Affairs/Department of Defense,[71] and international guidelines.[72] Meta-analyses assessing benzodiazepines for the treatment of alcohol withdrawal have shown them to be effective at reducing symptoms of alcohol withdrawal and reducing incidence of alcohol withdrawal seizures,[73,74] although the analyses were limited by marked heterogeneity in the studies included. Symptom-triggered therapy using benzodiazepines is the most common medication regimen and strategy used in the US.[75,76]

Although there are limited data supporting the choice of specific benzodiazepine used, long-acting benzodiazepines. Diazepam or chlordiazepoxide are generally preferred to short-acting benzodiazepines as their active metabolites theoretically allow for a smoother alcohol withdrawal course. Diazepam has an additional benefit for hospital use in that it can be given through multiple routes (oral, intramuscular (IM), and intravenous [IV]) and is rapidly acting to address symptoms. A noted exception in the preference for long-acting benzodiazepine is in patients with significant hepatic functional impairment, that is, those with Child–Pugh Class C, for whom lorazepam is preferred.[77] Table 8.7 outlines the pharmacologic properties of medications commonly used for hospital-based alcohol withdrawal management.

TABLE 8.7

Pharmacologic Properties of Medications Commonly Used for Hospital-Based Alcohol Withdrawal Management

Medication	Class	Time to peak	Half-life (hours)	Active metabolites (half-life)
Chlordiazepoxide	Benzodiazepine	PO: 0.5–2 h	24–48 h	Yes (14–95 h)
Carbamazepine	Anticonvulsant	PO tablet: 4–5 h PO Suspension: 1.5 h	35–65 h	Yes (25–43 h)
Diazepam	Benzodiazepine	IV: 1 min IM: 1 h PO: 15 min–2.5 h	IV: 33–45 h IM: 60–72 h PO: 44–48 h	Yes (IV: 87 h IM: 152–174 h PO: 100 h)
Lorazepam	Benzodiazepine	IV: 1–3 min[b] IM: ≤3 h PO: 2 h	IV: 14 h IM: 13–18 h PO: 12 h	No
Gabapentin	Anticonvulsant	PO: 2–4 h	PO: 5–7 h	No
Phenobarbital	Barbiturate	IV: 12–60 min[a] IM: 2–8 h[a] PO: 2–4 h	79 h	No

All values per Lexicomp unless otherwise specified.

[a]Trinka E. Phenobarbital in Status epilepticus—Rediscovery of an effective drug. *Epilepsy Behav*. 2023;141:109104.

[b]Ghiasi N, Bhansali RK, Marwaha R. Lorazepam. [Updated May 25, 2024]. In: *StatPearls* [Internet]. StatPearls Publishing; 2025 Jan–. https://www.ncbi.nlm.nih.gov/books/NBK532890/

Principle 4: In High-Risk Patients, Treatment Should Be Proactive

In patients deemed to be high risk for developing complicated alcohol withdrawal or those at risk of medical decompensation due to alcohol withdrawal symptoms, a proactive treatment strategy should be employed. Alcohol withdrawal complications generally progress over the course of days, thus, proactive treatment strategies utilize frequent or higher initial doses of long-acting medication to quickly capture symptoms and reduce symptom progression. This is generally accomplished through "front-loading" therapy with benzodiazepines or barbiturates.

Front-Loading Benzodiazepines

Front-loading of benzodiazepines is the treatment strategy recommended for patients at high risk of complicated alcohol withdrawal in the 2020 ASAM guidelines.[34] In this strategy, a long-acting benzodiazepine is given at higher doses than for patients with a lower risk of complicated alcohol withdrawal. For example, diazepam may be given intravenously at 10 mg to 20 mg every hour until symptoms are well controlled (CIWA-Ar <8) or the patient is mildly sedated. This strategy takes advantage of the rapid onset and long duration of diazepam to both quickly control alcohol withdrawal symptoms and to prevent complications due to the long duration of action. Front-loading is generally followed by additional symptom-triggered therapy (often at a lower dose and less frequent than the loading dose) to ensure symptoms remain well controlled throughout the course of hospitalization.

Barbiturates

Barbiturates, specifically phenobarbital, are gaining prominence as an alternative medication option for a front-loading regimen. One theoretical advantage to barbiturate use is that it addresses multiple neurobiologic mechanisms for alcohol withdrawal. Similar to benzodiazepines, barbiturates potentiate the effect of GABA at the $GABA_A$ receptor, facilitating the chloride ion channel's opening and hyperpolarizing the cell, increasing inhibitory effects of unopposed glutamate activity. In contrast to benzodiazepines, barbiturates also directly bind to the $GABA_A$ receptor. The latter action allows phenobarbital to activate the $GABA_A$ receptor in the absence of the GABA neurotransmitter, which may make it more effective to treat alcohol withdrawal in people who exhibit benzodiazepine resistance.[67–69] Barbiturates also act as an NMDA receptor antagonist and effectively antagonize glutamate's excitatory effects in the brain, which contribute to alcohol withdrawal symptoms.[78,79]

Safety Profile of Barbiturates

Barbiturates have a long history of use for the treatment of alcohol withdrawal[80] but fell out of favor due to concerns about a narrow therapeutic window and greater risk of adverse events, including overdose, compared to benzodiazepines. The narrow therapeutic index is due to barbiturates' ability to bypass the GABA neurotransmitter to open chloride ion channels directly. Phenobarbital toxicity presents as dizziness, confusion, nystagmus, respiratory depression, coma, and death with symptoms generally beginning at levels of >30 to 40 μg/mL[81,82] and progressing as levels increase.

Current Use of Barbiturates

The use of phenobarbital, often using a front-loading strategy, has recently reemerged as a treatment regimen in the ED[83,84] or ICU[65,85,86] settings. Phenobarbital regimens in these studies are variable but often involve phenobarbital administration as three separate doses for a total loading dose of 10 to 15 mg/kg of ideal body weight based on a pharmacokinetic dosing model published in the early 1990s.[87] While some studies show benefits of a phenobarbital-based treatment strategy, they are limited by comparisons to heterogeneous treatment regimens, small samples sizes, and observational study designs, making generalizability limited.[88] One of the largest observational studies to date found similar outcomes between a phenobarbital loading protocol and a benzodiazepine protocol although the authors noted the phenobarbital group had a higher proportion of patients with a history of complication from alcohol withdrawal.[89]

Phenobarbital loading appears to be a feasible alternative to benzodiazepines in carefully selected high risk patients; however, several unanswered questions remain about its use. While studies often utilize a single or multistep phenobarbital loading dose, whether additional phenobarbital is given after the load is variable.[65,85] Phenobarbital levels can be monitored, but unlike in status epilepticus, there remains no clear therapeutic level for the treatment of alcohol withdrawal.[90] Phenobarbital also comes with the added drawbacks—active hepatic metabolites, renal clearance,[81] and significant medication interactions through cytochrome p450 induction—which may cause prolonged increases in medication metabolism including that of methadone.[91]

A reasonable approach to phenobarbital use in patients at high risk for complicated alcohol withdrawal or who have a history of benzodiazepine resistance, described below, is to give a loading dose of 10 to 15 mg/kg ideal body weight followed by close monitoring of continued withdrawal symptoms using a validated symptoms scale, concomitant monitoring of potential phenobarbital side effects (eg, bradycardia, sedation), with additional "as-needed" phenobarbital doses available in case of continued withdrawal symptoms. Although there is limited evidence supporting these practices, capping the maximum phenobarbital dose to 25 mg/kg and evaluation with phenobarbital blood levels to ensure levels do not approach previously defined toxic levels of >30 to 40 μg/mL[81] can be an adjunct to serial monitoring to reduce the risk of unintentional overdose. Phenobarbital-based treatment, particularly with loading doses, should be reserved for clinicians comfortable with its use and loading doses should only be given in settings where patients can be closely monitored (ie, ED, step-down unit, ICU) (Tables 8.6 and 8.7, Figure 8.6).

Inclusion Criteria

- Patient with active AWS
- Patient must be in the critical care areas (intensive care unit, emergency department), or step-down unit to initiate phenobarbital therapy

Exclusion Criteria

- If patient received >20 mg lorazepam equivalents (≈100 mg of diazepam or 40 mg midazolam) in the last 8–12 hours then avoid phenobarbital and consider alternative therapy
- Patients initiated on phenobarbital for treatment of AWS or for other indications

Yale New Haven Health System Phenobarbital for Alcohol Withdrawal Guidelines

Due to the risk of additive side effects, concomitant benzodiazepines are NOT recommended for the management of AWS
Discontinue any standing and PRN benzodiazepine orders

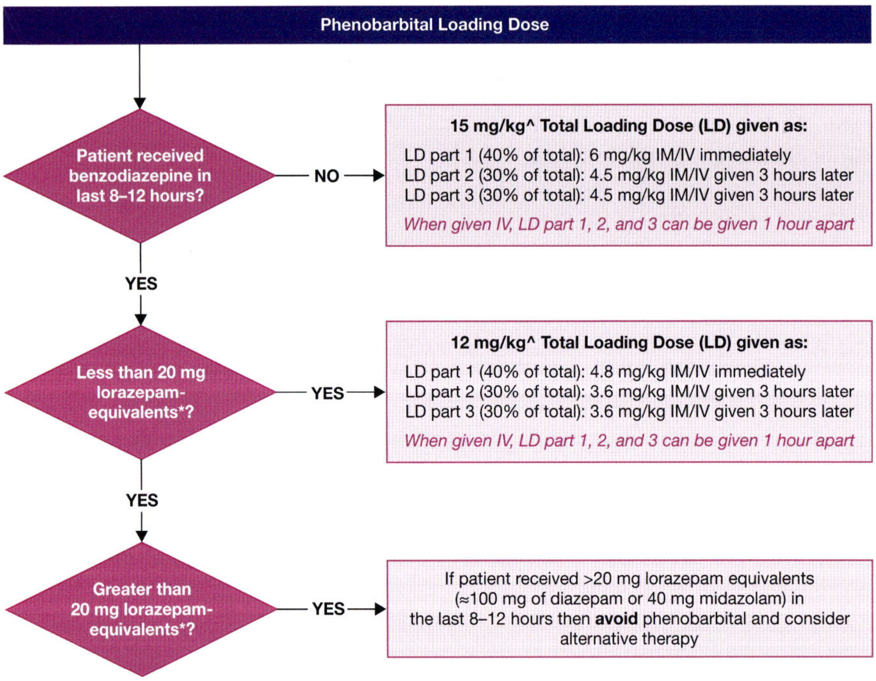

*20 mg lorazepam equivalent is ≈100 mg of diazepam and 50 mg midazolam

^ Other dosing and administration caveats:

- Dose based on **ideal body weight (IBW)** unless patient actual body weight is less than IBW then use actual body weight.
- IM route is preferred to minimize side effects (oversedation and respiratory compromise), but can be given IV.
- If given IV and patient is tolerating the dose (no oversedation or respiratory compromise) patient can receive LD part 2 or part 3 every hour.
- If total LD (15 mg/kg) was not given and there are no side effects but patient is still experiencing AWS symptoms, consider administering remainder of LD so that total of 15 mg/kg is given. See Appendix.

Monitoring (Day 1):

- **IV loading dose:** Vital signs (blood pressure, heart rate, and respiratory status) 15 minutes after dose administration then every 1 hour while receiving loading dose and recheck 1 hour after completion of the total loading dose.
- **IM loading dose:** Vital signs (blood pressure, heart rate, and respiratory status) 15 minutes after dose administration then every 2 hours while receiving loading dose and recheck 2 hours after completion of the total loading dose.
- Hold therapy if blood pressure <90/50 mm Hg, heart rate <50 bpm, respiratory rate <10 bpm, or RASS score <–2.

Figure 8.6: Example phenobarbital dosing guidance from Yale New Haven Health System.

Symptoms Worsen After Loading Dose

The maximum peak effect of phenobarbital is ≈5 hours for IM (15 minutes for IV). If patient's AWS symptoms worsen based on CIWA noncritical care units) and MINDS (critical care) assessment 5 hours post phenobarbital total LD administration, consider administering additional doses of Phenobarbital as follows (***only for patients who tolerated the LD, no hypotension or respiratory compromise***):

Patient received initial phenobarbital LD 12 mg/kg (IBW)? → **YES** and symptoms worsen after 5 hours (IM) or 15 minutes (IV) → **Give 3 mg/kg phenobarbital (IBW) for a total of 15 mg/kg (IBW)**

↓

Patient received cumulative phenobarbital LD 15 mg/kg (IBW)? → **YES** and symptoms worsen after 5 hours (IM) or 15 minutes (IV) → **Give 2 mg/kg phenobarbital (IBW)**
May repeat every 3 hours for a maximum total dose 25 mg/kg (IBW)

Patient received cumulative phenobarbital LD 15 mg/kg (IBW)? → **YES** and symptoms worsen after 5 hours (IM) or 15 minutes (IV) → **Give 2 mg/kg phenobarbital (IBW)**
May repeat every 3 hours for a maximum total dose 25 mg/kg (IBW)

Management of alcohol withdrawal symptoms while on phenobarbital:

A. If **continuous sedation** is indicated or **RASS ≥2** after receiving entire total LD:
- Consider dexmedetomidine if clinically appropriate
- Due to the risk of additive side effects, avoid propofol or continuous benzodiazepine infusion for sedation

B. Emergency Symptoms:
- **Agitation/anxiety:** consider non-benzodiazepine alternatives:
  - Quetiapine 12.5–25 mg PO every 6–12 hours as needed for agitation or anxiety
  - Haloperidol 2.5–5 mg IV every 6 hours as needed for agitation or anxiety
  - Trazodone 12.5–25 mg PO every 12 hours as needed for agitation or anxiety
- **Tachycardia:** consider beta-blockers as clinically appropriate
- **Hypertension:** consider clonidine as clinically appropriate

↓

Taper/Maintenance Dosing (Day 2–5)*

Day 2 and 3	Phenobarbital 64.8 mg IM/IV/PO every 12 hours for four doses
Day 4 and 5	Phenobarbital 32.4 mg IM/IV/PO every 12 hours for four doses

*The phenobarbital maintenance taper regimen should be stated approximately 8 hours after the LD is completed (after completion of third dose of the LD)

For IV/IM administration, round up to the nearest administrable dose based on vial size, eg, 32.4 mg round up to 39 mg

Monitoring (Day 2–5):
- Monitor vital signs (blood pressure, heart rate, and respiratory status) every 4 hours while receiving phenobarbital maintenance taper regimen. Hold therapy if blood pressure <90/50 mm Hg, heart rate <50 bpm, respiratory rate <10 bpm, or RASS score less than −2.
- CIWA (noncritical care units) and MINDS (critical care) can be used to assess patient's withdrawal severity but not to determine dosing during use of phenobarbital.
- Maintenance regimen should not be delayed in the event that phenobarbital serum level has not resulted.

Discontinuation of therapy and discharge:
- Given phenobarbital's long half-life, discontinuation of phenobarbital taper earlier in the hospital course can occur in patients no longer experiencing withdrawal symptoms.
- A full 5-day admission to complete the detox is not always necessary.
- Patients should **not be continued** on the phenobarbital upon discharge from the hospital, including those patients who leave before completing medical treatment, eg, self-directed discharge.
- If patient self-directs their discharge, patient should be warned of a greater potential for intoxication due to higher sensitivity to alcohol after phenobarbital therapy.

Appendix:
- Phenobarbital LD can be given intramuscularly (IM) or intravenously (IV). Administration of LD via the IM route is encouraged to decrease the risk of adverse events (oversedation and respiratory compromise). IM administration can be given in deltoid or gluteus muscles. Give LD IV if platelet <50,000 per microliter, INR >2 or if patient is therapeutically anticoagulated.
- Drug interactions: Phenobarbital is metabolized hepatically via cytochrome P450. Contact pharmacy for relevance of any cytochrome P450 drug–drug interactions. Avoid administering phenobarbital with clozapine, cronedarone, itraconazole, nifedipine, nimodipine, ranolazine, rivaroxaban, and voriconazole.
- Caution use of phenobarbital in patients with hepatic dysfunction (AST/ALT >5x UNL).
- Avoid the use of phenobarbital in patients with decompensated liver cirrhosis, Child–Pugh class C, or acute liver failure, including acetaminophen overdose.

Figure 8.6: *(Continued)*

Principles 5: When Symptoms Escalate, Escalate Care

A subset of patients will require more intensive treatment due to lack of response to the currently chosen therapy and/or progression to complicated alcohol withdrawal. These patients require closer monitoring (every 1- to 2-hour evaluations) and more intensive therapy necessitating admission to a step-down unit or an ICU. As these patients may be *unable* to participate in symptom assessment due to delirium or severe illness, use of a validated scale less reliant on patient report (ie, MINDS, RASS) is more suitable (Table 8.4).

Selection of the appropriate treatment regimen within this group requires consideration of the reason for complication and the lack of treatment response. As the risk stratification used above is an imperfect science with imperfect negative prediction, some patient will be assessed as low risk when they are in fact at higher risk. In addition, there may be an unaddressed neurobiologic reason for nonresponse or progression of symptoms. As noted above, alcohol withdrawal, and particularly complicated alcohol withdrawal, may be the result of the combination of reduced GABA stimulation and excessive glutamatergic tone[33] and tailoring treatment to address both factors may be needed. A subgroup of patients who do not respond to increasing benzodiazepine doses are described in the literature as both "resistant alcohol withdrawal" or "benzodiazepine-resistant alcohol withdrawal." Criteria used to define this concept typically include progression of symptoms despite receiving a specific dose of benzodiazepines over a set period of time (eg, 40 mg IV diazepam in 1 hour or 200 mg diazepam in 4 hours).[34,68]

For patients who were initially deemed low risk and started on symptom-triggered benzodiazepine therapy at admission, but who do not respond or have progression of symptoms, escalation of medications can be accomplished by transitioning to regimens similar to the proactive treatment described for high-risk patients. Higher, more frequent doses of IV long-acting benzodiazepines, similar to doses used in the front-loading approach (ie, diazepam 10 mg to 20 mg every hour until symptoms are well controlled or the patient is mildly sedated), can be used to attempt symptom control. Alternatively, transitioning to phenobarbital is a reasonable option that may have significant advantages. While data remain limited to single-center studies with heterogeneous comparators limiting generalizability, a recent mixed methods study of patients requiring ICU care for alcohol withdrawal found that transitioning to a phenobarbital loading–based protocol was well accepted, feasible, and significantly reduced rates of physical restraint use, while also decreasing hospital length of stay with a nonsignificant trend toward reduced use of mechanical ventilation.[85] If a patient has received a significant dose of benzodiazepines prior to transition to phenobarbital loading, lower loading doses split over a longer period of time can be considered to reduce the risk of adverse events related to the use multiple CNS depressants.

Alternatively, in patients ill enough to require intubation, propofol, a common sedative used during intubation, is a reasonable choice for both sedation and alcohol withdrawal management.[92]

Adjunctive Medications to Manage Severe or Complicated Alcohol Withdrawal

Beyond the use of benzodiazepines or phenobarbital, and propofol for those who require intubation, other medications can be used adjunctively. These medications should not be used as monotherapy due to lack of supportive data in preventing and treating complicated alcohol withdrawal.

Alpha-2 Agonists

Clonidine and dexmedetomidine work by decreasing sympathetic tone and have been studied in the treatment of alcohol withdrawal. Dexmedetomidine, used in addition to benzodiazepines or phenobarbital, is frequently used as a component of treatment alcohol withdrawal treatment protocols for patients requiring intensive care.[33,85]

Beta Blockers

Beta blockers (eg, propranolol) can similarly be used to address markers of increased sympathetic tone, tachycardia, and hypertension, but do not address the underlying neurobiologic mechanisms of alcohol withdrawal and should never be used as monotherapy. There is some concern that these medications may mask continued symptoms of alcohol withdrawal without being effective at preventing complications. They should only be used in combination with adequately dosed benzodiazepines or phenobarbital.[34]

Ketamine

Ketamine, an NMDA receptor antagonist, can be used as an adjunctive medication to address the excess glutamatergic activity at NMDA receptors contributing to alcohol withdrawal. Its use has been evaluated in several small single-center observational studies as an adjunct to benzodiazepines often in the ICU setting[93–95] with highly variable dosing strategies where its addition was associated with reduced benzodiazepine administration and, in one study, reduced intubations.[93] It should be reserved for institutions familiar with its use and monitoring. Ketamine should only be used in combination with adequately dosed benzodiazepines or phenobarbital.

Antipsychotics

Antipsychotic medications deserve particular attention for their use for agitation and hallucinations, causing psychological distress that are not adequately addressed by benzodiazepines or barbiturates. First-generation antipsychotics, other than haloperidol, should be avoided due to reduction in seizure threshold.[96] Dosing is similar to antipsychotic use for other causes of agitation.

Medications to Avoid

Oral or IV alcohol should be avoided due to lack of supportive data favoring its use. While alcohol administration has historically been described to manage withdrawal, it is not recommended.[34,56,70,97] Administration of oral or IV alcohol has no proven efficacy, no accepted protocols, and known toxicity.[56,70]

Phenytoin is also ineffective in preventing the recurrence of an alcohol withdrawal-related seizure and is not recommended unless the patient is being treated for a concomitant underlying seizure disorder.[31,34,98]

In contrast to the use of oral or IV alcohol, or the use of phenytoin for alcohol withdrawal seizures, the use of benzodiazepines for alcohol withdrawal management allows for a predictable onset of action and duration of treatment, which improve patient outcomes, as outlined above.

Reassessment for Other Etiologies

A lack of treatment response and/or escalation to complicated withdrawal should always prompt a reassessment for other etiologies of the current symptoms, with a workup dependent on exhibited symptoms. For fevers, while it may be a result of alcohol withdrawal or a progression to DTs, other etiologies should be considered and ruled out. For DTs in particular, workups should be broad, and general supportive care, including frequent reorientation, should be provided.

Principle 6: Address Associated Comorbidities

In addition to treating the symptoms of alcohol withdrawal, effective hospital-based management should include screening and treatment of associated comorbidities. Laboratory assessment on admission should include electrolyte testing, comprehensive metabolic panel (CMP) and other liver assessments, and a complete blood count (CBC).

Expected Electrolyte Abnormalities in People With Chronic Alcohol Use

Electrolyte derangements, specifically hypomagnesemia, hypokalemia, and hypophosphatemia, are common in people with AUD and those presenting to the hospital for alcohol withdrawal.[99] Electrolytes should be aggressively repleted and reassessed until normalized. Likewise, as inadequate nutrition is a common contributor to these derangements, attention should be paid to dietary intake and nutritional status during and after acute hospitalization.

Expected Liver Function Abnormalities in People With Chronic Alcohol Use

Alcohol use is associated with both acute liver injury (alcohol-induced hepatitis) and chronic liver disease (alcohol-associated liver disease). On admission, liver function testing should include assessment for acute inflammation with transaminase levels as well as synthetic function testing with bilirubin, both of which are generally included in a CMP. Coagulation testing to assess synthetic function is also reasonable, particularly given increasing rates of hospitalization for alcohol-induced hepatitis in which coagulation testing, specifically international normalized ratio (INR), is used to determine if treatment with steroids is indicated.[100] If there is concern for liver disease, further workup, including ultrasound assessment of the liver, should be dictated by the patient's symptomatology.

Expected CBC Abnormalities and Coagulopathies in People With Chronic Alcohol Use

Hematologic abnormalities, specifically cytopenias, related to alcohol use are common and often multifactorial. Alcohol has a directly toxic effect on the bone marrow, impairing the creation of all cell lines and leading to anemia, leukopenia, and thrombocytopenia.[101] Bone marrow toxicity that has not yet led to cytopenias may still lead to macrocytosis of red blood cells.[102]

Beyond suppressing cell production, alcohol can lead to anemia and thrombocytopenia through splenomegaly in the context of alcohol-associated liver disease.[101] The risk of gastrointestinal bleeding is higher in those with chronic alcohol use, further contributing to the risk of anemia as well.[103]

Expected Nutritional Abnormalities and Associated Pathologies in People With Chronic Alcohol Use

B1/Thiamine Deficiency and Wernicke–Korsakoff Syndrome

Vitamin deficiencies, most notably vitamin B1 or thiamine, are also more common in people with AUD.[104] Wernicke–Korsakoff syndrome (WKS), a neuropsychiatric disease caused by vitamin B1 deficiency, is of particular importance.[105] WKS is a spectrum of illness beginning with Wernicke encephalopathy, a reversible syndrome marked by three cardinal symptoms: confusion, oculomotor dysfunction, and ataxia. If not treated, the disease progresses to Korsakoff syndrome, an irreversible condition marked by dementia and retrograde amnesia.

Given higher likelihood of thiamine depletion in people with AUD, all patients admitted with alcohol withdrawal should be assessed for WKS and treated either prophylactically or therapeutically with thiamine. Wernicke encephalopathy is clinically diagnosed by the presence of the three cardinal symptoms, though diagnostic accuracy is generally poor. An autopsy study attempting to improve diagnostic accuracy of Wernicke encephalopathy suggests that the identification of malnutrition accompanied by any of the three cardinal symptoms may improve rates of diagnosis.[106]

Given the morbidity caused by WKS, the low risks of treatment, and the relatively low cost of treatment,[107] there should be a low threshold to administer *treatment doses* of thiamine rather than *prophylactic doses*. Treatment doses for concern of Wernicke's is 200 to 500 mg of thiamine intravenously every 8 hours for a minimum of 3 days followed by daily dosing.[108,109] Prophylactic thiamine should be given to all other patients and consists of 100 mg IV/IM daily for 3 to 5 days.[34] IV or IM routes are preferred during hospitalization, and especially among patients with poor nutritional status, malabsorption, or who are known to have severe complications of alcohol withdrawal, as oral absorption of thiamine is poor.[34] Figure 8.7 outlines recommendations for thiamine treatment in patients with chronic alcohol use.

Folate

Folate should be administered for patients with chronic alcohol use during hospitalization as well. Routine prescription of oral thiamine, folate, and other vitamins on discharge does not have clear supportive evidence particularly given poor oral absorption of thiamine.[110] In order to prioritize the

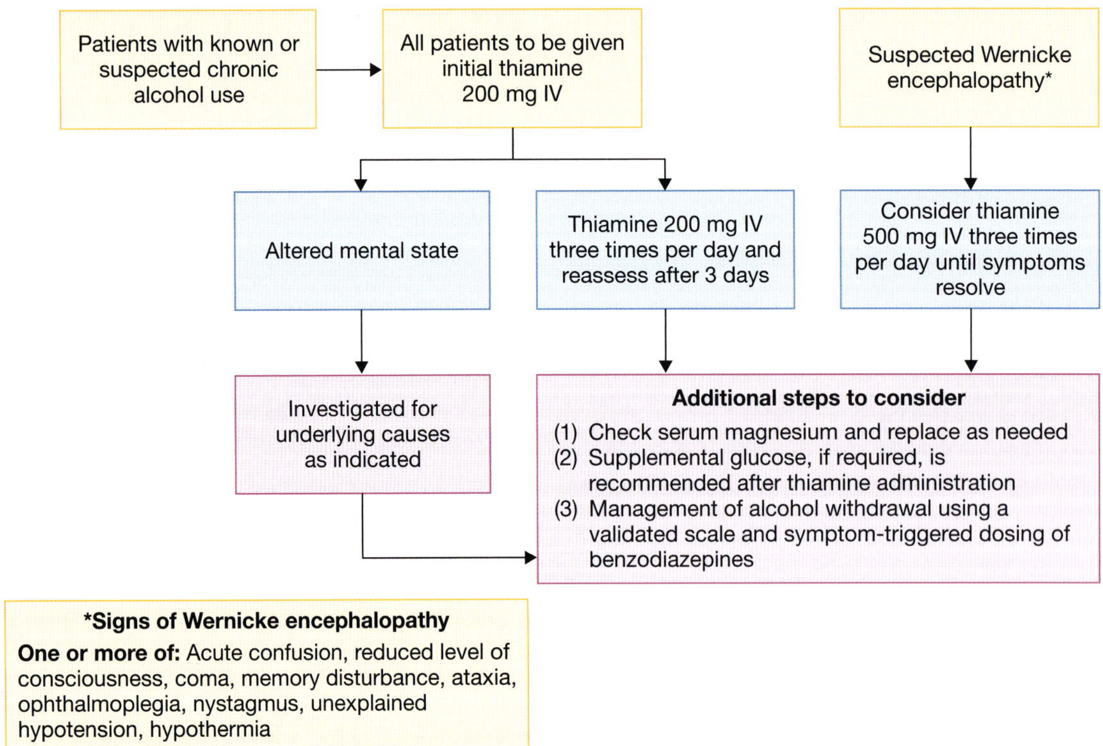

Figure 8.7: Recommendations for thiamine administration in people with unhealthy alcohol use.

prescription of effective medications and reduce pill burden, the focus on discharge should be on prescription of effective medications to treat AUD.

Biomarkers to Assess Alcohol Use

There are several laboratory tests that can be used as an assessment of alcohol use, both by measuring alcohol or its metabolites and by assessing for effects of alcohol (eg, macrocytosis). For the care of the hospitalized patient with AUD, direct measurement of alcohol is recommended.

Blood Alcohol Levels and Concentration

Recent alcohol use (ie, use within the last several hours) can be directly measured through breathalyzer or a BAL or a blood alcohol concentration (BAC). BAC and BAL both refer to BALs in the bloodstream. BAL refers to the ratio of alcohol to blood in the bloodstream and is reported in grams per deciliter (g/dL), milligrams per deciliter (mg/dL), or millimoles per liter (mmol/L). A BAC is represented as percentage. For example, a BAC of 0.08% means there are 8 g of alcohol per liter of blood, which is the legal limit for driving in the US. BAC levels above 0.4% (4 g/L) can be potentially fatal.[111,112] These tests can be useful in the context of risk stratification for complicated alcohol withdrawal as higher BAL on admission at the time of onset of withdrawal symptoms likely signifies that withdrawal will continue to worsen as the alcohol level continues to decrease. It is important to note that an alcohol level of zero on admission/evaluation does not preclude AUD or signify that there is no risk for impending alcohol withdrawal.

Phosphatidyl Ethanol, Carbohydrate-Deficient Transferrin, Ethylglucoronide, and Ethyl Sulfate

Other markers of alcohol use can include blood testing for phosphatidyl ethanol (PEth)[113] and carbohydrate-deficient transferrin (CDT)[114] as well as urine testing for ethylglucoronide (EtG) and ethyl sulfate (EtS).[113] PEth testing is increasingly being used as a tool for determining etiology of liver injury, detecting recent alcohol use, and others, suggesting PEth is an effective tool to assess for alcohol use in liver transplant candidates.[115–118] CDT is a biomarker for chronic alcohol use. It is highly specific, but has low sensitivity, making it an unsuitable test to screen for heavy alcohol use in the general population.[119] EtG and EtS are nonvolatile, water soluble, stable, and are detectable long after complete elimination of alcohol. EtG and EtS are concentrated by almost 200 times in the urine as compared to serum, therefore their window of detection in urine is up to 90 hours.[120]

PEth, CDT, and EtG and EtS are generally used for testing trends of alcohol use as part of a long-term treatment plan for AUD. They tend to have a longer processing time compared to a BAL/BAC and their utility in hospitalized patients is less clear.

Other Medical Complications of Chronic Alcohol Use

Other medical complications related to chronic alcohol use, such as alcohol-related cardiomyopathy, alcohol-related pancreatitis, cirrhosis, and gastrointestinal bleeding, should be assessed in the context of current symptoms suggestive of the disease.

As the hospitalized patient stabilizes from the treatment of their alcohol withdrawal, the next step should include discussing initiation of evidence-based treatment for AUD.

Behavioral Management of AUD

This section reviews indications for AUD treatment, how to define treatment goals, and how to decide among the various behavioral and pharmacologic options. Patterns of alcohol consumption fall along a spectrum from abstinence to minimal or moderate use, to unhealthy or “risky” alcohol use, and finally AUD, which is rated as mild, moderate, or severe. With increasing awareness that there is no “safe” level of alcohol consumption,[121] it is reasonable to consider some form of intervention, however small, for any and all persons who consume alcohol, though data for interventions geared toward patients who drink less than “at-risk” levels are lacking. For those drinking above at-risk levels, and those with mild AUD, specific evidence-based behavioral interventions (described below) are recommended, while those exhibiting more moderate to severe forms of AUD, and those hospitalized with alcohol-related complications, should be offered the full spectrum of treatment options. The intensity of these interventions depends upon the severity of AUD, patient preference, and treatment goals. The intensity of available treatment options ranges from a 5- to 10-minute “brief intervention” for patients exhibiting unhealthy drinking patterns, to combinations of behavioral and pharmacologic treatments such as longitudinal cognitive-behavioral therapy (CBT) sessions and oral or injectable medications designed to suppress alcohol cravings for people with moderate to severe AUD. Treatment should not be denied to patients with mild AUD, or to those with unhealthy alcohol use, based on extensive safety and efficacy data.

Defining Treatment Goals

Conversations about treatments for AUD should be driven by patient-centered goals. While clinicians might see complete abstinence as the only way forward for patients with severe AUD, patients are unlikely to adhere to treatment plans if they do not share this same goal. Instead, every effort should be made by the clinician to elicit patient goals, and to tailor treatment options accordingly.[122] While many patients may feel that abstinence is the best course of action, others may desire to cut back on their alcohol use, or to engage in safer practices around their alcohol use (eg, never drinking while driving). Prior research confirms that nonabstinent reductions in alcohol use can be a sustainable treatment goal[123] that is associated with reductions in alcohol-related consequences and mental health symptoms,[124] improvements in social functioning and quality of life,[125,126] and reductions in mortality.[124,127] By eliciting and understanding patient's goals, clinicians are "meeting patients where they are," and ensuring that conversations about treatment options are realistic, practical, and ultimately more likely to be achieved. Additional short-term goals may include promoting retention in treatment and adherence to prescribed pharmacotherapy, while longer-term goals may focus on more explicit reduction or cessation of alcohol.

Behavioral Strategies

The most well-studied behavioral treatments for AUD include CBT, motivational enhancement therapy (and its briefer derivative—Motivational Interviewing), and Mutual Support Programs, for example, 12-step facilitation. For an in-depth review of behavioral treatments for SUD, see Chapter 15: Behavioral and Psychosocial Treatments in the Hospital Setting.

Cognitive-Behavioral Therapy

Based on Social Learning Theory principles, CBT is an evidence-based behavioral intervention that helps patients to explore and mitigate the root causes of ongoing substance use. It is designed to help patients identify specific triggers and responses that lead to substance use, while equipping patients with relapse-prevention strategies such as assertiveness training, coping skills, and interpersonal skill development. Patients are often given homework between sessions, and sessions can be conducted face to face or asynchronously with the assistance of digital technology (eg, computer-based training for CBT or CBT4CBT).[128] In the largest meta-analysis to date, including 53 randomized trials of CBT versus usual care for the treatment of SUD (23 specifically for alcohol), CBT was found to have a small to moderate effect size on a range of alcohol use outcomes, with the authors concluding that "58% of patients receiving CBT fared better than patients in the comparison condition."[129]

Motivational Enhancement Therapy (MET)

In the Transtheoretical Model of change,[130] individuals are described as moving along a spectrum from highly resistant to change, that is, "precontemplative stage," to ready to employ specific strategies to make a change, that is, "action stage." Contrasted with a paternalistic approach in which individuals are simply told that they *should* make a change, MET is an evidence-based strategy designed to enhance patients' internal motivations to make behavioral changes, by helping patients to recognize potential links between their alcohol use and alcohol-related problems in the patient's life (eg, interpersonal conflict, gastroesophageal reflux). After eliciting the pros and cons of ongoing alcohol use, the patient's willingness to reduce his or her alcohol use is assessed, using nonjudgmental language. Finally, if appropriate, the clinician then negotiates with the patient to define specific, achievable goals that can be followed up at the next visit.

Derived from MET principles, motivational interviewing (MI) sessions may be quite brief, as little as a single 10-minute intervention, or may involve multiple sessions over time. MI skills can be learned through brief training sessions and can be effectively employed by a range of health care professionals. In a 2023 Cochrane Review that included 93 studies with 22,776 participants, with interventions ranging from 10 to 148 minutes, MI was found to be modestly more effective than no intervention with regard to postintervention substance use.[131]

Mutual Support

The most widely utilized and widely recognized mutual self-help program, with an estimated two million members representing nearly 180 countries, is Alcoholics Anonymous (AA)—an organization founded in 1935 by a physician and a lawyer.[132] As the name implies, membership is wholly anonymous, free, and readily available in most cities and towns throughout North America. Rooted in the "12-steps" believed within this community to be essential to the recovery process, AA meetings frequently reference Judeo-Christian principles. While AA's 12-step model is the most widely studied and widely available mutual support option, the past 20 years have seen a rapid proliferation of mutual self-help offerings that cater to individuals from diverse spiritual backgrounds (eg, Celebrate Recovery, Refuge Recovery, Recovery Dharma), explicitly secular CBT-based approaches (eg, Smart Recovery), harm-reduction–based programs that embrace a diversity of treatment goals (eg, Medication-Assisted Recovery Anonymous, Moderation Management), and groups geared toward integrating physical activity into mutual support principles (eg, The Phoenix, Yoga for 12-Step Recovery). While inherently difficult to study, the totality of evidence suggests that mutual support programs are moderately effective on a host of alcohol-related outcomes. A 2020 Cochrane Review of 27 studies with 10,565 participants concluded that there is high-quality evidence suggesting that 12-step programs like AA, particularly when facilitated by a licensed clinician using manualized therapy called 12-step facilitation, are more effective at promoting continuous abstinence than other established behavioral interventions such as CBT and MET (continuous abstinence at 12 months, risk ratio [RR] = 1.21; 95% confidence interval (CI), 1.03–1.42), with effect sizes that persisted for up to 36 months.[132] With this well-documented efficacy, for an intervention that is readily available and low risk, clinicians should encourage all patients with unhealthy drinking patterns to explore mutual support group options in their region. Of note, 12-step facilitation requires a trained facilitator, so unlike mutual support groups, it may be less available and typically requires reimbursement.

AUD Levels of Care and Treatment Settings

ASAM developed a framework for determining the appropriate level of care for people with SUD, using a care continuum model. These levels include the highest level, hospital-based treatment, followed by nonhospital inpatient residential treatment, followed by intensive outpatient treatment or high-intensity outpatient treatment, followed by outpatient treatment. Once a person leaves hospital or residential treatment, they may move into a recovery residence.[133]

Hospital Treatment or Medically Managed Intensive Inpatient Services

This level of care involves hospital care or less intensive nonhospital inpatient level of care. The hospital provides 24-hour nursing care and daily clinician visits. People in this level of care need daily physician monitoring, along with 24-hour oversight. This care can be provided in the hospital setting or in an inpatient treatment facility that supports this level of care. The less intensive level of care called "medically managed high-intensity inpatient treatment" is intended for people who need intensive medical or psychological monitoring in a 24-hour setting but do not need daily clinician interaction.[133]

Residential Treatment

Residential treatment, sometimes referred to as, "inpatient rehab," provides patients with a 24-hour substance-free environment, for varying lengths of time, from 4 weeks to 12 months or longer. "Best practice" treatment programs typically include mutual support meetings, individual counseling, varied therapeutic activities, and deliberate community reintegration efforts that ensure patients continue with treatments after their residential stay, while creating new therapeutic connections in the community. As the most intensive intervention for SUD, residential treatment is highly time intensive and costly.[133]

A meta-analysis of 23 studies (only 3 of which were randomized controlled trials [RCTs]) of residential SUD treatment programs yielded moderate-quality evidence that residential treatment has positive effects on some SUD outcomes, though high rates of attrition at follow-up and wide variation in treatment duration limit interpretation.[134] There are no consistent data suggesting that residential treatment is superior to outpatient treatment, drawing into question the cost-benefit of expensive residential SUD treatment options.

A lower level of care is "partial hospitalization" in which a person receives care and behavioral therapy for at least 20 hours a week, but less than 24 hours a day. People in partial hospitalization programs will often sleep at home but will spend their day in SUD treatment. This level of care provides structure and daily oversight for people who need daily monitoring, but not 24/7 care.[133]

Intensive Outpatient Treatment

These programs consist of SUD treatment that is at least 9 hours per week and no more than 20 hours per week of treatment. This level of care is appropriate for people with less severe SUD, or as a step-down from more intensive services.[133]

Outpatient Treatment

These programs consist of SUD treatment that is less than 9 hours per week. Services generally include groups, individuals counseling, medication management, and monitoring. Outpatient SUD treatment is appropriate for people with less severe SUD, or as a step-down from more intensive services.[133] Primary care practices can also provide outpatient SUD care that focuses on medication management and monitoring.

Recovery Residence

A recovery residence is a supportive, nonmedical living environment for individuals recovering from SUD. These residences provide a safe, sober space to help people transition from treatment, build recovery skills, and begin to live independently. They are often referred to as sober living houses or recovery homes. Recovery residences can be peer-run with minimal staff supervision, focusing on self-accountability and peer support. They can be monitored, with a house manager or staff member who oversees operations and ensures residents adhere to house rules and guidelines. They can be supervised, where there is more staff supervision and on-site support services like counseling or therapy. Finally, they can be treatment recovery residences, where clinical treatment services are offered directly within the residence.[135]

Pharmacotherapy for AUD

Food and Drug Administration (FDA)-approved medications for AUD (MAUD) include acamprosate, disulfiram, and naltrexone (see Table 8.8). There are also several medications which have not been FDA approved specifically for AUD, but which have strong efficacy and safety data (eg, topiramate and gabapentin). While abstinence from alcohol is often a key primary outcome in studies of MAUD, any reduction in alcohol consumption (ie, average number of drinks per day, number of days of heavy drinking per month), are worthy, commonly reported outcomes. MAUD research also often includes direct physiologic targets such as liver inflammation markers (AST, GGT), retention in treatment, health care utilization measures such as ED visits, hospitalizations, and others. Of note, the optimal duration of therapy for MAUD has not been firmly established, though the majority of studies investigating MAUD have provided medications for at least 3 months or more.

Despite several decades of research highlighting the safety and efficacy of MAUD, these medications remain grossly underutilized. It is estimated that fewer than 10% of patients with AUD are offered MAUD, with fewer than 1% actually receiving a prescription.[1] Efficacy data for MAUD, often measured as "number needed to treat" (NNT) shows that medications used to treat AUD are comparably more effective than countless medications widely prescribed by clinicians. For example, the estimated NNT for acamprosate to promote alcohol abstinence at 12 weeks is 11,[136] while the use of antibiotics to achieve clinical cure of acute sinusitis is 17[137] and that of a statin to prevent one nonfatal myocardial infarction is 104.[138] Many theories have been offered to explain this treatment gap, including lack of awareness of MAUD by patients, lack of training for clinicians, stigma and attitudes toward SUD, absence of direct-to-consumer advertising, and socioeconomic factors that serve as barriers to accessing treatment.[139]

National guidelines recommend and promote the use of MAUD for all patients with moderate to severe AUD.[71,122,140] The American Psychiatric Association recommend naltrexone and acamprosate as first-line agents for AUD while the Department of Veterans Affairs (VA/DoD) and the National Institute for Health and Care Excellence (NICE) in the United Kingdom include topiramate among this list of first-line agents. The APA and VA/DoD designate

TABLE 8.8

Medications for Alcohol Use Disorder

	Evidence supports[b]	Pill burden	Cost	Side effects
Acamprosate[a]	Abstinence, reduction in use	High	Intermediate	Diarrhea
Supervised disulfiram[a]	Abstinence	Low	Low	Hepatitis, neuropathy
Naltrexone oral[a]	Abstinence, Reduction in use	Low	Low	Nausea, rare hepatotoxicity
Naltrexone intramuscular[a]	Reduction in use	N/A	High	Nausea, injection site reaction
Topiramate	Reduction in use	Intermediate	Low	Gastrointestinal, cognitive issues, paresthesias
Gabapentin	Abstinence	High	Low	Fatigue, cognitive issues, nausea
Baclofen	Abstinence	Intermediate	Low	Dizziness, fatigue

[a]FDA-approved for AUD.

[b]See the following for evidentiary data:

McPheeters M, O'Connor EA, Riley S, et al. Pharmacotherapy for alcohol use disorder: a systematic review and meta-analysis. *JAMA*. 2023; 330(17):1653–1665.

Bahji A, Bach P, Danilewitz M, et al. Pharmacotherapies for adults with alcohol use disorders: a systematic review and network meta-analysis. *J Addict Med*. 2022;16(6):630–638.

gabapentin, and disulfiram as second-line agents, though some have questioned the rationale for disulfiram's second-line status.[141] Evidence for the use of MAUD and their potential adverse effects are listed below.

Disulfiram

In 1949, disulfiram became the first medication to be approved for the treatment of AUD,[142] shortly after it was discovered that men exposed to disulfiram while working in a rubber factory (disulfiram was a chemical used in the rubber-manufacturing process) had unintentionally become intolerant of alcohol.[143] By virtue of its inhibition of acetaldehyde dehydrogenase—a key step in the metabolism of alcohol—ingestion of disulfiram leads to the accumulation of an early metabolite of alcohol, acetaldehyde. Acetaldehyde, in turn, causes the "alcohol disulfiram reaction" (ADR), characterized by flushing, nausea and vomiting, headache, tremulousness, tachycardia, and malaise. Fear of this ADR, whether based on experience, or hearsay, serves as a deterrent to the consumption of alcohol. For this reason, it has been proposed that disulfiram is a medication-facilitated *behavioral* intervention, as the medication itself has no direct neuropsychiatric properties that influence cravings.[141,142]

Most early studies of disulfiram utilized double-blinded RCT trials, the gold standard study design when investigating medication interventions. However, many experts have argued that double-blinded trials undermine the efficacy of disulfiram since both treatment and placebo arms experience the same deterrent effect of disulfiram, thus diluting outcome data.[144] In contrast, when analyzing only open-labeled RCTs, the totality of high-quality open-labeled studies of disulfiram demonstrates that disulfiram is consistently superior for patients seeking to maintain abstinence from alcohol, as compared with control conditions including naltrexone and acamprosate comparison groups (Hedge's g effect size = .70; 95% CI, .46–.93). Importantly, the strongest data for disulfiram comes from studies that have utilized a "supervised disulfiram" approach wherein a supportive third party (eg, friend or family member) assists/encourages the patient to take their disulfiram each day.[144]

Disulfiram is typically administered as 250 mg once daily. Interestingly, numerous countries in Europe and elsewhere have employed a strategy of subcutaneous implantation of disulfiram tablets, with annual reimplantation, with remarkable success (this is not available in the US).[145] Patients taking disulfiram should be advised to avoid alcohol-based mouthwashes, alcohol-based foods, etc. Side effects for disulfiram, in addition to the ADR itself, include nausea, neuropathy, and rare hepatotoxicity. Liver failure may occur at a rate of one per million patients,[146] and disulfiram is contraindicated in those with Child–Pugh Class B and C. It should also be avoided in those with significant cardiac disease in light of the potential severity of the ADR, which could exacerbate underlying cardiac ischemia.

Naltrexone

While initially FDA approved for the treatment of opioid use disorder (OUD) in 1984, oral naltrexone was later approved for AUD as well in 1994. To bolster adherence to daily oral naltrexone, an extended-release injectable formulation was developed and approved in 2006, under the trade name, Vivitrol. As an opioid antagonist with irreversible binding to mu-opioid receptors, its role in the treatment of AUD may seem counterintuitive. Naltrexone's efficacy in suppressing cravings for alcohol is driven by a deeper understanding of alcohol's effects on beta-endorphin release and dopaminergic pathways in the mesocorticolimbic system. When consumed, alcohol binds to $GABA_A$ receptors, as described earlier in this chapter, with detrimental effects on level of alertness, coordination, and decision making. Alcohol also leads to the direct release of beta-endorphins (endogenous opioids) in the pituitary and hypothalamus, which fuel the reinforcing, pleasant effects of alcohol consumption—"the buzz." By taking naltrexone, which blocks the binding of beta-endorphins to mu-opioid receptors, the link between drinking alcohol and experiencing this pleasurable effect is uncoupled, which ultimately leads to less cravings to drink, and less alcohol consumed when patients do drink.

In contrast with disulfiram, data for naltrexone suggests it is most effective at reducing alcohol consumption and percentage of heavy drinking days, rather than promoting abstinence. Two large meta-nalyses conducted in recent years yielded somewhat different results in terms of efficacy data for naltrexone. McPheeters et al included 49 studies of oral or injectable naltrexone with at least 12 weeks of outcomes data and found a modest treatment size for oral naltrexone, with an NNT of 18 (RR = 0.93; 95% CI, 0.87–0.99) to prevent return to drinking, with no improvement in abstinence rates for injectable naltrexone. There was slight improvement in rates of return to *heavy* drinking with oral naltrexone, with an NNT of 11 (RR = 0.81; 95% CI, 0.72–0.90). The only significant outcome for injectable naltrexone was a reduction in percentage of drinking days and heavy drinking days, compared with placebo (weighted mean difference = −4.99 days; 95% CI, −9.49–−0.49 days).[136] In one RCT of hospitalized patients with AUD, the initiation of either oral or injectable naltrexone at the time of hospital discharge was associated with substantial reductions in percentage of heavy drinking days, regardless of formulation (MAUD initiation in hospital settings is discussed further below).[147]

A second meta-analysis with slightly different inclusion and exclusion criteria yielded 58 naltrexone studies with somewhat better efficacy data in terms of abstinence rates relative to placebo with oral naltrexone (RR = 0.84; 95% CI, 0.74–0.96) and injectable naltrexone (RR = 0.61; 95% CI, 0.38–0.98), as well as for reductions in heavy drinking (oral naltrexone RR = 0.81; 95% CI, 0.73–0.89) compared with placebo.[148]

Oral naltrexone is prescribed as one 50- to 100-mg tablet daily. Extended-release injectable naltrexone is administered as one monthly 380-mg intragluteal injection, a 4-cm^3 volume. For patients with mild AUD, some argue for the use of "as-needed" or targeted oral naltrexone, taking the medication only when high-risk situations and alcohol consumption are anticipated.[149]

While initial concerns were raised about naltrexone's potential hepatotoxicity, subsequent studies examining patients with and without advanced liver disease revealed that naltrexone is remarkably safe at recommended doses (50 to 100 mg daily), even in patients with Child–Pugh Class B and C.[150] These data led to the removal of a hepatotoxicity black box warning for naltrexone in 2013. Some studies suggest that markers of hepatotoxicity (AST, GGT) are more likely to *improve* than worsen while taking naltrexone, presumably due to reductions in alcohol consumption (safety of MAUD in advanced liver disease is discussed further below).[151]

The most common side effects of naltrexone are nausea and vomiting, dizziness, and, for the injectable form, injection site reactions. While rare, intragluteal injections of naltrexone can lead to a painful IM phlegmon, or an abscess, and patients should be cautioned to contact their treatment team if severe pain and fever develops following an intragluteal naltrexone injection. As an opioid antagonist, all forms of naltrexone are contraindicated in patients on opioids, including methadone, though injectable naltrexone may be a reasonable treatment option for patients with co-occurring OUD and AUD if abstinence from all opioids can be achieved for at least 7 to 10 days before administering the injection.

Acamprosate

Acamprosate, FDA approved for treatment of AUD in 2004, represents the last agent the FDA approved for the treatment of AUD in over 20 years—an indication of the paucity of commercial investment in addiction pharmacotherapies by the pharmaceutical industry. While the precise mechanism of action of acamprosate remains somewhat elusive, it is hypothesized to act by rebalancing GABA and glutamate neurotransmitter systems in the brain, ultimately attenuating alcohol cravings.

Efficacy data for acamprosate somewhat mirrors that of naltrexone. In a meta-analysis of 35 placebo-controlled RCTs, acamprosate was associated with improved rates of abstinence (RR = 1.33; 95% CI, 1.16–1.54) and reductions in heavy drinking (RR = 0.78; 95% CI, 0.71–0.85).[148] In a second meta-analysis that included 23 studies of acamprosate, acamprosate was associated with a lower risk of returning to drinking (RR = 0.88; 95% CI, 0.83–0.93), NNT = 11, with moderate evidence of a reduction in percentage of drinking days (weight mean difference = −8.3; 95% CI, −12.2–−4.4).[136]

Acamprosate is prescribed as two 333-mg tablets taken three times daily, which may limit adherence as compared with once daily regimens such as disulfiram and oral naltrexone. As acamprosate is renally cleared, it is safe even with the most advanced forms of decompensated cirrhosis. Patients with creatinine clearance (CrCl) 30 to 50 mL/min should take one 333-mg tablet three times daily, and those with CrCl ≤30 mL/min should use an alternative agent. Diarrhea is the most common adverse reaction.

Topiramate

As mentioned above, there are several well-studied medications, approved for other indications, that have shown great promise in the treatment of AUD. Among these, the anticonvulsant, topiramate has received significant attention and has been endorsed as a first-line treatment by the Department of Veterans Affairs.[71] Similar to acamprosate, topiramate acts via a rebalancing of GABA-ergic and glutamatergic neurotransmitter systems, while also attenuating the dopaminergic response to alcohol consumption.[152]

A recent meta-analysis of 13 RCTs and 1,397 patients demonstrated moderate effect sizes favoring topiramate over placebo, with significant reductions in number of heavy drinking days, and number of drinks per day, and serum GGT levels.[153] A second meta-analysis showed topiramate, with a moderate strength of evidence, was moderately effective at preserving abstinence (RR = 1.41; 95% CI, 1.07–1.87). Topiramate has also been demonstrated to improve several important physical health and quality-of-life measures, including blood pressure control, liver enzyme levels, and psychosocial well-being.[154]

Unlike the FDA-approved MAUD, achieving therapeutic doses of topiramate necessitates a gradual dose escalation over a period of 8 or more weeks, starting with 25 mg twice daily for 1 week, and advancing by 25-mg increments each week to a goal regimen of 100 to 150 mg twice daily. The primary limitation of topiramate, in addition to the complex and lengthy titration schedule, is the relatively high rate of unpleasant side effects including cognitive disturbances, gastrointestinal upset, taste perversion, and other paresthesias, which lead to treatment discontinuation twice as often as placebo.[148] Topiramate doses should be adjusted in those with CrCl less than 70 mL/min.

Gabapentin

Well known to clinicians, gabapentin has been available since 1993 for the treatment of seizure disorder, postherpetic neuralgia, and restless legs syndrome, among others. While not approved for AUD, gabapentin has been extensively studied for both alcohol withdrawal management and maintenance pharmacotherapy for AUD.

In a 12-week, double-blind, placebo-controlled RCT of 150 patients with AUD, gabapentin was associated with an abstinence rate of 17.0% (95% CI, 8.9%–30.1%) in the 1,800-mg group compared with 4.1% (95% CI, 1.1%–13.7%) in the placebo group (NNT = 8).[155] The "no heavy drinking" rate was 22.5% (95% CI, 13.6%–37.2%) in the placebo group and 44.7% (95% CI, 31.4%–58.8%) in the 1,800-mg group (NNT = 5). Subsequent studies have less compelling results, with "low strength of evidence for benefit" according to a recent meta-analysis,[136] but nonetheless suggest that gabapentin is most effective for patients who have experienced any alcohol withdrawal symptoms when trying to quit or cut back.[156] In this population, gabapentin has been highly linked to reductions in heavy drinking days ($P < .02$; NNT = 3.1) and preservation of abstinence ($P = .003$; NNT = 2.7).

Gabapentin can be quickly titrated up to 600 mg three times daily over 3 to 5 days. Concerns have been raised about the misuse of gabapentin with increasing numbers of documented accounts of gabapentin overdose, addiction, and diversion, though this has been seen predominantly in patients with other SUD, rather than AUD.[157]

Baclofen

Baclofen is a selective gamma-aminobutyric acid-B (GABA-B) receptor agonist. The use of this drug remains controversial, in part due to uncertainty regarding dosing and efficacy, alongside concerns about safety.[158] Data supporting baclofen for the treatment of AUD has been equivocal.

One large meta-analysis with 14 RCTs of baclofen (30 mg/d) found baclofen was effective in promoting abstinence (RR = 1.93; 95% CI, 1.47–2.52), with moderate evidence supporting a reduction in heavy drinking (RR = 0.57; 95% CI, 0.44–0.73).[148] A subsequent meta-analysis, however, found only low strength of evidence that baclofen promoted abstinence (RR = 0.83; 95% CI, 0.70–0.98).[136] A recent Cochrane Review of 17 studies and 1,818 participants, with baclofen dose ranges from 30 to 300 mg/d, found moderate evidence that baclofen decreases the risk of returning to drinking, relative to placebo (RR = 0.87; 95% CI, 0.77–0.99), but has little effect on number of drinks among those who are actively drinking.[157]

Baclofen is often touted as the first-line option for patients with advanced liver disease, due to safety data in this population, and efficacy in promoting abstinence.[136] However, with increasing data supporting the safety of naltrexone even in advanced liver disease, most experts still relegate baclofen to second-line status. Like topiramate, the primary limitation of baclofen is a relatively high rate of cognitive side effects, particularly dizziness and drowsiness.[136]

Other Medications

Additional medications that have been extensively studied, with some success, include nalmefene, varenicline, and gamma-hydroxybutyrate (GHB) (also known as sodium oxybate).

While nalmefene has garnered enthusiasm in Europe, it remains unavailable in the US. Interestingly, nalmefene, similar to naltrexone, has been promoted as an "as-needed" medication, to be taken by patients when they experience cravings, or in anticipation of cravings, with compelling data suggesting this approach can decrease the number of heavy drinking days per month with accompanying reductions in liver enzyme elevations.[159]

A recent meta-analysis of varenicline, with 22 RCTs and 1,421 participants found that varenicline, a medication commonly used to treat tobacco use disorder, did not impact abstinence rates or percentage of drinking days but was associated with reductions in other alcohol-related outcomes such as number of drinks per drinking day and intensity of cravings.[160]

While consistent data for GHB have been lacking, a recent large meta-analysis suggests that GHB may be particularly effective for patients with more severe AUD, with its use associated with significantly higher rates of abstinence compared with placebo (RR = 3.16; $P = 0.004$).[161] Concerns have been raised regarding GHB's risk of misuse, addiction, seizure, and overdose.

Hospital Initiation of MAUD

Periods of hospitalization for acute alcohol-related medical issues represent an opportune time to initiate maintenance treatment, once the acute issues have been addressed. Patients tend to be highly motivated when faced with direct, acute harms of their alcohol use, and thus are more likely to be willing to consider the full spectrum of treatment options. In one proof-of-concept study, investigators provided a 1-hour training session on the use of naltrexone for treating AUD to internal medicine residents.[162] As a result of this simple educational intervention, rates of naltrexone prescription at the time of discharge increased from 0% preintervention to 64% postintervention, while 30-day readmissions among patients with documented AUD at the index admission dropped from 23.4% to 8.2%. A more recent study of 6,794 patients demonstrated that the initiation of pharmacotherapy at the time of discharge led to a 42% reduction in the composite outcome of all-cause mortality and 30-day return to hospital.[11] With these benefits in mind, every effort should be made during acute hospitalizations to discuss the menu of options available, initiate pharmacotherapy as appropriate, and facilitate connections to longitudinal outpatient treatment programs.

Combinations of Pharmacotherapy and Behavioral Interventions

Various combinations of MAUD, including, for example, acamprosate and disulfiram,[163] or naltrexone and prazosin,[164] have been studied with some promising results. However, the majority of these studies have either utilized weak study designs or have small sample sizes that make extrapolation to a larger population difficult. In one of the largest multisite AUD trials, the addition of acamprosate to naltrexone was found to confer no additional benefit beyond naltrexone alone.[165]

In contrast, the combination of behavioral treatments with pharmacotherapy has yielded some modestly positive results in the treatment of SUD more broadly. A meta-analysis of 30 RCTs (15 of which involved patients with AUD) found that the addition of CBT to pharmacotherapy, compared with "usual care" and pharmacotherapy, yielded positive results on a range of alcohol-related outcomes.[166] Importantly, CBT was not found to be superior to other evidence-based behavioral treatments (eg, MET or 12-step facilitation). A second systematic review identified that a majority of studies demonstrated that pharmacotherapy provided added benefit to psychotherapy, but only three of nine studies demonstrated a benefit from the reverse—adding psychotherapy to pharmacotherapy compared to pharmacotherapy alone.[167] These data suggest that pharmacotherapy should remain the mainstay of treatment for AUD, but that adding an evidence-based behavioral treatment may confer additional benefits with no clear associated harms.

Special Populations

Pregnancy and Breastfeeding

Pregnancy presents a unique challenge in the management of AUD, with limited data on the safety of MAUD in this setting, and little evidence that current efforts are effective in curbing alcohol use.[168] Pregnant patients have largely been excluded from studies investigating both behavioral and pharmacologic interventions, and, in practice, medications are rarely prescribed during pregnancy, leaving little concrete evidence with which to guide clinicians.[168,169] Guidelines do recommend a focus on behavioral interventions during pregnancy, though acknowledge that the well-established risks of alcohol consumption during pregnancy, namely fetal alcohol spectrum disorder (FASD), may justify the use of MAUD when behavioral interventions are unsuccessful.[122] Patients in need of withdrawal management require consultation with an obstetrician and should ideally be referred for hospital-based management.[34] To date, data on the safety and efficacy of MAUD has largely been derived from animal studies, retrospective cohort studies, or case series.[170] Despite these limitations, expert consensus generally favors the use of benzodiazepines or barbiturates for alcohol withdrawal, and naltrexone or acamprosate for maintenance pharmacotherapy, while strictly avoiding disulfiram and topiramate in this setting.[34,122]

Advanced Liver Disease

Unhealthy alcohol use, with or without a formal AUD diagnosis, invariably leads to some degree of liver injury, which influences decisions around MAUD. This may include mild steatohepatitis, bouts of acute alcohol-related hepatitis, or the irreversible changes that accompany cirrhosis. As naltrexone, disulfiram, and topiramate are all metabolized in the liver, these medications were traditionally avoided in patients with advanced liver disease, in favor of acamprosate or gabapentin, which are exclusively cleared by the kidney.

However, more recent data highlighted the safety of naltrexone and topiramate, in particular, in patients with advanced forms of liver disease, emphasizing the known toxicity of alcohol and the well-established efficacy of these medications in reducing alcohol consumption.[150] In a large retrospective cohort study that included 9,635 individuals with AUD, the use of MAUD was associated with a reduced risk of developing alcohol-related liver disease (adjusted odds ratio [aOR]) = 0.37; 95% CI, 0.31–0.43; $P < .001$) and a lower risk of hepatic decompensation in patients with a known history of cirrhosis (aOR = 0.35; 95% CI, 0.23–0.53, $P < .001$).[151] This reduced risk of developing alcohol-related liver disease was seen in patients taking naltrexone, gabapentin, topiramate, or baclofen, while the reduced risk of hepatic decompensation, even in patients who started MAUD *after* the cirrhosis diagnosis was made, was seen with naltrexone and gabapentin. Likewise, one retrospective cohort study involving 9,131 individuals with alcohol-associated cirrhosis and ongoing alcohol consumption found that exposure to MAUD (naltrexone or acamprosate) was associated with improved survival, as compared to those without MAUD exposure (hazard ratio = 0.80; 95% CI, 0.67–0.97, $P = .024$).[12]

With these data in mind, it is advisable to still consider MAUD, with naltrexone,[171] acamprosate, topiramate, gabapentin, or baclofen, for patients with advanced liver disease, including Child–Pugh Class A, B, and C liver disease. For patients with Child–Pugh C liver disease, clinicians should evaluate the limited risks of MAUD versus the known benefits of reduced alcohol use in liver disease; naltrexone can be considered in these cases. Disulfiram can be used cautiously for patients with Child–Pugh Class A liver disease.

Co-occurring Opioid Use Disorder

While extended-release naltrexone is FDA approved for the treatment of both OUD and AUD, the presence of co-occurring OUD in patients with AUD often precludes the use of naltrexone for people who are on medications for OUD, including methadone or buprenorphine. For the majority of patients with OUD, the requirement to abstain from all opioids for a period of several days to a week in order to start naltrexone, an opioid antagonist, often makes this a less desirable option compared with the alternatives described above. However, for patients who are interested, and motivated, extended-release naltrexone can be a good treatment option for individuals with AUD and OUD.

Future Directions and Conclusion

Future directions in AUD treatment are evolving with advancements in research, technology, and societal understanding. Key trends include the following areas:

Personalized Medicine and Pharmacogenetics

In the 2015 study by Oslin et al, the researchers investigated the impact of a functional polymorphism (A118G) in the mu-opioid receptor gene (OPRM1) on the efficacy of naltrexone in treating AUD. The study found that individuals with AUD carrying at least one copy of the G allele (AG or GG genotypes) showed significantly better outcomes with naltrexone treatment compared to those with the AA genotype. These outcomes included lower rates of relapse and reduced heavy drinking. The findings support the idea of personalized medicine in the treatment of AUD, suggesting that genetic testing could help identify individuals who are more likely to benefit from naltrexone therapy.[172]

Novel Pharmacologic Agents

In the realm of pharmacotherapeutics, psilocybin, ketamine, and glucagon-like peptide-1 receptor agonists (GLP-1) are promising pharmacologic agents for the treatment of AUD.

Several studies have suggested that ketamine and psilocybin are effective in promoting alcohol abstinence when administered with guided psychotherapy. For example, a double-blinded RCT involving 95 patients with AUD assessed the efficacy of psilocybin-assisted psychotherapy in treating AUD.[173] Participants were randomized to either psilocybin or diphenhydramine (an active placebo), administered over two full-day sessions separated by 4 weeks, in concert with MET and CBT.[173] The treatment arm saw dramatic reductions in percent heavy drinking days over the 32 weeks of follow-up, as compared with the diphenhydramine group (9.7% vs 23.6%) with a mean difference of 13.9% (95% CI, 3.0–24.7; $P = .01$). In addition, the psilocybin group had lower mean daily alcohol consumption. These findings suggest that psilocybin with psychotherapy may be a promising treatment for reducing heavy drinking in individuals with AUD.[173]

Similarly, in a randomized clinical trial by Dakwar et al, participants with AUD received a single subanesthetic ketamine infusion (0.71 mg/kg) combined with MET. Participants receiving ketamine exhibited a higher likelihood of abstinence, longer time to relapse, and fewer heavy drinking days compared to those receiving midazolam, an active control. This one study suggests that ketamine, when integrated with behavioral therapy, may enhance treatment outcomes for individuals with AUD.[174] While promising, further study with larger-scale RCTs are needed before psychedelics can be routinely recommended.

GLP-1 agonists such as semaglutide are an active area of investigation with much excitement about their potential to curb cravings. Data in support of GLP-1 agonists in the treatment of AUD have largely come from animal studies, observational trials, or secondary analyses of weight loss or tobacco use disorder studies, with exceptions.[175,176] In a double-blind RCT by Hendershot et al, 48 adults with AUD were randomized into 2 groups receiving varying semaglutide doses or placebo. After 9 weeks, compared to the placebo group, the group receiving semaglutide had significantly reduced alcohol intake, decreased heavy drinking days, and lower alcohol cravings (measured using the Penn Alcohol Craving Scale). In a subgroup of individuals with tobacco use disorder, semaglutide also reduced tobacco consumption. Unsurprisingly, the semaglutide group also experienced an average weight loss of 5%. This study highlights semaglutide's potential as a treatment for AUD, though its small sample size and short duration suggest the need for larger, long-term, and real-world trials to confirm these findings.[177]

Digital Health and Telemedicine

In an article by Torous et al, the authors discussed how the COVID-19 pandemic created an urgent need to shift from traditional in-person mental health care to digital solutions, such as telepsychiatry, mobile apps, and digital therapy platforms. They argue that while the pandemic exposed gaps in access to mental health care, it also catalyzed innovation and adoption of digital tools at an unprecedented pace. The authors highlight key areas for improving digital mental health moving forward including building a strong digital infrastructure, for example, broadband access and device availability; ensuring equity in access, especially for marginalized and underserved populations; investing in clinician training for digital competencies and ethical digital practice; developing evidence-based tools that are not only engaging but also clinically effective; and encouraging collaboration between tech developers, researchers, and clinicians to cocreate solutions tailored to patient needs. In this article, the authors stress the importance of regulatory flexibility, data privacy, and outcomes-based evaluation to guide the safe and effective integration of digital tools into mainstream care.[178]

Interventional Neurostimulation and Brain-Based Therapies

A study by Mishra et al investigated the effectiveness of high-frequency repetitive transcranial magnetic stimulation (rTMS) targeting the right dorsolateral prefrontal cortex (DLPFC) in reducing alcohol cravings among participants with AUD. Conducted as a single-blind, sham-controlled trial, it involved 45 participants divided into active and sham rTMS groups. The active group showed significant reductions in craving scores compared to the sham group, as measured by the Alcohol Craving Questionnaire. The findings suggest that rTMS could be a promising strategy to manage alcohol cravings and prevent return to use for people with AUD; however, more extensive trials are needed to confirm the long-term efficacy, optimal protocols, and safety of rTMS in AUD treatment.[179]

Mindfulness and Behavioral Therapies

Mindfulness-based therapies have shown promising effectiveness in supporting recovery from AUD. Research indicates that these interventions can help individuals manage cravings, reduce substance use, and improve emotional regulation.[180] Techniques like mindfulness-based relapse prevention (MBRP) combine mindfulness practices with cognitive-behavioral strategies to enhance self-awareness and coping skills. Studies suggest that mindfulness-based interventions are as effective as other evidence-based treatments for AUD.[180] They offer a holistic approach by addressing both psychological and behavioral aspects of SUD. Future work should rigorously evaluate the effectiveness of mindfulness-based therapies.[181]

Conclusion

This chapter offers a comprehensive overview of the neurobiology, clinical manifestations, and evidence-based management of alcohol withdrawal and AUD in hospitalized patients. It emphasizes that hospitalization represents a critical opportunity to initiate both acute withdrawal management and long-term treatment for AUD. This chapter underscores the importance of risk stratification, appropriate pharmacologic interventions, and compassionate, patient-centered care for hospitalized patients with unhealthy alcohol use, AWS, and AUD. The story of Juan serves as a poignant reminder that behind every case lies a human life affected by SUD, and that even brief periods of sobriety can carry profound meaning for patients and their loved ones.

REFERENCES

1. Substance Abuse and Mental Health Services Administration. *Key Substance Use and Mental Health Indicators in the United States: Results from the 2023 National Survey on Drug Use and Health (HHS Publication No. PEP24-07-021, NSDUH Series H-59).* Center for Behavioral Health Statistics and Quality, Substance Abuse and Mental Health Services Administration; 2024. https://www.samhsa.gov/data/report/2023-nsduh-annual-national-report
2. US Center for Disease Control and Prevention. *Alcohol and Public Health: Alcohol-Related Disease Impact (ARDI).* Accessed January 14, 2025. https://nccd.cdc.gov/DPH_ARDI/Default/Report.aspx?T=AAM&P=F1F85724-AEC5-4421-BC88-3E8899866842&R=EACE3036-77C9-4893-9F93-17A5E1FEBE01&M=7F40785C-D481-440A-970F-50EFBD21B35B&F=&D=https://nccd.cdc.gov/DPH_ARDI/Default/Report.aspx?T=AAM&P=F1F85724-AEC5-4421-BC88-3E8899866842&R=EACE3036-77C9-4893-9F93-17A5E1FEBE01&M=7F40785C-D481-440A-970F-50EFBD21B35B&F=&D=
3. Rehm J, Gmel GE Sr, Gmel G, et al. The relationship between different dimensions of alcohol use and the burden of disease—an update. *Addiction.* 2017;112(6):968–1001.
4. The US Surgeon Generals Advisory. *Alcohol and Cancer Risk.* Accessed January 14, 2025. https://www.hhs.gov/sites/default/files/oash-alcohol-cancer-risk.pdf
5. Deutsch-Link S, Curtis B, Singal AK. COVID-19 and alcohol associated liver disease. *Dig Liver Dis.* 2022;54(11):1459–1468.
6. Ayyala-Somayajula D, Dodge JL, Leventhal AM, Terrault NA, Lee BP. Trends in alcohol use after the COVID-19 pandemic: a national cross-sectional study. *Ann Intern Med.* 2025;178(1):139–142.
7. Saitz R, Freedner N, Palfai TP, Horton NJ, Samet JH. The severity of unhealthy alcohol use in hospitalized medical patients. *J Gen Intern Med.* 2006;21(4):381–385.
8. Suen LW, Makam AN, Snyder HR, et al. National prevalence of alcohol and other substance use disorders among emergency department visits and hospitalizations: NHAMCS 2014–2018. *J Gen Intern Med.* 2022;37(10):2420–2428.
9. Steel TL, Matson TE, Hallgren KA, et al. Incidence of hospitalizations involving alcohol withdrawal syndrome in a primary care population. *JAMA Netw Open.* 2024;7(10):e2438128.
10. Englander H, Priest KC, Snyder H, Martin M, Calcaterra S, Gregg J. A call to action: hospitalists' role in addressing substance use disorder. *J Hosp Med.* 2020;15(3):184–187.
11. Bernstein EY, Baggett TP, Trivedi S, Herzig SJ, Anderson TS. Outcomes after initiation of medications for alcohol use disorder at hospital discharge. *JAMA Netw Open.* 2024;7(3):e243387–e243387.
12. Rabiee A, Mahmud N, Falker C, Garcia-Tsao G, Taddei T, Kaplan DE. Medications for alcohol use disorder improve survival in patients with hazardous drinking and alcohol-associated cirrhosis. *Hepatol Commun.* 2023;7(4):e0093.
13. Chartier K, Caetano R. Ethnicity and health disparities in alcohol research. *Alcohol Res Health.* 2010;33(1–2):152–60.
14. Mulia N, Ye Y, Greenfield TK, Zemore SE. Disparities in alcohol-related problems among white, black, and Hispanic Americans. *Alcohol Clin Exp Res.* 2009;33(4):654–62.
15. Witbrodt J, Mulia N, Zemore SE, Kerr WC. Racial/ethnic disparities in alcohol-related problems: differences by gender and level of heavy drinking. *Alcohol Clin Exp Res.* 2014;38(6):1662–1670.
16. Gilpin NW, Koob GF. Neurobiology of alcohol dependence: focus on motivational mechanisms. *Alcohol Res Health.* 2008;31(3):185–195.
17. Littleton J. Neurochemical mechanisms underlying alcohol withdrawal. *Alcohol Health Res World.* 1998;22(1):13–24.
18. Vazey EM, den Hartog CR, Moorman DE. Central noradrenergic interactions with alcohol and regulation of alcohol-related behaviors. *Handb Exp Pharmacol.* 2018;248:239–260.
19. Becker HC, Mulholland PJ. Neurochemical mechanisms of alcohol withdrawal. *Handb Clin Neurol.* 2014;125:133–156.
20. Hermann D, Hirth N, Reimold M, et al. Low μ-opioid receptor status in alcohol dependence identified by combined positron emission tomography and post-mortem brain analysis. *Neuropsychopharmacology.* 2017;42(3):606–614.
21. Gianoulakis C. Influence of the endogenous opioid system on high alcohol consumption and genetic predisposition to alcoholism. *J Psychiatry Neurosci.* 2001;26(4):304–318.
22. American Psychiatric Association, DSM-5 Task Force. *Diagnostic and Statistical Manual of Mental Disorders: DSM-5™* (5th ed.). American Psychiatric Publishing, Inc. 2013. https://doi.org/10.1176/appi.books.9780890425596
23. Schuckit MA, Danko GP, Smith TL, Hesselbrock V, Kramer J, Bucholz K. A 5-year prospective evaluation of DSM-IV alcohol dependence with and without a physiological component. *Alcohol Clin Exp Res.* 2003;27(5):818–825.
24. Saitz R. Introduction to alcohol withdrawal. *Alcohol Health Res World.* 1998;22(1):5–12.
25. Victor M. Treatment of alcoholic intoxication and the withdrawal syndrome: a critical analysis of the use of drugs and other forms of therapy. *Psychosomatic Medicine.* 1966;28(4):636–650.
26. Schuckit MA, Tipp JE, Reich T, Hesselbrock VM, Bucholz KK. The histories of withdrawal convulsions and delirium tremens in 1648 alcohol dependent subjects. *Addiction.* 1995;90(10):1335–1347.
27. Hillbom M, Pieninkeroinen I, Leone M. Seizures in alcohol-dependent patients: epidemiology, pathophysiology and management. *CNS Drugs.* 2003;17(14):1013–1030.
28. Victor M, Adams RD. The effect of alcohol on the nervous system. *Res Publ Assoc Res Nerv Ment Dis.* 1953;32:526–573.
29. Schuckit MA. Recognition and management of withdrawal delirium (delirium tremens). *N Engl J Med.* 2014;371(22):2109–2113.
30. Mainerova B, Prasko J, Latalova K, et al. Alcohol withdrawal delirium—diagnosis, course and treatment. *Biomed Pap Med Fac Univ Palacky Olomouc Czech Repub.* 2015;159(1):44–52.
31. Mayo-Smith MF, Beecher LH, Fischer TL, et al. Management of alcohol withdrawal delirium: an evidence-based practice guideline. *Arch Intern Med.* 2004;164(13):1405–1412.
32. Odlaug BL, Gual A, DeCourcy J, et al. Alcohol dependence, co-occurring conditions and attributable burden. *Alcohol Alcohol.* 2015;51(2):201–209.
33. Steel TL, Afshar M, Edwards S, et al. Research needs for inpatient management of severe alcohol withdrawal syndrome: an official American Thoracic Society research statement. *Am J Respir Crit Care Med.* 2021;204(7):e61–e87.
34. The ASAM clinical practice guideline on alcohol withdrawal management. *J Addict Med.* 2020;14(3S Suppl 1):1–72.
35. Banyal N, Dhillon HS, Sasidharan S. Risk factors associated with complicated alcohol withdrawal syndrome. *J Med Soc.* 2021;35(3):113–117.

36. Muncie HL Jr, Yasinian Y, Oge L. Outpatient management of alcohol withdrawal syndrome. *Am Fam Physician.* 2013; 88(9):589–95.
37. Tiglao SM, Meisenheimer ES, Oh RC. Alcohol withdrawal syndrome: outpatient management. *Am Fam Physician.* 2021; 104(3):253–262.
38. O'Connor PG, Gottlieb LD, Kraus ML, Segal SR, Horwitz RI. Social and clinical features as predictors of outcome in outpatient alcohol withdrawal. *J Gen Intern Med.* 1991; 6(4):312–316.
39. Hayashida M, Alterman AI, McLellan AT, et al. Comparative effectiveness and costs of inpatient and outpatient detoxification of patients with mild-to-moderate alcohol withdrawal syndrome. *N Engl J Med.* 1989;320(6):358–365.
40. Wagner E, Babaei M. *Provincial Guideline for the Clinical Management of High-Risk Drinking and Alcohol Use Disorder.* British Columbia Centre on Substance Use; 2019.
41. Maldonado JR, Sher Y, Das S, et al. Prospective validation study of the prediction of alcohol withdrawal severity scale (PAWSS) in Medically ill inpatients: a new scale for the prediction of complicated alcohol withdrawal syndrome. *Alcohol Alcohol.* 2015;50(5):509–518.
42. Cohen SM, Kashyap N, Steel TL, Edelman EJ, Fiellin DA, Joudrey PJ. Guideline concordance of electronic health record order sets for hospital-based treatment of alcohol withdrawal syndrome. *J Hosp Med.* 2025;20(6): 550–561.
43. Mo Y, Thomas MC, Laskey CS, Shcherbakova N, Bankert ML, Halloran RH. Current practice patterns in the management of alcohol withdrawal syndrome. *P T.* 2018;43(3): 158–162.
44. Heavner JJ, Akgün KM, Heavner MS, et al. Implementation of an ICU-specific alcohol withdrawal syndrome management protocol reduces the need for mechanical ventilation. *Pharmacotherapy.* 2018;38(7):701–713.
45. Melkonian A, Patel R, Magh A, Ferm S, Hwang C. Assessment of a hospital-wide CIWA-Ar protocol for management of alcohol withdrawal syndrome. *Mayo Clin Proc Innov Qual Outcomes.* 2019;3(3):344–349.
46. Duby JJ, Berry AJ, Ghayyem P, Wilson MD, Cocanour CS. Alcohol withdrawal syndrome in critically ill patients: protocolized versus nonprotocolized management. *J Trauma Acute Care Surg.* 2014;77(6):938–943.
47. Ng K, Dahri K, Chow I, Legal M. Evaluation of an alcohol withdrawal protocol and a preprinted order set at a tertiary care hospital. *Can J Hosp Pharm.* 2011;64(6): 436–445.
48. Pope S, Gustaw-Rothenberg K, Delos Reyes C. Linking orders in electronic medical records can improve the frequency with which recommended treatments are ordered as illustrated in the treatment of alcohol withdrawal. *J Psychiatr Pract.* 2016;22(1):64–67.
49. Institute of Medicine Committee on Standards for Developing Trustworthy Clinical Practice Guidelines. In: Graham R, Mancher M, Miller Wolman D, Greenfield S, Steinberg E, eds. *Clinical Practice Guidelines We Can Trust.* National Academies Press (US); 2011. https://www.ncbi.nlm.nih.gov/books/NBK209539/
50. Sullivan JT, Sykora K, Schneiderman J, Naranjo CA, Sellers EM. Assessment of alcohol withdrawal: the revised clinical institute withdrawal assessment for alcohol scale (CIWA-Ar). *Br J Addict.* 1989;84(11):1353–1357.
51. Rastegar DA, Applewhite D, Alvanzo AAH, Welsh C, Niessen T, Chen ES. Development and implementation of an alcohol withdrawal protocol using a 5-item scale, the Brief Alcohol Withdrawal Scale (BAWS). *Subst Abus.* 2017; 38(4):394–400.
52. DeCarolis DD, Rice KL, Ho L, Willenbring ML, Cassaro S. Symptom-driven lorazepam protocol for treatment of severe alcohol withdrawal delirium in the intensive care unit. *Pharmacotherapy.* 2007;27(4):510–518.
53. Gossop M, Keaney F, Stewart D, Marshall EJ, Strang J. A short alcohol withdrawal scale (SAWS): development and psychometric properties. *Addict Biol.* 2002;7(1):37–43.
54. Sessler CN, Gosnell MS, Grap MJ, et al. The Richmond Agitation-Sedation Scale: validity and reliability in adult intensive care unit patients. *Am J Respir Crit Care Med.* 2002; 166(10):1338–1344.
55. Wood E, Albarqouni L, Tkachuk S, et al. Will this hospitalized patient develop severe alcohol withdrawal syndrome?: the rational clinical examination systematic review. *JAMA.* 2018;320(8):825–833.
56. Wartenberg AA, Braun HM, Zimmerman C. Management of alcohol intoxication and withdrawal. In: Miller SC, Rosenthal RN, Levy S, Saxon AJ, Tetrault JM, Wakeman SE, eds. *The ASAM Principles of Addiction Medicine.* 7th ed. Lippincott Williams & Wilkins, a Wolters Kluwer Business; 2024.
57. Rastegar DA, Applewhite D, Alvanzo AAH, Welsh C, Niessen T, Chen ES. Development and implementation of an alcohol withdrawal protocol using a 5-item scale, the brief alcohol withdrawal scale (BAWS). *Subst Abus.* 2017;38(4): 394–400.
58. Sullivan JT, Sykora K, Schneiderman J, Naranjo CA, Sellers EM. Assessment of alcohol withdrawal: the revised clinical institute withdrawal assessment for alcohol scale (CIWA-Ar). *Br J Addict.* 1989;84(11):1353–1357.
59. DeCarolis DD, Rice KL, Ho L, Willenbring ML, Cassaro S. Symptom-driven lorazepam protocol for treatment of severe alcohol withdrawal delirium in the intensive care unit. *Pharmacotherapy.* 2007;27(4):510–518.
60. Sessler CN, Gosnell MS, Grap MJ, et al. The Richmond Agitation-Sedation Scale: validity and reliability in adult intensive care unit patients. *Am J Respir Crit Care Med.* 2002;166(10):1338–1344.
61. Gossop M, Keaney F, Stewart D, Marshall EJ, Strang J. A short alcohol withdrawal scale (SAWS): development and psychometric properties. *Addict Biol.* 2002;7(1): 37–43.
62. Goodson CM, Clark BJ, Douglas IS. Predictors of severe alcohol withdrawal syndrome: a systematic review and meta-analysis. *Alcohol Clin Exp Res.* 2014;38(10):2664–2677.
63. Wetterling T, Weber B, Depfenhart M, Schneider B, Junghanns K. Development of a rating scale to predict the severity of alcohol withdrawal syndrome. *Alcohol Alcohol.* 2006;41(6):611–615.
64. Adinoff B, O'Neill HK, Ballenger JC. Alcohol withdrawal and limbic kindling: a hypothesis of relapse. *Am J Addict.* 1995;4(1):5–17.
65. Ammar MA, Ammar AA, Rosen J, Kassab HS, Becher RD. Phenobarbital monotherapy for the management of alcohol withdrawal syndrome in surgical-trauma patients. *Ann Pharmacother.* 2021;55(3):294–302.
66. Saitz R, Mayo-Smith MF, Roberts MS, Redmond HA, Bernard DR, Calkins DR. Individualized treatment for alcohol withdrawal. A randomized double-blind controlled trial. *JAMA.* 1994;272(7):519–523.
67. Langlois H, Cormier M, Villeneuve E, Hoffman RS, Longo C, Gosselin S. Benzodiazepine resistant alcohol withdrawal: what is the clinician's preferred definition? *CJEM.* 2020; 22(2):165–169.
68. Hack JB, Hoffmann RS, Nelson LS. Resistant alcohol withdrawal: does an unexpectedly large sedative requirement identify these patients early? *J Med Toxicol.* 2006;2(2): 55–60.

69. Wong A, Benedict NJ, Lohr BR, Pizon AF, Kane-Gill SL. Management of benzodiazepine-resistant alcohol withdrawal across a healthcare system: benzodiazepine dose-escalation with or without propofol. *Drug Alcohol Depend.* 2015;154: 296–299.
70. Mayo-Smith MF. Pharmacological management of alcohol withdrawal. A meta-analysis and evidence-based practice guideline. American Society of Addiction Medicine Working Group on pharmacological management of alcohol withdrawal. *JAMA.* 1997;278(2):144–151.
71. Perry C, Liberto J, Milliken C, et al. The management of substance use disorders: synopsis of the 2021 U.S. Department of Veterans Affairs and U.S. Department of Defense Clinical Practice Guideline. *Ann Intern Med.* 2022;175(5):720–731.
72. National Clinical Guideline Centre (UK). *Alcohol Use Disorders: Diagnosis and Clinical Management of Alcohol-Related Physical Complications [Internet].* Royal College of Physicians (UK); 2010.
73. Holbrook AM, Crowther R, Lotter A, Cheng C, King D. Meta-analysis of benzodiazepine use in the treatment of acute alcohol withdrawal. *CMAJ.* 1999;160(5):649–655.
74. Amato L, Minozzi S, Vecchi S, Davoli M. Benzodiazepines for alcohol withdrawal. *Cochrane Database Syst Rev.* 2010;(3):Cd005063.
75. Steel TL, Malte CA, Bradley KA, Hawkins EJ. Benzodiazepine treatment and hospital course of medical inpatients with alcohol withdrawal syndrome in the Veterans Health administration. *Mayo Clin Proc Innov Qual Outcomes.* 2022;6(2): 126–136.
76. Ronan MV, Gordon KS, Skanderson M, et al. Contemporary management and outcomes of veterans hospitalized with alcohol withdrawal: a multicenter retrospective cohort study. *J Addict Med.* 2024;18(4):389–396.
77. Sud P, Lee DC. Sedative–hypnotics. In: Nelson LS, Howland MA, Lewin NA, Smith SW, Goldfrank LR, Hoffman RS, eds. *Goldfrank's Toxicologic Emergencies. 11th ed.* McGraw-Hill Education; 2019.
78. Löscher W, Rogawski MA. How theories evolved concerning the mechanism of action of barbiturates. *Epilepsia.* 2012;53(Suppl 8):12–25.
79. Enna SJ. The GABA receptors. In: Enna SJ, Möhler H, eds. *The GABA Receptors.* Humana Press; 2007:1–21.
80. Kramp P, Rafaelsen OJ. Delirium tremens: a double-blind comparison of diazepam and barbital treatment. *Acta Psychiatr Scand.* 1978;58(2):174–190.
81. Metcalf CS, Smith MD, Wilcox KS. Pharmacotherapy of the epilepsies. In: Brunton LL, Knollmann BC, eds. *Goodman & Gilman's: The Pharmacological Basis of Therapeutics.* 14th ed. McGraw-Hill Education; 2023.
82. Pagana KD, Pagana TJ. *Mosby's Manual of Diagnostic and Laboratory Tests-E-Book.* Elsevier Health Sciences; 2017.
83. Hendey GW, Dery RA, Barnes RL, Snowden B, Mentler P. A prospective, randomized, trial of phenobarbital versus benzodiazepines for acute alcohol withdrawal. *Am J Emerg Med.* 2011;29(4):382–385.
84. Rosenson J, Clements C, Simon B, et al. Phenobarbital for acute alcohol withdrawal: a prospective randomized double-blind placebo-controlled study. *J Emerg Med.* 2013; 44(3):592–598.e2.
85. Bosch NA, Crable EL, Ackerbauer KA, et al. Implementation of a phenobarbital-based pathway for severe alcohol withdrawal: a mixed-method study. *Ann Am Thorac Soc.* 2021;18(10):1708–1716.
86. Oks M, Cleven KL, Healy L, et al. The safety and utility of phenobarbital use for the treatment of severe alcohol withdrawal syndrome in the medical intensive care unit. *J Intensive Care Med.* 2020;35(9):844–850.
87. Ives TJ, Mooney AJ III, Gwyther RE. Pharmacokinetic dosing of phenobarbital in the treatment of alcohol withdrawal syndrome. *South Med J.* 1991;84(1):18–21.
88. Steel TL, Bradley KA. Improving care for inpatient alcohol withdrawal syndrome: addressing the lack of rigorous research on a common condition. *Ann Am Thorac Soc.* 2021;18(10):1622–1623.
89. Nisavic M, Nejad SH, Isenberg BM, et al. Use of Phenobarbital in alcohol withdrawal management—a retrospective comparison study of phenobarbital and benzodiazepines for acute alcohol withdrawal management in general medical patients. *Psychosomatics.* 2019;60(5):458–467.
90. Tangmose K, Nielsen MK, Allerup P, Ulrichsen J. Linear correlation between phenobarbital dose and concentration in alcohol withdrawal patients. *Dan Med Bull.* 2010;57(8):A4141.
91. Terasaki D, Kulick B, Calcaterra S, Ray L. Phenobarbital for alcohol withdrawal in the context of the opioid epidemic: a neglected caveat. *Addiction.* 2023;118(7):1198–1200.
92. Sohraby R, Attridge RL, Hughes DW. Use of propofol-containing versus benzodiazepine regimens for alcohol withdrawal requiring mechanical ventilation. *Ann Pharmacother.* 2014;48(4):456–461.
93. Pizon AF, Lynch MJ, Benedict NJ, et al. Adjunct ketamine use in the management of severe ethanol withdrawal. *Crit Care Med.* 2018;46(8):e768–e771.
94. Shah P, McDowell M, Ebisu R, Hanif T, Toerne T. Adjunctive use of ketamine for benzodiazepine-resistant severe alcohol withdrawal: a retrospective evaluation. *J Med Toxicol.* 2018;14(3):229–236.
95. Wong A, Benedict NJ, Armahizer MJ, Kane-Gill SL. Evaluation of adjunctive ketamine to benzodiazepines for management of alcohol withdrawal syndrome. *Ann Pharmacother.* 2015;49(1):14–19.
96. Hedges D, Jeppson K, Whitehead P. Antipsychotic medication and seizures: a review. *Drugs Today (Barc).* 2003;39(7): 551–557.
97. Department of Veterans Affairs. VA/DoD clinical practice guideline for the management of substance use disorders. Department of Veterans Affairs and Department of Defense (eds) Version; 2015;3.
98. Bråthen G, Ben-Menachem E, Brodtkorb E, et al. EFNS guideline on the diagnosis and management of alcohol-related seizures: report of an EFNS task force. *Eur J Neurol.* 2005;12(8):575–581.
99. Baj J, Flieger W, Teresiński G, et al. Magnesium, calcium, potassium, sodium, phosphorus, selenium, zinc, and chromium levels in alcohol use disorder: a review. *J Clin Med.* 2020;9(6):1901.
100. Wakil A, Mohamed M, Tafesh Z, et al. Trends in hospitalization for alcoholic hepatitis from 2011 to 2017: a USA nationwide study. *World J Gastroenterol.* 2022;28(34):5036–5046.
101. Ballard HS. The hematological complications of alcoholism. *Alcohol Health Res World.* 1997;21(1):42–52.
102. Seppä K, Laippala P, Saarni M. Macrocytosis as a consequence of alcohol abuse among patients in general practice. *Alcohol Clin Exp Res.* 1991;15(5):871–876.
103. Askgaard G, Christensen AI, Nordestgaard B, Grønbæk M, Tolstrup JS. Alcohol and risk of non-traumatic bleeding events requiring hospital care in the general population: a prospective cohort study. *Alcohol.* 2020;87:73–78.
104. Chamorro AJ, Rosón-Hernández B, Medina-García JA, et al. Differences between alcoholic and nonalcoholic patients with Wernicke encephalopathy: a multicenter observational study. *Mayo Clin Proc.* 2017;92(6):899–907.
105. Sechi G, Serra A. Wernicke's encephalopathy: new clinical settings and recent advances in diagnosis and management. *Lancet Neurol.* 2007;6(5):442–455.

106. Caine D, Halliday GM, Kril JJ, Harper CG. Operational criteria for the classification of chronic alcoholics: identification of Wernicke's encephalopathy. *J Neurol Neurosurg Psychiatry.* 1997;62(1):51–60.
107. Thomson A, Guerrini I, Marshall EJ. Incidence of adverse reactions to parenteral thiamine in the treatment of Wernicke's encephalopathy, and recommendations. *Alcohol Alcohol.* 2019;54(6):609–614.
108. Day E, Bentham PW, Callaghan R, Kuruvilla T, George S. Thiamine for prevention and treatment of Wernicke-Korsakoff syndrome in people who abuse alcohol. *Cochrane Database Syst Rev.* 2013;2013(7):CD004033.
109. Flannery AH, Adkins DA, Cook AM. Unpeeling the evidence for the banana bag: evidence-based recommendations for the management of alcohol-associated vitamin and electrolyte deficiencies in the ICU. *Crit Care Med.* 2016;44(8): 1545–1552.
110. DeFries T, Leyde S, Haber LA, Martin M. Things We Do for No Reason™: prescribing thiamine, folate and multivitamins on discharge for patients with alcohol use disorder. *J Hosp Med.* 2021;16(12):751–753.
111. Koob GF, Arends MA, Le Moal M. Chapter 6: Alcohol. In: Koob GF, Arends MA, Le Moal M, eds. *Drugs, Addiction, and the Brain.* Academic Press; 2014:173–219.
112. Vonghia L, Leggio L, Ferrulli A, Bertini M, Gasbarrini G, Addolorato G. Acute alcohol intoxication. *Eur J Intern Med.* 2008;19(8):561–567.
113. Mazhar A, Cheung A. Blood testing for phosphatidylethanol. *JAMA.* 2024;331(23):2039–2040.
114. Harris JC, Leggio L, Farokhnia M. Blood biomarkers of alcohol use: a scoping review. *Curr Addict Rep.* 2021;8(4): 500–508.
115. Andresen-Streichert H, Beres Y, Weinmann W, et al. Improved detection of alcohol consumption using the novel marker phosphatidylethanol in the transplant setting: results of a prospective study. *Transpl Int.* 2017;30(6):611–620.
116. Ulwelling W, Smith K. The PEth blood test in the security environment: what it is; why it is important; and interpretative guidelines. *J Forensic Sci.* 2018;63(6):1634–1640.
117. Lindenger C, Castedal M, Schult A, Åberg F. Long-term survival and predictors of relapse and survival after liver transplantation for alcoholic liver disease. *Scand J Gastroenterol.* 2018;53(12):1553–1561.
118. Fleming MF, Smith MJ, Oslakovic E, et al. Phosphatidylethanol detects moderate-to-heavy alcohol use in liver transplant recipients. *Alcohol Clin Exp Res.* 2017;41(4): 857–862.
119. Golka K, Wiese A. Carbohydrate-deficient transferrin (CDT)—a biomarker for long-term alcohol consumption. *J Toxicol Environ Health B Crit Rev.* 2004;7(4):319–337.
120. Shukla L, Sharma P, Ganesha S, et al. Value of ethyl glucuronide and ethyl sulfate in serum as biomarkers of alcohol consumption. *Indian J Psychol Med.* 2017;39(4):481–487.
121. Grummon AH, Hall MG. Updated health warnings for alcohol—informing consumers and reducing harm. *N Engl J Med.* 2022;387(9):772–774.
122. Reus VI, Fochtmann LJ, Bukstein O, et al. The American Psychiatric Association practice guideline for the pharmacological treatment of patients with alcohol use disorder. *Am J Psychiatry.* 2018;175(1):86–90.
123. Witkiewitz K, Kranzler HR, Hallgren KA, et al. Stability of drinking reductions and long-term functioning among patients with alcohol use disorder. *J Gen Intern Med.* 2021; 36(2):404–412.
124. Witkiewitz K, Hallgren KA, Kranzler HR, et al. Clinical validation of reduced alcohol consumption after treatment for alcohol dependence using the World Health Organization risk drinking levels. *Alcohol Clin Exp Res.* 2017;41(1):179–186.
125. Henssler J, Müller M, Carreira H, Bschor T, Heinz A, Baethge C. Controlled drinking-non-abstinent versus abstinent treatment goals in alcohol use disorder: a systematic review, meta-analysis and meta-regression. *Addiction.* 2021; 116(8):1973–1987.
126. Witkiewitz K, Kranzler HR, Hallgren KA, et al. drinking risk level reductions associated with improvements in physical health and quality of life among individuals with alcohol use disorder. *Alcohol Clin Exp Res.* 2018;42(12): 2453–2465.
127. Roerecke M, Gual A, Rehm J. Reduction of alcohol consumption and subsequent mortality in alcohol use disorders: systematic review and meta-analyses. *J Clin Psychiatry.* 2013; 74(12):e1181–e1189.
128. Carroll KM, Ball SA, Martino S, et al. Computer-assisted delivery of cognitive-behavioral therapy for addiction: a randomized trial of CBT4CBT. *Am J Psychiatry.* 2008;165(7): 881–888.
129. Magill M, Ray LA. Cognitive-behavioral treatment with adult alcohol and illicit drug users: a meta-analysis of randomized controlled trials. *J Stud Alcohol Drugs.* 2009;70(4): 516–527.
130. Raihan N, Cogburn M. Stages of change theory. [Updated 2023 Mar 6]. In: StatPearls [Internet]. Treasure Island (FL): StatPearls Publishing; 2025 Jan-. https://www.ncbi.nlm.nih.gov/books/NBK556005/
131. Schwenker R, Dietrich CE, Hirpa S, et al. Motivational interviewing for substance use reduction. *Cochrane Database Syst Rev.* 2023;12(12):CD008063.
132. Kelly JF, Humphreys K, Ferri M. Alcoholics Anonymous and other 12-step programs for alcohol use disorder. *Cochrane Database Syst Rev.* 2020;3(3):Cd012880.
133. American Society of Addiction Medicine. *The ASAM Criteria.* Accessed April 20, 2025. https://www.asam.org/asam-criteria/about-the-asam-criteria
134. de Andrade D, Elphinston RA, Quinn C, Allan J, Hides L. The effectiveness of residential treatment services for individuals with substance use disorders: a systematic review. *Drug Alcohol Depend.* 2019;201:227–235.
135. Legislative Analysis and Public Policy Association. Recovery Residences. 2022. Accessed January 14, 2025. https://legislativeanalysis.org/wp-content/uploads/2022/07/Recovery-Residences-Fact-Sheet.pdf
136. McPheeters M, O'Connor EA, Riley S, et al. Pharmacotherapy for alcohol use disorder: a systematic review and meta-analysis. *JAMA.* 2023;330(17):1653–1665.
137. Lemiengre MB, van Driel ML, Merenstein D, Liira H, Mäkelä M, De Sutter AI. Antibiotics for acute rhinosinusitis in adults. *Cochrane Database Syst Rev.* 2018;9(9): CD006089.
138. Taylor F, Huffman MD, Macedo AF, et al. Statins for the primary prevention of cardiovascular disease. *Cochrane Database Syst Rev.* 2013;2013(1):CD004816.
139. Venegas A, Donato S, Meredith LR, Ray LA. Understanding low treatment seeking rates for alcohol use disorder: a narrative review of the literature and opportunities for improvement. *Am J Drug Alcohol Abuse.* 2021;47(6): 664–679.
140. National Collaborating Centre for Mental H. National Institute for Health and Care Excellence: Guidelines. *Alcohol-Use Disorders: Diagnosis, Assessment and Management of Harmful Drinking and Alcohol Dependence.* British Psychological Society (UK) Copyright © 2011, The British Psychological Society & The Royal College of Psychiatrists; 2011.

141. Holt SR. Supervised disulfiram should be considered first-line treatment for alcohol use disorder. *J Addict Med.* 2024;18(6):614–616.
142. Mutschler J, Grosshans M, Soyka M, Rösner S. Current findings and mechanisms of action of disulfiram in the treatment of alcohol dependence. *Pharmacopsychiatry.* 2016;49(4): 137–141.
143. Williams E. Effects of alcohol on workers with carbon disulfide. *JAMA.* 1937;109(109):1472–1473.
144. Skinner MD, Lahmek P, Pham H, Aubin HJ. Disulfiram efficacy in the treatment of alcohol dependence: a meta-analysis. *PLoS One.* 2014;9(2):e87366.
145. Sezgin B, Sibar S, Bulam H, Findikcioglu K, Tuncer S, Dogan B. Disulfiram Implantation for the treatment of alcoholism: clinical experiences from the plastic surgeon's point of view. *Arch Plast Surg.* 2014;41(5):571–575.
146. Gopalakrishna H, Ghabril M, Gu J, et al. Drug-induced liver injury due to medications for alcohol use disorder: results from the DILIN prospective study. *J Addict Med.* 2024;19(3):314–321.
147. Magane KM, Dukes KA, Fielman S, et al. Oral vs Extended-release injectable naltrexone for hospitalized patients with alcohol use disorder: a randomized clinical trial. *JAMA Intern Med.* 2025;185(6):635–645.
148. Bahji A, Bach P, Danilewitz M, et al. Pharmacotherapies for adults with alcohol use disorders: a systematic review and network meta-analysis. *J Addict Med.* 2022;16(6): 630–638.
149. Sinclair JD. Evidence about the use of naltrexone and for different ways of using it in the treatment of alcoholism. *Alcohol Alcohol.* 2001;36(1):2–10.
150. Bolton M, Hodkinson A, Boda S, et al. Serious adverse events reported in placebo randomised controlled trials of oral naltrexone: a systematic review and meta-analysis. *BMC Med.* 2019;17(1):10.
151. Vannier AGL, Shay JES, Fomin V, et al. Incidence and progression of alcohol-associated liver disease after medical therapy for alcohol use disorder. *JAMA Netw Open.* 2022; 5(5):e2213014.
152. Blodgett JC, Del Re AC, Maisel NC, Finney JW. A meta-analysis of topiramate's effects for individuals with alcohol use disorders. *Alcohol Clin Exp Res.* 2014;38(6): 1481–1488.
153. Fluyau D, Kailasam VK, Pierre CG. A Bayesian meta-analysis of topiramate's effectiveness for individuals with alcohol use disorder. *J Psychopharmacol.* 2023;37(2):155–163.
154. Johnson BA, Rosenthal N, Capece JA, et al. Improvement of physical health and quality of life of alcohol-dependent individuals with topiramate treatment: US multisite randomized controlled trial. *Arch Intern Med.* 2008;168(11):1188–1199.
155. Mason BJ, Quello S, Goodell V, Shadan F, Kyle M, Begovic A. Gabapentin treatment for alcohol dependence: a randomized clinical trial. *JAMA Intern Med.* 2014;174(1):70–77.
156. Anton RF, Latham P, Voronin K, et al. Efficacy of gabapentin for the treatment of alcohol use disorder in patients with alcohol withdrawal symptoms: a randomized clinical trial. *JAMA Intern Med.* 2020;180(5):728–736.
157. Murnion B, Schaffer A, Cairns R, Brett J. Gabapentinoids: repeating mistakes of the past? *Addiction.* 2022;117(12): 2969–2971.
158. de Beaurepaire R, Sinclair JMA, Heydtmann M, et al. The use of baclofen as a treatment for alcohol use disorder: a clinical practice perspective. *Front Psychiatry.* 2018;9: 708.
159. Mann K, Bladström A, Torup L, Gual A, van den Brink W. Extending the treatment options in alcohol dependence: a randomized controlled study of as-needed nalmefene. *Biol Psychiatry.* 2013;73(8):706–713.
160. Phimarn W, Sakhancord R, Paitoon P, Saramunee K, Sungthong B. Efficacy of varenicline in the treatment of alcohol dependence: an updated meta-analysis and meta-regression. *Int J Environ Res Public Health.* 2023;20(5):4091.
161. Guiraud J, Addolorato G, Aubin HJ, et al. Sodium oxybate for alcohol dependence: a network meta-regression analysis considering population severity at baseline and treatment duration. *Alcohol Alcohol.* 2023;58(2):125–133.
162. Wei J, Defries T, Lozada M, Young N, Huen W, Tulsky J. An inpatient treatment and discharge planning protocol for alcohol dependence: efficacy in reducing 30-day readmissions and emergency department visits. *J Gen Intern Med.* 2015;30(3):365–370.
163. Besson J, Aeby F, Kasas A, Lehert P, Potgieter A. Combined efficacy of acamprosate and disulfiram in the treatment of alcoholism: a controlled study. *Alcohol Clin Exp Res.* 1998; 22(3):573–579.
164. Simpson TL, Achtmeyer C, Batten L, et al. Naltrexone augmented with prazosin for alcohol use disorder: results from a randomized controlled proof-of-concept trial. *Alcohol Alcohol.* 2024;59(5):agae062.
165. Anton RF, O'Malley SS, Ciraulo DA, et al. Combined pharmacotherapies and behavioral interventions for alcohol dependence: the COMBINE study: a randomized controlled trial. *JAMA.* 2006;295(17):2003–2017.
166. Ray LA, Meredith LR, Kiluk BD, Walthers J, Carroll KM, Magill M. Combined pharmacotherapy and cognitive behavioral therapy for adults with alcohol or substance use disorders: a systematic review and meta-analysis. *JAMA Netw Open.* 2020;3(6):e208279.
167. van Amsterdam J, Blanken P, Spijkerman R, van den Brink W, Hendriks V. The added value of pharmacotherapy to cognitive behavior therapy and vice versa in the treatment of alcohol use disorders: a systematic review. *Alcohol Alcohol.* 2022;57(6):768–775.
168. Minozzi S, Ambrosi L, Saulle R, et al. Psychosocial and medication interventions to stop or reduce alcohol consumption during pregnancy. *Cochrane Database Syst Rev.* 2024;4(4): CD015042.
169. Deflorimonte C, Glissendorf V, Hofer J, et al. National Provider Survey: use of naltrexone for pregnant individuals with substance use disorders. *J Addict Med.* 2023;17(6): 736–738.
170. Wachman EM, Saia K, Bressler J, Werler M, Carter G, Jones HE. Case series of individuals treated with naltrexone during pregnancy for opioid and/or alcohol use disorder. *J Addict Med.* 2024;18(3):288–292.
171. Kee DP, Buyske JJ, Calcaterra SL. Things We Do for No Reason™: avoiding naltrexone for alcohol use disorder in liver disease. *J Hosp Med.* 2024;20(7):768–771.
172. Oslin DW, Berrettini W, Kranzler HR, et al. A functional polymorphism of the μ-opioid receptor gene is associated with naltrexone response in alcohol-dependent patients. *Neuropsychopharmacology.* 2003;28(8):1546–1552.
173. Bogenschutz MP, Ross S, Bhatt S, et al. Percentage of heavy drinking days following psilocybin-assisted psychotherapy vs placebo in the treatment of adult patients with alcohol use disorder: a randomized clinical trial. *JAMA Psychiatry.* 2022; 79(10):953–962.
174. Dakwar E, Nunes EV, Hart CL, et al. A single ketamine infusion combined with mindfulness-based behavioral modification to treat cocaine dependence: a randomized clinical trial. *Am J Psychiatry.* 2019;176(11):923–930.

175. Probst L, Monnerat S, Vogt DR, et al. Effects of dulaglutide on alcohol consumption during smoking cessation. *JCI Insight*. 2023;8(22):e170419.
176. Aranäs C, Edvardsson CE, Shevchouk OT, et al. Semaglutide reduces alcohol intake and relapse-like drinking in male and female rats. *EBioMedicine*. 2023;93:104642.
177. Hendershot CS, Bremmer MP, Paladino MB, et al. Once-weekly semaglutide in adults with alcohol use disorder: a randomized clinical trial. *JAMA Psychiatry*. 2025;82(4): 395–405.
178. Torous J, Myrick KJ, Rauseo-Ricupero N, Firth J. Digital mental health and COVID-19: using technology today to accelerate the curve on access and quality tomorrow. *JMIR mental health*. 2020;7(3):e18848.
179. Mishra BR, Nizamie SH, Das B, Praharaj SK. Efficacy of repetitive transcranial magnetic stimulation in alcohol dependence: a sham-controlled study. *Addiction*. 2010;105(1):49–55.
180. Korecki JR, Schwebel FJ, Votaw VR, Witkiewitz K. Mindfulness-based programs for substance use disorders: a systematic review of manualized treatments. *Subst Abuse Treat Prev Policy*. 2020;15(1):51.
181. Goldberg SB, Pace B, Griskaitis M, et al. Mindfulness-based interventions for substance use disorders. *Cochrane Database Syst Rev*. 2021;10(10):CD011723.

9

Tobacco Use Disorder in the Hospital Setting

Erica Heiman, Alyssa Cheng, Stephen Baldassarri

I'll never forget seeing the patient walking slowly down the long hallway in his hospital gown. It was the fall of 2009, and I was a medical intern not more than a few months out of medical school. The patient headed for the door with purpose, opened it, and walked through. He strolled into the courtyard outside, hands in his pockets as he walked. Then, he did the unthinkable—he lit up a cigarette. *No!* I thought. *How could this be possible*? Here he was, admitted to the hospital with an acute medical problem, engaging in perhaps the most harmful health behavior imaginable (possibly even the *exact* behavior that had created his acute problem). Didn't he realize how bad this was? And why was no one here to stop him?

At the time, I didn't yet have the conceptual framework to understand what I had witnessed. It wouldn't be until many years later that I would come to more deeply understand this patient (and many like him) and the complex problem of tobacco use disorder. I didn't yet understand some of the complicating factors driving the behavior—nicotine withdrawal, smoking cravings, depressed mood, past traumas, and chronic pain, among a host of other problems. I decided to study tobacco use disorder in earnest while I was pursuing fellowship training in pulmonary and critical care medicine. I was confronted with many difficult clinical situations in the intensive care unit—a patient with aggressive and widely metastatic lung cancer; another with end-stage chronic obstructive pulmonary disease (COPD), attached permanently to a ventilator, struggling to breathe each time sedation was reduced; a young person with an acute opioid overdose and the resulting severe anoxic brain injury. Each of them, on the verge of death, had something in common—tobacco use disorder. It wasn't just one patient that impacted me. There were *so many* individuals who had this problem. And there seemed to be so many patients suffering from it. Yet, what could I do to help?

As I gained experience as a physician, I started to notice some of the other patterns in my patients with tobacco use disorder—the ever-present psychosocial stress; the underlying psychiatric illnesses that no doubt contributed to their addiction; the past severe traumas that created a persistent experience of chronic stress; the frequent desire to leave the hospital prematurely during hospitalizations, possibly in an attempt to relieve withdrawal symptoms and cravings; and the other psychoactive substances they frequently used to cope. These days, I hardly ever see a patient who is *just* smoking cigarettes. The electronic health record problem lists for patients are long, with a multitude of medical and psychiatric comorbidities. Their urine drug toxicology panels frequently return *positive* for multiple substances (cannabinoids and opioids in particular). Our patients, especially those admitted to the hospital with substance use disorders (SUD), are *hurting*—psychologically and physically.

I've come to understand addiction to cigarettes as something much more than just a compulsion to light a piece of paper on fire, inhale tobacco smoke, and consume nicotine. I've come to understand it as a way that many patients mitigate life's stresses. I've come to understand it as a way patients medicate for a whole host of symptoms.[1] And I've come to understand it as a *reflection* of life's hardships, and perhaps as a reflection of the very fabric of our society itself—a frank portrayal of the human struggle for equanimity. The hospital setting is a place where the costs of the maladaptive behavior are acutely revealed. Sometimes, tobacco use disorder is clearly the culprit of acute illness, such as in cases of acute coronary syndromes or acute exacerbations of asthma or COPD. Yet, in other cases, the addiction may appear as a subtle bystander lurking in the background—perhaps not directly responsible for a patient's acute decompensation, but instead a marker of general unwellness and stress, and potentially a harbinger of future health problems to come.

It can be very difficult to see things from our patient's point of view. Certainly, as a medical professional, it's been very difficult for me to understand why our patients smoke. They must know it's bad, right? And yet, they continue to do it. I've spent many years seeking answers to this vexing question. Yet as I've opened my mind and heart to our patients, I've discovered a paradoxical logic to such a seemingly maladaptive behavior. It is easy now to imagine for myself—if I felt bad, wouldn't I want to take something that made me feel *better,* too? Sure, it might cause me problems tomorrow. But, I want to feel better *today. Right now.*

As a physician, managing addiction is complicated. We do the best with the tools we have, but ultimately, these tools are limited, and the problems underlying addiction are vast. Even so, I still believe there are a lot of positive things we can do for our patients to ease their suffering, engage them in effective treatments, and leverage the resources of our health system to improve their outcomes.

—Stephen Baldassarri

Key Points

- **Tobacco use disorder is the leading preventable cause of death in the United States (US) and worldwide, and commonly results in hospitalization among people who use tobacco and nicotine.**
- **Tobacco use disorder is highly prevalent among people with other substance use disorders (SUD).**
- **Acute nicotine withdrawal may complicate hospital treatment and should be addressed at the time of hospital admission.**
- **Drug–drug interactions and the presence of other SUD create challenges for hospital treatment.**
- **Tobacco cessation interventions started in the hospital are effective, especially when continued for at least 1 month after hospital discharge, and that include a combination of behavioral and pharmacologic interventions.**
- **Linkage of tobacco cessation interventions from hospital to outpatient is vital to increase abstinence, promote continuation of tobacco use disorder treatment, and decrease return to tobacco use.**

This chapter will examine tobacco use disorder in the hospital setting, focusing on cigarette use—the leading cause of tobacco-related morbidity and mortality. The chapter will first examine the scope of the problem. Then it will turn to hospital-specific issues for this patient population, focusing on mitigating the effects of acute nicotine withdrawal, use of multiple substances, drug–drug interactions, and initiating standard treatments in the hospital setting. Finally, the chapter will examine care transitions from hospital to outpatient settings and will explore how hospitals may benefit from optimizing substance use disorder (SUD) treatment for our patients. With great awareness and focus, the chapter aims to support health care professionals making a major positive impact on the lives of their patients with tobacco use disorder.

Tobacco use disorder, like other SUD, is a chronic medical condition characterized by periods of relapse and remission.[2] Given the strong relationship between cigarette use and both physical and psychiatric illnesses, health care clinicians commonly encounter patients who smoke in hospital settings. The pathogenesis of the disorder is complex and includes environmental factors, structural and chemical brain changes, and hereditary susceptibility.[3,4] Tobacco use disorder typically begins in late childhood or adolescence, during a time of rapid brain development.[5–8] There are many reasons for initiation. Among them, trauma, psychosocial stress, dysphoria, and anxiety may be among the most important. Social forces also play a role, as peer pressure and societal norms influence rates of tobacco initiation. An earlier age of onset makes tobacco cessation later in life more challenging, as the neural development pathways become more hardwired for smoking at a younger age.[9]

Tobacco use disorder is more common among those with psychiatric disorders, including depression, anxiety, and cognitive disorders.[10–12] The cause-and-effect relationship between this observation is not entirely clear, though it is well established that coping for a variety of ailments likely plays an important role.[1] Many studies have shown high rates of relapse, also known as return to use, among people who smoke seeking abstinence from tobacco,[13–15] likely related to severity of nicotine withdrawal and the persistence of cravings over a prolonged period of time.[16,17] Consequently, patients typically benefit from persistent and longitudinal care to manage the issue and address comorbidities.

Tobacco cigarettes are highly potent nicotine delivery systems. Nicotine is the primary addictive chemical in cigarettes, though there are thousands of other chemicals present in smoke, some of which are also psychoactive.[18,19] In addition to tobacco cigarettes, other inhaled products delivering nicotine have emerged. Electronic nicotine delivery systems (ENDS) are a newer class of products that aerosolize nicotine via heating of a liquid nicotine solution (ie, "e-liquid").[20] ENDS are addictive given their ability to rapidly delivery nicotine to the brain.[21] ENDS use is typically referred to as "vaping". Vaping is the inhalation of a heated, aerosolized substance. The main difference between vaping and smoking is that smoking occurs at much higher temperatures (ie, >1,000 °F) compared with vaping (250 °F to 500 °F). Consequently, smoking leads to a much more toxic and complex mixture of chemicals as compared with vaping on a puff-for-puff basis.[22] Thus, while ENDS aerosol is inherently toxic, it is exceedingly less so than combustible cigarettes when comparing the products puff-for-puff.[22] Importantly, however, the long-term health effects of ENDS use are currently unknown. While ENDS use has risen in the past decade (particularly among adolescents and young adults),[23] tobacco cigarette smoking remain the dominant form of nicotine consumption worldwide and is the leading cause of preventable death in the United States (US).[24] For this reason, the chapter focuses on tobacco cigarette use as the primary manifestation of tobacco use disorder.

Why do people use nicotine, despite its known risks? Nicotine acts on "nicotinic" receptors, a subset of cholinergic receptors, whose endogenous ligand is acetylcholine.[25,26] Binding of nicotine to nicotinic receptors modulates release of multiple neurotransmitters including dopamine, gamma-aminobutyric acid, and glutamate.[19] The effects of these neurotransmitters in midbrain structures such as the ventral tegmental area and nucleus accumbens are thought to lead to reinforcement and recurrent use.[19] Dopamine in particular is a well-established mediator of pleasure and reward, and is required for the reinforcing effects that lead to substance self-administration in animal models.[27] As such, dopaminergic signaling is believed to be key in the pathogenesis of many SUD and compulsive behaviors, including nicotine.

Clinically, nicotine use results in complex effects on the central nervous system (CNS), many of which are perceived as beneficial to individuals using the substance. When used acutely, nicotine may relieve anxiety, reduce perception of pain,[28] improve symptoms of depression,[29] and induce a sense of well-being.[30] In the short run, nicotine use typically also improves cognitive performance, increases focusing, and results in a state of arousal.[31] In the gut, nicotine acts as a promotility agent and may relieve constipation. The neural changes that occur from chronic nicotine exposure can be very long lasting. For example, alterations in nicotine receptor levels in rats exposed in utero persist until adult life.[32] The adolescent brain may be particularly sensitive to long-term alterations induced by nicotine,[33] which may account for the sensitivity of adolescents to develop tobacco use disorder. Persistent changes in the brain may also account for the high risk of return to use even after periods of prolonged abstinence.

Cigarette smoking is more complex than physical dependence to nicotine. There are substantial behavioral and environmental factors that play a role in perpetuating the SUD.[18,19] Smoking typically becomes associated with specific cues, settings, and people, creating a "habitual" component to the maladaptive behavior. Nicotine has been demonstrated to increase both the intensity of operant conditioning as well as its persistence.[34,35] Furthermore, nicotine use is associated with other SUD (particularly opioid, cannabis, and alcohol).[36,37] Thus, the development of tobacco use disorder involves the combination of physical dependence on nicotine, conditioned behaviors, and adaptation to environmental stress.

Epidemiology and Scope of the Problem Related to the Hospital Setting

Great strides by public health programs have led to an impressive reduction in US adult smoking prevalence from over 40% in 1965, to 20% in 2005, to 11% in 2023.[38,39] Worldwide there is a similar trend toward reduction in smoking prevalence, from 22.7% in 2007 to 17.5% in 2019.[40] Despite these changes, smoking continues to be the leading cause of preventable death in the US and worldwide. This is unlikely to peak until 2030 in the US, due to an aging US population and lag time between smoking cessation and development of serious health complications.[41] Estimates put health care spending attributable to cigarette smoking at almost 9% of all US health care costs, or greater than $289 billion.[42]

The epidemiology of tobacco use disorder, and its sequelae, parallels that of other health conditions that are strongly correlated with social determinants of health.[43] Tobacco use disorder is more prevalent among people with lower socioeconomic status—much as preventable hospitalizations for chronic illnesses are more frequent among this demographic group, versus those within higher income brackets.[44] People of American Indian and Alaska Native heritage have been shown to have higher rates of tobacco use disorder than others, putting them at high risk for dangerous sequelae.[45] Black Americans, though demonstrating similar rates of tobacco use disorder, have lower quit rates than non-Hispanic White people.[46] The decreases in tobacco use disorder prevalence observed over the past several decades are most applicable to higher-income and more highly educated individuals, with those of lower income and lower education levels lagging behind with regard to cessation rates.[47,48] Any successful attempt to address tobacco use disorder must prioritize social, economic, and cultural determinants of health.

Hospitalized populations have been recognized to have higher prevalence of tobacco use disorder than general populations, often by a magnitude of two- to threefold.[49,50] The reasons for this are complex, including causal associations between tobacco use disorder and development of acute conditions; and increases in likelihood of hospitalization, and prolongation of hospitalization, among conditions that are not directly caused by tobacco use disorder. Among the former category, incident lung cancers are thought to be 80% to 90% attributable to tobacco use disorder, and cases of COPD are 70%.[51,52] Among the latter: surgical complications, from surgeries as disparate as intra-abdominal, neurologic, and orthopedic, have a higher incidence among people with a history of tobacco use disorder, which can lead to readmissions and prolonged hospitalizations.[53–55] Hospital outcomes are similarly poorer among people with sepsis with tobacco use disorder, compared to those who do not have tobacco use disorder,[56] and tobacco use disorder may predispose younger patients to development of acute respiratory distress syndrome (ARDS), which poses risk of prolonged hospitalizations.[57]

Screening Patients for Tobacco Use

Screening for tobacco use can be accomplished at the time of hospital admission by any qualified medical team member (ie, nurse, physician, pharmacist, respiratory therapist, etc). A simple question regarding current tobacco use and vaping behavior (ie, "Do you currently smoke cigarettes?" and "Do you currently vape electronic cigarettes?") typically establishes the presence or absence of the behavior. The quantity of use is also typically asked (ie, "How many cigarettes do you smoke daily?"), but reported "cigarettes per day" do not necessarily accurately reflect the true amount of smoke exposure (since one person may smoke the entire cigarette rod, while another many take only a few puffs before putting the cigarette out). The use of other drugs (ie, opioids, cannabis, alcohol) can also be screened at this time. As a rule of thumb, the presence of other SUD (especially opioid use disorder) increases the odds that the patient currently has tobacco use disorder. Many electronic health records (EMR) now track smoking status, and smoking status may be considered a "vital sign" in clinical settings.[58] Anecdotally, EMR documentation of smoking status may be unreliable, as misclassification commonly occurs (ie, the EMR classifies a patient as a "former smoker" when they still currently smoke) given the relapsing and remitting course of tobacco use disorder. Thus, it is important to ask about current smoking status during each encounter. While the use of a "quit date" has been commonly used,[59] there is some evidence that a gradual approach to smoking cessation (smoking reduction) can also be effective.[60–63] In hospital settings, "quit dates" may be irrelevant if hospital policies mandate smoking abstinence. The main challenge here will be developing a strategy to maintain abstinence after hospital discharge (see *Discharge Planning* section below).

Addressing Tobacco Use Disorder in the Hospital

Hospitalization creates unique challenges in caring for patients with tobacco use disorder. As described above, tobacco use disorder is a complex phenomenon that includes both chronic brain changes, environmental factors, and hereditary susceptibility. In the context of hospitalization, there are four key changes that may impact patients: (1) an acute illness; (2) an acute change in nicotine use; (3) an acute change in use of other substances that commonly co-occur with nicotine (ie, alcohol, cannabis, opioids, etc); and (4) a change in environment. This section considers several hospital-specific issues relating to these changes including (1) acute nicotine withdrawal; (2) concomitant other SUD; (3) drug–drug interactions; (4) standard treatments for tobacco use disorder; and (5) severe acute pulmonary illnesses associated with cigarette smoking and electronic cigarette vaping.

Acute Nicotine Withdrawal

Hospitals commonly do not permit admitted patients to smoke cigarettes. (The hospital described in the introduction story above no longer permits patients to smoke as of 2025.) Consequently, for patients who are accustomed to smoking routinely and without restriction, a hospital admission creates the conditions for acute nicotine withdrawal if patients are not adequately treated.

Acute nicotine withdrawal is a complex phenomenon involving disruptions to multiple neurotransmitter systems including acetylcholine, dopamine, opioids, serotonin, and glutamate.[64] Consequently, there are a wide range of clinical signs and symptoms

TABLE 9.1

Acute Nicotine Withdrawal Symptoms

Category	Symptom	Description
Affective	Irritability or frustration	Increased sensitivity to stress, easily annoyed
	Anxiety	Feelings of worry or unease, sometimes with physical symptoms
	Depressed mood	Sadness, lack of motivation, dysphoria
	Restlessness	Inability to relax or sit still
	Difficulty concentrating	Trouble focusing or staying on task, reduced cognitive performance
Somatic	Increased appetite	Craving for food, weight gain
	Sleep disturbance	Insomnia, fragmented sleep, or vivid dreams
	Headache	Dull or throbbing head pain
	Fatigue	Low energy
	Gastrointestinal discomfort	Constipation
	Coughing or sore throat	Possibly exacerbated by concomitant menthol withdrawal
Other	Cravings for nicotine	Strong urge to smoke or vape
	Increased stress perception	Everyday stressors may feel more overwhelming
	Slower reaction time	Reduced cognitive and motor performance

that patients may experience after abrupt smoking cessation (Table 9.1). Acute nicotine withdrawal syndrome has various combinations of somatic symptoms (ie, gastrointestinal discomfort, increased appetite, fatigue) and affective symptoms (ie, mood disturbances, anxiety, depression, cognitive deficits, and craving).[65–67] Acute withdrawal symptoms can be easily quantified and assessed using a validated scale such as the Wisconsin Smoking Withdrawal Scale or Cigarette Withdrawal Scale.[68,69] The presence of these symptoms can be predictive of treatment failure or return to use.[70,71] Symptoms can range from mild to severe, depending on prior heaviness of smoking and host factors. Onset of symptoms can occur within hours after the last cigarette, peak after several days, and can persist for many weeks.[72,73] Withdrawal symptoms may be complicated in patients who use multiple substances in addition to cigarettes. Clinically, acute nicotine withdrawal may be underrecognized if behavioral disturbances dominate the presentation. Patients may be perceived by staff as "difficult" or unpleasant, creating challenges for optimizing patient care. The desire of a patient to leave the hospital prematurely may be a common but underrecognized sign of an acute withdrawal syndrome. The desire to leave may represent the patient's perceived need to "escape" in order to smoke and relieve unpleasant symptoms, so treating withdrawal promptly may be key to preventing this outcome. Thorough history taking to identify the presence of the underlying tobacco use disorder, recognizing the potential for acute withdrawal, and medicating promptly with nicotine replacement (and additional medications for other substance withdrawal syndromes) to minimize unpleasant symptoms may improve patient engagement and reduce risk for premature discharge.

Role of Other SUD

Rates of tobacco use disorder among people with other SUD are estimated at two to four times those of the general population.[74] Although the emphasis of SUD treatment for hospitalized patients may be more focused on opioids, alcohol, or stimulants, tobacco use exacerbates and heightens the morbidity and mortality of people with comorbid SUD. Tobacco use disorder–related illnesses are responsible for an estimated 50% of the morbidity of people with opioid use disorders[75] and concordant focus on tobacco cessation is thus appropriate, as a component of comprehensive hospital-based SUD care. Due to the complex neurologic interplay between substances with addictive potential, people with comorbid tobacco use disorder and other SUD may have a different experience than people withdrawing from nicotine alone. Studies observe more severe nicotine withdrawal scores among people with comorbid SUD, among those undergoing nicotine withdrawal in the hospital setting.[76,77] However, the previously-accepted theory that concordantly quitting smoking alongside alcohol, opioids, or other substances would make it more difficult for individuals to stay abstinent from these other "harder" substances, has subsequently been put to rest. In fact, evidence supports efficacy of concurrent treatment of tobacco use disorder alongside other SUD treatments.[78] Smoking cessation may actually enhance efforts toward alcohol cessation, given how commonly people engage in both behaviors concurrently.[79] Even when they do not lead to long-term smoking cessation, smoking cessation interventions for people with other SUD have been linked to a 25% decrease in use of alcohol and other nonprescribed substances.[80]

Drug–Drug Interactions

Comprised of over 7,000 chemicals, tobacco smoke is a mixture of metals, gases, insoluble particles, and biologically active alkaloids such as nicotine, anatabine, and anabasine.[81,82] Some tobacco smoke components are known toxins, such as polycyclic aromatic hydrocarbons (PAHs).[83] PAHs are inducers of metabolism of hepatic enzymes cytochrome P450 (CYP) 1A1 and 1A2. Nicotine is metabolized primarily by CYP 2A6 in humans.[84,85]

PAH induction of CYP 1A1 and 1A2 may lead to faster systemic clearance of some commonly used medications such as antipsychotics (eg, clozapine, olanzapine, risperidone, haloperidol, chlorpromazine), antidepressants (eg, mirtazapine, trazodone, duloxetine, fluvoxamine), warfarin, clopidogrel, propranolol, ropinirole, tizanidine, and estrogen.[83,86–90] This enzymatic induction is underlying the insufficient dosing of these medications among people who smoke, as well as medication-related toxicity in the context of smoking cessation and downregulation of CYP enzyme activation.[91–94] Consideration for dose reduction of CYP 1A2 metabolized medications, especially those with a narrow therapeutic windows such as clozapine and warfarin, should be considered upon cessation of smoking, as the upregulatory properties of cigarette smoke have been shown to diminish within 4 days of cessation.[95]

In addition to pharmacokinetic interactions, nicotine and other substances in tobacco smoke appear to have pharmacodynamic interactions with other substances. Evidence for a modulatory effect of nicotine on opioid signaling comes from studies examining smoking and use of opioid agonists. In one trial, smoking and nicotine use were shown to decrease opioid withdrawal scores, indicating a synergistic reinforcement effect. In the same trial, the converse was also true: nicotine withdrawal scores were decreased with methadone use.[96]

Hepatic and Renal Effects

Many people with tobacco use disorder have comorbid renal dysfunction and hepatic dysfunction. Tobacco use disorder has been associated with development of and poor outcomes associated with chronic kidney disease.[97] Tobacco use disorder has been linked with increases in the incidence of nonalcoholic fatty liver disease (NAFLD), after controlling for confounders such as weight and alcohol use[98]; as well as increased risk of advanced fibrosis and hepatocellular carcinoma in people with chronic viral hepatitis.[99] From a treatment perspective, varenicline and bupropion require dose reduction in renal dysfunction, and bupropion requires dose reduction in hepatic dysfunction. Because of decreased clearance of nicotine in both hepatic and renal dysfunction, nicotine replacement products may need to be dose reduced, particularly in more advanced disease, though no firm guidelines exist.[100] Clinicians can consider a 50% decrease in initial dose, with upward adjustments as necessary.

General Treatment Principles

Treatment for hospitalized patients with tobacco use disorder should generally follow the 2008 Tobacco Treatment Guidelines, which are applicable to all individuals with tobacco use disorder.[59] Vaping addiction may also respond to these treatments, but there is not yet a robust base of evidence from clinical trials among people who vape. Decisions regarding which treatments to offer may depend on available workforce (ie, trained staff), pharmacy formulary, and patient preference. Many clinical trials and meta-analyses have demonstrated efficacy of counseling/behavioral therapy, pharmacologic treatment, and combination therapy for tobacco use disorder treatment in the general population.[59,101–104] An advantage to hospital-based treatment is that patients are generally in a controlled environment and are relieved from many daily stressors that occur in day-to-day life, which may allow greater receptivity to treatment. Notably, the *combination* of behavioral and pharmacologic treatments is superior to either modality alone.[59]

The Importance of Motivation

Modification of behavioral patterns through behavioral therapy and counseling have been shown to be effective for smoking cessation either alone or in combination with pharmacologic treatment.[59,104] The initial approach to behavioral treatment depends on the individual's baseline level of motivation. **Motivation** is generally a prerequisite for behavioral change, as the unmotivated individual is highly unlikely to spontaneously stop smoking.[105,106] It is therefore important to assess and optimize motivation prior to initiating treatment. The hospital setting may provide a natural form of motivation if the individual perceives their acute medical problem to be caused by smoking. This "teachable moment" may give the clinician a window to promote behavioral change. As such, motivation for smoking cessation in this setting may be stimulated via negative reinforcement (ie, removing smoking to avoid future illness).

The Ambivalent Patient

The approach to the unmotivated or ambivalent patient (ie, an individual lacking a desire to stop smoking) begins with **motivational interviewing (MI)**.[107] MI is a collaborative, person-centered communication style designed to help individuals explore and resolve ambivalence about making behavioral changes.[108,109] The techniques can be used to support any behavioral change, and there is robust evidence that it is effective for promoting smoking cessation, can be delivered by a range of trained clinicians including physicians and nonphysician health professionals, and may have a dose–response relationship to achieving the desired outcome.[107] The core principles of MI are to: (1) express empathy; (2) develop discrepancy; (3) roll with resistance; and (4) support self-efficacy. The object is to allow an individual to discover and express their own reasons for smoking cessation (as opposed to being told why it's important). **Expressing empathy** helps to create a nonjudgmental space where individuals feel understood ("You've been through a lot this past week. I can only imagine how difficult it has been.") Expressing empathy builds trust between the patient and clinician. **Developing discrepancy** helps individuals identify gaps between their current behavior and their goals or values. A hospitalization provides a key opportunity to developing discrepancy if clinicians are able to link the acute illness to tobacco use disorder ("Do you think smoking might have triggered this illness?"). **Resistance to change** is normal, and when a clinician **rolls with a patient's resistance** to change it can show respect for patient autonomy and build trust ("I hear that you may not be ready to stop smoking now. That is okay. I'm here to help you in any way that I can.") Finally, **supporting self-efficacy** promotes the patient's autonomy, expresses belief in their ability to change, and encourages them to take control of their own health, emphasizing their strengths and past successes ("You've had some success before with smoking cessation using nicotine patches. I know you can be successful again, and I'm here to help.") Ultimately, the patient is responsible for making the decisions necessary to achieve a smoke-free life, while the medical clinician's role is to facilitate this process.

There are multiple techniques utilized in MI to shift individuals from the unmotivated state to the motivated state. **Open-Ended Questions** allow individuals to freely associate and explore their thoughts and feelings about smoking ("How do you feel smoking impacts your life?") **Affirmations** emphasize a person's strengths to help them build confidence ("You've had a lot of success before, so it seems you are definitely capable of making changes.") **Reflections** demonstrate understanding and engagement by restating what the patient says ("I'm hearing that you are concerned about how you're going to manage stress once you stop smoking.") And, **summarizing** helps to create clarity, demonstrates clinician engagement, and reinforces motivation ("So to summarize, you're very interested in quitting smoking, but you're concerned about how you'll manage stressful events without cigarettes.") Read more about MI in Chapter 15.

The Motivated Patient

Patients who are motivated for behavioral change are typically receptive to further behavioral and/or pharmacologic interventions offered by health care clinicians. Generally speaking, intervention effectiveness (similar to MI) is dose responsive (ie, greater levels of support lead to greater smoking quit rates).[102,110,111] The intensity of the intervention will vary depending on the needs of the patient and locally available resources. **Brief clinician advice** to stop smoking is simple, effective, and can be delivered in any setting (hospital or outpatient).[59,112] The idea is to influence behavioral change through encouragement, support, and a simple message supporting the patient's intention to stop smoking. The hospital setting may be particularly advantageous for this approach, especially if the patient's reason for admission is related to tobacco use disorder (ie, exacerbation of COPD, coronary artery disease, etc). The advice can be initiated after inquiring into current and past tobacco use.

In programs and settings with the resources capable of delivering more robust behavioral therapy, two key general strategies can be pursued: **practical counseling** and **supportive treatment**.[59] **Practical counseling** assists individuals in recognizing situations that increase the risk of smoking or relapse, and to develop adaptive coping skills to manage these situations. Common scenarios that can interfere with smoking cessation efforts includes psychosocial stress, other substance use, exposure to cues associated with smoking (ie, certain locations or habitual patterns), and social aspects (ie, being around others who smoke). The main goal of counseling is to identify which situations are most pertinent for an individual patient and to then develop the necessary skills and strategies needed for coping. Common strategies that patients can employ include anticipating and avoiding certain situations, reducing stress through other lifestyle changes (ie, exercise, meditation, engagement in pleasurable hobbies), or reducing exposure to smoking cues. Cognitive-behavioral techniques can be used to disrupt common thoughts and behaviors that lead to smoking by creating awareness of the triggers and providing a plan of action to deal with challenging situations. The hospital setting presents a good opportunity for the patient to think through how to "reset" their daily routines in a way that improves their odds of sustaining smoking cessation once they return home.

Supportive treatment provides encouragement and empathy during the counseling process, and its techniques can overlap with those used during MI. Encouragement promotes smoking cessation by identifying personalized reasons for quitting and emphasizing the effectiveness of treatment. It is important to identify the patient's specific motivation, since there are many different reasons patients may want to make behavioral change. Positive message framing (ie, discussing benefits of smoking cessation) is thought to be more effective than negative message framing (ie, discussing harms of continued smoking or using scare tactics) in most cases.[113–115] Empathy and expression of caring involves an expression of support for the patient's feelings and concerns about the quitting process. Patients may express fear of withdrawal symptoms, weight gain, and management of stress, among other challenges. Exploration of these concerns is important at the beginning of therapy and as treatment progresses beyond the hospital setting, since patients are at high risk for relapse into smoking after initial periods of abstinence.

Pharmacologic Treatment Overview

Pharmacologic treatment for tobacco use disorder works synergistically with behavioral therapy. It can be delivered in hospital settings and continued after hospital discharge. There are currently seven Food and Drug Administration (FDA)-approved pharmacologic treatment options for tobacco use disorder: nicotine replacement therapy (NRT) (five formulations: transdermal nicotine patch, nicotine gum, nicotine lozenge, nicotine inhaler, nicotine nasal spray [Table 9.2]), varenicline, and bupropion.[59] Treatment decisions typically account for the patient's current conditions and medications (ie, drug–drug interactions or contraindications), patient preferences, and medication availability (ie, pharmacy formulary and local considerations). All patients should be monitored for neuropsychiatric symptoms (ie, depression or suicidal ideation) regardless of which treatment is selected. The large EAGLES clinical trial examining the safety of smoking cessation interventions found that the overall rate of severe neuropsychiatric events was approximately 2% and 6% for individuals with or without a known psychiatric history, respectively.[116] Some of these events may have been due to nicotine withdrawal, as opposed to the effects of the medications themselves. There were

TABLE 9.2

Nicotine Replacement Therapy (NRT) Formulations

NRT product	Route of administration	Typical dosing	Approx. cost (USD)	OTC	Notes/contraindications
Nicotine patch	Transdermal	21 mg/24 h, 14 mg/24 h, 7 mg/24 h	\$30–\$50 (2–4 wk supply)	Yes	Start with 21 mg/24 h for people smoking 10 cigarettes or more per day, and 14 mg/24 h for people smoking less than that. Many people will need dose adjustments May cause skin irritation or vivid dreams; avoid in people with dermatitis or adhesive allergy
Nicotine gum	Oral (buccal absorption)	2 mg or 4 mg; 1 piece every 1–2 h PRN	\$30–\$50 (100 pieces)	Yes	Avoid in patients with jaw disorders; must chew and park for effective absorption
Nicotine lozenge	Oral (buccal absorption)	2 mg or 4 mg; 1 lozenge every 1–2 h PRN	\$30–\$45 (72-count package)	Yes	May cause mouth irritation or hiccups; avoid swallowing whole; acidic beverages reduce effect
Nicotine nasal spray	Intranasal	0.5 mg per spray (1 mg/dose); 1–2 doses/h PRN	~\$60–\$90 (10 mL bottle)	No	Can cause nasal irritation; avoid in chronic nasal conditions (eg, rhinitis, sinusitis). Fastest nicotine delivery, but generally less well tolerated than other NRT forms
Nicotine inhaler	Oral (inhaled vapor)	10 mg/cartridge (delivers 4 mg); 6–16/d	~\$45–\$80 (42 cartridges)	No	Avoid in bronchospastic diseases (eg, asthma, COPD); may cause throat irritation

no differences in the rate of events across treatment groups. The next sections consider each treatment individually and in combination.

Nicotine Replacement Therapy

Nicotine binds to α4β2 nicotinic acetylcholine receptors and is the primary addictive component of tobacco cigarette smoke.[19,117] NRT comes in various different forms (Table 9.2) and provides nicotine to the brain more slowly through alternative routes as compared with cigarette smoking. As a result, NRT has substantial potential to reduce smoking-related harm and has very low abuse liability. The nicotine patch is a transdermal nicotine delivery system that provides controlled release of nicotine into venous blood over the course of a 24-hour period. Multiple randomized controlled trials and meta-analyses have shown that the patch is efficacious and increases odds of smoking cessation.[59,101,102] Since the patch releases nicotine slowly, it is typically combined with other faster-acting nicotine delivery systems such as nicotine gum, lozenge, inhaler, or nasal spray to help with craving.

Nicotine gum and lozenges deliver nicotine through the buccal mucosa and are used to relieve smoking cravings as needed. They can be consumed as 2- or 4-mg pieces and used as frequently as needed to relieve smoking cravings. The most effective way to take nicotine gum is via a method called "park and chew" where the patient chews the gum a few times and then "parks" it between their cheek and the space below their teeth. The patient holds the gum there for about 1 minute to let the nicotine absorb in the body. Then the patient repeats the process until the tingling stops (about 30 minutes). This can help prevent intolerance of nicotine gum. Nicotine lozenges should similarly be placed between your gums and cheek and allowed to slowly dissolve over 20 to 30 minutes, moving it around from one side of the mouth to the other.

The nicotine inhaler delivers an aerosol, while the nasal spray provides nicotine through the nasal mucosa. Like the patch, these forms of nicotine delivery can be used as monotherapy but are more commonly and effectively used in combination with the patch or other cessation medications. It is important to note that none of the NRT products deliver nicotine as fast as a cigarette, which somewhat limits effectiveness as a nicotine substitute for people who smoke.[118–121] The decision regarding which type of NRT to use depends on local availability, patient preference, and relevant comorbidities (Table 9.2).

NRT is safe and generally well tolerated, including in those with stable cardiovascular disease.[122–124] Nicotine toxicity may result in nausea, vomiting, abdominal pain, heart palpitations, dizziness, and anxiety. Since people who smoke cigarettes typically titrate their nicotine levels to the desired physiologic effect,[19] fatal nicotine overdose does not occur with NRT, even in the setting of ongoing smoking. Other symptoms and side effects of nicotine delivery systems typically reflect the route of administration. Oral forms of nicotine may have more prominent gastrointestinal symptoms, hiccups, mouth soreness, and jaw ache, while the transdermal patch can cause skin irritation. Local irritation to the nose and throat are specific to the nasal spray and inhaler.

Varenicline

Varenicline is a partial agonist of the α4β2 nicotinic acetylcholine receptor.[125,126] Varenicline reduces nicotine withdrawal and relieves craving symptoms in individuals who stop smoking through its action at this receptor site.[126,127] Several studies have demonstrated the efficacy of varenicline for smoking cessation, and the current data suggest that varenicline is the pharmacotherapy of choice for patients receiving *monotherapy*.[128] It has equivalent efficacy to dual NRT (patch plus gum or lozenge),[102] and it can also be used in conjunction with NRT or bupropion.[129,130] Treatment can be started prior to a planned quit date and is titrated up gradually to 1 mg twice daily.[59] The hospital is an ideal setting to start treatment because medication titration can occur during hospitalization along with monitoring for side effects. Although the minimum duration of treatment is 14 weeks, the medication has been shown to be safe and efficacious when used for up to a year.[131,132] Longer durations of treatment may be required for many individuals given the chronic nature of tobacco use disorder. Varenicline can be initiated in hospital settings and continued as an outpatient.

Nausea is a commonly reported side effect of varenicline that may subside with continued use.[128] Other common side effects include sleep disturbances and vivid dreams. In some cases, these effects may be related to nicotine withdrawal and may reflect restoration of normal sleep patterns. Meta-analyses have shown that there was no greater incidence in suicides or other psychiatric symptoms with varenicline treatment in psychiatric populations as compared with usual care controls.[128,133–135] Most notably, a recent large trial showed no significant increase in neuropsychiatric symptoms from varenicline or bupropion relative to the nicotine patch or placebo.[136]

Bupropion SR

Bupropion SR is an antidepressant medication that acts as a neuronal reuptake inhibitor of dopamine and norepinephrine.[137] It is effective for tobacco use disorder treatment as monotherapy or in combination with other tobacco use disorder treatments.[138] Bupropion is typically initiated at a dose of 150 mg daily before the target quit date and titrated up after 3 days to a full treatment dose of 150 mg twice daily. While generally less effective than varenicline as monotherapy,[139] bupropion can be used as part of a combination therapy regimen or in those who are unable to tolerate varenicline. Bupropion may cause weight loss or delay weight gain associated with smoking cessation, which may be advantageous in patients who are obese or overweight.[140,141] Sleep disturbances and dry mouth are the most common side effects of bupropion. Bupropion is associated with a small increased risk of seizure and should therefore be avoided in those with seizure disorders or heavy alcohol use.[138]

Combination Therapy

Combined behavioral and pharmacologic therapy for tobacco use disorder is optimal and is recommended in most cases whenever possible.[59] A multimodal approach may be required to control withdrawal symptoms and relieve cravings for many patients. There are no specific evidence-based algorithms available to determine which combination of medications to use, so much of this decision derives from individual clinical situations. Generally, combination pharmacotherapies (ie, varenicline plus NRT) perform better than monotherapies.[142] However, medication choices must consider the specific circumstances of the patient. NRT typically combines different forms together. For example, the nicotine patch (long-acting drug) can be used with a shorter-acting form of nicotine replacement (ie, gum, lozenge, etc).[143,144] Other studies have shown effectiveness in the use of two or more long-acting drugs (ie, combinations of nicotine patch, varenicline, and bupropion).[143,145] The initial choice of therapy will consequently be determined by the patient's comorbidities and preference based on prior experience.

Severe Acute Pulmonary Illnesses Associated With Cigarette Smoking and Electronic Cigarette Vaping

Much of the morbidity and mortality caused by tobacco use disorder relates to chronic, longstanding use that occurs over many years. Chronic disease complications of these behaviors (ie, asthma, COPD, CAD, and cancer) are typically what result in hospital admission. However, cases of severe acute lung injury do occur sporadically and warrant attention. For example, cigarette smoking is thought to be a cause of acute eosinophilic pneumonia (AEP), a rare acute lung injury that clinically resembles the acute respiratory distress syndrome.[146] AEP may be more likely to occur shortly after initiating smoking or reinitiating smoking after a period of abstinence, as opposed to after many years of stable use.[147] The cause of AEP is not entirely clear but is thought to be a severe hypersensitivity reaction to an aversive stimulus (in this case, cigarette smoke).[148] Bronchoalveolar lavage fluid typically shows an abundance of eosinophils (>25%), distinguishing it from other causes of acute lung injury. Patients with AEP commonly become critically ill and may temporarily require mechanical ventilation pending resolution of the acute lung injury. Clinical response to corticosteroids is typically rapid and robust.

A similar phenomenon of acute lung injury involving electronic cigarette use was discovered more recently and is referred to as "e-cigarette, or vaping, product use associated lung injury" (EVALI).[149] The condition typically presents with shortness of breath, cough, constitutional symptoms, and prominent gastrointestinal symptoms (ie, nausea or vomiting; 80% of affected individuals). In case series, the acute illness led to mechanical ventilation in one third of cases and (similar to AEP) clinically resembled the acute respiratory distress syndrome.[150] The reported range of pathologic findings during the peak of the EVALI epidemic was variable, making it difficult to identify a clear precipitant and disease mechanism. However, the largest EVALI series found that 84% of the cases involved the vaping of tetrahydrocannabinol (THC), the psychoactive chemical in cannabis.[150] Vitamin E acetate, an oil-based cutting agent added to THC oils, was discovered by Centers for Disease Control and Prevention (CDC) in many of the bronchoalveolar lavage (BAL) samples analyzed and is suspected to have played an important role in the outbreak.[151] Like AEP, EVALI appears to be steroid responsive.

Effective Interventions and Discharge Planning

Data suggest that 93% of patients with tobacco use disorder and who are admitted to the hospital return to smoking within 6 to 12 months. However, if they participate in smoking cessation interventions while hospitalized that rate can be reduced to 87%.[142] Robust data exist to suggest that the type and intensity of intervention offered can significantly increase the likelihood that a patient may remain abstinent. A recent study to evaluate a hospital-initiated tobacco use disorder treatment which involved a combination of interventions (automatic referral to tobacco use disorder specialized care including pharmacotherapy and behavioral support) throughout hospital stay and telephone support 6 months after discharge resulted 79.4% of patient accepting the support and at 6 months, 35.1% of successfully contacted patients reported smoking cessation.[143] In pooled estimates, enacting interventions that start in the hospital, and last at least 1 month after hospitalization, increase smoking cessation rates by 36% versus no interventions.[144] Taken together, every effort should be made to offer evidence-based interventions during the "teachable moment" that the hospitalization represents.[145]

Because the benefit of smoking cessation interventions is most effective with posthospital follow-up, thoughtful care coordination is vital. A randomized controlled trial shows that the intensity of linkage to postdischarge care adds to the likelihood of continued engagement in tobacco cessation, which in turn is linked to higher rates of abstinence. For example, the addition of a "warm handoff," defined as a phone call made while admitted to a counseling or quit line intervention, initiated by the clinician and with the involvement of the patient, may result in higher engagement in postdischarge recovery activities, versus simple referrals placed without active involvement on the part of the patient.[146,147] Per meta-analysis, the efficacy of quit line referrals is uncertain, though in a single head-to-head randomized trial, quit line referrals and continued counseling delivered through the health system resulted in similar tobacco quit rates at 1 and 3 months after discharge.[148] The strongest meta-analysis data from a single intervention comes from individual counseling focused on skills and techniques to avoid return to smoking, delivered by nurses, physicians, and health educators that are begun in the hospital with a session lasting at least 15 minutes, and then continued for at least 1 month after discharge.[144]

As discussed above, medications for tobacco cessation are effective. The addition of medication to counseling interventions increases success of quitting by up to 30%, with the highest level of evidence existing for NRT.[149] In one study examining factors increasing use of medications after hospital discharge, the receipt of the medication while hospitalized was associated with a discharge script written, suggesting that starting the medication—whether NRT or varenicline or bupropion—may be best during the hospitalization, for best chances of continued adherence postdischarge.[151] A summary of meta-analysis data for hospital-based interventions for smoking cessation is shown in Table 9.3.

Cost Effectiveness

Coordinated efforts to screen, begin treatment, and continue tobacco use disorder cessation efforts after hospital discharge have been shown to be cost effective. A cohort of 1,641 patients admitted to the Medical

TABLE 9.3

Summary of Hospital-Based Interventions for Tobacco Use Disorder

Intervention category		Risk ratio of quitting smoking	(95% confidence interval)	Level of certainty
Counseling				
	Counseling in the hospital—continued for >1 mo	1.36	1.24, 1.49	High
	In-hospital counseling <15 min	1.52	0.80, 2.89	Very low
	Counseling in hospital—continued <1 mo	1.04	0.90, 1.20	Very low
	In-hospital only counseling >15 min	1.27	1.02, 1.58	Moderate[a]
Pharmacotherapy				
	Nicotine replacement therapy	1.33	1.05, 1.67	High
	Varenicline	1.29	0.96, 1.75	Moderate[a]
	Bupropion	1.11	0.86, 1.43	Low
Posthospitalization support				
	Counseling and pharmacotherapy with postdischarge support	1.23	1.09, 1.38	High
	Real-time counseling without pharmacotherapy	1.23	0.95, 1.60	Low
	Unscheduled counseling without pharmacotherapy	0.97	0.83, 1.14	Low
Quitline-related interventions				
	Postdischarge telephone counseling vs tobacco quitline referral	1.23	1.00, 1.51	Low[a]
	Tobacco quitline referral vs control	1.17	0.70, 1.96	Low[a]

[a]Denotes imprecision in estimate.

Data extrapolated from Streck JM, Rigotti NA, Livingstone-Banks J, et al. Interventions for smoking cessation in hospitalised patients. *Cochrane Database Syst Rev*. 2024;5(5):CD001837.

University of South Carolina (MUSC) Hospital, identified via an integrated program and followed for 1 year, were shown to have a reduction in costs of over $7,000 versus those not enrolled in the program.[152] Indeed, in a meta-analysis of hospital-based tobacco cessation programs, all nine examined were found to be highly cost effective in terms of incremental cost-effectiveness ratio (ICER) measurements. All of them suggested a return on investment far superior to WHO-accepted standards for life years, and quality-adjusted life years.[153]

REFERENCES

1. Khantzian EJ. The self-medication hypothesis of substance use disorders: a reconsideration and recent applications. *Harv Rev Psychiatry.* 1997;4(5):231–244.
2. Joseph AM, Fu SS, Lindgren B, et al. Chronic disease management for tobacco dependence: a randomized, controlled trial. *Arch Intern Med.* 2011;171(21):1894–1900.
3. Volkow ND, Koob GF, McLellan AT. Neurobiologic advances from the brain disease model of addiction. *N Engl J Med.* 2016;374(4):363–371.
4. Lewis M. Brain change in addiction as learning, not disease. *N Engl J Med.* 2018;379(16):1551–1560.
5. Escobedo LG, Anda RF, Smith PF, Remington PL, Mast EE. Sociodemographic characteristics of cigarette smoking initiation in the United States. Implications for smoking prevention policy. *JAMA.* 1990;264(12):1550–1555.
6. Gilpin EA, Lee L, Evans N, Pierce JP. Smoking initiation rates in adults and minors: United States, 1944–1988. *Am J Epidemiol.* 1994;140(6):535–543.
7. Dierker L, Swendsen J, Rose J, He J, Merikangas K; Tobacco Etiology Research Network. Transitions to regular smoking and nicotine dependence in the Adolescent National Comorbidity Survey (NCS-A). *Ann Behav Med.* 2012;43(3):394–401.
8. National Center for Chronic Disease Prevention and Health Promotion (US) Office on Smoking and Health. *Preventing Tobacco Use Among Youth and Young Adults: A Report of the Surgeon General.* Centers for Disease Control and Prevention; 2012.
9. Crews F, He J, Hodge C. Adolescent cortical development: a critical period of vulnerability for addiction. *Pharmacol Biochem Behav.* 2007;86(2):189–199.
10. Lasser K, Boyd JW, Woolhandler S, Himmelstein DU, McCormick D, Bor DH. Smoking and mental illness: a population-based prevalence study. *JAMA.* 2000;284(20):2606–2610.
11. Kalman D, Morissette SB, George TP. Co-morbidity of smoking in patients with psychiatric and substance use disorders. *Am J Addict.* 2005;14(2):106–123.
12. Myles N, Newall HD, Curtis J, Nielssen O, Shiers D, Large M. Tobacco use before, at, and after first-episode psychosis: a systematic meta-analysis. *J Clin Psychiatry.* 2012;73(4):468–475.
13. Garvey AJ, Bliss RE, Hitchcock JL, Heinold JW, Rosner B. Predictors of smoking relapse among self-quitters: a report from the Normative Aging Study. *Addict Behav.* 1992;17(4):367–377.
14. Hughes JR. Tobacco withdrawal in self-quitters. *J Consult Clin Psychol.* 1992;60(5):689–697.
15. Ward KD, Klesges RC, Zbikowski SM, Bliss RE, Garvey AJ. Gender differences in the outcome of an unaided smoking cessation attempt. *Addict Behav.* 1997;22(4):521–533.
16. Killen JD, Fortmann SP. Craving is associated with smoking relapse: findings from three prospective studies. *Exp Clin Psychopharmacol.* 1997;5(2):137–142.
17. Norregaard J, Tonnesen P, Petersen L. Predictors and reasons for relapse in smoking cessation with nicotine and placebo patches. *Prev Med.* 1993;22(2):261–271.
18. Benowitz NL. Pharmacology of nicotine: addiction, smoking-induced disease, and therapeutics. *Annu Rev Pharmacol Toxicol.* 2009;49:57–71.
19. Benowitz NL. Nicotine addiction. *N Engl J Med.* 2010;362(24):2295–2303.
20. National Academies of Sciences, Engineering, and Medicine; Board on Population Health and Public Health Practice; Committee on the Review of the Health Effects of Electronic Nicotine Delivery Systems; Eaton DL, Kwan LY, Stratton K. *Public Health Consequences of E-Cigarettes.* The National Academies Press; 2018:774.
21. Baldassarri SR, Bernstein SL, Chupp GL, Slade MD, Fucito LM, Toll BA. Electronic cigarettes for adults with tobacco dependence enrolled in a tobacco treatment program: a pilot study. *Addict Behav.* 2018;80:1–5.
22. Goniewicz ML, Knysak J, Gawron M, et al. Levels of selected carcinogens and toxicants in vapour from electronic cigarettes. *Tob Control.* 2014;23(2):133–139.
23. Arrazola RA. Notes from the field: tobacco product use among adults—United States, 2017–2023. *MMWR Morb Mortal Wkly Rep.* 2025;74(7):118–121.
24. National Center for Chronic Disease Prevention and Health Promotion (U.S.) Office on Smoking and Health. Reports of the Surgeon General. *The Health Consequences of Smoking—50 Years of Progress: A Report of the Surgeon General.* Centers for Disease Control and Prevention (US); 2014.
25. Gotti C, Clementi F. Neuronal nicotinic receptors: from structure to pathology. *Prog Neurobiol.* 2004;74(6):363–396.
26. Drenan RM, Lester HA. Insights into the neurobiology of the nicotinic cholinergic system and nicotine addiction from mice expressing nicotinic receptors harboring gain-of-function mutations. *Pharmacol Rev.* 2012;64(4):869–879.
27. Leslie FM, Mojica CY, Reynaga DD. Nicotinic receptors in addiction pathways. *Mol Pharmacol.* 2013;83(4):753–758.
28. Pomerleau OF. Nicotine as a psychoactive drug: anxiety and pain reduction. *Psychopharmacol Bull.* 1986;22(3):865–869.
29. McClernon FJ, Hiott FB, Westman EC, Rose JE, Levin ED. Transdermal nicotine attenuates depression symptoms in nonsmokers: a double-blind, placebo-controlled trial. *Psychopharmacol (Berl).* 2006;189(1):125–133.
30. Henningfield JE, Miyasato K, Jasinski DR. Abuse liability and pharmacodynamic characteristics of intravenous and inhaled nicotine. *J Pharmacol Exp Ther.* 1985;234(1):1–12.
31. Heishman SJ, Kleykamp BA, Singleton EG. Meta-analysis of the acute effects of nicotine and smoking on human performance. *Psychopharmacol (Berl).* 2010;210(4):453–469.
32. Slotkin TA, Ryde IT, Seidler FJ. Additive and synergistic effects of fetal nicotine and dexamethasone exposure on cholinergic synaptic function in adolescence and adulthood: Implications for the adverse consequences of maternal smoking and pharmacotherapy of preterm delivery. *Brain Res Bull.* 2010;81(6):552–560.
33. Goriounova NA, Mansvelder HD. Short- and long-term consequences of nicotine exposure during adolescence for

prefrontal cortex neuronal network function. *Cold Spring Harb Perspect Med.* 2012;2(12):a012120.
34. Davis JA, Gould TJ. Associative learning, the hippocampus, and nicotine addiction. *Curr Drug Abuse Rev.* 2008; 1(1):9–19.
35. Guy EG, Fletcher PJ. Nicotine-induced enhancement of responding for conditioned reinforcement in rats: role of prior nicotine exposure and $\alpha 4\beta 2$ nicotinic receptors. *Psychopharmacol (Berl).* 2013;225(2):429–440.
36. Harton MR, Adams ZW, Parker MA. Associations of alcohol use disorder, cannabis use disorder, and nicotine dependence with concurrent opioid use disorder in U.S. adults. *Exp Clin Psychopharmacol.* 2023;31(6):998–1004.
37. Baldassarri SR, Fiellin DA, Savage ME, et al. Electronic cigarette and tobacco use in individuals entering methadone or buprenorphine treatment. *Drug Alcohol Depend.* 2019;197: 37–41.
38. Schiller JS, Norris T. *Early Release of Selected Estimates Based on Data From the 2022 National Health Interview Survey.* Division of Health Interview Statistics. National Health Interview Survey Early Release Program. 2023.
39. Statistics NCfH. *Percentage of Current Cigarette Smoking for Adults Aged 18 and Over, United States, 2019–2023.* Accessed December 27, 2024. https://wwwn.cdc.gov/NHISDataQueryTool/SHS_adult/index.html
40. World Health Organization. *WHO Report on the Global Tobacco Epidemic 2021: Addressing New and Emerging Products. 2021.* Accessed December 1, 2024. https://iris.who.int/bitstream/handle/10665/343287/9789240032095-eng.pdf
41. Le TTT, Mendez D, Warner KE. New estimates of smoking-attributable mortality in the U.S. from 2020 through 2035. *Am J Prev Med.* 2024;66(5):877–882.
42. Xu X, Bishop EE, Kennedy SM, Simpson SA, Pechacek TF. Annual healthcare spending attributable to cigarette smoking: an update. *Am J Prev Med.* 2015;48(3):326–333.
43. Yearby R, Clark B, Figueroa JF. Structural racism in historical and modern US Health Care Policy. *Health Aff (Millwood).* 2022;41(2):187–194.
44. Doshi RP, Aseltine RH Jr, Sabina AB, Graham GN. Racial and ethnic disparities in preventable hospitalizations for chronic disease: prevalence and risk factors. *J Racial Ethn Health Disparities.* 2017;4(6):1100–1106.
45. Odani S, Armour BS, Graffunder CM, Garrett BE, Agaku IT. Prevalence and disparities in tobacco product use among American Indians/Alaska Natives—United States, 2010–2015. *MMWR Morb Mortal Wkly Rep.* 2017;66(50): 1374–1378.
46. Jones MR, Joshu CE, Navas-Acien A, Platz EA. Racial/ethnic differences in duration of smoking among former smokers in the national health and nutrition examination surveys. *Nicotine Tob Res.* 2018;20(3):303–311.
47. Meza R, Cao P, Jeon J, Warner KE, Levy DT. Trends in US adult smoking prevalence, 2011 to 2022. *JAMA Health Forum.* 2023;4(12):e234213.
48. Nguyen-Grozavu FT, Pierce JP, Sakuma KK, et al. Widening disparities in cigarette smoking by race/ethnicity across education level in the United States. *Prev Med.* 2020;139:106220.
49. Benowitz NL, Schultz KE, Haller CA, Wu AH, Dains KM, Jacob P III. Prevalence of smoking assessed biochemically in an urban public hospital: a rationale for routine cotinine screening. *Am J Epidemiol.* 2009;170(7):885–891.
50. Srivastava AB, Ramsey AT, McIntosh LD, et al. Tobacco use prevalence and smoking cessation pharmacotherapy prescription patterns among hospitalized patients by medical specialty. *Nicotine Tob Res.* 2019;21(5):631–637.
51. Pesch B, Kendzia B, Gustavsson P, et al. Cigarette smoking and lung cancer–relative risk estimates for the major histological types from a pooled analysis of case-control studies. *Int J Cancer.* 2012;131(5):1210–1219.
52. Centers for Disease Control and Prevention. Smoking-attributable mortality, years of potential life lost, and productivity losses—United States, 2000–2004. *MMWR Morb Mortal Wkly Rep.* 2008;57(45):1226–1228.
53. Shin YS, Lee Y. Associations between smoking and postoperative complications following elective craniotomy. *J Neurosurg Sci.* 2021;65(6):642–647.
54. Teng S, Yi C, Krettek C, Jagodzinski M. Smoking and risk of prosthesis-related complications after total hip arthroplasty: a meta-analysis of cohort studies. *PLoS One.* 2015;10(4): e0125294.
55. Selvarajah S, Ahmed AA, Schneider EB, et al. Cholecystectomy and wound complications: smoking worsens risk. *J Surg Res.* 2014;192(1):41–49.
56. Alroumi F, Abdul Azim A, Kergo R, Lei Y, Dargin J. The impact of smoking on patient outcomes in severe sepsis and septic shock. *J Intensive Care.* 2018;6:42.
57. Hsieh SJ, Zhuo H, Benowitz NL, et al. Prevalence and impact of active and passive cigarette smoking in acute respiratory distress syndrome. *Crit Care Med.* 2014;42(9): 2058–2068.
58. Fiore MC, Jorenby DE, Schensky AE, Smith SS, Bauer RR, Baker TB. Smoking status as the new vital sign: effect on assessment and intervention in patients who smoke. *Mayo Clinic Proc.* 1995;70(3):209–213.
59. 2008 PHS Guideline Update Panel, Liaisons, and Staff. Treating tobacco use and dependence: 2008 update U.S. Public Health Service Clinical Practice Guideline executive summary. *Respir Care.* 2008;53(9):1217–1222.
60. Wang D, Connock M, Barton P, Fry-Smith A, Aveyard P, Moore D. 'Cut down to quit' with nicotine replacement therapies in smoking cessation: a systematic review of effectiveness and economic analysis. *Health Technol Assess.* 2008;12(2): iii–iv, ix–xi, 1–135.
61. Ebbert JO, Hughes JR, West RJ, et al. Effect of varenicline on smoking cessation through smoking reduction: a randomized clinical trial. *JAMA.* 2015;313(7):687–694.
62. Lindson-Hawley N, Aveyard P, Hughes JR. Reduction versus abrupt cessation in smokers who want to quit. *Cochrane Database Syst Rev.* 2012;11:CD008033.
63. Hughes JR, Carpenter MJ. Does smoking reduction increase future cessation and decrease disease risk? A qualitative review. *Nicotine Tob Res.* 2006;8(6):739–749.
64. Kenny PJ, Markou A. Neurobiology of the nicotine withdrawal syndrome. *Pharmacol Biochem Behav.* 2001;70(4): 531–549.
65. Jackson KJ, Muldoon PP, De Biasi M, Damaj MI. New mechanisms and perspectives in nicotine withdrawal. *Neuropharmacology.* 2015;96(Pt B):223–234.
66. Hughes JR, Hatsukami D. Signs and symptoms of tobacco withdrawal. *Arch Gen Psychiatry.* 1986;43(3):289–294.
67. Hughes JR, Hatsukami DK, Pickens RW, Krahn D, Malin S, Luknic A. Effect of nicotine on the tobacco withdrawal syndrome. *Psychopharmacology.* 1984;83(1):82–87.
68. Welsch SK, Smith SS, Wetter DW, Jorenby DE, Fiore MC, Baker TB. Development and validation of the Wisconsin Smoking Withdrawal Scale. *Exp Clin Psychopharmacol.* 1999; 7(4):354–361.
69. Etter JF. A self-administered questionnaire to measure cigarette withdrawal symptoms: the Cigarette Withdrawal Scale. *Nicotine Tob Res.* 2005;7(1):47–57.
70. Toll BA, O'Malley SS, McKee SA, Salovey P, Krishnan-Sarin S. Confirmatory factor analysis of the Minnesota Nicotine Withdrawal Scale. *Psychol Addict Behav.* 2007; 21(2):216–225.

71. al'Absi M, Hatsukami D, Davis GL, Wittmers LE. Prospective examination of effects of smoking abstinence on cortisol and withdrawal symptoms as predictors of early smoking relapse. *Drug Alcohol Depend.* 2004;73(3):267–278.
72. Hughes JR. Effects of abstinence from tobacco: valid symptoms and time course. *Nicotine Tob Res.* 2007;9(3):315–327.
73. Ward MM, Swan GE, Jack LM. Self-reported abstinence effects in the first month after smoking cessation. *Addict Behav.* 2001;26(3):311–327.
74. Guydish J, Passalacqua E, Pagano A, et al. An international systematic review of smoking prevalence in addiction treatment. *Addiction.* 2016;111(2):220–230.
75. Druckrey-Fiskaaen KT, Madebo T, Daltveit JT, et al. Integrated nicotine replacement and behavioral support to reduce smoking in opioid agonist therapy: a randomized clinical trial. *JAMA Psychiatry.* 2025;82(4):406–414.
76. Soyster P, Anzai NE, Fromont SC, Prochaska JJ. Correlates of nicotine withdrawal severity in smokers during a smoke-free psychiatric hospitalization. *Prev Med.* 2016;92:176–182.
77. Weinberger AH, Desai RA, McKee SA. Nicotine withdrawal in U.S. smokers with current mood, anxiety, alcohol use, and substance use disorders. *Drug Alcohol Depend.* 2010;108(1–2):7–12.
78. Baca CT, Yahne CE. Smoking cessation during substance abuse treatment: what you need to know. *J Subst Abuse Treat.* 2009;36(2):205–219.
79. Kalman D, Kahler CW, Garvey AJ, Monti PM. High-dose nicotine patch therapy for smokers with a history of alcohol dependence: 36-week outcomes. *J Subst Abuse Treat.* 2006;30(3):213–217.
80. Prochaska JJ, Delucchi K, Hall SM. A meta-analysis of smoking cessation interventions with individuals in substance abuse treatment or recovery. *J Consult Clin Psychol.* 2004;72(6):1144–1156.
81. Schmeltz I, Hoffmann D. Nitrogen-containing compounds in tobacco and tobacco smoke. *Chem Rev.* 1977;77(3):295–311.
82. Elsherbiny ME, Brocks DR. The ability of polycyclic aromatic hydrocarbons to alter physiological factors underlying drug disposition. *Drug Metab Rev.* 2011;43(4):457–475.
83. Anderson GD, Chan LN. Pharmacokinetic drug interactions with tobacco, cannabinoids and smoking cessation products. *Clin Pharmacokinet.* 2016;55(11):1353–1368.
84. Hukkanen J, Jacob P III, Peng M, Dempsey D, Benowitz NL. Effect of nicotine on cytochrome P450 1A2 activity. *Br J Clin Pharmacol.* 2011;72(5):836–838.
85. Smith GB, Harper PA, Wong JM, et al. Human lung microsomal cytochrome P4501A1 (CYP1A1) activities: impact of smoking status and CYP1A1, aryl hydrocarbon receptor, and glutathione S-transferase M1 genetic polymorphisms. *Cancer Epidemiol Biomarkers Prev.* 2001;10(8):839–853.
86. Ursing C, von Bahr C, Brismar K, Röjdmark S. Influence of cigarette smoking on melatonin levels in man. *Eur J Clin Pharmacol.* 2005;61(3):197–201.
87. Pakkir Maideen NM. Tobacco smoking and its drug interactions with comedications involving CYP and UGT enzymes and nicotine. *World J Pharmacol.* 2019;8:14–25.
88. Zhou SF, Yang LP, Zhou ZW, Liu YH, Chan E. Insights into the substrate specificity, inhibitors, regulation, and polymorphisms and the clinical impact of human cytochrome P450 1A2. *AAPS J.* 2009;11(3):481–494.
89. Lind AB, Reis M, Bengtsson F, et al. Steady-state concentrations of mirtazapine, N-desmethylmirtazapine, 8-hydroxymirtazapine and their enantiomers in relation to Cytochrome P450 2D6 genotype, age and smoking behaviour. *Clin Pharmacokinet.* 2009;48(1):63–70.
90. Berlin I, Gasior MJ, Moolchan ET. Sex-based and hormonal contraception effects on the metabolism of nicotine among adolescent tobacco-dependent smokers. *Nicotine Tob Res.* 2007;9(4):493–498.
91. Zullino DF, Delessert D, Eap CB, Preisig M, Baumann P. Tobacco and cannabis smoking cessation can lead to intoxication with clozapine or olanzapine. *Int Clin Psychopharmacol.* 2002;17(3):141–143.
92. Juergens TM. Adverse effects of ropinirole-treated restless leg syndrome (RLS) during smoking cessation. *J Clin Sleep Med.* 2008;4(4):371–372.
93. Tomko JR, Ahmed N, Kuntz C, Zick J. A reasonable alternative to clozapine in the chronically relapsing smoking patient? A retrospective analysis. *Hosp Pharm.* 2016;51(10):834–840.
94. Bondolfi G, Morel F, Crettol S, Rachid F, Baumann P, Eap CB. Increased clozapine plasma concentrations and side effects induced by smoking cessation in 2 CYP1A2 genotyped patients. *Ther Drug Monit.* 2005;27(4):539–543.
95. Faber MS, Fuhr U. Time response of cytochrome P450 1A2 activity on cessation of heavy smoking. *Clin Pharmacol Ther.* 2004;76(2):178–184.
96. Elkader AK, Brands B, Selby P, Sproule BA. Methadone-nicotine interactions in methadone maintenance treatment patients. *J Clin Psychopharmacol.* 2009;29(3):231–238.
97. Carter BD, Abnet CC, Feskanich D, et al. Smoking and mortality–beyond established causes. *N Engl J Med.* 2015; 372(7):631–640.
98. Marti-Aguado D, Clemente-Sanchez A, Bataller R. Cigarette smoking and liver diseases. *J Hepatol.* 2022;77(1): 191–205.
99. Rutledge SM, Asgharpour A. Smoking and liver disease. *Gastroenterol Hepatol (N Y).* 2020;16(12):617–625.
100. Sandhu A, Hosseini SA, Saadabadi A. Nicotine replacement therapy. *StatPearls [Internet].* StatPearls Publishing. 2025.
101. Stead LF, Perera R, Bullen C, Mant D, Lancaster T. Nicotine replacement therapy for smoking cessation. *Cochrane Database Syst Rev.* 2012;11:CD000146.
102. Cahill K, Stevens S, Lancaster T. Pharmacological treatments for smoking cessation. *JAMA.* 2014;311(2):193–194.
103. Cahill K, Stead LF, Lancaster T. Nicotine receptor partial agonists for smoking cessation. *Cochrane Database Syst Rev.* 2012;4:Cd006103.
104. Lancaster T, Stead LF. Individual behavioural counselling for smoking cessation. *Cochrane Database Syst Rev.* 2005; (2):CD001292.
105. Fiore M, Jae'n C, Baker T. *Treating tobacco dependence: 2008 Update. Clinical Practice Guideline.* US Department of Health and Human Services; 2008. https://www.ncbi.nlm.nih.gov/books/NBK63952/
106. Hughes JR, Keely J, Naud S. Shape of the relapse curve and long-term abstinence among untreated smokers. *Addiction.* 2004;99(1):29–38.
107. Lai DT, Cahill K, Qin Y, Tang JL. Motivational interviewing for smoking cessation. *Cochrane Database Syst Rev.* 2010; (1):CD006936.
108. Hettema J, Steele J, Miller WR. Motivational interviewing. *Ann Rev Clin Psychol.* 2005;1:91–111.
109. Rollnick S, Miller WR. What is motivational interviewing? *Behav Cognitive Psychotherapy.* 1995;23(4):325–334.
110. Lindson N, Thompson TP, Ferrey A, Lambert JD, Aveyard P. Motivational interviewing for smoking cessation. *Cochrane Database Syst Rev.* 2019;7(7):CD006936.
111. Lancaster T, Stead LF. Individual behavioural counselling for smoking cessation. *Cochrane Database Syst Rev.* 2017; 3(3):CD001292.
112. Russell MA, Wilson C, Taylor C, Baker CD. Effect of general practitioners' advice against smoking. *Br Med J.* 1979; 2(6184):231–235.

113. Toll BA, Rojewski AM, Duncan LR, et al. "Quitting smoking will benefit your health": the evolution of clinician messaging to encourage tobacco cessation. *Clin Cancer Res.* 2014;20(2):301–309.
114. Gallagher KM, Updegraff JA. Health message framing effects on attitudes, intentions, and behavior: a meta-analytic review. *Ann Behav Med.* 2012;43(1):101–116.
115. Toll BA, O'Malley SS, Katulak NA, et al. Comparing gain- and loss-framed messages for smoking cessation with sustained-release bupropion: a randomized controlled trial. *Psychol Addict Behav.* 2007;21(4):534–544.
116. Anthenelli RM, Benowitz NL, West R, et al. Neuropsychiatric safety and efficacy of varenicline, bupropion, and nicotine patch in smokers with and without psychiatric disorders (EAGLES): a double-blind, randomised, placebo-controlled clinical trial. *Lancet.* 2016;387(10037):2507–2520.
117. Henningfield JE, Stapleton JM, Benowitz NL, Grayson RF, London ED. Higher levels of nicotine in arterial than in venous blood after cigarette smoking. *Drug Alcohol Depend.* 1993;33(1):23–29.
118. Russell MA, Feyerabend C, Cole PV. Plasma nicotine levels after cigarette smoking and chewing nicotine gum. *Br Med J.* 1976;1(6017):1043–1046.
119. Lunell E, Curvall M. Nicotine delivery and subjective effects of Swedish portion snus compared with 4 mg nicotine polacrilex chewing gum. *Nicotine Tob Res.* 2011;13(7):573–578.
120. Esterlis I, Mitsis EM, Batis JC, et al. Brain β2*-nicotinic acetylcholine receptor occupancy after use of a nicotine inhaler. *Int J Neuropsychopharmacol.* 2011;14(3):389–398.
121. Shiffman S, Fant RV, Buchhalter AR, Gitchell JG, Henningfield JE. Nicotine delivery systems. *Expert Opin Drug Deliv.* 2005;2(3):563–577.
122. Nicotine replacement therapy for patients with coronary artery disease. Working group for the study of transdermal nicotine in patients with coronary artery disease. *Arch Intern Med.* 1994;154(9):989–995.
123. Meine TJ, Patel MR, Washam JB, Pappas PA, Jollis JG. Safety and effectiveness of transdermal nicotine patch in smokers admitted with acute coronary syndromes. *Am J Cardiol.* 2005;95(8):976–978.
124. Mohiuddin SM, Mooss AN, Hunter CB, Grollmes TL, Cloutier DA, Hilleman DE. Intensive smoking cessation intervention reduces mortality in high-risk smokers with cardiovascular disease. *Chest.* 2007;131(2):446–452.
125. Jorenby DE, Hays JT, Rigotti NA, et al. Efficacy of varenicline, an alpha4beta2 nicotinic acetylcholine receptor partial agonist, vs placebo or sustained-release bupropion for smoking cessation: a randomized controlled trial. *JAMA.* 2006;296(1):56–63.
126. Hays JT, Ebbert JO. Varenicline for tobacco dependence. *N Engl J Med.* 2008;359(19):2018–2024.
127. Coe JW, Brooks PR, Vetelino MG, et al. Varenicline: an α4β2 nicotinic receptor partial agonist for smoking cessation. *J Med Chem.* 2005;48(10):3474–3477.
128. Cahill K, Lindson-Hawley N, Thomas KH, Fanshawe TR, Lancaster T. Nicotine receptor partial agonists for smoking cessation. *Cochrane Database Syst Rev.* 2016;2016(5):CD006103.
129. Weeks GR, Gobarani RK, Abramson MJ, et al. Varenicline and nicotine replacement therapy for smokers admitted to hospitals: a randomized clinical trial. *JAMA Netw Open.* 2024;7(6):e2418120.
130. Vogeler T, McClain C, Evoy KE. Combination bupropion SR and varenicline for smoking cessation: a systematic review. *Am J Drug Alcohol Abuse.* 2016;42(2):129–139.
131. Tonstad S, Tonnesen P, Hajek P, Williams KE, Billing CB, Reeves KR. Effect of maintenance therapy with varenicline on smoking cessation: a randomized controlled trial. *JAMA.* 2006;296(1):64–71.
132. Williams KE, Reeves KR, Billing CB Jr, Pennington AM, Gong J. A double-blind study evaluating the long-term safety of varenicline for smoking cessation. *Curr Med Res Opin.* 2007;23(4):793–801.
133. Kishi T, Iwata N. Varenicline for smoking cessation in people with schizophrenia: systematic review and meta-analysis. *Eur Arch Psychiatry Clin Neurosci.* 2015;265(3):259–268.
134. Tsoi DT, Porwal M, Webster AC. Interventions for smoking cessation and reduction in individuals with schizophrenia. *Cochrane Database Syst Rev.* 2013;2013(2):CD007253.
135. Tonstad S, Davies S, Flammer M, Russ C, Hughes J. Psychiatric adverse events in randomized, double-blind, placebo-controlled clinical trials of varenicline: a pooled analysis. *Drug Saf.* 2010;33(4):289–301.
136. Anthenelli RM, Benowitz NL, West R, et al. Neuropsychiatric safety and efficacy of varenicline, bupropion, and nicotine patch in smokers with and without psychiatric disorders (EAGLES): a double-blind, randomised, placebo-controlled clinical trial. *Lancet.* 2016;387(10037):2507–2520.
137. Ascher JA, Cole JO, Colin J-N, et al. Bupropion: a review of its mechanism of antidepressant activity. *J Clin Psychiatry.* 1995;56(9):395–401.
138. Hughes JR, Stead LF, Lancaster T. Antidepressants for smoking cessation. *Cochrane Database Syst Rev.* 2004;(4):CD000031.
139. Gonzales D, Rennard SI, Nides M, et al. Varenicline, an alpha4beta2 nicotinic acetylcholine receptor partial agonist, vs sustained-release bupropion and placebo for smoking cessation: a randomized controlled trial. *JAMA.* 2006;296(1):47–55.
140. Croft H, Houser TL, Jamerson BD, et al. Effect on body weight of bupropion sustained-release in patients with major depression treated for 52 weeks. *Clin Ther.* 2002;24(4):662–672.
141. Filozof C, Fernández Pinilla MC, Fernández-Cruz A. Smoking cessation and weight gain. *Obesity Rev.* 2004;5(2):95–103.
142. Thomas KH, Dalili MN, López-López JA, et al. Comparative clinical effectiveness and safety of tobacco cessation pharmacotherapies and electronic cigarettes: a systematic review and network meta-analysis of randomized controlled trials. *Addiction.* 2022;117(4):861–876.
143. Piper ME, Smith SS, Schlam TR, et al. A randomized placebo-controlled clinical trial of 5 smoking cessation pharmacotherapies. *Arch Gen Psychiatry.* 2009;66(11):1253–1262.
144. Cahill K, Stevens S, Perera R, Lancaster T. Pharmacological interventions for smoking cessation: an overview and network meta-analysis. *Cochrane Database Syst Rev.* 2013;2013(5):CD009329.
145. Koegelenberg CF, Noor F, Bateman ED, et al. Efficacy of varenicline combined with nicotine replacement therapy vs varenicline alone for smoking cessation: a randomized clinical trial. *JAMA.* 2014;312(2):155–161.
146. Allen J. Acute eosinophilic pneumonia. *Semin Respir Crit Care Med.* 2006;27(2):142–147.
147. Uchiyama H, Suda T, Nakamura Y, et al. Alterations in smoking habits are associated with acute eosinophilic pneumonia. *Chest.* 2008;133(5):1174–1180.
148. De Giacomi F, Vassallo R, Yi ES, Ryu JH. Acute eosinophilic pneumonia. Causes, diagnosis, and management. *Am J Respir Crit Care Med.* 2018;197(6):728–736.

149. Outbreak of Lung Disease Associated with E-Cigarette Use, or Vaping. Centers for Disease Control and Prevention; 2019. Accessed January 27, 2020. https://archive.cdc.gov/www_cdc_gov/tobacco/basic_information/e-cigarettes/severe-lung-disease.html
150. Layden JE, Ghinai I, Pray I, et al. Pulmonary illness related to e-cigarette use in Illinois and Wisconsin—final report. *N Engl J Med*. 2020;382(10):903–916.
151. Blount BC, Karwowski MP, Morel-Espinosa M, et al. Evaluation of bronchoalveolar lavage fluid from patients in an outbreak of e-cigarette, or vaping, product use-associated lung injury–10 states, August-October 2019. *MMWR Morb Mortal Wkly Rep*. 2019;68(45):1040–1041.
152. Cartmell KB, Dismuke CE, Dooley M, et al. Effect of an evidence-based inpatient tobacco dependence treatment service on 1-year postdischarge health care costs. *Med Care*. 2018;56(10):883–889.
153. Lee D, Lee YR, Oh IH. Cost-effectiveness of smoking cessation programs for hospitalized patients: a systematic review. *Eur J Health Econ*. 2019;20(9):1409–1424.

10

Other Substance Use: Evaluation and Management

Paxton Bach, Brittany Dennis

It was nearing the end of my shift on the Addiction Medicine Consultation Service when I received a call from the emergency department (ED) physician. "We have a young man in bay seven who's not responding as expected to naloxone. He was found down, unresponsive, and required multiple doses of naloxone. We started a naloxone infusion, but something isn't adding up. Can you take a look?"

I made my way to the ED, pushing past the usual flurry of activity—nurses calling out orders, patients groaning in discomfort, and the steady beeping of monitors tracking vital signs. As I approached bay seven, I found David, a 20-year-old man I had seen multiple times before, lying in a hospital bed, his body slick with sweat.

According to paramedics, he was found unresponsive in a tent encampment under the highway overpass. Bystanders flagged down paramedics after noticing he was cyanotic and barely breathing. On arrival, they found him with pinpoint pupils and a respiratory rate of two breaths per minute. They immediately administered naloxone—one dose, then another. When he still showed no response, they escalated to a third, and finally, a fourth dose of naloxone, before transporting him to the hospital, where a naloxone infusion was started.

Now, as I examined him, it was clear something wasn't right. His Glasgow Coma Scale (GCS) score was 8—he was barely responsive, only groaning when I performed a sternal rub. But at the same time, his body told a different story. His pupils were no longer constricted but enlarged, his heart was racing at 120 beats/min, and his blood pressure was elevated at 170/90. His skin was clammy, and he had piloerection—goosebumps covering his arms. He was diaphoretic, with active lacrimation and rhinorrhea—classic signs of opioid withdrawal.

David was experiencing florid opioid withdrawal, but paradoxically, he remained profoundly sedated. Given his history—multiple presentations for opioid overdoses and prior attempts at medications for opioid use disorder—it was unquestionable that opioids had played a role in his condition. However, this wasn't just opioids. The persistence of his sedation despite repeated doses of naloxone, the prolonged obtundation, and the severity of his withdrawal pointed to another contributing factor. In the current climate, this was almost certainly related to another substance such as illicitly manufactured high-potency benzodiazepines contaminating the unregulated drug supply.

I discussed his case with the ED team. We agreed that while his opioid withdrawal needed to be managed, abruptly stopping the naloxone infusion risked resedation. At the same time, continuing the naloxone infusion at high doses would worsen his opioid withdrawal symptoms, increasing his agitation and cardiovascular instability. We opted for a cautious approach—gradually tapering the naloxone infusion while introducing symptom-based management for his opioid withdrawal with hydromorphone and clonidine. Given the suspected benzodiazepine toxicity, we avoided flumazenil, knowing it could precipitate seizures in someone with long-term benzodiazepine exposure. Instead, we supported his airway, monitored his vitals closely, and ensured he had access to symptomatic care as he stabilized.

David's case was yet another stark reminder of the unpredictability of the modern unregulated substance supply. Fentanyl, once the primary driver of overdose deaths, is now increasingly adulterated with substances like xylazine and illicit benzodiazepines, making unintentional overdose reversal more complex and withdrawal more severe. Without access to evidence-based treatment, patients like David are caught in a relentless cycle of overdose and withdrawal, with few options to break free.

I stayed by his bedside as he began to stir, his eyes fluttering open. His voice was hoarse as he murmured, "Where am I?"

"You're in the hospital, David," I said gently. "You had an overdose, but you're safe now."

His brows furrowed. "Not again," he whispered. "We're here to help," I assured him.

—Brittany Dennis

Key Points

- **Substances reviewed in this chapter include stimulants, cannabis, sedative hypnotics, kratom, dissociative substances, cathinones, hallucinogens, and inhalants.**
- **All of these substances are reinforcing while exhibiting a broad range of mechanisms of action affecting the adrenergic system, the GABAergic system, the serotonergic system, and the dopaminergic system.**
- **Some of these substances are approved as medical therapies to manage mental health conditions, withdrawal, and physical conditions; others have no approved medical use.**
- **Medical management of intoxication and withdrawal syndromes mostly involve supportive care in a monitored setting and hospital-based clinicians are well suited to provide this care.**

This chapter explores a range of substances beyond opioids and alcohol, including stimulants, cannabis and synthetic cannabinoids, sedative hypnotics, kratom, dissociative substances like ketamine and phencyclidine (PCP), cathinones, hallucinogens including psilocybin and dimethyltryptamine (DMT), "club drugs" including gamma-hydroxybutyrate (GHB) and methylenedioxymethamphetamine (MDMA), and inhalants. This chapter describes the epidemiology and basics of these substances, their clinical presentation, and hospital-based management. The chapter also describes potential for physical and psychological harm, physical dependence, the development of substance use disorders (SUD), and interactions with other substances. The chapter also highlights the legal and regulatory frameworks governing their distribution and use, stressing the importance of responsible use and medical oversight. In addition, the chapter examines the impact of these substances on behavior and cognitive function, noting how use can lead to impairment and long-term health consequences. Strategies for prevention and treatment are also covered, including education and harm-reduction efforts.

Stimulants

Stimulants consist of a broad class of psychoactive substances that mimic the effects of the sympathetic nervous system, described as "sympathomimetic," as a part of their mechanism of action. Broadly, use of sympathomimetic substances leads to physiologic changes including increased heart rate and cardiac output, elevated blood pressure, pupil dilation, decreased gastrointestinal mobility, and urinary retention.[1] Collectively, they are the second most popular class of illicit substance used around the world, second only to cannabis.[2] While there are dozens of different chemicals with stimulant-like properties that would fit within this class, the most common nonprescribed stimulants used in North America are cocaine and amphetamine-type substances (ATS), which includes methamphetamine. Cocaine, ATS, and other psychoactive substances that lead to excitatory effects on the central nervous system (CNS) are also commonly referred to and classified as psychostimulant substances.

The prevalence and impact of stimulant use and stimulant use disorder is rapidly increasing in North America, with the rates of overdose deaths involving both opioids and stimulants rising from 0.6% in 2010 to 32.3% in 2021.[3] The recent rapid increase in stimulant use in North America has been described as "the 4th wave" of the opioid overdose crisis.[3] The increase in popularity of stimulant use and its related consequences are mirrored in other settings[4] resulting in a dramatic increase in SUD treatment admissions for methamphetamine[5] and a 15-fold increase in methamphetamine-related emergency department (ED) encounters and hospitalizations over the past two decades.[6–8] While rates of cocaine use have remained more stable, cocaine is still implicated in overdose deaths with increasingly regularity.[3] For these reasons, the acute management of stimulant intoxication and its consequences is an important area of knowledge for hospital-based clinicians.

Cocaine

Cocaine is a psychoactive stimulant compound extracted from the coca leaf (*Erythroxylum coca*), endemic to parts of South America and used in some settings as a traditional Indigenous medication. It is commonly consumed in either its salt form (cocaine hydrochloride, ie, "powdered" cocaine) or its base form ("crack" or "freebase"). The cocaine salt is highly water soluble and lends itself best to insufflation or dissolution in water and intravenous injection. The base form is much less water soluble and seldom injected, but sublimates easily and is rapidly and efficiently absorbed via smoking.[9] Cocaine is by far the most popular illicit stimulant used in North America, with 10% to 12% of the adult population reporting use at some point in their lifetime, and up to 3% reporting past year use.[10,11]

Mechanism of Action

Cocaine exerts its effect on the CNS as a monoamine neurotransmitter reuptake inhibitor, thereby increasing neurotransmitter activity at the postsynaptic receptors. Cocaine is rapidly and efficiently absorbed, with a time to peak effect of seconds if smoked, 1 to 3 minutes if injected intravenously, and 10 to 15 minutes if insufflated.[12] Once it bypasses the blood–brain barrier, it leads to the rapid accumulation of neurotransmitters such as epinephrine, norepinephrine, and dopamine within the synaptic cleft via presynaptic reuptake blockade. This results in increased sympathetic tone and feelings of alertness, increased focus, and euphoria. It has a relatively short duration of action, with a terminal half-life of approximately 0.7 to 1.5 hours.[9] This may lead to a high frequency of usage, especially among those who meet criteria for a stimulant use disorder.

Amphetamine-Type Substances

ATS are a common form of psychostimulant used around the world, with an estimated 36 million individuals having taken some form of nonprescribed amphetamine in 2021 alone.[2] Their discovery can be traced back to the discovery of the natural stimulant ephedrine, first isolated from plants of the *Ephedra* genus in the late 1800s, and subsequently developed into a variety of synthesized ATS that were widely prescribed by physicians throughout the early and middle parts of the 20th century.[13] While nonprescribed ATS use has historically been less prevalent than cocaine in North America, approximately 1% to 2% of the general population still report lifetime use, and patterns are rapidly changing with dramatic increases being seen in many settings.[5,10,11] This category includes both amphetamines as well as methamphetamine, along with other commonly prescribed stimulant medications such as dextroamphetamine, lisdexamfetamine, and mixed amphetamine salts.

Mechanism of Action

ATS have a similar mechanism of action as cocaine, also serving to enhance the signaling of monoamine neurotransmitters in the CNS. They achieves this effect through three mechanisms. First, ATS promote the efflux of dopamine, serotonin, and norepinephrine into the synaptic cleft, thereby increasing their activity at the postsynaptic receptors. Next, similar to cocaine, ATS decrease the reuptake of dopamine, serotonin, and norepinephrine, further increasing the amount of neurotransmitter available to bind to, and activate, the postsynaptic receptors. Third, ATS decrease the metabolism of dopamine, serotonin, and norepinephrine, increasing the amount of neurotransmitter available to activate the postsynaptic receptors.[14]

ATS are highly water soluble and can be used efficiently via many routes including smoking, insufflation, injection, oral consumption, or administration per rectum. They have a similarly rapid onset of action to cocaine, depending on the route of use, however are characterized by a much longer duration of action, with acute subjective effects lasting for approximately 4 hours, and a terminal plasma half-life of approximately 10 hours.[15] For this reason, doses are often taken less frequently than cocaine, though patterns may vary substantially between individuals.

Clinical Indications for Stimulant Prescribing

Both cocaine and ATS are available in prescription form and have evidence-based indications for their clinical use, albeit ones that are generally limited to very specific situations.

Cocaine Hydrochloride

Cocaine hydrochloride is predominantly available in 4% liquid formulations for use in acute care settings (including the hospital and ED), often due to its vasoconstrictive properties. It is most commonly used as a topical anesthetic prior to nasal or other mucous membrane procedures, though it can also be a tool to decrease bleeding and enhance coagulation in the context of refractory epistaxis.[16] It has similar anesthetic properties when applied topically to the eye prior to ophthalmologic procedures, and can be used for the diagnosis of Horner syndrome, where the lack

intoxication may mask other acute medical issues that may or may not be directly related to the stimulant use, thus a broad approach is still recommended.

Initial investigations should include a complete blood count and metabolic panel, liver enzymes, troponin, creatine kinase (for signs of cardiac and skeletal muscle injury, respectively), and an electrocardiogram if the patient endorses chest pain or has tachycardia. If the patient demonstrates persistent hyperadrenergic symptoms, then telemetry may be considered until symptoms resolve.

Once clinical and psychiatric stability are established, then the clinician should obtain a detailed substance use history to guide ongoing treatment planning.[21] The majority of above-described care can be administered in an ED or hospital settings. In the event patients present with severe stimulant toxicity with symptoms of autonomic dysregulation (ie, hyperthermia), metabolic derangement (ie, rhabdomyolysis), or psychosis and severe agitation refractory to treatment with benzodiazepines, higher-level monitoring in critical care settings may be required.

Stimulant-Induced Psychosis

One of the most vexing challenges associated with stimulant use is the presentation of stimulant-induced psychosis, which can occur with either cocaine or ATS, but is much more common with the latter. While the rates of stimulant-induced psychosis have not been directly compared between patients using illicit, unregulated stimulants (ie, cocaine, methamphetamine) and those using prescribed ATS medications (ie, lisdexamphetamine), rates of new-onset psychosis among young adult populations with ADHD prescribed stimulant medications remains very low (1 in 660 patients).[26] In contrast, it is estimated that more than 40% of people who meet criteria for stimulant use disorder related to methamphetamine, for instance, may eventually display signs of stimulant-induced psychosis.[33]

Though a person exhibiting stimulant intoxication will retain insight or awareness into their environment, a person exhibiting stimulant-induced psychosis will lose insight or awareness into their environment. It can be challenging to distinguish stimulant-induced psychosis from an underlying primary psychotic disorder, however, there are key features on presentation that may assist with this distinction. A person is less likely to present with stimulant-induced psychosis if they have a past history of psychotic disorder, a timeline that is inconsistent with stimulants as the sole cause, or the presence of negative symptoms of psychosis (which are far more common in primary psychotic disorders).[14] In the short term, cases presenting with features of psychosis should be treated with an antipsychotic medication, though there are limited data to suggest a preferred choice. In general, chlorpromazine and clozapine are not recommended, as they may decrease seizure thresholds.[21] A 2021 meta-analysis suggested that olanzapine or quetiapine may be preferred agents in these scenarios, however noted that the evidence supporting this is low.[34]

Distinguishing Stimulant-Induced Psychosis From Underlying Psychotic Disorder

Making a clear distinction between the diagnoses of stimulant-induced psychosis versus underlying psychotic disorder can often only be accomplished after a sustained period of abstinence. These cases should be managed with longitudinal involvement of psychiatry (especially with the use of antipsychotic agents). As a general recommendation, the indication for ongoing antipsychotic treatment should be revisited no later than 6 months after initiation of a neuroleptic, and discontinuation may be considered any time in those with no ongoing symptoms of a psychotic disorder.[35] Prognostication is equally challenging for such cases, but data suggest that persistent psychotic symptoms will be present for more than 1 month in at least 25% of individuals presenting with methamphetamine-associated psychosis.[36] It is also important to note there are some data that suggest neuroleptic agents can also promote cravings and relapse to ATS over time due to their antidopaminergic effects, thus a careful balancing of risks and benefits is warranted.[35]

Stimulant Withdrawal

While stimulant withdrawal may not present in as specific or identifiable fashion as opioid or alcohol withdrawal, the potential for withdrawal symptoms following abrupt discontinuation or reduction in stimulant use is well characterized and can be incredibly uncomfortable and distressing. Symptoms of stimulant withdrawal are characterized by an acute phase that begins within the first 12 to 24 hours following cessation of use, peaks around 2 to 3 days, and largely resolves within 4 to 7 days. This period is characterized profound fatigue, physical discomfort, increased appetite, somnolence, low mood, and irritability.

The acute withdrawal phase may be followed by a subacute withdrawal phase, which presents as low energy, difficulty focusing, anxiety, extreme cravings for stimulants, and mood issues that may last for several weeks. A late and more insidious protracted phase characterized by mild memory and executive function issues may persist for weeks to months following cessation of use, depending on the duration and intensity of stimulant use.[37]

For patients withdrawing from other substances (ie, opioids, alcohol, sedatives), reliance on objective clinical exam findings may be helpful to support accurate assessments and delineate between various toxidromes and withdrawal syndromes. For instance, patients with stimulant use disorder may be experiencing fatigue and somnolence secondary to stimulant withdrawal, however for patients with concurrent OUD being titrated onto opioid agonist treatment, symptoms of somnolence may indicate opioid toxicity. In this situation, examination of the patients' pupils (ie, miosis), and respiratory assessments (ie, respiratory rate of <10) would support delineation between stimulant withdrawal versus opioid toxicity, with the above-described findings favoring opioid toxicity.

There is little evidence to support best practices in the treatment of acute or subacute stimulant withdrawal, and treatment is generally limited to supportive care and behavioral interventions, along with regular assessment for underlying medical or psychiatric diagnoses that may be contributing to (or exacerbated by) the symptoms of stimulant withdrawal. Many medications have been studied in small clinical trials, though none have demonstrated a consistent utility in this setting and pharmacotherapy is generally not recommended.[21,37] Within a hospital-based setting, supportive measures may include the following: (1) ensuring access to adequate oral hydration and nutrition (ie, ordering double meal portions); (2) providing a quiet, low-stimulation environment to facilitate rest in periods of acute/subacute withdrawal with hypersomnia (ie, arranging for a single room, or areas with lower light/sound potentially away from nursing stations); (3) symptom management with appropriate as-needed medications.

Other Acute Presentations and Medical Complications of Stimulant Use

Medical consequences of acute and chronic stimulant use are wide ranging and may present across many different organ systems. It is important to be aware of these complications as their presence may be masked in a patient who is presenting acutely intoxicated on stimulants, however given the breadth of potential complications, not all are discussed in detail here. Some common acute issues associated with stimulant use include an increased risk of seizures, fluid and electrolyte imbalances, metabolic acidosis, rhabdomyolysis, and risk of infection (skin and soft tissue, complex endovascular, and sexually transmitted and bloodborne infections). Clinicians should monitor carefully for these consequences in anyone presenting to the hospital with a history of stimulant use, however no specific treatments are recommended for these complications in the context of active stimulant use and they should generally be managed as per usual clinical care.[21,37] There are specific presentations that may require tailored interventions, which are highlighted in greater detail below.

Acute Coronary Syndrome

The use of psychostimulants induces a strong, immediate sympathomimetic response, which may provoke cardiovascular events on its own, or exacerbate existing conditions. Acute strokes or other infarcts in any organ system can be triggered by the profound catecholaminergic response that is often precipitated by use of these substances, especially in those with longstanding use or with other risk factors or comorbidities. In addition, chronic use of stimulants can lead to premature development of atherosclerotic disease.[13] Stimulant-induced myocardial infarction (MI) can occur by a variety of mechanisms including plaque rupture (type 1 MI) as well as by increasing metabolic demands and/or the causing coronary artery spasms in those with or without pre-established cardiovascular disease (type 2 MI).[38]

In patients presenting with chest pain in the context of acute simulant use, GABAergic medications such as benzodiazepines are recommended for initial management.[21] In the absence of a response to treatment of the intoxication, or if there is a high degree of suspicion for acute coronary syndrome (ACS), treatment should proceed as per the standard of care for ACS. There has been controversy around the safety of beta blockade in the context of active stimulant use, especially with cocaine, out of a concern for the potential of unopposed alpha-receptor stimulation and subsequent hypertension and/or decreased coronary artery perfusion.[39] More recent evidence suggests that this concern is exaggerated, and recommendations now generally state that beta blockers should be prescribed if indicated. The preferential use of beta blockers that possess additional alpha-blocking properties (eg, carvedilol, labetalol) is recommended to mitigate any remaining theoretical risk.[21,40]

Arrythmia

Stimulant use is well established as a risk factor for arrythmia, with several described mechanisms. First, cocaine has a direct inhibitory effect on sodium and potassium channels in the heart and has a modulating effect on calcium-related channels leading to prolonged QT and QRS intervals as well as repolarization abnormalities. ATS can affect the function and expression of various ion channels directly leading to a wide variety of ECG abnormalities, including prolonged QTC intervals. Second, both cocaine and ATS are known to cause myocyte cell death and fibrosis, leading to structural remodeling of the heart, increasing the risk of arrythmia. Last, an increase in circulating catecholamines, as well as stimulant-induced MI, may result in an increased risk of both atrial and ventricular tachyarrhythmias. In addition, various degrees of AV block and other bradyarrhythmias have been described, though much more rarely.[41]

Management of stimulant-related arrhythmias is complex and should involve expertise from cardiology. Sodium bicarbonate is felt to be an antidote for cocaine's sodium blocking properties based on its ability to reverse QRS widening in the context of cocaine intoxication, and should be administered prophylactically if QRS widening is detected.[41] If unavailable, 3% hypertonic saline is recommended as an alternative option.[21] ATS-associated arrhythmias have no specific antidotes, however the use of benzodiazepines may counteract the increased sympathetic tone.[41]

Cardiomyopathy

Chronic stimulant use, most commonly methamphetamine, can lead to the development of stimulant-induced cardiomyopathies. While estimates of prevalence and absolute risk in people who use methamphetamine are lacking, a dramatic rise in incidence has been described in several settings. One California study described a 585% percent increase in hospitalizations due to methamphetamine-related heart failure between 2008 and 2018.[42] The etiology remains poorly understood, but may be multifactorial due to a direct toxic effect of stimulants on the myocardium, recurrent ischemic insults, and/or prolonged exposure to high levels of circulating catecholamines.[13,42]

Goal-directed medical therapy (GDMT) remains the gold standard for stimulant-related cardiomyopathies with a good prognosis with cessation of stimulant use.[42] While historically an avoidance of beta blockers has been recommended in the context of ongoing stimulant use, more recent data has not borne this risk out, and they should be incorporated into the GDMT as indicated.[40]

Small Vessel Vasculitis

Levamisole is a veterinary antiparasitic medication with a similar texture to powdered cocaine commonly added to cocaine as a buffing agent to decrease its purity. It was previously used as a medication in humans due to its immunomodulating properties, however, was removed from market in the United States in 1999 due to risk of neutropenia, agranulocytosis, and antineutrophil cytoplasmic antibodies (ANCA)-positive vasculitis. Levamisole-induced vasculitis due to adulterated cocaine is a rare but well-described phenomenon that hospital-based clinicians should be aware of when caring for patients who use cocaine. Patients may report weight loss, fevers, headaches, arthralgias, and cutaneous manifestations. Investigations may show neutropenia, agranulocytosis, and/or high titers of p-ANCA, and physical exam may reveal hallmark purpuric plaques that can progress to significant skin necrosis on any body part, but commonly noted on the ears, cheeks, nasal tip, and limbs. Skin biopsies generally reveal a small vessel leukocytoclastic vasculitis, and the presentation may be accompanied by concurrent glomerulonephritis, and more rarely pulmonary hemorrhage.[43]

No specific interventions are recommended in these cases other than avoidance of the offending agent, and if there are concerns about a persistent neutropenia or other features of small vessel vasculitis, then early involvement of hematology is suggested.

Opioid Overdose

Stimulants contaminated by illicit opioids are commonly associated with opioid overdose, with approximately one-third of opioid overdose deaths in North America involving codetection of a stimulant.[3] The precise role that the stimulant drugs are playing in these deaths, and whether they are directly continued to an increased risk of overdose death, remains unclear. Inadvertent exposure to high-potency synthetic agents such as fentanyl in those who primarily use stimulants and who are opioid naïve can have devastating consequences.[44]

Harm-reduction counseling should always be included in any care visit for someone using unregulated stimulants. This includes offering or prescribing naloxone at hospital discharge and providing resources for safer substance use. Safer substance use education can be provided by any member of the hospital team, including the clinician, nurse, social worker, or peer counselor.

Stimulant Use Disorder Treatment

In the context of any hospitalization involving substance use, once the acute medical issues resolve, the clinician must obtain further substance use history, explore goals with the patient, and offer and initiate treatment, if appropriate. Current medication treatment options for the acute and long-term management of stimulant use disorder are limited and treatment is largely focused on nonpharmacologic interventions. Figure 10.2 outlines the management and treatment of stimulant use disorder.

Contingency Management

Contingency management (CM) is the only treatment demonstrating robust outcomes for people with stimulant use disorder, including reduction or cessation of substance use and longer retention in treatment. CM is a

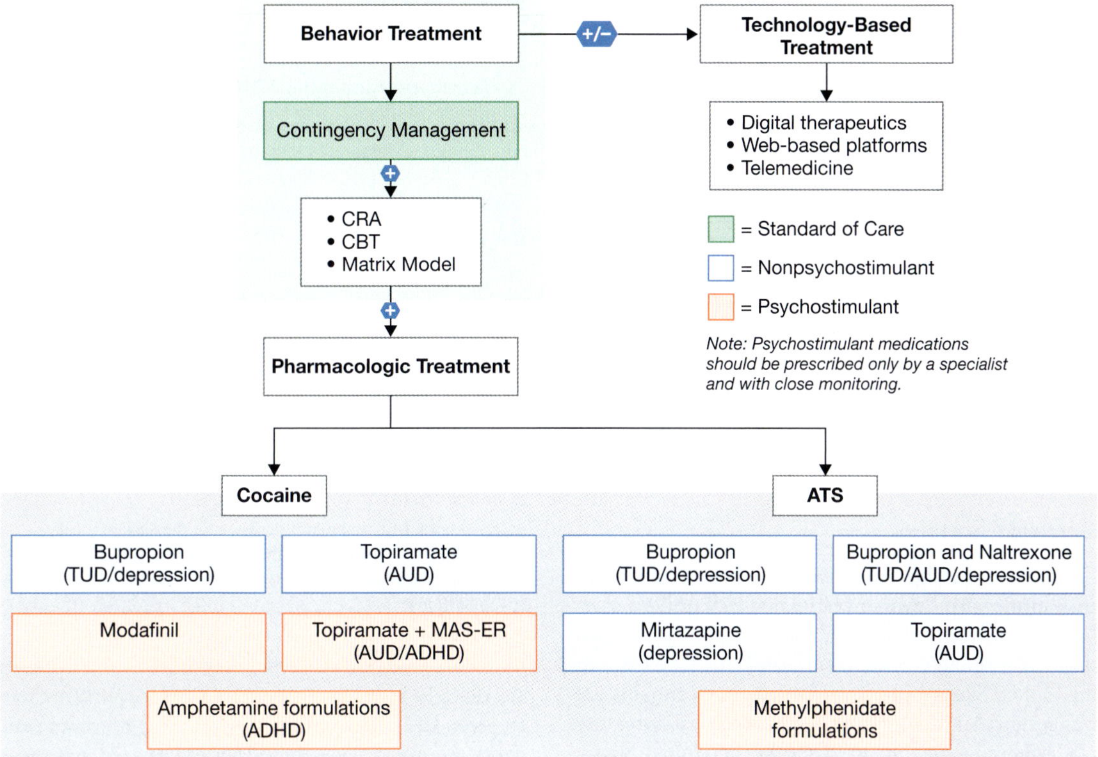

Parentheses contain co-occuring disorders for which the medication has demonstrated efficacy. Clinicians can give additional consideration to these medications for patients presenting with these comorbidities.

ADHA, attention-deficit/hyperactivity disorder; **ATS**, amphetamine-type stimulant; **AUD**, alcohol use disorder; **CBT**, cognitive behavioral therapy; **CRA**, community reinforcement approach; **MAS-ER**, extended-release mixed amphetamine salts; **TUD**, tobacco use disorder

Figure 10.2: Management of stimulant use disorder. The ASAM/AAAP clinical practice guideline on the management of stimulant use disorder, 2024.[21]

behavioral intervention that seeks to incentivize changes such as a reduction or cessation in stimulant use through the use of positive reinforcement, most commonly in the form of monetary incentives.[45] CM has been extensively described in the outpatient setting, with data suggesting that it can be highly effective in helping to promote abstinence from stimulants in the short term, with a number needed to treat as compelling as 4 to 5.[46] The durability of its effects, however, remains in question, as meta-analyses have failed to show positive outcomes at longest follow-up. More recently examples of CM have been described in hospital, targeted at improving outcomes such as reduction of stimulant use, in-hospital retention, and completion of antibiotic therapy.[47,48] Further evaluation and best practices for its implementation of CM in hospital settings is needed.

Cognitive Behavioral Therapy and the Matrix Model

Other behavioral treatment options, such as cognitive behavioral therapy and the Matrix Model, a structured, integrated outpatient treatment program, are supported by limited evidence and may be recommended as treatment options in some contexts, but have less applicability to the hospital setting.[21] Referrals to such programs may be made as available on hospital discharge, as a part of a comprehensive follow-up plan.

Pharmacotherapy

To date, there are no medications approved by the Food and Drug Administration (FDA) to treat stimulant use disorder. While there has been extensive research into pharmacotherapy for simulant use disorder, only a few medications have demonstrated benefit, and these may also be considered as off-label options for treatment. These nonpsychostimulant medication options include bupropion (with or without naltrexone), topiramate, and mirtazapine. More recently, the American Society of Addiction Medicine (ASAM)/American Academy of Addiction Psychiatry (AAAP) recommended the consideration of prescribed psychostimulants as off-label use for the treatment of stimulant use disorder in the context of ADD/ADHD. These medications include modafinil, extended-release mixed amphetamine salts (with or without topiramate), amphetamine formulations (dextroamphetamine, lisdexamfetamine), or methylphenidate.[21] The latter are strongly recommended to be used only by physicians with specific training, certification, and experience in the management of stimulant use disorders. While no medications have been specifically studied for their impact in the hospital setting, it is reasonable to offer these medications in select cases, especially when a clear follow-up plan is in place and the patient is motivated to reduce their stimulant use (Figure 10.1).

Cannabis and Synthetic Cannabinoids

Natural Cannabis

Cannabis is one of the most commonly used substances around the world, with an estimated 219 million users (or 4.3% of the global population) in 2021. The legal status of cannabis varies significantly in Canada and the United States.[2] In Canada, medicinal cannabis use was legalized in 2001, and recreational cannabis use was legalized for adults in 2018. In the United States, its legal status varies state to state and is evolving rapidly. At the beginning of 2025, cannabis was fully legal in 24 US states, legal for medicinal use or in other restricted circumstances in another 20 states, and fully illegal in the remaining 6 states.

According to the National Survey on Drug Use and Health (NSDUH), 22% of Americans used cannabis within the past year, with the highest percentage among young adults aged 18 to 25 years old (37%), and 63% of Canadians endorsed past year use.[10,11] Slightly over 16 million people in the United States are thought to meet criteria for cannabis use disorder, with the highest proportion among young adult males.[49]

The effects of cannabis use vary widely and include pleasurable sensations of relaxation, euphoria, loss of inhibitions, and altered sense of time, along with increased appetite, difficulty concentrating, and impairment of psychomotor coordination and short-term memory. At higher doses, it can result in unpleasant effects including dysphoria, paranoia, anxiety, hallucinations, and psychosis. Physical signs of cannabis intoxication include tachycardia, dry mouth, and a characteristic conjunctival injection.[49,50]

Mechanism of Action

Cannabis refers specifically to dried flowers harvested from the plant *Cannabis sativa,* which contains over 500 different chemical compounds, many with unique pharmacologic effects. The best studied cannabinoids are delta-9-THC and cannabidiol (CBD), but there are over 100 other cannabinoids.[50] The effects of cannabis are exerted via the endocannabinoid receptors of the central and peripheral nervous system (primarily CB1 and CB2 receptors), a complex system whose intrinsic functions remain incompletely understood.[50] Table 10.2 lists the major components in cannabis and their physiologic effects.

TABLE 10.2
Components of Cannabis and Their Effects

Δ^9-Tetrahydrocannabinol (THC)[a]	Cannabidiol (CBD)
Euphoria	Analgesic
Psychosis	Antianxiety
Antiemetic	Antipsychotic effects
Appetite stimulant	Anti-inflammatory
Analgesic	Antiseizure
Impairs judgement	Antispasmodic
Cognitive impairment	Neuroprotective
Reduced coordination and balance	Bradycardia
Tachycardia	

[a]Delta-8-tetrahydrocannabinol (Δ8) is also psychoactive with similar pharmacology to Δ^9 but less potent.

Source: Metrik J. Cannabis and alcohol use. The Systematically Testing the Evidence on Marijuana Project. May 2022. https://www.cannabisevidence.org/clinician-resources/clinician-briefs/cannabis-and-alcohol-use/

Cannabis can be smoked, ingested, vaporized, used topically, or used rectally.[51] It is available in plant form, edible form as brownies, cookies, candy or beverages, tinctures, oils, resins (ie, hash), and dabs (ie, "wax," "shatter," butane hash oil). The effects of these formulations may vary widely depending on the concentrations and specific compounds in a given sample. For instance, typical cannabis flowers may contain THC levels anywhere between 16% and 21%, whereas concentrated forms like tinctures, edibles, and dabs can achieve levels as high as 90% to 95%.[49]

Depending on how it is consumed, the peak onset of psychoactive effects is experienced within minutes, longer if ingested orally, and most psychoactive effects resolve by 6 to 8 hours after intake. THC is detectable in the body for days to weeks after last exposure, potentially up to 60 days, and detection depends on the frequency, duration, and nature of exposure, as well as the type of analytical method used for detection.[52]

Synthetic Cannabinoids

In contrast to natural cannabinoids extracted from the *Cannabis* plant, synthetic cannabinoids use has increased in North America. Much like synthetic cathinones and other new designer drugs, these fall under the broader category of "novel psychoactive substances" (NPS) and are the most commonly reported substances within this category.[53] Often sold under names such as "spice" or "K2," synthetic cannabinoids share structural or functional similarities with THC and were originally designed for research purposes in the 1970s. Since the early 2000s, they have become primarily recreational substances often sold as legal alternatives to cannabis (and one that does not test positive for THC on UDTs).[54] Synthetic cannabinoids are commonly sprayed onto inert plant material and may be smoked or ingested similar to natural cannabis.

The prevalence of synthetic cannabinoid use in the general population is much lower than for natural cannabis products, with lifetime use in the United States estimated to be between 0.2% and 4% (primarily in males in their late teens and early twenties).[54] Compared to natural cannabinoid use, synthetic cannabinoid use carries a 30-fold increase in the relative risk of requiring emergency medical care.[55]

Mechanism of Action

Like natural cannabis, synthetic cannabinoids bind to receptors in the endocannabinoid system, which are present throughout the body, their effects can be much more unpredictable, leading to episodes of dissociation, hallucinations, delirium, and frank psychosis.

Clinical Indications for Cannabis

People report using cannabis (or isolated CBD) for a wide range of issues, and a significant industry promotes its proposed benefits for a variety of common medical conditions. Though the current evidence base remains limited, it is growing rapidly, and the list of potential areas where cannabis products may provide benefit includes a broad range of conditions such neuropathic chronic pain, insomnia, seizure disorders, anxiety, muscle spasticity, multiple sclerosis, urinary incontinence, and anorexia.[56] While approved indications remain few, up to 27% of Americans have reported lifetime use of cannabis for medical conditions.[57]

Nabilone and dronabinol, the latter which may be either synthesized or extracted from the cannabis plant directly, are the two synthetic cannabinoids approved for medical use and function as partial agonists at cannabinoid receptors. They are approved for use in a limited number of indications, including anorexia in patients with AIDS and nausea and vomiting associated with chemotherapy.[58] An in-depth exploration of the evidence supporting clinical use is beyond the scope of this chapter, though it remains an interesting and important area of research.

Cannabis Intoxication/Overdose

Clinical Presentation

Patients presenting to the hospital with acute cannabis intoxication may fall broadly into two categories: (1) those who intentionally consumed cannabis or a cannabis-containing product and are experiencing undesirable effects, or (2) those who were unintentionally exposed and present with distressing and unexplained symptoms including anxiety, dysphoria, paranoia, palpitations, and ataxia, or more concerning presentations include hallucinations, delirium, psychosis, and dysrhythmias. Cannabis poisoning in children may be more severe, including seizures, respiratory depression, coma, and even death. Rates of cannabis poisoning remain generally low across North America, though increases have been seen in the context of legalization.[59]

Diagnostic Testing

Depending on available history, the differential diagnosis for someone presenting with symptoms related to cannabis intoxication may be broad. UDTs with point-of-care immunoassays may be helpful in making a diagnosis of cannabis intoxication, though many limitations must be considered. First, while UDTs are highly sensitive and specific for THC, they cannot be relied upon to diagnose exposure to prescribed or nonprescribed synthetic cannabinoids. Second, as is always the case with immunoassays, they cannot provide information on the dose, frequency, or timing of exposure(s) to cannabis. This is uniquely important in the context of THC. Due to the lipophilicity of the THC molecule, cannabis does not have a reliable half-life when it comes to UDT testing and can be detected in the urine for days or even weeks after last exposure. A positive point-of-care immunoassay for cannabis means that the person used cannabis, but it does not provide any information about the timing of the cannabis use.[54]

Management of Cannabis Intoxication

The primary treatment for cannabis intoxication is supportive care, though in extreme cases, especially involving altered levels of consciousness and/or youth or adolescents, consultation with a local toxicologist may be needed. Outside of severe complications such as seizure or coma, the symptoms should resolve on their own within several hours. Screening for an underlying diagnosis of cannabis use disorder is recommended once a patient has clinically stabilized.

Cannabis Withdrawal

Clinical Presentation

The development of physical dependence and withdrawal symptoms following chronic cannabis exposure is well documented, particularly in those with a history of daily use, concurrent cannabis and tobacco use, and/or other SUD.[60] Common symptoms include anxiety, irritability, aggression, disturbed sleep, low mood, and poor appetite. In more extreme cases, especially in individuals who habitually use high-potency cannabis products, more specific physical signs and symptoms may occur including chills, headaches, tachycardia, diaphoresis, and abdominal pain. Symptoms will generally appear 24 to 48 hours after cessation of use, and typically peak between day 2 to day 6 before resolving, though in those with a history of heavier use, symptoms may persist for up to 2 to 3 weeks.[61]

Management of Cannabis Withdrawal

Cannabis withdrawal can be quite distressing but is seldom dangerous and generally does not require hospitalization in the absence of other complicating factors. The greatest risk for those experiencing cannabis withdrawal is return to cannabis use itself. While there is minimal evidence to guide management in cannabis withdrawal, the approach includes supportive care, psychoeducation on the course and symptoms of withdrawal, coping with craving exercises, physical activity, and sleep hygiene. There may be added benefit of motivational approaches and/or cognitive behavioral therapy, as available.[61]

There are no approved pharmacologic approaches to symptom management of cannabis withdrawal, though a number of medications have shown some benefit in small clinical trials or have been used off-label. These include cannabinoid receptor agonists such as nabilone, dronabinol, and/or nabiximols, diazepam, antiemetics, hyoscine, antipsychotics, and other sedative-hypnotics such as zolpidem and gabapentin.[61] These agents may be considered in more severe cases, though data on effectiveness and adverse effects is limited, and they should be used judiciously.

Other Medical Complications of Cannabis Use

Cannabinoid Hyperemesis Syndrome

Hospital-based clinicians should be aware of other medical conditions associated with long-term cannabis use that may lead to hospitalization. Cannabinoid hyperemesis syndrome (CHS) is a cyclical vomiting syndrome linked to heavy cannabis and first described in 2004.[62] CHS presents with intermittent episodes of profound nausea, vomiting, and abdominal pain that may last up to a week in duration, are temporarily relieved by bathing in hot water, a feature that is almost pathognomonic for CHS.[63] Exact estimates about the prevalence of this disorder are unknown because the picture is clouded by rising rates of cannabis use among those who have other cyclic vomiting syndromes. However, incidence has dramatically increased in recent years from 15 to 32 ED visits per 100,000 population between 2017 and 2021.[64] The etiology of this increase may be related to the legalization of cannabis in many North American jurisdictions as well as the availability of higher-potency cannabinoids, though it is unclear how much of a role increased recognition and diagnosis may also be contributing.

Diagnosis of Cannabinoid Hyperemesis Syndrome

The underlying pathophysiology of CHS is not fully understood and a number of models have been suggested for its underlying causes, though supportive data is lacking for most. Diagnostic criteria are defined by the "Rome IV Criteria for Cyclic Vomiting in Adults" and include acute episodes of nausea and vomiting each lasting less than 1 week, at least three episodes in the past year and two within the past 6 months, occurring at least 1 week apart, the absence of vomiting between these episodes (other mild symptoms may be present), a history of prolonged cannabis use, and relief of vomiting episodes occurring with sustained abstinence from cannabis.[65] The presence of epigastric pain and temporary relief with exposure to hot water are not a part of the diagnostic criteria but are strong supporting features.

Management of Cannabinoid Hyperemesis Syndrome

Beyond symptom management with antiemetics and fluid resuscitation, the only definitive treatment for CHS is sustained cessation of cannabis use. It may take up to 6 months of cannabis cessation, or the equivalent of the total duration of three typical vomiting cycles, for symptoms to resolve.[65] The literature around pharmacotherapy is limited to case reports and several small clinical trials, though in totality it does suggest a potential role for benzodiazepines, dopamine antagonists such as haloperidol and droperidol, propranolol, and aprepitant in the acute management of symptoms.[63,65,66] Topical capsaicin cream has shown a modest benefit in both acute and long-term management of symptoms, whereas tricyclic antidepressants such as amitriptyline may provide some benefit in reducing the frequency of attacks and can be started prior to hospital discharge.[65] If patients are unable to abstain from cannabis use, they should be counselled to reduce their use and track their symptoms, with the goal of reducing the frequency of severe hyperemesis episodes requiring hospitalization.

Cannabis Use Disorder Treatment Options

Once a diagnosis of cannabis use disorder is made, treatment may be initiated during hospitalization, though there are few evidence-based options for management. Psychosocial interventions are considered first line for treatment, including cognitive behavioral therapy and motivational enhancement therapy (with some evidence suggesting that they are more effective when combined). CM programs focused on cannabis abstinence may also be effective adjuncts for treatment. Pharmacologic options are limited, with scant evidence supporting a role for N-acetylcysteine, cannabinoid agonists, CBD, gabapentin, and topiramate. Given the lack of strong evidence or clinical guidelines in this area, the decision to initiate pharmacotherapy is best left to clinicians with some experience and expertise in this area.[49]

For those who meet criteria for a cannabis use disorder and who are precontemplative about cannabis cessation, or for those who use cannabis regularly but do not meet diagnostic criteria for a use disorder, harm-reduction conversations should also occur. A helpful series of recommendations has been proposed outlining evidence-based lower-risk cannabis use, which can be used by hospital-based clinicians to help guide this conversation (Table 10.3).[67]

Cannabis use disorder is more common among people with other psychiatric conditions, including other SUD.[49] Regardless, a comprehensive assessment for other substance use, a thorough exploration of patient preference and goals, psychoeducation about risks, and initiation of other treatments, as appropriate, is recommended in all patients with psychiatric conditions.

TABLE 10.3

Canada's Lower-Risk Cannabis Use Guidelines[67]

Abstinence

1. The most effective way to avoid the risks of cannabis use is to abstain from use.

Age of initial use

2. Delaying cannabis use, at least until after adolescence, will reduce the likelihood or severity of adverse health outcomes.

Choice of cannabis products

3. Use products with low THC content and high CBD: content.

4. Synthetic cannabis products, such as K2 and Spice, should be avoided.

Cannabis use methods and practices

5. Avoid smoking burnt cannabis and choose safer inhalation methods including vaporizers, e-cigarette devices, and edibles.

6. If cannabis is smoked, avoid harmful practices such as inhaling deeply or breath-holding.

Frequency and intensity of use

7. Avoid frequent or intensive use, and limit consumption to occasional use, such as only 1 day a week or on weekends, or less.

Cannabis use and driving

8. Do not drive or operate other machinery for at least 6 h after using cannabis. Combining alcohol and cannabis increases impairment and should be avoided.

Special-risk populations

9. People with a personal or family history of psychosis or substance use disorders, as well as pregnant women, should not use cannabis at all.

Combining risks for risk behaviors

10. Avoid combining any of the risk factors related to cannabis use. Multiple high-risk behaviors will amplify the likelihood or severity of adverse outcomes. For example, early age onset of cannabis use, combined with frequent use of high-potency cannabis, is likely to disproportionately increase the risks of experiencing both acute and chronic problems.

Sedative Hypnotics—Benzodiazepines

History of Benzodiazepines

Benzodiazepines are a class of gamma-aminobutyric acid (GABA) adrenergic medications with psychoactive effects, primarily used for their anxiolytic, sedative, muscle relaxant, and anticonvulsant properties.[68–70] Originally synthesized in the 1956 by Austrian Scientist Leo Sternbach, benzodiazepines were adopted as sedative hypnotic agents with an improved safety profile that distinguished them from existing sedative hypnotics such as barbiturates like phenobarbital.[68] Developed as a safer alternative to barbiturates, they gained popularity due to their lower risk of respiratory depression in overdose.[69] Throughout the 1960s and 1970s, benzodiazepines were widely prescribed for conditions such as anxiety, insomnia, seizures, and acute alcohol withdrawal syndrome.[68] Broad prescribing practices and long-term use raised concerns due to the risk of dependence, tolerance, and withdrawal symptoms.[70] Over time, medical guidelines emphasized cautious prescribing,[71–73] reserving benzodiazepines for short-term or intermittent use for restricted indications.[74] Despite this, benzodiazepines remain widely used and likely prescribed beyond their indication,[75,76] which has triggered concerns for the potential for misuse and dependence, centering them as an ongoing focus of public health discussions.

Epidemiology of Benzodiazepine Use

Benzodiazepine use is prevalent globally and remains one of the most widely prescribed psychotropic medications in middle-to-high income countries. Past-year prevalence of benzodiazepine use for individuals over 18 years or older in North America is estimated to be between 5% and 10%.[77–79] Past-year nonmedical use of benzodiazepine was far lower at 0.5% of the population.[78,79] It is estimated that approximately 4% of the general population will use benzodiazepines for nonmedical reasons at some point in their lifetime.[80]

Major depression is the most common comorbidity among patients taking benzodiazepines. High rates of coprescribing benzodiazepines and antidepressants are observed among populations with major depressive disorder. The 2002 Canadian Community Health Survey identified that 49% of individuals who reported major depressive episode within the past 12 months were coprescribed benzodiazepines and antidepressants.[81] Prescribing differences varied by gender, whereby women had higher rates of benzodiazepine use[77,82,83] However, evaluation of yearly trends in Canada suggests that men are increasingly being prescribed sedative medications, including benzodiazepines.[82] Prescription data from the United States demonstrates that long-term benzodiazepine use is more prevalent among adults aged 65 years and older (31%) compared to adults aged 18 to 35 years old (15%).[77]

Mechanism of Action

Benzodiazepines exert their physiologic effects by enhancing the action of GABA, the brain's primary inhibitory neurotransmitter, through binding to $GABA_A$ receptors.[84] Binding of $GABA_A$ receptors leads to increased propagation of ionic currents through the ligand-gated chloride channel, ultimately resulting in sedation, reduced anxiety, and muscle relaxation.[84] Upon repeated use, neuroadaptive changes lead to downregulation of $GABA_A$ receptors, disrupting the balance between excitatory and inhibitory neurotransmission, contributing to tolerance and dependence as well as withdrawal syndromes upon abrupt cessation.[85]

Considering the compensatory mechanism between GABA and glutamatergic neurotransmission, withdrawal of benzodiazepines will lead to increase in excitatory neurotransmission mediated by glutamate, which is no longer balanced by enhanced GABA activity.[85] Disruption in the GABA and glutamate balance leads to an increase in excitatory glutaminergic neurotransmission. This is marked by subjective reports of anxiety and insomnia and objective signs of autonomic hyperactivity, including tachycardia, hypertension, and diaphoresis. Collectively, these symptoms characterize symptoms of benzodiazepine withdrawal and contribute to the complexities of managing benzodiazepine dependence and use disorders.

Benzodiazepine Use Disorder

Benzodiazepine use disorder, characterized by ongoing unhealthy use despite physical harms and significant social consequences, affects an estimated 1% of the general population.[80] Among individuals who reported using benzodiazepines for nonmedical use, the life-time prevalence of benzodiazepine use disorder was much higher at 26%.[80] Risk factors for developing a benzodiazepine use disorder include: female sex, long-term use of high benzodiazepine doses, any use of short-acting benzodiazepines, previous history of SUD, history of insomnia or chronic dysphoria, passively dependent personalities, older age, and Caucasian ethnicity.[86,87]

The growing recognition of these risks has prompted efforts to implement safer prescribing practices, such as limiting the duration of use, employing gradual tapering strategies, and offering nonbenzodiazepine alternatives for anxiety and insomnia. The selection of the type of benzodiazepine prescribed and used is important. Compared to other commonly prescribed benzodiazepines, alprazolam and clonazepam have a higher potential for misuse and are associated with the highest number of substance-related ED encounters.[88] ED encounters or hospitalizations related to alprazolam are more than double that of clonazepam,[88] though this may be attributed to higher prescribing rates of alprazolam compared to clonazepam.[89] In 2009, more than 44 million alprazolam prescriptions were dispensed, more than double the number of clonazepam prescriptions dispensed that same year.[89]

Illicitly Manufactured Benzodiazepines

The US Drug Enforcement Agency (DEA) has identified synthetic compounds known as "designer" benzodiazepines as the adulterants of major concern emerging within the illicit fentanyl supply.[90,91]

Research demonstrates that illicit fentanyl combined with unregulated psychoactive substances, including illicitly manufactured benzodiazepines, is responsible for rising overdose deaths.[92–98] The proliferation of illicitly manufactured synthetic adulterants has been noted among illicit substance surveillance programs across the United States.[99,100]

Commonly identified illicitly manufactured benzodiazepines include clonazolam, deschloroetizolam, diclazepam, etizolam, flubromazepam, flubromazolam, and meclonazepam.[101–104] Illicitly manufactured benzodiazepines potentiate the sedating effects of fentanyl, causing heavy sedation, amnesia, rapid development of tolerance, atypical withdrawal syndromes.[102–104] Furthermore, illicitly manufactured benzodiazepines are often dosed in microgram quantities, leading to substantial variability in their effects, increasing risks of overdose and other side effects. Overall, these synthetic contaminants are implicated as a source of increasing rates of oversedation, respiratory depression, and naloxone-resistant overdose.[105,106]

Benzodiazepine-involved overdoses have steadily increased since 2015[107,108] and were implicated in 12,500 deaths in 2021. Of these deaths, 70% involved fentanyl, a stark rise from 20% in 2015.[107] Overall, the emergence of fentanyl and its associated contaminants has created a uniquely challenging and deadly substance supply, with correspondingly difficult to manage SUD characterized by increased opioid tolerance[109] and more complex withdrawal.[110] It is anticipated that rates of benzodiazepine use disorder and associated harms resulting from use will rise, given the increasing presence of illicitly manufactured benzodiazepines.

Clinical Indications for Benzodiazepine Prescribing

Benzodiazepines were initially conceptualized as a safer alternative to barbiturates for anxiety and insomnia treatment. Their broad clinical indications, which include generalized anxiety, sleep disturbance, seizures, and withdrawal, and overall perceived safety profile contributed to widespread use, often for extended durations. Over time, growing awareness of their potential for dependence, misuse, and adverse effects, particularly in older adults and those with comorbid SUD, led to a significant shift in prescribing practices. Today, benzodiazepine use is guided by more restrictive clinical indications, such as short-term management of acute anxiety or severe insomnia and is often reserved for situations where other therapeutic options have proven ineffective. Benzodiazepine prescribing stewardship emphasizes careful patient selection, limited duration of use, regular reassessment, and consideration of nonpharmacologic alternatives, reflecting a broader effort to mitigate risks and promote safer benzodiazepine prescribing practices. Table 10.4 includes a full list of indications for benzodiazepine prescribing.

In the hospital setting, benzodiazepines are commonly used for acute alcohol withdrawal syndrome, sedation for procedures, and severe agitation. Benzodiazepines are contraindicated to treat agitation or agitation in elderly patients, given higher risks for falls, delirium, and mortality.[111]

Benzodiazepine Toxicity/Overdose

Clinical Presentation

Benzodiazepine toxicity occurs when a person is exposed to excessive amounts of benzodiazepines leading to CNS depression. Benzodiazepine toxicity or "overdose" presents as sedation, slurred speech, ataxia, drowsiness, and impaired cognition. In severe cases, respiratory depression, hypotension, and coma can occur, particularly when benzodiazepines are combined with other CNS depressants such as alcohol, opioids, or other sedatives (ie, xylazine). Unlike other sedative agents, isolated benzodiazepine overdose rarely leads to fatal respiratory compromise and is thought to stem from the low density of binding sites in the brainstem respiratory center for orally ingested benzodiazepines.[112] The risk of life-threatening toxicity increases significantly in polysubstance ingestions, which are becoming more common with sedating adulterants in the toxic, unregulated substance supply. Table 10.5 includes signs and symptoms of benzodiazepine toxicity/overdose.

Diagnostic Testing

While the patient's clinical history will likely be the most important aspect in confirming benzodiazepine consumption, additional tests can support the assessment for patients presenting with prolonged sedation and encephalopathy. Diagnostic work-up should include a complete blood count, complete metabolic panel, blood gases (if hypoxic or encephalopathic), noncontrast CT scan of the brain if encephalopathic, electroencephalogram (EEG), a chest radiograph if hypoxic, and UDT followed by urine GC-MS for confirmatory analysis if the UDT is positive. Last, consider an electrocardiogram to rule out cardiac causes of encephalopathy.

Urine Drug Testing

The UDT will be helpful in determining exposure to some benzodiazepines, but most point-of-care tests may not detect clonazepam and emerging, unregulated synthetic benzodiazepines (ie, etizolam).

TABLE 10.4

Indications for Benzodiazepine Prescribing

Indication	Type of benzodiazepine prescribed	Duration of use
Anxiety	**Short acting:** Lorazepam, alprazolam **Long-acting:** Diazepam, clonazepam	Short-term (2–4 wk) to manage acute symptoms; not recommended for long-term use due to risk of physical dependence. Often used in situational anxiety: panic attacks, exposure to panic-inducing fear (airplane ride).
Generalized anxiety disorder (GAD)	**Short acting:** Alprazolam **Long acting:** Clonazepam	Not recommended for long-term treatment of GAD.[113] In general, short-term (2–4 wk) to address acute symptoms; long-term management should rely on nonbenzodiazepine therapies like cognitive behavioral therapy or other pharmacologic agents including selective serotonergic reuptake inhibitors.
Insomnia	**Short acting:** Temazepam, triazolam	Short-term (7–10 d); intermittent use preferred to minimize risk of tolerance and physical dependence. Usually context specific.
Acute alcohol withdrawal syndrome	**Long acting:** Diazepam, chlordiazepoxide	Recommended for management in patients with history of complicated acute withdrawal syndrome. Typical treatment is 3–7 d, discontinued when withdrawal symptoms subside.
Benzodiazepine withdrawal	**Long acting:** Diazepam, clonazepam	Gradual taper over weeks to months depending on severity of withdrawal and prior dose; individualized to prevent withdrawal seizures or rebound anxiety.[113]
Seizure episode	**Short acting:** Lorazepam	Used for emergency management of seizures. This is the first-line treatment for abortion of seizures
Seizure disorders	**Long acting:** Clonazepam, diazepam	While far less common now, in certain conditions, benzodiazepines can be prescribed long-term for seizure management; periodic evaluation needed to assess continued appropriateness.
Panic disorder	**Short acting:** Lorazepam, alprazolam **Long acting:** Clonazepam	Short-term for acute attacks or bridging therapy while initiating long term treatments (eg, serotonergic reuptake inhibitors); re-evaluate use after 4–6 wk.
Muscle spasms	**Long acting:** Diazepam	Short-term use (2–4 wk) to manage acute muscle spasms; ongoing use typically not recommended unless other treatments fail.
Sedation (procedural)	**Short acting:** Midazolam	Single use for procedural sedation or preoperative anxiety; not intended for routine or prolonged use.
Catatonia	**Short acting:** Lorazepam	Can be used short-term (days to weeks) to manage symptoms; monitor for clinical response and taper as condition improves.
Agitation in acute care	**Short acting:** Lorazepam, midazolam	Short-term as needed during acute episodes, often in hospital settings; use should be reassessed frequently.
Stimulant intoxication	**Short acting:** Lorazepam, midazolam	Single or short-term use (hours to 1–2 d) to manage acute agitation, anxiety, or seizures associated with stimulant intoxication.

Furthermore, a positive UDT result for benzodiazepine should not be interpreted as diagnostic for benzodiazepine toxicity, as the UDT only confirms a benzodiazepine exposure at some point in the recent past. The quantity and timing of exposure cannot be confirmed through a UDT. Figure 10.3 highlights the metabolism of commonly used benzodiazepines.

The hospital clinician should review the patient's medical history, active prescriptions, and chart for any medications given during the hospitalization as these may confound the interpretation. Ultimately, in this context, GC-MS will be helpful in determining the exact substances an individual is exposed to; however, this test can take time and will not available during initial stages of in-hospital symptom management.

Serum Drug Testing

Assessment of serum benzodiazepine concentrations is not recommended due to limited availability in most hospital settings. Serum testing for benzodiazepine levels takes time, limiting the ability for

TABLE 10.5

Signs and Symptoms of Benzodiazepine Toxicity/Overdose

Sign	Description	Typical duration
Sedation	Reduced alertness and responsiveness to external stimuli.	Hours to a day, depending on dose and half-life.
Drowsiness	Excessive sleepiness, often with difficulty staying awake.	Hours, can persist longer in overdose situations.
Slurred speech	Impaired articulation and slowed or unclear speech.	Hours to a day, depending on drug clearance.
Ataxia	Loss of coordination, unsteady gait, and balance issues.	Hours, may persist until drug levels decrease.
Confusion	Disorientation, difficulty thinking clearly, and impaired cognition.	Hours to a day, usually resolves as drug is metabolized.
Hypotonia	Decreased muscle tone leading to generalized weakness.	Hours, resolves with drug elimination.
Respiratory depression	Slowed or shallow breathing due to CNS depression.	Can persist for hours to days, especially with coingestants.
Coma	Profound unresponsiveness with no reaction to external stimuli.	Variable, depends on severity and treatment response.

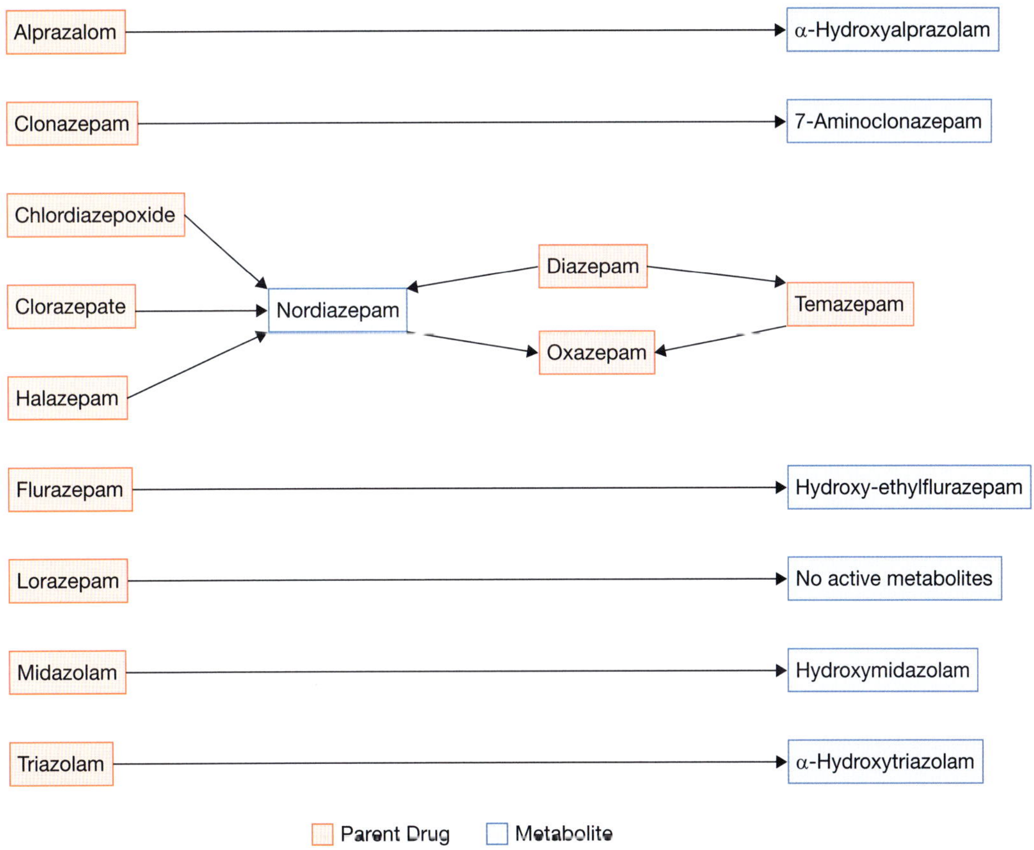

Figure 10.3: Benzodiazepine metabolism. (Price JW. Benzodiazepines and workplace safety: an examination of postaccident urine drug tests. *J Addict Med.* 2014;8(5):333–337.)

real-time correlation with clinical findings. However, in certain contexts, serum concentrations can serve as confirmatory forensic tests, with specific examples including unintentional exposures through targeted poisoning, such as in cases of sexual assault.

Management of Benzodiazepine Overdose

Management of benzodiazepine overdose requires hospitalization and supportive care with airway protection and monitoring of vital signs. Patients should be placed in a monitored area with telemetry, continuous oxygen monitoring, and frequent general and neurologic vital assessments (eg, every hour) until the patient is alert and oriented. In cases of severe CNS depression, flumazenil, a benzodiazepine receptor antagonist, may be administered. Its use is somewhat limited due to the risk of provoking seizures, particularly in patients with benzodiazepine dependence or coingestion of proconvulsant substances. In patients where prolonged exposure to benzodiazepines is suspected (ie, patients on prescribed benzodiazepines, patients with documented history of daily exposure to illicitly manufactured fentanyl in regions where unregulated benzodiazepines are prevalent), flumazenil is more likely to precipitate seizure. Whenever possible, administer naloxone to patients presenting with an overdose to determine if the overdose is related to an opioid or co-use of an opioid and benzodiazepine.

Management Following Resolution of Overdose Symptoms

Upon resolution of benzodiazepine toxicity, further discussions should be undertaken to determine whether the patient meets criteria for benzodiazepine use disorder. Intentional versus unintentional use must be discerned with appropriate harm-reduction counseling for patients presenting with overdose from unintentional exposure to benzodiazepines in the illicit substance supply. Emphasis should be placed on promoting safer substance use practices, including where possible: provision of naloxone for co-use of opioids and benzodiazepines, using drug checking services, consuming unregulated substances in overdose prevention sites, or if not available in the community, suggest co-use with a trusted individuals who would be willing and able to call emergency services in the event of an overdose.

Considerations for Patients Experiencing Benzodiazepine Toxicity from Prolonged Parenteral Exposure to Benzodiazepines

Patients experiencing benzodiazepine toxicity following prolonged exposure to intravenous benzodiazepines, namely diazepam or lorazepam, are at risk for propylene glycol toxicity. Diazepam and lorazepam contain propylene glycol as a diluent. Frequent and large volume exposures to propylene glycol can lead to an anion gap metabolic acidosis (AGMA). If a patient receiving prolonged intravenous diazepam or lorazepam develops an AGMA, rule out other causes with a blood gas and basic chemistries, and if none are identified, discontinue the intravenous diazepam or lorazepam and switch to an oral benzodiazepine or an alternative intravenous benzodiazepine.

Benzodiazepine Withdrawal

Clinical Presentation

Benzodiazepine withdrawal occurs when people who are regularly exposed to benzodiazepines, particularly at high doses or over extended periods, reduce or abruptly stop their use. Benzodiazepine withdrawal is characterized by a range of physical and psychological symptoms that develop in response to adaptations in the CNS secondary to long-term benzodiazepine exposure. Symptoms are driven by rebound hyperactivity and imbalance of excitatory and inhibitory neurotransmission, favoring excitatory processes.

Early symptoms of benzodiazepine withdrawal include restlessness, irritability, agitation, and anxiety.[114] Neurologic symptoms often manifest in 16 to 24 hours from time of last benzodiazepine use and include tremors, sensitivity to light, and paresthesia. Severe symptoms are collectively referred to as "complicated withdrawal" and include seizures, hallucinosis, psychosis, and delirium, like delirium tremens in acute alcohol withdrawal syndrome.[114,115] Autonomic hyperactivity includes diaphoresis, tachycardia, hypertension, and gastrointestinal upset including nausea and vomiting. Complicated withdrawal (ie, seizures, delirium) manifests at later stages among patients withdrawing from benzodiazepines in comparison to alcohol, but can start as early as 24 hours or up to 1 week or longer after cessation.[116] Complicated withdrawal involving seizures and psychosis are reported in less than 7% of all cases.

Benzodiazepine withdrawal timing and severity are related to the pharmacokinetic parameters of the benzodiazepine being used, with earlier and more severe withdrawal experienced among those with regular use of short-acting benzodiazepines (eg, alprazolam, lorazepam).[114,117,118] Long-term use of high-potency benzodiazepines (eg, alprazolam, clonazepam, etizolam) can lead to more severe and difficult-to-treat withdrawal manifestations compared to low-potency benzodiazepines such as diazepam. For patients chronically exposed to short-acting benzodiazepines, symptoms will often begin 12 to 24 hours after the last dose. In contrast, withdrawal onset is delayed among patients chronically exposed to long-acting benzodiazepines (eg, diazepam, clonazepam), typically arising within 24 to 72 hours after the last dose. Life-threating and complicated withdrawal typically resolves within 5 to 10 days, however protracted withdrawal symptoms, including anxiety, insomnia, and mood disturbances, can persist for weeks to months.

Clinical Management of Benzodiazepine Withdrawal

Hospitalized patients experiencing benzodiazepine withdrawal require frequent evaluation, including physical and neurologic vital assessments. Patients experiencing complicated withdrawal such as seizure or delirium may require admission to critical care settings. Table 10.6 includes a summary of the supportive measures required for optimal benzodiazepine withdrawal management.

Use of Long-Acting Benzodiazepines

Long-acting benzodiazepines are used to manage benzodiazepine withdrawal in hospitalized patients. A clinical trial evaluated differences in outcomes for hospitalized patients experiencing benzodiazepine withdrawal receiving fixed taper or symptom-triggered (Clinical Institute Withdrawal Assessment Scale—Benzodiazepines [CIWA-B]) benzodiazepine dosing protocols to guide long-acting benzodiazepine administration.[119] The authors concluded there was no difference between the two approaches in clinical outcomes, length of stay, or total benzodiazepine doses received.[119] Benzodiazepine sparing approaches achieved through symptom-triggered protocols are preferred for management of benzodiazepine withdrawal.

Administration of the CIWA-B scale is a validated tool to assess signs and symptoms of benzodiazepine withdrawal.[120] The hospital-based clinician orders the assessment tool at hospital admission if there is a clinical suspicion withdrawal. Nursing staff administers the CIWA-B scale by assessing subjective and objective signs and symptoms of withdrawal. Based on the patient's withdrawal severity and score, clear parameters direct the timing and dosage of the benzodiazepine for administration.

The frequency of CIWA-B assessment decreased overtime as the withdrawal severity lessens and the scale is no longer triggering benzodiazepine administration. Once a patient reaches a stable benzodiazepine

TABLE 10.6

Summary of Supportive Measures Required During Hospital-Based Management of Benzodiazepine Withdrawal

Supportive measure	Description	Frequency/context
Airway, breathing, and circulation (ABCs)	Rapidly assess airway, breathing, and circulation. Provide supplemental oxygen as needed and establish IV access for severe cases.	Immediately on presentation or deterioration.
Monitoring vital signs and neurologic status	Check vital signs and neurologic status frequently (every 1–2 h), with continuous cardiac and pulse oximetry monitoring in severe cases.	Every 1–2 h, continuously in severe withdrawal.
Volume status	Treat volume depletion (eg, vomiting, diaphoresis) or rhabdomyolysis with intravenous crystalloid fluids.	As needed for dehydration or rhabdomyolysis.
Nausea and vomiting management	Administer antiemetics to control nausea and vomiting. Antiemetics may include ondansetron or dimenhydrinate.	When nausea and vomiting are reported.
Severity scoring and assessment	Use scoring systems like CIWA-B to assess severity and response to interventions	Regularly throughout treatment to guide interventions.
Seizure management	Postictal care includes airway suctioning, recumbent positioning, and seizure precautions (pads on bedside rails, bed at lowest position).	If seizures occur or postictal state is observed.
Hyperthermia management	Manage hyperthermia caused by psychomotor agitation with rapid cooling (eg., ice immersion, evaporative spray) if temperature exceeds 40.5 °C. Should be transferred to critical care level setting.	When hyperthermia is detected, especially >40.5 °C.

TABLE 10.7

Benzodiazepine Approximate Dose Equivalents to 10 mg Oral Diazepam[a]

Benzodiazepine	ATC[b] Therapeutic class	VA/DoD SUD CPG (2021)[c,d]	Ashton Manual (2002)[e,f]
Alprazolam	Anxiolytic	1	0.5
Chlordiazepoxide	Anxiolytic	25	25
Clonazepam	Antiepileptic	1	0.5
Clorazepate	Anxiolytic	15	15
Diazepam	Anxiolytic	10	10
Estazolam	Sedative-hypnotic	1	1–2
Flurazepam	Sedative-hypnotic	15	15–30
Lorazepam	Anxiolytic	2	1
Oxazepam	Anxiolytic	30	20
Quazepam	Sedative-hypnotic	10	20
Temazepam	Sedative-hypnotic	15	20
Triazolam	Sedative-hypnotic	0.25	0.5

[a]Approximate dose equivalents of various BZD medications to a 10-mg dose of oral diazepam as determined by the VA/DoD SUD guideline and The Ashton Manual.

[b]ATC, Anatomical therapeutic chemical classification system.

[c]DoD, US Department of Defense; SUD, substance use disorder; VA, US Department of Veterans Affairs; CPG, clinical practice guideline.

[d]**Source:** Department of Veterans Affairs, Department of Defense. VA/DoD Clinical Practice Guideline for the Management of Substance Use Disorders. 2021.

[e]**Source:** Ashton CH. *Benzodiazepines: How They Work and How to Withdraw (The Ashton Manual).* Institute of Neuroscience, Newcastle University; 2002.

[f]Same equivalents in Ashton H. *Benzodiazepine Equivalence Table* [Online]. Revised April 2007. https://www.benzo.org.uk/bzequiv.htm and Ashton CH. The diagnosis and management of benzodiazepine dependence. *Curr Opin Psychiatry*. 2005;18(3):249–255.

dose (when scores are below 9), the hospital-based clinician will prescribe an initial total daily taper dose that is equivalent to, or less than, the dose required during the stabilization phase.

If a hospitalized patient is using high doses of a short-acting benzodiazepine, that is, alprazolam, either unprescribed use or prescribed use, and the goal is to dose reduce or fully discontinue the benzodiazepine, it is recommended to switch the patient from the shorter-acting benzodiazepine to a longer-acting benzodiazepine, that is, diazepam. Use of a longer-acting benzodiazepine will increase the time between peaks and valleys of the drug's effect. Use of a benzodiazepine dose equivalent calculator or a table with dose equivalence to manually calculate the benzodiazepine dose is recommended. Table 10.7 lists many commonly used benzodiazepines and their dose equivalents to 10 mg of oral diazepam, which can be used to transition patients from shorter to longer-acting benzodiazepines.

Benzodiazepine Taper

When initiating a benzodiazepine taper, the taper can begin in the hospital or upon transition to the community. If using a symptom-triggered approach is used to manage benzodiazepine withdrawal in the hospital, described above, then the discharge taper should begin with the last stable benzodiazepine dose required during the stabilization phase and prior to hospital discharge. If the hospital-based physician instead uses a fixed-dose benzodiazepine taper during hospitalization, then the in-hospital benzodiazepine dose decrease may be approximately 10% to 20% per day. If a fixed-dose taper is initiated in the hospital, it is important to still use a symptom-triggered approach to ensure that there are no breakthrough benzodiazepine withdrawal symptoms that go unassessed and unmanaged.

When the patient transitions to the community, it is essential that the patient has an outpatient clinician who agrees to manage the benzodiazepine taper. This is because people with benzodiazepine dependence are often unable to taper off completely from a symptom-triggered protocol in less than 10 days. Many of the benzodiazepines that patients become physically dependent on have long half-lives and active metabolites (eg, diazepam, clonazepam, and/or alprazolam) and these drugs take longer to clear, leading to a protracted postacute withdrawal period. Furthermore, patients using high quantities of nonprescribed benzodiazepines can develop an exceedingly high tolerance, which is usually determined through their CIWA-B dose requirements. This high tolerance often limits the ability for safe, comfortable, tapering in hospital-based settings. See Table 10.8 for example strategies to

TABLE 10.8

Example Benzodiazepine Taper Plan for Hospital and Outpatient Settings

Patient is taking 2 mg alprazolam three times a day (equals 6 mg total daily dose)

Step 1. Transition from alprazolam to diazepam

- 1 alprazolam = 10 diazepam using the VA/DoD SUD Clinical Practice Guidelines[b]
- 6 alprazolam = 60 diazepam total daily dose, split into a 20-mg dose three times per day
- Use symptom-triggered protocol (ie, CIWA-B[c]) to provide additional benzodiazepines for break through symptoms[c]
- Use as needed, supportive medications (ie, clonidine, gabapentin, hydroxyzine)

Step 2. Prescribe in-hospital diazepam taper (approximately 10–20% decrease per day*)

*Example includes a 3-day hospitalization:

Hospital day 1	20 mg AM	20 mg at noon	20 mg PM	+ symptom-triggered dosing of benzodiazepines
Hospital day 2	15 mg AM	15 mg at noon	20 mg PM	
Hospital day 3	10 mg AM	15 mg at noon	15 mg PM	+ supportive medications

Step 3. Planning for hospital discharge

- To facilitate a safe hospital discharge, wait until the patient's symptoms are within the mild withdrawal range using a validated withdrawal scale (ie, CIWA-B score of ≤10[2])
- Communicate with the outpatient clinician and verify they are willing to take over the benzodiazepine taper
- Plan for an outpatient taper of approximately 5–10% per week; prescribe a sufficient supply of medication to bridge patient to outpatient follow-up appointment
- Provide the patient with the taper plan in writing to reduce confusion and gain buy-in
- Anticipate an outpatient follow-up appointment within 5 d of hospital discharge

Patient's CIWA-B score is ≈5 with a total daily dose of 40 mg of diazepam on discharge (includes PRN diazepam using the CIWA-B symptom-triggered protocol)

Home: Day 4–8	10 mg AM	15 mg at noon	15 mg PM	+ supportive medications

Patient follows up with an outpatient clinician who begins a prolonged taper ≈10% dose reduction/week until the patient is off benzodiazepines[a,d,e]

Week 1	10 mg	10 mg	15 mg	
Week 2	10 mg	10 mg	10 mg +2 mg	
Week 3	10 mg	10 mg	10 mg	
Week 4	10 mg	10 mg	5 mg + 2 mg	
Week 5	10 mg	5 mg + 2 mg	5 mg + 2 mg	
Week 6	5 mg + 2 mg	5 mg + 2 mg	5 mg + 2 mg	
Week 7	5 mg + 2 mg	5 mg + 2 mg	5 mg	
Week 8	5 mg + 2 mg	5 mg	5 mg	
Week 9	5 mg	5 mg	5 mg	+ supportive medications
Week 10	5 mg	5 mg	2 mg	
Week 11	5 mg	2 mg	2 mg	
Week 12	2 mg	2 mg	2 mg	
Week 13	2 mg	2 mg	1 mg	
Week 14	2 mg	1 mg	1 mg	
Week 15	1 mg	1 mg	1 mg	
Week 15	1 mg	-	1 mg	
Week 16	1 mg	-	-	
Week 17	-	-	-	Patient completes taper

[a]Outpatient taper plan is meant to be flexible, with patient–clinician discussion about the frequency of clinic visits and if there are times when the taper should be slowed down (ie, stressful times in a person's life) or accelerated (ie, if the patient feels they are ready to do so).

[b]Department of Veterans Affairs, Department of Defense. VA/DoD Clinical Practice Guideline for the Management of Substance Use Disorders. 2021.

[c]Busto UE, Sykora K, Sellers EM. A clinical scale to assess benzodiazepine withdrawal. *J Clin Psychopharmacol.* 1989;9(6):412–416.

[d]Ashton CH. *Benzodiazepines: How They Work and How to Withdraw (The Ashton Manual).* Institute of Neuroscience, Newcastle University. 2002.

[e]Joint Clinical Practice Guidelines. *Benzodiazepine Tapering: Considerations when Benzodiazepines Risks Outweigh Benefits.* American Society of Addiction Medicine; 2024. https://www.asam.org/quality-care/clinical-guidelines/benzodiazepine-tapering

transition a patient from a shorter-acting to a longer-acting benzodiazepine with a faster dose reduction in the hospital (monitored by the hospital-based physician) and a slower dose reduction in the community setting (monitored by an outpatient clinician).

Use of Phenobarbital

Fixed-dose phenobarbital protocols have been described for the management of acute benzodiazepine withdrawal in hospital-based settings; however, the evidence to date is largely based on retrospective chart review. In benzodiazepine withdrawal refractory to use of benzodiazepines, patients who have failed prior attempts at monitored outpatient taper, or in situations where an outpatient benzodiazepine taper is not possible, use of a phenobarbital taper may be considered. The use of phenobarbital should be measured against the potential harms of its use, but it may be the safest option for individuals without durable access to outpatient benzodiazepine taper.[121]

Yale New Haven Hospital Phenobarbital Withdrawal Management for Benzodiazepine Withdrawal

Population: Enteral phenobarbital for acute benzodiazepine withdrawal may be considered for patients who are not candidates for an extended benzodiazepine taper, including those who have experienced paradoxical effects from benzodiazepine, a high risk for seizure, or prior failure of a benzodiazepine taper related to poor access to successful benzodiazepine taper strategies or other complicating mental health or substance use disorders.

Exclusion Criteria: Age >65, severe liver disease (Child–Pugh class C), concomitant treatment for alcohol use disorder, or prescribed phenobarbital use for another indication.

Dosing:

- **Day 1:** Phenobarbital 194.4 mg PO × 1, then starting in 4 hours Phenobarbital 97.2 mg PO every 4 hours × 5 doses **(Initial dose restricted to critical care areas)**
- **Day 2:** Phenobarbital 64.8 mg PO every 4 hours × 4 doses
- **Day 3:** Phenobarbital 64.8 mg PO every 8 hours × 3 doses
- **Day 4:** Supportive care only, no additional phenobarbital or benzodiazepines

Use of Adjunctive Medications

Adjunctive medication can be used to support withdrawal management in addition to benzodiazepines. These include gabapentin, clonidine, mirtazapine, and other agents to support with sleep and other mental health symptoms experienced during the acute withdrawal period.[122,123] In patients with a known history of complicated withdrawal, avoiding any medications that may mask symptoms of withdrawal (ie, gabapentin, clonidine) in early stages (24 to 48 hours) is essential.

Important Considerations

Hospital-based clinicians should be vigilant about concurrent withdrawal from opioids, which can present as diaphoresis, tachycardia, headache, and GI upset and will confound the assessment of benzodiazepine withdrawal. Frequent monitoring and assessment of the patient's response to individual medications (ie, benzodiazepines, short-acting opioids) will help to determine which intervention the patient is responding to. Repeat assessments following administration of multiple medications will lead to diagnostic uncertainty.

Management of Benzodiazepine Use Disorder

Closely monitored, medically supervised tapering of benzodiazepines after acute stabilization is the recommended standard of care to facilitate cessation of benzodiazepines for individuals with benzodiazepine use disorder.[113,114] The medically supervised taper is typically done with a longer-acting benzodiazepines such as diazepam or clonazepam. The ASAM offers additional examples of how this can be done in the outpatient setting.[113] Dose reductions will widely vary based on interindividual factors, however typically reductions of 10% to 25% every 2 to 3 weeks are used.[124] The hospital-based clinician should communicate with the patient's outpatient clinician to ensure the patient has access to ongoing benzodiazepine management in the outpatient setting. If outpatient management is not available, shorter hospital-based tapers may be necessary, though these are typically poorly tolerated by patients.

Treatment Considerations When Illicitly Manufactured Benzodiazepines Are Involved

For patients with benzodiazepine use disorder exposed to illicitly manufactured benzodiazepines, clinicians should consider the unpredictable potency and pharmacologic profiles of these benzodiazepines. As indicated above, treatment of benzodiazepine use disorder involves the use of a closely monitored extended benzodiazepine taper to reduce the risk of return to use. In the case of illicitly manufactured benzodiazepines, it may be challenging to convert the illicit benzodiazepine dose to a safe prescribed benzodiazepine dose.[125] Patients exposed to illicit benzodiazepines may require higher doses of prescribed benzodiazepines for withdrawal management due to cross tolerance, particularly if the nonprescribed agents have atypical half-lives or binding affinities. A reasonable and safe first step may be acute withdrawal management with phenobarbital while patients are in the hospital setting followed by a prolonged taper of prescribed benzodiazepines in the outpatient setting.

Kratom

Mitragyna speciosa is a Southeast Asian tree known locally as "kratom" and is used as a traditional medicine for its mild stimulant and euphoric effects. Kratom is commonly found in Thailand, where up to 15% of Thai citizens self-reported having tried kratom in their lifetime, with past year use approximately 2%.[126] In contrast, its prevalence in North America is much lower, with an estimate of lifetime use at 1.3% and past year use 0.8% in a large cross-sectional survey.[127] Nonetheless, there are signals that it is becoming more popular in North America, including a dramatic rise in the number of calls to the National Poison Data System from 18 in 2011 to 357 in the first 7 months of 2018, potentially due at least in part to the fact that it is not a scheduled substance under the Controlled Substance Act in the United States.[128]

Kratom is often consumed by chewing or swallowing dried preparations of the leaves of the *Mitragyna* plant, though preparation of a tea or smoking are also potential routes of use. The main active compound is mitragynine, an alkaloid whose primary mechanism of action is on the mu, delta, and kappa opioid receptors of the CNS. It appears to demonstrate a dose-response effect, with mild stimulating and euphoric effects at low doses, and analgesia and mild sedation at higher doses.[126] Reasons for kratom use vary widely as well, including everything from pain relief, improved mental acuity, management of mood disorders, help to manage opioid withdrawal syndromes, help abstain from use of other substances, or use as an alternative to traditional forms of opioid agonist treatment.[129]

Kratom Intoxication/Overdose

Clinical Presentation

Kratom overdose can occur with higher doses, and the incidence of presentations to the hospital for kratom toxicity in the United States has been increasing steadily. Patients may present with a breadth of features including agitation, tachycardia, drowsiness, vomiting, and confusion. Rarer complications include seizures, hallucinations, withdrawal syndromes, respiratory depression, coma, and respiratory or cardiac arrest. Deaths due to acute kratom toxicity are rare without concurrent use of other substances or prescribed medications but have been described.[126,128] Kratom has been associated with complications in individual case reports including intrahepatic cholestasis, hepatitis, liver failure, adult respiratory distress syndrome (ARDS), hypothyroidism, hyperprolactinemia, and posterior reversible encephalopathy syndrome, though a direct causal link for these rare cases has not been established.[126,130]

Diagnostic Testing

Mitragynine is not detected on point-of-case urine immunoassays, thus a presentation that is consistent with opioid overdose and an accompanying negative UDT should prompt consideration of kratom overdose as a part of the differential diagnosis. Importantly, kratom overdose will respond to naloxone, which can be helpful both in diagnosis and management.

Management of Kratom Overdose

Management of kratom overdose is similar to other opioid intoxications, requiring supportive care and naloxone as needed for respiratory depression or decreased level of consciousness. The pharmacokinetic parameters of mitragynine in humans are not well established, however it has a half-life of 23 to 40 hours.[131] Monitoring patients with kratom overdose in the hospital for 24 hours following a presentation for acute intoxication is recommended.

Kratom Withdrawal

Clinical Presentation

Kratom tolerance can develop after a period of regular use of several weeks and resembles opioid withdrawal with cessation. These symptoms are described in up to 50% of people who use kratom regularly.

Management of Kratom Withdrawal

As with other opioid receptor agonists, prolonged exposure can lead to physical dependence and a withdrawal syndrome upon sudden cessation. Kratom withdrawal phenomenon associated with kratom use resembles traditional opioid withdrawal and includes restlessness, anxiety, body aches, and diarrhea, however, it is generally more mild than opioid withdrawal related to heroin or fentanyl.[132] Acute management involves supportive care and symptomatic management with medications such as acetaminophen, ibuprofen, dimenhydrinate, loperamide, or clonidine. Consideration can be given to initiation of buprenorphine, both to help manage acute symptoms as well as a form of longer-term treatment.

Treatment Options

"Kratom use disorder" is not specifically defined within the DSM-5, though individuals who use kratom may meet criteria for an OUD.[132] Buprenorphine can successfully treat individuals who use kratom. Buprenorphine initiation occurs as with other opioids and doses range widely with titration to patient's needs, though generally effective buprenorphine doses are less than needed for individuals who use heroin or fentanyl. The use of full opioid receptor agonists, such as methadone, are not described in the literature but could be considered for select patients when buprenorphine is not an option and who have sufficient opioid tolerance.[133] While there are no data to support recommendations around psychosocial treatment, this may be considered based on local resources. Referral to outpatient addiction services for assessment is recommended.

Substances With Stimulant-Like Properties

Natural Cathinones

Cathinones are a group of compounds with stimulant-like properties originally derived from *Catha edulis*, a natural shrub known locally as "khat" or "miraa" that is often chewed or brewed into teas in East Africa and the Arabian Peninsula for its mild stimulant and euphoric effects. It is estimated that over 20 million people in this geographic region chew khat on a daily basis, with estimated dependence rates of 5% to 15% or higher, though it is currently illegal to import khat into North America and its use in this continent is much less common.[134]

Synthetic Cathinones

In contrast, synthetic cathinones such as mephedrone, methcathinone, methylone, and other related chemicals are more commonly sold in North America under labels such as "bath salts" or "plant food," and marketed as "not for human consumption" in order to circumvent legal restrictions.[135] A number of these substances are currently listed as Schedule 1 substances in the United States, yet a wide array of slightly modified versions have been introduced to bypass law enforcement. As a group, synthetic cathinones include a variety of related chemicals with stimulant-like properties, many of which have potent and unpredictable effects.

Synthetic cathinones can be ingested orally, smoked, insufflated, or injected, and are known to cause potent sympathomimetic and euphoric effects. They may also cause adverse effects including agitation, paranoia, confusion, hallucinations, tachycardia, palpitations, hypertension, myoclonus, serotonin syndrome, mydriasis, vomiting, hyperthermia, seizures, and death.[135] Synthetic cathinones are not detected by immunoassays and should be a part of the differential diagnosis for anyone exhibiting signs of stimulant intoxication or stimulant-induced psychosis with a negative UDT for ATS or cocaine.

Mechanism of Action

Like other commonly used stimulants, natural and synthetic cathinones exert their effects through promoting the release and/or preventing reuptake of monoamine neurotransmitters including dopamine, serotonin, and norepinephrine.[135]

Cathinone Intoxication

The clinical presentation and management of a patient with acute cathinone intoxication is like other presentations of stimulant intoxication or stimulant-induced psychosis. Clinical management involves behavioral and environmental interventions, supportive care, and the use of benzodiazepines and other GABAergic agents to manage significant agitation.[21] While persistent psychotic symptoms are common in patients presenting with cathinone intoxication (up to 38%), it is not clear how much of this is related to selection bias given higher rates of use in those with underlying psychiatric disorders.[136] Antipsychotics may be used judiciously for symptoms of psychosis based on clinical context, though caution is recommended due to the potential for lowered seizure threshold and lack of evidence on long-term effects of cathinone exposure and our inability to prognosticate for such patients.

Of note, the antidepressant bupropion is chemically related to the cathinone family and exerts its function primarily through inhibition of the reuptake of dopamine and norepinephrine. Bupropion has potential for nonprescribed use, especially in settings where access to substances is limited, such as incarcerated populations, and can be swallowed, insufflated, or injected intravenously. Like other cathinones, bupropion intoxication may present with signs of increased sympathetic tone including hypertension, tachycardia, agitation, delirium, generalized tonic–clonic seizures, arrhythmia, cardiogenic shock, and death. Management of bupropion intoxication should include supportive care, benzodiazepines for severe agitation and/or seizures, as well as the involvement of toxicology for more significant cases. If possible antipsychotics should be avoided due to the risk of lowered seizure threshold.[137]

Long-Term Management of Cathinone Use

There are no specific long-term treatment recommendations for patients presenting with cathinone intoxication or a history suggestive of an underlying use disorder. Harm-reduction counseling and refer to outpatient behavioral resources as available is recommended, like other stimulant use disorders.

Dissociative and Hallucinogenic Substances

Dissociative and hallucinogenic substances comprise a diverse group of psychoactive drugs that characteristically alter perception, mood, and cognition, while also inducing changes in consciousness and sensory experience. These substances include dissociatives, for example, ketamine and PCP, which enable dissociation and detachment from reality. They also include hallucinogens, for example, psilocybin and DMT, which evoke vivid sensory distortions, and for some, "mystical experiences." GHB and MDMA are particularly unique, with GHB being both a sedative and a recreational "club drug" with dissociative properties, and MDMA acting as an entactogen that blends stimulant and mild hallucinogenic effects. This section will describe the pharmacologic mechanisms, epidemiology and patterns of use, hospital presentations associated with common dissociative and hallucinogenic substances, and emerging hospital-based approaches to acute stabilization and treatment for patients taking these substances. Table 10.9 summarizes dissociative and hallucinogenic substances.

Dissociative Substances

Ketamine

Ketamine hydrochloride is a nonbarbiturate dissociative anesthetic used in medical settings for pain management and sedation, but it is widely known as a recreational substance used for its hallucinogenic effects, where it is referred to colloquially as "K" or "Special K."[138] Ketamine can cause dissociation and detachment from reality, and vivid sensory distortions.

Ketamine use is most common among young adults in nightlife environments, with increasing global prevalence in recent years. Data from 2015–2019 NSDUH demonstrated 0.13% of adults reporting past-year use of ketamine, with highest rates among young adult males.[139] Estimates of the global prevalence of ketamine use disorder are not known, but expected to be low. Ketamine, similar to other hallucinogenic and dissociative substances, does not produce neuroadaptive changes in the brain's reward system that commonly drive SUD.[140] Animal models comparing behaviors consistent with SUD in mice receiving ketamine demonstrate ketamine as less likely to cause SUD than cocaine.[141] This is thought to be driven by shorter bursts of dopamine released in response to ketamine use in comparison to cocaine.[140]

Mechanism of Action

Ketamine is a noncompetitive antagonist of N-methyl-D-aspartate (NMDA) receptors, affecting glutamate activity and neurotransmission to dopamine and opioid pathways. Its intricate effect across multiple neurotransmitter pathways is responsible for its anesthetic, dissociative, and psychoactive properties. Disruption of glutamatergic neurotransmission and partial agonism of opiate mu-receptors facilitates dissociation and analgesia during painful procedures.[138,142]

Routes and Indications for Use

Ketamine can be administered intravenously, intramuscularly, orally, and intranasally; each associated with different onset of action and peak plasma concentration timings. Intravenous and intramuscular routes of administration have a rapid onset of action, typically within 1 to 5 minutes, and achieve peak plasma concentrations within 5 to 30 minutes.[138] Due to first-pass hepatic metabolism, oral ketamine has profoundly lower bioavailability (16% to 29%). Intranasal administration has slightly better bioavailability at 45% to 50%.[138] As an anesthetic, ketamine is effective for brief procedural sedation that does not require skeletal muscle relaxation.[138] It is also used as a preanesthetic for induction of general anesthesia combined with other anesthetizing agents. For individuals in the perioperative setting, ketamine can be a useful form of multimodal analgesia, particularly for individuals with high opioid tolerance. Additional indications for ketamine use are under review by the FDA and include treatment-resistant depression, suicidal ideation, and refractory status epilepticus.[138]

Ketamine Toxicity and Withdrawal

Clinical Presentation

Acute toxicity from ketamine often presents with confusion, agitation, tachycardia, hypertension, and respiratory depression at high doses, as well as potential bladder dysfunction due to ketamine cystitis with chronic use. Death results from a lethal overdose of ketamine are unlikely due to its wide therapeutic range though it has been reported.[143,144] Physical harm resulting from ketamine toxicity usually occur

TABLE 10.9

Summary of Dissociative and Hallucinogen Substances

Drug name	Mechanism of action	Onset and peak effect	Toxidrome	Withdrawal syndrome	Treatments and special considerations
GHB (Gamma-Hydroxybutyrate) *"G"*	GABA-B receptor agonist; weak GABA-A activity	Onset: 15–30 min Peak: 1–2 h	CNS depression, respiratory depression, bradycardia, hypotension	Anxiety, insomnia, tremors, tachycardia. Severe withdrawal may include tremor, diaphoresis, autonomic dysregulation and complicated withdrawal (seizure, psychosis may resemble delirium tremens)	Supportive care, benzodiazepines for withdrawal, avoid flumazenil due to risk of seizures
MDMA (Methylenedioxymethamphetamine) *"Molly" "Ecstasy"*	Monoamine-releasing agent, neuromodulator of serotonin, dopamine, and norepinephrine	Onset: 30–60 min Peak: 75–120 min	Excitatory state: restlessness, agitation, diaphoresis, mydriasis, tachycardia, bruxism, and hypertension	Rare; may include general symptoms of dysphoria, insomnia, irritability, anxiety	Monitor for dehydration and serotonin syndrome in patients presenting with MDMA toxicity
Ketamine *"K" "Special K"*	NMDA receptor antagonist; affects dopamine and opioid systems	Onset: 5–10 min (IV); 10–20 min (IM) Peak: 30–60 min	Dissociative state, tachycardia, hypertension, agitation, hallucinations	Rare; may include cravings and dysphoria in chronic use	Supportive care for acute toxicity; benzodiazepines for agitation; monitor for urinary tract complications in chronic users
Psilocybin *"Shrooms"*	5-HT2A receptor agonist	Onset: 20–60 min Peak: 2–4 h	Serotonin toxicity (rare); hallucinations, anxiety, paranoia	Minimal to no physiologic withdrawal; may include psychological symptoms like anxiety or depression	Supportive care, benzodiazepines for agitation or anxiety; avoid antipsychotics unless absolutely necessary
PCP (Phencyclidine)	NMDA receptor antagonist; affects dopamine and serotonin systems	Onset: 5–15 min (smoked); 30–60 min (oral) Peak: 1–4 h	Dissociative state, violent behavior, nystagmus, hypertension, hyperthermia	Psychological cravings, depression, anxiety, irritability	Benzodiazepines for agitation; cooling measures for hyperthermia; avoid physical restraints to prevent rhabdomyolysis
DMT (Dimethyltryptamine)	5-HT2A receptor agonist	Onset: <1 min (smoked/inhaled) Peak: 2–5 min	Hallucinations, agitation, tachycardia, hypertension	No known withdrawal syndrome	Supportive care; benzodiazepines for agitation; effects are short lived due to rapid metabolism

secondary to ketamine-induced aggression and agitation or due to its dissociative effects leading to individuals to engage in high-risk behaviors (ie, jumping off building).[145] Overall, the understanding of ketamine toxicity secondary to recreational use is confounded by polysubstance use, whereby the majority of presentations for ketamine toxicity are associated with other substance ingestions.[146]

Management of Ketamine Toxicity and Withdrawal

Hospital-based supportive care includes vital sign assessments, neurologic monitoring, and management of agitation and confusion. All attempts should be made to limit visual and auditory stimulation until symptoms resolve.[145] Ketamine withdrawal symptoms can include anxiety, cravings, and sleep disturbances, reflecting its potential for SUD development. Typically, hospital-based monitoring is not required to manage and support patients during ketamine withdrawal.

Medical Complications of Ketamine Use

Ketamine-Induced Cystitis

Ketamine-induced cystitis (KIC) is a serious complication of chronic ketamine use. Up to 25% of individuals who use ketamine will experience some form of urinary symptoms, the experience of which is directly associated with quantity, frequency, and duration of ketamine use.[147] KIC is an inflammation and dysfunction of the bladder secondary to ketamine use. Symptoms include pelvic pain, dysuria, urinary frequency, urgency, hematuria, and, in its most severe forms, reduced bladder capacity and incontinence.[148]

The mechanism of KIC is not well understood but is thought to develop in response to exposure of ketamine and its metabolites on the urothelium leading to inflammatory and neurogenic changes.[148] Over time, exposure to toxic metabolites within the urothelium causes fibrosis and scarring of the bladder wall and can lead to irreversible damage.

Management of KIC is centered on ketamine cessation and is critical to stop disease progression. Additional treatments include the use of anti-inflammatory medications (ie, diclofenac), anticholinergics, pentosan polysulfate, bladder instillations, or surgical intervention.[148,149] Early identification and intervention are critical to prevent long-term complications, including chronic pain and bladder reconstruction. Patients presenting with ketamine toxicity and/or ketamine use disorder in the hospital should be screened for symptoms of KIC. If present, appropriate supportive treatments should be provided; in severe cases, consider a urologic consultation.

Phencyclidine

Phencyclidine (PCP) is a dissociative substance initially developed for medical use as an anesthetic but was discontinued due to severe adverse effects, including aggression, dysphoria, hallucination, and in some patients, prolonged psychosis.[150] PCP became notorious in the US media due to reports of extreme violence, self-mutilation, and murder among PCP exposed people.[151,152] Unlike the dissociative ketamine, PCP use is marked by a more severe side-effect profile including psychosis, light-headedness, vertigo, ataxia, and nystagmus during acute intoxication at high doses.[153]

The prevalence of PCP use is relatively low compared to other substances, with sporadic increases across specific regions and subpopulations. The highest prevalence of PCP use occurred in the 1980s with a steady decrease since then.[154] There is limited discussion in the literature describing PCP use, its associated side effects, and substance use outcomes, with the majority of studies dating before 1990.[154–156] Per reports, PCP use was concentrated in young Black men in Washington DC in the late 1980s.[155] However, more recent surveillance data suggests a possible resurgence of use. In 2011, 75,500 ED encounters due to PCP were reported in the United States in 2011, an increase of 400% from 2005.[150]

Mechanism of Action

Like ketamine, PCP acts as a noncompetitive antagonist at the NMDA receptor, disrupting glutamate-mediated neurotransmission, contributing to its dissociative properties including altered perception, detachment from reality, and euphoria. PCP inhibits the uptake of dopamine and norepinephrine, leading to sympathomimetic effects and autonomic hyperactivity.[150] PCP can be administered through multiple routes including oral ingestion, intravenous, insufflation, and inhalation.[151]

PCP Toxicity and Withdrawal

Clinical Presentation

PCP toxicity manifests as a range of symptoms, from mild agitation to severe, life-threatening complications including psychosis and seizure.[150] Acute toxicity is associated with an excitatory state with behavioral disturbances such as agitation, aggression, and paranoia. Hallucinations are often present among patients experiencing toxicity. Hallmark physical signs of acute intoxication include autonomic hyperactivity, for example, tachycardia, hypertension, rotational nystagmus, muscle rigidity, and hyperthermia.[150] In its most severe form, toxicity from PCP can lead to seizures, rhabdomyolysis, or coma. PCP withdrawal is less well characterized, but includes symptoms such as dysphoria, fatigue, restlessness, and anxiety.

Management of PCP Toxicity and Withdrawal

Management of PCP toxicity and withdrawal requires supportive care, ensuring a calm and safe environment to minimize agitation or self-harm. In episodes of toxicity, short-term use of benzodiazepines can be employed to control severe agitation, anxiety, or seizures, while antipsychotics may be considered for psychotic symptoms and severe aggression. Monitoring for hyperthermia among patients presenting with autonomic dysregulation is recommended with cooling measures including intravenous fluids and cooling blankets. Rhabdomyolysis is a known complication of PCP toxicity and is observed in patients with severe muscle rigidity. Rhabdomyolysis can be diagnosed using standard basic metabolic profiles and creatinine kinase (CK) during periods of active symptoms. Early intervention is key to preventing long-term cognitive and psychological consequences associated with PCP use.

Dimethyltryptamine

Dimethlytryptamine (DMT) is an indole alkaloid that occurs naturally in plants and is produced endogenously in small quantities by primates.[157–159] Plants containing DMT include *Delosperma, Phalaris, Desmodium, Mimosa, Acacia, Virola, and Psychotria*, in addition, other relatively innocuous sources like citrus plant leaves.[160] DMT is a key psychoactive compound found in traditional South American ceremonial brews such as ayahuasca, hoasca, and yagé.[161] When ingested at higher concentrations, DMT is a hallucinogenic substance known for causing altered perceptions of time and space and brief vivid visual hallucinations, contributing to its often referred to name as the "spirit molecule."[162]

DMT distinguishes itself from other traditional hallucinogenic substances such as psilocybin and lysergic acid diethylamide (LSD) through its relatively short duration of action and lack of tachyphylaxis with repeated use.[157,163,164] While rates of DMT consumption are thought to be far less than traditional hallucinogenic substances such as LSD or psilocybin, a global drug surveillance survey conducted in 2012 reported lifetime prevalence of DMT use was 9% and a past year prevalence of 5%.[165] Interestingly, the global drug surveillance survey indicated DMT was most often smoked and associated with relatively few side effects, and was reported to have a larger proportion of new users compared with the other substances.[165] Rising prevalence of DMT use may be driven by growing consumption in niche communities seeking spiritual exploration and experimental therapies.

Mechanism of Action

DMT's mechanism of action involves serotonergic pathways through nonselective activities across serotonin 5-hydroxytryptamine (5-HT) receptors. DMT is also known to interact with a broad range of receptors, including ionotropic and metabotropic glutamate receptors, dopamine, acetylcholine, trace amine-associated receptor (TAAR), and sigma-1 receptors.[158] DMT's agonist action at 5-HT2a receptors is thought to be the primarily mechanism driving its key hallucinogenic properties.[166]

DMT Toxicity

DMT toxicity is rare due to its high therapeutic index and brief duration of action. Adverse effects include intense anxiety, paranoia, and disorientation during or shortly after use. DMT has been known to produce sympathomimetic effects including tachycardia and hypertension which is dose dependent.[158,167] Serious complications, such as persistent psychosis or hallucinogen persisting perception disorder (HPPD), are extremely rare and typically occur in individuals with underlying mental health conditions or those consuming other substances in conjunction with DMT.[168,169]

Management of DMT toxicity focuses on limiting psychological distress through creating a calm and supportive environment and removing any distracting stimuli that may contribute to anxiety and/or aggression. In more severe cases, benzodiazepines can be used, but efforts should be taken to avoid repeated and long-term use of benzodiazepines in patients presenting with recurrent DMT toxicity.

DMT Withdrawal

Withdrawal symptoms associated with DMT cessation are not well known or documented in the literature. This may be in part due to the pharmacologic properties of DMT, which do not facilitate tolerance and physical dependence.

Management of DMT Use

Encourage patients who use DMT and/or other psychedelic compounds to seek support from medical practitioners who are licensed and experienced in using psychedelic compounds for therapeutic purposes. Harm-reduction education on safe use practices, including a focus on staging and preparation, is critical for minimizing adverse effects, particularly for individuals who use DMT in therapeutic or ritualistic contexts. This approach emphasizes the importance of preparing a safe, supportive, and controlled environment and ensuring that the person's mindset gamma-hydroxybutyrate (GHB) is conducive to a positive experience.

Gamma-Hydroxybutyrate

Gamma-hydroxybutyrate (GHB) goes by various names including: "G", "liquid G", "liquid X", "easy lay", "Georgia home boy", "juice", "liquid ecstasy", and "mils".[170–172] Its use is often associated with nightlife and party or "club" settings where it is consumed for its euphoric and disinhibiting effects.[170,173] GHB is also known to enhance sexual performance, referred to as "chem sex" or "party and play."[174] GHB use is far less common compared to other illicit "party" substances. Current estimates from the 2015–2020 National Survey of Drug Use and Health report 0.05% of US adults endorse consuming GHB in the past year.[175] Those aged 35 to 49 years, gay, and bisexual communities report disproportionally greater levels of GHB use compared to younger, heterosexual cohorts.[175]

GHB use is also associated with bodybuilders due to its perceived growth hormone-stimulating effects and was historically marketed and sold as a prodrug in products for the gym as a "performance-enhancer dietary supplement."[176] Desired effects from GHB for body-builder communities included sleep management, mood enhancement, and vigilance.[176]

A very low therapeutic index is responsible for many of the complications seen from GHB use, especially high risk of overdose and sedation.[177] GHB was easily accessible until the year 2000, when it was listed as a Schedule I drug within the Rape Drug Prohibition Act in response its associated use in substance-facilitated sexual assaults.[178]

Mechanism of Action

GHB occurs naturally within the body as an endogenous water-soluble tetracarbon neurotransmitter. It is a CNS depressant that acts as both neurotransmitter and neuromodulator, binding to GHB-specific and $GABA_B$ receptors in the brain, leading to sedative, euphoric, and anesthetic effects.[170,179] GHB's distinct effect on $GABA_B$ receptors distinguishes it from other sedative hypnotics such as alcohol and benzodiazepines, which primarily act on $GABA_A$ receptors. GHB is medically approved for narcolepsy (marketed as sodium oxybate).

GHB Toxicity

GHB toxicity leads to CNS depression with sedation and drowsiness progressing to loss of consciousness or coma.[180] Other concerning signs associated with GHB-induced CNS depression include shallow or slowed breathing and respiratory depression, which can be life threatening. Autonomic symptoms to monitor for include hypotension, hypothermia, and seizures. A characteristic pattern seen in GHB toxicity includes intermittent somnolence and agitation. While patients may present as unresponsive, they can become extremely agitated with abrupt awakening and combativeness as the substance wears off.[181]

Based on pharmacokinetics of GHB, toxicity often resolves within a few hours,[182,183] but the risk of aspiration, anoxic brain injury, and death associated with toxicity and significant CNS depression underscores the need for immediate medical intervention. Due to the narrow safety margin, accidental poisoning is common with use.

There is no antidote to reverse GHB toxicity. Management of GHB toxicity involves monitoring and supportive care. Like management of benzodiazepine toxicity, patients should be monitored in the hospital where frequent general and neurologic vital assessments are conducted until the patient is alert and oriented and can protect their airway. Use of continuous pulse oximetry and telemetry is recommended to monitor the patient for respiratory depression, hypoxia, and coma.

GHB Withdrawal

GHB withdrawal is characterized by a range of physical and psychological symptoms that emerge within hours of cessation, particularly in individuals with chronic, high-dose use. Common features of GHB withdrawal include restlessness, anxiety, agitation, and insomnia. Given GHB's similar mechanism of action to benzodiazepines, GHB withdrawal is also characterized by rebound hyperactivity and imbalance of excitatory and inhibitory neurotransmission, favoring excitatory processes. Autonomic hyperactivity in response to GBH cessation includes tachycardia, hypertension, diaphoresis, and nausea. Severe cases can progress to symptoms noted in complicated withdrawal from alcohol and benzodiazepines, including hallucinations, delirium, and seizures.[184–186]

Management of GHB requires hospitalization, supportive care, and often the use CNS depressants like benzodiazepines to control symptoms and prevent complications. Because GHB withdrawal occurs rapidly and intensely after cessation, early recognition and intervention are crucial. GHB is managed in the hospital and treated with short- and/or long-acting benzodiazepines.[185,187]

Standardized protocols for GHB withdrawal management are not available, but administration of benzodiazepines using a CIWA symptom-triggered protocol is reported in the literature.[188] The effectiveness of benzodiazepines for GHB withdrawal management is variable, with many reports of benzodiazepine refractory GHB withdrawal.[184,185,188] Limitations of benzodiazepine effectiveness are thought to be driven by their primary mechanism of action, with preferential binding affinity of $GABA_A$ versus $GABA_B$ receptors. The use of benzodiazepines for optimization of GHB withdrawal can lead to significant challenges including complications related to the use of high doses of benzodiazepines, for example, sedation, respiratory depression, and inability to protect the airway.[186]

Given the mechanism of action of GHB with primary binding affinity for $GABA_B$ receptors, trials of baclofen treatment, an antispasmodic $GABA_B$ receptor agonist, have been used to manage GHB withdrawal with success.[184] While baclofen is often reported as an adjunctive therapy or a benzodiazepine sparing agent, some case reports have reported success using baclofen as a monotherapy for GHB withdrawal management.[188]

Management of GHB Use Disorder

There are currently no FDA-approved medications for long-term treatment of GHB use disorder. Research studies have examined medications that target the GABAergic and glutamatergic systems, such as baclofen, which is the most promising treatment. There is one open-label, nonrandomized trial demonstrating a reduction in return to GHB use among patients receiving 45 to 60 mg of baclofen daily when compared to patients receiving treatment as usual.[189] Similar findings are also reported in a recent case series.[190] Standard of care for GHB use disorder is psychosocial support and behavioral treatments.

3,4-Methylenedioxymethamphetamine

3,4-Methylenedioxymethamphetamine (3,4-MDMA), commonly referred to as "molly," and "ecstasy," is a synthetic psychoactive substance that produces stimulant and hallucinogenic effects. MDMA is commonly associated with the club and rave scene, where it is used to enhance social interaction and the sensory experience of music and lights.[191] MDMA is typically consumed orally with an onset action of 30 to 60 min and with peak effects within 75 to 120 minutes of use.[192] MDMA can also be insufflated.

MDMA use is most prevalent among adolescents and young adults in nightlife settings, with usage patterns varying by region and culture.[191,193] Current estimates of the incidence of MDMA use disorder remain unknown, however, it is thought to be largely uncommon due to subjective experiences reported by individuals who use it, namely the unpleasant side effects experienced 24 hours after use, coupled with the phenomena of diminished positive experiences with successive doses.[194,195]

While typically considered less likely to cause SUD than traditional stimulants like cocaine or methamphetamine, chronic MDMA use can lead to neurotoxic effects, particularly in the serotonergic system, and may result in cognitive impairments, mood disturbances, and other health risks. In recent years, MDMA gained attention in clinical research for its potential therapeutic applications in treating conditions like posttraumatic stress disorder (PTSD), though these uses remain investigational.

MDMA is a monoamine releasing agent which primarily acts as a neuromodulator of serotonin, dopamine, and norepinephrine in the brain. While MDMA exerts effects on multiple neurotransmitters, its effect on serotonin release is most pronounced. Increasing levels of serotonin cause by MDMA consumption leads to heightened sensory perception, emotional openness, empathy, and euphoria.[196]

Management of MDMA Toxicity

Clinical Presentation

While rare, MDMA toxicity presents as an excitatory state, including restlessness, agitation, and in rare cases, confusion. Autonomic hyperactivity can occur with tachycardia, diaphoresis, mydriasis, and hypertension. In severe cases, patients may experience hyperthermia, seizures, rhabdomyolysis, and multiorgan failure, particularly kidney and liver dysfunction.

One concerning complication resulting from excessive MDMA consumption includes serotonin syndrome characterized by altered mental status, autonomic dysregulation (eg, hyperthermia, sweating), and neuromuscular hyperactivity (eg, tremors, clonus).[197,198] Serotonin syndrome has not occurred in any clinical trials evaluating MDMA for clinical indications and is only documented in 22 cases in FDA adverse event reporting system, of which all patients reported using one or more substances with serotonergic properties, in addition to MDMA.[197]

Hyponatremia resulting from excessive water intake with MDMA use combined with the drug's effects on antidiuretic hormone is another known complication which can lead to cerebral edema and seizures.[199] Prompt recognition and supportive management, including cooling measures, hydration, and symptomatic treatment, are critical to mitigating the potentially fatal consequences of MDMA toxicity, especially presentations marked by autonomic hyperactivity.

MDMA Withdrawal

MDMA is not known to lead to physical dependence or neuroadaptive changes that produce severe withdrawal syndromes. However, general symptoms of dysphoria, irritability, insomnia, and anxiety are reported in the literature.[195] Supportive care measures can address the short-term symptoms that occur (ie, acetaminophen for headache, melatonin for sleep). MDMA withdrawal symptoms are anticipated to be short lived, and caution should be taken when managing mood symptoms including anxiety and depression with serotonergic antidepressants.

Hallucinogens

Psilocybin and Lysergic Acid Diethylamide

Psilocybin and Lysergic Acid Diethylamide (LSD) are hallucinogenic substances characterized by their traditional properties with profound effects on sensorium, perception, and cognition.[157,200] Both substances are referred to colloquially as, "psychedelics," a term coined by Humphrey Osmond in 1957 to describe their mind-manifesting capabilities.[201]

While psilocybin is a naturally occurring compound found in mushroom species, LSD is synthetically derived from ergot alkaloids.[157,200] Rates of lifetime psychedelic use is highest among individuals aged 30 to 34 years, whereby 20% report using hallucinogenic substances in their lifetimes, with higher proportions in males (26% in males vs 15% in females).[202] Similar to other substances with hallucinogenic properties, that is, ketamine and MDMA, psilocybin and LSD have low potential for development of SUD because they do not exert effects on the traditional dopamine reward pathways.

Mechanism of Action

Psilocybin and LSD are agonists at the serotonin 5-HT2A receptors, with preferential activity on 5-HT2A receptors.[200] Agonism of the serotonergic pathway is thought to be responsible for their characteristic effects of altered sensory perception, heightened introspection, and changes in thought patterns. Figure 10.4 demonstrates similarities between the molecular structure of psilocin, a metabolite of psilocybin, and serotonin.

Psilocybin and LSD Toxicity

Despite low potential for physical dependence, use of psilocybin and LSD carry risks, including the experience of "bad trips," characterized by anxiety or paranoia.[203] Physical symptoms of toxicity include nausea, dizziness, and mild increases in heart rate and blood pressure. Severe complications, such as prolonged psychosis or HPPD, are rare but more likely in individuals with a history of mental illness.

Management of toxicity typically focuses on supportive care with reassurance and a calm and safe environment to alleviate psychological distress. In cases of severe agitation or paranoia, benzodiazepines may be used. Hospitalization is rarely needed but may be warranted in cases involving psychosis or self-harm risk. Education about "set" (mindset) and "setting" (environment) is essential to reduce the risk of adverse experiences during use, particularly in therapeutic or experimental contexts.

Withdrawal symptoms are not commonly associated with psilocybin or LSD, as these substances do not produce physical dependence.

Inhalants

Inhalants represent any substance whose vapors can be inhaled to produce a range of intoxicating effects including euphoria, stimulation, disinhibition, sedation, or dissociation. Common substances in this class include solvents, for example, gasoline, toluene, acetone, and gases, for example, butane and propane. There are hundreds of chemicals that may cause similar psychoactive effects. Many common household products can be repurposed for these effects, including paint thinner, insect repellants, glue, aerosol cans, and fuel canisters. Commonly, the product is concentrated in a ballon or plastic bag, soaked into a rag, or it can be directly inhaled from the container itself. Alkyl nitrates and nitrous oxide are other psychoactive substances often distinguished from other inhalants and are inhaled.

Youth and adolescent populations most commonly use inhalants. Use is higher in youth and adolescents who have co-occurring mental illness, financial hardship, and/or are involved in the criminal legal system. More than 22 million Americans have used inhalants in the past, with more than half occurring for the first time before the end of ninth grade. Most people

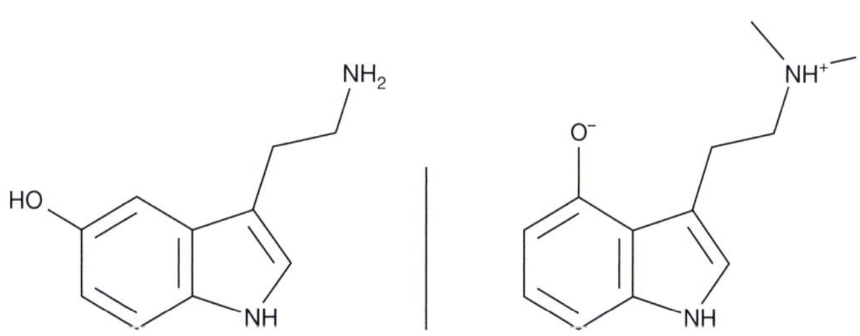

Serotonin
(5-Hydroxytryptamine)

Psilocin
(4-Hydroxy-N,N-Dimethyltrymptamine)

Figure 10.4: Psilocybin is metabolized to psilocin which closely resembles serotonin's molecular structure. (Innerbloom Ketamine Therapy. *Ketamine, Psilocybin, and Microdosing for Depression and Mental Health Treatment*. November 6, 2024. Accessed March 30, 2025. https://innerbloom-ketamine.com/blog/ketamine-psilocybin-and-microdosing-for-depression-and-mental-health-treatment/)

discontinue inhalant use quickly, though anywhere from <10% to almost 50% may meet criteria for an inhalant use disorder, depending on the population sampled.[204]

Mechanism of Action

Inhalants exert their actions at a range of receptors in the CNS. Because there are many substances within this class, there are variable effects depending on the substance used. Inhalants act as a positive modulator of the GABA system, they demonstrate NMDA blocking activity with inhibition of glutamate, and they increase dopamine release.[205,206] They tend to be very short acting in their effects leading to frequent dosing intervals to obtain desired result.

Inhalant Intoxication

Clinical Presentation

Presentation to the hospital due to the immediate effects of an inhalant will be rare, given their short half-lives. A patient would most commonly present with a transient decreased or altered state of consciousness, though traumatic injury related to acute intoxication may be a common alternative presentation. Although the acute intoxication typically resolves quickly (and there are no reversal agents), inhalant use can lead to numerous serious medical complications that may present in the hospital and require their own investigations.

Inhalant Withdrawal

Inhalant withdrawal symptoms in those with long-term inhalant use have been described and may occur in as many as 1 in 5 people who use inhalants. Symptoms such as hypersomnia, fatigue, nausea, diaphoresis, and low mood were most common in the days after cessation of inhalant use.[207]

No specific diagnostic testing is recommended to diagnose inhalant intoxication or inhalant withdrawal. Instead, the medical work up should focus on the variety of potentially significant medical complications associated with inhalant use that require their own investigations.

Medical Comorbidities Related to Inhalant Use

Sudden Death

Sudden death sniffing syndrome (SDSS) is a rare but well-described consequence of inhalant use and can occur following the use of a range of substances. Most commonly it is thought that inhalant use leads to catecholamine surges leading to tachyarrhythmia, though bradycardia due to vagal depression and acute hypoxemia are likely etiologies. Alternatively, respiratory arrest due to aspiration and/or physical suffocation may also play a role in some cases. All patients with any history of inhalant use should be counseled on the risk of this devastating consequence, which can occur even with infrequent (or first time) inhalant use.[208]

Neurologic Impairment/Parkinsonism

Long-term inhalant use is associated with a variety of permanent neurologic deficits, including a range of motor, cognitive, and sensory effects. These deficits arise through multiple mechanisms that cause white matter degeneration, myelin loss, and polyneuropathy, manifesting as irritability, tremor, ataxia, nystagmus, slurred speech, reduced visual acuity, and even hearing loss.[209] While these deficits are mostly irreversible, a thorough physical exam and neurologic imaging is recommended for patients presenting with a history of inhalant use. Cases of psychotic disorders diagnosed following long-term solvent use have been described, however a causal link has not been established.[210]

Vitamin B12 Deficiency

Long-term use of nitrous oxide can lead to a profound vitamin B12 deficiency. This presents clinically as a presentation of pernicious anemia and is characterized by myelopathy, peripheral sensorimotor neuropathy, encephalopathy, and hematologic abnormalities such as macrocytic anemia, leukopenia, and hypersegmented neutrophils. Skin hyperpigmentation has also been described, and the diagnosis can be confirmed by checking B12 levels. In such cases, an MRI of the brain will often be normal, but MRI of the spine will show characteristic findings of the myelopathy, and nerve conduction studies will almost always be abnormal. Cessation of exposure to nitrous oxide is the most important treatment approach in such patients, however aggressive replacement of cobalamin is strongly recommended, and most patients will improve at least partially.[211]

Management of Inhalant Use Disorder

There are no specific evidence-based treatment options for the management of inhalant use other than addressing associated complications. The best available evidence suggests a focus on prevention and multimodal intervention is the most promising approach, though a number of antipsychotic agents and other medications have shown some signals of benefit in very small clinical trials.[204] In general, once the patient is stabilized, hospital-based clinicians should refer patients to comprehensive outpatient SUD treatment resources as available for a full assessment of their substance use, education, and exploration of available treatment options.

Emerging Evidence

This chapter covers many diverse substances, some of which have FDA-approved indications. Some of these substances may hold promise for the treatment of different conditions such as ketamine[212] for the treatment of refractory alcohol withdrawal; MDMA[213] and/or psilocybin[214] for the treatment of alcohol use disorder; MDMA[215] for the treatment of severe PTSD; and THC/CBD and/or ketamine for the management of chronic pain.[216] There are doubtless myriads of other conditions that could be managed using these substances that are not yet discovered. Research challenges include variation in state and federal laws governing controlled substances and obtaining approval for study.[217]

Conclusion

While use of some of the substances described in this chapter are rare and may not be seen by most hospital-based clinicians (eg, PCP intoxication), other substances described in this chapter are very common (eg, THC and CHS, cocaine and methamphetamine-related cardiomyopathy). Hospital-based clinicians should recognize the potential harms of both acute and chronic use of these substances and be familiar with best practices for managing the associated medical complications. When hospitalized patients present with symptoms consistent with stimulant or depressant intoxication, the evaluation is typically straightforward and relies on routine blood tests. Management is usually supportive—such as providing a quiet room to rest—and symptoms can be treated with standard medications including benzodiazepines, antiemetics, and intravenous fluids. Hospital-based clinicians are well equipped to provide this supportive care to most patients who present with acute substance intoxication and withdrawal management with referral to treatment after discharge.

REFERENCES

1. Barile FA. Sympathomimetics. In: *Barile's Clinical Toxicology*. CRC Press; 2019:203–223.
2. UNODC. *World Drug Report 2023*. United Nations Publication; 2023.
3. Friedman J, Shover CL. Charting the fourth wave: geographic, temporal, race/ethnicity and demographic trends in polysubstance fentanyl overdose deaths in the United States, 2010–2021. *Addiction*. 2023;118(12):2477–2485.
4. Han B, Compton WM, Jones CM, Einstein EB, Volkow ND. Methamphetamine use, methamphetamine use disorder, and associated overdose deaths among US adults. *JAMA Psychiatry*. 2021;78(12):1329–1342.
5. Jones CM, Olsen EO, O'Donnell J, Mustaquim D. Resurgent methamphetamine use at treatment admission in the United States, 2008–2017. *Am J Public Health*. 2020;110(4):509–516.
6. Crispo JAG, Liu L, Bach P, et al. Amphetamine-related emergency department visits in Ontario, Canada, 2003–2020. *Can J Psychiatry*. 2023;68(11):838–849.
7. Liu LJW, Crispo JAG, Bach P, et al. Amphetamine-related care in the USA, 2003-2014: cross-sectional analyses examining inpatient trends and factors associated with hospitalisation outcomes. *BMJ Open*. 2022;12(9):e059898.
8. Winkelman TNA, Admon LK, Jennings L, Shippee ND. Richardson CR, Bart G. Evaluation of amphetamine-related hospitalizations and associated clinical outcomes and costs in the United States. *JAMA Netw Open*. 2018;1(6):e183758.
9. Ciccarone D, Shoptaw S. Understanding stimulant use and use disorders in a new era. *Med Clin North Am*. 2022;106(1):81–97.
10. Substance Abuse and Mental Health Services Administration. *Key Substance Use and Mental Health Indicators in the United States: Results from the 2023 National Survey on Drug Use and Health (HHS Publication No. PEP24-07-021, NSDUH Series H-59)*. Center for Behavioral Health Statistics and Quality, Substance Abuse and Mental Health Services Administration; 2024.
11. Canadian Substance Use Survey – Summary of Results 2023. Government of Canada. Health Canada. *Controlled Substances and Overdose Response Directorate*. Office of Drug Research and Surveillance; 2024.
12. Volkow ND, Wang G-J, Fischman MW, et al. Effects of route of administration on cocaine induced dopamine transporter blockade in the human brain. *Life Sci*. 2000;67(12):1507–1515.
13. Vearrier D, Greenberg MI, Miller SN, Okaneku JT, Haggerty DA. Methamphetamine: history, pathophysiology, adverse health effects, current trends, and hazards associated with the clandestine manufacture of methamphetamine. *Dis Mon*. 2012;58(2):38–89.
14. Panenka WJ, Procyshyn RM, Lecomte T, et al. Methamphetamine use: a comprehensive review of molecular, preclinical and clinical findings. *Drug Alcohol Depend*. 2013;129(3):167–179.
15. Cruickshank CC, Dyer KR. A review of the clinical pharmacology of methamphetamine. *Addiction*. 2009;104(7):1085–1099.
16. Saif AM, Farboud A, Delfosse E, Pope L, Adke M. Assessing the safety and efficacy of drugs used in preparing the nose for diagnostic and therapeutic procedures: a systematic review. *Clin Otolaryngol*. 2016;41(5):546–563.
17. Kardon RH, Denison CE, Brown CK, Thompson HS. Critical evaluation of the cocaine test in the diagnosis of Horner's syndrome. *Arch Ophthalmol*. 1990;108(3):384–387.
18. CADDRA—Canadian ADHD Resource Alliance. *Canadian ADHD Practice Guidelines, 4.1 Edition*, CADDRA; 2020.
19. Maski K, Trotti LM, Kotagal S, et al. Treatment of central disorders of hypersomnolence: an American Academy of Sleep Medicine clinical practice guideline. *J Clin Sleep Med*. 2021;17(9):1881–1893.

20. Wolraich ML, Hagan JF, Allan C, et al. Clinical practice guideline for the diagnosis, evaluation, and treatment of attention-deficit/hyperactivity disorder in children and adolescents. *Pediatrics.* 2019;144(4):e20192528.
21. Clinical Guideline Committee (CGC) Members; ASAM Team; AAAP Team; IRETA Team. The ASAM/AAAP Clinical Practice Guideline on the Management of Stimulant Use Disorder. *J Addict Med.* 2024;18(1S Suppl 1):1–56.
22. Hardy SE. Methylphenidate for the treatment of depressive symptoms, including fatigue and apathy, in medically ill older adults and terminally ill adults. *Am J Geriatr Pharmacother.* 2009;7(1):34–59.
23. Lavretsky H, Reinlieb M, St. Cyr N, Siddarth P, Ercoli LM, Senturk D. Citalopram, methylphenidate, or their combination in geriatric depression: a randomized, double-blind, placebo-controlled trial. *Am J Psychiatry.* 2015;172(6):561–569.
24. Piper BJ, Ogden CL, Simoyan OM, et al. Trends in use of prescription stimulants in the United States and Territories, 2006 to 2016. *PLoS One.* 2018;13(11):e0206100.
25. Xu G, Strathearn L, Liu B, Yang B, Bao W. Twenty-year trends in diagnosed attention-deficit/hyperactivity disorder among US children and adolescents, 1997–2016. *JAMA Netw Open.* 2018;1(4):e181471.
26. Moran LV, Ongur D, Hsu J, Castro VM, Perlis RH, Schneeweiss S. Psychosis with methylphenidate or amphetamine in patients with ADHD. *N Engl J Med.* 2019;380(12):1128–1138.
27. Zhang Le, Li L, Andell P, et al. Attention-deficit/hyperactivity disorder medications and long-term risk of cardiovascular diseases. *JAMA Psychiatry.* 2024;81(2):178–187.
28. Brown H, Pollard KA. Drugs of abuse: sympathomimetics. *Crit Care Clin.* 2021;37(3):487–499.
29. Kale N. Urine drug tests: ordering and interpreting results. *Am Fam Physician.* 2019;99(1):33–39.
30. Smith MP, Bluth MH. Common interferences in drug testing. *Clin Lab Med.* 2016;36(4):663–671.
31. Pope JD, Drummer OH, Schneider HG. False-positive amphetamines in urine drug screens: a 6-year review. *J Anal Toxicol.* 2023;47(3):263–270.
32. Honour JW. Gas chromatography—mass spectrometry. *Methods Mol Biol.* 2006;324:53–74.
33. Lecomte T, Dumais A, Dugré JR, Potvin S. The prevalence of substance-induced psychotic disorder in methamphetamine misusers: a meta-analysis. *Psychiatry Res.* 2018;268:189–192.
34. Srisurapanont M, Likhitsathian S, Suttajit S, et al. Efficacy and dropout rates of antipsychotic medications for methamphetamine psychosis: a systematic review and network meta-analysis. *Drug Alcohol Depend.* 2021;219:108467.
35. Hartel-Petri R, Krampe-Scheidler A, Braunwarth WD et al. Evidence-based guidelines for the pharmacologic management of methamphetamine dependence, relapse prevention, chronic methamphetamine-related, and comorbid psychiatric disorders in post-acute settings. *Pharmacopsychiatry.* 2017;50(3):96–104.
36. Voce A, Calabria B, Burns R, Castle D, McKetin R. A systematic review of the symptom profile and course of methamphetamine-associated psychosis (substance use and misuse). *Subst Use Misuse.* 2019;54(4):549–559.
37. Li MJ, Shoptaw SJ. Clinical management of psychostimulant withdrawal: review of the evidence. *Addiction.* 2023;118(4):750–762.
38. Boarescu I, Boarescu PM. Drug-induced myocardial infarction: a review of pharmacological triggers and pathophysiological mechanisms. *J Cardiovasc Dev Dis.* 2024;11(12):406.
39. Lange RA, Cigarroa RG, Yancy CW, et al. Cocaine-induced coronary-artery vasoconstriction. *N Engl J Med.* 1989;321(23):1557–1562.
40. Wilson T, Pitcher I, Bach P. Avoidance of beta-blockers in patients who use stimulants is not supported by good evidence. *Can Med Assoc J.* 2022;194(4):E127–E128.
41. Dominic P, Ahmad J, Awwab H, et al. Stimulant drugs of abuse and cardiac arrhythmias. *Circ Arrhythm Electrophysiol.* 2022;15(1):e010273.
42. Manja V, Nrusimha A, Gao Ya, et al. Methamphetamine-associated heart failure: a systematic review of observational studies. *Heart.* 2023;109(3):168–177.
43. Nolan AL, Jen KY. Pathologic manifestations of levamisole-adulterated cocaine exposure. *Diagn Pathol.* 2015;10:48.
44. Patel P, Guzman S, Lysyshyn M, et al. Identifying cocaine adulteration in the unregulated drug supply in British Columbia, Canada. *Can J Addict.* 2021;14(4):6–13.
45. Ronsley C, Nolan S, Knight R, et al. Treatment of stimulant use disorder: a systematic review of reviews. *PLoS One.* 2020;15(6):e0234809.
46. De Crescenzo F, Ciabattini M, D'Alò GL, et al. Comparative efficacy and acceptability of psychosocial interventions for individuals with cocaine and amphetamine addiction: a systematic review and network meta-analysis. *PLoS Med.* 2018;15(12):e1002715.
47. Appa A, Baral S, Stein B, et al. The IMPACT (infection management plus addiction care together) pilot: a case series of combined contingency management for substance use disorders and antibiotic adherence in the hospital setting. *J Addict Med.* 2024;18(2):138–143.
48. Bach P, Garrod E, Robinson K, Fairbairn N. An acute care contingency management program for the treatment of stimulant use disorder: a case report. *J Addict Med.* 2020;14(6):510–513.
49. Le Foll B, Tang VM, Rueda S, Trick LV, Boileau I. Cannabis use disorder: from neurobiology to treatment. *J Clin Invest.* 2024;134(20):172887.
50. Bukowska B. Current and potential use of biologically active compounds derived from cannabis sativa L. in the treatment of selected diseases. *Int J Mol Sci.* 2024;25(23):12738.
51. Cannabis basics. *Systematically Testing the Evidence on Marijuana.* US Department of Veterans Affairs and the Center for Evidence-based Policy at Oregon Health & Science University. Updated June 2023. Accessed April 28, 2025. https://www.cannabisevidence.org/clinician-resources/cannabis-basics/
52. Mørland J, Bretteville-Jensen AL, Bramness JG. On the duration of cannabis effects and the presence of THC in the body. *Addiction.* 2023;118(2):390–391.
53. Taflaj B, La Maida N, Tittarelli R, Di Trana A, D'Acquarica I. New psychoactive substances toxicity: a systematic review of acute and chronic psychiatric effects. *Int J Mol Sci.* 2024;25(17):9484.
54. Loeffler G, Delaney E, Hann M. International trends in spice use: prevalence, motivation for use, relationship to other substances, and perception of use and safety for synthetic cannabinoids. *Brain Res Bull.* 2016;126(Pt 1):8–28.
55. Winstock A, Lynskey M, Borschmann R, Waldron J. Risk of emergency medical treatment following consumption of cannabis or synthetic cannabinoids in a large global sample. *J Psychopharmacol.* 2015;29(6):698–703.
56. Montagner P, de Salas Quiroga A, Ferreira AS, et al. Charting the therapeutic landscape: a comprehensive evidence map on medical cannabis for health outcomes. *Front Pharmacol.* 2024;15:1494492.
57. Leung J, Chan G, Stjepanović D, Chung JYC, Hall W, Hammond D. Prevalence and self-reported reasons of cannabis use for medical purposes in USA and Canada. *Psychopharmacology (Berl).* 2022;239(5):1509–1519.

58. Bajtel A, Kiss T, Tóth B, et al. The safety of dronabinol and nabilone: a systematic review and meta-analysis of clinical trials. *Pharmaceuticals (Basel)*. 2022;15(1):100.
59. Allaf S, Lim JS, Buckley NA, Cairns R. The impact of cannabis legalization and decriminalization on acute poisoning: a systematic review. *Addiction*. 2023;118(12):2252–2274.
60. Bahji A, Stephenson C, Tyo R, Hawken ER, Seitz DP. Prevalence of cannabis withdrawal symptoms among people with regular or dependent use of cannabinoids: a systematic review and meta-analysis. *JAMA Netw Open*. 2020;3(4):e202370.
61. Connor JP, Stjepanović D, Budney AJ, Le Foll B, Hall WD. Clinical management of cannabis withdrawal. *Addiction*. 2022;117(7):2075–2095.
62. Allen JH, de Moore GM, Heddle R, Twartz JC. Cannabinoid hyperemesis: cyclical hyperemesis in association with chronic cannabis abuse. *Gut*. 2004;53(11):1566–1570.
63. Stjepanović D, Kirkman J, Hall W. Rare but relevant: cannabinoid hyperemesis syndrome. *Addiction*. 2025;120(2): 380–384.
64. Andrews CN, Rehak R, Woo M, et al. Cannabinoid hyperemesis syndrome in North America: evaluation of health burden and treatment prevalence. *Aliment Pharmacol Ther*. 2022;56(11-12):1532–1542.
65. Rubio-Tapia A, McCallum R, Camilleri M. AGA clinical practice update on diagnosis and management of cannabinoid hyperemesis syndrome: commentary. *Gastroenterology*. 2024;166(5):930–934.
66. Senderovich H, Patel P, Jimenez Lopez B, Waicus S. A systematic review on cannabis hyperemesis syndrome and its management options. *Med Princ Pract*. 2022;31(1):29–38.
67. Fischer B, Russell C, Sabioni P, et al. Lower-risk cannabis use guidelines: a comprehensive update of evidence and recommendations. *Am J Public Health*. 2017;107(8):e1–e12.
68. Kang M, Galuska MA, Ghassemzadeh S. Benzodiazepine toxicity [Updated 2023 Jun 26]. In: *StatPearls [Internet]*. StatPearls Publishing; 2024. https://www.ncbi.nlm.nih.gov/books/NBK482238
69. Araújo ÉJFD, Rezende-Júnior LM, Lima LKF, et al. Pathophysiological investigations, anxiolytic effects and interaction of a semisynthetic riparin with benzodiazepine receptors. *Biomed Pharmacother*. 2018;103:973–981.
70. Schmitz A. Benzodiazepine use, misuse, and abuse: a review. *Ment Health Clin*. 2016;6(3):120–126.
71. American Geriatrics Society 2012 Beers Criteria Update Expert Panel. American Geriatrics Society updated Beers Criteria for potentially inappropriate medication use in older adults. *J Am Geriatr Soc*. 2012;60(4):616–631.
72. McLeod PJ, Huang AR, Tamblyn RM, Gayton DC. Defining inappropriate practices in prescribing for elderly people: a national consensus panel. *CMAJ*. 1997;156(3):385–391.
73. American Psychiatric Association Task Force on Benzodiazepine Dependency. *Benzodiazepine Dependence, Toxicity, and Abuse*. American Psychiatric Publishing; 1990.
74. Kennedy KM, O'Riordan J. Prescribing benzodiazepines in general practice. *Br J Gen Pract*. 2019;69(680):152–153.
75. Islam MM, Conigrave KM, Day CA, Nguyen Y, Haber PS. Twenty-year trends in benzodiazepine dispensing in the Australian population. *Intern Med J*. 2014;44(1):57–64.
76. Davies J, Rae TC, Montagu L. Long-term benzodiazepine and Z-drugs use in England: a survey of general practice. *Br J Gen Pract*. 2017;67(662):e609–e613.
77. Olfson M, King M, Schoenbaum M. Benzodiazepine use in the United States. *JAMA Psychiatry*. 2015;72(2):136.
78. Government of Canada. *Canadian Alcohol and Drug Use Monitoring Survey (CADUMS): Summary of Results for 2012 [Internet]*. 2014. http://www.hc-sc.gc.ca/hc-ps/drugs-drogues/stat/_2012/summary-sommaire-eng.php
79. Murphy Y, Wilson E, Goldner EM, Fischer B. Benzodiazepine use, misuse, and harm at the population level in Canada: a comprehensive narrative review of data and developments since 1995. *Clin Drug Investig*. 2016;36(7):519–530.
80. Huang B, Dawson DA, Stinson FS, et al. Prevalence, correlates, and comorbidity of nonmedical prescription drug use and drug use disorders in the United States: results of the National Epidemiologic Survey on alcohol and related conditions. *J Clin Psychiatry*. 2006;67(7):1062–1073.
81. Sanyal C, Asbridge M, Kisely S, Sketris I, Andreou P. The utilization of antidepressants and benzodiazepines among people with major depression in Canada. *Can J Psychiatry*. 2011;56(11):667–676.
82. Vozoris NT, Leung RS. Sedative medication use: prevalence, risk factors, and associations with body mass index using population-level data. *Sleep*. 2011;34(7):869–874.
83. Petitjean S, Ladewig D, Meier CR, Amrein R, Wiesbeck GA. Benzodiazepine prescribing to the Swiss adult population: results from a national survey of community pharmacies. *Int Clin Psychopharmacol*. 2007;22(5):292–298.
84. Charney DS, Mihic SJ, Harris RA. Hypnotics and sedatives. In: Brunton LL, Lazo JS, Parker KL, eds. *Goodman & Gilman's the Pharmacological Basis of Therapeutics*. 11th ed. McGraw-Hill; 2006:401–427.
85. Allison C, Pratt JA. Neuroadaptive processes in GABAergic and glutamatergic systems in benzodiazepine dependence. *Pharmacol Ther*. 2003;98(2):171–195.
86. Winstock AR. *Psychoactive Drug Misuse*. Elsevier; 2012: 439–462.
87. Cook B, Creedon T, Wang Ye, et al. Examining racial/ethnic differences in patterns of benzodiazepine prescription and misuse. *Drug Alcohol Depend*. 2018;187:29–34.
88. Centers for Disease Control and Prevention (CDC). Emergency department visits involving nonmedical use of selected prescription drugs—United States, 2004–2008. *MMWR Morb Mortal Wkly Rep*. 2010;59(23):705–709.
89. Greenblatt DJ, Harmatz JS, Shader RI, Psychotropic drug prescribing in the United States: extent, costs, and expenditures. *J Clin Psychopharmacol*. 2011;31(1):1–3.
90. Department of Justice. *Drug Enforcement Agency. Public Safety Alert U.S. DEA Reports Widespread Threat of Fentanyl Mixed with Xylazine*. Accessed March 12, 2024. https://dea.gov/alert/dea-reports-widespread-threat-fentanyl-mixed-xylazine
91. Department of Justice. *Drug Enforcement Administration. Report: Five Synthetic Benzodiazepine Drugs Deemed Imminent Hazard to Public Safety*. DEA's Diversion Control Division. Published September 25, 2023. Accessed March 13, 2024. https://www.dea.gov/stories/2023/2023-09/2023-09-25/five-synthetic-benzodiazepine-drugs-deemed-imminent-hazard-public
92. Friedman J, Akre S. COVID-19 and the drug overdose crisis: Uncovering the deadliest months in the United States, January–July 2020. *Am J Public Health*. 2021;111(7):1284–1291.
93. Friedman J, Montero F, Bourgois P, et al. Xylazine spreads across the US: a growing component of the increasingly synthetic and polysubstance overdose crisis. *Drug Alcohol Depend*. 2022;233:109380.
94. Reyes JC, Negrón JL, Colón HM, et al. The emerging of xylazine as a new drug of abuse and its health consequences among drug users in Puerto Rico. *J Urban Health*. 2012; 89(3):519–526.
95. Jalal H, Buchanich JM, Roberts MS, Balmert LC, Zhang K, Burke DS. Changing dynamics of the drug overdose epidemic in the United States from 1979 through 2016. *Science (1979)*. 2018;361(6408):eaau1184.
96. Ciccarone D. The rise of illicit fentanyls, stimulants and the fourth wave of the opioid overdose crisis. *Curr Opin Psychiatry*. 2021;34(4):344–350.

97. United States Drug Enforcement Agency. 2024. *One Pill Can Kill Campaign*. https://www.dea.gov/onepill
98. Moses J, Korona-Bailey J, Mukhopadhyay S. Exploring trends in benzodiazepine-positive fatal drug overdoses in Tennessee, 2019–2021. *Ann Med.* 2023;55(2):2287194.
99. Russell E, Sisco E, Thomson A, et al. Rapid analysis of drugs: a pilot surveillance system to detect changes in the illicit drug supply to guide timely harm reduction responses—Eight Syringe Services Programs, Maryland, November 2021–August 2022. *MMWR Morb Mortal Wkly Rep.* 2023;72:458–462.
100. Park JN, Serafinski R, Ujeneza M, et al. Xylazine awareness, desire, use and exposure: preliminary findings from the Rhode Island community-based drug checking cohort study. *Drug Alcohol Depend Rep.* 2024;11:100247.
101. Carpenter JE, Murray BP, Dunkley C, Kazzi ZN, Gittinger MH. Designer benzodiazepines: a report of exposures recorded in the National Poison Data System, 2014–2017. *Clin Toxicol.* 2019;57(4):282–286.
102. Edinoff AN, Nix CA, Odisho AS, et al. Novel designer benzodiazepines: comprehensive review of evolving clinical and adverse effects. *Neurol Int.* 2022;14(3):648–663.
103. Stahl SM. *Stahl's Essential Psychopharmacology: Neuroscientific Basis and Practical Applications*. Cambridge University Press; 2021.
104. O'Connell CW, Sadler CA, Tolia VM, Ly BT, Saitman AM, Fitzgerald RL. Overdose of etizolam: the abuse and rise of a benzodiazepine analog. *Ann Emerg Med.* 2015;65(4):465–466.
105. D'Orazio J, Nelson L, Perrone J, Wightman R, Haroz R. Xylazine adulteration of the heroin-fentanyl drug supply: a narrative review. *Ann Intern Med.* 2023;176(10):1370–1376.
106. Choi S, Irwin MR, Kiyatkin EA. Xylazine effects on opioid-induced brain hypoxia. *Psychopharmacology (Berl).* 2023;240(7):1561–1571.
107. National Institute on Drug Abuse. *Drug Overdose Death Rates—Trends and Statistics*. Accessed March 13, 2024. https://nida.nih.gov/research-topics/trends-statistics/overdose-death-rates#:~:text=Benzodiazepines%20were%20involved%20in%2012%2C499,%2C%2020%25%20also%20involved%20fentanyl
108. Tori ME, Larochelle MR, Naimi TS. Alcohol or benzodiazepine co-involvement with opioid overdose deaths in the United States, 1999–2017. *JAMA Netw Open.* 2020;3(4):e202361.
109. Bromley L, Kahan M, Regenstreif L, Srivastava A, Wyman J. *Methadone Treatment for People Who Use Fentanyl: Recommendations*. META:PHI; 2021. www.metaphi.ca
110. Spadaro A, O'Connor K, Lakamana S, et al. Self-reported xylazine experiences: a mixed methods study of reddit subscribers. *medRxiv.* 2023.
111. Markota M, Rummans TA, Bostwick JM, Lapid MI. Benzodiazepine use in older adults: dangers, management, and alternative therapies. *Mayo Clin Proc.* 2016;91(11):1632–1639.
112. Potokar J, Coupland N, Wilson S, Rich A, Nutt D. Assessment of GABA(A)benzodiazepine receptor (GBzR) sensitivity in patients on benzodiazepines. *Psychopharmacology (Berl).* 1999;146(2):180–184.
113. Benzodiazepine tapering. American Society of Addiction Medicine. Accessed April 28, 2025. https://www.asam.org/quality-care/clinical-guidelines/benzodiazepine-tapering
114. Pétursson H. The benzodiazepine withdrawal syndrome. *Addiction.* 1994;89(11):1455–1459.
115. Schöpf J. Withdrawal phenomena after long-term administration of benzodiazepines. A review of recent investigations. *Pharmacopsychiatria.* 1983;16(1):1–8.
116. Fialip J, Aumaitre O, Eschalier A, Maradeix B, Dordain G, Lavarenne J. Benzodiazepine withdrawal seizures: analysis of 48 case reports. *Clin Neuropharmacol.* 1987;10(6):538–544.
117. Busto U, Sellers EM, Naranjo CA, Cappell H, Sanchez-Craig M, Sykora K. Withdrawal reaction after long-term therapeutic use of benzodiazepines. *N Engl J Med.* 1986;315(14):854–859.
118. Rickels K, Schweizer E, Case WG, Greenblatt DJ. Long-term therapeutic use of benzodiazepines. I. Effects of abrupt discontinuation. *Arch Gen Psychiatry.* 1990;47(10):899–907.
119. McGregor C, Machin A, White JM. In-patient benzodiazepine withdrawal: comparison of fixed and symptom-triggered taper methods. *Drug Alcohol Rev.* 2003;22(2):175–180.
120. Busto UE, Sykora K, Sellers EM. A clinical scale to assess benzodiazepine withdrawal. *J Clin Psychopharmacol.* 1989;9(6):412–416.
121. Kawasaki SS, Jacapraro JS, Rastegar DA. Safety and effectiveness of a fixed-dose phenobarbital protocol for inpatient benzodiazepine detoxification. *J Subst Abuse Treat.* 2012;43(3):331–334.
122. Leung E, Ngo DH, Espinoza JA, et al. A retrospective study of the adjunctive use of gabapentin with benzodiazepines for the treatment of benzodiazepine withdrawal. *J Psychiatr Pract.* 2022;28(4):310–318.
123. Chandrasekaran PK. Employing mirtazapine to aid benzodiazepine withdrawal. *Singapore Med J.* 2008;49(6):e166–e167.
124. Vicens C, Bejarano F, Sempere E, et al. Comparative efficacy of two interventions to discontinue long-term benzodiazepine use: cluster randomised controlled trial in primary care. *Br J Psychiatry.* 2014;204(6):471–479.
125. Hauck TS, Rochon S, Bahra P, Selby P. Outpatient treatment of chronic designer benzodiazepine use: a case report. *J Addict Med.* 2022;16(2):e137–e139.
126. Corkery JM, Streete P, Claridge H, et al. Characteristics of deaths associated with kratom use. *J Psychopharmacol.* 2019;33(9):1102–1123.
127. Schimmel J, Amioka E, Rockhill K, et al. Prevalence and description of kratom (Mitragyna speciosa) use in the United States: a cross-sectional study. *Addiction.* 2021;116(1):176–181.
128. Eggleston W, Stoppacher R, Suen K, Marraffa JM, Nelson LS. Kratom use and toxicities in the United States. *Pharmacotherapy.* 2019;39(7):775–777.
129. Henningfield JE, Grundmann O, Huestis MA, Smith KE. Kratom safety and toxicology in the public health context: research needs to better inform regulation. *Front Pharmacol.* 2024;15:1403140.
130. Alsarraf E, Myers J, Culbreth S, Fanikos J. Kratom from head to toe—case reviews of adverse events and toxicities. *Curr Emerg Hosp Med Rep.* 2019;7:141–168.
131. Trakulsrichai S, Sathirakul K, Auparakkitanon S, et al. Pharmacokinetics of mitragynine in man. *Drug Des Devel Ther.* 2015;9:2421–2429.
132. Smith KE, Panlilio LV, Feldman JD, Grundmann O, Dunn KE. Ecological momentary assessment of self-reported kratom use, effects, and motivations among US adults. *JAMA Netw Open.* 2024;7(1):e2353401.
133. Smith KE, Epstein DH, Weiss ST. Controversies in assessment, diagnosis, and treatment of kratom use disorder. *Curr Psychiatry Rep.* 2024;26(9):487–496.
134. Silva B, Soares J, Rocha-Pereira C, Mladěnka P, Remião F. Khat, a cultural chewing drug: a toxicokinetic and toxicodynamic summary. *Toxins (Basel).* 2022;14(2):71.
135. Riley AL, Nelson KH, To P, et al. Abuse potential and toxicity of the synthetic cathinones (i.e., "Bath salts"). *Neurosci Biobehav Rev.* 2020;110:150–173.
136. Daswani RR, Choles CM, Kim DD, Barr AM. A systematic review and meta-analysis of synthetic cathinone use and psychosis. *Psychopharmacology (Berl).* 2024;241(5):875–896.

137. Costa R, Oliveira NG, Dinis-Oliveira RJ. Pharmacokinetic and pharmacodynamic of bupropion: integrative overview of relevant clinical and forensic aspects. *Drug Metab Rev.* 2019; 51(3):293–313.
138. Rosenbaum SB, Gupta V, Patel P, et al. Ketamine. [Updated January 30, 2024]. In: *StatPearls [Internet]*. StatPearls Publishing; 2024. https://www.ncbi.nlm.nih.gov/books/NBK470357/
139. Yockey RA. Past-year ketamine use: evidence from a United States population, 2015–2019. *J Psychoactive Drugs.* 2023;55(2):134–140.
140. Campbell R, Lobo MK. A short burst of reward curbs the addictiveness of ketamine. *Nature.* 2022;608(7922):271–272.
141. Simmler LD, Li Y, Hadjas LC, Hiver A, van Zessen R, Lüscher C. Dual action of ketamine confines addiction liability. *Nature.* 2022;608(7922):368–373.
142. Nichols KA, Paciullo CA. Subdissociative ketamine use in the emergency department. *Adv Emerg Nurs J.* 2019;41(1): 15–22.
143. Sinner B, Graf BM. Ketamine. *Handb Exp Pharmacol.* 2008; (182):313–333.
144. Chaves TV, Wilffert B, Sanchez ZM. Overdoses and deaths related to the use of ketamine and its analogues: a systematic review. *Am J Drug Alcohol Abuse.* 2023;49(2):141–150.
145. Kalsi SS, Wood DM, Dargan PI. The epidemiology and patterns of acute and chronic toxicity associated with recreational ketamine use. *Emerg Health Threats J.* 2011;4(1):7107.
146. Abstracts of the 2008 North American Congress of Clinical Toxicology Annual Meeting, September 11–16, 2008, Toronto, Canada. *Clin Toxicol.* 2008;46(7):591–645.
147. Winstock AR, Mitcheson L, Gillatt DA, Cottrell AM. The prevalence and natural history of urinary symptoms among recreational ketamine users. *BJU Int.* 2012;110(11): 1762–1766.
148. J. Anderson D, Zhou J, Cao D, et al. Ketamine-induced cystitis: a comprehensive review of the urologic effects of this psychoactive drug. *Health Psychol Res.* 2022;10(3):38247.
149. Chu PS-K, Ma W-K, Wong SC-W, et al. The destruction of the lower urinary tract by ketamine abuse: a new syndrome? *BJU Int.* 2008;102(11):1616–1622.
150. Journey JD, Bentley TP. Phencyclidine toxicity. In: *StatPearls [Internet]*. StatPearls Publishing Copyright © 2024, StatPearls Publishing LLC: 2024.
151. Bertron JL, Seto M, Lindsley CW. DARK Classics in Chemical neuroscience:hencyclidine (PCP). *ACS Chem Neurosci.* 2018;9(10):2459–2474.
152. Morgan JP, Kagan D. The dusting of America: the image of phencyclidine (PCP) in the popular media. *J Psychedelic Drugs.* 1980;12(3-4):195–204.
153. Pradhan SN. Phencyclidine (PCP): some human studies. *Neurosci Biobehav Rev.* 1984;8(4):493–501.
154. Garey RE, Daul GC, Samuels MS, Ragan FA, Hite SA. PCP abuse in New Orleans: a six-year study. *Am J Drug Alcohol Abuse.* 1987;13(1–2):135–144.
155. Thombs DL. A review of PCP abuse trends and perceptions. *Public Health Rep.* 1989;104(4):325–328.
156. Davis BL. The PCP epidemic: a critical review. *Int J Addict.* 1982;17(7):1137–1155.
157. Nichols DE. Psychedelics. *Pharmacol Rev.* 2016;68(2):264–355.
158. Carbonaro TM, Gatch MB. N-dimethyltryptamine. *Brain Res Bull.* 2016;126(Pt 1):74–88.
159. Saavedra JM, Axelrod J. Psychotomimetic N-methylated tryptamines: formation in brain in vivo and in vitro. *Science (1979).* 1972;175(4028):1365–1366.
160. Servillo L, Giovane A, Balestrieri ML, Cautela D, Castaldo D. N-methylated tryptamine derivatives in citrus genus plants: identification of N,N,N-trimethyltryptamine in bergamot. *J Agric Food Chem.* 2012;60(37):9512–9518.
161. Pochettino ML, Cortella AR, Ruiz M. Hallucinogenic snuff from northwestern Argentina: microscopical identification of anadenanthera colubrina var. cebil (Fabaceae) in powdered archaeological material. *Econ Bot.* 1999;53(2):127–132.
162. Strassman R. *DMT: The Spirit Molecule: A Doctor's Revolutionary Research into the Biology of Near-Death and Mystical Experiences.* Simon and Schuster; 2000.
163. Strassman RJ. Human psychopharmacology of N,N-dimethyltryptamine. *Behav Brain Res.* 1996;73(1-2):121–124.
164. Strassman RJ, Qualls CR, Berg LM. Differential tolerance to biological and subjective effects of four closely spaced doses of N,N-dimethyltryptamine in humans. *Biol Psychiatry.* 1996; 39(9):784–795.
165. Winstock AR, Kaar S, Borschmann R. Dimethyltryptamine (DMT): prevalence, user characteristics and abuse liability in a large global sample. *J Psychopharmacol.* 2014;28(1):49–54.
166. Cozzi NV, Gopalakrishnan A, Anderson LL, et al. Dimethyltryptamine and other hallucinogenic tryptamines exhibit substrate behavior at the serotonin uptake transporter and the vesicle monoamine transporter. *J Neural Transm (Vienna).* 2009;116(12):1591–1599.
167. Strassman RJ, Qualls CR. Dose-response study of N,N-dimethyltryptamine in humans. I. Neuroendocrine, autonomic, and cardiovascular effects. *Arch Gen Psychiatry.* 1994; 51(2):85–97.
168. Barbic D, Fernandes J, Eberdt C, Chakraborty A. N,N-Dimethyltryptamine: DMT-induced psychosis. *Am J Emerg Med.* 2020;38(9):1961.e1–1961.e2.
169. dos Santos RG, Bouso JC, Hallak JEC. Ayahuasca, dimethyltryptamine, and psychosis: a systematic review of human studies. *Ther Adv Psychopharmacol.* 2017;7(4):141–157.
170. Busardo F, Jones A. GHB pharmacology and toxicology: acute intoxication, concentrations in blood and urine in forensic cases and treatment of the withdrawal syndrome. *Curr Neuropharmacol.* 2015;13(1):47–70.
171. Brunt T, Amsterdam J, Brink W. GHB, GBL and 1,4-BD addiction. *Curr Pharm Des.* 2014;20(25):4076–4085.
172. Zvosec DL, Smith SW, Porrata T, Strobl AQ, Dyer JE. Case series of 226 γ-hydroxybutyrate-associated deaths: lethal toxicity and trauma. *Am J Emerg Med.* 2011;29(3):319–332.
173. Sumnall HR, Woolfall K, Edwards S, Cole JC, Beynon CM. Use, function, and subjective experiences of gamma-hydroxybutyrate (GHB). *Drug Alcohol Depend.* 2008;92(1–3): 286–290.
174. Giorgetti R, Tagliabracci A, Schifano F, Zaami S, Marinelli E, Busardò FP. When "Chems" Meet Sex: a rising phenomenon called "ChemSex". *Curr Neuropharmacol.* 2017;15(5): 762–770.
175. Palamar JJ. Prevalence and correlates of GHB use among adults in the United States. *J Psychoactive Drugs.* 2023; 55(3):268–273.
176. Giorgetti A, Busardò FP, Giorgetti R. Toxicological characterization of GHB as a performance-enhancing drug. *Front Psychiatry.* 2022;13:846983.
177. Miró O, Nogué S, Espinosa G, To-Figueras J, Sánchez M. Trends in illicit drug emergencies: the emerging role of gamma-hydroxybutyrate. *J Toxicol Clin Toxicol.* 2002;40(2): 129–135.
178. White CM. Pharmacologic, pharmacokinetic, and clinical assessment of illicitly used γ-hydroxybutyrate. *J Clin Pharmacol.* 2017;57(1):33–39.
179. Wong CGT, Chan KFY, Gibson KM, Snead OC. Gamma-hydroxybutyric acid: neurobiology and toxicology of a recreational drug. *Toxicol Rev.* 2004;23(1):3–20.
180. Aronsen AC, Brekke M, Vallersnes OM. Acute poisoning with gamma-hydroxybutyrate. *Tidsskr Nor Laegeforen.* 2020; 140(10).

181. Van Sassenbroeck DK, De Neve N, De Paepe P, et al. Abrupt awakening phenomenon associated with gamma-hydroxybutyrate use: a case series. *Clin Toxicol.* 2007;45(5):533–538.
182. Liechti ME, Quednow BB, Liakoni E, et al. Pharmacokinetics and pharmacodynamics of γ-hydroxybutyrate in healthy subjects. *Br J Clin Pharmacol.* 2016;81(5):980–988.
183. Schep LJ, Knudsen K, Slaughter RJ, Vale JA, Mégarbane B. The clinical toxicology of γ-hydroxybutyrate, γ-butyrolactone and 1,4-butanediol. *Clin Toxicol.* 2012;50(6):458–470.
184. LeTourneau JL, Hagg DS, Smith SM. Baclofen and gamma-hydroxybutyrate withdrawal. *Neurocrit Care.* 2008; 8(3):430–433.
185. Dyer JE, Roth B, Hyma BA. Gamma-hydroxybutyrate withdrawal syndrome. *Ann Emerg Med.* 2001;37(2):147–153.
186. Miotto KRB. *GHB Withdrawal Syndrome.* In: *Texas: TCADA: Texas Commission on Alcohol and Drug Abuse*; 2001.
187. Delic M. Inpatient management of GHB/GBL withdrawal. *Psychiatr Danub.* 2019;31(Suppl 3):354–356.
188. Habibian S, Ahamad K, McLean M, Socias ME. Successful management of gamma-hydroxybutyrate (GHB) withdrawal using baclofen as a standalone therapy: a case report. *J Addict Med.* 2019;13(5):415–417.
189. Beurmanjer H, Kamal RM, de Jong CAJ, Dijkstra BAG, Schellekens AFA. Baclofen to prevent relapse in gamma-hydroxybutyrate (GHB)-dependent patients: a multicentre, open-label, non-randomized, controlled trial. *CNS Drugs.* 2018;32(5):437–442.
190. Kamal RM, Loonen AJM, Dijkstra BAG, De Jong CAJ. Baclofen as relapse prevention in the treatment of gamma-hydroxybutyrate dependence: a case series. *J Clin Psychopharmacol.* 2015;35(3):313–318.
191. Strote J, Lee JE, Wechsler H. Increasing MDMA use among college students: results of a national survey. *J Adolesc Health.* 2002;30(1):64–72.
192. Kalant H. The pharmacology and toxicology of "ecstasy" (MDMA) and related drugs. *CMAJ.* 2001;165(7):917–928.
193. Boyd CJ, McCabe SE, d'Arcy H. Ecstasy use among college undergraduates: gender, race and sexual identity. *J Subst Abuse Treat.* 2003;24(3):209–215.
194. Peroutka SJ, Newman H, Harris H. Subjective effects of 3,4-methylenedioxymethamphetamine in recreational users. *Neuropsychopharmacology.* 1988;1(4):273–277.
195. Degenhardt L, Bruno R, Topp L. Is ecstasy a drug of dependence? *Drug Alcohol Depend.* 2010;107(1):1–10.
196. Baylen CA, Rosenberg H. A review of the acute subjective effects of MDMA/ecstasy. *Addiction.* 2006;101(7):933–947.
197. Makunts T, Jerome L, Abagyan R, de Boer A, Reported cases of serotonin syndrome in MDMA users in FAERS database. *Front Psychiatry.* 2021;12:824288.
198. Mueller PD, Korey WS, Death by "Ecstasy": the serotonin syndrome? *Ann Emerg Med.* 1998;32(3):377–380.
199. Elkattawy S, Mowafy A, Younes I, Tucktuck M, Agresti J. Methylenedioxymethamphetamine (MDMA)-induced hyponatremia: case report and literature review. *Cureus.* 2021;13(5): e15223.
200. Nichols DE. Hallucinogens. *Pharmacol Ther.* 2004;101(2): 131–181.
201. Osmond H. A review of the clinical effects of psychotomimetic agents. *Ann N Y Acad Sci.* 1957;66(3):418–434.
202. Krebs TS, Johansen P-Ø. Over 30 million psychedelic users in the United States. *F1000Res.* 2013;2:98.
203. Martinotti G, Santacroce R, Pettorruso M, et al. Hallucinogen persisting perception disorder: etiology, clinical features, and therapeutic perspectives. *Brain Sci.* 2018;8(3):47.
204. Howard MO, Bowen SE, Garland EL, Perron BE, Vaughn MG. Inhalant use and inhalant use disorders in the United States. *Addict Sci Clin Pract.* 2011;6(1):18–31.
205. MacIver MB. Abused inhalants enhance GABA-mediated synaptic inhibition. *Neuropsychopharmacology.* 2009;34(10): 2296–2304.
206. Riegel A, Zapata A, Shippenberg T, et al. The abused inhalant toluene increases dopamine release in the nucleus accumbens by directly stimulating ventral tegmental area neurons. *Neuropsychopharmacol.* 2007;32:1558–1569.
207. Perron B, Glass JE, Ahmedani B, Vaughn MG, Roberts DE, Wu LT. The prevalence and clinical significance of inhalant withdrawal symptoms among a national sample. *Subst Abuse Rehabil.* 2011;2011(2):69–76.
208. Radparvar S. The clinical assessment and treatment of inhalant abuse. *Perm J.* 2023;27(2):99–109.
209. Brouette T, Anton R. Clinical review of inhalants. *Am J Addict.* 2001;10(1):79–94.
210. Byrne A, Kirby B, Zibin T, Ensminger S. Psychiatric and neurological effects of chronic solvent abuse. *Can J Psychiatry.* 1991;36(10):735–738.
211. De Halleux C, Juurlink DN. Diagnosis and management of toxicity associated with the recreational use of nitrous oxide. *Can Med Assoc J.* 2023;195(32):E1075–E1081.
212. Goldfine CE, Tom JJ, Im DD, et al. The therapeutic use and efficacy of ketamine in alcohol use disorder and alcohol withdrawal syndrome: a scoping review. *Front Psychiatry.* 2023;14:1141836.
213. McDonagh MS, Morasco BJ, Wagner J, et al. Cannabis-based products for chronic pain: a systematic review. *Ann Intern Med.* 2022;175(8):1143–1153.
214. Bogenschutz MP, Ross S, Bhatt S, et al. Percentage of heavy drinking days following psilocybin-assisted psychotherapy vs placebo in the treatment of adult patients with alcohol use disorder: a randomized clinical trial. *JAMA Psychiatry.* 2022;79(10):953–962.
215. Mitchell JM, Ot'alora GM, van der Kolk B, et al. MDMA-assisted therapy for moderate to severe PTSD: a randomized, placebo-controlled phase 3 trial. *Nat Med.* 2023;29:2473–2480.
216. Hocking G, Cousins MJ. Ketamine in chronic pain management: an evidence-based review. *Anesth Analg.* 2003; 97(6):730–1739.
217. Mann B. Trump team revokes $11 billion in funding for addiction, mental health care. *NPR.* March 27, 2025. Accessed March 30, 2025. https://www.npr.org/2025/03/27/nx-s1-5342368/addiction-trump-mental-health-funding

11

Infectious Complications of Substance Use Disorders

Laura R. Marks, Madeline McCrary

In 2017, Molly was brought to her local hospital by her boyfriend for fevers, back pain, and inability to walk. She was found to have a methicillin-resistant *Staphylococcus aureus* (MRSA) bacteremia resulting in a spinal epidural abscess and infective endocarditis. She was emergently airlifted to the State's tertiary care center.

In addition to antibiotics, she underwent emergency spinal surgery to decompress the spinal epidural abscess and perform a laminectomy. The vegetation on her heart valve was small enough that she did not require heart valve replacement surgery. Her antibiotic course was straightforward—she needed at least 6 weeks of antibiotics for a complicated MRSA infection with multiple sites of infection. She did not have stable housing and she was too complicated for nursing facilities to accept her, so she needed to remain at the hospital to complete her antibiotic course and repeat imaging.

On admission, Molly disclosed that she had been using opioids and injecting substances prior to her admission. Molly was 22 years old and devastated by this infection. She reported she had started experimenting with substances in high school and eventually went to pills that turned out to be pressed fentanyl. Her use spiraled and she started injecting substances about a year ago. She was very interested in starting buprenorphine and was seen by the Addiction Medicine Consult service.

In addition to addressing her opioid use disorder (OUD), Molly was also screened for human immunodeficiency virus (HIV), hepatitis C virus (HCV), hepatitis B virus (HBV), syphilis, gonorrhea, and chlamydia. She was found to have active HCV (detectable HCV RNA) and was not immune to HBV. She also had a positive RPR with a titer of 1:64 and no known past history of syphilis. Since she had a prolonged hospital stay ahead of her, authorization for HCV treatment was obtained and she was started on direct-acting antivirals in the hospital. She completed 5 of 8 weeks of treatment inpatient. Since she was HBV nonimmune, she was able to receive both doses of HBV vaccine 1 month apart while admitted. And finally, she received a full course of three weekly injections of intramuscular penicillin G benzathine.

At the time of discharge, she had reunited with her mother who offered to stay with her posthospital discharge. She continued buprenorphine via telemedicine and was ultimately linked to a local clinician who could also provide primary care. Since she lived 3 hours away, she followed up with infectious diseases via telemedicine. She completed the remainder of her HCV treatment and achieved sustained virologic response or HCV cure.

While Molly's infection was devastating and life changing, it was also an opportunity to address many other health issues. She started medication for OUD for the first time, cured her HCV, was vaccinated for HBV, and treated for late latent syphilis. Molly was appreciative of being able to have these issues addressed while she was convalescing in the hospital and helped keep her motivated to stay to have her bacterial infection treated.

I last saw Molly 2 years ago, when she was admitted to the hospital after delivery of her newborn son. At that time she was stable on buprenorphine, and reported ongoing engagement with local community supports and outpatient clinics. She was grateful that early screening during her prior admission was able to identify and cure her HCV and syphilis infections prior to becoming pregnant so they would not be passed on to her son.

—Madeline McCrary

Key Points

- **People with substance use disorders (SUD) are at increased risk of blood-borne viruses, invasive bacterial or fungal infections, and sexually transmitted infections (STIs).**
- **Hospitalizations for infectious complications of SUD should prompt initiation of medications for SUD and harm-reduction education.**
- **Shared decision making about antibiotic treatment approaches should be pursued, particularly when patients cannot stay in the hospital for the full course of treatment.**
- **Multidisciplinary hospital-based teams are an effective framework to address and optimize the care of complex infectious complications of SUD.**
- **Hospitalizations offer people with SUD an important opportunity to provide comprehensive screening for blood-borne viruses and STIs, along with immunizations for vaccine-preventable diseases.**

People who use substances and with substance use disorders (SUD) are at increased risk of a wide range of invasive bacterial and fungal infections[1] in addition to blood-borne viruses such as human immunodeficiency virus (HIV), viral hepatitis, and other STIs.[1–3] Hospitalizations for infections related to substance use, particularly from injection substance use, having been drastically[4,5] increasing over the past two decades. For example, hospitalizations for substance use–associated infective endocarditis and related cardiac surgeries increased by more than 12-fold from 2010 to 2017 in North Carolina.[5] Hospitalizations, however, can be an opportunity to offer SUD treatment, harm-reduction education and screening for, diagnosis, treatment and prevention of other infectious complications of substance use, such as HIV, viral hepatitis and STIs.

This chapter will describe the pathogenesis, clinical syndromes, and models of treatment for common infectious complications among people who use substances and have SUD.

Pathogenesis of Infections

Pathogens may be introduced at many points during substance preparation and consumption. A careful history from people who use substances who are presenting with fevers or other symptoms concerning for infection should include details on substances consumed and how, any substance preparation steps and equipment used.[6] Preparation steps between substances may differ and can influence the types of pathogens that may be introduced. A careful substance use history may also identify opportunities for discussion of harm-reduction techniques.

Infectious complications of substance use can occur through several mechanisms. Direct inoculation of pathogens into the bloodstream can occur when either substances, diluents, preparation materials or substance use equipment becomes contaminated with infectious pathogens. Table 11.1 outlines potential opportunities for pathogen introduction during substance preparation and use, along with different strategies for approaching harm-reduction conversations.

Contaminated Substance Supply

Bacterial spores are resistant to heat or desiccation and can be recovered from contaminated substance supplies.[7–9] Spore-forming pathogens commonly include *Bacillus* species and *Clostridium* species[10–12] and can cause toxin-mediated diseases, resulting in sporadic outbreaks within substance use networks.[13,14] Outbreaks among people who inject substances from direct contamination of opioids or other substances have included clusters of Anthrax from contaminated heroin in Scotland in 2009–2010,[15] and tetanus outbreaks in both the United Kingdom[10–12] and sporadic cases in the United States.[16]

Solvent-Associated Infections

Dissolving substances in liquid prior to injection represents another opportunity for pathogen introduction. Bacterial pathogens frequently associated with contaminated water systems such as *Escherichia coli, Enterobacter* species, *Pseudomonas aeruginosa*, and *Serratia marcescens* may be introduced during this process. Other pathogens classically associated with this step can include *Candida* species introduced when lemon juice is used to acidify the solution as aid with dissolving substances.[17–19] The resulting candidemia can manifest as severe systemic infections causing ocular,[20,21] osteoarticular as well as endovascular infections such as infective endocarditis.[22]

TABLE 11.1

Common Pathogens and Targeted Harm-Reduction Practices

Opportunities for pathogen entry	Pathogen	Recommended harm-reduction practice
Contaminated substances	*Spore-forming Bacilli:* *Clostridia species* *Bacillus species*	■ Update tetanus immunization
Liquids used to dissolve substances	*Water-loving gram negatives: Pseudomonas aeruginosa, Serratia marcescens, Escherichia coli*	■ Encourage use of sterile water or use of sterile saline sachets
Skin flora introduced during nonsterile injection practices Some skin flora such as *S. aureus* may persist on reused equipment acting as fomites	*Skin flora: Staphylococcus species, Streptococcus pyogenes*	■ Encourage handwashing prior to substance preparation or substance use ■ Clean injection sites with alcohol swabs ■ Discard any used injection equipment, particularly if materials were injected into a site with active infection
Oral flora introduced from saliva by licking needles	*Oral anaerobes: Streptococcus mutans, Eikinella, Prevotella, Veilonella, "mixed microbes"*	■ Avoid introducing saliva into injection process ■ Avoid reuse of needles
Equipment reuse transmits blood-borne pathogens	Human immunodeficiency virus (HIV) Hepatitis A virus (HAV) Hepatitis B virus (HBV) Hepatitis C virus (HCV)	■ Avoid sharing needles ■ Link patients to syringe service programs ■ Immunize against HAV and HBV if nonimmune ■ Offer pre-exposure prophylaxis for HIV

Nonsterile Injection Practices

For people who use substance via an intravenous route, the physical act of injecting substances presents another moment during which pathogens can be introduced into the body. Nonsterile injection technique increases the risk of injection site infection with skin flora such as *Staphylococcus aureus*, coagulase-negative staphylococci, or *Streptococcus pyogenes*.[23–25] In some cases, saliva[22] used to lubricate dull needles may lead to the direct inoculation of oral pathogens, including streptococci, into the bloodstream.[26,27] Saliva may also come into contact with injection equipment when people lick needles or other equipment to gauge the strength of the substance preparation.[28] Saliva contains a number of aerobic and anaerobic pathogens which cause bloodstream infections and associated endovascular and osteoarticular complications. Common oral flora causing endovascular and osteoarticular infections among people who inject substances include *Eikenella, Haemophilus, Prevotella,* and Viridans group streptococci.[27,29]

Reuse of Drug Preparation Equipment

Finally, the shared use or reuse of substance preparation and injection equipment represents another crucial nidus for pathogens, as *S. aureus* can remain viable on environmental surfaces for a prolonged period of time,[30] and the presence of residual blood in shared needles or works can allow for transmission of blood-borne viral infections such as HIV, hepatitis B virus (HBV), or hepatitis C virus (HCV).[1,3] Shared needles, syringes, or other paraphernalia propagate outbreaks of blood-borne pathogens within communities of people who inject substances. People who inject substances should be instructed to avoid reuse of substances and drug preparation equipment where possible, to reduce the risk of both recurrent staphylococcal infections and the acquisition or transmission of blood-borne viruses.

Harm-Reduction Counseling

Harm-reduction counseling for people with SUD presenting with acute infectious complications should focus on education about the mechanism of their specific infection and a tailored discussion of methods to reduce their risk of similar recurrent infections in the future. For example, a harm-reduction conversation with an individual admitted with *S. aureus* bacteremia might focus on handwashing, cleaning injection sites, and avoiding reuse of equipment that might serve as a nidus for recurrent infections. In contrast, harm-reduction conversations for an individual admitted with a *Streptococcus mutans* bloodstream infection might focus more on avoiding the introduction of saliva into the injection process, either by avoiding licking needles, or licking their fingers after testing potency. For both individuals, that discussion should be supplemented by a referral to nearby needle exchange facilities where available. If access to new sterile supplies is limited, clinicians should educate on avoiding needle sharing and best practices for cleaning supplies using bleach to reduce harm from both the transmission of viral infections and persistence of bacterial pathogens.[31,32] As route of substance use can also influence the likelihood of infection acquisition, people with SUD should also be counseled on reducing the use of subcutaneous injection "skin popping" and intramuscular injection, both of which have a higher risk of skin and soft tissue infections.[33–36]

Clinical Syndromes

Skin and Soft Tissue Infections

The most frequently described infectious complication of injection substance use is skin and soft tissue infection, including skin abscesses,[37,38] with lifetime incidence of up to 68%.[39] Many people who inject substances describe self-treating abscesses by draining them themselves,[40] seeking antibiotics from friends, or delaying care until an infection becomes too severe to ignore.[41] Infections can also include septic tenosynovitis, often in the hands, which require a longer course of antibiotics than simple abscesses and sometimes surgery. Injection site skin and soft tissue infections are most commonly caused by gram-positive organisms related to skin flora including *S. aureus* and *S. pyogenes* which may be introduced during nonsterile injection procedures if skin is not cleaned with alcohol swabs or handwashing is not performed.[23] Empiric antibiotic therapy for skin and soft tissue infections should therefore be primarily directed toward gram-positive bacteria including MRSA and *S. pyogenes* with additional organisms such as oral anaerobes included if indicated by specific risk factors, such as licking needles, are elicited during a substance use history. Clinicians should have a low threshold to broaden antimicrobial therapy in settings where patients are not responding to first-line antimicrobial regimens given higher risk of polymicrobial and gram-negative organisms among people who inject substances.[23]

Wound Botulism and Tetanus

People who inject substances are at increased risk for toxin-mediated infections caused by bacillus and clostridium species. The anaerobic environment provided by subcutaneous injection of substances, or skin popping, is a risk factor for toxin-mediated infections, particularly wound botulism and tetanus.[10,42]

Wound botulism may develop several days after injecting substances contaminated with *Clostridium botulinum* spores. Initial symptoms may include double/blurred vision, speech and swallowing difficulties, muscle weakness, and eventually respiratory collapse.[43,44] Treatment consists of surgical debridement of the wound with irrigation as well as prompt administration of antibiotics. In severe cases, early administration of antitoxin has been associated with improved outcomes.[45] People who inject substances are also at increased risk for tetanus and outbreaks can occur due to contaminated substance batches.[11,46] Tetanus presents with muscle spasms, with jaw muscle spasms classically called trismus, accompanied by autonomic instability. Tetanus is a vaccine-preventable illness and all people who inject substances should be immunized, with boosters recommended every 5 years for patients presenting with necrotizing fasciitis. Other clostridial infections caused by toxin-mediated illnesses include necrotizing fasciitis and toxic-shock syndromes secondary to *C. perfringens* and *C. sordellii*.[47,48] These syndromes often begin as pain out of proportion to exam prior to rapid decompensation and septic shock. Early recognition and surgical debridement with appropriate antimicrobial coverage is critical.

Xylazine-Related Wounds

Xylazine is an $alpha_2$-agonist and common adulterant in the fentanyl supply[49] that can be associated with chronic necrotic skin and soft tissue wounds. Wounds are often on the extensor surfaces of limbs, can progress to becoming large ulcerations with eschar and slough,[50] and can be very painful. While most associated with injection substance use, particularly subcutaneous injection, wounds can occur among people who use substance via noninjection routes.[50,51] While xylazine-associated wounds can be associated with superinfections and sloughing can look like purulence, these wounds are noninfectious in nature, and many heal with regular wound care, including enzymatic debridement.[51,52] Antibiotics are only needed in cases of secondary infections like cellulitis or when the wound has progressed to underlying.[51]

Bloodstream Infections With No Evident Focus

There is a broad range of other causative organisms, including many discussed under the "Pathogenesis of Infections" section above. Many bacterial or fungal organisms, if directly injected into the bloodstream in sufficient quantities due to nonsterile substances, diluents, equipment or injection-related practices can cause a bloodstream infection. The most common other organisms that may be identified in people who inject substances with isolated bloodstream infections include Staphylococcus species including *S. aureus, S. epidermidis, S. capitis* or other coagulase-negative staphylococci. *B. cereus* and other bacilli can often contaminate substance supplies and cause bloodstream infections with no evident focus. Oral anaerobes and facultative anaerobes such as *Streptococcus mutans* can also present as isolated bacteremias. Similarly, gram-negative organisms such as pseudomonas or Serratia may also present this way. Candida can also manifest with isolated bloodstream infections in people who inject substances.

However, almost all these organisms are also capable of causing infective endocarditis particularly if the inoculum is large enough, or the patient has a damaged heart valve or prosthetic heart valve. As a result, clinicians need to maintain a high index of suspicion for infective endocarditis or other metastatic sites of disease among people who inject substances who present with bacteremia or fungemia. In people who inject substances presenting with fever and no clear focus, at least two sets of blood cultures should be taken, plus a thorough clinical evaluation including detailed history and physical examination, with targeted imaging.

Infective Endocarditis

The usual route of acquisition of infective endocarditis among people with SUD is via intravenous substance use, therefore it is generally assumed to be predominantly right sided (since the veins lead directly to the right atrium,[53] with the majority occurring on the tricuspid valve.[54] Endocarditis in the context of injection substance use is most frequently presents as an acute illness, with recent onset of fevers, a new or changing heart murmur, and occasionally signs of embolic or metastatic infection.[55] For right-sided endocarditis, this includes parenchymal lung infection, pleural effusions, and lung abscesses, which are usually multiple. For left-sided endocarditis, metastatic infection can include polymicrobial septic arthritis, septic infarcts of fingers and toes, septic emboli to the spleen or acute cerebrovascular accident.[56,57]

In 2022, the American Heart Association published an updated scientific statement on the management of infective endocarditis among people who inject substances.[58] The scientific statement discussed specific management[58] strategies in this unique population including implementing multidisciplinary care teams for complex decision making, starting SUD treatment, addressing antimicrobial treatment, and offering cardiac valve surgery (text box). Multidisciplinary teams for complex infectious disease management are discussed in the next section.

Summary of American Heart Association Recommendations for Individuals With Infective Endocarditis Related to Injection Substance Use[58]

- Develop multidisciplinary teams to optimize patient outcomes.
- Offer medication treatment for SUD and harm-reduction education to all individuals with infective endocarditis related to SUD.
- Consider peripherally inserted central catheters and outpatient parenteral antibiotic therapy (OPAT) for some patients with infective endocarditis related to SUD.
- Consider oral antibiotics or long-acting lipoglycopeptides as alternative treatments for individuals who are unable to complete prolonged antibiotic courses.
- Facilitate close outpatient follow-up for patients, even in cases of premature hospital discharge.
- Offer cardiac surgery in accordance with general recommendations for infective endocarditis that is not related to SUD.

Osteoarticular Infections

As in the general population, bone and joint infections in people who inject substances can be divided into native joint septic arthritis, osteomyelitis, and prosthetic joint infection. Native joint septic arthritis most commonly affects the large joints such as hips, knees, and wrists, and is more likely to be polyarticular and may be associated with infective endocarditis. It presents with an acute onset of a painful, hot swollen joint with a limited range of motion. An aspirate of synovial fluid from the joint is the key diagnostic test, and in the presence of septic arthritis has a high white cell count (usually >50,000/high powered field), which are predominantly neutrophils, combined with bacterial growth from culture (with or without organisms seen on Gram stain).[59] Although typical large joints are still the most common focus in people who inject substance with septic arthritis, the sternoclavicular and sacroiliac joints are other potential sites of infection.[60,61]

Vertebral osteomyelitis presents with back pain, usually associated with midline point tenderness at the affected level on examination, raised inflammatory markers in blood (such as C-reactive protein) and vertebral endplate inflammation on CT or MRI scan. Vertebral osteomyelitis can be complicated by (or coexist with) spinal epidural abscess. Spinal epidural abscess, in addition to back pain, can present with neurologic manifestations, including radiculopathy and signs of direct cord compression such as bladder and bowel involvement, limb pain, and weakness, and sensory loss below the involved level. In a cohort study of people who inject substance with vertebral osteomyelitis, approximately 30% were associated with epidural abscess, and required neurosurgical intervention.[62]

Inhalation-Related Infections

Inhalation use of any substances including cannabis, stimulants, and opioids, predisposes to pulmonary infections due to impaired mucociliary clearance. The mucociliary system is a key innate immune defense in the lungs and dysfunction can lead to chronic inflammation, obstructive pulmonary disease, and recurrent bacterial pneumonia.[63] There are also preclinical studies suggesting cannabis,[64,65] stimulants,[66,67] and opioids[68,69] may cause immune system dysfunction thereby increasing risk for infections or increasing replication of HIV.

Beyond bacterial pneumonias, inhalation of cannabis has been associated with invasive fungal infections[70] and sharing smoking supplies used for inhalation of substances like cocaine and methamphetamine may be associated with transmission of blood-borne viruses, in particular HCV.[71,72] Cracked or cut lips and oral sores from hot pipes used to smoke substances may leave blood and virus on the pipe. If smoking supplies are then shared, viral transmission could theoretically occur. Further research is needed in this area. Harm reduction through distribution of safe smoking supplies and safe smoking sites[73] may help curb community transmission of HCV.

Sexually Transmitted Infections

People with SUD are at higher risk of acquiring and transmitting STIs. While we traditionally think more of HIV with injection substance use, people with SUD are also at increased risk for other STIs like syphilis, gonorrhea, chlamydia, and trichomonas. For example, pregnant persons with congenital syphilis outcomes were four to six times more likely to report substance use than persons without congenital syphilis outcomes. The reasons for this are complex and involve the interactions of interweaving factors like population prevalence, transmission fitness of the organism itself, and the impact of substances on sexual behavior. To address this, the CDC issued guidance through a 2012 Morbidity and Mortality Weekly Report recommending integrated services for SUD treatment and the treatment and prevention of STIs, HIV, and viral hepatitis. Unfortunately, people with SUD face barriers to accessing outpatient health care including stigma and difficulty navigating the health care system. Inpatient hospitalization however has been shown to be an opportunity to screen for, diagnose, and treat STIs or offer pertinent prevention services.

Multidisciplinary Management of Complex SUD-Related Infections

Many infectious complications of injection substance use are medically and surgically complex and involve multiple organ systems. Acute pain, physical debility, high nursing needs, psychosocial needs, social determinants of health, and SUD are also components that add to this complexity. Multidisciplinary hospital-based teams have been developed as one model of care to address, organize, and optimize complex care.[74,75] Operating like a tumor board for cancer management, these teams exist in several hospitals around the United States. The teams are also recommended by professional organizations such as the American Heart Association for the management of infective endocarditis.[58] Involved disciplines could include any of the following: hospital medicine, infectious disease, cardiac surgery, neurology, addiction medicine or addiction psychiatry, cardiology, psychiatry, anesthesia, ethics, palliative care, nursing, case management, social work, and patient advocates. One model called the "Multidisciplinary Endocarditis Evaluation Team (MEET)" is described in Figure 11.1. These models could be adapted to other infectious complications like osteomyelitis as well.

Blood-Borne Viruses

Transmission of HIV and viral hepatitis outbreaks within networks of people who inject substances is well described.[3,76–80]

Human Immunodeficiency Virus

People with SUD can be exposed to HIV through both sex and shared use of needles, syringes, or other drug equipment. All people with ongoing substance use should receive routine screening for HIV at least annually, or more frequently if needed based on exposures, and be offered pre-exposure prophylaxis (PrEP) for HIV if testing is negative.[81,82] PrEP offers the highest level of protection against sexual acquisition of HIV but also reduces the likelihood of acquisition from substance use.[83] People with SUD who are diagnosed with a new HIV infection should be offered linkage to care and offered "rapid start" of antiretroviral therapy (ART).[84] For patients with SUD who are currently hospitalized, this should include initiation of ART during the hospital stay accompanied by a prescription for ongoing ART at the time of

MEET members

- Agree to respect the opinions and roles of the other team members
- Approach the treatment of injection drug use–related infective endocarditis (IDU-IE) with the same principles of treatment as non–IDU-IE
- Acknowledge addiction is a chronic medical disease
- Understand hospitalization is a reachable moment when effective treatments for addiction can and should be offered and initiated
- Employ principles of trauma-informed care and harm reduction
- Advocate for patient-centered care
- Respect patient autonomy
- Support patient-centered goals
- Integrate harm-reduction principles into treatments and longitudinal care
- Appreciate the importance of connection to ongoing medical and addiction treatment for treatment success

Addiction medicine	Anesthesia	Cardiac surgery	Cardiology	Infectious disease	Medicine	Social work	Nursing, care management
-Substance use disorder (SUD) assessment -Initiate medication treatment for SUD -Connection to ongoing addiction treatment -Provide harm reduction education -Provide follow-up monitoring and care	-Perioperative pain evaluation and treatment -ICU treatment	-Surgical assessment -Surgical intervention -Cardiac care during hospitalization -Postoperative outpatient follow-up at 30 days and 6 months	-Cardiac imaging assistance -Cardiac management of arrhythmia or heart failure -Postdischarge hospital follow-up	-Infectious disease evaluation for antibiotic selection, length and setting -Arrange outpatient parental therapy options -Provide harm reduction education -Follow in the outpatient setting to monitor antibiotic treatment	-May be the admitting team for patients -Evaluation and treatment of underlying medical conditions	-Social work evaluation for homelessness and other psychosocial needs -Engage with partners and families for patient support -Collaboration with addiction medicine for posthospital addiction services	-Provide daily bedside support and treatment -Coordination of posthospitalization care including discharge to nursing facilities, home, or other locations

Patient needs, values, and treatment goals

Figure 11.1: Multidisciplinary team model for complex infections: The Multidisciplinary Endocarditis Evaluation Team (MEET). (Weimer MB, Falker CG, Seval N, et al. The need for multidisciplinary hospital teams for injection drug use-related infective endocarditis. *J Addict Med*. 2022;16(4):375–378.)

discharge with close outpatient HIV clinic follow-up. For people living with HIV who may also have an opioid use disorder (OUD), an increasing number of HIV clinics offer buprenorphine in an effort to provide colocated care for both HIV and OUD.[85]

Hepatitis B Virus Infection

Hepatitis B immunization was incorporated into the pediatric immunization schedule in the United States in the early 1990s. The vaccine is extremely safe and has an efficacy of >90%.[86] Universal immunization of children has helped reduce the incidence of HBV infections in the United States.[87] However, many individuals who were born prior to its introduction into the immunization schedule may be nonimmune. Nonimmune people with SUD are at increased risk of HBV infection from sharing injection equipment and have a higher overall prevalence than the general population. Chronic HBV infection has been identified in between 3% and 20% of people who use substances in a variety of settings, and 22% of people who use substances have evidence of past infection. Because of this increased risk, routine screening for HBV with a hepatitis B surface antigen is recommended for all people with SUD. Nonimmune people with SUD, those with a negative surface antibody, should be offered HBV immunization. For individuals diagnosed with HBV infection, the WHO guidelines offer an algorithm[88,89] for the assessment, treatment, and monitoring of people with chronic HBV infection. First-line treatment for chronic HBV includes antiviral therapy with well tolerated antivirals such as tenofovir or entecavir. Treatment should be offered to all adults including people with SUD who have evidence of significant fibrosis or cirrhosis, or HBV DNA >2,000 and ALT above the upper limit of normal, or the presence of a coinfection (HIV, HDV, HCV), family history of liver cancer or cirrhosis, immunosuppression, extrahepatic manifestations of HBV, or comorbidities such as diabetes. Treatment should be tailored to their liver injury status. Active SUD including active injection substance use is not a contraindication to treatment.

Strategies to promote and sustain adherence to long-term antiviral therapy including peer counselors, mobile text reminders, cognitive behavioral therapy, and medication adherence training are all evidence based.

For individuals who are interested in PrEP for HIV, and who are found to have chronic HBV infection, a PrEP modality that includes a tenofovir-based component such as tenofovir disoproxil fumarate (TDF) and emtricitabine (FTC), or tenofovir alafenamide fumarate (TAF) and emtricitabine (FTC) will provide concurrent HBV treatment[89] and HIV prevention.

Hepatitis C Virus Infection

Like both HIV and HBV, HCV is a blood-borne virus. It is primarily transmitted through the parenteral route and shared use of injection substance use equipment is the most common means of transmission in the United States. Globally, estimates suggest that over half of current people with SUD have been exposed to HCV.[90] The advent of direct-acting antivirals over the last two decades has transformed HCV care, with more than 95% of patients achieving sustained virologic response or cure. Importantly, neither a history of SUD nor current SUD should be considered a contraindication to treatment for HCV. While there has previously been reluctance among clinicians to initiate HCV treatment for people with SUD, guidelines from the American Association for the Study of Liver Diseases, and the Infectious Diseases Society of America note that ongoing SUD is not a contraindication to HCV treatment.[91] Research has consistently demonstrated that people with SUD are motivated to complete treatment and successfully adhere to medication plans[92] with low posttreatment reinfection rates among people with SUD. For hospitalized patients with SUD, the hospital stay offers a unique opportunity to obtain pretreatment labs, screen for cirrhosis, and initiate antivirals either during the hospital admission or immediately following discharge.[93]

Hepatitis A Virus Infection

While hepatitis A does not cause a chronic viral infection the way HBV or HCV do, it can cause outbreaks. Recent person-to-person transmission of hepatitis A has occurred across the country, with some of the largest outbreaks occurring among people with SUD. Both injection and noninjection routes of substance use have been prevalent in outbreaks.[94] People with SUD are at increased risk for hepatitis A virus (HAV) infection and are recommended to be immunized against HAV infection.[95] More than 95% of adults will develop protective antibodies within 4 weeks of a single dose of vaccine, and nearly 100% will seroconvert after receiving two doses. Serologic testing for immunity is not recommended prior to vaccination, particularly in outbreak settings where attaining 80% immunity in a population can stop outbreaks.[96] HAV infection should be considered in people with SUD who present with nonspecific gastrointestinal symptoms including nausea, vomiting, abdominal pain, diarrhea, particularly in outbreak settings.[97]

Latent Tuberculosis

People with SUD are at increased risk for acquiring latent tuberculosis infection (LTBI).[98–100] Unhoused status and incarceration are also exposures that put people with SUD at risk for LTBI. Substance use including substances and alcohol, malnutrition, and HIV are risk factors for LTBI reactivation into active disease. People with SUD, particularly those experiencing homelessness or with histories of incarceration,[101] should be screened for LTBI.[102] Screening should typically be done with an interferon-gamma release assay (IGRA). Tuberculin skin testing (TST) can also be done but requires two visits 48 to 72 hours apart whereas an IGRA is a single blood draw. If the IGRA or TST is positive, active disease should be ruled out and a chest x-ray should be obtained. However, these are screening tests for latent infection only and a negative result does not exclude active disease.[103] Caution should be taken when interpreting LTBI screening in patients hospitalized with septic emboli. Patients with positive testing should be linked to care.

Leveraging Hospitalizations

Hospitalization of people with SUD with an invasive bacterial or fungal infection represents a critical opportunity to screen for a variety of communicable diseases, as well as engage people with SUD with SUD care. Hospitalization can be a transformative, reachable moment for patients if acute medical care is paired with highly effective treatments for their SUD.[104] All patients who are hospitalized should be offered evidence-based SUD treatments while hospitalized and transitioned to ongoing treatment at the time of discharge. For many people with SUD who have limited access to routine preventative medical care, this interaction with the health care system may also represent the only opportunity for preventative health care measures such as immunizations. A comprehensive list of testing and care measures recommended for people with SUD presenting with injection substance use–related infections is outlined in Table 11.2.

Management of Long-Course Durations of Antimicrobial Treatment

Many of the invasive bacterial and fungal infection syndromes described above require prolonged

TABLE 11.2

List of Testing and Care Measures for People With SUD

	Recommendations
Screening tests	
Human immunodeficiency virus (HIV)	Screen at initial visit, offer repeat screening regularly if ongoing substance use Link patients with HIV diagnoses to infectious diseases care. Rapid start of antiretrovirals is preferred
Hepatitis B virus (HBV)	HBV surface antigen at initial visit. Evaluate immunity with HBV surface antibody and immunize if nonimmune. Link patients with active HBV to infectious diseases or hepatology care
Hepatitis C virus (HCV)	HCV antibody at initial visit. If positive, obtain HCV RNA and link to HCV treatment for viremic patients
Syphilis	RPR or T pallidum (as determined by hospital syphilis algorithm testing protocols) should be assessed at initial visit. Additional testing as indicated by sexual health history
Gonorrhea and Chlamydia	Gonorrhea and Chlamydia nucleic acid amplification testing (urine) at initial visit. Additional testing (throat and rectum) can be considered based on sexual health history. Consider testing for other infections such as trichomonas and bacterial vaginosis
Tuberculosis	Assess for latent tuberculosis at initial visit with periodic rescreening based on individual risk
Immunizations and preventive health care	
Pre-exposure prophylaxis (PrEP) for HIV	Counsel all people with SUD who use injection substances and offer PrEP
Hepatitis A and B	Immunize all patients with SUD for hepatitis A and B
Influenza vaccine	Offer yearly
Tetanus	Immunize at initial visit then every 10 y, or every 5 y for patients with necrotizing skin and soft tissue infections
Sexually transmitted infection prevention	Besides vaccination against HBV, Human papilloma virus (HPV), and PrEP, condoms are the most effective way of preventing STI transmission and acquisition. Condoms should be offered to all people who use substances in addition to routine STI screening For patients who identify as gay, bisexual, or other men who have sex with men or transgender women, doxycycline postexposure prophylaxis (Doxy PEP) should[105] be offered to prevent acquisition of bacterial STIs like syphilis, chlamydia, and gonorrhea. Patients should take doxycycline 200 mg within 72 h of oral, vaginal, or anal sex with routine STI screening of anatomic sites of exposure every 3–6 mo
Contraception	As with all people of reproductive[106] potential, people who use substances should be offered and counseled on the risks and benefits of various contraceptive methods including condoms and more effective contraception such as long-acting reversible contraception. People who use substances should also be counseled on emergency contraception
Substance use disorder interventions	
Overdose education	Provide take-home naloxone and education on opioid overdose prevention
Harm-reduction counseling	Educate on safer injection techniques including cleaning injection sites, use of sterile works, and location of needle exchange facilities See www.safersubstanceuse.org[107]
Offer medications for opioid use disorder (MOUD)	All people with opioid use disorder should be offered initiation of MOUD (methadone, intramuscular naltrexone or buprenorphine) and linkage to ongoing outpatient care

HIV, human immunodeficiency virus; HAV, hepatitis A virus; HBV, hepatitis B virus; HCV, hepatitis C virus; PrEP, pre-exposure prophylaxis for HIV; RPR, rapid plasma regain.

durations of antibiotic therapy which can present unique challenges for hospitals, clinicians, and people with SUD. Current Infectious Diseases Society of America (IDSA) guidelines for both bacterial and fungal infections causing endocarditis, septic arthritis, epidural abscess, or osteomyelitis recommend intravenous antibiotics for a period of between 4 and 6 weeks depending on pathogen and clinical syndrome. Full details of antimicrobial regimens for specific conditions are delineated in professional guidelines and are generally not unique for people with SUD.[108] With the increasing prevalence of injection substance use–associated infective endocarditis, the American Heart Association has published a scientific statement to help guide clinicians through the available evidence for alternative models of antibiotic therapy when guideline-directed IV antibiotics are not feasible for the patient or the health care team.[58] This approach can be used as a guide for other clinical syndromes.

Clinicians should be aware of both standard-of-care approaches to people with SUD with injection-related infections as well as be willing to integrate emerging high bioavailability antibiotic alternatives. While some small programs exist to offer people with SUD access to outpatient parenteral antibiotic therapy (OPAT), that may not be feasible in all locations or in scenarios where individuals do not have stable housing or other patient factors preclude use of that option. In such situations, the default may be prolonged hospitalizations for supervised IV antibiotics. While this can offer a high standard of care for patients, it may not always be in line with a patient's individual goals. In those situations, clinicians should assess the severity of the infection, along with emerging literature surrounding the safety and efficacy of long-acting lipoglycopeptides or high bioavailability oral antibiotics.[58]

For patients who elect not to continue standard antibiotic treatment regimens, clinicians are encouraged to offer an alternative option for infection treatment to prevent morbidity and mortality. A patient-centered approach to this complex decision making has been described by Sikka et al. in a program called "OPTIONS-DC" and has shown positive outcomes (Figure 11.2).[109–111] Programs like these generally engage multiple disciplines through a care conference model to evaluate safe, harm-reduction–based, and patient-centered antibiotic treatment options for individuals with SUD and long-term antibiotic needs.

In addition, for patients with OUD and injection-related infections, it is of the utmost importance that they are offered MOUD in addition to antimicrobial treatment. Patients with OUD who are treated with MOUD and OPAT have had improved clinical outcomes, higher odds of completing antibiotic treatments, and shorter hospital length of stay.[112]

Prolonged hospitalization for patients with injection-related infection can be challenging. Clinicians are encouraged to offer supportive care, counseling, and other services to help patients tolerate prolonged hospitalization. Whenever possible, less restrictive environments like skilled nursing facilities can be sought as safe alternatives. For all patients, evidence-based approaches to support patients' SUD and mental health should be provided. As above, if patients decline prolonged hospitalization for parental antibiotics, they can and should be offered a safe alternative option such as oral antibiotics or long-acting lipoglycopeptides.

Outpatient Parenteral Antibiotic Therapy

Invasive infections often require prolonged courses of antibiotics for which parenteral or intravenous antibiotics may be the "gold standard." OPAT allows patients to continue their intravenous antibiotics outside the hospital setting such as in the home or in a nursing facility, thereby reducing hospital length of stay[113] and reducing health care costs.[114] However, people with SUD have typically been excluded from consideration for OPAT. Recent literature suggests that if otherwise an OPAT candidate (eg, stable and safe discharge location, access to a phone, transportation), people with SUD have similar OPAT outcomes and venous access manipulation was rare.[112,115,116] If patients have OUD, pairing OPAT with medications for OUD should be pursued.[112,117]

Long-Acting Lipoglycopeptides

Long-acting lipoglycopeptides offer an attractive mode of antibiotic therapy for gram-positive invasive infections, particularly *S. aureus*. These agents allow patients to receive a therapeutic level of antibiotics for weeks after a single intravenous infusion.[118] The two commercially available drugs, dalbavancin and oritavancin, are based on the chemical structure of vancomycin.[119] While only specifically approved by the US FDA for complex acute bacterial skin and skin structure infections, an increasing body of research demonstrates their utility in clinical syndromes ranging from infective endocarditis to osteomyelitis.[120–122] Most commonly they are used following a period of initial IV antibiotics, where the long-acting lipoglycopeptide infusion is administered after a patient is clinically stable and has had source control of any metastatic sites of infection.[123] In this scenario they may be used to achieve the last several weeks of antibiotic therapy and thus

Introductory Script: "Thank you for taking time to attend this conference. OPTIONS-DC is a structured multidisciplinary conference with a goal to review all aspects of OPAT and discuss the best and safest options for this patient to receive treatment for their infection. I will ask each discipline to weigh in on specific questions. It is vital that we consider patient preferences in discharge planning and treatment decisions. As we proceed, I ask that everyone approach this discussion with the following ethical principles in mind:

- How much is paternalism playing a role in this decision-making process?
- What is beneficent in this patient's situation?
- What is nonmaleficient in this patient's situation?
- What autonomy does this patient have in the current situation?"

Because the language we use when talking about addiction can reduce stigma and improve care, we want to take an opportunity to remind people to use person-first, nonstigmatizing language (eg, avoiding the term "abuse"). Folks are encouraged to gently remind one another about this as we are all learning."

Topic (responsible participant)	**Specific considerations for review**
1. Infection type and management (ID)	Therapeutic options (drug, dose, route, frequency)
	Recommended duration of therapy
2. Antibiotic administration and setting safety (OPAT, ID, CM) • Which route (IV, long acting, PO)? • What setting (hospital, home infusion, infusion center, SNF)?	Living environment: *Access to running water, refrigeration, heat in winter, nonabusive/safe environment*
	Provider ability to reach patient after discharge: *Working personal cell phone, available emergency contact*
	Patient ability to self-manage care; social supports
	Insurance coverage in outpatient settings
	Transportation
3. Substance use history (ACS)	Substance, severity, use practices
	Engagement with ACS in hospital
	Medication treatment for SUD
	Peer support and engagement
	Potential use triggers, including PICC line
4. Patient goals and preferences (all; commonly ACS peer provides unique insights)	Understanding of seriousness of infection and possibility of progression if not fully treated
	Other patient-identified priorities (eg, parenting, work)
5. Stability for discharge (primary team)	Skilled nursing needs
	Physical or occupational therapy needs
	Wound care needs
6. Access to outpatient care (primary team, ID, ACS)	Established primary care provider
	Plan for continuing SUD care after discharge
	Ongoing additional mental health needs and follow-up
	Plan for ID follow-up including imaging needs

Figure 11.2: Example format of a multidisciplinary conference to discuss alternative antibiotic regimens for individuals needing longer courses of antibiotics. (Sikka MK, Gore S, Vega T, et al. "OPTIONS-DC", a feasible discharge planning conference to expand infection treatment options for people with substance use disorder. *BMC Infect Dis*. 2021;21:772.)

expedite hospital discharge.[124] A single dose provides approximately 2 weeks of systemic levels, with longer durations achieved with multiple-dose protocols. If a multiple-dose protocol is chosen, the health care team should ensure that the patient has a way to return for subsequent doses and that intravenous access is easily obtained.

Transitions to Oral Antibiotics

Use of oral antibiotics as an alternative to IV antibiotics and long-acting lipoglycopeptides is an active area of research. There has been a substantial body of work comparing published serum antimicrobial levels after both oral and IV administration determining that safe levels of commonly used oral antibiotics can be achieved orally.[125] Randomized clinical trials in infective endocarditis have demonstrated that oral step-down therapy is at least as effective as intravenous antimicrobial therapy in right-sided, left-sided, or prosthetic valve IE.[126–128] Multiple retrospective and observational studies have demonstrated similar outcomes.[129–135] If oral antibiotics are chosen, best practices are to wait until after patients have achieved clinical stability with intravenous regimens, source control has been achieved,[136] and an initial period of intravenous antibiotics has been given for patients with associated bacteremias.[137] If oral antibiotics are chosen, then antibiotics with high bioavailability should be chosen.

Case Examples

Case 1

John was admitted for low back and right leg pain. He was found to have a large lumbar epidural abscess requiring surgical drainage, as well as MRSA bacteremia and tricuspid valve endocarditis. He cleared his bacteremia soon after abscess drainage and his endocarditis did not require surgical intervention. John lived 3 hours away and did not have health insurance. He stated he could stay in the hospital for 4 weeks but then needed to get home to his family and job. John was offered either oral antibiotics or a dose of dalbavancin prior to discharge to finish the remaining 2 weeks of treatment and to complete a 6-week course for his infection. He reported having difficulty remembering to take oral medications so opted for the long-acting lipoglycopeptide.

Considerations:

- Long-acting lipoglycopeptides are excellent options for patients with gram-positive infections *and* source control of any abscesses. Drainage of any infection is important in use of these agents as they have a prolonged "tail" that may result in development of resistance if large pockets of infection are not addressed.
- Discussing options and feasibility of that plan with the patient is important. In John's case, he needed to go home after 4 weeks and while we could have transitioned to oral antibiotics, he reported difficulty remembering to take medications. Thus, oral antibiotics would not have been the best choice and a long-acting lipoglycopeptide ensures he receives the remainder of his course.

Case 2

Tia presented with several days of severe left knee pain, swelling, and redness. She was found to have a septic joint as well as early osteomyelitis of the distal femur. She underwent surgery to drain and debride the joint. Cultures grew MRSA susceptible to oral antibiotics including trimethoprim/sulfamethoxazole, doxycycline, and linezolid. She reported a sulfa drug allergy (anaphylaxis). Tia stated she needed to leave as soon as possible due to family responsibilities. By day 7 postop, she was walking, and her knee swelling, warmth, and pain were substantially reduced. She was transitioned from IV antibiotics to doxycycline for 5 weeks to complete a 6-week course to cover both septic arthritis and osteomyelitis. Tia states that she lives several hours away and may have trouble coming to clinic for follow-up but is willing to do phone follow-up. She also reports that she has trouble getting blood draws or IV's placed when she is an outpatient and that when she is in the hospital they have to use an ultrasound to draw blood or place IVs.

Considerations:

- When selecting antibiotics, several factors are important: (1) antibiotic coverage of the bacteria and whether it reaches effective concentrations in the infected space (eg, blood, bone, tissue); (2) drug interactions; (3) drug toxicities; (4) drug allergies or intolerances; and (5) any needed safety monitoring. In this patient's case, she had an MRSA osteoarticular infection without bacteremia. The MRSA isolate was susceptible to trimethoprim/sulfamethoxazole, doxycycline, and linezolid. The patient however had a reported an allergy to sulfa drugs, so trimethoprim/sulfamethoxazole cannot be used. Linezolid can have increased toxicities with courses longer than 2 weeks, thus laboratory monitoring after 2 weeks is preferred, and she has 5 weeks of treatment left and reported difficulty with getting labs as an outpatient due to difficult venous access, making a regimen with less safety monitoring preferred. Doxycycline is safe and well tolerated for prolonged durations with excellent bone penetration. Out of the options, doxycycline would be the best based on her allergies and its relative safety profile.
- Transitioning to oral antibiotics can be considered once the patient is clinically stable and improved, and if the patient is bacteremic, once they have cleared their bacteremia. Sometimes patients with osteoarticular infections require multiple surgical interventions to achieve adequate source control, so ensuring clinical improvement prior to discharge is important. In this patient's case, she improved postoperatively and after working with physical therapy was able to be safe at home after 7 days. Transitioning to oral antibiotics at this juncture can be considered.
- While dalbavancin might have been an excellent option for her, if more than 2 weeks of additional antibiotic therapy is needed then a multidose series would be required. Because she reports that IV access requires an ultrasound for her, it is unlikely that an infusion center will be able to place an IV to administer a second dalbavancin dose as an outpatient. She also lives several hours away from clinic which makes transportation to clinic to get dalbavancin more challenging.

Conclusions

Infectious complications of injection substance use represent the most common reasons that people with SUD may require hospitalization. Identification of an underlying SUD is a critical first step in addressing both the acute infection, preventing future complications, and reducing mortality. Harm-reduction efforts should be tailored to a patient's substance use practices to prevent future infectious complications. With an increasing array of antimicrobial treatment options available, clinicians should make every attempt to ensure that people with SUD are provided with flexible antimicrobial options to complete infectious diseases treatment and achieve clinical cure. Clinicians should be attuned to the unique risks for comorbid infections among people with SUD and prepared to offer comprehensive screening, as well as initiation of SUD treatment and linkage to outpatient treatment resources.

REFERENCES

1. Ronan MV, Herzig SJ. Hospitalizations related to opioid abuse/dependence and associated serious infections increased sharply, 2002–12. *Health Aff (Millwood)*. 2016;35:832–837.
2. Hansel M. As HIV cluster investigation moves into second month, health officials increase opportunities to test. *NKyTribune*. 2018. Accessed January 30, 2026. https://nkytribune.com/2018/02/as-hiv-cluster-investigation-moves-into-second-month-health-officials-increase-opportunities-to-test/
3. Golden MR, Lechtenberg R, Glick SN, et al. Outbreak of human immunodeficiency virus infection among heterosexual persons who are living homeless and inject drugs—Seattle, Washington, 2018. *MMWR Morb Mortal Wkly Rep*. 2019;68:344–349.
4. Sredl M, Fleischauer AT, Moore Z, Rosen DL, Schranz AJ. Not just endocarditis: hospitalizations for selected invasive infections among persons with opioid and stimulant use diagnoses-North Carolina, 2010–2018. *J Infect Dis*. 2020;222:S458–S464.
5. Schranz AJ, Fleischauer A, Chu VH, Wu LT, Rosen DL. Trends in drug use-associated infective endocarditis and heart valve surgery, 2007 to 2017: a study of statewide discharge data. *Ann Intern Med*. 2019;170:31–40.
6. Seval N, Eaton E, Springer SA. Beyond antibiotics: a practical guide for the infectious disease physician to treat opioid use disorder in the setting of associated infectious diseases. *Open Forum Infect Dis*. 2020;7:ofz539.
7. Benusic MA, Press NM, Hoang LM, Romney MG. A cluster of Bacillus cereus bacteremia cases among injection drug users. *Can J Infect Dis Med Microbiol*. 2015;26:103–104.
8. Mc LJ, Mithani V, Bolton FJ, et al. An investigation into the microflora of heroin. *J Med Microbiol*. 2002;51:1001–1008.
9. Cole C, Jones L, McVeigh J, Kicman A, Syed Q, Bellis M. Adulterants in illicit drugs: a review of empirical evidence. *Drug Test Anal*. 2011;3:89–96.
10. Peak CM, Rosen H, Kamali A, et al. Wound botulism outbreak among persons who use black tar heroin—San Diego County, California, 2017–2018. *MMWR Morb Mortal Wkly Rep*. 2019;67:1415–1418.
11. Centers for Disease Control and Prevention. Tetanus among injecting-drug users—California, 1997. *MMWR Morb Mortal Wkly Rep*. 1998;47:149–151.
12. Waltenburg MA, Larson VA, Naor EH, et al. Notes from the field: botulism type B after intravenous methamphetamine use—New Jersey, 2020. *MMWR Morb Mortal Wkly Rep*. 2020;69:1425–1426.
13. Palmateer NE, Hope VD, Roy K, et al. Infections with spore-forming bacteria in persons who inject drugs, 2000–2009. *Emerg Infect Dis*. 2013;19:29–34.
14. Shooting Up: infections among people who inject drugs in the UK. *GOV.UK*. 2023. Accessed January 30, 2026. https://www.gov.uk/government/publications/shooting-up-infections-among-people-who-inject-drugs-in-the-uk
15. Ramsay CN, Stirling A, Smith J, et al. An outbreak of infection with Bacillus anthracis in injecting drug users in Scotland. *Euro Surveill*. 2010;15(2):19465.
16. Pichlinski EM, Hoff E, Epperson LC, et al. Tetanus: a rare complication of black tar heroin use. *Open Forum Infect Dis*. 2021;9(3):ofab613.
17. Miró JM, De La Bellacasa JP, Odds FC, et al. Systemic Candidiasis in Spanish heroin addicts: a possible source of infection. *J Infect Dis*. 1987;156:857–858.
18. Podzamczer D, Fernández-Viladrich P, Ribera M, Arruga J, de Celis G, Gudiol F. Systemic candidiasis in drug addicts. *Eur J Clin Microbiol Infect Dis*. 1985;4:509–512.
19. Shankland G, Richardson M, Dutton G. Source of infection in candida endophthalmitis in drug addicts. *Br Med J (Clin Res Ed)*. 1986;292:1106.
20. Aboltins CA, Allen P, Daffy JR. Fungal endophthalmitis in intravenous drug users injecting buprenorphine contaminated with oral Candida species. *Med J Aust*. 2005;182:427.
21. Cassoux N, Bodaghi B, Lehoang P, Edel Y. Presumed ocular candidiasis in drug misusers after intravenous use of oral high dose buprenorphine (Subutex). *Br J Ophthalmol*. 2002;86:940–941.
22. Poowanawittayakom N, Dutta A, Stock S, Touray S, Ellison RT III, Levitz SM. Reemergence of Intravenous drug use as risk factor for Candidemia, Massachusetts, USA. *Emerg Infect Dis*. 2018;24:631–637.
23. Jenkins TC, Knepper BC, Jason Moore S, et al. Microbiology and initial antibiotic therapy for injection drug users and non-injection drug users with cutaneous abscesses in the era of community-associated methicillin-resistant Staphylococcus aureus. *Acad Emerg Med*. 2015;22:993–997.
24. Phillips KT, Anderson BJ, Herman DS, Liebschutz JM, Stein MD. Risk factors associated with skin and soft tissue infections among hospitalized people who inject drugs. *J Addict Med*. 2017;11:461–467.
25. Murphy EL, DeVita D, Liu H, et al. Risk factors for skin and soft-tissue abscesses among injection drug users: a case-control study. *Clin Infect Dis*. 2001;33:35–40.
26. Raucher B, Dobkin J, Mandel L, Edberg S, Levi M, Miller M. Occult polymicrobial endocarditis with Haemophilus parainfluenzae in intravenous drug abusers. *Am J Med*. 1989;86:169–172.
27. Kannangara DP, Pandya D. Infections in injection drug users: the significance of oral bacteria and a comparison with bacteria originating from skin and environmental sources. *Drug Drug Abuse*. 2020:1–5.
28. Oh S, Havlen PR, Hussain N. A case of polymicrobial endocarditis caused by anaerobic organisms in an injection drug user. *J Gen Intern Med*. 2005;20:C1–C2.
29. McCarthy NL, Baggs J, See I, et al. Bacterial infections associated with substance use disorders, large cohort of United States hospitals, 2012–2017. *Clin Infect Dis*. 2020;71:e37–e44.

30. Desai R, Pannaraj PS, Agopian J, Sugar CA, Liu GY, Miller LG. Survival and transmission of community-associated methicillin-resistant Staphylococcus aureus from fomites. *Am J Infect Control.* 2011;39:219–225.
31. Dolan KA, Wodak AD, Hall WD. A bleach program for inmates in NSW: an HIV prevention strategy. *Aust N Z J Public Health.* 1998;22:838–840.
32. Thomas G. Harm reduction policies and programs for persons involved in the criminal justice system. *CCSA.* 2005.
33. Sanchez DP, Tookes H, Pastar I, Lev-Tov H. Wounds and skin and soft tissue infections in people who inject drugs and the utility of syringe service programs in their management. *Adv Wound Care (New Rochelle).* 2021;10:571–582.
34. Freibott CE, Phillips KT, Anderson BJ, Stewart C, Liebschutz JM, Stein MD. Under the skin: the relationship between subcutaneous injection and skin infections among people who inject drugs. *J Addict Med.* 2022;16:164–168.
35. Phillips KT, Stein MD. Risk practices associated with bacterial infections among injection drug users in Denver, Colorado. *Am J Drug Alcohol Abuse.* 2010;36:92–97.
36. Brown PD, Ebright JR. Skin and soft tissue infections in injection drug users. *Curr Infect Dis Rep.* 2002;4:415–419.
37. Larney S, Peacock A, Mathers BM, Hickman M, Degenhardt L. A systematic review of injecting-related injury and disease among people who inject drugs. *Drug Alcohol Depend.* 2017;171:39–49.
38. See I, Gokhale RH, Geller A, et al. National Public Health burden estimates of endocarditis and skin and soft-tissue infections related to injection drug use: a review. *J Infect Dis.* 2020;222:S429–S436.
39. Binswanger IA, Kral AH, Bluthenthal RN, Rybold DJ, Edlin BR. High prevalence of abscesses and cellulitis among community-recruited injection drug users in San Francisco. *Clin Infect Dis.* 2000;30:579–581.
40. Marks LR, Durkin MJ, Ayres K, Ellis M. Drug preparation, injection-related infections, and harm reduction practices among a national sample of individuals entering treatment for opioid use disorder. *Harm Reduct J.* 2024;21:16.
41. Harris RE, Richardson J, Frasso R, Anderson ED. Experiences with skin and soft tissue infections among people who inject drugs in Philadelphia: a qualitative study. *Drug Alcohol Depend.* 2018;187:8–12.
42. Passaro DJ, Werner SB, McGee J, Mac Kenzie WR, Vugia DJ. Wound botulism associated with black tar heroin among injecting drug users. *JAMA.* 1998;279:859–863.
43. Centers for Disease Control and Prevention (CDC). *Injection Drug Use and Wound Botulism.* Accessed March 1, 2025. https://www.cdc.gov/botulism/risk-factors/wound-botulism.html
44. Yuan J, Inami G, Mohle-Boetani J, Vugia DJ. Recurrent wound botulism among injection drug users in California. *Clin Infect Dis.* 2011;52:862–866.
45. Sandrock CE, Murin S. Clinical predictors of respiratory failure and long-term outcome in black tar heroin-associated wound botulism. *Chest.* 2001;120:562–566.
46. Hahné SJ, White JM, Crowcroft NS, et al. Tetanus in injecting drug users, United Kingdom. *Emerg Infect Dis.* 2006;12(4):709–710.
47. Kimura AC, Higa JI, Levin RM, Simpson G, Vargas Y, Vugia DJ. Outbreak of necrotizing fasciitis due to Clostridium sordellii among black-tar heroin users. *Clin Infect Dis.* 2004;38:e87–e91.
48. Bangsberg DR, Rosen JI, Aragon T, Campbell A, Weir L, Perdreau-Remington F. Clostridial myonecrosis cluster among injection drug users: a molecular epidemiology investigation. *Arch Intern Med.* 2002;162(5):517–522.
59. Kariisa M, O'Donnell J, Kumar S, Mattson CL, Goldberger BA. Illicitly manufactured fentanyl-involved overdose deaths with detected xylazine—United States, January 2019–June 2022. *MMWR Morb Mortal Wkly Rep.* 2023;72:721–727.
50. Lutz L, McFadden R, Xu L, et al. Wound characteristics among patients exposed to xylazine. *JAMA Dermatol.* 2025; 161:75–80.
51. Jawa R, Ismail S, Shang M, et al. Drug use practices and wound care experiences in the age of xylazine adulteration. *Drug Alcohol Depend.* 2024;263:112390.
52. McFadden R, Wallace-Keeshen S, Petrillo Straub K, et al. Xylazine-associated wounds: clinical experience from a low-barrier wound care clinic in Philadelphia. *J Addict Med.* 2024; 18:9–12.
53. Moreillon P, Que YA. Infective endocarditis. *Lancet.* 2004; 363:139–149.
54. Pericas JM, Llopis J, Athan E, et al. Prospective cohort study of infective endocarditis in people who inject drugs. *J Am Coll Cardiol.* 2021;77:544–555.
55. Cecchi E, Corcione S, Lupia T, et al. Infective endocarditis in people who inject drugs: report from the Italian Registry of Infective Endocarditis. *J Clin Med.* 2022;11(14):4082.
56. Anavekar NS, Tleyjeh IM, Anavekar NS, et al. Impact of prior antiplatelet therapy on risk of embolism in infective endocarditis. *Clin Infect Dis.* 2007;44:1180–1186.
57. Snygg-Martin U, Gustafsson L, Rosengren L, et al. Cerebrovascular complications in patients with left-sided infective endocarditis are common: a prospective study using magnetic resonance imaging and neurochemical brain damage markers. *Clin Infect Dis.* 2008;47:23–30.
58. Baddour LM, Weimer MB, Wurcel AG, et al. Management of infective endocarditis in people who inject drugs: a scientific statement from the American Heart Association. *Circulation.* 2022;146:e187–e201.
59. Margaretten ME, Kohlwes J, Moore D, Bent S. Does this adult patient have septic arthritis? *JAMA.* 2007;297:1478–1488.
60. Gobao VC, Alfishawy M, Smith C, et al. Risk factors, screening, and treatment challenges in Staphylococcus aureus native septic arthritis. *Open Forum Infect Dis.* 2021;8:ofaa593.
61. Ross JJ, Ard KL, Carlile N. Septic arthritis and the opioid epidemic: 1465 cases of culture-positive native joint septic arthritis from 1990–2018. *Open Forum Infect Dis.* 2020; 7:ofaa089.
62. Ananda RA, Attwood LO, Lancaster R, et al. Clinical and financial burden of spinal infections in people who inject drugs. *Intern Med J.* 2022;52:1741–1748.
63. Chinnapaiyan S, Unwalla HJ. Mucociliary dysfunction in HIV and smoked substance abuse. *Front Microbiol.* 2015; 6:1052.
64. Maggirwar SB, Khalsa JH. The link between cannabis use, immune system, and viral infections. *Viruses.* 2021;13:1099.
65. Milad N, Fantauzzi MF, McGrath JJC, et al. Cannabis smoke suppresses antiviral immune responses to influenza A in mice. *ERJ Open Res.* 2023;9(6):00219-2023.
66. Aouizerat BE, Garcia JN, Domingues CV, et al. Frequent cocaine use is associated with larger HIV latent reservoir size. *JAIDS.* 2024;97:156–164.
67. Prakash MD, Tangalakis K, Antonipillai J, Stojanovska L, Nurgali K, Apostolopoulos V. Methamphetamine: effects on the brain, gut and immune system. *Pharmacol Res.* 2017; 120:60–67.
68. Madhuravasal Krishnan J, Kong L, Meeds HL, et al. The synthetic opioid fentanyl increases HIV replication in macrophages. *PLoS One.* 2025;20:e0298341.
69. Bettinger JJ, Friedman BC. Opioids and immunosuppression: clinical evidence, mechanisms of action, and potential therapies. *Palliat Med Rep.* 2024;5:70–80.
70. Benedict K, Thompson GR III, Jackson BR. Cannabis use and fungal infections in a commercially insured population, United States, 2016. *Emerg Infect Dis.* 2020;26:1308–1310.

71. Macias J, Palacios RB, Claro E, et al. High prevalence of hepatitis C virus infection among noninjecting drug users: association with sharing the inhalation implements of crack. *Liver Int.* 2008;28:781–786.
72. Scheinmann R, Hagan H, Lelutiu-Weinberger C, et al. Non-injection drug use and hepatitis C Virus: a systematic review. *Drug Alcohol Depend.* 2007;89:1–12.
73. Shannon K, Ishida T, Morgan R, et al. Potential community and public health impacts of medically supervised safer smoking facilities for crack cocaine users. *Harm Reduct J.* 2006;3:1.
74. Weimer MB, Falker CG, Seval N, et al. The need for multidisciplinary hospital teams for injection drug use-related infective endocarditis. *J Addict Med.* 2022;16(4):375–378.
75. O'Donnell M, Englander H, Strnad L, Bhamidipati CM, Shalen E, Riquelme PA. Expanding the team: optimizing the multidisciplinary management of drug use-associated infective endocarditis. *J Gen Intern Med.* 2022;37(4):935–939.
76. Tookes H, Bartholomew TS, Geary S, et al. Rapid identification and investigation of an HIV risk network among people who inject drugs—Miami, FL, 2018. *AIDS Behav.* 2020;24:246–256.
77. Ramachandran S, Thai H, Forbi JC, et al. A large HCV transmission network enabled a fast-growing HIV outbreak in rural Indiana, 2015. *EBioMedicine.* 2018;37:374–381.
78. Alpren C, Dawson EL, John B, et al. Opioid use fueling HIV transmission in an urban setting: an outbreak of HIV infection among people who inject drugs—Massachusetts, 2015–2018. *Am J Public Health.* 2020;110:37–44.
79. Tong SY, Davis JS, Eichenberger E, Holland TL, Fowler VG Jr. Staphylococcus aureus infections: epidemiology, pathophysiology, clinical manifestations, and management. *Clin Microbiol Rev.* 2015;28:603–661.
80. Minnesota Department of Health. *Health Advisory: HIV Outbreak in Persons Who Inject Drugs (PWID).* 2020. Accessed March 1, 2025. https://www.health.mn.gov/communities/ep/han/2020/feb3hiv.pdf
81. CDC Health Alert Network (HAN). *Health Advisory: Increase in Fatal Drug Overdoses Across the United States Driven by Synthetic Opioids Before and During the COVID-19 Pandemic.* 2020. Accessed January 30, 2026. https://stacks.cdc.gov/view/cdc/98848
82. Centers for Disease Control and Prevention HAN. *Recent HIV Clusters and Outbreaks Across the United States Among People Who Inject Drugs and Considerations During the COVID-19 Pandemic-CDCHAN-00436.* 2020.
83. Centers for Disease Control and Prevention. *Preventing HIV with PrEP.* 2024. Accessed April 15, 2025. https://www.cdc.gov/hiv/prevention/prep.html
84. Panel on Antiretroviral Guidelines for Adults and Adolescents. *Guidelines for the Use of Antiretroviral Agents in Adults and Adolescents with HIV.* Department of Health and Human Services. Accessed March 14, 2025. https://clinicalinfo.hiv.gov/en/guidelines/adult-and-adolescent-arv
85. Oldfield BJ, Munoz N, McGovern MP, et al. Integration of care for HIV and opioid use disorder. *AIDS.* 2019;33:873–884.
86. Meireles LC, Marinho RT, Van Damme P. Three decades of hepatitis B control with vaccination. *World J Hepatol.* 2015;7:2127–2132.
87. Centers for Disease Control and Prevention (CDC). Hepatitis B virus: a comprehensive strategy for eliminating transmission in the United States through universal childhood vaccination. Recommendations of the Immunization Practices Advisory Committee (ACIP). *MMWR Recomm Rep.* 1991;40:1–25.
88. World Health Organization (2024). Guidelines for the prevention d, care and treatment for people with chronic hepatitis B infection. Accessed March 17, 2025. https://www.who.int/publications/i/item/9789240090903
89. Szabo I, Szantho A, Papp Z. Uterine sarcoma: diagnosis with multiparameter sonographic analysis. *Ultrasound Obstet Gynecol.* 1997;10:220–221.
90. Degenhardt L, Peacock A, Colledge S, et al. Global prevalence of injecting drug use and sociodemographic characteristics and prevalence of HIV, HBV, and HCV in people who inject drugs: a multistage systematic review. *Lancet Glob Health.* 2017;5:e1192–e1207.
91. Ghany MG, Morgan TR, Panel A-IHCG. Hepatitis C Guidance 2019 update: American Association for the Study of Liver Diseases-Infectious Diseases Society of America Recommendations for testing, managing, and treating hepatitis C virus infection. *Hepatology.* 2020;71:686–721.
92. Haber P, Schillie S. 2021. *Pinkbook: Hepatitis B.* Centers for Disease Control and Prevention. Retrieved February 24, 2025. https://www.cdc.gov/pinkbook/hcp/table-of-contents/chapter-10-hepatitis-b.html
93. Midgard H, Finbraten AK, Malme KB, et al. Opportunistic treatment of hepatitis C virus infection (OPPORTUNI-C): study protocol for a pragmatic stepped wedge cluster randomized trial of immediate versus outpatient treatment initiation among hospitalized people who inject drugs. *Trials.* 2020;21:524.
94. Hofmeister MG, Asher A, Jones CM, et al. Prevalence and types of drugs used among hepatitis a patients during outbreaks associated with person-to-person transmission, Kentucky, Michigan, and West Virginia, 2016–2019. *J Appalach Health.* 2022;4:51–60.
95. Nelson NP, Link-Gelles R, Hofmeister MG, et al. Update: recommendations of the Advisory Committee on immunization practices for use of hepatitis a vaccine for postexposure prophylaxis and for preexposure prophylaxis for international travel. *MMWR Morb Mortal Wkly Rep.* 2018;67:1216–1220.
96. McMahon BJ, Beller M, Williams J, Schloss M, Tanttila H, Bulkow L. A program to control an outbreak of hepatitis A in Alaska by using an inactivated hepatitis A vaccine. *Arch Pediatr Adolesc Med.* 1996;150:733–739.
97. US Centers for Disease Control and Prevention. Clinical screening and diagnosis for hepatitis A. Updated January 11, 2025.
98. Armenta RF, Collins KM, Strathdee SA, et al. Mycobacterium tuberculosis infection among persons who inject drugs in San Diego, California. *Int J Tuberc Lung Dis.* 2017;21:425–431.
99. Nagot N, Hai VV, Dong TTT, et al. Alarming tuberculosis rate among people who inject drugs in Vietnam. *Open Forum Infect Dis.* 2022;9:ofab548.
100. Armenta RF, Collins KM, Strathdee SA, et al. Mycobacterium tuberculosis infection among persons who inject drugs in San Diego, California. *Int J Tuberc Lung Dis.* 2017;21(4):425–431.
101. Force USPST, Mangione CM, Barry MJ, et al. Screening for latent tuberculosis infection in adults: US Preventive Services Task Force Recommendation Statement. *JAMA.* 2023;329:1487–1494.
102. Visconti AJ, Sell J, Greenblatt AD. Primary care for persons who inject drugs. *Am Fam Physician.* 2019;99:109–116.
103. Centers for Disease Control and Prevention (CDC). *Clinical Testing Guidance for Tuberculosis: Tuberculin Skin Test. Tuberculosis (TB).* 2025. Accessed January 30, 2026. https://www.cdc.gov/tb/hcp/testing-diagnosis/tuberculin-skin-test.html
104. Englander H, Weimer M, Solotaroff R, et al. Planning and designing the Improving Addiction Care Team (IMPACT) for hospitalized adults with substance use disorder. *J Hosp Med.* 2017;12:339–342.
105. Bachmann LH, Barbee LA, Chan P, et al. CDC clinical guidelines on the use of doxycycline postexposure prophylaxis for

bacterial sexually transmitted infection prevention, United States, 2024. *MMWR Recomm Rep*. 2024;73:1–8.
106. Centers for Disease Control and Prevention. (2024). *Contraception and Birth Control Methods*. Accessed April 15, 2025. https://www.cdc.gov/contraception/about/index.html
107. Chan CA, Minahan-Rowley R, Biegacki ET, Sue KL, Weimer MB. Development of a patient and clinician informed website on injection drug use related infective endocarditis. *Subst Use Addctn J*. 2025;46(2):280–290.
108. Baddour LM, Wilson WR, Bayer AS, et al. Infective endocarditis in adults: diagnosis, antimicrobial therapy, and management of complications: a scientific statement for healthcare professionals from the American Heart Association. *Circulation*. 2015;132:1435–1486.
109. Strnad L, Douglass A, Young K, et al. 742. The development, implementation, and feasibility of multidisciplinary treatment planning conference for individuals with unstable substance use disorders and active infections requiring prolonged antimicrobial therapy: the OPTIONS-DC Model. *Open Forum Infect Dis*. 2019;6:S331–S332.
110. Eaton EF, Mathews RE, Lane PS, et al. A 9-point risk assessment for patients who inject drugs and require intravenous antibiotics: focusing inpatient resources on patients at greatest risk of ongoing drug use. *Clin Infect Dis*. 2019;68:1041–1043.
111. Conte M, Schneider B, Varley CD, Streifel AC, Sikka MK. Description and outcomes of patients with substance use disorder with serious bacterial infections who had a multidisciplinary care conference. *Ther Adv Infect Dis*. 2022;9:20499361221117974.
112. Fanucchi LC, Walsh SL, Thornton AC, Nuzzo PA, Lofwall MR. Outpatient parenteral antimicrobial therapy plus buprenorphine for opioid use disorder and severe injection-related infections. *Clin Infect Dis*. 2020;70:1226–1229.
113. Loesch GH, Cruz JAW, Gasparetto J, Oliveira DDS, Telles JP, Tuon FF. Cost minimization analysis of outpatient parenteral/oral antibiotic therapy at a trauma hospital: public health system. *Infect Control Hosp Epidemiol*. 2021;42:1445–1450.
114. Chapman AL, Dixon S, Andrews D, Lillie PJ, Bazaz R, Patchett JD. Clinical efficacy and cost-effectiveness of outpatient parenteral antibiotic therapy (OPAT): a UK perspective. *J Antimicrob Chemother*. 2009;64:1316–1324.
115. Dalai AS, Leung W, Johnson H, Bai AD. Management of people who inject drugs with serious injection-related infections in an outpatient setting: a scoping review. *Open Forum Infect Dis*. 2024;11:ofae613.
116. Suzuki J, Johnson J, Montgomery M, Hayden M, Price C. Outpatient parenteral antimicrobial therapy among people who inject drugs: a review of the literature. *Open Forum Infect Dis*. 2018;5:ofy194.
117. Pineo T, Goldman JD, Swartzentruber G, Kanderi T, Qurashi H, Dimech C. An observational study on the use of long acting buprenorphine (Sublocade) and a Tamper resistant PICC for outpatient IV antibiotic administration in patients with serious infections and opioid use disorder; The STOP OUD project. *Drug Alcohol Depend Rep*. 2022;2:100020.
118. Dunne MW, Puttagunta S, Sprenger CR, Rubino C, Van Wart S, Baldassarre J. Extended-duration dosing and distribution of dalbavancin into bone and articular tissue. *Antimicrob Agents Chemother*. 2015;59:1849–1855.
119. Brade KD, Rybak JM, Rybak MJ. Oritavancin: a new lipoglycopeptide antibiotic in the treatment of gram-positive infections. *Infect Dis Ther*. 2016;5:1–15.
120. Morrisette T, Miller MA, Montague BT, Barber GR, McQueen RB, Krsak M. Long-acting lipoglycopeptides: "lineless antibiotics" for serious infections in persons who use drugs. *Open Forum Infect Dis*. 2019;6(7):ofz274.
121. Krsak M, Morrisette T, Miller M, et al. Advantages of outpatient treatment with long-acting lipoglycopeptides for serious gram-positive infections: a review. *Pharmacotherapy*. 2020;40:469–478.
122. Tobudic S, Forstner C, Burgmann H, et al. Dalbavancin as primary and sequential treatment for gram-positive infective endocarditis: 2-year experience at the General Hospital of Vienna. *Clin Infect Dis*. 2018;67:795–798.
123. Leanza GM, Rando E, Frondizi F, et al. A systematic review of dalbavancin efficacy as a sequential therapy for infective endocarditis. *Infection*. 2025;53:15–23.
124. Suarez M, Perez-Landeiro A, Sanjurjo A, et al. Comparison of dalbavancin with standard of care in the management of infective endocarditis: efficacy, safety, and cost analysis. *Int J Infect Dis*. 2024;138:41–45.
125. Brown E, Gould FK. Oral antibiotics for infective endocarditis: a clinical review. *J Antimicrob Chemother*. 2020;75:2021–2027.
126. Heldman AW, Hartert TV, Ray SC, et al. Oral antibiotic treatment of right-sided staphylococcal endocarditis in injection drug users: prospective randomized comparison with parenteral therapy. *Am J Med*. 1996;101:68–76.
127. Iversen K, Ihlemann N, Gill SU, et al. Partial oral versus intravenous antibiotic treatment of endocarditis. *N Engl J Med*. 2019;380:415–424.
128. Stamboulian D, Bonvehi P, Arevalo C, et al. Antibiotic management of outpatients with endocarditis due to penicillin-susceptible streptococci. *Rev Infect Dis*. 1991;13(Suppl 2):S160–S163.
129. Marks LR, Liang SY, Muthulingam D, et al. Evaluation of partial oral antibiotic treatment for persons who inject drugs and are hospitalized with invasive infections. *Clin Infect Dis*. 2020;71(10):e650–e656.
130. Tissot-Dupont H, Gouriet F, Oliver L, et al. High-dose trimethoprim-sulfamethoxazole and clindamycin for Staphylococcus aureus endocarditis. *Int J Antimicrob Agents*. 2019;54:143–148.
131. Mzabi A, Kerneis S, Richaud C, Podglajen I, Fernandez-Gerlinger MP, Mainardi JL. Switch to oral antibiotics in the treatment of infective endocarditis is not associated with increased risk of mortality in non-severely ill patients. *Clin Microbiol Infect*. 2016;22:607–612.
132. Dworkin RJ, Lee BL, Sande MA, Chambers HF. Treatment of right-sided Staphylococcus aureus endocarditis in intravenous drug users with ciprofloxacin and rifampicin. *Lancet*. 1989;2:1071–1073.
133. Colli A, Campodonico R, Gherli T. Early switch from vancomycin to oral linezolid for treatment of gram-positive heart valve endocarditis. *Ann Thorac Surg*. 2007;84:87–91.
134. Chayakul P, Akaravinake A, Yipintsoi T. Streptococcal endocarditis treated with two-week antibiotic regimen: preliminary report of a partial oral regimen. *J Med Assoc Thai*. 1993;76:374–379.
135. Wildenthal JA, Atkinson A, Lewis S, et al. Outcomes of partial oral antibiotic treatment for complicated Staphylococcus aureus bacteremia in people who inject drugs. *Clin Infect Dis*. 2023;76:487–496.
136. Spellberg B, Aggrey G, Brennan MB, et al. Use of novel strategies to develop guidelines for management of pyogenic osteomyelitis in adults: a WikiGuidelines Group Consensus Statement. *JAMA Netw Open*. 2022;5:e2211321.
137. McDonald EG, Aggrey G, Aslan AT, et al. Guidelines for diagnosis and management of infective endocarditis in adults: a WikiGuidelines Group Consensus Statement. *JAMA Netw Open*. 2023;6:e2326366.

12 Substance Use Disorders in Pregnancy and Peripartum

Miriam T.H. Harris, Ximena A. Levander, Cecily M. Barber, Elisha M. Wachman, Phaedra Moore

Time has a way of taking a horrific story and unveiling its true beauty. Like a time-lapse video of a lily blooming—something unrecognizable and maybe disturbing erupts into perfect glory. The longer time has to unfold, the more delicate and profound the story becomes. For me, it has softened memories of my home and of family who have died. Memories that used to be too sharp to touch have receded into soft focus. What started as great periods of anguish and magical thinking has evolved into gentle nostalgia and homesickness.

Time has changed my recovery too. It's been 6 years since I've had a drink or a drug. I don't wake up sick anymore. I don't fear getting text messages from random drug dealers checking to see where I've been. My bills are mostly paid, my relationships are mostly healthy, and I no longer spend the day wondering how I will stay clean. Things that were profoundly difficult in the beginning have become automatic with practice, while other things that were never a problem have become challenges to my sanity. One of those things is my propensity to parent out of guilt.

For the first 7 years of my daughter's life, I was deeply sick; habituated to the daily cycle of getting and using drugs. On hard days, all I see are the ways my addiction robbed my daughter of her own set of soft-focus memories. And so, I try to pack in enough "clean time" memories to outweigh that absence. I feel compelled to make all of her hopes and aspirations real, even when she hasn't articulated them to me. In those cases, I just guess. Blindly trying to understand what an emotionally mysterious 13-year-old girl needs to mend a mom-sized hole in her fabric.

Today I was shopping in Boston, hoping that the pulse of the city would vibrate in her small body the way it vibrates in mine. Shops overflowing with ultraexpensive, rustic crafts; tinctures and tins in windows crowded with plush dolls and trinkets, and games, and candles, and things everywhere. And people everywhere. And me, everywhere—trying to impose cheer on my anxious kid who chips a bit every time a stranger bumps into her until she's covered in invisible slights that only she can count. We were in the process of grabbing a bite to eat from a food truck (whimsical, right?) when I looked to my left and found her crying, silently. She got a text from her friends who were hanging out without her, and she crumbled.

Thirteen. Far too many adults in her life. No siblings because, honestly, she wasn't planned, and I was too busy getting high to understand the magnitude of time; to plan for the long game. To think, I better give her a tribe or else she's going to be lonely and cerebral and awkward and so, so lovely.

Watching her cry, all at once, I was looking through time to the miles of mistakes that led to this moment. I saw her loneliness and peculiarity (because of all those hours playing alone while mom was…). I saw her clumsy and sometimes selfish approach to friendship (because playdates don't happen when mom is…). I saw the fear of being left behind (because one day, when she was seven, mom had to leave and …). I'm always aching to be the parent she needs. To lay hard boundaries. To take things in stride. To have sound advice. To be cool and motherly. To cook brownies from scratch and know how to make popular kids like you or, better yet, to teach you not to care. And I'm always worried I will come up short because I screwed up so badly, and every time I come up short, I always worry I'm dooming her future. It's very easy to get tripped up by yesterday's wreckage and tomorrow's terror. It's easy to forget the power of the choices we can make right now.

Like the choice to change perspective when hard things happen, the choice to shrug off a slight or to lean into a fight—now is what builds the future. I think I know that on most days—and I know that addiction is what taught me that—but, it's harder to trust when it's her future I have to have blind faith in.

In the end, after we got home, I insisted that she lie in her bed next to me and cry over the injustice of being left out. When I was 13, crying wasn't allowed and that helped carve an addict out of me. After that, I reminded her that it's also okay that her friends hung out without her. Two things can be true. They can love you and hang out without you. It can hurt, and it can be okay. I can be a recovering drug addict and a great mother. The past can be a field of fire, the future can be uncertain, and I can still show up right now.

For me, the long game has everything to do with the quality of now. How good are your right nows? How much empathy are you holding, right now? How much tough love? How much accountability are you taking, right now? How much fun are you having? How much do you love, right now? What are you planting?

Thirteen years ago, in the grips of debilitating addiction, I planted a seed. Now, it's no longer just my story of addiction and recovery. It's her story of survival and the rebirth of trust, one little now at a time. I get to be a part of that. I get to watch and wait. That's the long game, and I'm happy to say, I'm addicted to it.

—Phaedra Moore

Key Points

- **Substance use is a leading cause of maternal morbidity and mortality in the United States.**
- **Screening for substance use disorder (SUD) in the peripartum period is recommended by medical and public health organizations.**
- **Toxicology testing can have unintended and severe repercussions in substance-exposed dyads—its use must be disclosed with clinical justification.**
- **Treating substance withdrawal and SUD is lifesaving, has maternal and neonatal benefits, and though there are some important treatment nuances, management is similar to that of the general, nonpregnant population.**
- **Harm-reduction approaches should be universally incorporated in SUD treatment plans for peripartum individuals with SUD.**
- **Transparency about mandated reporting practices is critical, and child custody loss is associated with adverse maternal outcomes like overdose.**
- **Breastfeeding is recommended for individuals who are not actively using nonprescribed substances and is safe with most SUD treatments.**
- **Hospitals should have consistent policies for the care of opioid-exposed newborns that include neonatal abstinence syndrome (neonatal opioid withdrawal syndrome [NOWS]) assessment and management guidelines that utilize both nonpharmacologic and pharmacologic approaches.**

The United States (US) is experiencing a maternal health crisis, ranking lowest in maternal health outcomes among high-income countries and being one of only eight nations with worsening maternal mortality from 2000 to 2020.[1,2] Mental health and substance use disorder (SUD) are major contributors to this crisis, with SUD being a leading cause of maternal morbidity and mortality.[3] Pregnant and parenting individuals* with SUD experience greater sociodemographic disadvantages, preexisting health conditions, and comorbid psychiatric diagnoses than their counterparts.[4] They are also more likely to utilize acute care services, such as the emergency department or hospital, during the antenatal period, and are less likely to utilize prenatal health care services.[4] Pregnant and parenting individuals with SUD face higher rates of maternal and neonatal complications, such as postpartum depression, overdose, death,[5] preterm birth, low birth weight, and neonatal

*We recognize and acknowledge the changing nature of language in the reproductive health literature. In this chapter, the term pregnant and postpartum individuals is mostly used. The authors use the terms "women" or "females" or "maternal" to be consistent with the language found in the reference material. The authors acknowledge that not all postpartum individuals may identify as women or females, and these terms are not inclusive of all gender identities in this context.

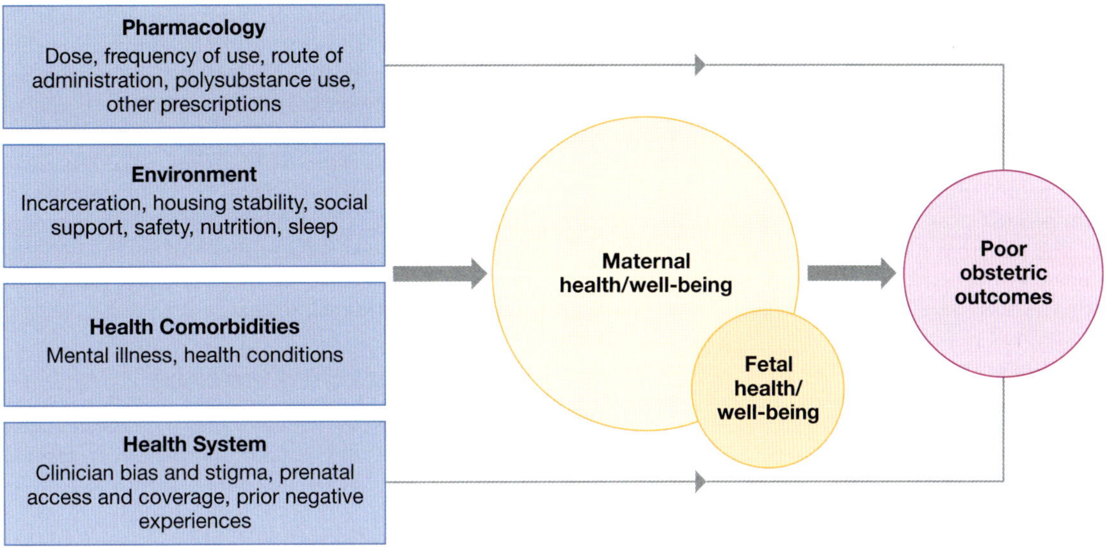

Figure 12.1: Factors contributing to maternal and fetal adverse health outcomes among substance-exposed dyads. (Wakeman B, Kremer M, Schulkin J. The application of harm reduction to methamphetamine use during pregnancy: a call to arms. *Am J Obstet Gynecol MFM*. 2021;3(5):100418.)

mortality.[4] Compounding these disparities is clinician bias attributed to the clinician's lack of education, resources, and training in SUD management.[6] For example, women with SUD report not feeling heard, feeling judged by perinatal clinicians, and receiving insufficient education about maternal SUD care and the effects of substance use and SUD treatment on child development.[7] A visual summary of the varying factors contributing to maternal and fetal adverse health outcomes among substance-exposed dyads is presented in Figure 12.1. This chapter aims to comprehensively review SUD diagnoses and treatment in pregnant and parenting individuals, designed for hospital-based clinicians.

Epidemiology

Between 2010 and 2019, 11.4% of maternal deaths were substance-related, marking an increase of 190% during this time period (Figure 12.2).[8] Driven by illicit fentanyl and psychostimulants (eg, methamphetamine), fatal overdoses in pregnant and postpartum individuals continue to increase.[5,9] Overdose deaths are considered preventable because overdose prevention strategies (eg, naloxone) and SUD treatment are highly effective, though they remain underutilized.[10] Less than half of pregnant women with opioid use disorder (OUD) receive medications for opioid use disorder (MOUD), the standard of care for OUD treatment, and among those who do, roughly a third discontinue treatment in the postpartum period.[11–13] While studies use different definitions of early and late postpartum periods, overdose risk tends to be greatest further out from delivery, up to 1 year postpartum, and lowest during the third trimester and early postpartum periods.[5,14] Fluctuations in overdose risk throughout the peripartum period could indicate

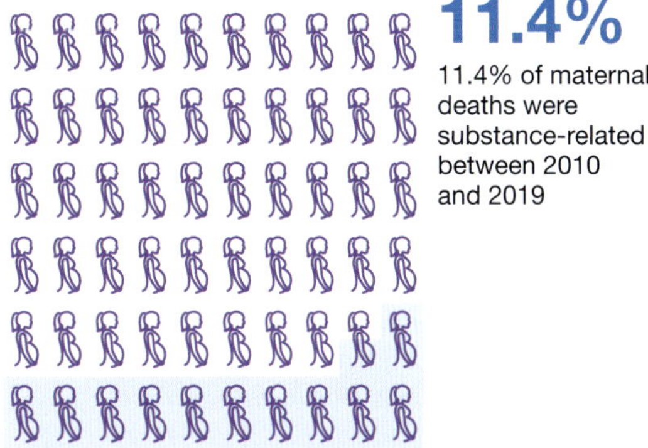

Figure 12.2: Substance-related maternal deaths between 2010 and 2019. (Data from Margerison CE, Roberts MH, Gemmill A, Goldman-Mellor S. Pregnancy-associated deaths due to drugs, suicide, and homicide in the United States, 2010–2019. *Obstet Gynecol*. 2022;139(2):172–180.)

the protective nature of increased engagement in care during pregnancy and early postpartum that can taper off or abruptly end in later postpartum due to transitions of care and termination of insurance coverage. In addition, competing demands of caring for a new family and child custody removal are associated with mental and SUD-related crises in the postpartum period.[15]

The maternal substance use crisis has disproportionately impacted communities that experience other forms of structural marginalization. Black, Indigenous, Latine,* and rural communities face higher rates of substance use and related harms and have poorer access to needed services.[2,16,17]

Data from the 2023 National Survey of Drug Use and Health (NSDUH) estimates past-month use of illicit substances, including cannabis, to be 21% among nonpregnant reproductive-age females aged 15 to 44 years old and 4.9% among pregnant reproductive-age females aged 15 to 44 years old.[18] The prevalence of past-month illicit substance use by pregnant females decreased from 9.6% in 2022 and remained stable in nonpregnant reproductive-age females.[18] Estimates of past-month nicotine product use, including cigarettes, vaping products, etc, were 14% among nonpregnant females, and 9.4% among pregnant, reproductive-age females, aged 15 to 44, the latter slightly up from 8.4% in 2022.[18] Estimates of past-month alcohol use were 51% among nonpregnant females, and 8.4% among pregnant reproductive-age females, aged 15 to 44, the latter decreased from 11% in 2022.[18] In summary, approximately 22% of pregnant individuals used an illicit substance, a nicotine product, and/or alcohol in the past month.

Despite persistently high rates of substance use during the peripartum period, pregnant and parenting individuals with SUD continue to face substantial barriers to SUD treatment. This is due to the limited availability of services equipped to care for them, the siloing of obstetric and SUD treatment services, fears of legal repercussions or custody loss, comorbid mental health conditions, stigma, and feelings of guilt and shame.[19–21] Nationally, there is vast state variability in SUD treatment access for peripartum patients with SUD. A recent study of Medicaid claims data from 39 states demonstrated a wide range of SUD treatment access, with a low of 19% of people with SUD receiving treatment in Kansas to a high of 79% of people with SUD receiving treatment in Maine (average 55%).[22]

*In this chapter, the authors use the term Black to refer to Black and/or African American individuals. The authors use the gender-neutral term Latine to refer to Hispanic and/or Latino/a/e/x individuals. The authors also use the term Women of Color to be consistent with language found in the reference text.

However, pregnancy can motivate many women to seek SUD care.[23] Thus, increasing access to high-quality SUD services is critical for peripartum individuals. Evidence demonstrates that programs designed to meet the specific needs of pregnant and postpartum individuals with SUD reduce access barriers and increase engagement with SUD treatment and prenatal care.[24,25] This chapter covers best practices in SUD diagnosis and treatment across the peripartum period, particularly as they pertain to the care of patients in the hospital setting.

Summary of the Evidence

Screening for SUD with the use of evidence-based instruments in the peripartum period is recommended by medical and public health organizations. However, toxicology testing (maternal urine substance testing or neonatal umbilical cord, blood, urine, or meconium testing) is not equivalent to, nor is it a substitute for, evidence-based screening instruments and can have unintended and severe repercussions for substance-exposed dyads. Given that polysubstance use is common among peripartum individuals with SUD, it is important to screen and address all substances. Treating substance withdrawal is critical for peripartum individuals with SUD. Though there are some treatment nuances, management of substance withdrawal is similar to that of the general population. However, medically managed withdrawal is not SUD treatment, and without ongoing treatment, that is, initiation of MOUD in the instance of OUD, is associated with an increased risk of overdose. Therefore, SUD treatment should be universally offered to peripartum individuals with SUD and is associated with maternal and neonatal benefits. Harm-reduction approaches should also be universally incorporated in SUD treatment plans. Team-based care models can facilitate SUD treatment in the hospital and outpatient setting, as well as address co-occurring mental health conditions and socioeconomic barriers to care. The postpartum period is a particularly vulnerable time for adverse SUD outcomes, such as treatment cessation, relapse, and overdose. Specifically, child custody loss is associated with adverse maternal outcomes like overdose. Thus, transparency about mandated reporting practices is critical throughout the peripartum period. Breastfeeding is recommended for individuals who are not actively using nonprescribed substances and reduces the severity of neonatal abstinence syndrome (NAS). Most medications for SUD are compatible with breastfeeding. Clinicians caring for birthing dyads affected by substance use should be prepared to address NAS. This umbrella diagnosis also includes neonatal opioid withdrawal syndrome (NOWS). NOWS requires standardized hospital protocols for diagnosis, monitoring, and treatment, emphasizing nonpharmacologic care (eg, rooming-in, breastfeeding, caregiver presence) as first-line therapy, with pharmacologic treatment reserved for severe cases.

Clinical Guidance

Screening for Substance Use Disorders

Clinicians cannot appropriately diagnose, intervene, and treat pregnant patients with SUD without first being aware of the patient's experience with substances. Screening for SUD with the use of evidence-based instruments in the peripartum period is recommended by medical and public health organizations.[26] These recommendations are informed by the prevalence of substance use, particularly polysubstance use, and SUD, among peripartum individuals.[18] It is critical that all pregnant patients undergo screening as early as possible, and that screening is protocolized as part of the standard of care to reduce the likelihood of clinician and staff bias, the possibility of missed cases, and patient perceptions of discrimination and stigma.[27] Screening should be voluntary and without coercion.[28] The importance of SUD screening must be balanced with the knowledge that a positive screen requires further investigation and is not a diagnosis of a SUD (high false-positive rate).[29] Screening must also come with the recognition of the real misgivings and fears patients may have around disclosing use, particularly of illegal substances, while pregnant, to members of the health care system.[30] Clinicians and staff should be competent in best practices in the use of nonstigmatizing and nonjudgmental language and in asking for patient permission to inquire about potentially sensitive topics such as substance use. They should also be aware of disclosure requirements in their state and be transparent with patients about mandated reporting. Pregnant individuals should be screened for SUD ideally during their first visit to prenatal care.[31] However, many patients with SUD are not engaged in prenatal care, so hospital teams should be prepared to screen and refer to treatment (screening with brief intervention and referral to treatment [SBIRT]) as part of routine care. Given the fragmentation of health care systems in SBIRT, innovative approaches to improving screening rates are necessary (see case example).

> **Case Example to Improve Substance Screening Among Pregnant Individuals**
>
> The Colorado Maternal Mortality Review Committee, convened by the Colorado Department of Public Health and Environment, established a three-prong approach to reduce state-wide preventable maternal mortality. The first approach includes a cost-free learning collaborative and hospital guidelines with protocols to implement universal screening with brief intervention and referral to treatment (SBIRT) for unhealthy substance use and the use of evidence-based screening tools to identify patients at risk of perinatal mood and anxiety disorders. This intervention led to a 38% increase in screening from baseline after bundle implementation.[32]

Validated Screening Instruments

There are numerous validated and recommended screening instruments and tools for unhealthy substance use among nonpregnant adults and less validated screening tools for pregnant individuals.[33] Two studies were conducted as direct comparisons of self-reported SUD screening instruments for use during pregnancy.[29,33] The first study examined three tools—the 4 P's Plus, the NIDA Quick Screen-ASSIST (Modified Alcohol, Smoking, and Substance Involvement Screening Test), and the SURP-P (Substance Use Risk Profile-Pregnancy).[29] The authors found that the 4 P's Plus (sensitivity 90.2 [84.5–93.8], negative predictive value [NPV] 83.0 [73.4–88.9]) and SUPR-P (sensitivity 92.4 [87.6–95.8], NPV 82.3 [72.1–90.0]) had higher sensitivity with similar NPVs compared to the NIDA Quick Screen-ASSIST (sensitivity 79.7 [71.2-84.2], NPV 86.9 [81.3–89.7]). The second study compared five tools—the SURP-P, the CRAFFT (five-item screener related to car use, relax, alone, forget, friends, and trouble), the 5 P's (parents, peers, partner, pregnancy, past), the WIDUS (Wayne Indirect Drug Use Screener), and the NIDA Quick Screen.[33] In that study, no one tool had both high sensitivity and specificity; thus, no one tool was deemed better than another to accurately screen for all unhealthy substance use. Table 12.1 summarizes the three most commonly used screening tools and their limitations. Even a brief version of the first two questions from the 4 P's, such as "Have you used alcohol or drugs during this pregnancy?" and "Have you had a problem with alcohol or drug use in the past?", can serve as a valuable starting point for discussion.

When a Patient Screens Positive for Unhealthy Substance Use

Pregnant patients who screen positive for unhealthy substance use should undergo a formal evaluation

TABLE 12.1

Summary of Screening Tools for Unhealthy Substance Use Among Pregnant Individuals

Tool	Sensitivity	Limitations	Access information
4 P's Plus	87%[33] 90.2%[29]	Must be purchased	https://www.ntiupstream.com/4psabout
SURP-P	Low risk: 80–100%[33] High risk: 48–100%[33] 92.4%[29]	Only asks about cannabis and alcohol	http://www.mass.gov/doc/substance-use-risk-profile-pregnancy-scale-pdf/download
NIDA Quick Screen and ASSIST	79.7%[29]	Potentially a two-part questionnaire; can be lengthy Not initially validated for prenatal screening	https://www.drugabuse.gov/sites/default/files/pdf/nmassist.pdf

SURP-P, Substance use risk profile—pregnancy; NIDA, National Institute on Drug Abuse.

Adapted from Wakeman B, Kremer M, Schulkin J. The application of harm reduction to methamphetamine use during pregnancy: a call to arms. *Am J Obstet Gynecol MFM*. 2021;3(5):100418, with permission from Elsevier.

with a clinician to assess for SUD using the Diagnostic and Statistical Manual of Mental Disorders, 5th Edition (DSM-5)[34] with a determination of SUD severity (ie, mild, moderate, severe). Patients who meet DSM-5 criteria for SUD should be offered referral to SUD treatment. Pregnant patients who do not meet DSM-5 criteria for SUD, but who report unhealthy substance use, should receive brief intervention, counseling, and continued monitoring with follow-up assessments.

Pregnant patients with SUDs are vulnerable to other medical, behavioral, and psychosocial stressors. Therefore, it is recommended that they should also be screened for co-occurring conditions, including mood and anxiety disorders.[35] When pregnant patients screen positive for these conditions, they should be offered referral to behavioral or medical treatment. All pregnant patients (regardless of SUD status) should be screened for, and provided resources for, intimate partner violence (IPV) and for social determinants of health, including housing and food insecurity.[36,37]

Toxicology Testing

Verbal screening is the only validated screening tool for unhealthy substance use among pregnant patients. The diagnosis of SUD relies on meeting DSM-5 criteria. While data exists to support urine drug testing of patients with known SUD to monitor treatment and support recovery, little data exists to support the role of urine drug testing in the pregnant patient without a diagnosis of SUD.[26,38] Concurrently, multiple studies have demonstrated maternal and fetal harm from urine drug testing, including deterrence from prenatal care and racial bias in testing.[39–43]

Toxicology testing (maternal and infant) has a long history of being misused—often it is incorrectly used as a substitute for true, validated screening. Thus, it is important to identify what the exact goal of toxicology testing is, which should include the clinical indication, before proceeding. Furthermore, toxicology test interpretation is particularly complex during the prenatal period due to changes in peripartum physiology. For example, in maternal toxicology due to physiologic changes of pregnancy involving metabolism and fat sequestration, there can be impaired illicit fentanyl clearance in pregnancy that complicates result interpretation.[44] In addition, the time of substance detection varies greatly across substances, and both false-positive and false-negative results are common in screening urine drug tests.[45,46] Thus, the American Society of Addiction Medicine (ASAM) recommendations are clear that definitive testing (ie, gas chromatography-mass spectrometry [GC-MS]) are required "when the results will inform a decision with major clinical or nonclinical implications for the patient" which, given the child reporting complexities in the peripartum period, apply to all toxicology tests in pregnancy, especially during the birthing hospitalization.[47] Furthermore, it is well documented that multiple medications, like labetalol, commonly used in pregnancy and during the delivery hospitalization, are associated with false-positive urine toxicology tests.[48] Table 12.2 lists commonly used medications associated with false positives in urine toxicology screening tests (Note: Table 12.2 is not an exhaustive or all-inclusive list).

Despite the significant limitations of toxicology testing to correctly identify use of unprescribed substances, they are often utilized in the hospital setting. Strong recommendations from obstetrics and

TABLE 12.2

Medications Associated With False Positives by Urine Toxicology Screen[a,b]

Toxicology screen	Medications that may cause false positives	Common medication class
Amphetamine/ methamphetamine	Bupropion, labetalol, metformin, promethazine, trazodone	Antidepressant, antihypertensive, diabetes medication, antihistamine/antiemetic
Benzodiazepine	Sertraline (>150 mg)	Antidepressant (SSRI)
Barbiturate	Fioricet/Fiorinal[c]	Combination analgesic (contains butalbital)
Methadone	Bupropion, diphenhydramine, quetiapine (≥125 mg)	Antidepressant, antihistamine, antipsychotic
Fentanyl	Labetalol, loperamide, risperidone	Antihypertensive, antidiarrheal, antipsychotic

[a]Lab-specific immunoassays are subject to change over time.

[b]Amphetamine immunoassays generally have ~10% cross-reactivity.

[c]Fioricet contains butalbital (a barbiturate).

gynecology (OBGYN) and addiction organizations state that informed consent is necessary for any toxicology testing to occur.[49,50] However, studies suggest that this is infrequently performed or documented.[51] Clinicians should be honest and transparent regarding how information is obtained from either screening (ie, immunoassay) or confirmatory (GC-MS) testing and how it may be shared with external agencies, including child welfare. Table 12.3 summarizes considerations for toxicology testing in the peripartum period.

Substance Use Disorder and Treatment

This section reviews medically managed withdrawal, stabilization, treatment, and substance-related harms for alcohol, opioids, benzodiazepines and other sedatives, stimulants, cannabis, tobacco, and nicotine. The adverse outcomes associated with nonprescribed substance use are reviewed in Table 12.4, and medically managed withdrawal as well as SUD treatments are summarized in Table 12.5. It is important to keep in mind the dynamic and unstable nature of the illicit substance supply that can further complicate withdrawal management and SUD treatment. In addition, roughly 18% of pregnant and parenting individuals with SUD use multiple substances.[52] Thus, there is a need to screen and treat for all substances patients are using when presenting to the hospital.[52] The highest prevalence of substance use during pregnancy is during the first trimester, indicating the importance of connecting with patients early when possible.[14]

Alcohol

Despite public health efforts, alcohol use among persons of childbearing age and during pregnancy has remained unchanged for the past few decades in the

TABLE 12.3

Summary of Considerations for Toxicology Testing in Pregnant and Postpartum Individuals

- Toxicology testing is never equivalent to or a substitute for evidence-based validated screening instruments
- Immunoassay toxicology screening tests are limited with a high rate of false positives
- Toxicology confirmatory testing (ie, gas chromatography-mass spectrometry) is required for unexpected positive results with major clinical or nonclinical implications
- Immunoassay screening (with confirmatory testing) should be used to:
  - Evaluate the efficacy of recovery treatment for patients with a known SUD
  - Detect recent ingestion of a potentially harmful substance for purposes of patient safety and education
- Toxicology testing can have unintended and severe repercussions in pregnant/parenting persons who use substances
  - Clearly describe the clinical indication for toxicology testing with the patient
  - Document the reason and reasoning behind toxicology testing in the medical record
    - This will minimize bias, discrimination, and punitive use of urine toxicology
  - Obtain proper consent
  - Be transparent about potential consequences of legal family system involvement

TABLE 12.4

Adverse Maternal and Fetal Outcomes Associated with Nonprescribed Substance Use During Pregnancy

Substance	Maternal outcomes	Fetal/neonatal outcomes
Alcohol	Increased risk of miscarriage[53] Nutritional deficiencies[53]	FAS (leading modifiable cause of intellectual disability and developmental delay)[54] Preterm birth[53] Increased risk of SUID when co-used with tobacco[55]
Opioids	Increased maternal morbidity and ICU admissions[56] Cesarean delivery complications[57]	Low birth weight[56,57] Preterm delivery[56,57] NOWS[56,57] Possible congenital malformations (lower with buprenorphine vs methadone)[57,58]
Kratom	Withdrawal symptoms similar to opioid withdrawal[59]	Case reports of neonates with in utero kratom exposure developing NOWS-like symptoms[60]
Sedative-Hypnotics	Increased risk of cesarean delivery[61]	Increased risk of spontaneous abortion[62] Preterm birth[4] Low birth weight[63] SGA[63] Low Apgar scores at 5 min[61] Increased risk of NOWS with co-opioid exposure[64]
Stimulants	Maternal morbidity[65] Gestational hypertension[65] Cardiovascular risks: heart failure, arrhythmias, stroke, etc[66,67]	Preterm birth[65,68] SGA[65,68] Fetal death[65,68] Increased NICU admissions[65]
Cannabis	Preeclampsia[69,70] Gestational hypertension[69,70]	Preterm birth[69,70] SGA[69,70] Cognitive and sociobehavioral developmental concerns[69,70]
Tobacco/ Nicotine	Obstetric complications: placental abruption, premature labor[71] Nutritional deficiencies[71]	Stillbirth[71,72] Low birth weight[71,72] SGA[71,72] Congenital malformations[71,72] SUID[71,72]

FAS, fetal alcohol syndrome; NOWS, neonatal opioid withdrawal syndrome; SGA, small for gestational age; SUID, sudden unexplained infant death.

US.[73,74] The 2023 NSDUH estimated that 8.4% of pregnant individuals reported past-month alcohol use, while the Behavioral Risk Factor Surveillance Survey indicated that from 2018 to 2020, nearly 14% of pregnant individuals reported drinking, and 5% reported past 30-day binge alcohol use.[75] This inconsistency suggests that alcohol use among pregnant individuals may be underestimated. Rates of any alcohol use and alcohol use disorder (AUD) are low among pregnant individuals, but are similarly likely underestimated.[75] Alcohol is an established teratogen, and the safe, lower limit of alcohol exposure remains unknown. Fetal alcohol syndrome (FAS) is the leading modifiable cause of intellectual disability and developmental delay in the US, with a similar rate to Down syndrome, and 20 times more common in the US (1.95/1,000) than in Europe (0.08/1,000).[54] Maternal tobacco and alcohol use is associated with an increased risk of sudden unexplained infant death (SUID) in the postpartum period.[55]

Alcohol Withdrawal Management in Pregnancy

All individuals who report alcohol use should be evaluated for alcohol withdrawal and AUD. When a

TABLE 12.5

Medically Managed Withdrawal and SUD Treatment Recommendations in Pregnant Individuals

Medication	Mechanism	Indication	Dosing considerations	Neonatal considerations	Recommendation
Sedative hypnotics					
Phenobarbital	GABA neuromodulator and agonist	Alcohol withdrawal	Lowest effective dose, for shortest period	Crosses the placenta, known teratogen, associated with increased fetal malformations[76,77]	Consider using in severe alcohol withdrawal refractory to benzodiazepines
Benzodiazepines	GABA-A receptor agonist	Alcohol withdrawal, benzodiazepine withdrawal, and use disorder treatment	Symptom-triggered dosing for alcohol withdrawal symptoms using a validated tool (ie, CIWA-Ar, MINDS)[78,79] Symptom-triggered dosing and/or scheduled tapers for benzodiazepine withdrawal using a validated tool (ie, CIWA-B)[80] Lowest effective dose, for shortest period	Case series and cohort studies show associations with adverse neonatal outcomes (eg, preterm delivery),[61] increased risk of NOWS in setting of polysubstance use[64,81]	Appropriate for withdrawal and benzodiazepine use disorder management
Acamprosate	Glutamate/GABA neuromodulator	AUD	666 mg TID	Animal studies show adverse fetal effects, small cohort studies found no increases in fetal malformation[82]	Use shared decision making to guide treatment decisions
Disulfiram	ADH inhibitor	AUD	Disulfiram works by inhibiting ADH, thus, any ingestion of alcohol causes alcohol toxicity	Animal studies show adverse fetal outcomes, limited clinical data[83]	Not recommended
Naltrexone	Nonselective opioid receptor antagonist	AUD	Oral 50-100 mg daily XR 380 mg every 28 days	Limited safety data	Shared decision making of benefits, risks, and limitations of available data
Topiramate	GABA A receptor agonist	AUD		Crosses the placenta, known teratogen, associated with increased fetal malformations[76,84]	Not recommended
Opioids					
Clonidine	Central alpha-antagonist	Opioid detoxification and/or adjunct during MOUD induction	Lowest effective dose, for shortest period 0.1-0.2 mg TID PRN	Cohort studies found no increases in fetal malformation[85,86]	Appropriate to use for short durations
Methadone	Full mu-agonist and weak NMDA receptor antagonist	Opioid withdrawal, detoxification, OUD	High-dose inductions can be pursed in the inpatient setting Split dosing in pregnancy is associated with decrease in maternal symptoms and possible decrease in NOWS[87,88]	Higher association with NOWS and congenital abnormalities than buprenorphine[89]	Recommended for OUD Restricting dose in an attempt to decrease NOWS is discouraged

(*continued*)

TABLE 12.5

Medically Managed Withdrawal and SUD Treatment Recommendations in Pregnant Individuals (*Continued*)

Medication	Mechanism	Indication	Dosing considerations	Neonatal considerations	Recommendation
Buprenorphine (BUP)	Partial mu-agonist with a high affinity for the mu-opioid receptor	Opioid withdrawal, detoxification, OUD	Monthly XR formulations contain N-Methyl-2-pyrrolidone (NMP)[90] Low dose buprenorphine initiation approaches can be used in pregnant individuals who are using fentanyl[91,92]	Lower association with NOWS compared to methadone[89]	Sublingual (SL) mono or combination (buprenorphine-naloxone) is equivocal, focus should be on stability There is limited data on maternal, fetal, and child outcome data for XR-bup products Available monthly formulations contain NMP, shared decision making should be used for XR-bup
Naltrexone	Nonselective opioid-receptor antagonist	OUD	Oral 50-100 mg daily XR 380 mg every 28 days	Similar safety profile to other MOUD but data far more limited[93]	Shared decision making of benefits, risks, and limitations of available data
Nicotine/tobacco					
Nicotine replacement therapy (NRT)	Nicotine agonist	Smoking cessation	NRT type and duration should be determined by clinical needs	Maybe associated with adverse birth and neonatal outcomes (eg, small for gestational age [SGA], preterm delivery [PTD]), but data are conflicting[94–96]	Benefits outweigh the risks compared to ongoing tobacco product use
Varenicline	Partial nicotine agonist	Smoking cessation		Limited safety data available[97,98]	Use shared decision making based on the severity of tobacco use
Bupropion	Aminoketone antidepressant, some nicotine receptor–blocking activity	Smoking cessation, methamphetamine use disorder	XR product is used for smoking cessation	It may be associated with congenital heart defects[99,100]	After shared decision making, bupropion can be used for smoking cessation treatment
Stimulants					
Topiramate	GABA-A receptor agonist	Cocaine use disorder		Crosses the placenta, known teratogen, associated with increased fetal malformations[76,84]	Not recommended
Mirtazapine	Noradrenergic and serotonergic activity, antagonizing alpha receptors and blocking serotonin receptors	Methamphetamine use disorder	Titrate as tolerated up to 30 mg orally once daily	Cohort studies are reassuring but some conflicting results for fetal malformations[101]	Use shared decision making based on the severity of methamphetamine use

pregnant patient is at risk for alcohol withdrawal, the hospital-based clinician should initiate medication management to prevent progression to severe alcohol withdrawal, which can be life threatening. Untreated alcohol withdrawal is associated with a nearly 5% yearly mortality rate.[102] ASAM recommends hospital-based management for individuals at risk of severe withdrawal, which includes pregnant patients.[103] Benzodiazepines and phenobarbital, medications used to treat alcohol withdrawal, are likely safe in short courses in pregnant individuals. The risks of morbidity or mortality from untreated alcohol withdrawal outweigh the theoretical risks of short-term exposure to these medications.

There are limited and conflicting data on phenobarbital exposure in pregnancy and the risk of congenital malformations. The data are limited in their applicability to acute alcohol withdrawal management, as much of the data are derived from chronic exposure associated with epilepsy treatment, as opposed to short-term use, for alcohol withdrawal management.[76,77] Longer exposure to anticonvulsants and higher doses is associated with greater teratogenic risk.[76,77] Given the risk of congenital malformations seen in chronic use of phenobarbital, it is recommended to use benzodiazepines as first-line treatment for alcohol withdrawal, particularly in the first trimester of pregnancy. However, the benefits of short-term use of phenobarbital (at the lowest possible total dose) for acute life-saving management of alcohol withdrawal outweigh the potential risks to the fetus.

Although in utero exposure to benzodiazepines does not suggest teratogenicity or negative effects on neurocognitive development in children, extended in utero exposure can cause neonatal withdrawal symptoms similar to opioids and is associated with longer NOWS treatment, especially in the context of methadone.[104,105] Alcohol withdrawal management alone is not sufficient treatment for AUD. The mainstay treatment for AUD is medication combined with behavioral interventions.[106,107] Behavioral interventions alone are associated with high rates of return to use.[106,107]

Medications for Alcohol Use Disorder in Pregnancy

A recent study showed that receipt of medication for any alcohol-related diagnosis in pregnant individuals is rare (~10%), and pregnant patients were more likely to receive medications for alcohol withdrawal rather than medications for AUD.[108] Data suggest that state-level pregnancy-specific alcohol policies—mandatory warning signs, priority treatment—are largely ineffective in decreasing alcohol use during pregnancy or decreasing adverse obstetric outcomes and may be harmful to public health outcomes like maternal engagement in prenatal and infant health care.[109]

Disulfiram, Acamprosate, and Naltrexone

There are three approved medications for AUD: disulfiram, an aldehyde dehydrogenase (ADH) inhibitor, acamprosate, a glutamate/GABA neuromodulator, and naltrexone, a mu-opioid receptor antagonist. The safety and efficacy of these medications are well established in nonpregnant adults,[110] but due to the exclusion of pregnant individuals from medication trials, there is limited evidence regarding the safety and effectiveness of these medications in pregnancy.[111] For nonpregnant individuals, the American Psychiatric Association (APA) recommends acamprosate or naltrexone (reviewed in greater detail in Table 12.5) as first-line treatment for moderate-to-severe AUD, with disulfiram considered second-line therapy under close supervision.[112] Disulfiram works by inhibiting ADH, one of the enzymes responsible for the metabolism of alcohol.[113] Any ingestion of alcohol while taking disulfiram causes alcohol toxicity, thus, it is not recommended in pregnancy. Though there are limited safety data, given the known adverse effects and harm of untreated AUD and fetal alcohol exposure, naltrexone and acamprosate should be seriously considered in the clinical care of pregnant and postpartum individuals with AUD.[114]

Opioids

From 1999 to 2014, the rate of OUD complicating birth increased between 4- to 10-fold across the US, yet OUD treatment remains stigmatized and underutilized.[115,116] Opioid use during pregnancy is associated with complications. These include high rates of maternal morbidity, low infant birth weight, preterm delivery, maternal and neonatal intensive care unit admission, and NOWS,[56] all of which result in substantially higher associated health care costs.[26,57] Despite public health and professional society recommendations supporting MOUD,[26] pregnant and postpartum individuals with OUD continue to face barriers to treatment, including stigma,[117] discrimination, lack of access to clinicians who treat OUD,[118] and misinformation about NOWS. Only 50% of pregnant individuals admitted to specialty SUD treatment programs receive medications,[119] and there are marked racial inequities in medication receipt, type, and dose.[120] Black pregnant women are less likely to receive medications compared to White pregnant women.[12] Even among those who receive methadone, mean daily doses are higher for White (144.9 mg) compared to Black (97.5 mg) pregnant women.[120]

Available data regarding negative fetal effects of opioids are inconsistent, and much of the literature is observational. In a recent large cohort study comparing methadone to buprenorphine for treatment of OUD, the risk of major congenital malformations overall was lower in buprenorphine-exposed infants compared to methadone-exposed infants.[89] These study results can guide shared decision making for pregnant patients with OUD, acknowledging that untreated OUD is associated with serious maternal health risks.

Opioid Withdrawal Management in Pregnancy

Medically supervised opioid withdrawal alone is not recommended in pregnancy. Medically supervised withdrawal from nonprescribed opioids or MOUD is not treatment, is linked to a return to use and fatal overdose, and does not reduce the risk of NOWS.[85,121] However, it is important to respect patient autonomy, and medically supervised opioid withdrawal may be attempted after shared decision making with counseling on the safety and the risk of return to use.[122] Studies show clonidine use is reasonable in opioid withdrawal management or for use as an adjunctive agent during MOUD initiation.[85,86]

Medications for OUD in Pregnancy

Methadone, Buprenorphine, and Naltrexone

All three Federal Drug Administration (FDA)-approved medications for OUD should be offered to pregnant individuals with OUD. Methadone, a full mu-agonist and weak NMDA receptor antagonist, buprenorphine, a partial mu-agonist with a high affinity for the mu-opioid receptor, and naltrexone, a nonselective opioid receptor antagonist, save lives and are the standard OUD treatment among pregnant and postpartum individuals.[115] MOUD improves both SUD and pregnancy outcomes and decreases overdose risk compared with no treatment. Evidence for the safety and efficacy of methadone and buprenorphine is the strongest, including the safety and efficacy of the buprenorphine-naloxone combination product.[123] When approaching MOUD treatment in pregnancy, if a patient is stable and in recovery, it is not recommended to switch MOUD (eg, from methadone to buprenorphine-naloxone).[124] If a patient is on MOUD and still using nonprescribed opioids, offering titration of their current medication (ie, increasing the dose), is an important strategy. Switching treatments can be destabilizing. MOUD dose (methadone or buprenorphine) is not correlated with NOWS,[125] however, buprenorphine products are associated with a lower incidence and severity of NOWS compared to methadone.[126]

Extended-Release Medications: Buprenorphine

Injectable, extended-release buprenorphine products have multiple formulations, some last for 1 week while others last up to 28 days. There are two available extended-release buprenorphine products currently available for use in nonpregnant individuals: Sublocade® and Brixadi®. Sublocade, a once monthly, injectable formulation, was FDA approved in November 2017 and contains N-methyl-2-pyrrolidone (NMP). In preclinical studies, NMP was associated with adverse pregnancy and fetal outcomes[90] and NMP's use in pregnancy is not advised. However, accumulating observational data on the use of Sublocade® during pregnancy does not indicate an increased risk of adverse neonatal outcomes.

Brixadi® is an extended-release buprenorphine product that is available in a weekly and monthly injectable formulation. Brixadi® has been available in Europe and Australia for several years and was approved by the FDA in May 2023. Brixadi does not contain NMP but does include ethanol as a solvent. According to data from an ongoing randomized multisite outpatient clinical trial, a pregnant person on the highest Brixadi dose would be exposed to the equivalent of a fraction of one standard alcohol-containing drink over the entire pregnancy.[127] The Medication treatment for Opioid use disorder in expectant MotherS (MOMS) study is examining the use of weekly Brixadi® during pregnancy and when breastfeeding.[128] Weekly and monthly extended-release buprenorphine products are not contraindicated in pregnancy. In summary, clinicians should always use shared decision making with their pregnant patients to weigh the risks and benefits of extended-release buprenorphine (Brixadi® and Sublocade®) versus sublingual buprenorphine versus methadone.[127]

Naltrexone

Naltrexone is available in oral and extended-release formulations (injectable and implants, which are only available in Europe), and the extended release formulation has comparable safety data to other forms of MOUD.[93] One small retrospective study found that urogenital anomalies were more frequent in naltrexone implant-exposed fetuses compared with methadone or buprenorphine exposed fetuses, however, the study was underpowered.[129] Injectable naltrexone is currently being studied in pregnancy and postpartum in an ongoing multisite trial.[130] Although specific data are limited, the established limitations of naltrexone, such as the need for complete detoxification before initiation, lower retention rates, and potential increased overdose risk after stopping, also apply to pregnant populations.[131,132] Naltrexone may be a reasonable option for pregnant patients with comorbid AUD or a remote history of OUD, particularly if they are stable in recovery, not actively using opioids, and engaged in ongoing care. Naltrexone, particularly extended-release naltrexone, can be considered after a shared decision making process that reviews the benefits, risks, and limitations of available data in pregnant individuals.[57,93]

Behavioral Supports for OUD

Behavioral interventions such as contingency management, cognitive behavioral therapy, and family therapy are helpful for OUD treatment,[133] but absence of, or nonadherence, with behavioral interventions should not be used as justification to withhold MOUD.[10] MOUD discontinuation postpartum is common and is associated with increased rates of return to use, overdose, and death.[134] Clinicians should be aware of community resources, including peer recovery support services and "12-step programs" because use of peer services is associated with increased engagment in care.[135] Recent qualitative studies suggest that peer services are valued among pregnant and postpartum individuals with OUD and are increasingly accessible online.[136]

Kratom

"Kratom" refers to both *Mitragyna speciosa,* a tree native to Southeast Asia, and to products derived from its leaves that are marketed as herbal supplements.[137] There is minimal rigorous research on kratom use during pregnancy, including its impact on fetal, maternal, and neonatal outcomes, and on the development and subsequent treatment of kratom use disorder in the peripartum period. In the US, kratom is neither a controlled substance nor is it regulated by the Drug Enforcement Administration (DEA), though some states have placed regulations or controls on its distribution or sale.[138]

Kratom is known to have a dose-dependent effect. At lower doses, it has stimulant-like properties, including increased alertness and tachycardia. At higher doses, it has opioid-like properties, including pain relief and sedation. The active compounds found in kratom, particularly mitragynine and 7-hydroxymitragynine, act as partial agonists on the mu- and delta-opioid receptors.[139] Pregnant individuals have reported the use of kratom to treat pain and opioid withdrawal symptoms.[60]

Physical dependence to kratom can occur with potential for the development of OUD. Kratom withdrawal symptoms are similar to opioid withdrawal symptoms.[59] Given the similarity to opioid withdrawal, OUD related to kratom use can be treated with MOUD, particularly buprenorphine/buprenorphine-naloxone products.[59] There are no reports of fetal anomalies in humans related to kratom use during pregnancy.[139] However, there are case reports of neonates with in utero kratom exposure developing symptoms consistent with NOWS and responding to NOWS treatment.[60] More research is needed to guide treatment recommendations for prenatal kratom use. Hospital-based clinicians should ask about kratom use in the peripartum period and ask patients about kratom use if symptoms consistent with opioid withdrawal are noted in the peripartum person or neonate and the patient denies other regular opioid use.

Sedative-Hypnotics

Data on the prevalence of sedative-hypnotic (benzodiazepines, barbiturates, gabapentin, and z-drugs such as zolpidem, zaleplon, and zopiclone, etc) use disorders in pregnancy are lacking, but in the general population, prescribed sedative-hypnotic use is more common among women than men.[140] Data suggest that the use of sedative-hypnotics (prescribed and nonprescribed) affects 1.9% of pregnancies globally,[141] and rates of nonprescribed use and use disorders affect about 2% of US women.[142,143] A Swedish study conducted between 1996 and 2011 found that sedative-hypnotics were the third most commonly used central nervous system–active drugs during pregnancy, following antidepressants and opioids, with 4.6% of infants exposed to these medications.[63] Reviews and limited meta-analyses[61] demonstrate that benzodiazepines and z-drugs are not teratogenic, and the risk for significant adverse child neurodevelopment is low.[144] However, adverse perinatal outcomes are associated with antenatal benzodiazepine exposure, including increased risk for spontaneous abortion,[62] preterm birth,[4] low birth weight,[63] small for gestational age (SGA),[63] low Apgar scores at 5 minutes,[61] and increased risk of NOWS.[64]

Benzodiazepine Withdrawal Management

Addressing and treating sedative-hypnotic use during pregnancy is critical as abrupt discontinuation or dose reduction can result in severe, life threatening, withdrawals, such as seizures.[145] Benzodiazepines are the most commonly prescribed and nonprescribed sedative-hypnotic used among women, and much of the literature in pregnancy focuses on benzodiazepines. Therefore, this section highlights benzodiazepine withdrawal and use disorder. Differences in benzodiazepine half-lives result in significant differences in the duration of withdrawal symptoms, often necessitating frequent dose adjustments for effective withdrawal management in the acute period. In the hospital setting, benzodiazepine withdrawal during pregnancy should be managed similarly to that in nonpregnant individuals, using moderate-to-long–acting benzodiazepines. Depending on the clinical context, treatment approaches include symptom-triggered benzodiazepine dosing using evidence-based withdrawal assessment tools, scheduled tapering using benzodiazepines or phenobarbital, front-loading using benzodiazepines or phenobarbital, or continuous infusion protocols using benzodiazepines.[146] While symptom-triggered protocols may minimize overall fetal benzodiazepine exposure, tapering with a moderate-to-long–acting benzodiazepine different than the one the patient is regularly using may facilitate a smoother benzodiazepine withdrawal experience for the pregnant person, which may help with relapse prevention.[146] In the context of large quantities of reported benzodiazepine use, it may be beneficial to use a scheduled benzodiazepine taper concurrently with a symptom-triggered protocol with use of benzodiazepine breakthrough withdrawal symptoms.[146] The use of these protocols is discussed in detail in Chapter 10.

Treatment of Sedative Hypnotic or Benzodiazepine Use Disorder

There is little guidance on how to treat sedative-hypnotic or benzodiazepine use disorders for people with SUDs in general, and even less among pregnant individuals. Expert opinion guidelines, which were developed to address prescribed benzodiazepine misuse, recommend dose reductions of 10% to 25% every 1 to 2 weeks, resulting in extended tapers.[147] For patients with other SUDs using nonprescribed benzodiazepines, rapid hospital-based tapers are most often utilized.[148] However, rapid tapers do not treat protracted benzodiazepine withdrawal symptoms that can last weeks to months and have lower rates of long-term benzodiazepine cessation compared to longer tapers.[148] If safe and possible,[149] extended benzodiazepine tapers should be offered to pregnant individuals through shared decision making where the risks of benzodiazepine exposures are reviewed. Chapter 10 describes best practices in benzodiazepine taper management with detailed taper protocols.

Stimulants

Stimulants, including cocaine, ecstasy, methamphetamines, and prescription stimulants, are the second most widely used and misused illicit substances in North American.[150] Stimulant-related diagnoses (excluding cocaine) at the time of delivery have substantially increased since 2010.[65] Stimulant use during pregnancy is associated with maternal morbidity, gestational hypertension, and increased need for neonatal intensive care unit admission, preterm birth, SGA, and fetal death.[65,68] Patients with chronic cocaine and methamphetamine use are at increased risk for various cardiovascular, cardiopulmonary, and cerebrovascular complications, including diastolic and systolic heart failure, arrhythmias, pulmonary hypertension, cardiomyopathy, atherosclerosis, and stroke.[66,151] Chapter 10 describes complications related to stimulant use. Pregnant patients with stimulant use are at increased risk for severe and often unrecognized cardiovascular disease thought to be due to pregnancy-related hemodynamic changes (eg, increased plasma volume, high cardiac output).[67] Despite the known increased risk for cardiac disease in pregnant patients with stimulant use, there are no clinical guidelines directing when or how to screen pregnant patients for cardiac disease with regular stimulant use. The index of suspicion for underlying cardiac disease in the hospitalized pregnant or postpartum patient with stimulant use should be high, and there should be a low threshold for cardiac evaluation (eg, transthoracic echocardiography) and cardiology consultation. Patients do benefit and see improvement in cardiac function with abstaining from stimulant use.[152]

Stimulant Intoxication

Acute intoxication due to stimulants frequently presents with varied symptomatology, particularly in hospitalized pregnant patients with co-occurring SUDs and medical and/or psychiatric comorbidities.[153,154] Stimulant intoxication can be life-threatening and is managed with benzodiazepines and/or antipsychotics in nonpregnant patients, and though there is limited data, a similar approach should be used for pregnant patients. Stimulant withdrawal is not life threatening, but untreated increases the risk of relapse.[153]

Stimulant Withdrawal

Treatment for stimulant withdrawal includes allowing the patient to sleep and ensuring adequate food and water intake. Chapter 10 describes management of stimulant withdrawal.

Treatment of Stimulant Use Disorder

There are no FDA-approved medications available to treat stimulant use disorder. Non-FDA pharmacotherapy approaches for stimulant use disorder treatment may also help address withdrawal symptoms,[155] including bupropion, naltrexone, topiramate, and mirtazapine.[156] However, there are limited data on pharmacotherapy for stimulant use disorder treatment in pregnancy. Topiramate, a mood stabilizer and antiepileptic, readily crosses the placenta and is associated with preterm delivery, SGA, and neonatal seizures.[157] Though less teratogenic than other anticonvulsants, topiramate is not recommended for stimulant use disorder treatment in pregnancy. Mirtazapine, a tetracyclic antidepressant commonly used for methamphetamine use disorder treatment, has not been associated with adverse maternal or fetal outcomes, but results on congenital malformations and spontaneous abortion are conflicting, and data quality is poor.[101] Mirtazapine may be an appropriate tool to support methamphetamine use disorder treatment in pregnancy through a shared decision-making process.

The mainstay of treatment for stimulant use disorders is behavioral interventions, particularly contingency management.[158] The effectiveness of behavioral interventions for SUD, including for stimulant use disorders, has not been extensively studied in pregnant patients, with the best-published evidence to support contingency management being for smoking cessation during pregnancy and postpartum.[159] Contingency management has not been extensively studied in the hospital setting, though there are a few programs that have adapted it for use in the hospital.[160,161] Chapter 10 describes the evidence for various stimulant use disorder treatment options.

Cannabis

Cannabis is the most frequently used nonlegal (at the US federal level) substance by pregnant people in the US.[18] As more states in the US legalize cannabis, an increasing number of patients report cannabis use during pregnancy, corresponding to a rise in cannabis-related hospitalizations.[162] Pregnant and postpartum individuals may use cannabis to self-medicate because of barriers to SUD treatment or to manage pregnancy-related symptoms such as nausea, insomnia, and mood changes[163,164] and due to perceptions that it is a natural, safer alternative to pharmaceuticals.[164]

Increasing prevalence of cannabis use perinatally is particularly concerning, as there is a growing body of research demonstrating associated risks for maternal complications, including preeclampsia and gestational hypertension, neonatal/fetal complications, including preterm birth and SGA, and childhood cognitive and sociobehavioral developmental concerns.[69,70] National organizations universally recommend against cannabis use prior to conception, during pregnancy, or while breastfeeding, given these and potential unknown/undescribed risks.[165] However, patients report an overall lack of counseling about cannabis cessation/abstinence recommendations by clinicians, which may give the perception that cannabis is less risky.[163]

There are no approved medication treatments for cannabis withdrawal or cannabis use disorder.[166] There is some evidence to support behavioral interventions for cannabis use disorder in pregnant patients, including cognitive behavioral therapy and motivational enhancement therapy.[167]

Nicotine and Tobacco

Nicotine and tobacco product use, including cigarettes and vaping products, remains the most commonly used substance during pregnancy, affecting roughly 10% of pregnant individuals.[18] Though the prevalence of use has decreased in high-income countries, it is increasing in low- and middle-income countries.[168] In addition, US data suggest that nicotine vaping product use may be on the rise.[169] There are well-documented adverse maternal and neonatal outcomes associated with tobacco use. For pregnant individuals, these include an increased risk of obstetric complications (eg, placental abruption, premature labor) and nutritional deficiencies compared to those who do not use nicotine or tobacco.[71] Neonatal risks include an increased risk of stillbirth, low birth weight, SGA, congenital malformations, and sudden unexpected infant death (SUID) in infancy.[71,72] Smoking cessation reduces these risks, especially if achieved within the first 20 weeks of pregnancy.[170] Challenges like stress, violence, and limited health care access that affect SUD treatment generally also hinder tobacco use disorder treatment.[170] In addition, many women are unaware of nicotine and tobacco use risks or treatment options due to a lack of attention in health care settings.[171] Thus, the hospital setting is an opportunity for the hospital-based clinician to address tobacco use disorder and initiate treatment.

Pharmacotherapy Used to Support Smoking Cessation

Nicotine replacement therapy (NRT), bupropion, and varenicline are the three evidence-based pharmacotherapies used for tobacco use disorder treatment. Among nonpregnant individuals, the most effective tobacco use disorder treatment is a combination of

NRT (nicotine patches, gum, etc) and medication (varenicline or bupropion) treatments.[172,173] In pregnancy, there is less data on combination pharmacologic approaches. A fixed-effect meta-analysis of seven studies (six on NRT, one on bupropion) with 1,386 participants found that pharmacotherapy nearly doubled tobacco use disorder treatment success in pregnant women compared to usual care (relative risk [RR] 1.80; 95% confidence interval [CI] 1.32–2.44).[174]

Nicotine Replacement Therapy

NRT is the best-studied tobacco use disorder treatment approach in pregnancy, and while the risks of nicotine exposure remain (similar to nicotine-containing products),[94] there is consensus that the benefits outweigh the risks compared to ongoing tobacco product use.[71] A 2020 Cochrane meta-analysis showed NRT increased smoking cessation rates by 40% (RR 1.41, 95% CI 1.03–1.93) without increased harms.[175] NRT is available in short- and long-acting formulations, including gum, lozenges, nasal spray, oral inhalers, and transdermal patches, and the type of NRT used should be determined by the clinical needs.

Varenicline

Varenicline, a partial nicotine agonist, is the most effective treatment for tobacco use disorder, but there are limited safety data available for its use during pregnancy. Cohort studies found that varenicline was not associated with an increased risk of adverse birth outcomes such as preterm birth and SGA.[97,98] Data on other adverse birth outcomes, such as stillbirth and congenital anomalies, are lacking. There are no randomized controlled trials (RCT) assessing varenicline effectiveness in pregnancy, but observational studies show that it is associated with smoking cessation.[176] The decision to use varenicline should be pursued through shared decision making based on the severity of tobacco use disorder and the clinical context.

Bupropion

Bupropion, an aminoketone antidepressant, has some nicotine receptor-blocking activity, and the sustained-release formulation is an effective tobacco use disorder treatment.[177] There is limited evidence describing the effectiveness of bupropion to treat tobacco use disorder in pregnancy. A single RCT showed it to be more effective (RR 3.33, 95% CI 1.06–10.49) compared to no treatment.[174] It may be associated with a higher risk of congenital heart defects in case-control studies, but bupropion has not been associated with other fetal or maternal complications.[99,100] After shared decision making, bupropion can be used for tobacco use disorder treatment.

Harm-Reduction Approaches

Vaping or electronic nicotine delivery systems are used as a harm-reduction smoking cessation approach in nonpregnant individuals in contexts where first-line treatments have not helped or in settings where patients remain precontemplative.[178] A 2022 RCT with more than 1,000 women who smoked cigarettes compared NRT to e-cigarette use showed similar quit rates and safety profiles for both study products.[95] In light of these findings, it may be reasonable to use e-cigarettes as a harm-reduction approach to reduce cigarette product use during pregnancy for patients who remain ambivalent about tobacco use disorder treatment.

Behavioral Interventions

There is also evidence for behavioral interventions alone, and in combination with, pharmacotherapy to support smoking cessation. Contingency management, social supports, counseling, such as health education, and motivational interviewing improve cessation, though their evidence for relapse prevention is less robust.[71] All patients should receive nonjudgmental information education about smoking and, if available, offered behavioral interventions to support smoking cessation.

Harm Reduction in Peripartum Individuals

Peripartum individuals, like other individuals with SUD, may not be able to achieve abstinence from substance use, or may not wish to. For these individuals, harm-reduction strategies can help minimize the risks of substance use while fostering health, self-worth, and dignity. The public health approach of harm reduction aims to reduce the adverse effects of substance use with an emphasis on health and well-being.[179] Chapter 19 provides an in-depth overview of harm reduction.

Limited research exists on the utilization of harm reduction during the peripartum period.[52,180] Studies from specialized OB-GYN and SUD clinics that employed harm-reduction techniques demonstrate reductions in adverse SUD-related outcomes in pregnancy, improved engagement with prenatal care, and reductions in low birth weight for infants.[181,182] A qualitative study of pregnant or recently pregnant women who used substances found that many women independently adopted harm-reduction methods.[183] Such techniques include reducing substance use, substituting substances that were perceived as less harmful (eg, cannabis), prioritizing eating and sleeping, and changing their social circle to distance themselves from family, friends, or neighbors who used substances.[183]

Global harm-reduction strategies, such as counseling on reducing substance use, should be discussed with peripartum patients, including:

- Switching to a safer method of substance use (eg, smoking instead of injecting)
- Identifying ways to stay safe when using substances (eg, never using alone, substance checking, use of fentanyl/xylazine test strips)
- Use of skin cleaning techniques and clean syringes to reduce the risk of skin bacterial and blood-borne infections
- Importance of carrying naloxone at all times for overdose reversal

Given the increase in intentional and unintentional illicit fentanyl use, pregnant and postpartum individuals and their supports should be counseled on the increased risk of overdose, the need for immediate naloxone (short-acting opioid antagonist that rapidly reverses opioid overdose) administration in case of overdose, and to call emergency medical services because multiple doses of naloxone and/or oxygen support may be needed.[184]

There are increasing reports of xylazine (alpha-2 adrenergic agonist) in the illicit substance supply. Xylazine, a sympatholytic, causes severe sedation, respiratory depression, and bradycardia, complicating overdose prevention and management. Patient education about the toxic supply and xylazine-complicated overdoses (naloxone resistance or prolonged respiratory depression) is important.[185]

However, peripartum individuals with SUD require specific considerations, including a greater focus on food, nutrition, safety, sleep during pregnancy, as well as planning for childcare while parenting if using substances. The Academy of Perinatal Harm Reduction has a comprehensive patient-facing pregnancy harm-reduction toolkit that is an excellent resource to provide patients.[186] Shifting the focus away from substance use and toward care that supports health and well-being during the prenatal period may help reduce adverse pregnancy outcomes.[187] Table 12.6 summarizes harm-reduction practices for use during the peripartum period.

Birthing Hospitalization

Prior experiences of discrimination in health care settings, concern about pain management, and fear regarding child welfare intervention make the birthing hospitalization a stressful time for pregnant individuals with SUD.[188] Ideally, clinicians should discuss options for pain control during delivery throughout prenatal care and upon admission to the birthing hospitalization using a trauma-informed approach founded upon shared decision making.

Management of MOUD

MOUD should be continued throughout the birthing hospitalization.[38,189] The hospital-based clinician or pharmacist should verify the patient's buprenorphine dose through medical record review and prescription drug monitoring program; the methadone dose must be verified directly with the patient's opioid treatment program. When taken routinely, the patient's maintenance MOUD dose is their "baseline dose" and does not provide sufficient analgesia for child delivery. Pregnant individuals with OUD will likely require higher doses of opioid pain medications compared to pregnant individuals without OUD due to increased tolerance and opioid-induced hyperalgesia.[190] This is not the case for nonopioid analgesia. Some pregnant patients may have concerns or fear about how opioid analgesia will impact their recovery and may prefer to avoid opioids altogether, so early ascertainment of patient preference for pain management is paramount.

Methadone and buprenorphine should be continued perioperatively for scheduled cesarean delivery to decrease the risk for return to use and for a difficult transition back to MOUD after acute pain has resolved.[191] Research shows reduced postoperative pain scores, morphine equivalents (MEQs) consumed, and use of adjunct analgesics for patients continued on buprenorphine or methadone, and therefore highlights the importance of continuing therapeutic doses of both medications for OUD during the perioperative period.[192,193] Patients on buprenorphine and methadone have better reported pain control with protocols that account for increased pain sensitivity and higher opioid tolerance in patients with OUD.[194]

If a pregnant patient is maintained on extended-release naltrexone during their pregnancy with success in recovery, then it should be continued during the delivery. Case studies of naltrexone use at the time of nonobstetric operative procedures show significant challenges with postoperative pain control, with poor pain capture even with high-dose opioids, but success after adding medications such as ketamine. In nonobstetric planned procedures, it is recommended to transition to oral naltrexone and allow for at least 72-hour washout period perioperatively. However, such an approach is not recommended in pregnancy because delivery is often unpredictable, even in the case of scheduled C-sections, and changes to naltrexone that are supporting a patient's recovery risk

TABLE 12.6

Harm-Reduction Recommendations for Peripartum Individuals

Harms associated with substance use in pregnancy	Application of harm-reduction practices	Screening tools and guides
General substance use	Discuss reduction in substance use frequency, dosing, or binging[195] Discuss switching to a safer method of use (eg, oral/smoking vs injection)[195] Avoid polysubstance use[52,195]	See table 12.1
Overdose	Counsel against using substances alone[196] Offer naloxone[184] Utilization of substance checking services[197] Counsel/offer fentanyl and xylazine test strips[196]	
Mandate reporting	Be transparent about mandated reporting practices[41] Obtain consent for urine toxicology testing[51]	
Adverse childhood experiences	Screening[198]	ACOG Committee Opinion No. 498: screening for sexual violence
Intimate partner violence	Screening: once per trimester of pregnancy and once after delivery[36]	ACOG Committee Opinion No. 518: sample intimate partner violence screening questions
Mental health needs	Screening for psychiatric comorbidities[35] and support access or referral to mental health care providers[35]	Edinburgh Postnatal Depression Scale
Social supports	Inquire about social and structural determinants of health: employment, immigration status, and access to safe and secure housing[199] Screen for food insecurities[199] Refer to relevant social support services[199,200] Partner with social workers, local community advocates, medical–legal teams[199]	ACOG Committee no. 729: sample screening tool; Health Leads Screening Toolkit
Infectious risk from injection substance use	Education on safe injection practices[195,201] Utilization of needle and syringe programs[195,201]	National Harm Reduction Coalition training guide: Getting off right: a safety manual for injection drug users
Unsafe sexual practices	Safe sex education[195,201] Distribution of condoms[195,201]	
Sexually transmitted blood-borne infections	Infectious disease testing—HIV, syphilis, HCV, HBV, HAV[202,203] HBV and HAV vaccinations among those nonimmune Offer PrEP for HIV prevention[204,205]	Centers for Disease Control (CDC) Clinical Guidance for PrEP
Lack of sleep	Education on the importance of sleep during pregnancy[201]	
Nutrition	Education on the importance of nutrition and hydration during pregnancy[201]	
Oral health	Education on the importance of basic dental health[201]	

ACOG, American College of Obstetricians and Gynecologists; HCV, hepatitis C virus; HBV, hepatitis B virus; HAV, hepatitis A virus; SURP-P, Substance Use Risk Profile—Pregnancy.

Adapted from Wakeman B, Kremer M, Schulkin J. The application of harm reduction to methamphetamine use during pregnancy: a call to arms. *Am J Obstet Gynecol MFM*. 2021;3(5):100418, with permission from Elsevier.

destabilization. Early involvement with anesthesiology to facilitate multimodal pain control, including topical, regional, and systemic approaches, is recommended for patients on naltrexone for OUD (pain management strategies described below).

Pain Management

Suboptimal predelivery pain management can have long-term psychological and physical sequelae. This is further amplified in patients with SUD due to the risk of return to use triggered by untreated pain or possibly by inadequate preparation and discussion around use of opioids for pain control.[206,207] Short-acting opioids can be safely prescribed for all patients on MOUD, including those on injectable naltrexone, for both vaginal and cesarean deliveries.[208] For all patients, post-partum approaches should typically include a fixed regimen of acetaminophen and nonsteroidal anti-inflammatory agents.[208] For cesarean deliveries, there is limited research addressing the potential role of supplemental abdominal wall blocks for optimizing pain management in patients with OUD, however, labor analgesia should be multimodal and should consider topical, regional, and systemic approaches. Pharmacologic adjunct analgesics such as short courses of gabapentin and ketamine can also be considered and discussed with anesthesia colleagues prior to delivery admission.[192]

Pain Control After Hospital Discharge

The hospital-based clinician should discuss postoperative pain management with the patient and inquire about the patient's preference for pain control. Some patients may prefer opioids for pain management during hospitalization, but may not feel it is necessary upon hospital discharge. Other patients may prefer an opioid prescription at hospital discharge. In this scenario, the clinician and patient should identify a safety plan for having opioids in their home if needed. This may include using a lock box, having additional support from the clinical team (calls/check-ins about short-acting opioid management), or family involvement in medication dispensing. Short-acting opioids can be safely prescribed and coused with MOUD. All people who may witness or are at high risk of an overdose, including people with OUD and those receiving MOUD, should be coprescribed naloxone upon hospital discharge.[31,208]

Team-Based Care and Care Coordination

Given the significant prevalence of co-occurring mental health issues, trauma, and social and structural inequities among pregnant individuals with SUD, comprehensive prenatal and SUD care can aid in stabilizing substance use prior to delivery and support recovery postpartum.[20,209] Hospital settings offer an opportunity to initiate treatment and connect women with SUD services. Examples of tailored SUD programming in the hospital include addiction consultation services supporting hospitalized perinatal patients, maternal–fetal medicine programs with SUD expertise, and social work and peer staff integrated within OB or SUD treatment teams to support patients during hospitalizations and with care transitions to community settings.

In the outpatient setting, interdisciplinary care models that incorporate mental health services, SUD treatment, case management, and social support alongside prenatal care have demonstrated improved obstetric and neonatal outcomes.[210,211] While various models exist, dyadic approaches—programs that cater to both parents and children—offer particular advantages.[24] These programs emphasize interdisciplinary service delivery, case management, community outreach, housing assistance, and legal support. Integrated programs enhance SUD treatment retention, reduce parenting stress, lower levels of substance use and relapse, boost self-esteem, and improve parenting knowledge.[212]

Involvement of doulas and peer-recovery specialists in the care team in the hospital and outpatient setting may improve patient outcomes. A doula is a trained professional who provides physical, emotional, and informational support before, during, and after birth.[213] Among the general population, doula support is associated with improved birth outcomes such as increased self-efficacy and decreased preterm delivery.[213,214] Among women with SUD, doula engagement is linked with increased health literacy, reduced stigma, and enhanced self-advocacy.[215] Peer support specialists are similarly associated with improved outcomes among peripartum women with SUD, including reductions in nonprescribed substance use and enhanced trust with health care clinicians.[216]

Breastfeeding

Breastfeeding guidance and support a critical aspects of the postpartum period for all patients, but there are specific considerations for substance-exposed parental–infant dyads. In addition to the general well-documented benefits,[217] breastfeeding reduces the severity of NOWS by decreasing the need for pharmacologic treatment and shortening infant hospitalization.[218] Breastfeeding may also help parents bond with their infants, aiding recovery.[219] However, breastfeeding can also pose risks for infants in the presence of parental nonprescribed substance use, such as diminished responsiveness to infant feeding cues and potential for infant substance exposure through breastmilk. Infant exposure to nonprescribed substances through breastmilk may lead to acute toxicity, may hinder breastfeeding effectiveness, and could disrupt neonatal brain development.[220,221] Thus, breastfeeding recommendations must be highly individualized according to the clinical context (reviewed in detail below and Table 12.7).

Discussing breastfeeding throughout the peripartum period is important to support shared decision making around when breastfeeding is safe and beneficial for the parent and infant or when it should be avoided. Such discussions should occur within the context of active, nonprescribed substance use, as well as treatment and recovery. They should address the benefits, risks, and challenges of breastfeeding in the setting of substance use and SUD treatment (summarized in Table 12.7) to adequately prepare patients and reduce feelings of guilt or shame that can arise. The relative infant dose (RID) estimates infant drug exposure and is dependent on drug pharmacology, maternal exposure, metabolism into breastmilk, and infant gastric absorption and metabolism. The RID is helpful to inform some SUD treatment discussions. Medications with RID values less than 10% are generally considered safe for breastfeeding while those with RID values of greater than 25% should be avoided. Such communication is critical because studies indicate that one of the most common reasons for not initiating breastfeeding or for early discontinuation of breastfeeding is concern about neonatal exposure to medications or substances, even in cases where evidence supports the safety of breastfeeding.[222,223] Individuals with SUD remain less likely to initiate and maintain breastfeeding than those without SUD[224,225] related to misinformation, pharmacotherapy that interferes with milk production, active nonprescribed substance use, pain during breastfeeding, and histories of physical or sexual trauma that complicate the breastfeeding experience.[226,227] In addition, infant factors, such as NOWS, may create difficulty with latching, necessitate the use of formula supplementation due to weight loss, and result in greater parent–infant separation, further challenging breastfeeding.[223,228,229] Rooming-in models of care and skin-to-skin positioning throughout the perinatal hospital stay can promote improved parent–infant bonding and lead to higher breastfeeding rates.[230] Other in-hospital breastfeeding supports include providing person-centered, customized lactation support to help build practical breastfeeding skills.

Breastfeeding recommendations should use a shared decision-making approach that provides individualized recommendations regarding the specific

TABLE 12.7

Breastfeeding Recommendations in Substance-Exposed Parent–Infant Dyads

Condition	Breastfeeding recommendation	Monitoring	Additional information
Nonprescribed substance use	Individuals who discontinue nonprescribed substance use by delivery should be supported in breastfeeding[231]	Ongoing postpartum multidisciplinary lactation support and SUD treatment needed to facilitate breastfeeding safety[231]	If evidence of recent nonprescribed substance use, individuals can express milk to establish supply and discard until sufficient time has passed to allow for substance clearance
HIV	Use shared decision making achieving and maintaining viral suppression through ART during pregnancy, delivery, and after birth decreases risk of transmission through breastfeeding to <1%, but not 0%[232]	If mothers choose to breastfeed, clinicians should emphasize the importance of taking ART postpartum as directed and sustaining an undetectable HIV viral load[232]	Clinicians can consult the National Perinatal HIV/AIDS Hotline (1-888-448-8765) with questions about infant feeding by individuals with HIV
HCV	Compatible, except when the mother has cracked, damaged, or bleeding nipples, or in the context of HIV coinfection[233]	Recheck HCV RNA after delivery to assess for spontaneous clearance[233]	
HBV	Compatible, if infants born to HBV-positive mothers are vaccinated, but there is no need to delay breastfeeding until the infant is fully immunized	Infants should receive HBIG and the first dose of the HBV vaccine within 12 h of birth, test for HBV after completion of the vaccine series	

TABLE 12.7

Breastfeeding Recommendations in Substance-Exposed Parent–Infant Dyads (*Continued*)

Condition	Breastfeeding recommendation	Monitoring	Additional information
SUD treatment	**Breastfeeding recommendation**	**Monitoring**	**Additional information**
Methadone	Compatible with breastfeeding, regardless of dose	During uptitration, infants should be monitored for sedation[231]	RID: 1.9–6.5%[113]
Buprenorphine	Compatible with breastfeeding, regardless of dose[231]; however, safety data for injectable ER buprenorphine formulations are lacking[231]		SL Bup RID: 0.1–2.5%[113]
Naltrexone	Injectable and oral formulations are compatible and recommended[231]		RID: 1%[113]
Acamprosate	Breastfeeding appears compatible, but there is little evidence, pursue a risk–benefit discussion[231]		No data on the transfer of acamprosate into breastmilk Due to its low molecular weight and lack of protein binding, it is possible that it could readily enter breastmilk; however, it has low oral absorption[113]
Disulfiram	Not compatible, not recommended, consider other AUD treatments[231]	Ingestion of alcohol while taking disulfiram causes alcohol toxicity, thus, in breastfeeding, it could potentially cause toxicity in the infant	RID: unknown
Nicotine replacement therapy	Compatible and is recommended[231] The type of NRT should be determined by the clinical needs of the breastfeeding mother[231]		RID: unknown
Varenicline	Clinicians should pursue a risk–benefit discussion based on the severity of tobacco use[231]	Animal data suggests there may be some harms associated with varenicline exposure through breastmilk and to monitor for seizures in exposed infants, through clinical data is lacking[231]	RID: unknown
Bupropion	Compatible and is recommended[231]	Data on infant harms is mixed, with some studies finding no adverse effects, while others found seizure-like events[234]	RID: 2.0–11%[113,234] A randomized controlled trial assessing bupropion for smoking cessation among postpartum women is underway which will provide more specific insights into its harms and benefits[235]

SUD, substance use disorder; HIV, human immunodeficiency virus; ART, antiretroviral therapy; HCV, hepatitis C virus; HBV, hepatitis B virus; SUD, substance use disorder; RID, relative infant dose (substances with RID <10% are safe for breastfeeding, RID 11-25% pursue risk benefit discussion, RID >25% should be avoided while breastfeeding); ER, extended release; SL, sublingual; AUD, alcohol use disorder; NRT, nicotine replacement therapy.

benefits and potential risks of breastfeeding based on the presence of nonprescribed substance use, SUD treatments, and other factors such as HIV (see Table 12.7 for detailed recommendations). In general, individuals who stop nonprescribed substance use by the delivery hospitalization can be supported in breastfeeding initiation with appropriate follow-ups such as lactation support and postpartum SUD care.[236,237] Patients motivated to breastfeed who report recent nonprescribed substance use and/or have positive toxicology testing postpartum should be supported in expressing milk to establish milk production. The decision of whether to give expressed milk to the infant and when to start breastfeeding should be made using a multidisciplinary shared decision-making approach. Ideally, before breastfeeding, sufficient time should pass to allow for substance clearance from breastmilk.[113]

Neonatal Abstinence Syndrome/Neonatal Opioid Withdrawal Syndrome

Clinicians caring for birthing dyads affected by SUD or substance use should be prepared to address NAS, the umbrella diagnosis that also includes NOWS. NAS is defined by signs and symptoms of withdrawal that infants develop after in utero exposure to substances.[238,239] In the US, the estimated NAS rate increased significantly from 4.0 per 1,000 birth hospitalizations (95% CI 3.3–4.7) in 2007 to 7.3 per 1,000 birth hospitalizations (95% CI 6.8–7.7) in 2017.[240] Rural and tribal areas have experienced steeper increases in the rate of NAS, as have infants enrolled in Medicaid.[241] Evidence suggests that the recent increases in NAS have been primarily driven by in utero exposure to opioids.[242] Infants exposed to nonopioid substances alone, such as cocaine, amphetamines, benzodiazepines, psychiatric medications (eg, selective serotonin reuptake inhibitors [SSRIs]), alcohol, and cannabis, do not require any specific monitoring, scoring, or neonatal treatment protocol. This section will focus on NOWS diagnosis and treatment.

NOWS Diagnosis

Based on expert consensus, the following two criteria are required for the diagnosis of NOWS[239,243]: (1) evidence of in utero chronic opioid exposure (by maternal history, plus or minus toxicology testing) with or without the presence of other psychotropic substances; and (2) presence of at least two of the most common clinical signs characteristic of withdrawal (excessive crying, fragmented sleep, tremors, increased muscle tone, gastrointestinal dysfunction). Importantly, the diagnosis is not dependent on the infant receiving pharmacologic treatment for NOWS. The American Academy of Pediatrics (AAP) recommends hospital monitoring for 4 to 7 days for opioid-exposed infants for signs of NOWS.[239] Infants exposed to short-acting opioids can be monitored for a minimum of 3 to 5 days.

The primary signs and symptoms of NOWS reflect central nervous system irritability, autonomic overstimulation, and gastrointestinal tract dysregulation.[244] Infants often have problems interacting with their environment, with dysregulation in motor control, state control, or sensory processing.[244] The primary clinical manifestations of NOWS are shown in Table 12.8.

NOWS Assessment Methods

All infants with known prenatal opioid exposure should be assessed every 3 to 4 hours, in coordination with infant care and feeding times, for signs and symptoms of NOWS. The infant should remain in the room with the parent during assessments and should be conducted after feeds to ensure hunger is not a contributing factor. These assessments should begin at birth and continue until the monitoring

TABLE 12.8

Clinical Manifestations of Neonatal Opioid Withdrawal Syndrome

Neurologic	Autonomic	Gastrointestinal and respiratory
Altered sleep	Sweating	Difficulty feeding
Irritability	Sneezing	Excessive weight loss
Excessive crying	Mottled skin	Vomiting
Sensitivity to stimuli	Fever	Gassiness
High muscle tone	Nasal stuffiness	Loose stools
Tremors	Frequent yawning	
Increased startle response	Tachypnea	

period is complete. It is recommended that hospitals utilize a standardized training program to ensure interrater reliability between clinicians.[239,245]

There are two commonly utilized NOWS assessment tools, the Finnegan Neonatal Abstinence Scoring Tool (FNAST), and the Eat, Sleep, Console (ESC) Care Approach. Over the past decade, the FNAST has become less utilized in favor of the ESC Care approach.[246,247] The ESC Care approach is a function-based assessment that relies on the infant's ability to eat expected amounts for gestational and postnatal age, sleep expected amounts for age, and the level of support required to console the infant to guide management is expected for gestational and postnatal age. In a 26-centered cluster-randomized clinical trial, the ESC Care approach was associated with shorter length of hospital stay by 6.7 days and a 30% decrease in pharmacologic treatment in comparison to infants cared for with the FNAST approach.[246]

Contributors of NOWS Severity

The timing of presentation of NOWS depends on infant and maternal factors. For the infant, the type of opioid exposure, as well as the duration and proximity to delivery, are important. Infants exposed to short-acting opioids demonstrate opioid withdrawal within 24 hours after delivery, while withdrawal from longer-acting opioids typically begins 48 to 72 hours after delivery.[239,245] In most infants, NOWS symptoms peak 2 to 4 days after delivery, with the acute signs and symptoms of withdrawal subsiding within 1 to 2 weeks. Other factors that influence the severity of NOWS include infant sex,[248] gestational age,[249] genetic factors, and epigenetic factors.[250] Maternal factors that are associated with more severe NOWS include untreated SUD, polysubstance use, nicotine use, use of sedative-hypnotics (eg, benzodiazepines, gabapentin), and use of other psychotropic treatments (eg, SSRIs).[64,251] Thus, in addition to anticipatory guidance about NOWS and treatment of SUDs, where clinically appropriate, reducing polypharmacy and/or titrating to the lowest effective dose of sedative-hypnotics and psychotropic medications may reduce NOWS incidence and severity.

NOWS Hospital Policies and Guidelines

Hospitals are encouraged to have consistent policies regarding the care of opioid-exposed newborns. These policies should be consistent with the care of all pregnant individuals at the institution to decrease clinician bias and variability in care practices.[252] Recommended policies surrounding infants with NOWS should include the following topics: criteria for toxicology testing for birthing individuals and infants, breastfeeding in the setting of birthing person SUD, social work consultation and involvement, child protective services policies that are consistent and transparent, and NOWS assessment and management guidelines. In addition to the primary pediatric care team, the following consultants and ancillary team members should be involved in the care of an opioid-exposed newborn for optimal care: social work, lactation, nutrition, occupational and/or physical therapy, and ancillary nonpharmacologic clinicians as available.[253–256]

Nonpharmacologic NOWS Care

Nonpharmacologic care is considered the first line of therapy for infants with NOWS. In recent years, due to the implementation of quality improvement measures aimed at improving nonpharmacologic care, the average length of hospitalization for infants with NOWS is between 10 to 14 days. Essential components to all nonpharmacologic care bundles include promotion of rooming-in, caregiver presence, breastmilk, and breastfeeding.[238,239,257]

The current standard of care for infants being monitored for NOWS is a rooming-in model with the parent, with zero separation being the ultimate goal.[230] Numerous studies have examined the role of rooming-in on NOWS outcomes and have consistently demonstrated a reduction in the receipt of pharmacologic treatment (20% to 60%), a decrease in the total opioid treatment days, and a shortened length of hospitalization (1 to 2 weeks).[230,238] Additional components of a nonpharmacologic care bundle include environmental modifications such as ensuring a quiet environment with limited excessive stimulation, and clustering of care to avoid overstimulation and disruptions in sleep. Caring for infants outside of an intensive care setting has been well demonstrated to improve NOWS outcomes.[230,258]

Opioid-exposed infants who receive breastmilk have reduced severity of NOWS.[218,259] Due to increased metabolic demands as well as feeding difficulties, infants with NOWS may require additional caloric support or nasogastric tube feedings if unable to meet their feeding goals. In the case of formula feeding in term infants, there is no consensus on the first-line formula. Studies examining low lactose or partially hydrolyzed formulas compared with standard infant formulas have not demonstrated any differences in NOWS outcomes.[260,261] A randomized control trial of high-calorie versus standard-calorie formula found no significant differences in NOWS pharmacologic treatment rates or length of stay.[262]

TABLE 12.9

NOWS Pharmacologic Treatment Regimens

First-line agents		
Morphine	**Methadone**	**Buprenorphine**
PRN dosing: 0.03–0.05 mg/kg/dose orally every 3–4 h	PRN dosing: 0.07 mg/kg/dose orally every 6–8 h	PRN dosing: Has not been studied
Standing dosing: 0.3–1.0 mg/kg/d orally divided every 3–4 h	Standing dosing: 0.2–0.9 mg/kg/d orally divided every 6–12 h	Standing dosing: 13–40 µg/kg/d sublingual divided every 8 h
Weaning: 10% per day down to 10–20% maximum dose	Weaning: 10% per day down to 10–20% of maximum dose, or space interval until every 24 h	Weaning: 10% per day until down to 10% of maximum dose
Second-line agents		
Phenobarbital		**Clonidine**
Loading doses: 20 mg/kg/dose orally for initial, subsequent loads of 10 mg/kg/dose		Standing dose: 1 µg/kg orally every 4 h
Standing dosing: 5–8 mg/kg/d orally in 1–2 divided doses		
Weaning: 20% every 3–7 d after being off of primary agent		Weaning: Increase dosing interval from every 4 to every 8 to every 12 h
Levels: Ideal serum levels 20–30 mg/mL		

Pharmacologic NOWS Treatment

Approximately 30% to 50% of infants with prenatal opioid exposure receive medication treatment for NOWS. With the ESC Care approach, medication treatment is indicated if the infant is unable to eat, sleep, and/or console effectively due to NOWS after optimizing nonpharmacologic care.[263] A summary of recommended pharmacologic treatment protocols for NOWS is included below in Table 12.9.

Recommend first-line medication treatment is use of an opioid medication, most commonly morphine or methadone.[238] Randomized trials have demonstrated that methadone is associated with fewer opioid treatment days and shorter length of hospitalization compared to morphine.[264] Sublingual buprenorphine has also been trialed as a first-line agent with promising results from initial studies.[265,266] Studies comparing buprenorphine to morphine or methadone indicated shorter duration of treatment in the buprenorphine group.[267] For infants on scheduled opioids, the most common approach is to wean by 10% of the maximum daily dose every 24 hours. For methadone, spacing out the interval is also a standard approach to weaning.[268,269] The opioid medication is typically stopped when at 10% to 20% of the maximum dose, with subsequent monitoring for 24 to 48 hours prior to discharge. Alternatively, using symptom-triggered or "PRN" dosing for opioids is being increasingly used, with preliminary studies indicating significantly shorter lengths of treatment. Both PRN morphine and PRN methadone have been examined in single-center studies, with infants requiring, on average, two doses of medication.[270,271]

For infants on maximum doses of a primary agent who continue to have worsening withdrawal, a secondary pharmacologic agent is indicated. Phenobarbital and clonidine are currently approved secondary agents.[245] Phenobarbital is the most commonly used second-line agent, with some evidence to suggest it is superior to clonidine for NOWS outcomes.[272] Phenobarbital often requires monitoring of serum levels. Typically, phenobarbital weaning begins 48 to 72 hours after the infant completes the wean off of their opioid medication.[264] Phenobarbital can be weaned as an outpatient and may be better for polypharmacy-exposed infants, such as those exposed to opioids and benzodiazepines and/or psychotropic medications (eg, SSRIs).[273] There is concern that prolonged use of phenobarbital may put infants at risk for neurodevelopmental delays.[274]

NOWS Discharge Preparation

All opioid-exposed newborns should be monitored in a hospital setting for 4 to 7 days for long-acting opioid exposure and 3 to 5 days for short-acting opioid exposure if they do not require pharmacologic treatment, and 24 to 48 hours after the last dose of opioid medication if they do require treatment.[239] Infants should be past the peak of their withdrawal prior to discharge. In addition, infants should have stable weight and adequate oral intake and be able

TABLE 12.10

Hospital Discharge Checklist for Infants with NOWS

Full-term infant routine care discharge checklist per the American Academy of Pediatrics[281]
3–7 d of monitoring, and/or 24–48 h after the final dose of opioids for the treatment of NOWS
Social work evaluation and/or child protective services evaluation if indicated
Family care plan completion
Early intervention referral
Hepatitis C follow-up if prenatally exposed
Stable weight gain and oral intake
Safe sleep education
Hand-off to the outpatient primary care clinician with follow-up appointment scheduled within 1–2 d
Consider ophthalmology referral
Consider developmental follow-up referral

to self-console with low levels of caregiver support, including being able to sleep independently in a crib.

It is important to note that substance-exposed newborns are at higher risk for SUID compared to nonexposed infants.[275] A Family Care Plan should be completed with clinicians, including an evaluation of available support systems and outpatient services, including subspecialist referrals if needed.[276] Opioid-exposed newborns are at higher risk for growth delays, behavioral and developmental difficulties due to multiple risk factors.[277,278] They are specifically at higher risk for eye abnormalities such as strabismus and refractive errors, thus a referral to ophthalmology for a routine exam is recommended at 4 to 6 months of age.[279] In addition, >50% of birthing persons with OUD have hepatitis C virus (HCV) with a risk of perinatal transmission of 4% to 8%.[280] Recommended laboratory testing for HCV-exposed infants includes HCV antibody testing at 15 to 18 months, though serum quantitative HCV RNA testing can also be done beginning at 2 to 6 months.[281] A summary of discharge recommendations for infants with NOWS is included below in Table 12.10.

Child Abuse Prevention and Treatment Act (CAPTA)

In 2025, 25 states and the District of Columbia require reporting of substance use during pregnancy to child welfare agencies, and in three states (Minnesota, South Dakota, and Wisconsin), drug use in pregnancy can lead to civil commitment.[282] Hospital-based clinicians and social workers should familiarize themselves with state statutes, but should not propagate the misconception that substance use during pregnancy necessarily leads to child abuse or neglect. Reporting practices can differ significantly by county and hospital. Therefore, hospital-based clinicians should collaborate with pediatric and social work teams to understand local reporting practices.

Pregnant individuals living in states with more punitive reporting policies (eg, mandatory reporting) are more likely to present later to prenatal care and less likely to be engaged in SUD treatment.[22,41] Over the past decade, more states have enacted punitive policies (eg, criminal persecution) for substance use while pregnant (12 states in 2000 to 26 states in 2017).[283] These punitive policies are associated with elevated rates of NAS[283,284] and other harms, including delays in prenatal care.[285] Decreased access to reproductive self-determination and prosecution of reproductive complications (eg, miscarriages) could further exacerbate adverse outcomes among pregnant individuals with SUD.[286] In addition, unintended negative impacts of child welfare involvement on both parents and children are well-documented and contribute to racial disparities, with Black and American Indian children being removed at 2 to 10 times the rate of White children in cases involving parental substance use.[287–289] Losing custody, whether temporarily or permanently, increases the risk of discontinuing SUD treatment and has been linked to pregnancy-related deaths from overdose during periods of destabilization.[15,290]

Clinicians should approach conversations about substance use and mandated reporting with empathy and transparency.[291,292] Affirming that the patient and their infant have a right to medical care regardless of reporting decisions is of utmost importance. It is critical to be clear and upfront about hospital-mandated reporting practices before disclosures to child services are made. Explain what information must be reported under state law, under what circumstances, and what the process looks like.[293] Ideally, these conversations happen several times and well in advance of delivery. If a report must be made, inform the patient before it happens and offer to include the patient in the conversation with child services. Whenever possible, involve social workers, peer advocates, or doulas early to help navigate systems, support difficult conversations, and minimize trauma.

Postpartum Period

The postpartum period is a time of increased vulnerability to return to substance use, overdose, and

TABLE 12.11

National Resources That Support Substance-Exposed Dyads in the Postpartum Period

Resource	Available at:	Application
Movement for Family Power	https://www.movementforfamilypower.org/	Advocacy, Legal, Policy
Drug Policy Alliance	https://drugpolicy.org/	Advocacy, Legal, Policy
Academy of Perinatal Harm Reduction	https://www.perinatalharmreduction.org/	Advocacy, Clinical
Center on Parenting and Opioids	https://cpo.uoregon.edu/	Clinical, Policy
Substance Abuse and Mental Health Services Administration (SAMHSA)	https://store.samhsa.gov/sites/default/files/d7/priv/sma18-5054.pdf	Clinical, Legal
National Network of Perinatal Quality Collaboratives (NNPQC)	https://www.cdc.gov/reproductivehealth/maternalinfanthealth/nnpqc.htm	Clinical
National Clinical Consultation Center: Substance Use Warmline	Substance Use Warmline (855)-300-3595, https://nccc.ucsf.edu/clinical-resources/substance-use-resources/	Clinical

Barber CM, Terplan M. Principles of care for pregnant and parenting people with substance use disorder: the obstetrician gynecologist perspective. *Front Pediatr*. 2023;11:1045745.

overdose death.[294] Health care interactions, which were primarily focused on the pregnant individual, become less frequent and shift from mother to infant and from medical to nonmedical domains. In some US states, insurance changes, including the termination of Medicaid coverage, occur. This loss of insurance contributes to health care discontinuation, especially for SUD treatment.[134,295] A recent review of Medicaid data demonstrated that individuals with OUD had a six-fold higher incidence of death at 1 year postpartum compared to other pregnant individuals.[294] In this review, opioid overdose was the leading cause of postpartum deaths among individuals with OUD, and postpartum use of MOUD was associated with 60% lower odds of opioid overdose death.[294] Rates of MOUD discontinuation are as high as 50% at 6 months among postpartum individuals with OUD.[134] In some states, there are didactic (mother–baby) residential treatment models or care programs that facilitate family-based SUD care in the postpartum period. Sustained focus on SUD treatment in the postpartum period is critical. Table 12.11 reviews some national resources to support patients and clinicians caring for substance-exposed dyads in the postpartum period.

Structural Considerations and Vulnerabilities

In addition to the structural vulnerabilities created by CAPTA and insurance lapses, pregnant and parenting individuals with SUD also face greater socioeconomic challenges, exposure to violence (eg, IPV), violence while using substances or engaging in sex work, and criminal legal involvement. In general, studies suggest that IPV may increase in frequency and severity during pregnancy among those who have a history of IPV.[296] Exposure to violence during pregnancy is associated with poor maternal and neonatal outcomes (eg, low birth weight, miscarriage, postpartum depression, and death).[296] Rates of violence among women with SUD are three times higher than those of the general population[296] and violence is associated with adverse SUD outcomes like overdose and return to substance use.[297,298] Despite the risk of IPV, only 25% to 50% of pregnant women report ever being screened for, or counseled on, IPV.[296] Clinicians, social workers, or nurses should assess all pregnant and parenting patients for violence in the hospital setting. If a patient reports violence, the hospital social worker should connect the patient with services, such as IPV programs or sex worker services.

Understanding the patient's socioeconomic context is important in treatment planning. For example, a lack of housing may inform the medical team and social worker's decisions about prioritizing SUD residential treatment and placement from the hospital for pregnant patients or dyads. Fear of punitive actions, such as the involvement of child protective services or legal consequences, discourages many pregnant and postpartum individuals from disclosing their survival needs or criminal legal involvement.[299] A team-based approach, such as working with hospital-based social work or addiction teams, can facilitate discussions about structural vulnerabilities and connections to appropriate services.

Structural racism intersects and compounds other forms of structural marginalization that contextualize substance use during pregnancy. Black, Latine, and Indigenous women have been subjected to a long history of reproductive coercion, forced sterilization, and trauma from the medical and judicial systems.[300,301] Structural racism means that Women of Color often experience greater socioeconomic barriers, higher rates of IPV, and greater criminal legal involvement.[302,303] Recognizing such inequities can help mitigate reinforcing structural racism in the hospital setting (eg, biased toxicology testing practices).

Emerging Evidence and Future Directions

There remains a dearth of research that focuses on pregnant and parenting individuals with SUD. Future research should prioritize evaluating the safety and efficacy of SUD treatments during pregnancy and breastfeeding, particularly AUD treatments. There is a need to develop and integrate tailored harm-reduction and overdose prevention interventions into the clinical care for pregnant and parenting individuals with SUD. Emerging evidence suggests that team-based models, including the integration of peers and doulas, can improve outcomes during pregnancy and postpartum, warranting further research and investment in these innovative care approaches. In addition, stigma and punitive policies continue to act as major barriers to care, underscoring the need for interventions at the individual, system, and structural levels that promote more supportive and equitable care. Finally, expanding access to SUD treatment for pregnant individuals is essential, especially in light of the escalating maternal health crisis in the US.

REFERENCES

1. Trends in Maternal Mortality 2000 to 2020: Estimates by WHO, UNICEF, UNFPA, World Bank Group, and UNDESA/Population Division. Executive Summary. World Health Organization; 2023.
2. *White House Blueprint for Addressing the Maternal Health Crisis*. The Biden-Harris Administration; 2022.
3. Trost S, Beauregard J, Chandra G, et al. *Pregnancy-Related Deaths: Data From Maternal Mortality Review Committees in 36 US States, 2017–2019*. Centers for Disease Control and Prevention, US Department of Health and Human Services; 2022. https://www.cdc.gov/maternal-mortality/php/data-research/mmrc-2017-2019.html
4. Kotelchuck M, Cheng ER, Belanoff C, et al. The prevalence and impact of substance use disorder and treatment on maternal obstetric experiences and birth outcomes among singleton deliveries in Massachusetts. *Matern Child Health J*. 2017;21(4):893–902.
5. Bruzelius E, Martins SS. US trends in drug overdose mortality among pregnant and postpartum persons, 2017–2020. *JAMA*. 2022;328(21):2159–2161.
6. van Boekel LC, Brouwers EPM, van Weeghel J, Garretsen HFL. Stigma among health professionals towards patients with substance use disorders and its consequences for healthcare delivery: systematic review. *Drug Alcohol Depend*. 2013;131(1–2):23–35.
7. Kuo C, Schonbrun YC, Zlotnick C, et al. A qualitative study of treatment needs among pregnant and postpartum women with substance use and depression. *Subst Use Misuse*. 2013;48(14):1498–1508.
8. Margerison CE, Roberts MH, Gemmill A, Goldman-Mellor S. Pregnancy-associated deaths due to drugs, suicide, and homicide in the United States, 2010–2019. *Obstet Gynecol*. 2022;139(2):172–180.
9. Han B, Compton WM, Einstein EB, Elder E, Volkow ND. Pregnancy and postpartum drug overdose deaths in the US before and during the COVID-19 pandemic. *JAMA Psychiatry*. 2024;81(3):270–283.
10. National Academies of Sciences, Engineering, and Medicine; Health and Medicine Division; Board on Health Sciences Policy; Committee on Medication-Assisted Treatment for Opioid Use Disorder. In: Mancher M, Leshner AI, eds. *Medications for Opioid Use Disorder Save Lives*. National Academies Press (US); 2019. Accessed January 7, 2025. http://www.ncbi.nlm.nih.gov/books/NBK538936/
11. Krans EE, Kim JY, James AE, Kelley D, Jarlenski MP. Medication-assisted treatment use among pregnant women with opioid use disorder. *Obstet Gynecol*. 2019;133(5):943–951.
12. Schiff DM, Nielsen T, Hoeppner BB, et al. Assessment of racial and ethnic disparities in the use of medication to treat opioid use disorder among pregnant women in Massachusetts. *JAMA Netw Open*. 2020;3(5):e205734.
13. Xu KY, Jones HE, Schiff DM, et al. Initiation and treatment discontinuation of medications for opioid use disorder in pregnant people compared with nonpregnant people. *Obstet Gynecol*. 2023;141(4):845–853.
14. Peltier MR, Roberts W, Verplaetse TL, et al. Licit and illicit drug use across trimesters in pregnant women endorsing past-year substance use: results from National Survey on Drug Use and Health (2009-2019). *Arch Womens Ment Health*. 2022;25(4):819–827.
15. Thumath M, Humphreys D, Barlow J, et al. Overdose among mothers: the association between child removal and unintentional drug overdose in a longitudinal cohort of marginalised women in Canada. *Int J Drug Policy*. 2021;91:102977.
16. Huang RS, Spence AR, Abenhaim HA. Non-obstetric maternal mortality trends by race in the United States. *Matern Child Health J*. 2024;28(5):895–904.
17. Wakeman SE, Bryant A, Harrison N. Redefining child protection: addressing the harms of structural racism and punitive approaches for birthing people, dyads, and families affected by substance use. *Obstet Gynecol*. 2022;140(2):167–173.
18. Substance Abuse and Mental Health Services Administration. *Results from the 2023 National Survey on Drug Use and Health: Detailed Tables*. U.S. Department of Health and Human Service; 2023. Accessed January 19, 2025. https://www.samhsa.gov/data/report/2023-nsduh-detailed-tables
19. Apsley HB, Brant K, Brothers S, et al. Pregnancy- and parenting-related barriers to receiving medication for opioid use disorder: a multi-paneled qualitative study of women in treatment, women who terminated treatment, and the professionals who serve them. *Womens Health Lond Engl*. 2024;20:17455057231224181.
20. Choi S, Rosenbloom D, Stein MD, Raifman J, Clark JA. Differential gateways, facilitators, and barriers to substance use disorder treatment for pregnant women and mothers: a scoping systematic review. *J Addict Med*. 2022;16(3):e185–e196.
21. Khachikian T, Amaro H, Guerrero E, Kong Y, Marsh JC. Disparities in opioid treatment access and retention among

women based on pregnancy status from 2006 to 2017. *Drug Alcohol Depend Rep*. 2022;2:100030.
22. Roberts T, Frederiksen, Saunders H, Salganicoff A. *Opioid Use Disorder and Treatment Among Pregnant and Postpartum Medicaid Enrollees*. KFF; 2023. Accessed January 30, 2025. https://www.kff.org/medicaid/issue-brief/opioid-use-disorder-and-treatment-among-pregnant-and-postpartum-medicaid-enrollees/
23. Bleasdale J, Morse DS, Cerulli C, et al. Women's motivators to engage in opioid use disorder treatment while enrolled in an opioid intervention court. *Subst Use Misuse*. 2022;57(7):1035–1042.
24. Stulac S, Bair-Merritt M, Wachman EM, et al. Children and families of the opioid epidemic: under the radar. *Curr Probl Pediatr Adolesc Health Care*. 2019;49(8):100637.
25. Sword W, Jack S, Niccols A, Milligan K, Henderson J, Thabane L. Integrated programs for women with substance use issues and their children: a qualitative meta-synthesis of processes and outcomes. *Harm Reduct J*. 2009;6:32.
26. Reddy UM, Davis JM, Ren Z, Greene MF; Opioid Use in Pregnancy, Neonatal Abstinence Syndrome, and Childhood Outcomes Workshop Invited Speakers. Opioid use in pregnancy, neonatal abstinence syndrome, and childhood outcomes: executive summary of a Joint Workshop by the Eunice Kennedy Shriver National Institute of Child Health and Human Development, American College of Obstetricians and Gynecologists, American Academy of Pediatrics, Society for Maternal-Fetal Medicine, Centers for Disease Control and Prevention, and the March of Dimes Foundation. *Obstet Gynecol*. 2017;130(1):10–28.
27. Kerker BD, Horwitz SM, Leventhal JM. Patients' characteristics and providers' attitudes: predictors of screening pregnant women for illicit substance use. *Child Abuse Negl*. 2004;28(2):209–223.
28. Barber CM, Terplan M. Principles of care for pregnant and parenting people with substance use disorder: the obstetrician gynecologist perspective. *Front Pediatr*. 2023;11:1045745.
29. Coleman-Cowger VH, Oga EA, Peters EN, Trocin KE, Koszowski B, Mark K. Accuracy of three screening tools for prenatal substance use. *Obstet Gynecol*. 2019;133(5):952–961.
30. Paris R, Herriott AL, Maru M, Hacking SE, Sommer AR. Secrecy versus disclosure: women with substance use disorders share experiences in help seeking during pregnancy. *Matern Child Health J*. 2020;24(11):1396–1403.
31. Alliance for Innovation on Maternal Health. Care for Pregnant and Postpartum People with Substance Use Disorder | AIM. Saferbirth.org. 2021. Accessed January 7, 2025. https://saferbirth.org/psbs/care-for-pregnant-and-postpartum-people-with-substance-use-disorder/
32. Johnson A, Swenson KS, Dillner E, et al. Addressing perinatal substance use: a triad approach led by the Colorado Perinatal Care Quality Collaborative. *J Midwifery Womens Health*. 2024;69(4):586–592.
33. Ondersma SJ, Chang G, Blake-Lamb T, et al. Accuracy of five self-report screening instruments for substance use in pregnancy. *Addict Abingdon Engl*. 2019;114(9):1683–1693.
34. American Psychiatric Association. *Diagnostic and Statistical Manual of Mental Disorders*. American Psychiatric Association; 2013.
35. American College of Obstetricians and Gynecologists. ACOG Committee Opinion No. 757: screening for perinatal depression. *Obstet Gynecol*. 2018;132(5):e208–e212.
36. Committee on Health Care for Underserved Women. ACOG Committee Opinion No. 554: reproductive and sexual coercion. *Obstet Gynecol*. 2013;121(2 Pt 1):411–415.
37. American College of Obstetricians and Gynecologists Committee on Health Care for Undeserved Women. ACOG Committee Opinion No. 343: psychosocial risk factors: perinatal screening and intervention. *Obstet Gynecol*. 2006;108(2):469–477.
38. Substance Abuse and Mental Health Services Administration. Clinical guidance for treating pregnant and parenting women with opioid use disorder and their infants | SAMHSA Publications and Digital Products. 2018. Accessed January 7, 2025. https://library.samhsa.gov/product/clinical-guidance-treating-pregnant-and-parenting-women-opioid-use-disorder-and-their
39. Tucker Edmonds B, Mckenzie F, Austgen MB, Carroll AE, Meslin EM. Women's opinions of legal requirements for drug testing in prenatal care. *J Matern Fetal Neonatal Med*. 2017;30(14):1693–1698.
40. Roberts SCM, Nuru-Jeter A. Women's perspectives on screening for alcohol and drug use in prenatal care. *Womens Health Issues*. 2010;20(3):193–200.
41. Austin AE, Naumann RB, Simmons E. Association of state child abuse policies and mandated reporting policies with prenatal and postpartum care among women who engaged in substance use during pregnancy. *JAMA Pediatr*. 2022;176(11):1123–1130.
42. Ellsworth MA, Stevens TP, D'Angio CT. Infant race affects application of clinical guidelines when screening for drugs of abuse in newborns. *Pediatrics*. 2010;125(6):e1379–1385.
43. Perlman NC, Cantonwine DE, Smith NA. Toxicology testing in pregnancy: evaluating the role of social profiling. *Obstet Gynecol*. 2020;136(3):607–609.
44. Huhn AS, Hobelmann JG, Oyler GA, Strain EC. Protracted renal clearance of fentanyl in persons with opioid use disorder. *Drug Alcohol Depend*. 2020;214:108147.
45. Moeller KE, Kissack JC, Atayee RS, Lee KC. Clinical interpretation of urine drug tests: what clinicians need to know about urine drug screens. *Mayo Clin Proc*. 2017;92(5):774–796.
46. Siegel MR, Mahowald GK, Uljon SN, et al. Fentanyl in the labor epidural impacts the results of intrapartum and postpartum maternal and neonatal toxicology tests. *Am J Obstet Gynecol*. 2023;228(6):741.e1–741.e7.
47. Jarvis M, Williams J, Hurford M, et al. Appropriate use of drug testing in clinical addiction medicine. *J Addict Med*. 2017;11(3):163–173.
48. Yee LM, Wu D. False-positive amphetamine toxicology screen results in three pregnant women using labetalol. *Obstet Gynecol*. 2011;117(2 Pt 2):503–506.
49. American College of Obstetricians and Gynecologists. Opposition to criminalization of individuals during pregnancy and the postpartum period. *Am Coll Obstet Gynecol*. 2020:12.
50. Baxter L Sr, Brown DL, Hurford DM, et al. Appropriate use of drug testing in clinical addiction medicine. *J Addict Med*. 2017;11:1–56.
51. Koenigs KJ, Chou JH, Cohen S, et al. Informed consent is poorly documented when obtaining toxicology testing at delivery in a Massachusetts cohort. *Am J Obstet Gynecol MFM*. 2022;4(4):100621.
52. Board A, D'Angelo DV, von Essen BS, et al. Polysubstance use during pregnancy: the importance of screening, patient education, and integrating a harm reduction perspective. *Drug Alcohol Depend*. 2023;247:109872.
53. Oei JL. Alcohol use in pregnancy and its impact on the mother and child. *Addiction*. 2020;115(11):2148–2163.
54. May PA, Baete A, Russo J, et al. Prevalence and characteristics of fetal alcohol spectrum disorders. *Pediatrics*. 2014;134(5):855–866.
55. Adgent MA. Environmental tobacco smoke and sudden infant death syndrome: a review. *Birth Defects Res B Dev Reprod Toxicol*. 2006;77(1):69–85.

56. Smith K, Lipari RN. *Women of Childbearing Age and Opioids*. Center for Behavioral Health Statistics and Quality, Substance Abuse and Mental Health Services Administration; 2017. https://www.samhsa.gov/data/sites/default/files/report_2724/ShortReport-2724.html
57. Sanjanwala AR, Lim G, Krans EE. Opioids and opioid use disorder in pregnancy. *Obstet Gynecol Clin North Am*. 2023; 50(1):229–240.
58. Zedler BK, Mann AL, Kim MM, et al. Buprenorphine compared with methadone to treat pregnant women with opioid use disorder: a systematic review and meta-analysis of safety in the mother, fetus and child. *Addiction*. 2016;111(12):2115–2128.
59. Weiss ST, Douglas HE. Treatment of kratom withdrawal and dependence with buprenorphine/naloxone: a case series and systematic literature review. *J Addict Med*. 2021;15(2): 167–172.
60. Wright ME, Ginsberg C, Parkison AM, Dubose M, Sherbondy M, Shores E. Outcomes of mothers and newborns to prenatal exposure to kratom: a systematic review. *J Perinatol*. 2021;41(6):1236–1243.
61. Grigoriadis S, Graves L, Peer M, et al. Pregnancy and delivery outcomes following benzodiazepine exposure: a systematic review and meta-analysis. *Can J Psychiatry*. 2020;65(12): 821–834.
62. Ban L, Tata LJ, West J, Fiaschi L, Gibson JE. Live and non-live pregnancy outcomes among women with depression and anxiety: a population-based study. *PLoS ONE*. 2012;7(8): e43462.
63. Källén B, Borg N, Reis M. The use of central nervous system active drugs during pregnancy. *Pharmaceuticals*. 2013;6(10): 1221–1286.
64. Huybrechts KF, Bateman BT, Desai RJ, et al. Risk of neonatal drug withdrawal after intrauterine co-exposure to opioids and psychotropic medications: cohort study. *BMJ*. 2017; 358:j3326.
65. Pippard NS, Bandoli G, Baer RJ. Trends and adverse pregnancy and birth outcomes associated with stimulant-related disorder diagnosis. *Addiction*. 2024;119(11):2006–2014.
66. Kevil CG, Goeders NE, Woolard MD, et al. Methamphetamine use and cardiovascular disease. *Arterioscler Thromb Vasc Biol*. 2019;39(9):1739–1746.
67. Evans K, Wu P, Mamas MA, et al. Substance use in pregnancy and its association with cardiovascular events. *JACC Adv*. 2023;2(8):100619.
68. Graves LE, Green CR, Robert M, Cook JL. Methamphetamine use in pregnancy: a call for action. *J Obstet Gynaecol Can*. 2021;43(8):1001–1004.
69. Lo JO, Shaw B, Robalino S, et al. Cannabis use in pregnancy and neonatal outcomes: a systematic review and meta-analysis. *Cannabis Cannabinoid Res*. 2024;9(2):470–485.
70. Lo JO, Hedges JC, Girardi G. Impact of cannabinoids on pregnancy, reproductive health, and offspring outcomes. *Am J Obstet Gynecol*. 2022;227(4):571–581.
71. Gould GS, Havard A, Lim LL, Kumar R. Exposure to tobacco, environmental tobacco smoke and nicotine in pregnancy: a pragmatic overview of reviews of maternal and child outcomes, effectiveness of interventions and barriers and facilitators to quitting. *Int J Environ Res Public Health*. 2020;17(6):2034.
72. Tappin D. The importance of permanent cessation for pregnant smokers. *Addiction*. 2016;111(6):991–992.
73. Centers for Disease Control and Prevention (CDC). Alcohol use among women of childbearing age–United States, 1991–1999. *MMWR Morb Mortal Wkly Rep*. 2002;51(13):273–276.
74. Alcohol use and binge drinking among U.S. men, pregnant and non-pregnant women ages 18–44: 2002–2017—Science Direct. Accessed January 25, 2025. https://www.sciencedirect.com/science/article/abs/pii/S0376871619303679
75. Gosdin LK, Deputy NP, Kim SY, Dang EP, Denny CH. Alcohol consumption and binge drinking during pregnancy among adults aged 18–49 years—United States, 2018–2020. *Morb Mortal Wkly Rep*. 2022;71(1):10–13.
76. Tomson T, Battino D, Bonizzoni E, et al. Comparative risk of major congenital malformations with eight different antiepileptic drugs: a prospective cohort study of the EURAP registry. *Lancet Neurol*. 2018;17(6):530–538.
77. Battino D, Tomson T, Bonizzoni E, et al. Risk of major congenital malformations and exposure to antiseizure medication monotherapy. *JAMA Neurol*. 2024;81(5):481–489.
78. Sullivan JT, Sykora K, Schneiderman J, Naranjo CA, Sellers EM. Assessment of alcohol withdrawal: the revised clinical institute withdrawal assessment for alcohol scale (CIWA-Ar). *Br J Addict*. 1989;84(11):1353–1357.
79. Trojand T, Morgan J, Shamoun CJ. Using the modified Minnesota Detoxification Scale to evaluate alcohol withdrawal syndrome: an integrative review. *Crit Care Nurse*. 2025;45(2):60–68.
80. Busto UE, Sykora K, Sellers EM. A clinical scale to assess benzodiazepine withdrawal. *J Clin Psychopharmacol*. 1989; 9(6):412–416.
81. Dave CV, Goodin A, Zhu Y, et al. Prevalence of maternal-risk factors related to neonatal abstinence syndrome in a commercial claims database: 2011–2015. *Pharmacotherapy*. 2019;39(10):1005–1011.
82. Kelty E, Tran D, Lavin T, Preen DB, Hulse G, Havard A. Prevalence and safety of acamprosate use in pregnant alcohol-dependent women in New South Wales, Australia. *Addiction*. 2019;114(2):206–215.
83. Helmbrecht GD, Hoskins IA. First trimester disulfiram exposure: report of two cases. *Am J Perinatol*. 1993;10(1):5–7.
84. Hernández-Díaz S, Smith CR, Shen A, et al. Comparative safety of antiepileptic drugs during pregnancy. *Neurology*. 2012;78(21):1692–1699.
85. Terplan M, Laird HJ, Hand DJ, et al. Opioid detoxification during pregnancy: a systematic review. *Obstet Gynecol*. 2018;131(5):803–814.
86. Lepreau FJ, Garvey B, Paull N, Stein MD. Opiate detoxification of pregnant women using clonidine: an observational cohort study. *J Womens Health*. 1995;4(4):381–386.
87. Jansson LM, Dipietro JA, Velez M, Elko A, Knauer H, Kivlighan KT. Maternal methadone dosing schedule and fetal neurobehaviour. *J Matern-Fetal Neonatal Med*. 2009; 22(1):29–35.
88. Wakeman SE, Larochelle MR, Ameli O, et al. Comparative effectiveness of different treatment pathways for opioid use disorder. *JAMA Netw Open*. 2020;3(2):e1920622.
89. Suarez EA, Bateman BT, Straub L, et al. First trimester use of buprenorphine or methadone and the risk of congenital malformations. *JAMA Intern Med*. 2024;184(3):242–251.
90. Jouyban A, Fakhree MAA, Shayanfar A. Review of pharmaceutical applications of N-methyl-2-pyrrolidone. *J Pharm Pharm Sci*. 2010;13(4):524–535.
91. Patel NB, Parilla BV. Buprenorphine induction using microdosing for the management of opioid use disorder in pregnancy. *AJP Rep*. 2024;14(1):e88–e90.
92. Reddy S, Martin CE. Low-dose buprenorphine initiation during pregnancy: a case report. *AJOG Glob Rep*. 2024;4(1): 100308.
93. Atluru S, Bruehlman AK, Vaughn P, Schauberger CW, Smid MC. Naltrexone compared with buprenorphine or methadone in pregnancy: a systematic review. *Obstet Gynecol*. 2024; 143(3):403–410.
94. Robijn AL, Tran DT, Cohen JM, et al. Smoking cessation pharmacotherapy use in pregnancy. *JAMA Netw Open*. 2024; 7(6):e2419245.

95. Hajek P, Przulj D, Pesola F, et al. Electronic cigarettes versus nicotine patches for smoking cessation in pregnancy: a randomized controlled trial. *Nat Med.* 2022;28(5):958–964.
96. Morales-Suárez-Varela M, Puig BM, Kaerlev L, Peraita-Costa I, Perales-Marín A. Safety of nicotine replacement therapy during pregnancy: a narrative review. *Int J Environ Res Public Health.* 2022;20(1):250.
97. Tran DT, Preen DB, Einarsdottir K, et al. Use of smoking cessation pharmacotherapies during pregnancy is not associated with increased risk of adverse pregnancy outcomes: a population-based cohort study. *BMC Med.* 2020;18(1):15.
98. Pedersen L, Petronis KR, Nørgaard M, et al. Risk of adverse birth outcomes after maternal varenicline use: a population-based observational study in Denmark and Sweden. *Pharmacoepidemiol Drug Saf.* 2020;29(1):94–102.
99. Hendrick V, Suri R, Gitlin MJ, Ortiz-Portillo E. Bupropion use during pregnancy: a systematic review. *Prim Care Companion CNS Disord.* 2017;19(5):17r02160.
100. Bupropion. In: *Mother To Baby | Fact Sheets.* Organization of Teratology Information Specialists (OTIS); 1994. Accessed March 14, 2025. http://www.ncbi.nlm.nih.gov/books/NBK582611/
101. Ostenfeld A, Lyngholm S, Christensen SE, et al. Mirtazapine in pregnancy and lactation: a systematic review of adverse outcomes. *Acta Psychiatr Scand.* 2025;151(1):6–32.
102. Campos J, Roca L, Gude F, Gonzalez-Quintela A. Long-term mortality of patients admitted to the hospital with alcohol withdrawal syndrome. *Alcohol Clin Exp Res.* 2011;35(6):1180–1186.
103. Crotty K, Freedman KI, Kampman KM. Executive summary of the focused update of the ASAM national practice guideline for the treatment of opioid use disorder. *J Addict Med.* 2020;14(2):99–112.
104. Grigoriadis S, Graves L, Peer M, et al. Benzodiazepine use during pregnancy alone or in combination with an antidepressant and congenital malformations: systematic review and meta-analysis. *J Clin Psychiatry.* 2019;80(4):18r12412.
105. Seligman NS, Salva N, Hayes EJ, Dysart KC, Pequignot EC, Baxter JK. Predicting length of treatment for neonatal abstinence syndrome in methadone-exposed neonates. *Am J Obstet Gynecol.* 2008;199(4):396.e1–e7.
106. Pettinati HM, Weiss RD, Dundon W, et al. A structured approach to medical management: a psychosocial intervention to support pharmacotherapy in the treatment of alcohol dependence. *J Stud Alcohol Suppl.* 2005;(15):170–178; discussion 168–169.
107. Anton RF, O'Malley SS, Ciraulo DA, et al; COMBINE Study Research Group. Combined pharmacotherapies and behavioral interventions for alcohol dependence: the COMBINE study: a randomized controlled trial. *JAMA.* 2006;295(17):2003–2017.
108. Roberts SC, Liu G, Terplan M. Medications for alcohol use disorder among birthing people with an alcohol-related diagnosis. *J Addict Med.* 2025;19(1):41–46.
109. Roberts SCM, Schulte A, Zaugg C, Leslie DL, Corr TE, Liu G. Association of pregnancy-specific alcohol policies with infant morbidities and maltreatment. *JAMA Netw Open.* 2023;6(8):e2327138.
110. Jonas DE, Amick HR, Feltner C, et al. Pharmacotherapy for adults with alcohol use disorders in outpatient settings: a systematic review and meta-analysis. *JAMA.* 2014;311(18):1889–1900.
111. Smith EJ, Lui S, Terplan M. Pharmacologic interventions for pregnant women enrolled in alcohol treatment. *Cochrane Database Syst Rev.* 2009;2009(3):CD007361.
112. Reus VI, Fochtmann LJ, Bukstein O, et al. The American Psychiatric Association practice guideline for the pharmacological treatment of patients with alcohol use disorder. *Focus (Am Psychiatr Publ).* 2019;17(2):158–162.
113. Hale TW, Krutsch K. *Hale's Medications & Mothers' Milk 2023: A Manual of Lactational Pharmacology.* Springer Publishing; 2022.
114. DeVido J, Bogunovic O, Weiss RD. Alcohol use disorders in pregnancy. *Harv Rev Psychiatry.* 2015;23(2):112–121.
115. Opioid use and opioid use disorder in pregnancy. Accessed January 22, 2025. https://www.acog.org/clinical/clinical-guidance/committee-opinion/articles/2017/08/opioid-use-and-opioid-use-disorder-in-pregnancy
116. Haight SC, Ko JY, Tong VT, Bohm MK, Callaghan WM. Opioid use disorder documented at delivery hospitalization—United States, 1999–2014. *MMWR Morb Mortal Wkly Rep.* 2018;67(31):845–849.
117. Terplan M, Kennedy-Hendricks A, Chisolm MS. Prenatal substance use: exploring assumptions of maternal unfitness. *Subst Abuse Res Treat.* 2015;9(Suppl 2):1–4.
118. Cleary EM, Smid MC, Charles JE, et al. Buprenorphine X-waiver exemption – beyond the basics for the obstetrical provider. *Am J Obstet Gynecol MFM.* 2021;3(6):100451.
119. Short VL, Hand DJ, MacAfee L, Abatemarco DJ, Terplan M. Trends and disparities in receipt of pharmacotherapy among pregnant women in publically funded treatment programs for opioid use disorder in the United States. *J Subst Abuse Treat.* 2018;89:67–74.
120. Rosenthal EW, Short VL, Cruz Y, et al. Racial inequity in methadone dose at delivery in pregnant women with opioid use disorder. *J Subst Abuse Treat.* 2021;131:108454.
121. Mattick RP, Breen C, Kimber J, Davoli M. Methadone maintenance therapy versus no opioid replacement therapy for opioid dependence. *Cochrane Database Syst Rev.* 2009;(3):CD002209.
122. Jones HE, Terplan M, Meyer M. Medically assisted withdrawal (detoxification): considering the mother-infant dyad. *J Addict Med.* 2017;11(2):90–92.
123. Ordean A, Tubman-Broeren M. Safety and efficacy of buprenorphine-naloxone in pregnancy: a systematic review of the literature. *Pathophysiology.* 2023;30(1):27–36.
124. Buprenorphine-naloxone versus buprenorphine for treatment of opioid use disorder in pregnancy. Accessed December 9, 2024. https://oce-ovid-com.liboff.ohsu.edu/article/01271255-202211000-00025?relatedarticle=y
125. Wong J, Saver B, Scanlan JM, et al. Does maternal buprenorphine dose affect severity or incidence of neonatal abstinence syndrome? *J Addict Med.* 2018;12(6):435–441.
126. Jones HE, Kaltenbach K, Heil SH, et al. Neonatal abstinence syndrome after methadone or buprenorphine exposure. *N Engl J Med.* 2010;363(24):2320–2331.
127. Lofwall MR, Young JL, Hansen Z, et al. What to expect with pregnant or postpartum prescribing of extended-release buprenorphine (CAM2038). *J Clin Gynecol Obstet.* 2023;12(3):110–116.
128. Winhusen T, Lofwall M, Jones HE, et al. Medication treatment for opioid use disorder in expectant mothers (MOMs): design considerations for a pragmatic randomized trial comparing extended-release and daily buprenorphine formulations. *Contemp Clin Trials.* 2020;93:106014.
129. Kelty E, Hulse G. A retrospective cohort study of birth outcomes in neonates exposed to naltrexone in utero: a comparison with methadone-, buprenorphine- and non-opioid-exposed neonates. *Drugs.* 2017;77:1211–1219.
130. Wachman EM, Saia K, Miller M, et al. Naltrexone treatment for pregnant women with opioid use disorder compared with matched buprenorphine control subjects. *Clin Ther.* 2019;41(9):1681–1689.
131. Morgan JR, Schackman BR, Weinstein ZM, Walley AY, Linas BP. Overdose following initiation of naltrexone and

buprenorphine medication treatment for opioid use disorder in a United States commercially insured cohort. *Drug Alcohol Depend.* 2019;200:34–39.

132. Ross RK, Nunes EV, Olfson M, et al. Comparative effectiveness of extended-release naltrexone and sublingual buprenorphine for treatment of opioid use disorder among Medicaid patients. *Addict Abingdon Engl.* 2024;119(11):1975–1986.
133. Terplan M, Ramanadhan S, Locke A, Longinaker N, Lui S. Psychosocial interventions for pregnant women in outpatient illicit drug treatment programs compared to other interventions. *Cochrane Database Syst Rev.* 2015;2015(4):CD006037.
134. Wilder C, Lewis D, Winhusen T. Medication assisted treatment discontinuation in pregnant and postpartum women with opioid use disorder. *Drug Alcohol Depend.* 2015;149:225–231.
135. Kleinman MB, Felton JW, Johnson A, Magidson JF. "I have to be around people that are doing what I'm doing": the importance of expanding the peer recovery coach role in treatment of opioid use disorder in the face of COVID-19 health disparities. *J Subst Abuse Treat.* 2021;122:108182.
136. Fallin-Bennett A, Elswick A, Ashford K. Peer support specialists and perinatal opioid use disorder: someone that's been there, lived it, seen it. *Addict Behav.* 2020;102:106204.
137. National Institute on Drug Abuse (NIDA). Kratom. 2022. Accessed April 24, 2025. https://nida.nih.gov/research-topics/kratom
138. *Kratom: Summary of State Laws.* Legislative Analysis and Public Policy Association; 2024.
139. Chomchai S, Phuditshinnapatra J, Mekavuthikul P, Chomchai C. Effects of unconventional recreational drug use in pregnancy. *Semin Fetal Neonatal Med.* 2019;24(2):142–148.
140. Kaufmann CN, Spira AP, Alexander C, Rutkow L, Mojtabai R. Trends in prescribing of sedative-hypnotic medications in the United States: 1993–2010. *Pharmacoepidemiol Drug Saf.* 2016;25(6):637–645.
141. Bais B, Molenaar NM, Bijma HH, et al. Prevalence of benzodiazepines and benzodiazepine-related drugs exposure before, during and after pregnancy: a systematic review and meta-analysis. *J Affect Disord.* 2020;269:18–27.
142. Substance Abuse Mental Health Services Administration. *Key Substance Use and Mental Health Indicators in the United States: Results from the 2019 National Survey on Drug Use and Health.* Center for Behavioral Health Statistics and Quality, Substance Abuse and Mental Health Services Administration; 2020. https://library.samhsa.gov/product/results-2019-national-survey-drug-use-and-health-nsduh-key-substance-use-and-mental-health
143. Votaw VR, Geyer R, Rieselbach MM, McHugh RK. The epidemiology of benzodiazepine misuse: a systematic review. *Drug Alcohol Depend.* 2019;200:95–114.
144. Vigod SN, Dennis CL. Benzodiazepines and the Z-Drugs in pregnancy—reasonably reassuring for neurodevelopment but should we really be using them? *JAMA Netw Open.* 2019;2(4):e191430.
145. Gopalan P, Moses-Kolko E, Valpey R, Shenai N, Smith E. Benzodiazepine withdrawal in pregnant women with opioid use disorders: an observational study of current clinical practices at a tertiary obstetrical hospital. *Gen Hosp Psychiatry.* 2019;57:29–33.
146. Gopalan P, Glance JB, Azzam PN. Managing benzodiazepine withdrawal during pregnancy: case-based guidelines. *Arch Womens Ment Health.* 2014;17(2):167–170.
147. Soyka M. Treatment of benzodiazepine dependence. *N Engl J Med.* 2017;376(12):1147–1157.
148. Peng L, Morford KL, Levander XA. Benzodiazepines and related sedatives. *Med Clin North Am.* 2022;106(1):113–129.
149. Laks J, Kim TW, Christine PJ, et al. Treating benzodiazepine withdrawal in a bridge clinic. *J Addict Med.* 2024;18(6):649–656.
150. SMID MC, Metz TD, Gordon AJ. Stimulant use in pregnancy—an under-recognized epidemic among pregnant women. *Clin Obstet Gynecol.* 2019;62(1):168–184.
151. Pergolizzi JV, Magnusson P, LeQuang JAK, Breve F, Varrassi G. Cocaine and cardiotoxicity: a literature review. *Cureus.* 2021;13(4):e14594.
152. Manja V, Nrusimha A, Gao Y, et al. Methamphetamine-associated heart failure: a systematic review of observational studies. *Heart.* 2023;109(3):168–177.
153. Priest KC, Balasanova AA, Levander XA, et al. Caring for hospitalized adults with methamphetamine use disorder: a proposed clinical roadmap. *Am J Med.* 2023;136(6):507–509.
154. Center for Substance Abuse Treatment. *Treatment for Stimulant Use Disorders.* Substance Abuse and Mental Health Services Administration (US); 1999. Accessed March 7, 2025. http://www.ncbi.nlm.nih.gov/books/NBK64333/
155. Acheson LS, Williams BH, Farrell M, McKetin R, Ezard N, Siefried KJ. Pharmacological treatment for methamphetamine withdrawal: a systematic review and meta-analysis of randomised controlled trials. *Drug Alcohol Rev.* 2023;42(1):7–19.
156. Li MJ, Shoptaw SJ. Clinical management of psychostimulant withdrawal: review of the evidence. *Addiction.* 2023;118(4):750–762.
157. Ornoy A, Zvi N, Arnon J, Wajnberg R, Shechtman S, Diav-Citrin O. The outcome of pregnancy following topiramate treatment: a study on 52 pregnancies. *Reprod Toxicol.* 2008;25(3):388–389.
158. Ronsley C, Nolan S, Knight R, et al. Treatment of stimulant use disorder: a systematic review of reviews. *PLoS One.* 2020;15(6):e0234809.
159. Higgins ST. Behavior change, health, and health disparities 2023: contingency management for treating substance use disorders and promoting health in vulnerable populations. *Prev Med.* 2023;176:107746.
160. Appa A, Baral S, Stein B, et al. The IMPACT (Infection Management Plus Addiction Care Together) pilot: a case series of combined contingency management for substance use disorders & antibiotic adherence in the hospital setting. *J Addict Med.* 2024;18(2):138–143.
161. Peng L, Titus H, Roellich P, Englander H. Adapting contingency management for hospitalized patients with stimulant use disorder. *J Addict Med.* 2023;17(5):580–586.
162. Washio Y, Mark K, Terplan M. Characteristics of pregnant women reporting cannabis use disorder at substance use treatment entry. *J Addict Med.* 2018;12(5):395–400.
163. Weisbeck SJ, Bright KS, Ginn CS, Smith JM, Hayden KA, Ringham C. Perceptions about cannabis use during pregnancy: a rapid best-framework qualitative synthesis. *Can J Public Health.* 2020;112(1):49–59.
164. Zaugg C, Terplan M, Mailman K, Roberts SCM. Reasons pregnant people use cannabis to self-treat health conditions during pregnancy: results from a US population-based survey. *Drug Alcohol Rev.* 2024;43(7):1742–1752.
165. Kobernik EK, Ford ND, Levecke M, et al. Marijuana use among pregnant and nonpregnant women of reproductive age, 2013–2019. *Subst Use Misuse.* 2024;59(5):690–698.
166. Kondo KK, Morasco BJ, Nugent SM, et al. Pharmacotherapy for the treatment of cannabis use disorder. *Ann Intern Med.* 2020;172(6):398–412.
167. Groff D, Bollampally P, Buono F, Knehans A, Spotts H, Bone C. Interventions addressing cannabis use during pregnancy: a systematic review. *J Addict Med.* 2023;17(1):47–53.

168. Lange S, Probst C, Rehm J, Popova S. National, regional, and global prevalence of smoking during pregnancy in the general population: a systematic review and meta-analysis. *Lancet Glob Health*. 2018;6(7):e769–e776. Epub 2018 May 31.
169. Nian H, Odland R, Mindlin S, et al. Demographic characteristics, perinatal smoking patterns, and risk for neonatal health complications among pregnant smokers in the united states who begin using electronic cigarettes during pregnancy: a descriptive study using population-based surveillance data. *Nicotine Tob Res*. 2024;26(11):1455–1462.
170. Prabhu N, Smith N, Campbell D, et al. First trimester maternal tobacco smoking habits and fetal growth. *Thorax*. 2010;65(3):235–240.
171. Baxter S, Everson-Hock E, Messina J, Guillaume L, Burrows J, Goyder E. Factors relating to the uptake of interventions for smoking cessation among pregnant women: a systematic review and qualitative synthesis. *Nicotine Tob Res*. 2010;12(7): 685–694.
172. Rigotti NA, Kruse GR, Livingstone-Banks J, Hartmann-Boyce J. Treatment of tobacco smoking: a review. *JAMA*. 2022;327(6):566–577.
173. Baker TB, Piper ME, Stein JH, et al. Effects of nicotine patch vs varenicline vs combination nicotine replacement therapy on smoking cessation at 26 weeks: a randomized clinical trial. *JAMA*. 2016;315(4):371–379.
174. Myung SK, Ju W, Jung HS, et al; Korean Meta-Analysis (KORMA) Study Group. Efficacy and safety of pharmacotherapy for smoking cessation among pregnant smokers: a meta-analysis. *BJOG*. 2012;119(9):1029–1039.
175. Claire R, Chamberlain C, Davey M, et al. Pharmacological interventions for promoting smoking cessation during pregnancy. *Cochrane Database Syst Rev*. 2020;3(3):CD010078.
176. Choi SKY, Tran DT, Kemp-Casey A, et al. The comparative effectiveness of varenicline and nicotine patches for smoking abstinence during pregnancy: evidence from a population-based cohort study. *Nicotine Tob Res*. 2021;23(10): 1664–1672.
177. Howes S, Hartmann-Boyce J, Livingstone-Banks J, Hong B, Lindson N. Antidepressants for smoking cessation. *Cochrane Database Syst Rev*. 2020;4:CD000031.
178. Hartmann-Boyce J, McRobbie H, Lindson N, et al. Electronic cigarettes for smoking cessation. *Cochrane Database Syst Rev*. 2020;10:CD010216.
179. Stancliff S, Phillips BW, Maghsoudi N, Joseph H. Harm reduction: front line public health. *J Addict Dis*. 2015;34(2–3): 206–219.
180. Wakeman B, Kremer M, Schulkin J. The application of harm reduction to methamphetamine use during pregnancy: a call to arms. *Am J Obstet Gynecol MFM*. 2021;3(5):100418.
181. Wright TE, Schuetter R, Fombonne E, Stephenson J, Haning WF. Implementation and evaluation of a harm-reduction model for clinical care of substance using pregnant women. *Harm Reduct J*. 2012;9:1–10.
182. Marshall SK, Charles G, Hare J, Ponzetti JJ, Stokl M. Sheway's services for substance using pregnant and parenting women: evaluating the outcomes for infants. *Can J Commun Ment Health*. 2005;24(1):19–34.
183. Rosenbaum M, Irwin K. Pregnancy, drugs, and harm reduction. In: *Harm Reduction: National and International Perspectives*. SAGE Publications, Inc.; 2000:89–110.
184. Blandthorn J, Bowman E, Leung L, Bonomo Y, Dietze P. Managing opioid overdose in pregnancy with take-home naloxone. *Aust N Z J Obstet Gynaecol*. 2018;58(4): 460–462.
185. Haffajee RL, Cherney S, Smart R. Legal requirements and recommendations to prescribe naloxone. *Drug Alcohol Depend*. 2020;209:107896.
186. Academy of Perinatal Harm Reduction, National Harm Reduction Coalition. Pregnancy and substance use: a harm reduction toolkit. APHR. October 2022. Accessed March 4, 2025. https://www.perinatalharmreduction.org/toolkit-pregnancy-substance-use
187. El-Mohandes A, Herman AA, Nabil El-Khorazaty M, Katta PS, White D, Grylack L. Prenatal care reduces the impact of illicit drug use on perinatal outcomes. *J Perinatol*. 2003;23(5):354–360.
188. King C, Laynor G, McNeely J, et al. Strategies to improve delivery of equitable and evidence-informed care for pregnant and birthing people with a substance use disorder in acute care settings: a scoping review protocol. *PLoS One*. 2024;19(3): e0300183.
189. Smid MC, Terplan M. What obstetrician-gynecologists should know about substance use disorders in the perinatal period. *Obstet Gynecol*. 2022;139(2):317–337.
190. Lim G, Soens M, Wanaselja A, et al. A systematic scoping review of peridelivery pain management for pregnant people with opioid use disorder: from the society for obstetric anesthesia and perinatology and society for maternal fetal medicine. *Anesth Analg*. 2022;135(5):912–925.
191. Buresh M, Ratner J, Zgierska A, Gordin V, Alvanzo A. Treating perioperative and acute pain in patients on buprenorphine: narrative literature review and practice recommendations. *J Gen Intern Med*. 2020;35(12):3635–3643.
192. Jones HE, Johnson RE, Milio L. Post-cesarean pain management of patients maintained on methadone or buprenorphine. *Am J Addict*. 2006;15(3):258–259.
193. Vilkins AL, Bagley SM, Hahn KA, et al. Comparison of post-cesarean section opioid analgesic requirements in women with opioid use disorder treated with methadone or buprenorphine. *J Addict Med*. 2017;11(5):397–401.
194. Veazie S, Mackey K, Peterson K, Bourne D. Managing acute pain in patients taking medication for opioid use disorder: a rapid review. *J Gen Intern Med*. 2020;35(Suppl 3):945–953.
195. National Harm Reduction Coalition. Principles of harm reduction. Published online. 2020.
196. Park JN, Tomko C, Silberzahn BE, Haney K, Marshall BDL, Sherman SG. A fentanyl test strip intervention to reduce overdose risk among female sex workers who use drugs in Baltimore: results from a pilot study. *Addict Behav*. 2020;110:106529.
197. Laing MK, Tupper KW, Fairbairn N. Drug checking as a potential strategic overdose response in the fentanyl era. *Int J Drug Policy*. 2018;62:59–66.
198. American College of Obstetricians and Gynecologists. Committee Opinion No. 498: adult manifestations of childhood sexual abuse. *Obstet Gynecol*. 2011;118(2 Pt 1):392–395.
199. Committee on Health Care for Underserved Women. ACOG Committee Opinion No. 729: importance of social determinants of health and cultural awareness in the delivery of reproductive health care. *Obstet Gynecol*. 2018;131(1):e43–e48.
200. Organization WH. *Guidelines for the Identification and Management of Substance Use and Substance Use Disorders in Pregnancy*. World Health Organization; 2015.
201. Pinkham S. Speeding up the response: a global review of the harm reduction response to amphetamines. *Harm Reduct Int Glob State Harm Reduct*. Published online. 2011:97–104.
202. Socias ME, Cui Z, Le Foll B, et al. Sexually transmitted and blood-borne infection risk reduction with methadone and buprenorphine/naloxone among people with prescription-type opioid use disorder: findings from a Canadian pragmatic randomized trial. *HIV Med*. 2024;25(7):817–825.
203. Gibson B, Hoff E, Haas A, et al. Overlapping needs for sexual and reproductive health and HIV prevention in women with substance use disorders. *Womens Health (Lond)*. 2022;18:17455065211070543.

204. Aaron E, Cohan D. Preexposure prophylaxis for the prevention of HIV transmission to women. *AIDS Lond Engl.* 2013;27(1):F1–F5.
205. Calabrese SK, Willie TC, Galvao RW, et al. Current US guidelines for prescribing HIV pre-exposure prophylaxis (PrEP) disqualify many women who are at risk and motivated to use PrEP. *J Acquir Immune Defic Syndr.* 2019;81(4):395.
206. Souzdalnitski D, Snegovskikh D. Analgesia for the parturient with chronic nonmalignant pain. *Tech Reg Anesth Pain Manag.* 2014;18(4):166–171.
207. Xiong PT, Poehlmann J, Stowe Z, Antony KM. Anxiety, depression, and pain in the perinatal period: a review for obstetric care providers. *Obstet Gynecol Surv.* 2021;76(11): 692–713.
208. Krans EE, Campopiano M, Cleveland LM, et al. National partnership for maternal safety: consensus bundle on obstetric care for women with opioid use disorder. *Obstet Gynecol.* 2019;134(2):365–375.
209. Harris MTH, Laks J, Stahl N, Bagley SM, Saia K, Wechsberg WM. Gender dynamics in substance use and treatment: a women's focused approach. *Med Clin North Am.* 2022;106(1):219–234.
210. Ganetsky VS, Heil J, Yates B, et al. A low-threshold comprehensive shared medical appointment program for perinatal substance use in an underserved population. *J Addict Med.* 2022;16(3):e203–e209.
211. Schiff DM, Partridge S, Gummadi NH, et al. Caring for families impacted by opioid use: a qualitative analysis of integrated program designs. *Acad Pediatr.* 2022;22(1): 125–136.
212. Moreland AD, McRae-Clark A. Parenting outcomes of parenting interventions in integrated substance-use treatment programs: a systematic review. *J Subst Abuse Treat.* 2018;89:52–59.
213. Ramey-Collier K, Jackson M, Malloy A, McMillan C, Scraders-Pyatt A, Wheeler SM. Doula care: a review of outcomes and impact on birth experience. *Obstet Gynecol Surv.* 2023;78(2):124–127.
214. Hodnett ED, Gates S, Hofmeyr GJ, Sakala C. Continuous support for women during childbirth. *Cochrane Database Syst Rev.* 2007;(3):CD003766.
215. Gannon M, Short V, Becker M, et al. Doula engagement and maternal opioid use disorder (OUD): experiences of women in OUD recovery during the perinatal period. *Midwifery.* 2022;106:103243.
216. Olarewaju O, Tundealao S. Pregnancy and the rising challenge of opioid dependency: a summary of potential solutions. *Subst Use Misuse.* 2025;60(2):306–309.
217. Victora CG, Bahl R, Barros AJD, et al. Breastfeeding in the 21st century: epidemiology, mechanisms, and lifelong effect. *Lancet.* 2016;387(10017):475–490.
218. Chu L, McGrath JM, Qiao J, et al. A meta-analysis of breastfeeding effects for infants with neonatal abstinence syndrome. *Nurs Res.* 2022;71(1):54–65.
219. Chapman SLC, Wu LT. Postpartum substance use and depressive symptoms: a review. *Women Health.* 2013;53(5): 479–503.
220. Rutherford H, Williams S, Moy S, Mayes L, Johns J. Disruption of maternal parenting circuitry by addictive process: rewiring of reward and stress systems. *Front Psychiatry.* 2011;2:37.
221. D'Apolito K. Breastfeeding and substance abuse. *Clin Obstet Gynecol.* 2013;56(1):202–211.
222. Yonke N, Jimenez EY, Leeman L, Leyva Y, Ortega A, Bakhireva LN. Breastfeeding motivators and barriers in women receiving medications for opioid use disorder. *Breastfeed Med.* 2020;15(1):17–23.
223. Hicks J, Morse E, Wyant DK. Barriers and facilitators of breastfeeding reported by postpartum women in methadone maintenance therapy. *Breastfeed Med.* 2018;13(4): 259–265.
224. Nidey N, Groh K, Agnoli A, et al. Breastfeeding initiation and continuation among women with substance and tobacco use during pregnancy: findings from the pregnancy risk assessment monitoring system 2016–2018. *Breastfeed Med.* 2022;17(6):544–549.
225. Rangmar J, Lilja M, Köhler M, Reuter A. Children who face development risks due to maternal addiction during pregnancy require extra medical and psychosocial resources. *Acta Paediatr.* 2019;108(1):101–105.
226. Cottler LB, Nishith P, Compton WM. Gender differences in risk factors for trauma exposure and post-traumatic stress disorder among inner-city drug abusers in and out of treatment. *Compr Psychiatry.* 2001;42(2):111–117.
227. Jansson LM, Velez ML, Butz AM. The effect of sexual abuse and prenatal substance use on successful breastfeeding. *J Obstet Gynecol Neonatal Nurs.* 2017;46(3):480–484.
228. Howard MB, Wachman E, Levesque EM, Schiff DM, Kistin CJ, Parker MG. The joys and frustrations of breastfeeding and rooming-in among mothers with opioid use disorder: a qualitative study. *Hosp Pediatr.* 2018;8(12):761–768.
229. Jansson LM, Velez M, Harrow C. Methadone maintenance and lactation: a review of the literature and current management guidelines. *J Hum Lact.* 2004;20(1):62–71.
230. MacMillan KDL, Rendon CP, Verma K, Riblet N, Washer DB, Volpe Holmes A. Association of rooming-in with outcomes for neonatal abstinence syndrome: a systematic review and meta-analysis. *JAMA Pediatr.* 2018;172(4):345.
231. Harris M, Schiff DM, Saia K, Muftu S, Standish KR, Wachman EM. Academy of Breastfeeding Medicine clinical protocol #21: breastfeeding in the setting of substance use and substance use disorder (revised 2023). *Breastfeed Med.* 2023;18(10):715–733.
232. Department of Health and Human Services (HHS). *Management of Unique & Key Populations With HCV Infection.* Office of AIDS Research Advisory Council; 2024. https://clinicalinfo.hiv.gov/en/guidelines/perinatal/infant-feeding-individuals-hiv-united-states
233. AASLD, IDSA. HCV Guidance: Recommendations for Testing, Managing, and Treating Hepatitis C. 2020. https://www.hcvguidelines.org/unique-populations/pregnancy#: ~:text=Breastfeeding%20is%20not%20contraindicated%20in, the%20context%20of%20HIV%20coinfection.
234. Anderson PO. Breastfeeding with smoking cessation products. *Breastfeed Med.* 2021;16(10):766–768.
235. Allen S, Thomas J, Harrison K, et al. Bupropion for postpartum smoking relapse: a remote protocol for a two-arm, double-blind, placebo-controlled randomized clinical trial. *Contemp Clin Trials.* 2021;105:106352.
236. Ordean A, Kim G. Cannabis use during lactation: literature review and clinical recommendations. *J Obstet Gynaecol Can.* 2020;42(10):1248–1253.
237. Harris M, Joseph K, Hoeppner B, et al. A retrospective cohort study examining the utility of perinatal urine toxicology testing to guide breastfeeding initiation. *J Addict Med.* 2021;15(4): 311–317.
238. Wachman EM, Schiff DM, Silverstein M. Neonatal abstinence syndrome: advances in diagnosis and treatment. *JAMA.* 2018;319(13):1362–1374.
239. Patrick SW, Barfield WD, Poindexter BB. Neonatal opioid withdrawal syndrome. *Pediatrics.* 2020;146(5):e2020029074.
240. Hirai AH, Ko JY, Owens PL, Stocks C, Patrick SW. Neonatal abstinence syndrome and maternal opioid-related diagnoses in the US, 2010–2017. *JAMA.* 2021;325(2):146–155.

241. Winkelman TNA, Villapiano N, Kozhimannil KB, Davis MM, Patrick SW. Incidence and costs of neonatal abstinence syndrome among infants with Medicaid: 2004–2014. *Pediatrics*. 2018;141(4):e20173520.
242. Patrick SW, Schumacher RE, Benneyworth BD, Krans EE, McAllister JM, Davis MM. Neonatal abstinence syndrome and associated health care expenditures: United States, 2000–2009. *JAMA*. 2012;307(18):1934–1940.
243. Jilani SM, Jones HE, Grossman M, et al. Standardizing the clinical definition of opioid withdrawal in the neonate. *J Pediatr*. 2022;243:33–39.e1.
244. Jansson LM, Patrick SW. Neonatal abstinence syndrome. *Pediatr Clin North Am*. 2019;66(2):353.
245. Mascarenhas M, Wachman EM, Chandra I, Xue R, Sarathy L, Schiff DM. Advances in the care of infants with prenatal opioid exposure and neonatal opioid withdrawal syndrome. *Pediatrics*. 2024;153(2):e2023062871.
246. Young LW, Ounpraseuth ST, Merhar SL, et al. Eat, sleep, console approach or usual care for neonatal opioid withdrawal. *N Engl J Med*. 2023;388(25):2326–2337.
247. Wachman EM, Houghton M, Melvin P, et al. A quality improvement initiative to implement the eat, sleep, console neonatal opioid withdrawal syndrome care tool in Massachusetts' PNQIN collaborative. *J Perinatol*. 2020;40(10):1560–1569.
248. Charles MK, Cooper WO, Jansson LM, Dudley J, Slaughter JC, Patrick SW. Male sex associated with increased risk of neonatal abstinence syndrome. *Hosp Pediatr*. 2017;7(6):328–334.
249. Allocco E, Melker M, Rojas-Miguez F, Bradley C, Hahn KA, Wachman EM. Comparison of neonatal abstinence syndrome manifestations in preterm versus term opioid-exposed infants. *Adv Neonatal Care*. 2016;16(5):329–336.
250. Vernovsky S, Herning A, Wachman EM. The role of genetics in neonatal abstinence syndrome. *Semin Perinatol*. 2025;49(1):152006.
251. Patrick SW, Dudley J, Martin PR, et al. Prescription opioid epidemic and infant outcomes. *Pediatrics*. 2015;135(5):842–850.
252. Shadowen C, Wheeler R, Terplan M. Patient and provider knowledge of and attitudes toward medical conditions and medication during pregnancy. *Addict Sci Clin Pract*. 2021;16(1):22.
253. Jackson HJ, López C, Miller S, Englehardt B. Neonatal abstinence syndrome: an integrative review of neonatal acupuncture to inform a protocol for adjunctive treatment. *Adv Neonatal Care*. 2019;19(3):165–178.
254. Oostlander SA, Falla JA, Dow K, Fucile S. Occupational therapy management strategies for infants with neonatal abstinence syndrome: scoping review. *Occup Ther Health Care*. 2019;33(2):197–226.
255. McGlothen-Bell K, Cleveland L, Recto P, Brownell E, McGrath J. Feeding behaviors in infants with prenatal opioid exposure: an integrative review. *Adv Neonatal Care*. 2020;20(5):374–383.
256. McCarty T, Braswell E. Implementation of interprofessional rounds decreases neonatal abstinence syndrome length of stay. *J Pediatr Pharmacol Ther*. 2022;27(2):157–163.
257. Pahl A, Young L, Buus-Frank ME, Marcellus L, Soll R. Non-pharmacological care for opioid withdrawal in newborns. *Cochrane Database Syst Rev*. 2020;12(12):CD013217.
258. Lembeck AL, Tuttle D, Locke R, et al. Outcome differences in neonates exposed in-utero to opioids managed in the NICU versus pediatric floor. *J Addict Med*. 2019;13(1):75–78.
259. McQueen K, Taylor C, Murphy-Oikonen J. Systematic review of newborn feeding method and outcomes related to neonatal abstinence syndrome. *J Obstet Gynecol Neonatal Nurs*. 2019;48(4):398–407.
260. Alsaleem M, Berkelhamer SK, Wilding GE, Miller LM, Reynolds AM. Effects of partially hydrolyzed formula on severity and outcomes of neonatal abstinence syndrome. *Am J Perinatol*. 2020;37(11):1177–1182.
261. Pandey R, Kanike N, Ibrahim M, et al. Lactose-free infant formula does not change outcomes of neonatal abstinence syndrome (NAS): a randomized clinical trial. *J Perinatol*. 2021;41(3):598–605.
262. Bogen DL, Hanusa BH, Baker R, Medoff-Cooper B, Cohlan B. Randomized clinical trial of standard- versus high-calorie formula for methadone-exposed infants: a feasibility study. *Hosp Pediatr*. 2018;8(1):7–14.
263. Wachman EM, Grossman M, Schiff DM, et al. Quality improvement initiative to improve inpatient outcomes for neonatal abstinence syndrome. *J Perinatol*. 2018;38(8):1114–1122.
264. Davis JM, Shenberger J, Terrin N, et al. Comparison of safety and efficacy of methadone vs morphine for treatment of neonatal abstinence syndrome: a randomized clinical trial. *JAMA Pediatr*. 2018;172(8):741–748.
265. Devlin LA, Young LW, Kraft WK, et al. Neonatal opioid withdrawal syndrome: a review of the science and a look toward the use of buprenorphine for affected infants. *J Perinatol*. 2022;42(3):300–306.
266. Kraft WK, Gibson E, Dysart K, et al. Sublingual buprenorphine for treatment of neonatal abstinence syndrome: a randomized trial. *Pediatrics*. 2008;122(3):e601–607.
267. Hall ES, Isemann BT, Wexelblatt SL, et al. A cohort comparison of buprenorphine versus methadone treatment for neonatal abstinence syndrome. *J Pediatr*. 2016;170:39–44.e1.
268. Brown MS, Hayes MJ, Thornton LM. Methadone versus morphine for treatment of neonatal abstinence syndrome: a prospective randomized clinical trial. *J Perinatol*. 2015;35(4):278–283.
269. Hall ES, Meinzen-Derr J, Wexelblatt SL. Cohort analysis of a pharmacokinetic-modeled methadone weaning optimization for neonatal abstinence syndrome. *J Pediatr*. 2015;167(6):1221–1225.e1.
270. Morrison TM, MacMillan KDL, Melvin P, et al. Neonatal opioid withdrawal syndrome: a comparison of as-needed pharmacotherapy. *Hosp Pediatr*. 2022;12(5):530–538.
271. Wachman EM, Minear S, Hirashima M, et al. Standard fixed-schedule methadone taper versus symptom-triggered methadone approach for treatment of neonatal opioid withdrawal syndrome. *Hosp Pediatr*. 2019;9(8):576–584.
272. Brusseau C, Burnette T, Heidel RE. Clonidine versus phenobarbital as adjunctive therapy for neonatal abstinence syndrome. *J Perinatol*. 2020;40(7):1050–1055.
273. Surran B, Visintainer P, Chamberlain S, Kopcza K, Shah B, Singh R. Efficacy of clonidine versus phenobarbital in reducing neonatal morphine sulfate therapy days for neonatal abstinence syndrome. A prospective randomized clinical trial. *J Perinatol*. 2013;33(12):954–959.
274. Czynski AJ, Davis JM, Dansereau LM, et al. Neurodevelopmental outcomes of neonates randomized to morphine or methadone for treatment of neonatal abstinence syndrome. *J Pediatr*. 2020;219:146–151.e1.
275. Makarious L, Teng A, Oei JL. SIDS is associated with prenatal drug use: a meta-analysis and systematic review of 4 238 685 infants. *Arch Dis Child Fetal Neonatal Ed*. 2022;107(6):617–623.
276. Deutsch SA, Donahue J, Parker T, Hossain J, Loiselle C, De Jong AR. Impact of plans of safe care on prenatally substance exposed infants. *J Pediatr*. 2022;241:54–61.e7.
277. Arter SJ, Tyler B, McAllister J, Kiel E, Güler A, Cameron Hay M. Longitudinal outcomes of children exposed to opioids in-utero: a systematic review. *J Nurs Scholarsh*. 2021;53(1):55–64.

278. Nelson LF, Yocum VK, Patel KD, Qeadan F, Hsi A, Weitzen S. Cognitive outcomes of young children after prenatal exposure to medications for opioid use disorder: a systematic review and meta-analysis. *JAMA Netw Open.* 2020;3(3):e201195.
279. Gill AC, Oei J, Lewis NL, Younan N, Kennedy I, Lui K. Strabismus in infants of opiate-dependent mothers. *Acta Paediatr.* 2003;92(3):379–385.
280. Epstein RL, Sabharwal V, Wachman EM, et al. Perinatal transmission of hepatitis C virus: defining the cascade of care. *J Pediatr.* 2018;203:34–40.e1.
281. Benitz WE; Committee on Fetus and Newborn, American Academy of Pediatrics. Hospital stay for healthy term newborn infants. *Pediatrics.* 2015;135(5):948–953.
282. Institute Guttmacher. Substance use during pregnancy. 2021. https://www.guttmacher.org/gpr/2000/12/state-responses-substance-abuse-among-pregnant-women
283. Haffajee RL, Faherty LJ, Zivin K. Pregnant women with substance use disorders—the harm associated with punitive approaches. *N Engl J Med.* 2021;384(25):2364–2366.
284. Faherty LJ, Kranz AM, Russell-Fritch J, Patrick SW, Cantor J, Stein BD. Association of punitive and reporting state policies related to substance use in pregnancy with rates of neonatal abstinence syndrome. *JAMA Netw Open.* 2019;2(11):1–12.
285. Carroll JJ, El-Sabawi T, Ostrach B. The harms of punishing substance use during pregnancy. *Int J Drug Policy.* 2021; 98(2):103433.
286. Aspinwall C, Bailey B, Yurkanin A. They lost pregnancies for unclear reasons. Then they were prosecuted. The Washington Post. September 1, 2022. https://www.washingtonpost.com/national-security/2022/09/01/prosecutions-drugs-miscarriages-meth-stillbirths/
287. Augenstein K. The real war on families—an examination on American Child Welfare Law in the shadow of drug prohibition. *Ohio State Legal Studies Research Paper No. 698.* 2022.
288. Harp KLH, Bunting AM. The racialized nature of child welfare policies and the social control of black bodies. *Soc Polit.* 2020;27(2):258–281.
289. Work EC, Muftu S, MacMillan KDL, et al. Prescribed and penalized: the detrimental impact of mandated reporting for prenatal utilization of medication for opioid use disorder. *Matern Child Health J.* 2023;27(Suppl 1):104–112.
290. Smid MC, Maeda J, Stone NM, et al. Standardized criteria for review of perinatal suicides and accidental drug-related deaths. *Obstet Gynecol.* 2020;136(4):645–653.
291. Stone R. Pregnant women and substance use: fear, stigma, and barriers to care. *Health Justice.* 2015;3(1):1–15.
292. Roberts SC, Pies C. Complex calculations: how drug use during pregnancy becomes a barrier to prenatal care. *Matern Child Health J.* 2011;15(3):333–341.
293. Patrick SW, Schiff DM; COMMITTEE ON SUBSTANCE USE AND PREVENTION. A public health response to opioid use in pregnancy. *Pediatrics.* 2017;139(3):e20164070.
294. Suarez EA, Huybrechts KF, Straub L, et al. Postpartum opioid-related mortality in patients with public insurance. *Obstet Gynecol.* 2023;141(4):657–665.
295. Admon LK, Zivin K, Kozhimannil KB. Perinatal insurance coverage and behavioural health-related maternal mortality. *Int Rev Psychiatry.* 2021;33(6):553–556.
296. Morrison PK, Pallatino-Trevelline C, Fusco R, et al. Co-occurring substance use and intimate partner violence in pregnant and postpartum women: a systematic literature review. *J Fam Violence.* 2025;40(2):353–367.
297. El-Bassel N, Marotta PL, Goddard-Eckrich D, et al. Drug overdose among women in intimate relationships: the role of partner violence, adversity and relationship dependencies. *PLoS One.* 2019;14(12):e0225854.
298. Harris MT, Goldenberg S, Cui Z, et al. Association of sex work and social-structural factors with non-fatal overdose among women who use drugs in Vancouver, Canada. *Int J Drug Policy.* 2023;112:103950.
299. Holcomb LA, Maldonado L, Nietert PJ, et al. Examining the role of social determinants of health in maternal mental health screening and treatment engagement during the perinatal period. *Biol Sex Differ.* 2025;16(1):11.
300. Terplan M. Substance use and use disorder in pregnancy and postpartum. *Int Rev Psychiatry.* 2021;33(6):501.
301. Knight KR, Duncan LG, Szilvasi M, Premkumar A, Matache M, Jackson A. Reproductive (In)justice—two patients with avoidable poor reproductive outcomes. *N Engl J Med.* 2019; 381(7):593–596.
302. Alexander M. *The New Jim Crow: Mass Incarceration in the Age of Colorblindness.* 10th Anniversary ed. The New Press; 2020.
303. Goldenberg SM, Perry C, Watt S, Bingham B, Braschel M, Shannon K. Violence, policing, and systemic racism as structural barriers to substance use treatment amongst women sex workers who use drugs: findings of a community-based cohort in Vancouver, Canada (2010–2019). *Drug Alcohol Depend.* 2022;237:109506.

13

Substance Use Disorder Management in Adolescents

Deepa R. Camenga, Molly M. Perri, Sivabalaji Kaliamurthy

Fresh out of training, my first consult was for a young woman named Shelby, a 15-year-old female admitted to our children's hospital for the treatment of pelvic inflammatory disease (PID). All I knew was that during the admission, the resident team noted that she reported daily use of "weed and pain pills." The residents had heard me, the new addiction medicine physician in town, give a noon conference during the previous week and the next morning I received my first consult as a brand-new attending.

As I used my shiny new badge to enter the pediatric unit, I was immersed in the familiar charms of the pediatric hospital—babies crying, brightly colored walls, and parents and nurses crowded around hospital cribs. My patient was in a corner room (that perhaps would not be noticed by hospital visitors and guests). The nurse was outside, rapidly typing on the computer. I introduced myself and said I was the new addiction medicine consultant, to which they replied, "She's not in a good mood today," and returned to her charting.

The room seemed hot and dark when I entered. Shelby was underneath the blankets, facing the window with a bag of antibiotics hanging from her IV pole. I sat down and noticed the stuffed animal on her pillow and the picture of her and what I presumed to be her mom happily posed on her cracked cell phone screen. She turned around and looked at me wide eyed but seemed to relax after I explained I was from the addiction medicine consult service and was just here to provide support.

Just as we were beginning, the cell phone rang with the name "Mama" on the screen. Shelby picked up and said, "The doctor is here." I asked if I could speak with her mom, and on speakerphone, again introduced myself and my role. Mom said, "they need more of you out there, an addiction specialist who treats kids." She reminded Shelby to be honest and asked me to call her after I was done.

Shelby was quiet at first but then told me how she started taking "percs" about 2 years ago. They helped her deal with a "bad situation," which I later learned was a sexual assault by an older family member. She had tried to stop but described intolerable withdrawal symptoms whenever she tried. In addition to opioids, she had a history of vaping nicotine, cannabis, and trying benzodiazepines, alcohol, psilocybin, and LSD. She also had a history of being hospitalized after a suicide attempt last year, but she was unable to locate an outpatient psychiatric clinician and was managed by her primary care pediatrician, who was prescribing her low-dose fluoxetine.

Her history was consistent with opioid use disorder (OUD), nicotine use disorder, and cannabis use disorder. She had not been using any other substances recently, so I was confident she was withdrawing only from opioids. The diagnosis was the easy part, now I had to figure out how to execute a basic treatment plan. I had done it a hundred times during fellowship but needed to figure out how to get it done at my new institution. I thanked her for speaking with me and said I would come back later with a plan to help her.

As I exited the room, I remembered that my office had a brand-new whiteboard with my first to-do list, #1 being to develop a protocol for OUD management in pediatric patients. The hospital did not have active protocols in place to adequately address opioid withdrawal symptoms, so I realized that my note and treatment plan would be the first prototype of one.

I ran to the workroom and asked the residents what they knew about OUD. They all talked about "a patient I saw in med school" but said they "never saw" a pediatric patient with OUD. I asked them to help me put in some orders and quickly learned that we had to send her urine sample to an external lab to test for the presence of fentanyl. I had them download a Clinical Opioid Withdrawal Scale (COWS) calculator on their phones and ran over the signs and symptoms of withdrawal. We decided to use clonidine to help alleviate some of her symptoms as it was available on formulary. After some investigation, I learned that buprenorphine was not on the hospital formulary and would require "special permission" from the Director of Pharmacy.

I did not know how to find that person, so I added that to my growing list of to dos. My next stop was the nurses. They quickly routed me to the nurse manager who explained to me that their nurses were not "trained" to use the COWS, and that we should transfer Shelby to another hospital. She must have been concerned with my expression, as she quickly told me to show her how to do it and she would make sure the bedside nurse would obtain the COWS every 4 hours.

The next 24 hours were filled with phone calls with what seemed like every director, manager, and department head within the hospital during which I uncovered the treatment gaps that hospitalized adolescents face every day. As Shelby received her last IV dose of antibiotics for PID, the case management team discovered that there were no evidence-based treatment programs for minors with OUD that accepted the patient's insurance. After Shelby's COWS scores started to downtrend (and with several back-and-forth emails with American Society of Addiction Medicine [ASAM] and American Academy of Pediatrics [AAP] clinical practice guidelines attached), the pharmacy team reported that if I entered a nonformulary order request, they could order the buprenorphine from an outside institution and have it ready by tomorrow. As Shelby eventually started asking to take walks outside of her room, I also learned that, unlike what was suggested by the other team members, she could not be transferred to a psychiatric bed because she did not present with an acute psychiatric concern. However, the case management team discovered that the resident clinic in psychiatry was willing to see Shelby if I continued managing the buprenorphine.

In the end, it was Shelby's mom, who also was in recovery, who advocated for Shelby to receive the standard of care. After multiple emails, 2 hours of phone calls, several impromptu "teaching rounds," and many, many thank yous, Shelby successfully initiated buprenorphine in the hospital. Her mother would bring Shelby to my new "Adolescent Clinic." With Shelby as my first patient, I checked off the #1 on my to-do list.

—Sivabalaji Kaliamurthy

Key Points

- **Despite declining prevalence of substance use among the general population of adolescents, hospitalizations for substance-related complications in adolescents have increased over time.**
- **Validated screening tools like Car-Relax-Alone-Forget-Friends-Trouble (CRAFFT), Screening to Brief Intervention (S2BI), and Brief Screener for Tobacco, Alcohol, and Other Drugs (BSTAD) can accurately identify adolescents at risk for substance use disorders (SUDs).**
- **Unique aspects of evaluating substance use in hospitalized adolescents include managing confidentiality and consent, involving parents, screening for co-occurring mental health disorders, and recognizing mandated reporting requirements.**
- **Evidence-informed treatment approaches for adolescents with SUD include psychoeducation, harm-reduction counseling, and pharmacologic treatments for specific substances (eg, buprenorphine for OUD, nicotine-replacement therapy [NRT] for nicotine).**
- **Hospital-based SUD screening and treatment models that are specific to adolescents are emerging to include screening, risk stratification, evaluation, hospital-based treatment and interventions, and referral to ongoing treatment.**

Adolescent substance use remains a leading public health problem that contributes to a high burden of preventable morbidity and mortality in this age group. Although the prevalence of alcohol and substance use are declining in this population (see Figure 13.1),[1,2] the overall morbidity and mortality related to adolescent substance use has increased over the past decade. Substance-related poisonings are now the third leading

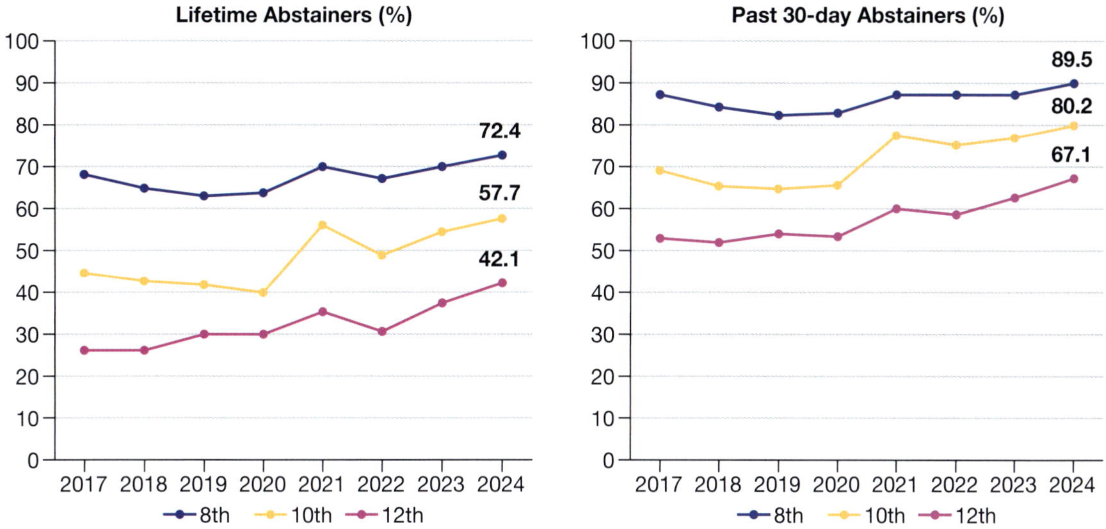

Figure 13.1: Prevalence of abstaining from all substances among 8th-, 10th-, and 12th-grade US students. (Data from Meich RA, Johnston LD, Patrick ME, O'Malley PM. *Monitoring the Future. National Survey Results on Drug Use, 1975–2024: Overview and detailed results for secondary school students*. 2025.)

cause of death in young people aged 10 to 19 years old in the United States.[3] Substance use also contributes to other leading causes of death in adolescents, including motor vehicle crashes and suicide.[4] Similar to adults, alcohol, cannabis, and nicotine are the most common substances used by youth in the United States.[5] In 2023, the prevalence of past month substance use among 12th graders was 41.7% for alcohol, 25.8% for cannabis, 21% for nicotine vaping, and 6.8% for any illicit substance other than cannabis.[5]

While many social and environmental factors contribute to adolescent substance use, the adolescent brain's unique vulnerability to both experimenting with and continuing to use substances makes this developmental period critical for prevention and intervention. During adolescence, the human brain undergoes considerable neuroplasticity and uneven maturation of the reward circuitry and the prefrontal cortex.[6] As a result, substance exposure during this time tends to enhance reward responses while diminishing aversive effects from substances, which amplifies the reinforcing effects of substances on the adolescent brain. Moreover, substance use can negatively impact neurodevelopment and impair crucial functions related to reward processing, decision making, and impulse control. These neurodevelopmental consequences are linked to an increased risk of SUDs, mental health disorders, and other health-risking behaviors.

Although most adolescents who try substances do not develop a SUD, in 2023, 8.5 million adolescents aged 12 to 17 years reported symptoms of a SUD.[5] Onset of substance use at younger ages strongly correlates with the increased severity and chronicity of SUDs that persist into adulthood.[7,8] Epidemiologic data also repeatedly demonstrate that a lower age of substance use initiation is associated with poorer health, occupational, social, and educational outcomes over the life course. For example, early initiation of substance use can lead to a series of interconnected challenges, including difficulty with memory and concentration, leading to poor school performance[9] and thus limited employment and future earning potential. Of note, over the past two decades, the mean age of initiation of substance use has increased.[10]

Even youth who do not have a SUD are at risk of experiencing harm related to substance use. The ubiquity of high-potency synthetic opioids like fentanyl in the unregulated substance supply, the emergence of counterfeit pills, and the increasing potency of nicotine and cannabinoid products, combined with the ease of accessing substances through online and digital sources, have led to substance-related complications rising in adolescents who are substance naive. Consequently, there is a consensus that there is no known "safe" level of substance use during the active neuromaturation that occurs during adolescence. In other words, during this critical developmental period, any amount of substance use, regardless of quantity, has the potential to harm health.

In general, substance use treatment services for adolescents are lacking across the care continuum. For example, whereas >90% of pediatricians report asking adolescents about substance use, less than half report using a validated screening tool (under review).[11] Nationally, about 40% of adolescents with a SUD had received any form of treatment in the past year.[6] Access to medications for SUD is limited for adolescents as well. Less than 5% of adolescents with opioid use disorder (OUD) receive medications for OUD (MOUD),[12] and less than 2% of adolescents who use tobacco or nicotine products receive NRT.[13] A study of 160 US residential substance use treatment facilities for adolescents found that only one in eight offered buprenorphine for OUD treatment.[14] Further, a 2022 survey of adolescent residential facilities that treat adolescent OUD found that 10 states and Washington DC do not have any facilities that provide MOUD.[15]

As such, hospitalizations present an important opportunity to intervene on adolescent substance use and SUD. Health care systems, especially hospitals, traditionally have not considered the identification and management of SUD as part of routine pediatric hospital care. As of 2024, no empirical data describes the landscape of screening, SUD treatment, or presence of addiction consultative services for hospitalized children in the United States. However, a 2024 study of nine Canadian children's hospitals found that addiction medicine–related hospital practices varied widely, including those related to screening, medications for SUD, and substance withdrawal management services.[16] This study also found that four of the surveyed Canadian children's hospitals had a consultative service that could potentially address substance use and SUD, with adolescent medicine being the most cited resource.[16]

This chapter will review the unique aspects of the inpatient management of adolescents admitted with substance-related complications and SUD. First, the chapter will summarize the published evidence outlining the epidemiology of SUD in hospitalized adolescents. The evidence review will focus on medical hospital settings. However, given the paucity of literature in this area, the findings from psychiatric inpatient settings will also be reviewed when directly relevant. Second, the chapter will discuss models of care and the unique aspects of caring for hospitalized adolescents, focusing on legal, ethical, and practical issues when treating minors. Finally, the chapter will summarize the clinical approach to common conditions that result in substance-related hospitalizations for adolescents. This chapter represents one of the first summaries of best practices for the care of adolescents admitted to hospitals with substance-related concerns. Because the application of hospital-based SUD treatment principles to pediatric hospital settings is relatively new, many of the management approaches outlined herein, like many clinical approaches within pediatrics, are guided by research conducted in adults and informed by expert experience and consensus.

Epidemiology of Substance Use Disorder and Related Hospitalizations among Adolescents

Overall, only a small percentage of adolescents who use substances will be admitted to the hospital with a primary substance-related diagnosis. However, data suggest that many adolescents hospitalized for other reasons may actually have a SUD. For example, a 2016 analysis of the Kids Inpatient Database, which includes a nationally representative sample of hospital discharges in the United States, found that nearly 10% of hospitalized patients aged 13 to 19 years had a SUD listed in their discharge diagnoses.[17] Unsurprisingly, with the escalating impact of substances on adolescent morbidity and mortality, substance-related emergency department (ED) visits, and hospitalizations have increased over the past decade for this patient population. In adolescents, SUD can contribute to hospitalizations for various reasons, including, but not limited to, substance-specific intoxication, alcohol or substance-related withdrawal, unintentional overdose, intentional overdose, respiratory complications, and exacerbation of mental health conditions.[18]

An analysis of 106,793 substance-related visits involving 84,632 youth within the Pediatric Hospital Inpatient Sample database found that between 2016 and 2021, substance-related visits increased by 47.9% across demographic groups, regions, and payors.[19] Much of this trend was attributed to the 82.4% increase in cannabis-related hospitalization. Overall, cannabis was the cause of 52.2% of all substance-related hospitalizations during this period, indicating that cannabis is the most common substance involved in substance-related hospitalizations in this age group. Of added concern, an analysis of claims data from >500,000 individuals in Canada found that a new diagnosis of cannabis use disorder during a hospitalization was associated with increased all-cause 5-year mortality, with especially high risk of death by suicide, opioid poisoning, or other drug poisoning.[20]

After cannabis, nicotine is the second most common substance involved in hospitalizations, accounting for about one in four adolescent substance-related presentations.[19] The emergence of electronic-cigarettes (e-cigarettes) has been correlated with an escalation in nicotine-related hospitalizations related to nicotine poisonings, e-cigarette or vaping-associated lung injuries, and exacerbations of other respiratory conditions, such as asthma.

Although alcohol is the most common substance used by US adolescents, it ranks third overall in causing ED visits and hospitalizations for this age group. This differs from adult data, where alcohol is the most frequently implicated substance in ED visits and hospitalizations.[21] Rates of alcohol use among adolescents have dropped significantly over the past few decades. For instance, in 1991, 77.7% of 12th graders reported consuming alcohol in the past year, whereas in 2023, less than half of 12th graders (45.7%) reported past-year alcohol use.[5] Reflecting this trend, there has not been a significant increase in alcohol-related hospitalizations among adolescents, despite an overall rise in substance-related hospitalizations.[19]

Opioid, stimulant, and hallucinogen-related hospital presentations have also increased over the past few years. The increase in hospital visits for opioids mirrors the rise in adolescent mortality from opioid overdose events.[13] As illicitly manufactured high-potency synthetic opioids like fentanyl have become more prevalent, there is a greater risk of opioid overdose events and death in adolescents due to exposure. There is also a risk of exposure through contamination of high-potency synthetic opioids in other substances.[22] Adolescent overdoses also commonly involve stimulants and sedative hypnotics.

Identification and Evaluation of Substance Use and SUD in the Hospitalized Adolescent

Identifying Adolescent Substance Use

Many adolescents with SUD have not been formally identified or diagnosed. As such, clinicians may not readily consider substance use as contributing to their initial hospital presentation, especially when patients present with an acute concern that is not immediately recognized as related to substance use. In addition, electronic health record (EHR) documentation of a patient's past substance use may not be accurate. A study conducted in a children's hospital found low concordance between EHR documentation and self-reported substance use (ie, concordance rates of 15% for nicotine, 18% for cannabis, 9% for alcohol, and 9% for illicit substances).[23] Thus, the first step in providing high-quality SUD care for hospitalized adolescents is to accurately identify patients who may be at risk for SUD or who have unhealthy substance use.

Validated Screening Tools Unhealthy Substance Use in Adolescents

Screening is a crucial component in identifying patients who may benefit from SUD evaluation and treatment. The American Academy of Pediatrics (AAP) and the American Academy of Child and Adolescent Psychiatry (AACAP) recommend screening adolescents for unhealthy substance use and SUD risk using validated, frequency-based screening tools.[24] The United States Preventive Services Task Force (USPSTF) does not yet recommend routine screening of adolescents for substance use, citing insufficient evidence.[25] To date, research has yet to validate substance use screening tools specifically for adolescents in the hospital setting. The discrepancies in professional guidance, along with gaps in workforce training and reimbursement for screening in the hospital setting, may contribute to the under recognition of substance use among hospitalized adolescents, even though recommendations for screening by AAP and AACAP have remained consistent for over a decade.

Nonetheless, there are potential benefits to implementing universal screening for substance use in all hospitalized adolescents. The HEADDSS (Home, Education, Activities, Drugs, Suicidality, Sex) and SSHADESS (**S**trength, **S**chool, **H**ome, **A**ctivities, **D**rugs/Substance Abuse, **E**motion/Depression, **S**exuality, **S**afety)[26,27] are overarching strengths-based frameworks to organize the adolescent psychosocial history. They are not validated screening tools and should not be used for SUD risk screening but can be used to gain a broad overview of the social–environmental context contributing to an individual's substance use. As part of psychosocial history, the clinician can use an interviewer- or self-administered validated questionnaire to screen for substance use. Screening tools such as the Screening to Brief Intervention (S2BI), Brief Screener for Tobacco, Alcohol, and Drugs (BSTAD), and tobacco, alcohol, prescription medication and other substance use (TAPS) are validated substance use screening tools for adolescents ages 12 to 17 years.[28–30] However, the validation studies for these tools were primarily conducted in pediatric primary care and outpatient specialty substance use clinics; more data are needed on their use in hospital settings. For patients who screen positive for any substance use, the additional Car-Relax-Alone-Forget-Family-Trouble (CRAFFT) screening tool can provide further information to determine risk levels and appropriate interventions.[31,32] Unlike the previously mentioned screening tools, the CRAFFT has been validated among adolescents in hospital-based adolescent clinics, as well as ED and inpatient settings.[33,34] To date, no studies have investigated whether hospital-based screening improves substance use or treatment outcomes.

There is a gap in training and preparedness to screen and treat adolescents for unhealthy substance use. Although pediatric clinicians in multiple treatment settings acknowledge the need to address adolescent substance use, they also cite barriers, including time constraints, inadequate staffing, and concerns about parental reactions to screening.[35] Despite the opportunity, clinicians infrequently or incompletely document the substance use history during hospital encounters for adolescents.[36,37] For example, in the ED, less than half of clinicians used a validated tool when screening adolescents for alcohol use.[38] Several studies in children's hospitals have shown that tobacco, alcohol, and cannabis use history is documented in less than 30% of adolescent patients' hospital admission notes.[37,39,40]

In 2007, the American College of Surgeons Committee on Trauma (ACS-COT) recommended that all adolescent trauma patients be universally screened for alcohol use during their hospital visit.[29] A systematic review of seven studies of pediatric trauma centers found that when accounting for all methods of identifying substance use (via a combination of biologic testing [$n = 5$ studies], clinician interview [$n = 2$ studies], and the validated CRAFFT screening tool [$n = 3$ studies]), 26% to 45% of pediatric trauma patients were screened for alcohol use and 10% to 47% for illicit substance use.[41] Of note, biologic testing is not recommended as the primary form of screening for substance use, although SUD risk screening protocols for pediatric trauma patients may incorporate this data.[42] An implementation study of seven pediatric trauma centers found that technical assistance activities (including the creation of a screening, brief intervention, and referral to treatment [SBIRT] policy for admitted adolescent trauma patients, an online curriculum, an in-person workshop, and monthly conference calls) increased SBIRT rates for eligible patients from 11% to 73%.[33] Institutions also have successfully improved the screening rate through didactics, performance feedback, external facilitation, and self-screening technology.[42–44]

Given the existing evidence, it is reasonable to use a validated frequency-based screening tool to identify unhealthy substance use among adolescents admitted to the hospital. As noted later in this chapter, the validated screening tools can be administered by various team members, including nurses, behavioral health clinicians, social workers, and medical clinicians. Although universal screening is suggested for adolescents in the outpatient settings, it is currently unclear whether universal screening of all admitted adolescents is more feasible or effective than targeted screening of higher-risk populations (ie, adolescents admitted with injuries, primary psychiatric concerns). Nonetheless, the data demonstrates that validated screening tools improve the rates of identifying unhealthy substance use, and it is reasonable to recommend their use in hospitalized adolescents.

Assessment of SUD in the Adolescent Patient

Confidentiality and Consent

Most hospitalized minors are accompanied by a parent who may have variable knowledge of the extent of the adolescent's substance use history. Confidentiality and consent are guided by a combination of federal and state laws.[45] On a national level, confidentiality around SUD treatment is governed by federal law 42 code of federal regulations (CFR) Part 2, which allows adolescents in states not requiring parental consent for SUD treatment who have not reached the legal age of majority (18 years in most states) to receive confidential treatment.[46] However, exceptions apply if there is an imminent risk of harm to the patient or others, including concerns of child abuse or neglect. Primary care clinicians' or hospital-based general clinicians' (eg, pediatricians, internists) documentation of the pertinent substance use information is protected by health insurance portability and accountability act (HIPAA) but is not covered by 42 CFR Part 2. Specialty addiction medicine or psychiatry clinicians' documentation of substance use for a patient in an outpatient federally funded health care setting does merit protection under the 42 CFR Part 2 confidentiality regulations. In the hospital setting, HIPAA applies to most clinicians, however addiction medicine consultative services may be covered under 42 CFR Part 2. Clinicians should consult with their institution to determine if this is appropriate for their local context.

In general, the ability to consent to SUD treatment follows from confidentiality.[45] As of 2022, 36 states allowed minors to consent for SUD treatment, 2 did not specify whether minors could consent, and 15 had minimum age requirements.[47] In addition, state-based laws may require parental notification for specific aspects of treatment (eg, use of medications) or that the adolescent assumes responsibility for the costs associated with confidential SUD care.[47] Thus, the treatment team should understand how confidentiality laws apply to the specific patient and setting, which may require consultation with risk management or hospital legal services.

That said, if an adolescent requires hospitalization for a substance-related concern, it most likely indicates that the adolescent's substance use is at a level that has resulted in harm, in which case it is highly recommended to involve a parent. There are also many practical reasons to involve parents in adolescent's health care, such as insurance barriers, transportation needs, and coordinating outpatient care. The use of patient portals adds an additional layer of complexity to maintaining confidentiality, as the 21st Century Cures Act prohibits "information blocking" and requires patients to be able to view their medical notes. Studies have shown that more than half of adolescents' patient portals are accessed by parents, suggesting that their medical notes are susceptible to confidentiality breaches.[48,49] Some EHRs allow for "chart segmentation," or the documentation of confidential aspects of care in sections of the EHR that are not shown on the patient portal. However, many health information systems remain without this functionality.

In summary, if an adolescent reports a history of substance use or SUD during a non–substance-related hospital admission, the clinician must weigh the risks and benefits of maintaining confidentiality in this setting. Maintaining confidentiality generally shows respect for the adolescent's growing autonomy and independence and improves the likelihood that the adolescent will provide an accurate history. On the other hand, parents have many practical reasons to be involved. As such, when working with an adolescent in this situation, the clinician should attempt to gauge how the adolescent believes their parents might react and whether the adolescent's safety may be compromised, as this can inform the timing and approach for involving family members.

Involving Families

When involving the parent or guardian in the initial consultation, it is important to honor the adolescents' privacy, autonomy, and decision-making abilities. Figure 13.2 presents an overview of the workflow of the substance use evaluation with an adolescent and a parent. The clinician might start the visit by explaining to the patient and parent why they have been asked to evaluate the adolescent. They might then explain that they will speak to the patient and parent individually and then discuss the plan with everyone. When meeting with the adolescent alone, the clinician should review the limits of confidentiality before obtaining the substance use history and performing any brief motivational interventions. They should also clarify with the adolescent which aspects of their history they can share with their parents, taking into account the limits of confidentiality. When meeting individually with the parent or caregiver (hereunto referred to as parent), the clinician can obtain collateral information related to the history of previous SUD treatment, listen to the parent's concerns, and confirm any personal or family history of SUD. Parents may express feelings of guilt, fear, or anger, and it is important for the clinician to provide empathy and support while also sharing evidence-based information to dispel myths and provide a clear understanding of adolescent SUD. Offering parents resources and tools, such as the Community Reinforcement and Family Training (CRAFT) model or the Partnership to End Addiction's online tools (available at https://drugfree.org/), can prepare them to support their child more effectively. In addition, directing parents to support groups like the National Alliance on Mental Illness, Al-Anon, and Narc-Anon can provide ongoing community support as they navigate their child's treatment journey.

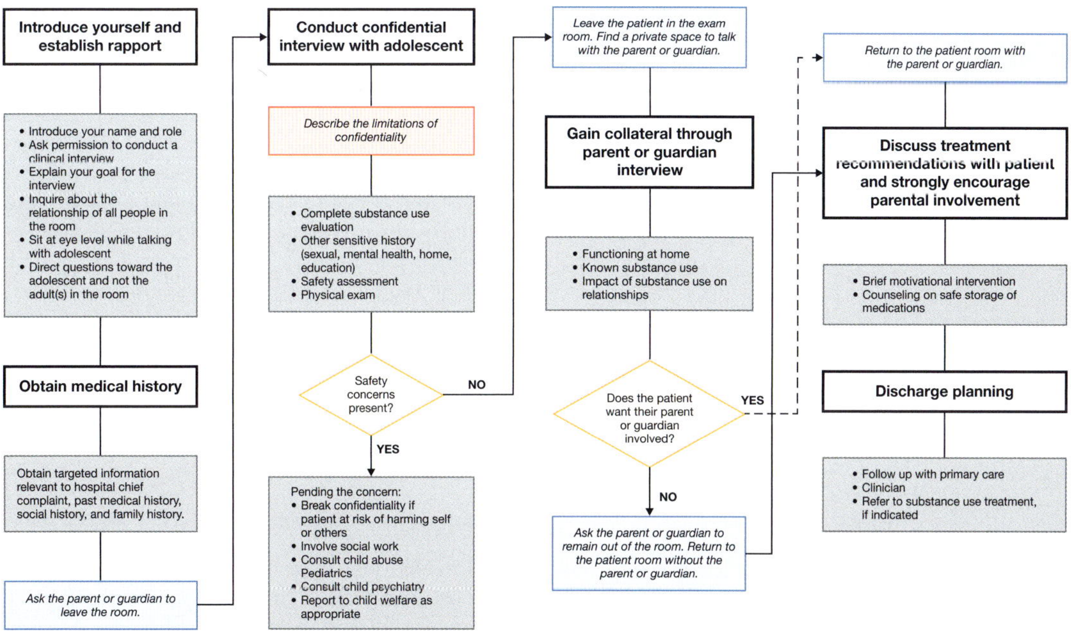

Figure 13.2: Suggested workflow for the adolescent evaluation in the hospital setting.

Diagnosing SUD

The clinician can use the Diagnostic and Statistical Manual of Mental Disorders-5 (DSM-5) criteria for SUD to determine whether an adolescent has mild, moderate, or severe SUD.[50] The criteria are the same for adolescents and adults, although some argue the DSM does not incorporate a developmental perspective into its criteria.[51] Traditionally, addiction practitioners viewed withdrawal symptoms as a phenomenon arising from prolonged substance use, and therefore, adolescents rarely experienced such symptoms. In the context of the current substance supply, wherein it is typical for adolescents to initiate substances with high potency (eg, nicotine, cannabis, and opioid products), our clinical experience suggests that adolescents do experience symptoms of withdrawal even after shorter periods of use. When assessing for negative consequences of substance use, some adolescents may minimize the impacts of their substance use on their function and relationships. Collateral information from parents may further clarify whether the adolescents' substance use is impacting school, activities, or family relationships. If the evaluation does not indicate any social consequences of use, the clinicians can weigh whether the lack of social consequences is secondary to parent permissiveness around substance use (eg, parents allowing the child to use substances) or parent enablement through consequence mitigation (eg, advocating for law enforcement not to ticket an adolescent who drives impaired).

In some cases, an adolescent may be hospitalized for a substance-related complication, but their presentation does not meet diagnostic criteria for SUD. For example, an individual may be admitted after a fentanyl overdose, but the history reveals that the overdose was secondary to fentanyl contamination of illicitly manufactured "prescription" medication and there is no evidence of OUD. Another example would be if an adolescent overconsumes alcohol during their first episode of drinking and sustains a significant injury while driving under the influence of alcohol. In general, if an adolescent presents with a substance-related complication without SUD, the clinician should provide psychoeducation and counseling (including overdose prevention counseling, if indicated) as outlined later in the chapter and use brief motivational strategies to enhance motivation to minimize/stop ongoing substance use.

Screening for Comorbid Mental Health Conditions

Comorbid mental health conditions are present in nearly half of hospital admissions attributed to substance use.[52] Similarly, SUD is present in 25% to 33% of adolescents admitted for psychiatric concerns.[48,53] Substance use can also trigger psychiatric emergencies, such as first-episode psychosis or the development of suicidal ideation.[54–56] Substance use also plays a role in the pathology of completed suicide; in 2021, 40% of suicide decedents who were tested for alcohol and substances had a positive toxicology for alcohol at the time of death.[57] Thus, if not already completed, any evaluation of SUD should concomitantly screen for depression and suicidality and consider screening for adverse childhood experiences and trauma, as these factors can significantly impact an adolescent's vulnerability to further escalation of substance use. Prompt involvement of child psychiatry may be needed if concern for suicidality arises during the substance use evaluation.

Concerns for Child Abuse/Neglect

In addition to assessing for suicidality, when completing the substance use evaluation with a minor, it is important to screen for any concerns of child abuse/neglect. The US Child Abuse Prevention and Treatment Act defines child abuse and neglect as: "Any recent act or failure to act on the part of a parent or caretaker which results in death, serious physical or emotional harm, sexual abuse or exploitation"; or "An act or failure to act which presents an imminent risk of serious harm." In all US states, if a health care clinician knows of or suspects child abuse or neglect, they are required by law as mandated reporters to report the alleged child maltreatment to child welfare agencies.[58] Asking about how the adolescent pays for substances may raise suspicion of gang involvement or exchanging sex for substances, all of which heighten concerns for child neglect and may necessitate the involvement of child welfare or other services. If safety concerns arise, collaboration with child and adolescent psychiatry, child abuse pediatrics, or social work professionals may be needed to create a treatment and discharge plan that addresses immediate risks and establishes a safe discharge environment that supports recovery.

Brief Interventions and Counseling Approaches

Evidence Supporting Brief Interventions

Brief interventions have been the most studied substance use intervention in the outpatient, emergency care, or psychiatric hospital setting.[43–45] A 2020 meta-analysis of brief behavioral interventions in these settings found that, compared to treatment as usual, motivational interviewing (MI)-based brief interventions reduced past-month alcohol use and heavy drinking days among adolescents, but did not impact cannabis use. The approach to MI with adolescents is largely similar to that used with adults, emphasizing the patient's autonomy and encouraging them to take ownership of their decisions by creating a nonjudgmental and empathetic environment. It is important to remember that for many hospitalized adolescents, the hospital admission may serve as the first encounter wherein they discuss their substance use with a health care clinician; therefore, it is natural that the young patient may need some support in identifying the pros and cons of substance use, as well as feasible and realistic goals around their substance use.

Because the American Academy of Surgeons' Committee on Trauma recommends that level 1 trauma centers integrate a brief intervention for adolescent trauma patients who screen positive for substance use,[59] many brief interventions for hospitalized adolescents have been piloted within ED-based trauma services. For example, one study of a hospital-based and nurse-delivered brief intervention demonstrated a significant change in trauma patients' belief that drinking alcohol will negatively affect health.[60] In the trauma setting, brief interventions have varied widely in duration, structure, and delivery mode. For example, interventions have been delivered by mental health professionals[51] or via computer[52,53] and have varied utility in reducing adolescent substance use.

Psychoeducation and Harm-Reduction Counseling

Harm-reduction strategies tailored for adolescents are another important component of care. Given the known neurodevelopmental risks associated with adolescent-onset substance use, a major focus of SUD treatment is on the cessation and reduction of substance use. However, a large portion of adolescents, like adults, may not aim to cease all substance use, but instead aim to minimize harms from use. Harm-reduction counseling can occur in parallel to providing clear advice about the harms of adolescent substance use and benefits of cessation. Table 13.1 includes potential messages that could be covered in the psychoeducation and harm-reduction education that can be provided to both the adolescent and their parent during SUD treatment counseling.

As outlined in Table 13.1, both the teen and the parent should be counseled to never drive under the influence of alcohol, cannabis, or other substances. Adolescents and young adults have the highest motor

TABLE 13.1

Psychoeducation and Harm-Reduction Education for Adolescents and Parents

Substance	Psychoeducation for adolescent and parents	Harm-reduction education for adolescent	Harm-reduction education for parents
Cannabis	■ Risks of adolescent cannabis use (links with mental health disorders, psychosis, and impacts on learning and memory, sleep) ■ Signs and symptoms of cannabis intoxication or overdose ■ Signs and expected time course of cannabis withdrawal ■ Difference between dispensary products vs nondispensary products ■ Variable quality and labeling of cannabis dispensary products ■ High potency of some cannabis products like tinctures, edibles, dabs ■ Contamination of drug supply with fentanyl	Strongly Recommend: ■ Never drive impaired ■ Do not ride with an impaired driver Recommend: ■ 2-wk tolerance break ■ No use of high-potency cannabis products like tinctures, dabs, and others	Strongly Recommend: ■ Never allow child to operate vehicle if using cannabis ■ Remove all cannabis products from home ■ Do not use cannabis around child

(continued)

TABLE 13.1

Psychoeducation and Harm-Reduction Education for Adolescents and Parents (*Continued*)

Substance	Psychoeducation for adolescent and parents	Harm-reduction education for adolescent	Harm-reduction education for parents
Nicotine (vaped or smoked)	▪ Risks of adolescent nicotine use (links with asthma, exercise intolerance, development of SUD, alternations in executive function) ▪ Signs and expected time course of nicotine withdrawal ▪ For vaping: variable quality and labeling of e-cigarette/vaping products	Suggest: ▪ 2-wk tolerance break ▪ Use of nicotine replacement therapy during school days, or on alternating days ▪ Commit to not buying a new tobacco product/vaping device	Recommend: ▪ Remove nicotine products from home ▪ Do not use nicotine products around children
Alcohol	▪ Risks of adolescent alcohol use (poisoning, intoxication associated with injuries, unwanted sexual contact, violence) ▪ If relevant, signs and expected time course of alcohol withdrawal	Strongly recommend: ▪ Never drive impaired ▪ Do not ride with an impaired driver Suggest: ▪ Preplanning for social events when alcohol may be present	Recommend: ▪ Never allow the child to operate a vehicle if drinking alcohol ▪ Remove alcohol products from home ▪ Do not use alcohol around children ▪ Encourage parents to support adolescents in calling for a ride without punishment
Opioids	▪ Contamination of drug supply (including counterfeit pills) with fentanyl ▪ Signs of opioid overdose ▪ Good Samaritan laws ▪ Availability of naloxone over the counter	Strongly recommend: ▪ Never use alone ▪ Carry naloxone and use it when needed ▪ Call 911 if you suspect an overdose ▪ Use of fentanyl test strips	Strongly recommend: ▪ Lock all over-the-counter and prescription medications in the home ▪ Carry naloxone and use it when needed
All substances	▪ Short- and long-term impacts of SUD on adolescent brain development ▪ How SUD develops and progresses without treatment ▪ Treatment options and expectations ▪ Contamination of drug supply with fentanyl ▪ For parents: educate on potential sources of substance acquisition (peers, social media, mail)	Avoidance of pills due to the risk of fentanyl contamination	Recommend: ▪ Family involvement in treatment ▪ Lock all over the counter and prescription medications in the home ▪ Consider monitoring social media use ▪ (If relevant) supervise adolescent during the administration of prescription medications

vehicle fatality rate of any age group, and alcohol is implicated in nearly 20% of fatalities,[61] highlighting the importance of encouraging parents to work with teens to arrange for sober drivers or rideshare. Regarding opioids, providing naloxone to both the adolescent and their parents and offering counseling on its use can be lifesaving and empower families to respond effectively in the prevention and care of overdose. Counseling on safe substance use practices and avoiding high-risk situations can further reduce harm. Parents have an important role in providing a safe home environment after hospital discharge, and they can be encouraged to remove all substances from the home, not use substances around their child, and lock all over the counter and prescription medications. Resources such as the Stanford Safety First Curriculum can aid these harm-reduction goals.[62]

SUD Treatment Linkage After Hospitalization

Determining the appropriate level of care for adolescent substance use, as recommended by the American Society of Addiction Medicine (ASAM) criteria, is an important role for clinicians providing hospital-based SUD care and connection to treatment. If available, options include office-based care, intensive outpatient or partial hospital programs for moderate needs, and residential treatment for those requiring a more structured environment. Ideally, treatment would address SUD and mental health treatment needs concurrently. A scoping review of 30 peer-reviewed studies examining studies of interventions for concurrent disorders in youth aged 10 to 29 years identified several promising interventions that impacted SUD and mental outcomes; however, due to the heterogeneity of the included studies it was not possible to determine which were most effective.[63] Regardless, the review identified several promising approaches for co-occurring disorders, such as cognitive behavioral therapy, motivational enhancement therapy, and family therapies (multidimensional family therapy, assertive community reinforcement approach coupled with assertive continuing care, functional family therapy). Further supporting this, a meta-analysis from 2020 of outpatient psychosocial treatments for adolescent substance use also concluded that these same therapies were most likely efficacious.[64]

Overall, there is a paucity of literature on effective methods of linking adolescents to appropriate SUD treatment after acute substance-related hospitalizations. At least one study has shown it is feasible for trained health promotion advocates to perform brief interventions and provide referrals and resources related to substance use.[65] There is also strong evidence base for the assertive continuing care model, which facilitates outpatient SUD treatment linkage for adolescents being discharged from residential SUD treatment.[66,67] This model uses weekly in-home case management visits to connect families to needed SUD outpatient services and adolescents to prosocial activities. These intensive models have not been modified for the hospital setting.

In reality, finding an appropriate level of SUD care is often a rate-limiting step for hospital discharge due to the lack of appropriate services in most geographic regions. Although the treatment gap is due to many factors, including stigma,[2] treatment readiness or willingness,[2,3] cost,[4] and public lack of confidence that treatment will be effective,[5] the overall lack of services for adolescent SUD treatment is a major barrier. Between 2021 and 2023, an analysis of the 2017 National Survey of Substance Abuse Treatment Services identified 3,527 facilities that provided programming for individuals less than age 18 years, of which >90% were SUD outpatient level of care.[68] Only 25% of the facilities accepted Medicaid or offered MOUD. Of those that offered MOUD, nearly 50% were located in the Northeast, indicating geographic disparities in SUD treatment access. As such, anyone providing SUD treatment in the hospital setting must understand the local landscape of adolescent SUD treatment services, including any eligibility criteria for admission.

Behavioral and Pharmacologic Treatment Considerations for Adolescents

Many aspects of the medical management of substance-related harms among adolescents in the hospital setting are similar to those of adults. This section will review the existing evidence around behavioral approaches and medications for SUD in adolescents less than age 18 years, with a focus on cannabis, nicotine, alcohol, and opioids. The behavioral approaches reviewed herein are specific to adolescents and limited to those that are most feasible to implement within a hospital setting. Because there are very few clinical trials that have tested medications for SUD in adolescents, with the exception of buprenorphine, all other medications have not been approved for SUD treatment.[10] Thus, the suggestions for pharmacotherapy are based on the small emerging evidence base and clinical experience. As most adolescents weigh enough not to need weight-based dosing, medication dosing suggestions are based on those for adults, with the caveat that younger patients tend to respond to the lower end of the dosing range. In all cases, clinicians should consider the use of the proposed medications on a case by case basis with shared decision making and clear education on the potential benefits and risks of any medications.[68]

Cannabis

Cannabis contributes to the majority of substance-related hospitalizations for adolescents in the United States, with common diagnoses including cannabis-induced psychosis, cannabinoid hyperemesis syndrome (CHS), or respiratory illnesses associated with smoking or vaping cannabis. In children, cannabis-induced psychosis is primarily managed by child

TABLE 13.2

Medication Options for Cannabis-Related Symptoms[a] and Cannabis Use Disorder

Medication	Dose range	Frequency	Notes
For vomiting associated with cannabinoid hyperemesis syndrome (CHS)			
Topical capsaicin cream	Strength 0.1%, apply pea size amount to the abdomen	Every 2–4 h	May cause initial burning sensation. Provides relief by desensitizing TRPV1 receptor
Droperidol	0.625–2.5 mg IV/IM	Every 4–6 h as needed	Antiemetic. Monitor for QTc prolongation, especially at higher doses
Haloperidol	0.5–5 mg IV/IM/PO	Every 6–12 h as needed	Antiemetic. Lower doses (0.5–1 mg) more effective for CHS. Higher doses may increase risk of extra pyramidal symptoms and QTc prolongation. Monitor for sedation and akathisia.
Lorazepam	0.5–1 mg IV/PO	Every 4–6 h as needed	Antiemetic, avoid if possible in children
Diazepam	1–2.5 mg IV/PO	Every 4–6 h as needed	Antiemetic, avoid if possible in children
Aprepitant	125 mg PO Day 1 80 mg PO Days 2–3	Once daily up to 3 d	Often needs prior authorization or may not be on hospital formulary
Amitriptyline or other tricyclic antidepressants	10–75 mg PO	At bedtime	To prevent recurrent CHS episodes. Monitor for anticholinergic side effects including but not limited to dry mouth, constipation, urinary retention, and sedation
For symptoms of Cannabis Withdrawal			
Gabapentin	300–1,800 mg/d PO	Divided three times a day	May help with anxiety, irritability, and sleep disturbances. Start low (eg, 200 mg TID) and titrate based on symptoms
Hydroxyzine	25–100 mg/d PO	Divided twice a day or three times a day	May help with insomnia, restlessness, and anxiety. Common doses: 25–50 mg QHS for sleep, 10–25 mg TID PRN for anxiety
For cannabis use disorder			
***N*-acetylcysteine (NAC)**	1,200–2,400 mg PO	Twice a day	May help with reducing cannabis use and cravings via modulation of glutamate homeostasis

[a]All suggested medications have been used by the authors off label for adolescents, on a case by case basis. Medications should only be prescribed after careful consideration of risks and benefits and using shared decision making with the adolescent and family.

TRPV1, transient receptor potential vanilloid 1.

psychiatry, although addiction medicine consults and generalists can collaborate on treatment planning around cannabis cessation and the management of withdrawal. Medications such as hydroxyzine or gabapentin may help alleviate cannabis withdrawal-related symptoms that arise during hospitalizations, such as sleep disturbances or anxiety (see Table 13.2).

Cannabinoid Hyperemesis Syndrome

A common indication for medical hospitalization is CHS. CHS is characterized by cyclic episodes of nausea, vomiting, and abdominal pain in the setting of regular cannabis use. A case series of 34 patients aged 13 to 20 years who were diagnosed with CHS found that, unlike in adults, there was a female predominance of presentations (60% female)[69] in the pediatric population. Among the 50% of patients with documented length of cannabis use, the median length was 42 months (range 3 to 93). Among the 70% of patients with documented frequency of cannabis use, the median frequency of use was 21 times per week. Amount and type of cannabis consumed, and method of consumption were rarely documented. The etiology, diagnosis, and management of cannabinoid hyperemesis are further discussed in Chapter 10.

As in adults, acute management of CHS in adolescents focuses on alleviating nausea, vomiting, and abdominal pain, which are key characteristics of this syndrome.[70] Strategies for acute management include fluid administration, electrolyte repletion, antiemetics, and the use of topical capsaicin cream. As symptoms improve, dietary intake can be gradually increased as tolerated. Ondansetron, droperidol, haloperidol, and benzodiazepines have been used as antiemetics. Aprepitant, a neurokinin 1 receptor antagonist commonly used for treating cyclical vomiting syndrome and chemotherapy-induced nausea and vomiting, has also been employed for treatment-refractory emesis in CHS.[38] The only known definitive treatment is cannabis cessation. A case series of 85 patients with CHS found that 62/62 patients with toxicology-confirmed cannabis cessation had complete resolution of symptoms, whereas 21 who did not abstain and 2 who did not have confirmatory urine testing had ongoing symptoms.[70] Finally, tricyclic antidepressants (TCAs) have often been used in the treatment of CHS due to significant overlap of symptoms with cyclical vomiting syndrome, a condition where TCAs (specifically amitriptyline) have shown benefit, there are no studies looking at their efficacy in patients with CHS.

In addition to medical stabilization, hospitalization offers an opportunity to educate patients about the hypothesized mechanisms of CHS (eg, regular cannabis use leading to endocannabinoid dysregulation) and emphasizes that cessation is the only known effective treatment. Adolescents may face recurrent CHS with ongoing cannabis use, which may or may not be linked to cannabis use disorder. Symptom misattribution (attributing symptoms to dietary choices or other medical causes), beliefs in strain-specific tolerance, the perception that episodes can be prevented by using certain levels or types of cannabis, and barriers to accessing cessation treatments may also contribute to continued cannabis use in the context of CHS. Besides treating gastrointestinal symptoms, hospital-based interventions may also include psychoeducation, MI, mental health assessments, and connections to outpatient SUD treatment and mental health services.

Cannabis Use Disorder Treatment

For adolescents who have developed cannabis use disorder, features of which include loss of control over use, physiologic dependence, failing social obligations, and continued use despite negative consequences, relevant interventions include MI, symptomatic treatment of cannabis withdrawal, and a referral to treatment for cannabis use disorder.

There is currently no Food and Drug Administration (FDA)-approved treatment for cannabis use disorder. To date, *N*-acetylcysteine (NAC) and topiramate are the only two medications that have been tested among adolescents with cannabis use disorder. An RCT of NAC (1,200 mg twice daily) combined with contingency management and brief weekly cessation counseling found increased cannabis abstinence among adolescents. Youth who received NAC were 2.4 times more likely to submit negative urine cannabinoid tests over the treatment period than those who received placebo.[71] Given its relatively low side-effect profile, NAC may be a safe adjunct to other therapeutic interventions for cannabis use disorder. Another RCT tested the impact of topiramate combined with motivational enhancement therapy in treatment seeking individuals (aged 15 to 24 years), but high-dropout rates due to topiramate's side effect burden limited the ability to study its effect. Importantly, both studies used behavioral treatments such as contingency management and motivational enhancement therapy. Referral to treatment after hospitalization should include programs that can offer these types of interventions in addition to management of co-occurring mental illness, if present, and medication treatment of cannabis use disorder. Programs that can monitor cannabis cessation via urine drug testing may also be helpful.

Nicotine

Adolescents can present to the hospital with complications arising from the use of a variety of tobacco products, including combustible cigarettes, cigars, and electronic nicotine delivery systems (ie, e-cigarettes or vapes). E-cigarettes are the most common tobacco product used among adolescents and can directly contribute to hospital admissions for e-cigarette or vaping product use–associated lung injury (EVALI). E-cigarettes and combustible tobacco products can also contribute to asthma exacerbations or other respiratory conditions. Finally, adolescents admitted for other reasons might also experience nicotine withdrawal symptoms due to forced abstinence.

Overall, the hospital-based evaluation of tobacco use among adolescents has several nuanced differences from that of adults. First, the original versions of the CRAFFT, S2BI, and BSTAD screening tools did not include questions around vaping. However, newer versions of the CRAFFT (the CRAFFT 2.1+N) do include vaping as an example of a tobacco product. Similarly, updated versions of the S2BI and BSTAD that include vaping in the examples of tobacco or cannabis use have been shown to accurately identify nicotine and cannabis vaping.[35] Thus, the clinician needs to be aware of the exact version of the screening tool that is used and confirm whether nicotine and cannabis exposures are from vaping, smoking, or oral products (pouches, cannabis edibles). Second, the

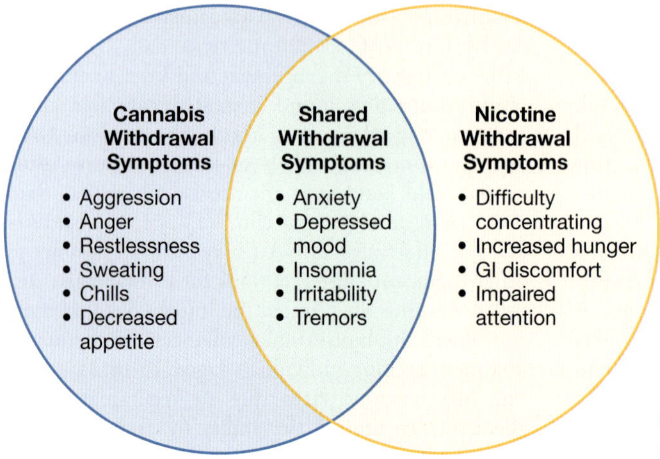

Figure 13.3: Cannabis and nicotine withdrawal symptoms.

co-use of cannabis (vaped or smoked) and nicotine (vaped or smoked) is very common in this population. Thus, when assessing for a use disorder or withdrawal, it is important to carefully evaluate whether the noted withdrawal symptoms may be secondary to cannabis or nicotine. Because the symptoms overlap considerably (see Figure 13.3), it can be helpful to ask the adolescent to describe how they experience withdrawal from nicotine versus cannabis and whether they think the symptoms they are experiencing in the hospital are due to nicotine, cannabis, or both. Finally, the amount of nicotine delivered into the body varies based on multiple factors. Due to these reasons, the amount of nicotine an adolescent is exposed to, the severity of tobacco use disorder, and the treatment of withdrawal symptoms can be challenging. See Chapter 9 for more information about tobacco use disorder treatment.

Substantial evidence supports the benefits of medications and behavioral interventions for smoking cessation among adults.[72] Of relevance to adolescents, the USPTF concluded in 2020 that the evidence is currently insufficient to assess the risks and benefits of tobacco cessation interventions for adolescents younger than 18 years.[73] Similarly, although multiple FDA-approved medications exist for adult tobacco use disorder, to date, there are no FDA-approved medications for the treatment of tobacco use disorder in adolescents.[72] Only three studies in the 2020 USPSTF systematic review evaluated the effectiveness of pharmacotherapy (bupropion and NRT) for tobacco use disorder among adolescents younger than 18 years.[73] In all three trials, there were no significant differences between intervention and control groups for tobacco abstinence. A double-blind RCT with 157 adolescents who smoked cigarettes comparing varenicline and placebo for tobacco use disorders similarly found that the groups randomized to varenicline and placebo did not differ in the primary outcome of cotinine-confirmed self-reported 7-day abstinence at the end of treatment.[74] The trials also did not show any safety concerns with the use of NRT in adolescents, however. Given the safety profile of NRT and the well-known consequences of untreated tobacco use disorder, this evidence base informed the AAPs' guidance recommending the prescription of NRT to adolescents with moderate or severe tobacco use disorder.[75]

Several published studies have started to examine approaches to nicotine-vaping cessation in youth. For example, an RCT of 1,503 adolescents aged 13 to 17 years found that a text messaging program (Truth Initiative's This is Quitting program) increased the point prevalence of self-reported e-cigarette abstinence from 28% among the control group to 37% in the intervention group.[75] A randomized clinical trial of 261 youth aged 16 to 24 years (mean age = 21.4 years) who vaped nicotine daily or near daily compared the effectiveness of varenicline with incentivized remote peer-delivered cognitive behavioral therapy–based counseling (peer support) and referral to a text messaging vaping cessation program (peer support), placebo with incentivized peer support and text messaging, or text messaging only.[76] Varenicline-randomized youth experienced substantially higher levels of biochemically confirmed abstinence than those randomized to placebo or text messaging only (51% vs 14% and 6%) during weeks 9 through 12, suggesting that varenicline may be effective for vaping cessation when combined with peer support.[76]

Taken together, these data indicate that several interventions can be offered to hospitalized adolescents with tobacco use disorder. Given the safety profile of NRT and the well-known consequences of untreated tobacco use, NRT can be offered to adolescents with moderate to severe tobacco use disorder,

TABLE 13.3

Medication Options for Adolescents With Nicotine Withdrawal Symptoms or Nicotine Use Disorder

Form of nicotine replacement therapy	Moderate dependence	Severe dependence
Nicotine transdermal patch	Start with 14 mg patch applied once daily and then step down	Start with 21 mg patch applied once daily and then step down
Nicotine lozenge	2 mg every 1–2 h as needed	4 mg every 1–2 h as needed
Nicotine gum		
Varenicline (for nicotine vaping cessation)	Can be titrated to 1 mg twice daily over 7 d (standard titration),[a] then 1 mg twice daily for 12 wk[a]	

[a]Tested in 1 RCT of 16–25-year-old youth.[76]

as defined by DSM-5 criteria. Further, at least one trial suggests that varenicline is effective for nicotine-vaping cessation in older adolescents and young adults.[76] Table 13.3 outlines NRT dosing recommendations from the AAP as well as varenicline dosing. Whereas NRT dosing is guided by cigarettes per day, the dosing of NRT for nicotine-vaping cessation is based on the severity of dependence symptoms, which can be measured with the Hooked on Nicotine Checklist, E-Cigarette Dependence Scale, or Modified Fagerstrom Tolerance Questionnaire.[77] Of note, NRT is available over the counter for adults aged 18+, however can be dispensed to minors with a prescription. Some adolescents may decline longer-term use of NRT; nonetheless, short courses of NRT can be offered to help with withdrawal symptoms that arise during hospitalization. Additionally, clinicians can recommend that hospitalized adolescents enroll in text-based vaping cessation programs or counseling services for tobacco cessation, if available. Additional clinical resources for youth tobacco cessation are available at Tobacco Use: Considerations for Clinicians (www.aap.org/cessation). This guide is based on expert consensus and reflects the current evidence on behavioral and pharmacologic options for youth tobacco use disorder.

Alcohol

Alcohol is a major contributor to hospitalizations among adults; however, it is a less common cause of hospitalization among adolescents. Key risk factors for alcohol withdrawal included daily alcohol use, previous alcohol withdrawal symptoms, early age of initiation, family history of alcohol use disorder (AUD), co-occurring psychiatric conditions, using multiple substances or nonethanol forms of alcohol, and poor nutritional status. Clinical literature on alcohol withdrawal syndrome management in adolescents is limited to a few case reports and series.[78–80] For example, the largest published case series of youth with alcohol withdrawal included 130 patients under age of 21 years, of whom 17 were between 14 and 17 years.[80] Overall, 77% of these patients were admitted for suicidality, 8.5% for trauma, and 4.6% for non–alcohol-related conditions. Within this sample, 22% required admission to an intensive care unit for alcohol withdrawal management, 40% received benzodiazepines, 2% developed delirium tremens, and 3.4% experienced seizures related to alcohol withdrawal.

Alcohol withdrawal in adolescents, similar to adults, is primarily monitored with the Clinical Institute Withdrawal Assessment for Alcohol, revised (CIWA-Ar) and managed using benzodiazepines, titrated based on withdrawal severity as assessed by the CIWA-Ar.[81] Case reports have described the use of phenobarbital in minors with benzodiazepine-refractory alcohol withdrawal; however, our clinical experience suggests that complicated withdrawal in this population is an uncommon occurrence.[78] At least one case report has described fixed-dose benzodiazepine tapers to prevent alcohol withdrawal in adolescents with AUD.[79]

In general, behavioral treatments are considered first-line for the treatment of AUD. All hospitalized adolescents should receive a brief intervention for alcohol use, and those with AUD should be linked to ongoing treatment at the needed level of care. To date, only one RCT has examined the effectiveness of medications for AUD among adolescents. This study tested NAC in treating AUD among 126 adolescents and young adults aged 13 to 25 years (mean age of 21 years).[82] Youth randomized to 1,200 mg NAC twice daily for 8 weeks reported drinking an average of 37.9 drinks during weeks 5 to 8, whereas those randomized to placebo drank 42.6 drinks. Two additional clinical trials have examined the effect of naltrexone on adolescent alcohol use, but did not require a diagnosis of AUD for participation. The first trial included 22 adolescents aged 15 to 19 years in a within-subject, randomized, double-blind, placebo-controlled crossover trial of 50-mg oral naltrexone.[83] This trial included adolescents who drank at least twice in the past month. Naltrexone use resulted in within-subjects reductions in the likelihood of drinking and heavy drinking and was generally well tolerated by participants. The second trial included data from 128 young adults aged 18 to 25 years who reported four or more binge drinking episodes per month.[84] In this trial, 25 mg oral naltrexone daily (+25 mg naltrexone once daily as needed prior to drinking) did not reduce drinking or binge drinking frequency, however the young adults in the naltrexone arm did report reduced numbers of drinks per drinking day, compared to young adults randomized to placebo (~5 vs ~6 drinks per drinking day). In practice, the rates of prescribing medications for AUD among adolescents are very low. An analysis of claims data from 3,669 Medicaid-enrolled youth aged 13 to 17 years with AUD, found that, between 2014 and 2019, <1% were prescribed either naltrexone, disulfiram, or acamprosate.[85]

In summary, alcohol withdrawal is rare in adolescents and is primarily treated with benzodiazepines. Adolescents with AUD should receive psychoeducation and harm-reduction counseling per Table 13.1, as well as referral to ongoing behavioral treatments, such as family-based therapies, MI, and CBT. Currently, there is not enough evidence to determine which medications are indicated for the treatment of AUD in adolescents. Due to the overall safety of NAC and naltrexone, it may be reasonable to offer these medications to hospitalized adolescents with the caveat that they are aware that there is limited data on their effectiveness long term. Currently, very few pediatric medical clinicians manage either of these medications in the outpatient setting, and if an adolescent is interested in continuing these medications as an outpatient, referral to addiction medicine or psychiatry specialists may be necessary.

Opioids

Adolescents admitted for opioid-related issues frequently present following unintentional or intentional overdoses, often involving synthetic opioids such as fentanyl. Hospitalizations may also occur for other complications of opioid withdrawal, such as malnourishment, dehydration, complicated detoxification, and injection-related infections. The Clinical Opioid Withdrawal Scale (COWS), though not validated in adolescents, is still of utility and can be used to assess opioid withdrawal symptoms. Opioid withdrawal is managed with a combination of pharmacologic and supportive interventions. Commonly used nonopioid medications for opioid withdrawal are outlined in Table 13.4.

Buprenorphine and methadone both treat opioid withdrawal and OUD. In the United States, buprenorphine is the only FDA-authorized medication for adolescents with OUD aged 16 through 17 years and therefore is considered a first-line treatment for OUD. It can also be used for younger children, provided state laws permit it. Three RCTs (with $n = 56$ participants <age 18 across all three trials) demonstrate the safety and efficacy of buprenorphine in reducing opioid use and improving treatment retention among adolescents with OUD in outpatient settings.[86–90] Despite the evidence, less than 5% of adolescents are prescribed buprenorphine, and Black and Hispanic adolescents are even less likely than their White counterparts to receive it. Furthermore,

TABLE 13.4

Medication Options for the Symptomatic Management of Opioid Withdrawal

Drug	Dosing		Targeted symptom
Clonidine	Taper option: 0.2 mg PO every (Q) 6 h × 4 d 0.1 mg PO Q6h × 2 d 0.05 mg PO Q12h × 1 d	As needed option: 0.1 mg PO Q4h COWS >10 (Do not exceed 1.2 mg/24 h)	Agitation, sympathetic overdrive
Loperamide	4 mg PO × 1, then 2 mg PO Q6h as needed (PRN)		Diarrhea
Dicyclomine	20 mg PO Q6h PRN		Abdominal cramps
Ondansetron	8 mg PO Q6h PRN		Nausea/vomiting
Prochlorperazine	10 mg PO Q6h PRN		Nausea/vomiting/anxiety
Ibuprofen	400 mg PO Q6h PRN		Myalgia
Acetaminophen	650 mg PO Q6h PRN		Myalgia
Hydroxyzine	25 mg PO Q6h PRN		Anxiety

unlike the trends observed for adults, overall rates of buprenorphine dispensing for adolescents decreased between 2015 and 2020, although rates increased slightly between 2020 and 2023.[12,91]

Thus, it is arguable that hospital admissions present one of the key access points for adolescents to initiate buprenorphine. At least one study has demonstrated the feasibility of pediatric hospitalists initiating buprenorphine on a pediatric medical unit within a safety net hospital.[92] The study reported on 46 hospital admissions among 12- to 21-year-old patients with OUD. Using a standard buprenorphine initiation protocol, 87% of these admissions resulted in patients successfully initiating buprenorphine, and 72% resulted in linkage to ongoing treatment occurring within 2 weeks. The buprenorphine initiation protocol recommended administering 8 mg of buprenorphine for COWS ≥8 and then administering additional 8 mg doses every 1 hour until the COWS score was <8.[92] It is currently unknown whether certain dosing strategies are more or less effective or appropriate for adolescents, and real-word clinical protocols for hospital-based buprenorphine initiation for adolescents can slightly vary (see Chapter 7 for examples of hospital-based buprenorphine initiation protocols).

Several studies have shown that methadone can be safely used in adolescents, and, like adults, it is effective in decreasing opioid use and increasing treatment retention.[86] However, the feasibility of integrating methadone into the treatment of hospitalized adolescents is limited. Federal guidelines require written consent from a parent/guardian before starting methadone for minors in opioid treatment programs (OTPs). Further, most OTPs do not offer methadone to minors. However, as of 2024, two unsuccessful withdrawal management attempts are no longer required for people under age 18 to be admitted to OTP services, making hospital-initiated methadone a potential treatment option if there is parental consent and an accepting OTP.[93] These nuances should be discussed with the patient and guardian as part of informed consent prior to initiating methadone. Extended-release naltrexone is another option with evidence supporting its use in adolescents, but due to the requirement of complete detoxification from opioids (a process that takes 5 to 10 days), it will likely be harder to treat adolescents with this treatment in the hospital setting.

Other Substance Use

Adolescents may also present to the hospital with medical complications arising from the use of other substances, such as amphetamines, hallucinogens, over-the-counter medication, or inhalants (gases containing nitrous oxide, butane, nitrites, aerosols, or volatile solvents). In these cases, management often focuses on the acute stabilization of any toxidromes and symptomatic management of anxiety, insomnia, irritability, and aggression while hospitalized. Evidence for the use of medications to treat SUD stemming from these substances is limited.

Additional Considerations When Prescribing Medications for Addictions in Adolescents

Availability of Medications on Hospital Formularies

No medication is FDA approved to treat SUD among patients younger than 16 years of age. As such, many pediatric hospitals do not have these medications in their formulary because many are only approved for patients over 18 years old, making them less of a priority for the general pediatric patient population. To address this, we recommend that clinician advocate for hospitals that serve children to include NRT, buprenorphine, methadone, naltrexone, and naloxone as a minimum on their formularies to support treatment of adolescent SUD.

Confidentiality and Consent for Pharmacotherapy

Even though most states allow adolescents to receive confidential care for SUD, some states require parental or guardian consent for the prescription of any medications. Further, adolescent confidentiality laws do not typically cover insurance claims and may reveal details of prescriptions or treatments. For some adolescents, notifying their parent of their SUD limits their willingness to receive a prescription. For young adults over 18 years old, prescribing medication does not require parental consent. However, if a young adult is dependent on their parent's health insurance, their parent may access information about medications or other treatments through the explanation of benefits. If an adolescent chooses to assume responsibility for treatment costs without parent or guardian insurance, they must pay out of pocket, and many adolescents do not have a sustainable income source.

Continuing Medications for SUD After Discharge

Another consideration when starting a medication for adolescents is the scarcity of outpatient prescribers. Of the outpatient SUD treatment that serves adolescents, very few prescribe MOUD.[8] In 2020, pediatricians made up only 1% of the prescribers writing buprenorphine prescriptions to patients less than 19 years old.[23] Historically, Family Medicine, Psychiatry, and Internal Medicine clinicians have written most buprenorphine prescriptions to patients less than 19 years old. However, now that the prescribing authority has been expanded to nurse practitioners and physician assistants,[24] the prescriber group writing the most buprenorphine prescriptions is nurse practitioners (27%).[23] Thus, nurse practitioners and physician assistants are essential partners in expanding adolescent SUD treatment in the hospital and as outpatient partners to continue treatment plans initiated in the hospital.

Models of Adolescent Hospital-Based SUD Screening and Treatment

There are no published comprehensive admission-to-discharge models of adolescent hospital-based SUD screening and treatment. A comprehensive model for hospitals presented below can be adapted to different programs depending on local context and resources. Case examples describe how the model could be applied in two settings: an academic children's hospital and a pediatric trauma center.

Overview of the Model

As seen in Figure 13.4, a model for hospital-based SUD care for adolescents includes five components: (1) screening, (2) risk stratification, (3) diagnostic evaluation, (4) intervention, (5) referral to treatment. When implementing the model, hospitals should consider where each domain may take place (ED, inpatient medical unit, inpatient psychiatric unit), who is responsible for each task, and what resources are available postdischarge to support ongoing care.

Hospital SUD treatments and interventions include brief counseling interventions, psychoeducation, and harm-reduction counseling. They can be delivered by a variety of team members and may include pharmacotherapy. In general, the literature supports the use of brief motivational interventions in the hospital setting.[94,95] Psychoeducation and harm-reduction counseling ideally would involve families (see Table 13.1). Finally, in preparation for discharge, all hospitalized adolescents with SUD should be referred for ongoing SUD treatment at the appropriate level of care. Discharge planning should include a discussion about safe substance use, storage, and disposal of medication after use, particularly if a patient is discharged with a controlled substance. It also includes counseling on harm-reduction, overdose-risk, and overdose-prevention education.

Case Examples

Herein, two examples are presented on how this model could be applied to two distinct settings (see Figure 13.5). The first example illustrates the workflow within a children's hospital in an academic medical center. The larger hospital serves adults and has dedicated pediatric units staffed by pediatric hospitalists and nurses, a consult liaison Child Psychiatry team, social workers trained in the SBIRT model, and an addiction medicine consult team that sees both adults and children. In this setting, all patients admitted to the children's hospital who are 12 years old or older are screened for SUD risk (universal screening). First nursing administers the S2BI questionnaire. The results of the screening triage patients into either a lower, tobacco use, or a higher-risk group. The higher-risk group is defined by the S2BI risk cut-offs for SUD, and includes patients who report monthly, weekly, or daily use of substances (other than tobacco) over the past 12 months. If a patient is in the tobacco use group, nursing will alert the primary pediatric team, who can access a detailed EHR-embedded clinical pathway with detailed guidance on the evaluation and treatment of tobacco and nicotine use disorder in adolescents. If a patient is in the higher-risk group, the nurse will place a social work consult. Social work will then meet with the patient, determine whether there are any substance-related problems (the CRAFFT) and complete screening for mental health, history of opioid use, history of overdose, prior illicit pill use, parental awareness of substance use, imminent risks to the patient's life, and prior/current SUD treatment. The social worker and primary team can then use the criteria outlined in Figure 13.4 to determine whether a consultation with Child Psychiatry and/or Addiction Medicine is necessary. The consultation criteria were jointly drafted by the Child Psychiatry and Addiction Medicine service based on local service capacity and expertise. If an addiction medicine consultant is involved, they conduct the brief intervention and recommend additional treatments, including pharmacotherapy. Child Psychiatry, on the other hand, takes primary responsibility for managing acute psychiatric concerns. Ultimately, all team members contribute to the discharge planning process.

The second example is based on a model that was implemented across 10 pediatric trauma centers to improve rates of screening and intervention for substance use (Figure 13.5).[42] This model is primarily implemented by nurses and social workers, although medical clinicians order urine and blood toxicology for pediatric trauma patients per pre-established trauma protocols.[59] This model only focuses on screening pediatric trauma patients for SUD risk and,

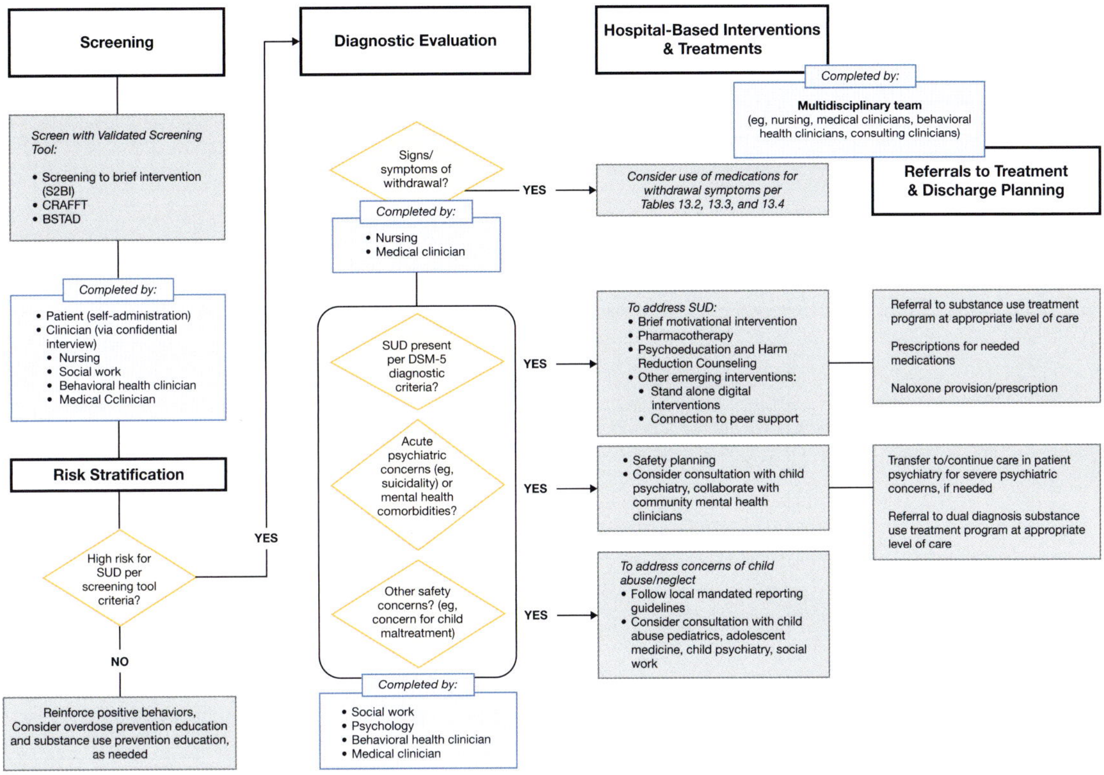

Figure 13.4: Model for hospital-based SUD care for adolescents.

therefore, uses a selective screening strategy. First, ED nurses administer the S2BI tool. If the patient reports any substance use over the past 12 months or has a positive toxicology result, then a social work consult is placed. The social worker interprets the results of the S2BI to stratify adolescents into low risk (used once or twice in the past year), mild–moderate risk (monthly use), or moderate–severe risk (weekly or daily use). Those who are mild moderate or moderate–severe risk receive a brief evaluation and brief motivational intervention. Social work also completes a safety assessment and provides counseling. Finally, adolescents with SUD risk are referred to outpatient follow-up either with their primary care clinician or a SUD specialist upon discharge. Interestingly, when this protocol was adapted for the 10 research sites, three made adjustments based on their staffing and existing workflows, highlighting the need for any model to be tailored to the specific hospital system.

Emerging Treatments and Interventions

The approach to treating hospitalized adolescents with SUD is continually changing. This change is motivated by the increasing need to address adolescent SUD amidst the rise of new substances and limited treatment infrastructure. With this in mind, emerging approaches focus on further removing barriers to SUD care.

Long-Acting Injectable Medications for SUD Treatment in Adolescents

A key opportunity for enhancing adolescent SUD treatment lies in employing long-acting injectable MOUD. Long-acting injectable formulations of buprenorphine and naltrexone offer several benefits over daily sublingual or oral options, such as better adherence and decreased risk of diversion. However, neither is FDA approved for individuals under 18 years due to insufficient safety and efficacy data. There is emerging data on the viability of injectable buprenorphine for adolescents with OUD. A case series involving six adolescents younger than age 18 years treated with long-acting injectable buprenorphine suggests that it is a safe, viable, and acceptable option that promotes OUD treatment retention and opioid abstinence.[84]

Parent Navigators

Engaging families in adolescent SUD treatment is critical and important to help with treatment retention.

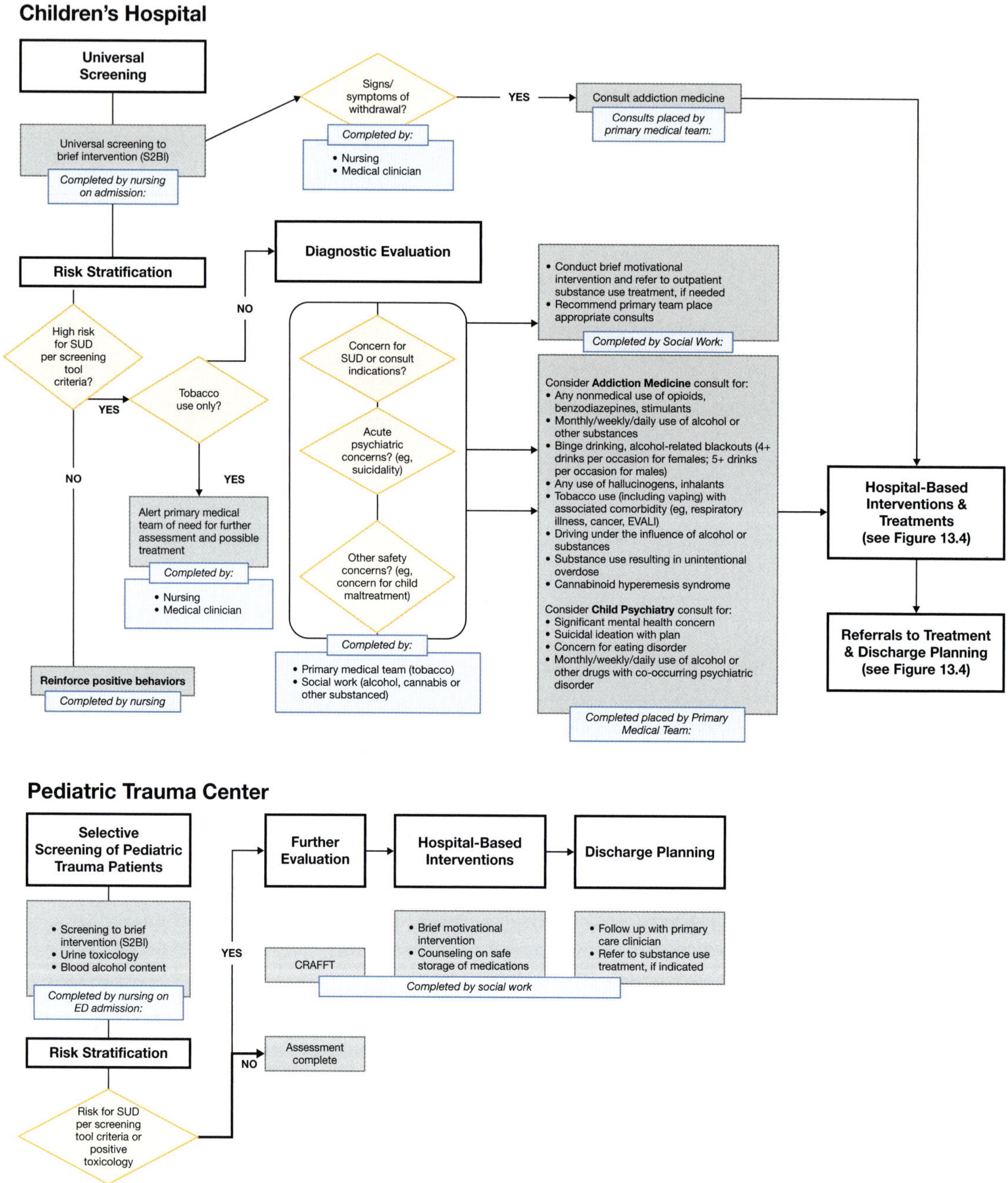

Figure 13.5: Overview of case examples.

Many parents struggle to navigate the health care system and access appropriate care for their child. Parent navigators have been used in mental health and other fields to support the care of children with chronic conditions.[96–98] These roles are filled by individuals who have lived experience supporting a child with a chronic mental health condition who are trained to provide peer-based support to parents, helping them understand treatment options, access services, and advocate for their child's care.[96] Hospital-based parent navigator programs have also been developed to support parents caring for children with complex health care needs.[97] These models are ripe for adaptation to SUD care and have the potential to reduce stigma and enhance families' self-efficacy, knowledge, and treatment linkage.

Peer Recovery Supports

Peer recovery coaches are individuals with lived experience of SUD who are in recovery[99] and are increasingly being integrated into hospital settings to provide real-time support to patients with SUDs. In the United States, each state has specific requirements for who can be certified as a peer recovery support specialist. Peers can often undergo additional training to specifically work with youth and their families. In EDs, peers can engage youth immediately after an overdose or substance-related crisis, a high-risk period for recurrence of use. In hospital and outpatient settings, they can serve as mentors and motivators, helping adolescents navigate early recovery, re-engage in education, and develop life skills. In the hospital, peers can play an important role with a warm-handoff approach, ensuring continuity of care as adolescents transition from the hospital to community-based treatment.

Summary

Though not widespread, hospital-based SUD screening and treatment can increase the capacity to address adolescent substance use and SUD. Many aspects of evaluating and treating adolescents in the hospital setting are similar to those of adults. Unique aspects of care include those related to screening, consent, confidentiality, and parent or guardian involvement. Harm reduction is an important cornerstone of hospital-based SUD care that can be tailored for adolescents and their parents. Overall, there is a lack of research addressing adolescent SUD interventions in the hospital setting; however, with increased subspecialty training and education, these interventions can expand to serve an important role in the care continuum for adolescents. Addressing unhealthy substance use in the hospital setting also prevents more severe health consequences in the future.

REFERENCES

1. Levy S, Campbell MD, Shea CL, DuPont CM, DuPont RL. Trends in substance nonuse by high school seniors: 1975–2018. *Pediatrics*. 2020;146(6):e2020007187.
2. Miech R, Patrick ME, Keyes K. Declines in adolescent substance use after the COVID-19 pandemic onset: the role of initiation in grades 7 and 9. *J Adolesc Health*. 2023;73(5):838–844.
3. Goldstick JE, Cunningham RM, Carter PM. Current causes of death in children and adolescents in the United States. *N Engl J Med*. 2022;386(20):1955–1956.
4. Richter LAS, Salmassi MLV, A. R. *Rethinking Substance Use Prevention: An Earlier and Broader Approach*; 2022. https://drugfree.org/reports/rethinking-substance-use-prevention-an-earlier-and-broader-approach/
5. Miech RA, Johnston LD, O'Malley PM. *Monitoring the Future National Survey Results on Drug Use, 1975–2024: Overview and Detailed Results for Secondary School Students*. Institute for Social Research, University of Michigan; 2024. https://monitoringthefuture.org/results/annual-reports/
6. Substance Abuse and Mental Health Services Administration. *Key Substance Use and Mental Health Indicators in the United States: Results from the 2023 National Survey on Drug Use and Health (HHS Publication No. PEP24-07-021, NSDUH Series H-59)*. 2024.
7. Richmond-Rakerd LS, Slutske WS, Wood PK. Age of initiation and substance use progression: a multivariate latent growth analysis. *Psychol Addict Behav*. 2017;31(6):664–675.
8. Jordan CJ, Andersen SL. Sensitive periods of substance abuse: early risk for the transition to dependence. *Dev Cogn Neurosci*. 2017;25:29–44.
9. Williams GC, Battista K, Leatherdale ST. An examination of how age of onset for alcohol, cannabis, and tobacco are associated with school outcomes in grade 12. *Addict Behav*. 2020;102:106215.
10. Alcover KC, Thompson CL. Patterns of mean age at drug use initiation among adolescents and emerging adults, 2004–2017. *JAMA Pediatr*. 2020;174(7):725–727.
11. Camenga DR, Hadland S, Zoucha K, Solmberg C, Burr W. Substance use screening practices among primary care pediatricians in the US: results from the 2021 AAP Periodic Survey. *Pediatric Academic Societies' Annual Meeting*. 2023. (Oral Presentation).
12. Terranella A, Guy GP, Mikosz C. Buprenorphine dispensing among youth aged #19 years in the United States: 2015–2020. *Pediatrics*. 2023;151(2):e2022058755.
13. Chadi N, Rodean J, Earlywine JJ, et al. Treatment for nicotine use disorder among Medicaid-enrolled adolescents and young adults. *JAMA Pediatr*. 2019;173(11):1103–1105.
14. King C, Beetham T, Smith N, et al. Treatments used among adolescent residential addiction treatment facilities in the US, 2022. *JAMA*. 2023;329(22):1983–1985.
15. King CA, Beetham T, Smith N, et al. Adolescent residential addiction treatment in the US: Uneven access, waitlists, and high costs. *Health Aff (Millwood)*. 2024;43(1):64–71.
16. Leslie K, Hosang S, Chadi N, et al. 04 Care for adolescents with substance use: a national survey of paediatric hospitals. *Paediatr Child Health*. 2024;29(Supplement_1):e2.
17. Alemu BT, Olayinka O, Beydoun HA. Prevalence and hospital resource usage associated with substance use disorder among hospitalized adolescents in the United States. *J Addict Dis*. 2023;41(3):233–241.
18. Masonbrink AR, Middlebrooks L, Gooding HC, et al. Substance use disorder visits among adolescents at children's hospitals during COVID-19. *J Adolesc Health Off Publ Soc Adolesc Med*. 2022;70(4):673–676.
19. Ball A, Hadland S, Rodean J, Hall M, Mendoza J, Ahrens K. Trends in substance-related visits among youth to US children's hospitals, 2016–2021: an analysis of the Pediatric Health Information System Database. *J Adolesc Health*. 2024;75(1):76–84.
20. Myran DT, Pugliese M, McDonald AJ, et al. Cannabis use disorder emergency department visits and hospitalizations and 5-year mortality. *JAMA Netw Open*. 2025;8(2):e2457852.
21. Suen LW, Makam AN, Snyder HR, et al. National prevalence of alcohol and other substance use disorders among emergency department visits and hospitalizations: NHAMCS 2014–2018. *J Gen Intern Med*. 2022;37(10):2420–2428.
22. Lim JK, Earlywine JJ, Bagley SM, Marshall BDL, Hadland SE. Polysubstance involvement in opioid overdose deaths in

adolescents and young adults, 1999–2018. *JAMA Pediatr.* 2021;175(2):194–196.
23. Masonbrink AR, Hunt JA, Bhandal A, et al. Self-reported and documented substance use among adolescents in the pediatric hospital. *Pediatrics.* 2021;147(6):e2020031468.
24. Levy SJL, Williams JF; American Academy of Pediatrics Committee on Substance Use and Prevention. Substance use screening, brief intervention, and referral to treatment. *Pediatrics.* 2016;138(1):e20161210.
25. Patnode CD, Perdue LA, Rushkin M, U.S O 'Connor EA. *Preventive Services Task Force Evidence Syntheses, Formerly Systematic Evidence Reviews. Screening for Unhealthy Drug Use in Primary Care in Adolescents and Adults, Including Pregnant Persons: Updated Systematic Review for the US Preventive Services Task Force.* Agency for Healthcare Research and Quality (US); 2020.
26. Ginsburg KR. Viewing our adolescent patients through a positive lens. *Contemp Pediatr.* 2007;24(1):65. Accessed January 8, 2025. https://scholar.google.com/scholar_lookup?title=Viewing%20our%20adolescent%20patients%20through%20a%20positive%20lens&author=KR%20Ginsburg&publication_year=2007&journal=Contemp%20Pediatr&volume=24&pages=65-76
27. Goldenring JM, Rosen DS. Goldenring: getting into adolescent heads: an essential update. *Contemp Pediatr.* 2004;21(1):64.
28. Levy S, Weitzman ER, Marin AC, Magane KM, Wisk LE, Shrier LA. Sensitivity and specificity of S2BI for identifying alcohol and cannabis use disorders among adolescents presenting for primary care. *Subst Abuse.* 2021;42(3):388–395.
29. Levy S, Weiss R, Sherritt L, et al. An electronic screen for triaging adolescent substance use by risk levels. *JAMA Pediatr.* 2014;168(9):822–828.
30. Kelly SM, Gryczynski J, Mitchell SG, Kirk A, O'Grady KE, Schwartz RP. Validity of brief screening instrument for adolescent tobacco, alcohol, and drug use. *Pediatrics.* 2014;133(5):819–826.
31. Knight JR, Sherritt L, Shrier LA, Harris SK, Chang G. Validity of the CRAFFT substance abuse screening test among adolescent clinic patients. *Arch Pediatr Adolesc Med.* 2002;156(6):607–614.
32. Mitchell SG, Kelly SM, Gryczynski J, et al. The CRAFFT cutpoints and DSM-5 criteria for alcohol and other drugs: a reevaluation and reexamination. *Subst Abus.* 2014;35(4):376–380.
33. Mello MJ, Bromberg J, Baird J, et al. Translation of alcohol screening and brief intervention guidelines to pediatric trauma centers. *J Trauma Acute Care Surg.* 2013;75(4 Suppl 3):S301–S307.
34. Johnson KN, Raetz A, Harte M, et al. Pediatric trauma patient alcohol screening: a 3 year review of screening at a Level I pediatric trauma center using the CRAFFT tool. *J Pediatr Surg.* 2014;49(2):330–332.
35. Ross JA, Minegishi M, Brogna M, Subramaniam G, Levy S, Weitzman E. Identifying adolescent vaping with screening to brief intervention and brief screener for tobacco, alcohol, and drugs screening tools. *J Adolesc Health.* 2024;75(1):196–199.
36. Kralik N, Roybal BO, Teitell SD, et al. Improving HEADSS assessments for inpatient adolescents: a quality improvement initiative. *J Adolesc Health.* 2023;72(3):S52.
37. Riese A, Tarr E, Baird J, Alverson B. Documentation of tobacco, alcohol, and drug screening in hospitalized adolescents. *Hosp Pediatr.* 2019;9(9):719–723.
38. Parvataneni S, Varela L, Vemuri-Reddy SM, Maneval ML. Emerging role of aprepitant in cannabis hyperemesis syndrome. *Cureus.* 2019;11(6):e4825.
39. Alexander A, Honan R, Molina A, Rahman AKMF, Walley SC. Tobacco screening and use in hospitalized adolescents at a children's hospital. *Hosp Pediatr.* 2021;11(6):605–612.
40. Pfaff N, Pantell MS, Kaiser SV. High-risk behavior screening and interventions in hospitalized adolescents. *Hosp Pediatr.* 2021;11(3):293–297.
41. Smith JR, Hazen EP, Kaminski TA, Wilens TE. Literature review: substance use screening and co-morbidity in medically hospitalized youth. *Gen Hosp Psychiatry.* 2020;67:115–126.
42. Mello MJ, Baird J, Spirito A, et al. Implementing screening, brief interventions, and referral to treatment at pediatric trauma centers: a step wedge cluster randomized trial. *J Pediatr Surg.* 2024;59(11):161618.
43. Ranney ML, Choo EK, Spirito A, Mello MJ. Adolescents' preference for technology-based emergency department behavioral interventions: does it depend on risky behaviors? *Pediatr Emerg Care.* 2013;29(4):475–481.
44. Wiley E, Kulkarni D, Dong H, Hwang LY. Quality improvement: a template-based approach to HEADSS assessments for hospitalized adolescents. *Hosp Pediatr.* 2023;13(7):588–596.
45. Chung RJ, Lee JB, Hackell JM, Alderman EM, Committee on Adolescence, Committee on Practice & Ambulatory Medicine. Confidentiality in the care of adolescents: technical report. *Pediatrics.* 2024;153(5):e2024066327.
46. 42 CFR Part 2–Confidentiality of substance use disorder patient records. Accessed January 8, 2025. https://www.ecfr.gov/current/title-42/part-2
47. Sharko M, Jameson R, Ancker JS, Krams L, Webber EC, Rosenbloom ST. State-by-state variability in adolescent privacy laws. *Pediatrics.* 2022;149(6):e2021053458.
48. Xie J, McPherson T, Powell A, et al. Ensuring adolescent patient portal confidentiality in the age of the cures act final rule. *J Adolesc Health.* 2021;69(6):933–939.
49. Ip W, Yang S, Parker J, et al. Assessment of prevalence of adolescent patient portal account access by guardians. *JAMA Netw Open.* 2021;4(9):e2124733.
50. American Psychiatric Association. *American Psychiatric Association: Diagnostic and Statistical Manual of Mental Disorders, Text Revision (DSM-5-TR).* 5th ed.; 2002.
51. Kaminer Y, Winters KC. DSM-5 criteria for youth substance use disorders: lost in translation? *J Am Acad Child Adolesc Psychiatry.* 2015;54(5):350–351.
52. Chisolm DJ, Kelleher KJ. Admission to acute care hospitals for adolescent substance abuse: a national descriptive analysis. *Subst Abuse Treat Prev Policy.* 2006;1:17.
53. Hollen V, Ortiz G. Mental health and substance use comorbidity among adolescents in psychiatric inpatient hospitals: prevalence and covariates. *J Child Adolesc Substance Abuse.* 2015;24(2):102–112.
54. Govender T, Yu J, Vidal-Ribas P, Gilman SE, Haynie DL. Adolescent substance use patterns and risk for suicidal thoughts and behaviors in young adulthood. *J Stud Alcohol Drugs.* 2023;84(6):892–901.
55. Beckmann D, Lowman KL, Nargiso J, McKowen J, Watt L, Yule AM. Substance-induced psychosis in youth. *Child Adolesc Psychiatr Clin N Am.* 2020;29(1):131–143.
56. Gobbi G, Atkin T, Zytynski T, et al. Association of cannabis use in adolescence and risk of depression, anxiety, and suicidality in young adulthood: a systematic review and meta-analysis. *JAMA Psychiatry.* 2019;76(4):426–434.
57. Nguyen BL, Lyons BH, Forsberg K, et al. Surveillance for violent deaths—national violent death reporting system, 48 states, the District of Columbia, and Puerto Rico, 2021. *MMWR Surveill Summ.* 2024;73(5):1–44.
58. Thomas R, Reeves M. *Mandatory Reporting Laws.* In: *StatPearls.* StatPearls Publishing; 2025. Accessed March 24, 2025. http://www.ncbi.nlm.nih.gov/books/NBK560690/
59. Kelleher DC, Renaud EJ, Ehrlich PF, Burd RS; Pediatric Trauma Society Guidelines Committee. Guidelines for

alcohol screening in adolescent trauma patients: a report from the Pediatric Trauma Society Guidelines Committee. *J Trauma Acute Care Surg*. 2013;74(2):671–682.

60. Brown WN, D'Errico E, Morrell HE. The youth alternative solutions program: evaluating a hospital-based intervention for adolescent substance use. *J Addict Nurs*. 2015;26(1): 32–40.
61. National Center for Statistics and Analysis. *2020 Report Young Drivers*. National Highway Traffic Safety Administration; 2020. Accessed March 29, 2025. https://crashstats.nhtsa.dot.gov/Api/Public/ViewPublication/813313
62. safetyfirst: Comprehensive Drug Education and Intervention Lessons. Halpern-Felsher REACH Lab. Accessed May 5, 2025. https://med.stanford.edu/halpern-felsher-reach-lab/preventions-interventions/Safety-First.html
63. Marshall T, Reeson M, Loverock A, et al. Evidence-based interventions for youth with concurrent mental health and substance use disorders: a scoping review: interventions fondées sur des données probantes pour les jeunes atteints de troubles concomitants de santé mentale et liés à l'usage de substances psychoactives: une étude de la portée. *Can J Psychiatry Rev Can Psychiatr*. 2025;70(5):347–371.
64. Hogue A, Henderson CE, Becker SJ, Knight DK. Evidence base on outpatient behavioral treatments for adolescent substance use, 2014–2017: outcomes, treatment delivery, and promising horizons. *J Clin Child Adolesc Psychol*. 2018;47(4): 499–526.
65. Bernstein J, Dorfman D, Lunstead J, et al. Reaching adolescents for prevention: the role of pediatric emergency department health promotion advocates. *Pediatr Emerg Care*. 2017;33(4): 223–229.
66. Henderson CE, Wevodau AL, Henderson SE, et al. An independent replication of the Adolescent-Community Reinforcement Approach with justice-involved youth. *Am J Addict*. 2016; 25(3):233–240.
67. Godley MD, Godley SH, Dennis ML, Funk RR, Passetti LL. The effect of assertive continuing care on continuing care linkage, adherence and abstinence following residential treatment for adolescents with substance use disorders. *Addiction*. 2007;102(1):81–93.
68. Alinsky RH, Hadland SE, Matson PA, Cerda M, Saloner B. Adolescent-serving addiction treatment facilities in the united states and the availability of medications for opioid use disorder. *J Adolesc Health*. 2020;67(4):542–549.
69. Lonsdale H, Kimsey KM, Brown JM, et al. Pediatric cannabinoid hyperemesis: a single institution 10-year case series. *J Adolesc Health Off Publ Soc Adolesc Med*. 2021;68(2): 255–261.
70. Sorensen CJ, DeSanto K, Borgelt L, Phillips KT, Monte AA. Cannabinoid hyperemesis syndrome: diagnosis, pathophysiology, and treatment—a systematic review. *J Med Toxicol*. 2017; 13(1):71–87.
71. Gray KM, Carpenter MJ, Baker NL, et al. A double-blind randomized controlled trial of N-acetylcysteine in cannabis-dependent adolescents. *Am J Psychiatry*. 2012;169(8):805–812.
72. United States Public Health Service Office of the Surgeon General, National Center for Chronic Disease Prevention and Health Promotion (US) Office on Smoking and Health. *Smoking Cessation: A Report of the Surgeon General*. US Department of Health and Human Services; 2020. Accessed March 26, 2025. http://www.ncbi.nlm.nih.gov/books/NBK555591/
73. Selph S, Patnode CD, Bailey SR, et al. *Primary Care Interventions for Prevention and Cessation of Tobacco Use in Children and Adolescents: A Systematic Review for the U.S. Preventive Services Task Force*. Agency for Healthcare Research and Quality (US); 2020. Accessed March 26, 2025. http://www.ncbi.nlm.nih.gov/books/NBK556871/
74. Gray KM, Baker NL, McClure EA, et al. Efficacy and safety of varenicline for adolescent smoking cessation: a randomized clinical trial. *JAMA Pediatr*. 2019;173(12):1146–1153.
75. Jenssen BP, Walley SC, Boykan R, Little Caldwell A, Camenga D; Section on Nicotine and Tobacco Prevention and Treatment, Committee on Substance Use and Prevention. Protecting children and adolescents from tobacco and nicotine. *Pediatrics*. 2023;151(5):e2023061806.
76. Evins AE, Cather C, Reeder HT, et al. Varenicline for youth nicotine vaping cessation: a randomized clinical trial. *JAMA*. 2025;333(21):1876–1886.
77. Morean ME, Krishnan-Sarin S, O'Malley SS. Assessing nicotine dependence in adolescent e-cigarette users: the 4-item patient-reported outcomes measurement information system (PROMIS) nicotine dependence item bank for electronic cigarettes. *Drug Alcohol Depend*. 2018;188:60–63.
78. Friedman N, Seltzer J, Harvey H, Ly B, Schneir A. Severe alcohol withdrawal in an adolescent male. *Toxicol Rep*. 2023; 10:428–430.
79. Moubayed D, Chadi N. An innovative inpatient protocol for alcohol withdrawal prevention in a 16-year-old adolescent: a case report. *J Med Case Rep*. 2023;17(1):179.
80. Unlu H, Yehia A, El-Gayar S, et al. Clinical characteristics and treatment outcomes of alcohol withdrawal syndrome in adolescents and young adults. *JAACAP Open*. 2024;3(2):216–231.
81. Sullivan JT, Sykora K, Schneiderman J, Naranjo CA, Sellers EM. Assessment of alcohol withdrawal: the revised clinical institute withdrawal assessment for alcohol scale (CIWA-Ar). *Br J Addict*. 1989;84(11):1353–1357.
82. Squeglia LM, Tomko RL, Baker NL, Kirkland AE, McClure EA, Gray KM. A randomized controlled trial of N-acetylcysteine for adolescent and young adult alcohol use disorder. *J Am Acad Child Adolesc Psychiatry*. 2025:S0890-8567(25)02088-X. Epub ahead of print.
83. Miranda R, Ray L, Blanchard A, et al. Effects of naltrexone on adolescent alcohol cue reactivity and sensitivity: an initial randomized trial. *Addict Biol*. 2014;19(5):941–954.
84. O'Malley SS, Corbin WR, Leeman RF, et al. Reduction of alcohol drinking in young adults by naltrexone: a double-blind, placebo-controlled, randomized clinical trial of efficacy and safety. *J Clin Psychiatry*. 2015;76(2):e207–e213.
85. Earlywine JJ, Bagley SM, Rodean J, et al. Medications for alcohol use disorder and retention in care in medicaid-enrolled youth, 2014–2019. *J Adolesc Health*. 2023;73(5):845–851.
86. Camenga DR, Colon-Rivera HA, Muvvala SB. Medications for maintenance treatment of opioid use disorder in adolescents: a narrative review and assessment of clinical benefits and potential risks. *J Stud Alcohol Drugs*. 2019;80(4):393–402.
87. Borodovsky JT, Levy S, Fishman M, Marsch LA. Buprenorphine treatment for adolescents and young adults with opioid use disorders: a narrative review. *J Addict Med*. 2018;12(3): 170–183.
88. Woody GE, Poole SA, Subramaniam G, et al. Extended vs short-term buprenorphine-naloxone for treatment of opioid-addicted youth: a randomized trial. *JAMA*. 2008;300(17): 2003–2011.
89. Marsch LA, Bickel WK, Badger GJ, et al. Comparison of pharmacological treatments for opioid-dependent adolescents: a randomized controlled trial. *Arch Gen Psychiatry*. 2005;62(10): 1157–1164.
90. Marsch LA, Moore SK, Borodovsky JT, et al. A randomized controlled trial of buprenorphine taper duration among opioid-dependent adolescents and young adults. *Addiction*. 2016;111(8):1406–1415.
91. Lee E, Rikard SM, Guy G Jr, Terranella A. Trends in buprenorphine dispensing among adolescents and young adults in the US. *JAMA*. 2025;333(5):425–427.

92. Trope LA, Stemmle M, Chang A. A novel inpatient buprenorphine induction program for adolescents with opioid use disorder. *Hosp Pediatr.* 2023;13(2):e23–e28.
93. Substance Abuse and Mental Health Services Administration. *Federal Guidelines for Opioid Treatment Programs.* 2024.
94. Brown RA, Abrantes AM, Minami H, et al. Motivational interviewing to reduce substance use in adolescents with psychiatric comorbidity. *J Subst Abuse Treat.* 2015;59:20–29.
95. Cunningham RM, Chermack ST, Ehrlich PF, et al. Alcohol interventions among underage drinkers in the ED: a randomized controlled trial. *Pediatrics.* 2015;136(4):783–793.
96. Hoagwood KE, Olin SS, Storfer-Isser A, et al. Evaluation of a train-the-trainers model for family peer advocates in children's mental health. *J Child Fam Stud.* 2018;27(4):1130–1136.
97. Carty CL, Soghier LM, Kritikos KI, et al. The Giving Parents Support Study: a randomized clinical trial of a parent navigator intervention to improve outcomes after neonatal intensive care unit discharge. *Contemp Clin Trials.* 2018;70:117–134.
98. Kutash K, Duchnowski AJ, Green AL, Ferron J. Effectiveness of the parent connectors program: results from a randomized controlled trial. *School Ment Health.* 2013;5(4):192–208.
99. Stack E, Hildebran C, Leichtling G, et al. Peer recovery support services across the continuum: in community, hospital, corrections, and treatment and recovery agency settings–a narrative review. *J Addict Med.* 2022;16(1):93–100.

14

Co-occurring Mental Illness and Substance Use Disorders

Morgan Zipperly, Erica Kirsten Rapp, Thida Thant

It's the first cases that always stick with you. I still remember the faces of many of the patients I took care of 15 years ago as a medical student. As time goes on, faces start to blend into one another, but when you see something new or striking, you always remember that person. As a consultation-liaison psychiatrist, several cases have stayed with me since fellowship and early practice: autoenucleation, autoamputation, self-inflicted gunshot wounds to the head, and a man in his mid-30s (let's call him M) whom I treated early in my attending years after he doused himself in gasoline and set himself on fire.

Of course, I'd heard of self-immolation, and I knew I'd see it at some point, especially when I took my first faculty job at a hospital with a large burn unit. But I wasn't prepared to walk into M's room and see him covered in wet yellow bandages from head to toe. There were gaps in the bandages for his eyes, but even his eyelids were burned. The room was so hot that I was sweating through my scrubs under my contact gown.

M was awake, and he watched me pull up a chair and sit down next to him. I asked him to talk to me about what had happened. He seemed willing to talk, but all he could tell me was that he'd done it in "protest." He wasn't able to tell me what he was protesting, just a vague injustice. I started asking him specific questions about his psychiatric history. To my surprise, he hadn't been having clear psychotic symptoms (most self-immolations in the United States are in the context of psychosis), nor had he clearly intended this as a suicide attempt. The only thing that was clearly positive in his history was that he used methamphetamine.

M was in the hospital for several months, so I had many hours of visits to gather information and refine my diagnosis. I was never able to get a clearer story of why M felt so strongly that he needed to set himself on fire or what he was protesting. Although he expressed vague suspicions about many things, he was never paranoid toward me or any other clinicians or hospital staff. He had a vague idea that there were bad things going on out there in the world. By the time of his hospital discharge months later, the best diagnosis I had was a cluster A personality disorder complicated by methamphetamine use disorder. I guessed that methamphetamine intoxication at the time of the event contributed to his self-immolation. As a result of his prolonged hospitalization, M had not used methamphetamine for months. As he neared hospital discharge, he expressed a strong desire to abstain from methamphetamine use. We discharged him with resources for substance use disorder (SUD) treatment, and unfortunately, due to his physical rehabilitation needs, he was unable to directly discharge to a residential SUD treatment program.

Over the next year, I thought about M often. I wondered how he was doing and whether or not he was in recovery from methamphetamine use. Just as I was starting to feel comfortable that he was probably doing well, about a year and a half after his hospital discharge, M was back in the hospital. He had used methamphetamine and self-immolated again.

concurrent psychiatric disorders and AUD diagnoses receive inpatient mental health treatment.[16]

In the hospital setting, estimates report that 44% to 61% of patients with a SUD had a current comorbid psychiatric disorder, with over 30% having at least two psychiatric diagnoses.[35,36] Among hospitalized patients with SUD, the most common co-occurring psychiatric disorders include MDD (26%) and PTSD (14%).[35,37] One study demonstrated that almost 45% of hospitalized patients with a SUD screened positive for current PTSD symptoms and 80% reported a history of at least one traumatic event.[38] The type of SUD is also associated with differing rates of concurrent psychiatric disorders. In the hospital setting, those with AUD (77%) and those with cannabis use disorder (CUD) (76%) have higher rates of comorbid psychiatric disorders compared to individuals with stimulant use disorder or opioid use disorder (OUD).[35]

Anxiety disorders are also common among hospitalized patients with SUD, particularly GAD and panic disorder,[39,40] as are cluster B personality disorders, such as borderline personality disorder and antisocial personality disorder, which are characterized by personality traits such as erratic and/or dramatic behaviors, impulsivity, unstable relationships, poor self-image, and emotional lability (Figure 14.1).[35,39]

Gender and age are also risk factors for dual diagnosis in inpatient settings. Women are more likely to have co-occurring psychiatric disorders (74%) compared to men (55%) with SUD, and younger patients are more likely to have a SUD concurrently with a severe psychiatric disorder.[35] In a study of Veterans Health Administration patients with SUD and co-occurring psychiatric disorder, social factors predictive

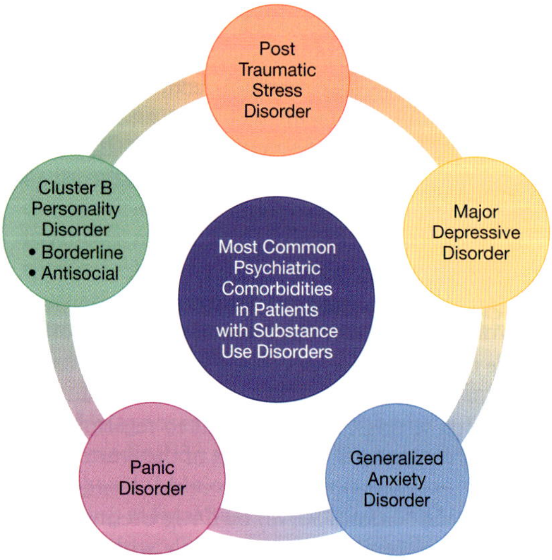

Figure 14.1: Most common psychiatric comorbidities in patients with substance use disorders.[35,37,39,40]

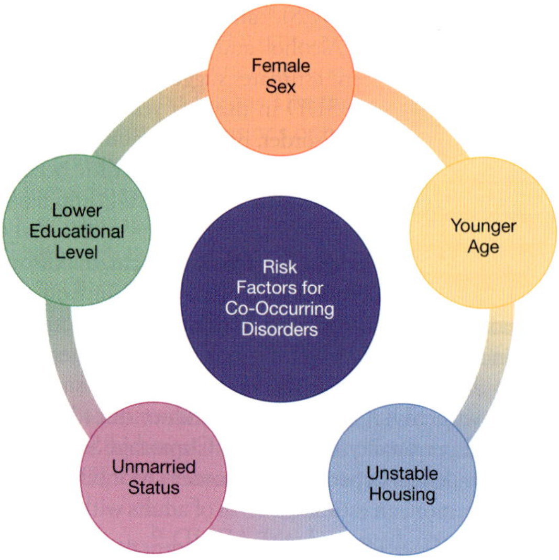

Figure 14.2: Risk factors for co-occurring disorders.[35]

of co-occurring disorders included unstable housing, unmarried status, and lower level of education.[41] These risk factors were associated with high inpatient utilization with similar use of psychiatric, medical, and SUD-related services[41] (Figure 14.2).

Though not inherently associated with psychiatric disorders, patients with dual diagnosis are more likely to demonstrate disruptive behavior during their hospitalization (ie, agitation), particularly in the acute intoxication and withdrawal periods, to have higher rates of patient-directed discharge (PDD), and to have higher rates of rehospitalization.[42,43]

Summary of the Evidence

Integrated Versus Parallel SUD and Mental Health Treatment

Historically, it was thought that SUD and psychiatric disorders should be treated separately for the patient to reap the full benefits of both treatment modalities.[29] More recent evidence demonstrates that patients with co-occurring psychiatric disorder and SUD often experience worse outcomes when these conditions are treated separately.[29] These findings contributed to updated recommendations emphasizing integrated treatment for this unique patient population, as outlined in Figure 14.3. Integrated treatment in an evidence-based treatment approach where both SUD and psychiatric disorders are addressed concurrently through multiple modalities and services such as medication, therapeutic modalities and behavioral treatments, and case management.[44] Integrated treatment is more effective in reducing both substance use and

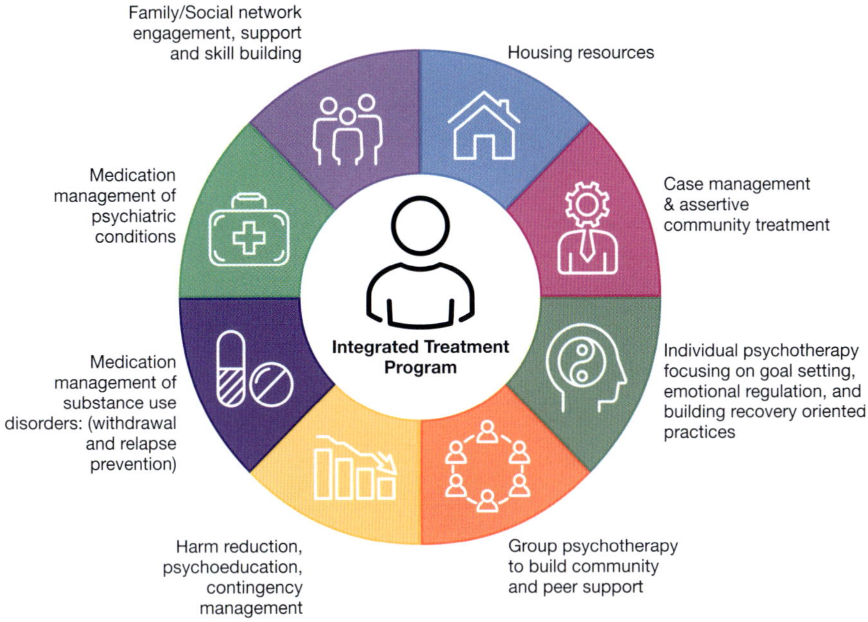

Figure 14.3: Elements of an integrated treatment program for co-occurring disorders.

psychiatric symptoms, lowering rehospitalizations, decreasing hospital length of stay (when admissions occur), increasing posttreatment employment and housing stability, and improving patients' adjustment to their communities and social functioning.[30–32,45,46] Furthermore, involvement in an integrated treatment program significantly reduces potential criminal–legal outcomes such as incidence of arrests, probation violations, length of incarceration, and number of convictions.[47] One analysis comparing parallel treatment (ie, separate, nonintegrated treatment) to integrated dual diagnosis treatment found that integrated treatment led to a reduction in hospitalization incidence (12.2% to 3.3%) and a reduction in total number of psychiatric hospitalization days (5.7 to 2.4) while parallel treatment resulted in an increase in both of these metrics,[46] highlighting the importance of integrated approaches when available.

It is also crucial not to defer treating a psychiatric condition until a SUD is resolved. Addressing both simultaneously prevents suffering, improves overall treatment adherence, and other outcomes as outlined in Table 14.1.[33]

Furthermore, some individuals use substances to "self-medicate" psychiatric symptoms.[16,24,25] Delaying mental health treatment in favor of prioritizing SUD treatment would likely be counterproductive. Both the American Society of Addiction Medicine (ASAM) and the American Academy of Addiction Psychiatry (AAAP) recommend treating both conditions concurrently using an integrated behavioral treatment approach, which, among people with stimulant use disorder, is more convenient, improves access to mental health care, and is often more cost-effective.[34]

Aspects of Integrated Treatment

As seen in Figure 14.3, integrated programs include a combination of pharmacologic treatment, intensive case management, motivational interviewing, individual and group psychotherapy, contingency management, and community reinforcement approaches, which are all tailored to the patient's stage of change and individual needs.[31,34,48] Intensive case management is a community-based care approach for individuals with complex needs, providing long-term intensive support to those with co-occurring psychiatric disorders and SUD with the goal of symptom reduction or remission and improved quality of life. Community reinforcement approaches within the integrated care

TABLE 14.1

Positive Benefits of Integrated SUD and Mental Health Treatment

- Reduction in both substance use and mental health symptoms
- Decrease in number of hospitalizations
- Decreased hospital length of stay
- Increase in posttreatment employment rates
- Reduction in criminal–legal outcomes
- Improved functional outcomes (social functioning, housing stability)
- Improved treatment adherence

References 30–33, 45–47.

model involve assisting individuals with co-occurring disorders in adopting healthy, rewarding habits and activities to build a balanced lifestyle without substances.[49] Motivational interviewing is an approach commonly employed in SUD treatment and assesses the patient's intrinsic reasoning for change. This is often combined with contingency management, a therapy that encourages positive behavioral change through the use of rewards and incentives. Both motivational interviewing and contingency management are discussed more in-depth in Chapter 15.

Several different types of psychotherapies, outlined in Table 14.2, may be used when treating patients with co-occurring disorders depending on the patient's primary struggles, motivation, and availability.[50–52] One specific type of psychotherapy, Integrated Group Therapy (IGT), is effective in treating patients with comorbid bipolar disorder and SUD by increasing the chance that a patient will abstain from substance use for three or more consecutive months. Unfortunately, these benefits were not observed with patients suffering from other psychiatric disorders, suggesting that specific approaches for different psychiatric disorders may provide greater benefit.[53,54] Availability of support systems, such as family involvement, housing, and case management are crucial for patient success within an integrated treatment program framework.[32,55] The following sections will present guidance for how to practically and effectively approach the clinical evaluation and management of hospitalized patients with co-occurring psychiatric disorders and SUD.

Clinical Guidance

Initial Assessment

An initial evaluation of a patient upon hospital admission should be completed by a hospital-based

TABLE 14.2

Types of Psychotherapy

Types of psychotherapy	Description	Indications
Cognitive behavioral therapy (CBT)	Therapy focusing on identifying and correcting distorted beliefs, thought patterns and behaviors	■ Depression, anxiety, trauma, substance use disorders, OCD, eating disorders, insomnia ■ Best suited for patients who are highly motivated and benefit from a problem-solving approach
Dialectical behavioral therapy (DBT)	Therapy focusing on emotional regulation, mindfulness, and acceptance	■ Most commonly used for borderline personality disorder or for patients with significant issues with emotional regulation
Acceptance and commitment therapy (ACT)	Focuses on accepting negative thoughts, emotions, and circumstances as opposed to eliminating them while committing to behaviors and changes that align with personal values	■ Anxiety, depression, chronic pain/medical illness, stress management.
Interpersonal therapy (IPT)	Focuses on interpersonal challenges that lead to psychological issues	■ Depression, grief, relationship problems, social isolation, eating disorders
Family therapy	Focuses on the family system including topics like communication, psychoeducation, impaired relationships, coping and problem solving	■ Family conflict, unhealthy substance use, behavioral issues in children. ■ Most appropriate when both family members and patient are willing to participate
Psychodynamic therapy	Focuses on developing insight and uncovering and exploring unconscious patterns of relationships, conflicts, desires, and how past experiences may influence a patient's current situation and challenges	■ Depression, anxiety, relationship issues, trauma, self-esteem, eating disorders, and personality disorders. ■ Often a more intensive form of therapy which requires patients that can reliably engage in more frequent sessions.
Group therapy	Involves a group of individuals sharing experiences and supporting each other under the guidance of a therapist, often focused on individuals with similar challenges	■ Social isolation, substance use, grief, anxiety, depression, medical illness

References 50–52.

**Integrated group therapy will simultaneously address both mental health and substance use concerns.*

clinician. Regardless of the medical specialty of the admitting service, the evaluation should include a detailed assessment of mental health symptoms, psychiatric history, history of SUD, and current/recent substance use (Table 14.3). This includes a careful assessment of the patient's mental health status, suicide risk, and overall stability (ie, severity, acuity and persistence of psychiatric symptoms).

TABLE 14.3

Overview of the Evaluation and Management of Co-occurring Disorders in Hospitalized Patients

↓

Initial evaluation and treatment of the patient with substance use presenting with psychiatric symptoms

Current/recent mental health symptoms

- Temporal relationship between substance use and onset/worsening of mental health symptoms (ie, did psychiatric symptoms exist/start prior to onset of substance use?)

Psychiatric risk assessment and safety history

- Insight into reason for admission, current/recent/past suicidal or homicidal thoughts, suicide attempts, or self-harming behaviors (cutting or burning self), access to lethal means (firearms, medication stockpiles)

Psychiatric history

- Diagnoses, medication trials, prior psychiatric hospitalizations, current access to mental health care

Current/recent substance use and treatment history

- Duration, frequency, and intensity of use, timeline of use and symptoms of intoxication/withdrawal
- Level of care (outpatient, intensive outpatient, residential, detox, etc)

Review/solicitation of additional data sources

- Chart review, collateral information from friends, family, or longitudinal treatment team member regarding history and timeline of symptoms, urine drug testing results

Evaluation considerations

- Serial evaluations may be needed to clarify diagnosis and need for treatment

Treatment considerations

- Consider medical comorbidities when choosing medications, particularly those with QTc prolongation concerns
- For longer-term treatment, consider metabolic concerns with atypical antipsychotics

↓ ↓ ↓ ↓

Next steps in Evaluation and Management of Co-Occurring Disorders in Hospitalized Patients Based on Symptom Timeline

Symptom timeline	Diagnostic considerations	Treatment considerations	Follow-up
Acute onset of psychiatric symptoms in the setting of substance use	***Substance-induced psychiatric disorder (depression, mania, psychosis)*** ▪ Symptoms often resolve or improve rapidly without significant intervention as intoxication/withdrawal resolves ▪ Depending on substance and specific lab test, often (but not always) associated with positive urine drug test; see Table 14.5	**If primary concern is agitation:** ▪ Consider fast-acting benzodiazepine (usually lorazepam) ± antipsychotic if additional medication required **If primary concern is manic and/or psychotic symptoms:** ▪ Consider antipsychotic (ie, olanzapine, risperidone, or haloperidol) ± benzodiazepine if concurrent agitation ▪ If patient is started on standing medications, should consider tapering off after acute symptoms have resolved **If primary concern is depression/anxiety:** ▪ No long-term medications are indicated ▪ Can use as-needed or daily/scheduled short-term hydroxyzine, clonidine, propranolol, or gabapentin	▪ Long-term medication management of psychiatric symptoms likely not indicated, more often used for symptomatic management during hospitalization ▪ May or may not need psychiatric follow-up in the ambulatory setting

(continued)

TABLE 14.3

Overview of the Evaluation and Management of Co-occurring Disorders in Hospitalized Patients (*Continued*)

Symptom timeline	Diagnostic considerations	Treatment considerations	Follow-up
	Acute intoxication or withdrawal ■ Typically associated with classic signs of substance-specific intoxication or withdrawal, including physical exam findings, ie, tremor or diaphoresis and vital sign abnormalities	■ Follow evidence-based guidelines for management of withdrawal. Symptomatically treating acute psychiatric symptoms during active withdrawal may mask severity of withdrawal and lead to undertreatment or delay in care, particularly in alcohol, opioid or sedative-hypnotic withdrawal. ■ If concerned for acute suicidal ideation (SI) in setting of recent substance use, intoxication or withdrawal, consider direct patient observation (such as bedside sitter) until acute intoxication/withdrawal has improved, then reassess SI before determining need/timing for more in-depth risk assessment	
	Altered mental status, encephalopathy, or delirium ■ Typically associated with disorientation, waxing/waning alertness and confusion; see Table 14.4	■ Rule out contribution from acute intoxication or withdrawal ■ Implement delirium precautions, work up additional causes ■ Medication is used primarily on an as-needed basis for acute symptom and behavioral management, such as disruptive agitation or distressing hallucinations ■ Avoid deliriogenic agents such as benzodiazepines	
Exacerbation of preexisting psychiatric symptoms in setting of substance use **Unclear** temporal relationship between psychiatric symptoms and substance use	Consider primary psychiatric condition (if meeting DSM-5 criteria) co-occurring with substance use disorder if no other medical or neurological contributor found/likely; see Table 14.4 ■ Rule out more urgent conditions such as acute intoxication/withdrawal or altered mental status/encephalopathy/delirium ■ Rule out other possible medical or neurological contributors/etiologies **If the above are ruled out, consider:** ■ Substance/medication induced psychiatric disorder (depression, mania, psychosis) ■ Primary psychiatric condition (if meeting DSM-5 criteria) co-occurring with substance use disorder	**If concerned for primary depressive/anxiety disorder:** ■ Consider initiation of antidepressant such as an SSRI or SNRI ■ Bupropion may be beneficial in patients with concurrent tobacco or stimulant use disorders ■ Should typically avoid benzodiazepines if concurrent SUD, particularly alcohol, sedative-hypnotic or opioid use disorders **If concerned for primary psychotic disorder:** ■ Recommend psychiatry consultation ■ If unavailable/while waiting, consider initiation of an antipsychotic, such as olanzapine, risperidone, or haloperidol **If concerned for primary bipolar disorder/mania:** ■ Recommend psychiatry consultation ■ If unavailable/while waiting, consider initiation of a mood stabilizer such as valproate/divalproex sodium, ± an atypical antipsychotic if psychosis is present **Other treatment considerations** ■ When considering medications for concurrent AUD, use caution with disulfiram given higher likelihood of ingesting alcohol in concurrent bipolar disorder or psychosis, as well as possibility of worsening underlying psychosis ■ Outside of acute mania or agitation, avoid benzodiazepines if concurrent substance use disorder, particularly alcohol, sedative–hypnotic or opioid use disorders	■ Long-term medication management of psychiatric symptoms may be indicated if symptoms persist or remain worsened outside of acute substance use period (including intoxication, withdrawal) ■ May need psychiatry follow-up in the ambulatory setting for ongoing management of preexisting and persistent psychiatric symptoms and disorders and/or for ongoing diagnostic clarity

Sometimes, patients may be unable to provide this information due to their level of impaired functioning secondary to their presentation. In these scenarios, a thorough chart review, review of urine drug testing (whereby a negative test may be more informative than a positive test), and collateral reports, including identifying and calling family, friends, or other people who know the patient, can be immensely helpful to gain an understanding of the patient's baseline mental health status compared to their current presentation.

Differential Diagnosis

In patients without a previously diagnosed psychiatric disorder, concurrent substance use often complicates the presentation and heightens diagnostic difficulty. For example, stimulant use can lead to mood swings, irritability, insomnia, and paranoia that can be confused with symptoms of a primary psychiatric disorder such as schizophrenia or bipolar disorder.[14] It is important to remember that an individual can experience psychotic symptoms, which can include hallucinations, paranoia, responding to internal stimuli, delusional ideation, and a break from reality, without meeting diagnostic criteria for a primary psychotic disorder. A patient presenting with such symptoms could be suffering from benzodiazepine or alcohol withdrawal, heavy cannabis use, a stimulant use disorder, acute stimulant intoxication, bipolar disorder, a psychotic disorder, or a combination of these. Overall, intoxication with alcohol, cannabis, hallucinogens, inhalants, sedative/hypnotic/anxiolytics, and stimulants and withdrawal from alcohol and sedative/hypnotic/anxiolytics have all been associated with psychotic symptoms.

Several medications may precipitate psychosis, including anesthetics and analgesics, anticholinergics, anticonvulsants, antihistamines, antihypertensive and cardiovascular medications, antimicrobials, antiparkinsonian agents, chemotherapeutics, corticosteroids, gastrointestinal medications, muscle relaxants, nonsteroidal anti-inflammatories, phenylephrine, pseudoephedrine, antidepressants, and disulfiram.[56] While a vast number of medications have been implicated in the onset of psychotic symptoms, these outcomes are rare and limited to a small number of case studies for most pharmacologic treatments; medications that are more commonly associated with psychosis are outlined in Table 14.4.[57–59]

Other toxins that may precipitate psychotic symptoms include anticholinesterases, organophosphates, nerve gases (eg, sarin), carbon monoxide, carbon dioxide, and volatile compounds (eg, paint, fuel).[56] Additional considerations in the differential diagnosis of psychiatric symptoms in patients with co-occurring disorders are included in Table 14.5.[60,61]

TABLE 14.4

Medications With Highest Risk of Psychosis

Medication class	Agents commonly associated with psychosis[a]
Dopaminergic agents	Pramipexole
	Ropinirole
	Amantadine
Corticosteroids	Prednisone
	Dexamethasone
Immunosuppressants	Cyclosporine
	Tacrolimus
Antihistamines	Diphenhydramine
Stimulants	Amphetamine/dextroamphetamine
	Methylphenidate
Antibiotics and antivirals	Isoniazid
	Efavirenz
	Mefloquine
Sympathomimetics	Pseudoephedrine
	Dextromethorphan

[a]Not a comprehensive list.

References 57–59.

Temporal Relationship Between Time of Last Use and Symptom Presentation

To improve diagnostic clarity, the clinician should consider the temporal relationship between psychiatric symptom onset and substance use, as well as the level of symptom severity. The clinician should inquire if the patient's psychiatric symptoms preceded their reported substance use. If so, a separate psychiatric disorder should be higher on the differential, and the patient's substance use may be a contributing factor to further destabilization. The clinician should inquire if the patient has a family history of psychiatric disorders. If so, then a primary psychiatric disorder should be considered more deeply.[62,63]

Next, the clinician should determine how long the psychiatric symptoms have persisted following intoxication or withdrawal from the patient's preferred or reported substance. For example, a patient who presents with concern for mania who reports remote cocaine use and has a negative urine drug test (UDT) is more likely experiencing a manic episode

TABLE 14.5

Differential Diagnosis of Psychiatric Symptoms in Patients With Co-occurring Disorders

Psychiatric symptom	Differential diagnosis[a]
Psychosis	**Substance induced:** ■ Stimulant intoxication/use ■ Hallucinogen use ■ Opioid intoxication/use ■ Alcohol intoxication or withdrawal ■ Sedative–hypnotic use or withdrawal **Psychiatric disorder:** ■ Mood disorder (depression or bipolar) ■ Psychotic disorder (schizophrenia, schizoaffective, brief psychotic disorder, delusional disorder) ■ Trauma ■ Personality disorders **Medical/neurologic:** ■ Delirium ■ Dementia ■ Medication related (ie, steroids, immunosuppressants, sympathomimetics) ■ Head injury or brain tumors/masses ■ Encephalitis ■ Postviral ■ Hypoxia
Depression	**Substance induced:** ■ Stimulant withdrawal ■ Opioid intoxication/use ■ Alcohol intoxication or withdrawal ■ Sedative–hypnotic use or withdrawal **Psychiatric disorder:** ■ Mood disorder (depression or bipolar) ■ Trauma ■ Personality disorders ■ Anxiety disorders **Medical/neurologic:** ■ Delirium ■ Dementia ■ Medication related (ie, steroids, immunosuppressants, interferon, sedative–hypnotics) ■ Head injury or brain tumor/masses ■ Encephalitis ■ Postviral ■ Cancer ■ Hypothyroidism ■ Syphilis ■ Multiple sclerosis
Mania	**Substance induced:** ■ Stimulants (ie, cocaine, methamphetamine, amphetamine) ■ Hallucinogen ■ PCP ■ Nicotine ■ Alcohol intoxication or withdrawal ■ Sedative–hypnotic use or withdrawal **Psychiatric disorder:** ■ Bipolar ■ Trauma ■ Personality disorders ■ Severe OCD **Medical/neurologic:** ■ Delirium ■ Dementia ■ Medication related (ie, steroids, immunosuppressants, human growth hormone, testosterone, sympathomimetics) ■ Head injury or brain tumors/masses ■ Encephalitis ■ Postviral ■ Hypertensive urgency ■ Hypercortisolemia, hyperaldosteronism ■ Hyperthyroidism

[a]Not a comprehensive list.

References 60, 61.

associated with bipolar disorder, rather than the direct effects of cocaine intoxication. On the other hand, if a patient has known recent methamphetamine use and presents with paranoia and psychotic features, the presentation could be a direct effect of the substance itself, or it could be related to an underlying psychotic disorder, and more time is needed for further assessments to determine the etiology of the psychotic symptoms.

According to the DSM-5, a patient's presentation is consistent with a substance- or medication-induced psychiatric disorder if (1) there is evidence that the symptoms occurred during or within 1 month of intoxication or withdrawal of a substance/medication and (2) the substance/medication being considered is known to cause the psychiatric symptoms.[56] Furthermore, the symptoms cannot be limited to an episode of delirium. If the presentation is associated with a substance- or medication-induced psychiatric disorder, in general, the associated symptoms should remit within approximately 1 month of cessation of the offending substance/medication. Clinical features of primary and secondary psychiatric disorders are summarized in Table 14.6.[64–69]

Prolonged Psychiatric Symptoms Related to SUD

There are notable exceptions when considering the expected timeline of symptomatic improvement of psychiatric symptoms related to substance cessation. For example, patients with benzodiazepine use disorder and physical benzodiazepine dependence can experience debilitating protracted benzodiazepine withdrawal symptoms such as anxiety, insomnia, irritability, and dysphoria for weeks to months to years after the last dose of benzodiazepine.[70–72] The most successful approach to reduce these symptoms is to initiate a prolonged benzodiazepine taper regimen with close clinician monitoring and frequent follow-up appointments. Tapers should be flexible with dose decreases informed by patient-centered decision making and clinician expertise.[73]

Patients experiencing a neurocognitive disorder (NCD) induced by alcohol, inhalants, or sedative–hypnotics/anxiolytics may also have protracted symptoms lasting beyond 1 month from their last substance use. Cognitive domains which may be affected with long-term sedative–hypnotic use include attention and concentration; problem solving; visuospatial; psychomotor

TABLE 14.6

A Comparison of the Clinical Features of Primary Psychiatric Disorders Versus Substance-Induced Psychiatric Symptoms

Primary psychiatric disorders	Substance-induced psychiatric symptoms
More insidious/subacute onset of symptoms	More acute or sudden onset of symptoms
Slower resolution of symptoms, often requires pharmacologic or psychological intervention	Rapid resolution of symptoms with or without pharmacologic or psychological intervention
Usually improves with medications	May or may not improve with medications
Lack of timeline correlation between substance use (both intoxication/withdrawal) and onset/resolution of psychiatric symptoms	Timeline correlation between substance use (both intoxication/withdrawal) and onset/resolution of psychiatric symptoms
Symptoms persist even during periods of abstinence	Symptoms resolve during periods of abstinence
Typical clinical presentation of psychiatric disorder (ie, age of onset, symptom timeline/duration, constellation of symptoms)	Atypical clinical presentation of psychiatric disorder (ie, unusual age of onset, abnormal symptom duration, does not meet diagnostic criteria for primary psychiatric disorder, association with episodes of confusion, waxing/waning presentations)
Positive psychiatric family history (especially for schizophrenia, bipolar disorder)	Negative psychiatric family history or positive family history of SUD
Prior psychiatric history, especially in absence of concurrent substance use	Negative psychiatric history
In primary psychotic disorders: presence of thought disorder, negative symptoms, predominant auditory hallucinations	Lack of thought disorder, intact insight, lack of negative symptoms, presence of visual, tactile, and/or olfactory hallucinations
Toxicology may or may not be positive	Toxicology generally positive for common substances (ie, opioids, stimulants, cannabis, alcohol)

Adapted from Refs. 64–69.

speed; general intelligence; sensory processing; verbal memory; nonverbal memory; speed of processing; motor control; working memory; and verbal reasoning. After withdrawal from these substances, patients often recover in many cognitive domains, but many patients have deficits when compared to control groups.[74]

Finally, if the patient used hallucinogens or dissociative substances in the past (ie, greater than 1 month), hallucinogen persisting perception disorder (HPPD) should be considered. HPPD is a condition in which someone with a history of substance use experiences persisting visual hallucinations and/or perceptual distortions that are similar to acute hallucinogen intoxication. HPDD is a rare condition and is more often diagnosed in people with a history of previous psychiatric disorder or SUD.[75] HPPD can arise in anyone, even after a single exposure to triggering substances. Notably, patients with HPDD demonstrate appropriate insight into their presentation, and reality testing would remain intact.

Other Considerations When Differentiating between Primary and Secondary Psychotic Symptoms

Intensity and Resolution of Psychiatric Symptoms

In addition to the time course, the clinician should consider the severity of psychiatric symptoms. For instance, are the psychiatric symptoms more pronounced than what would be expected considering the type, amount, route, and duration of substance use? This may be difficult to quantify, particularly if the patient has unknowingly used, or not reported use of substances not detected on standard UDTs, such as synthetic cannabinoids, cathinones, or illicitly manufactured benzodiazepines (see Chapter 10 for more information).

In contrast to primarily auditory hallucinations and complex delusions seen in primary psychotic disorders, drug-induced psychotic hallucinations generally involve more visual, tactile, or olfactory hallucinations.[76,77] Compared to people with primary psychotic disorders, people with substance-induced psychosis tend to have higher levels of insight into their condition.[63,76] Finally, drug-induced psychotic hallucinations generally improve with time once the patient is no longer acutely intoxicated or within the acute withdrawal phase (within a few days to weeks), whereas these symptoms are more persistent in those with primary psychiatric disorders.

Community Drug Supply

Regarding type of substance used and how this may impact presentation and accurate diagnostic assessment, laboratory testing, and knowledge of local use patterns, can be very helpful. This includes knowledge of the local illicit substance supply (including substance purity, potency, and common contaminants), preferred routes of substance administration, consistency in substance quality, and local rates of substance overdose and/or toxicity. There could be risk of contamination of which the patient is unaware, and which could result in the presenting symptoms. For example, a patient may report opioid use or have a known OUD, but present with elevated or irritable mood and insomnia, which could be due to unknown ingestion of cocaine along with their opioid supply. Other substances known to be commonly contaminated or appear as contaminants include hallucinogens and phencyclidine, respectively.[56] Resources such as the National Drug Early Warning System (NDEWS)[78] and the Researched Abuse, Diversion and Addiction-Related Surveillance (RADARS)[79] System can be useful for understanding national and local substance use trends and usage patterns.

Depressive Symptoms in the Setting of Concurrent SUD

People with SUD may present with depressive symptoms, suicidality, and anxiety that may be related to their substance use, an independent psychiatric disorder, or another medical condition. The clinician should follow the same general assessment outlined above to elucidate the etiology of the symptoms, determining the temporal course of symptom onset, severity of symptoms, history, and laboratory values. In addition to a UDT, other laboratory tests to consider include thyroid function tests, liver function tests, and possibly nutritional labs (eg, vitamin D, vitamin B12, folate, homocysteine, ferritin, iron panel) if there is concern for malnutrition.

In general, due to their mechanism of action in the brain and body, sedative–hypnotic/anxiolytic substances and alcohol are associated with significant depressive symptoms during intoxication. Conversely, withdrawal of these substances leads to an excitatory state, including anxiety, delirium, tactile and visual hallucinations, tremors, tongue fasciculations, tachycardia, hypertension, and occasionally fevers.[56]

Stimulants increase the effect of dopamine and norepinephrine in the brain which may lead to psychotic presentations with acute intoxication, as described above. Acute stimulant intoxication may also lead to substance-induced anxiety disorders and/or panic attacks. Stimulant withdrawal leads to a depletion of dopamine and norepinephrine and results in hypersomnia and depressive episodes during the acute withdrawal period. Some people report persistent dysphoria lasting weeks to months following cessation of chronic stimulant use, a known risk factor for returning to stimulant use.[56] Chapter 10 describes medical and psychiatric syndromes associated with acute intoxication and withdrawal of various substances.

Differentiating Between Primary and Secondary Mood Disorders

While a substance-induced mood or anxiety disorder should always be on the differential for a patient with a known history of substance use who is presenting with these symptoms, evidence suggests that the majority of affective and anxiety disorders that occur in patient populations who also use substances are not, in fact, substance induced. Results from the National Epidemiologic Survey on Alcohol and Related Conditions identified that less than 1% of patients who presented with a mood disorder who also used alcohol met diagnostic criteria for a substance-induced mood disorder.[9]

There are some reliable diagnostic tools that can be used to differentiate between primary (ie, not substance-induced) and secondary (ie, substance-induced) disorders in patients who present with psychiatric symptoms and who are known to use substances. One of these is the Psychiatric Research Interview for Substance and Mental Disorders (PRISM), a semistructured clinician-administered interview that measures the major, historical DSM-4 diagnoses of SUD and psychiatric disorders.[80,81] PRISM was designed to provide clear guidelines for differentiating between the expected effects of intoxication and withdrawal, substance-induced disorders, and primary psychiatric disorders and demonstrated a high reliability to diagnose primary depressive disorders, substance-induced MDD, and primary anxiety disorders.[82] The PRISM and other assessment tools can be useful to clinicians in the initial evaluation of patients with known substance use and psychiatric symptoms, whether that be during hospitalization or in other treatment settings. However, in cases where psychiatric illness is suspected, and psychiatric consultation services are available, specialists should be involved early on for evaluation and treatment planning.

Presentations With Cognitive Impairments and Deficits in Alertness and Attention

If a patient presents as confused with decreased alertness and deficits in cognitive domains and/or attention, this could be due to acute intoxication with a more sedating or dissociative substance, postacute withdrawal (ie, withdrawal symptoms that occur multiple days after last substance use and can last for weeks to years) but could also be due to acute delirium and/or an underlying NCD. When assessing a patient with decreased alertness or deficits in attention or cognition, the clinician should expand the differential diagnosis to include delirium, NCDs, and toxic metabolic leukoencephalopathy, all of which may cause neuropsychiatric symptoms that mimic a primary psychiatric illness, such as hallucinations, delusions, and mood changes.

Delirium

The DSM-5 diagnostic criteria for delirium include a significant reduction in attention and awareness, acute development of symptoms, fluctuation in symptoms over the course of a day, disturbances in cognition, and some evidence that these disturbances are secondary to another medical condition, substance use, toxin exposure, or a combination of these.[56] While delirium generally lasts hours to days, more persistent presentations can also occur and last on the scale of weeks to months; in hospital settings, delirium generally resolves after about 1 week.[56] Patients with delirium may also present with sleep–wake disturbances, emotional changes (including depressed mood and suicidality) and/or emotional lability, psychosis, and agitation.

In addition to a thorough laboratory work-up to screen for substances, for example, a UDT, and underlying medical conditions, for example, liver function tests, thyroid function, vitamin B12 levels, urinalysis, serum electrolytes, glucose, creatinine, and a complete blood count, an electroencephalography (EEG) can be useful for supporting a diagnosis of delirium, though it is not sensitive or specific enough to diagnose the condition on its own; generalized slowing is noted in most cases of delirium, though fast activity has also been reported in delirium caused by alcohol withdrawal.[56]

Neurocognitive Disorders

Neurocognitive Disorders (NCDs) include a wide range of conditions and etiologies and include Alzheimer disease; frontotemporal degeneration; Lewy body disease; vascular disease; traumatic brain injury; substance or medication intoxication; HIV infection; prion disease; Parkinson disease; Huntington disease; and other medical conditions or multiple etiologies. DSM-5 criteria used to diagnose a mild to severe NCD requires that the disease or syndrome is accompanied by a clinically significant behavioral disturbance, such as psychotic symptoms, mood disturbance, agitation, apathy, or other behavioral symptoms.

NCD should be considered in any patient who exhibits confusion that is not waxing and waning, especially in aging population and among people with SUD.[83] While there are many subtypes of NCDs with varied presentations that go beyond the scope of this chapter, these should be considered in older patients who may present with cognitive deficits in addition to paranoia, delusions, hallucinations, mood disturbances, agitation, apathy, sleep disturbances, disinhibition, and/or hyperphagia.[56] Some notable distinctions between psychotic features due to NCD compared to other psychotic or mood disorders include the lack of disorganized speech and behaviors and the higher likelihood of visual hallucinations in NCD causes.

Assessment for NCD etiology requires both subjective concern and objective evidence, usually in the form of formal neuropsychological testing, neuroimaging, cerebrospinal fluid analysis, family/genetic history, and bedside cognitive screens. NCDs can be substance or medication induced, in which case the cognitive impairments would need to persist outside of an episode of delirium and beyond what would be expected for substance intoxication or acute withdrawal.

There are several subtypes of substance-induced NCDs, most caused by alcohol, inhalants, or sedative–hypnotic/anxiolytics. Sedative–hypnotic/anxiolytic-induced NCD is often marked by greater deficits in memory compared to other cognitive domains.[56] Alcohol-induced NCDs can present with deficits in executive functioning, learning, and memory. In the amnestic confabulatory subtype of alcohol-induced NCD (ie, Korsakoff syndrome), patients present with amnesia, particularly with new information, and confabulation. This subtype can also present in conjunction with Wernicke encephalopathy if the patient also has thiamine deficiency, in which case they would also display nystagmus, ataxia, and lateral gaze paralysis.[56] On neuroimaging, patients with suspected NCD secondary to AUD may demonstrate cortical thinning, white matter loss, and enlargement of ventricles and sulci.[56] A history of SUD can also give rise to other types of NCD, such as vascular dementia in patients with a history of stimulant use disorder.

Toxic Metabolic Leukoencephalopathy

Toxic metabolic leukoencephalopathy is defined as a structural alteration of cerebral white mater in the central nervous system which may be caused by exposure to medications, illicit substances, organic solvents, or environmental toxins.[84] In leukoencephalopathy, myelin, the insulating sheath of surround nerve fibers in the white mater of the brain, suffers the most damage.

Leukoencephalopathy presents with cognitive impairment manifested as difficulty with thinking, memory and decision making; motor deficits including weakness, clumsiness, and difficulty with movement, language and vision problems, and personality changes including changes in mood, with emotional dysfunction, and changes in behavior and personality. Symptoms of confusion with inattention, memory loss, and emotional dysfunction may be mistaken for a psychiatric disorder, acute intoxication from an illicit substance, or a SUD.

Laboratory testing to consider includes urine substance use testing, if the exposure is recent, testing for toluene toxicity (ie, from huffing of volatile organic solvents) further described in Chapter 10, carboxyhemoglobin to test for carbon monoxide poisoning, and screening the urine for heavy metals, if available. The diagnosis requires that the clinician has a high index of suspicion, a documented exposure to a toxin, observed neurobehavioral deficits, and abnormalities identified on computed tomography (CT) or magnetic resonance imaging (MRI). Imaging of the brain is only indicated if deficits are detected on the mental-status examination or neuropsychological testing, described below.

Treatment for toxic metabolic leukoencephalopathy is limited and there is no uniform therapeutic approach. Prevention of ongoing iatrogenic or illicit exposure is critical to prevent further damage to the brain's white matter.

Cognitive Assessments and Neuropsychological Testing

Neuropsychological testing can be helpful in identifying cognitive impairments in several different domains, thereby narrowing the differential diagnosis and guiding treatment recommendations based on the cognitive processes that are affected. There are several short mental status scales that can be performed by clinicians at the bedside in the hospital setting. These include the Mini-Mental Status Examination (MMSE),[85] the Montreal Cognitive Assessment (MoCA),[86,87] and the Saint Louis University Mental Status Examination (SLUMS).[88–90] These examinations assess different cognitive domains such as memory, attention, language, visuospatial abilities, and executive functioning, and can be used to track changes in cognition over time.[91] However, these shorter assessments only provide a limited picture and are not sufficient in themselves to determine if a patient has a neurocognitive diagnosis.[92]

In patients with evidence of cognitive impairment requiring further characterization, formal neuropsychological testing may be indicated. This level of assessment is performed by a neuropsychologist and can take multiple hours, often distributed over several appointments in the outpatient setting. More formalized testing can provide greater insight into which brain areas and pathways may be affected based on their known involvement in different cognitive processes.[91,92]

When considered together, delirium, NCDs, and toxic metabolic leukoencephalopathy disease may cause neuropsychiatric symptoms that mimic a primary psychiatric disorder, such as hallucinations, delusions, and mood changes. Importantly, patients with neurocognitive deficits and/or delirium may not be able to provide accurate historical information and/or may have an unknown baseline of functioning. In these instances, collateral reports from people who are familiar with the patient's baseline state and medical and psychiatric history are key for determining how much the patient's current presentation differs from their baseline functional status.

Safety and Risk Assessment

Suicide Risk in People With Substance Use

In addition to honing the differential diagnosis for a patient who presents intoxicated with psychiatric symptoms, it is also important for the hospital-based clinician to conduct a thorough risk assessment. According to the DSM-5, there is increased risk of suicide in individuals who use substances, whether it be due to acute intoxication, withdrawal, or a substance-induced psychiatric disorder.[56] When considering patients who present to the emergency department with suicidal ideation (SI), one-third meet criteria for AUD.[93] Similarly, 43% of patients who present following a suicide attempt have an AUD, and this is the most common diagnosis among individuals who die by suicide.[94,95] Alcohol use influences suicide risk in patients diagnosed with PTSD,[96] bipolar disorder,[97] anxiety, and mood disorders.[98] Thus, AUD presents a significant risk factor for patient self-harm that should not be minimized. An accurate suicide safety assessment can be difficult to determine in acutely intoxicated patients and should be repeated once the individual is no longer intoxicated.

Safety Assessments

Table 14.7 outlines examples of how to approach a psychiatric safety assessment.[99–103] One tool that may be

TABLE 14.7

Steps to Performing a Psychiatric Risk Assessment

Can utilize free tools such as the SAFE-T, Columbia-Suicide Severity Rating Scale, or SAD PERSONS Scale to assist with evaluation

1. **Assess current suicidal ideation:** Okay to directly ask about suicidal thoughts as direct questioning is not associated with increased risk of suicide (ie, "*Are you having any thoughts about harming or killing yourself today? Are you having any thoughts that you would be better off dead or are okay with going to sleep and never waking up?*")
   a. **Ideation:** Similar to a physical symptom, ask about frequency, intensity, duration
   b. **Plan:** Ask about any preparatory acts (stockpiling extra pills, acquiring a firearm, buying rope or knives, etc.) as well as if they have had any thoughts about where/when they would try to hurt or kill themselves
   c. **Behaviors:** Ask about any prior suicide attempts, self-harming behavior, rehearsals, or aborted suicide attempts (ie, they held the gun to their head but then called a friend instead)
   d. **Intent:** Assess to what degree the person expects to carry out their suicide plan, as well as whether they believe the act to be lethal. Ask about any ambivalence/hesitation (ie, *"what causes you to not act on these thoughts? What are the reasons you think you should live? What are the reasons you think there is no point to living?"*)
2. **Specifically assess risk factors:** Often includes prior suicide attempts, substance/alcohol use, history of mental health concerns (especially mood disorders), access to lethal means, knowing someone who died by suicide (especially a family member), social isolation, chronic disease/disability, lack of access to mental health care, persistent feelings of hopelessness, gender (male is typically associated with higher risk), age (youth and older adults are typically associated with higher risk), loss of rational thought (ie, presence of psychosis, confusion, cognitive issues), presence of a specific, organized plan to harm self
3. **Specifically assess protective factors:** Often includes social connection, access to effective/helpful mental health care, ability to regulate emotions and behaviors, the presence of problem-solving and coping skills, cultural/spiritual/religious/personal beliefs against suicide, lack of access to lethal means, a sense of purpose
4. **Determine risk:**
   a. Can utilize online calculators and guides such as the SAFE-T and SAD PERSONS Scale to help determine risk:
      i. Typically involves weighing risk factors against protective factors to determine if a patient needs a higher level of care or monitoring to remain imminently safe
   b. Work with the patient to identify which risk factors could be modified through treatment, monitoring, or resources
   c. Engage in safety planning (can use free tools such as the Stanley–Brown Safety Plan)
   d. Provide crisis resources such as the 988 Suicide & Crisis Lifeline

Consider mental health/psychiatry consult for more in-depth assessment if patient at elevated risk of suicide

References and Resources 99–103.

helpful in approaching patients with SI is the five-step evaluation and triage (SAFE-T), which determines risk factors and protective factors and assists with risk level assessment and intervention.[99] The SAD PERSONS acronym is also a useful tool in directing these interactions[100,104] and serves as a reminder to consider the patient's Sex, Age, Depressive symptoms, Previous attempt(s), Ethanol use, Rational thinking loss, Social supports, and whether they have an Organized suicidal plan, No spouse, and/or Sickness.

Clinical Sobriety

Patients who present intoxicated and endorse SI may provide histories that are difficult to follow or are inaccurate, and they often are unable to actively participate in treatment and discharge planning.[105] While there are different approaches to suicide risk assessment in intoxicated patients, current standard practice is to assess the patient once they present as "clinically sober." Clinical sobriety is often determined by evaluating the patient's ambulation, coordination, speech patterns, concentration, short-term memory, orientation, level of alertness, and ability to engage in the interview.

Utility of Laboratory Tests to Assess Sobriety

It is helpful to collect laboratory blood alcohol content (BAC) on patients who appear intoxicated, which can not only confirm recent alcohol use, but also provide a guide for estimating one's timeline to sobriety. While the BAC is a useful data point in assessment, it is recommended to proceed with the safety evaluation based on clinical presentation rather than a specific nonzero BAC level, as patient presentation correlates inconsistently with BAC.[106,107] Some patients may appear to be at their baseline when they have high BAC levels, while other patients may present with a low BAC and appear quite intoxicated. While waiting until a patient has a BAC of zero is the most cautious approach and would confirm sobriety unequivocally, this could lead to longer hospital stays and/or acute withdrawal.[105] Furthermore, there are individual differences in the rate of alcohol metabolization, providing a limitation for time-based protocols for reassessment.[108]

Ensuring substances are no longer detectable on blood or urine test prior to assessing for SI may be generalized to other substances when a patient presents acutely intoxicated with SI. Thus, in the case where an SI assessment must be made rapidly, the clinician may place greater emphasis on a clinical assessment of sobriety in the absence of quantitative laboratory data. This is especially the case when patients are intoxicated with substances that may be metabolized more slowly, or where depressive symptoms are presenting in the setting of withdrawal or a substance-induced depressive or psychotic disorder. In this scenario, continued safety assessment in the emergency department may not be feasible, warranting hospitalization for continued observation.

While clinical assessment is currently recommended for determining sufficient sobriety for risk assessment, this could be complicated by the fact that the patient may be intoxicated with multiple substances, or that the patient may have preexisting cognitive impairment secondary to chronic substance use. Clinical assessment tools for this purpose are limited, and further research is needed to develop effective strategies to determine patients' level of impairment and ability to agree to psychiatric treatment and disposition.[105] In general, clinicians should utilize the aforementioned standard risk assessment tools and utilize specialty behavioral health services as available.

Trauma-Informed Care and Interview Considerations

Trauma-informed care will be discussed elsewhere in this book, but it is important to note that taking a trauma-informed approach when evaluating a patient is of utmost importance given the elevated rates of PTSD observed in patients with comorbid psychiatric and SUD. Trauma-informed care involves recognizing the impact of trauma and creating a safe environment that empowers patients and prevents further harm. In the hospital setting, it may be counterproductive to delve too deeply into the details of a prior or recent traumatic experiences, especially if mental health resources and longitudinal follow-up are limited and if the patient is reluctant to divulge this information, as patients may experience destabilization of mood and PTSD symptoms. Assessing distressing symptoms of PTSD and/or the presence of prior trauma can be done without soliciting details of the inciting traumatic event and allow for proactive management of symptoms while in the hospital, including modifying communication and team rounding styles for patients easily overwhelmed by lots of new people and conversations, considering door signs recommending against loud knocking or announcements for hypervigilant patients, and adjusting intervention schedules and giving advance notice for patients who struggle with unclear schedules and unexpected surprises.

Acute Treatment Considerations and Recommendations

Treatment protocols for co-occurring SUD and psychiatric disorders in the hospital setting should involve both integrated and concurrent treatment for best outcomes. Specifically, pharmacologic approaches should be used in conjunction with psychosocial interventions. For example, medications for OUD should be initiated without delay, even if psychiatric assessments are ongoing. Motivational interviewing approaches are also useful in encouraging patient engagement in treatment. Many of the approaches for treatment of specific SUD will be covered in other chapters. Therefore, the discussion presented here focus on the management of psychiatric symptoms in the setting of SUD, as well as specific treatments to consider and avoid in this unique patient population.

Management of Psychotic and Manic Symptoms

Antipsychotic Treatment: Initiation and Drug Selection

For patients who present with symptoms of psychosis or mania, initiation of treatment with an antipsychotic is often indicated to reduce these symptoms (see Table 14.8).[109,110] If a patient's presentation is concerning for psychosis or mania, the hospital-based clinician should consult psychiatry early in the hospital course for assistance with assessment and treatment planning. However, psychiatric consultation may not be readily available in some hospital settings, in which case a hospital-based clinician may start antipsychotic treatment to manage these symptoms. Generally, initial treatment with a second-generation antipsychotic is recommended, given this class of medications has a lower risk of extrapyramidal side effects (eg, akathisia, dystonia, parkinsonism). However, therapeutic effects are not significantly different between first- and second-generation antipsychotics. For a daily scheduled medication, aripiprazole or risperidone are recommended as initial options, given their more favorable side-effect profile and general tolerability.[111]

Antipsychotic Treatment: Special Considerations

There are certain cases where other medications may be more beneficial than beginning with a second-generation antipsychotic. For example, in patients struggling with insomnia and SUD, a more sedating antipsychotic may be preferred, such as quetiapine.

In patients with concurrent dementia and SUD, the threshold for initiating treatment with an antipsychotic is higher compared to other patient populations. In these patients, the use of an antipsychotic is reserved for those with severe neuropsychiatric symptoms that pose a safety risk or their symptoms are negatively impacting the patient's quality of life in a significant way. In these patients, antipsychotic treatment is associated with increased risk of stroke, myocardial infarction, and death, and their use for controlling behavioral symptoms is not approved by the FDA.[112] If necessary, initial considerations include olanzapine, quetiapine, and pimavanserin, with low starting doses and slow, cautious titration with careful monitoring for side effects such as orthostatic hypotension and sedation.[112]

In patients who are high-risk for metabolic side effects (eg, obesity, dyslipidemia, diabetes mellitus, cardiovascular disease, increased waist circumference), aripiprazole, lurasidone, and ziprasidone may be considered, given their lower risk of metabolic effects compared to other antipsychotics.[113] Metformin can also be added to counteract antipsychotic-induced weight gain,[114] and this may be particularly useful in cases where the above medications may be contraindicated or ineffective, requiring alternative antipsychotic agents.

Antipsychotic Treatment Duration and Considerations for Discontinuation

If a substance-induced condition is suspected, then the patient should be tapered off the antipsychotic medication after psychiatric symptoms have resolved.[34] If psychotic symptoms resolve rapidly and the patient is outside of the expected time window for acute intoxication and withdrawal, then antipsychotic treatment may be discontinued prior to hospital discharge. In some cases, substance-induced psychotic symptoms may be slower to resolve and deprescribing of the antipsychotic can occur in the outpatient setting after a period of stability. If continued assessment is more suggestive of a concurrent psychotic illness, then the clinician should titrate the antipsychotic to the lowest effective dose for controlling symptoms, and it should be continued upon hospital discharge. These patients will need a follow-up appointment with a mental health provider or psychiatrist within a few weeks from discharge.

Screening and Monitoring Recommendations With Antipsychotic Treatment

For patients started on an antipsychotic, it is important to collect a hemoglobin A1c, lipid panel, and electrocardiogram prior to, or at the time of, treatment initiation. These laboratory tests are important to establish a metabolic baseline, as antipsychotics can increase hemoglobin A1c and cause dyslipidemia.[115] Antipsychotics also increase the QTc, which in patients with a known prolonged QTc or who

TABLE 14.8

Recommended Dosing of Psychiatric Medications

Medications for management of acute agitation		
Medication	**Starting dose**	**Maximum dose/day**
Antipsychotics:		
Olanzapine		
Orally disintegrating tablets (ODT)	2.5–5 mg every 4–6 h	20 mg per 24 h
Intramuscular (IM)	2.5–10 mg for severe agitation	30 mg per 24 h
Note: IM olanzapine is contraindicated with IM/IV benzodiazepines		
Risperidone ODT (M-tabs)	0.5–1 mg every 6 h	4 mg per 24 h
Haloperidol		
Oral, IM, or intravenous (IV)	2.5–5 mg every 4–6 h	20 mg per 24 h
Note: Administration of diphenhydramine 50 mg with IM or IV haloperidol is recommended. IV use is common but is off label in the United States		
Benzodiazepines:		
Lorazepam PO, IM, or IV	1–2 mg every 4–6 h	Limited by vital signs, need to monitor for respiratory depression
Midazolam IV or IM	2.5 mg every 3–5 min (IV) or 5–10 min (IM) until adequate sedation or behavioral control	
Medications for long-term management		
Medication	**Starting dose**	**Maximum dose**
Antipsychotics:		
Olanzapine	2.5–5 mg nightly, divide if desired	20 mg total daily
Aripiprazole	5–10 mg daily	30 mg daily
Risperidone	1–2 mg nightly, divide if desired	8 mg total daily
Quetiapine	25–50 mg twice daily	800 mg total daily
Antidepressants:		
Bupropion	Extended release (XL) 150 mg daily	450 mg daily
Sertraline	25–50 mg daily	200 mg daily
Escitalopram	5–10 mg daily	20 mg daily
Venlafaxine	37.5–75 mg daily	225 mg daily
Mirtazapine	7.5–15 mg nightly	45 mg nightly
When mirtazepine used for sleep only, no additional benefit above 15 mg nightly		
Mood stabilizers:		Target levels:
Divalproex	250–500 mg twice daily	50–100 mcg/mL
Lithium	300 mg two to three times daily	0.8–1.2 mEq/L
Miscellaneous:		
Melatonin *(sleep)*	3 mg nightly	12 mg nightly
Hydroxyzine *(anxiety, sleep)*	10–25 mg every 4–6 h	400 mg total daily
Gabapentin *(anxiety, sleep)*	100–300 mg three times daily	3,600 mg total daily
Trazodone *(sleep)*	25–50 mg nightly	200–300 mg nightly
Clonidine *(anxiety)*	0.1 mg daily to twice daily	Limited by vital signs
Propranolol *(anxiety)*	10 mg three times daily	Limited by vital signs

References 109, 110.

TABLE 14.9

Common QTc-Prolonging Medications

QTc prolongation risk stratification	Commonly used medications
Low risk	Sertraline
	Venlafaxine
	Duloxetine (increased risk in overdose)
	Bupropion (except in overdose)
	Aripiprazole
	Olanzapine
	Psychostimulants
	Benzodiazepines
	Anticonvulsants
	Ondansetron (PO)
Moderate risk	Quetiapine
	Buprenorphine
	Risperidone
	Escitalopram
	Citalopram
	Ciprofloxacin
High risk	Methadone
	Haloperidol (IV)
	Ziprasidone (particularly IM/IV)
	Amisulpride

CYP450 inhibitors that can contribute to QTc prolongation by increasing serum levels: fluoxetine, paroxetine, sertraline, fluvoxamine, valproic acid, bupropion, duloxetine, citalopram, escitalopram, haloperidol.

References 117–119.

are on other QTc-prolonging medications (such as methadone), increases the risk of torsades des pointes. In patients who benefit from the antipsychotic (or methadone) with a persistently prolonged QTc, it is important to have a patient-centered, risk–benefit conversation before deprescribing the QTc prolonging medications. Common QTc-prolonging medications are reviewed in Table 14.9. Complications of QTc-prolonging treatments will be discussed in more detail later in the chapter.[116–119]

Long-Acting Antipsychotic Formulations

Long-acting injectable (LAI) antipsychotics may be a good option for patients who have difficulty taking a daily antipsychotic. LAIs duration of action is between 2 and 4 weeks depending on the medication. LAI use is often limited by expense and need for close outpatient follow-up for continued dosing. Patients often need to be in the hospital for several days to titrate the oral antipsychotic dosage to estimate the appropriate LAI loading and maintenance dose. Oral dosage titration and LAI loading dose administration often occur in the hospital setting, and patients are discharged with plans for follow-up for additional maintenance doses, which can be provided by an outpatient psychiatrist, the patient's primary care clinician, or the assertive community treatment (ACT) team. Despite the benefits of avoiding medication nonadherence, it is notable that, while LAI formulations have been shown to reduce relapse risk in clinical trials when compared with placebo, randomized controlled trials (RCTs) comparing oral and LAI antipsychotics have often failed to show advantages of LAIs over oral antipsychotics in terms of relapse and/or hospitalization risk.[120]

Management of Agitation

Behavioral Approaches for Managing Agitation

When treating patients who present with acute agitation or aggression, it is important to consider any causal factors (eg, delirium, NCDs, psychiatric illness, environmental causes) that go beyond acute intoxication and address all possible causes of agitation. Behavioral measures should always be first line for redirecting problematic behaviors and should be employed by all members of the treatment team. These can include verbal de-escalation strategies, approaching the patient calmly and actively listening to their concerns.[34,111] In addition, environmental modifications can also be of great benefit to reduce patient agitation, including minimizing environmental stimuli, providing adequate lighting, and creating a safe and quiet space for the patient.[121] For patients who may be agitated and/or delirious, it is recommended to employ a strategy that involves reorientation, cognitive stimulation, promoting good sleep hygiene (minimizing light and noise when appropriate), encouraging patient mobility, addressing any sensory impairments (ie, providing glasses, hearing aids), and making clocks available.[122]

Pharmacologic Management of Agitation

When behavioral measures alone are ineffective at controlling patient agitation, particularly in the setting of physical aggression, pharmacologic interventions are recommended to maintain patient and staff safety. Benzodiazepines are considered first line for managing substance-induced agitation, aggression, and/or confusion.[34] In these cases, a shorter-acting benzodiazepine is generally preferred, such as lorazepam or midazolam, which can be administered orally, intramuscularly, or intravenously.[123]

Antipsychotics can be useful for controlling psychotic agitation and aggression in the hospital setting, whether that be related to substance use or psychiatric illness.[111] In these cases, antipsychotics with orally disintegrating forms such as risperidone or olanzapine are helpful in assuring patient compliance with a quick onset of action. Intramuscular (IM) formulations can also be used for rapid control of behavior in situations where the patient declines oral options and patient or staff safety is of concern. If the patient has intravenous (IV) access, then IV haloperidol can also be used. In general, oral formulations are preferred because they are associated with lower risk of adverse effects. Coadministration of diphenhydramine or benztropine with an IM or IV antipsychotic is recommended to decrease the risk of extrapyramidal symptoms.[111] In cases of severe agitation, a combination of IM haloperidol (5 mg), lorazepam (2 mg), and diphenhydramine (50 mg) is often used.[111]

It is important to monitor the patient's QTc closely with regular antipsychotic administration, particularly in patients with co-occurring mental health and SUD diagnoses, who are likely to receive other QTc-prolonging medications and risk of QTc-prolongation can help guide medication choices. Table 14.9 lists medications that are associated with QTc prolongation.

Pharmacologic Considerations and Limitations

While having antipsychotic and benzodiazepine options available as-needed for agitation, it is important to remember that benzodiazepines should not be used in conjunction with IM olanzapine. The combination of benzodiazepine and IM olanzapine has a black box warning for respiratory depression which can be life-threatening.[124,125] This contraindication does not exist when olanzapine is administered orally, regardless of whether the benzodiazepine used is oral, IV, or IM. Chlorpromazine and clozapine should generally be avoided in patients with co-occurring illness due to the increased risk of seizures.[34] In cases of severe agitation that are not responsive to benzodiazepine and antipsychotic treatment, ketamine (IM, IV) or dexmedetomidine (SL, IV) can be considered. These medications are particularly useful when rapid control is required for patient and staff safety, though administration of these medications may not be permitted on a general medical floor and may require admission to a step-down unit or ICU for close monitoring and higher level-of-care.[34,111]

Management of Mood and Anxiety Symptoms

Considerations for the Pharmacologic Treatment of Depression

For depressive or anxiety symptoms, treatment should be considered based on severity and duration. It is common for patients who are acutely intoxicated or in postacute withdrawal to experience a dysphoric or anxious state. In this patient population, these symptoms may initially present as co-occurring MDD, GAD, or panic disorder. Careful examination of the temporal history of these symptoms should be considered before starting a daily medication, such as a selective serotonin reuptake inhibitor (SSRI) or serotonin norepinephrine reuptake inhibitor (SNRI), which would take weeks before the patient would experience any reduction in symptoms. If considering long-term treatment for depression, bupropion may be a good choice for patients with concurrent tobacco use disorder[126] or stimulant use disorder,[34,127] as this can address both mood symptoms and may decrease cravings, assisting with cessation.

Adjunctive and As-Needed Medications for Anxiety

As-needed anxiolytic medications are a key part of withdrawal management for many SUD. For many patients experiencing opioid withdrawal, hydroxyzine, an H_1 receptor inverse agonist, can be a helpful adjunctive medication to manage mild to moderate anxiety, in addition to the use of medications for OUD.[128] Clonidine, an alpha-2 adrenoceptor agonist, is often effective in managing anxiety and symptoms of autonomic hyperactivity in patients experiencing withdrawal from opioids, and it is likely also helpful in patients experiencing anxiety due to withdrawal from other substances.[129,130] Gabapentin may be used for concurrent anxiety and neuropathic pain and may even reduce cravings in patients with AUD.[131,132] For patients with contraindications to other options, propranolol can be helpful for reducing anxiety, specifically physical manifestations such as tachycardia, though should be avoided in patients who actively use cocaine or who are experiencing cocaine-associated chest pain. Use of propranolol in this population may result in an unopposed alpha-adrenergic stimulation, which can worsen coronary vasoconstriction, increase blood pressure, and cause severe complications.[133] More recently, some data suggests that propranolol may be useful in managing symptoms associated with severe cocaine withdrawal in certain patient populations, but more research is needed.[134] Finally, in patients who use benzodiazepines, other methods of controlling their anxiety may not be effective, so careful consideration of benzodiazepine treatment should be weighed against potential complications, particularly in patients with concomitant opioid use, given the additional risk of respiratory depression.[135] While benzodiazepines have a clear role in managing withdrawal and agitation in patients with AUD and/or sedative–hypnotic use disorder, these should be avoided outside of these clinical scenarios due to the risk of cross-dependence and relapse.

Management of Insomnia and Sleep Disturbances

Insomnia is a common symptom in hospitalized patients with comorbid psychiatric disorders and SUD. While patients may require medications for acute stabilization during their hospitalization, it is important to promote healthy sleep–wake cycles and encourage good sleep hygiene. Obtaining restful sleep in the hospital is challenging and every effort should be made to open the blinds during the day to expose the patient to natural sunlight, limit light exposure at night, reduce noise and blood draws at night, schedule mealtimes, and keep other daily routines as structured as possible.

Melatonin, as a treatment for insomnia, has minimal side effects.[34,136] It is available over the counter and can be continued following hospital discharge at the patient's discretion. Lower-risk medications to promote sleep include mirtazapine, an atypical antidepressant, and trazodone, an antidepressant. Both of these medications may provide some mood benefit in patients with MDD and have lower potential for misuse.[34,136] Trazodone promotes sleep while improving sleep architecture and mood.[137] Due to its antihistamine effects, hydroxyzine can cause sedation and may be used as needed nightly. It is particularly useful for patients who have a hard time falling asleep due to racing thoughts. Low-dose quetiapine may also be useful in patients with co-occurring psychiatric disorders and SUD[138] with a recommended starting dose of 25 mg nightly.[111] Benzodiazepines and other GABA-A agonists, including barbiturates (eg, phenobarbital), nonbenzodiazepine hypnotics (eg, zolpidem, zaleplon, zopiclone), and certain anesthetics (eg, propofol, etomidate), should generally be avoided in patients with co-occurring illness due to a risk of dependence and misuse, as well as increased risk of side effects.[136,138]

Given risk of polypharmacy, it is generally not recommended to discharge a patient with sleep medications for long-term use, aside from low-dose melatonin, instead promoting behavioral approaches, such as continued sleep hygiene and cognitive behavioral therapy for insomnia (CBT-I), if available.[139,140]

Treatment Selection: Special Considerations in Specific Populations

Aside from treating the presenting symptoms outlined above, there is limited evidence concerning long-term specific treatment choices for specific subgroups of patients with co-occurring psychiatric disorders and SUD. The following paragraphs will summarize existing knowledge and outline cases where specific medications may offer some benefit, or should be avoided, in this patient population. These recommendations are summarized in Figure 14.4.

Bipolar Disorder and SUD

Considering patients with comorbid bipolar disorder and SUD, substance use often leads to a more severe course of illness, with increased mood episode frequency, higher number of hospitalizations, worsened depression, and higher risk of self-harm and suicide attempts.[14,141–144] Ongoing substance use can also

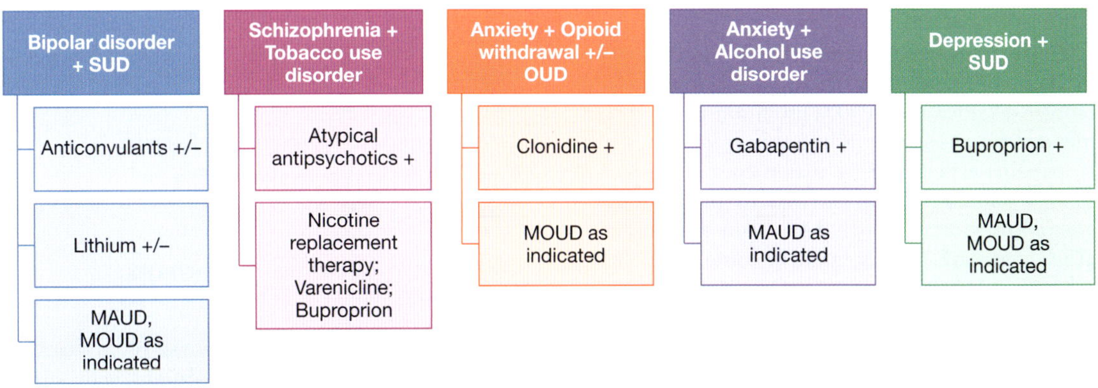

Figure 14.4: Preferred medications for specific diagnoses. MOUD, medications for opioid use disorder; MAUD, medications for alcohol use disorder.[126,127,129–132,145,146]

decrease the efficacy of mood-stabilizing medications, sometimes requiring higher doses in order to have desired clinical effect.[14] For this reason, patients with co-occurring bipolar disorder and SUD should be referred to psychotherapy to support their SUD treatment.

Medication Considerations for Co-occurring Bipolar Disorder and SUD

There are limited studies examining the efficacy of specific pharmacotherapy recommendations for patients with co-occurring bipolar disorder and SUD. One retrospective chart review of hospitalized patients with bipolar I disorder and a current manic episode found that those patients with co-occurring substance use who received an anticonvulsant, alone or in combination with lithium, were more likely to reach remission of their symptoms.[145] In patients with bipolar disorder without SUD, there were no significant differences in remission status between those treated with lithium alone, anticonvulsants alone, or the combination of the two. Importantly, while lithium is first-line treatment for bipolar spectrum illness, initiating treatment with this medication is not recommended without psychiatric consult, given lithium's narrow therapeutic index and the risks of toxicity.

Some evidence suggests that use of gabapentin as an add-on treatment for patients with bipolar disorder with a co-occurring AUD and panic disorder could reduce the severity of depressive episodes.[147] Thus, based on current evidence, treatment with anticonvulsants, either as monotherapy or as an adjunct to lithium, is superior to treatment with lithium alone in patients with co-occurring bipolar spectrum illness and SUD. When in doubt, treating a patient's psychiatric disorder and SUD with individual pharmacotherapies directed at these problems individually is still preferred to deferring treatment.

Medications to Avoid in Patients With Co-occurring Bipolar Disorder and SUD

There are some medications that should be avoided or used with caution in patients with co-occurring bipolar disorder and SUD. Disulfiram is not recommended for patients with impulsive tendencies, that is, patients experiencing a manic episode. Couse of alcohol and disulfiram will lead to the disulfiram-ethanol reaction with includes a rapid onset of headache, confusion, nausea, and, in some cases, hallucinations, delirium, seizures, coma, and potentially death.[14] Disulfiram should also be used with extreme caution in patients with bipolar disorder who have a history of psychotic features. Disulfiram inhibits dopamine-β-hydroxylase, which catalyzes the conversion of dopamine to norepinephrine.[14]

While treatment with naltrexone is generally thought to be safe and effective in patients with co-occurring bipolar disorder and AUD, there are two case reports of patients with bipolar disorder treated with divalproex who developed symptoms more consistent with opioid withdrawal following initiation of naltrexone treatment, although they had no known opioid use.[148]

Finally, one study demonstrated that quetiapine was ineffective in patients with co-occurring bipolar disorder and SUD, so other antipsychotics should be considered in this population.[149,150] While the evidence demonstrating adverse effects with the use of these medications in specific clinical scenarios is limited, whenever possible, it is recommended to choose other treatment options until further research is completed.

Schizophrenia Spectrum Disorders and SUD

Among patients with schizophrenia spectrum disorders, clozapine is particularly effective in addressing both psychotic symptoms and substance use, demonstrating efficacy in patient populations who use alcohol, cocaine, and cannabis.[150–157] Treatment with clozapine should only be initiated by or in collaboration with a psychiatrist, as this medication may lead to severe side effects and requires careful monitoring and cautious titration.

There is some evidence that bupropion may promote nicotine abstinence in patients with co-occurring schizophrenia and tobacco use disorder.[158] Interestingly, the use of atypical antipsychotics was more likely to result in smoking cessation in patients with schizophrenia and tobacco use disorder compared to typical antipsychotics, when both were combined with nicotine replacement therapy.[146] Furthermore, there is some evidence that interventional approaches, particularly repetitive transcranial magnetic stimulation (rTMS), a noninvasive brain stimulation technique using magnetic pulses is a promising treatment for patients with comorbid schizophrenia and SUD, particularly tobacco use disorder.[159,160]

Recommendations to Avoid Adverse Outcomes With Pharmacotherapy

Safety Considerations in Patients With a History of Self-harm

For all patients with an increased risk of self-harm or suicide, whenever possible, medications with serious side effects or lethality in overdose should be avoided. These include, but are not limited to, lithium, tricyclic antidepressants, sedative–hypnotics, venlafaxine, bupropion, quetiapine, olanzapine, ziprasidone, valproic acid, carbamazepine, and citalopram.[161] In cases where these medications are best practice, limit risk by prescribing 1 to 2 weeks of medication at a time to avoid medication stockpiling. When available, request a pill blister pack from the pharmacy, which may also be helpful to mitigate overdose risk.

Medications With Risk of Diversion

Medication diversion increases overdose risk both in the patient receiving the medication and among those living in the community. In general, patients should be treated with the medication that is indicated for their underlying conditions. However, if the "best" evidence-based medication is commonly diverted, the clinician must carefully considered the risks and benefits of the medication choice when building treatment plans.

Quetiapine is commonly misused for its sedative effects.[162–164] In correctional care settings, trazodone may be diverted to self-treat withdrawal symptoms or to enhance the effects of other substances.[164] Trazodone is generally considered safe to use in patients with co-occurring psychiatric disorders and SUD outside of the correctional setting.[164] Cyclobenzaprine can also be misused due to its sedating properties. There are some reports of people misusing venlafaxine and bupropion.[165] Finally, benzodiazepines and other sedative–hypnotics should be avoided in patients with SUD due to their risk of misuse, dependence, and risk of severe side effects and even death when used in combination with other substances.

Risks for QT Prolongation and Management

One common challenge to treating patients with co-occurring psychiatric disorder and SUD is polypharmacy. Patients with a psychiatric diagnosis and a SUD (ie, dual diagnosis) have a higher rate of being prescribed three or more medications, which can increase rates of hospitalization and negative health outcomes.[166] Patients with co-occurring disorders are often at higher risk for QTc prolongation, raising their risk of torsades de pointes, which can be lethal. This is due to the types of medications used to treat these disorders, many of which prolong QTc. Whenever possible, polypharmacy of multiple QTc-prolonging medications should be avoided. When initiating medications that prolong QTc, it is recommended to collect a baseline electrocardiogram. This should be followed by periodic electrocardiograms for continued QTc monitoring in patients taking multiple QTc-prolonging medications, in patients with hepatic impairment, and in patients who are also taking CYP450 inhibitors (ie, fluoxetine, paroxetine, sertraline, fluvoxamine, valproic acid, bupropion, duloxetine, citalopram, escitalopram, haloperidol), which can elevate serum levels of several QTc-prolonging medications.

Patients with AUD often experience hypokalemia and hypomagnesemia due to poor nutrient intake, which can exacerbate QTc prolongation risks. Always correct electrolytes before initiating higher-risk medications and monitor patient's metabolic panels periodically. Common QTc-prolonging medications are listed in Table 14.9.

General Contraindications in Patients With Co-occurring Disorders

Some medications are mostly contraindicated in patients with co-occurring psychiatric disorders and SUD due to their risk of exacerbating symptoms and/or their potential for misuse. Stimulant medications are generally contraindicated in patients who have a history of psychosis or stimulant use disorder. Some studies demonstrate benefit with the use of prescribed stimulants for patients with stimulant use disorder, described in Chapter 10, however this would be recommended in the outpatient setting with careful monitoring by an addiction psychiatrist or addiction medicine physician and is not recommended in the hospital setting. Scheduled benzodiazepines are not recommended for patients with psychiatric disorders and SUD due to the risk of misuse, physical dependence, diversion, and increased risk of side effects such as respiratory depression. However, if a patient has been taking long-term prescribed benzodiazepines, these should not be discontinued abruptly due to the risk of severe and/or protracted withdrawal. Instead, tapering these medications may occur in the outpatient setting over a period of months with careful monitoring and support.[70–73] There are cases when these medications are used to treat symptoms and may overall result in harm reduction, though these regimens must be considered cautiously and would be implemented in the outpatient setting by a clinician with whom the patient has good rapport and a stable long-term treatment relationship.

Peripartum Considerations

There is also often apprehension about treating comorbid psychiatric disorders and SUD in pregnant patients despite rising prevalence rates of SUD in the United States.[167] Though a nuanced and complicated topic, it is increasingly recognized that "whole patient" care and maternal health has significant impact on longer-term outcomes of the fetus and child[168] and that appropriate treatment for both psychiatric disorders and SUD should not be withheld.[169] Many resources exist to help guide treatment of these disorders during pregnancy, such as perinatal mental health access lines (maternal mental health leadership alliance [MMHLA]) and resources through organizations like MotherToBaby[170] and the American College of Obstetricians and Gynecologists (ACOG).[171] Chapter 12 addresses SUD in pregnancy.

Discharge Planning and Continuity of Care

At hospital discharge, patients with co-occurring psychiatric disorder and SUD must be linked to outpatient mental health and SUD treatment, support groups, and other recovery services. Patients with co-occurring disorders generally have a higher rate of return to substance use (40%) compared to those without concurrent psychiatric disorders (26%) at 3 months posttreatment.[172] Connecting these patients to appropriate care and follow-up is imperative for continued treatment success.[172] For further discussion of SUD-directed treatment and support involved in discharge planning, please refer to Chapter 20.

Dual Diagnosis Treatment and Programming

When planning dual-diagnosis treatment options, it is important to consider several factors for optimal patient experience and outcomes including patient eligibility; availability of, and patient openness to integrated care; treating facilities' culture around co-occurring diagnoses; and existing support systems for the individual once they are in treatment. When considering patient eligibility, the patient must have concurrent psychiatric disorder and SUD diagnoses, and the severity of each disorder should be significant enough to negatively impact the patient's daily functioning and overall prognosis. Elements of these diagnoses to consider include chronicity of symptoms; acuity; and level of functional impairment. Crucially, the patient's readiness and motivation for treatment are also paramount in this decision.[173,174] Though integrated co-occurring care is preferred, in some cases, such as acute psychosis, mania, or suicidality, psychiatric symptoms may be severe enough to warrant inpatient psychiatric care prior to SUD/co-occurring care.

Addressing Stigma in Access to Care

Unfortunately, though less common now, some SUD treatment programs will not accept patients taking psychiatric medications or will actively discourage patients from taking daily psychiatric medications in the name of avoiding using medication as a "crutch." This outdated practice is not evidence based and is often stigmatizing to the patient. Similarly, some mental health programs do not accept patients with co-occurring SUD and psychiatric disorders until the patient's SUD is addressed. Unsurprisingly, this creates barriers to receiving essential mental health care. Given these outdated practices, it is essential to assess the culture of a treatment facility when creating a discharge plan for patients with co-occurring psychiatric disorders and SUD. When this happens, clinicians may consider advocating against this stigmatizing treatment on their patients' behalf by filing an Americans with Disabilities Act (ADA) complaint to the US Department of Justice Civil Rights Division.[175] Insurance barriers and lack of mental health parity in insurance coverage also remain a significant problem, with some plans not providing coverage for higher levels of co-occurring care and others having mental health "carve-outs" to reduce costs and, as a result, provide less care and fewer services.[176] Fortunately, stigma is slowly decreasing around the treatment of co-occurring disorders, and there has been a concurrent rise of integrated treatment program options.

Emerging Evidence and Future Directions

There is a dearth of evidence assessing the effectiveness of specific pharmacotherapies or combinations of therapies in dual-diagnosis populations. This is also the case for guidance on best practices to approach and manage co-occurring psychiatric disorders and SUD in hospitalized patients. Thus, more controlled studies that include diverse patient populations are needed to better evaluate best treatment approaches when managing co-occurring illnesses.

In previous studies assessing utilization of SUD and mental health treatment,[16] survey data suggested that patients were more likely to interact with mental health clinicians than SUD-specific treatments. Thus, one way of increasing access to care specific to patients with co-occurring disorders may be to increase substance use-focused training for mental health and primary care clinicians. This approach may face difficulties given already demanding workloads and limited resources.[16,177] While recent policy changes aimed to increase access to behavioral health and SUD treatment, it is important to note that increasing access does not necessarily equate to improving the quality of care offered. A 2006 report from the Institute of Medicine suggested that integrated treatment for both psychiatric disorders and AUD was often not in accordance with established guidelines.[16] Medical training should include education on the medication management and behavioral interventions recommended for people living with SUD and psychiatric disorders.

In addition to efforts to improve access to and quality of care, increased treatment modalities are also needed to better address the needs of this patient population. Interventional psychiatry and neuromodulation approaches have shown promise in treating co-occurring psychiatric disorders and SUDs.

Repetitive transcranial magnetic stimulation (rTMS) is an intervention that targets the dorsolateral prefrontal cortex (DLPFC), a brain region involved in management of cognitive functions like executive function, memory, and attention as well as mood concerns like depression. rTMS reduces substance craving and consumption among people with SUD, especially following multiple stimulation sessions.[159,160] rTMS may be particularly helpful for people with SUDs and comorbid depression or schizophrenia spectrum illnesses, though more research is needed.[159,160,178,179]

Deep brain stimulation (DBS) is a surgical procedure that involves an electrode implantation in specific brain areas. DBS has been studied in small, uncontrolled studies targeting reward neurocircuitry and may be helpful for severe cases of SUD. DBS has been associated with prolonged abstinence from substance use, but its implementation is limited by its invasive nature, costs, and need for larger controlled trials.[180,181]

Transcranial direct current stimulation (tDCS) is a noninvasive brain stimulation technique using weak electrical currents. tDCS has been effective in reducing cravings and substance use, though less consistently than rTMS. Similar to DBS, larger trials are needed to confirm its safety and efficacy.[159,180,182] These newer approaches, rTMS, DBS, tDCS, may have increased efficacy and effectiveness when combined with traditional pharmacotherapy, such as antidepressants and medications for OUD,[183,184] though concomitant treatment with benzodiazepines and antipsychotics appears to interfere somewhat with therapeutic response.[183,185]

Another emerging technique is focused ultrasound (FUS), a noninvasive neuromodulation approach that has shown promise in treating patients with co-occurring SUD and psychiatric disorders, including schizophrenia, schizoaffective disorder, and MDD.[186–189]

Glucagon-like peptide-1 (GLP-1) receptor agonists may also be useful in addressing SUD, as well as treating weight gain and metabolic effects related to treatment with many psychiatric medications. While limited clinical studies have been completed thus far, current evidence demonstrates that GLP-1 agonists significantly decrease alcohol and nicotine use and may also reduce the risk of hospitalization as a result of AUD.[190–193]

Given the complexity and challenges in treating co-occurring disorders, these exciting new possibilities, along with increased integrated treatment programs, more nuanced and patient-centered medical and clinical education, and destigmatizing efforts in the medical field, bring much-needed hope to clinicians and patients alike.

REFERENCES

1. Harris MG, Bharat C, Glantz MD, Sampson NA, Al-Hamzawi A; World Health Organization's World Mental Health Surveys collaborators. Cross-national patterns of substance use disorder treatment and associations with mental disorder comorbidity in the WHO World Mental Health Surveys. *Addiction*. 2019; 114(8):1446–1459.
2. Morisano D, Babor TF, Robaina KA. Co-occurrence of substance use disorders with other psychiatric disorders: implications for treatment services. *Nord Stud Alcohol Drugs*. 2014;31(1):5–25.
3. Hjorthøj C, Østergaard MLD, Benros ME, et al. Association between alcohol and substance use disorders and all-cause and cause-specific mortality in schizophrenia, bipolar disorder, and unipolar depression: a nationwide, prospective, register-based study. *Lancet Psychiatry*. 2015;2(9):801–808.
4. Batki SL, Meszaros ZS, Strutynski K, et al. Medical comorbidity in patients with schizophrenia and alcohol dependence. *Schizophr Res*. 2009;107(2–3):139–146.
5. Benaiges I, Prat G, Adan A. Health-related quality of life in patients with dual diagnosis: clinical correlates. *Health Qual Life Outcomes*. 2012;10:106.
6. Mårtensson S, Düring SW, Johansen KS, Tranberg K, Nordentoft M. Time trends in co-occurring substance use and psychiatric illness (dual diagnosis) from 2000 to 2017—a nationwide study of Danish register data. *Nord J Psychiatry*. 2023;77(4):411–419.
7. Regier DA, Farmer ME, Rae DS, et al. Comorbidity of mental disorders with alcohol and other drug abuse. *JAMA*. 1990;264(19):2511–2518.
8. Kessler RC, Crum RM, Warner LA, Nelson CB, Schulenberg J, Anthony JC. Lifetime co-occurrence of DSM-III-R alcohol abuse and dependence with other psychiatric disorders in the National Comorbidity Survey. *Arch Gen Psychiatry*. 1997;54(4):313–321.
9. Grant BF, Stinson FS, Dawson DA, et al. Prevalence and co-occurrence of substance use disorders and independent mood and anxiety disorders: results from the National Epidemiologic Survey on Alcohol and Related Conditions. *Arch Gen Psychiatry*. 2004;61(8):807–816.
10. Hasin DS, Goodwin RD, Stinson FS, Grant BF. Epidemiology of major depressive disorder: results from the National Epidemiologic Survey on Alcoholism and Related Conditions. *Arch Gen Psychiatry*. 2005;62(10):1097–1106.
11. Hasin DS, Stinson FS, Ogburn E, Grant BF. Prevalence, correlates, disability, and comorbidity of DSM-IV alcohol abuse and dependence in the United States: results from the National Epidemiologic Survey on Alcohol and Related Conditions. *Arch Gen Psychiatry*. 2007;64(7):830–842.

12. Kessler RC, Nelson CB, McGonagle KA, Edlund MJ, Frank RG, Leaf PJ. The epidemiology of co-occurring addictive and mental disorders: implications for prevention and service utilization. *Am J Orthopsychiatry*. 1996;66(1):17–31.
13. Petersen SM, Toftdahl NG, Nordentoft M, Hjorthøj C. Schizophrenia is associated with increased risk of subsequent substance abuse diagnosis: a nation-wide population-based register study. *Addiction*. 2019;114(12):2217–2226.
14. Levin FR, Hennessy G. Bipolar disorder and substance abuse. *Biol Psychiatry*. 2004;56(10):738–748.
15. Kress CB, Schlesinger S. The prevalence of comorbidities and substance use disorder. *Nurs Clin North Am*. 2023;58(2): 141–151.
16. Edlund MJ, Booth BM, Han X. Who seeks care where? Utilization of mental health and substance use disorder treatment in two national samples of individuals with alcohol use disorders. *J Stud Alcohol Drugs*. 2012;73(4):635–646.
17. Grella CE, Karno MP, Warda US, Moore AA, Niv N. Perceptions of need and help received for substance dependence in a national probability sample. *Psychiatr Serv*. 2009; 60(8):1068–1074.
18. Urbanoski K, Inglis D, Veldhuizen S. Service use and unmet needs for substance use and mental disorders in Canada. *Can J Psychiatry*. 2017;62(8):551–559.
19. Harris KM, Edlund MJ. Use of mental health care and substance abuse treatment among adults with co-occurring disorders. *Psychiatr Serv*. 2005;56(8):954–959.
20. Han B, Compton WM, Blanco C, Colpe LJ. Prevalence, treatment, and unmet treatment needs of US adults with mental health and substance use disorders. *Health Aff*. 2017;36(10): 1739–1747.
21. Choi NG, DiNitto DM, Marti CN. Treatment use, perceived need, and barriers to seeking treatment for substance abuse and mental health problems among older adults compared to younger adults. *Drug Alcohol Depend*. 2014;145:113–120.
22. Ali MM, Teich JL, Mutter R. The role of perceived need and health insurance in substance use treatment: implications for the Affordable Care Act. *J Subst Abuse Treat*. 2015;54:14–20.
23. Manuel JI, Stebbins MB, Wu E. Gender differences in perceived unmet treatment needs among persons with and without co-occurring disorders. *J Behav Health Serv Res*. 2018; 45(1):1–12.
24. Khantzian EJ. The self-medication hypothesis of substance use disorders: a reconsideration and recent applications. *Harv Rev Psychiatry*. 1997;4(5):231–244.
25. Robinson J, Sareen J, Cox BJ, Bolton JM. Role of self-medication in the development of comorbid anxiety and substance use disorders: a longitudinal investigation. *Arch Gen Psychiatry*. 2011;68(8):800–807.
26. Levit KR, Kassed CA, Coffey RM, et al. Future funding for mental health and substance abuse: increasing burdens for the public sector. *Health Aff*. 2008;27(6):w513–w522.
27. Arya S, Delic M, Ruiz BII, et al. Closing the gap between training needs and training provision in addiction medicine. *BJPsych Int*. 2020;17(2):37–39.
28. Lundin RM, Hill H. The worrying, current state of addictions training in medicine. *Front Med (Lausanne)*. 2022;9: 1062096.
29. Watkins KE, Hunter SB, Burnam MA, Pincus HA, Nicholson G. Review of treatment recommendations for persons with a co-occurring affective or anxiety and substance use disorder. *Psychiatr Serv*. 2005;56(8):913–926.
30. Velasco J, Meyer A, Lippmann S. How to treat coexistent mental illness and substance abuse. *South Med J*. 1997; 90(2):180–183.
31. Brunette MF, Mueser KT. Psychosocial interventions for the long-term management of patients with severe mental illness and co-occurring substance use disorder. *J Clin Psychiatry*. 2006;67(7):10–17.
32. Drake RE, Mueser KT. Psychosocial approaches to dual diagnosis. *Schizophr Bull*. 2000;26(1):105–118.
33. Rundell KOR, Greco L, Cruzado EO. Caring for patients with co-occurring mental health and substance use disorders. *J Fam Pract*. 2019;68(7):400–404.
34. Clinical Guideline Committee (CGC) Members; ASAM Team; AAAP Team; IRETA Team. The ASAM/AAAP clinical practice guideline on the management of stimulant use disorder. *J Addict Med*. 2024;18(1S):1–56.
35. Chen KW, Banducci AN, Guller L, et al. An examination of psychiatric comorbidities as a function of gender and substance type within an inpatient substance use treatment program. *Drug Alcohol Depend*. 2011;118(2–3):92–99.
36. Ding K, Yang J, Cheng G, et al. Hospitalizations and hospital charges for co-occurring substance use and mental disorders. *J Subst Abuse Treat*. 2011;40:366–375.
37. Lai HMX, Huang QR. Comorbidity of mental disorders and alcohol- and drug-use disorders: analysis of New South Wales inpatient data. *Drug Alcohol Rev*. 2009;28:235–242.
38. Dore G, Mills K, Murray R, Teesson M, Farrugia P. Post-traumatic stress disorder, depression and suicidality in inpatients with substance use disorders. *Drug Alcohol Rev*. 2012; 31(3):294–302.
39. Skinstad AH, Swain A. Comorbidity in a clinical sample of substance abusers. *Am J Drug Alcohol Abuse*. 2001;27(1):45–64.
40. Kar H, Gania AM, Bandy A, ud din Dar N, Rafiq F. Psychiatric comorbidities and concurrent substance use among people who inject drugs: a single-centre hospital-based study. *Sci Rep*. 2023;13:19053.
41. Painter JM, Malte CA, Rubinsky AD, et al. High inpatient utilization among Veterans Health Administration patients with substance-use disorders and co-occurring mental health conditions. *Am J Drug Alcohol Abuse*. 2018;44(3):386–394.
42. Simon R, Snow R, Wakeman S. Understanding why patients with substance use disorders leave the hospital against medical advice: a qualitative study. *Subst Abus*. 2020;41(4):519–525.
43. Schorb A, Grunze H. Agitation due to substance use, abuse, and withdrawal. In: Zeller SL, Nordstrom K, Wilson MP, eds. *The Diagnosis and Management of Agitation*. Cambridge University Press; 2017:32–47.
44. Kelly TM, Daley DC. Integrated treatment of substance use and psychiatric disorders. *Soc Work Public Health*. 2013; 28(3–4):388–406.
45. McCoy ML, Devitt T, Clay R, et al. Gaining insight: who benefits from residential, integrated treatment for people with dual diagnosis? *Psychiatr Rehabil J*. 2003;27(2):140–150.
46. Mangrum LF, Spence RT, Lopez M. Integrated versus parallel treatment of co-occurring psychiatric and substance use disorders. *J Subst Abuse Treat*. 2006;30:79–84.
47. Judd PH, Thomas N, Schwartz T, Outcalt A, Hough R. A dual diagnosis demonstration project: treatment outcomes and cost analysis. *J Psychoactive Drugs*. 2003;35(1):181–192.
48. Tsuang J, Fong T. Treatment of patients with schizophrenia and substance abuse disorders. *Curr Pharm Des*. 2004; 10(18):2249–2261.
49. Meyers RJ, Roozen HG, Smith JE. The community reinforcement approach: an update of the evidence. *Alcohol Res Health*. 2011;33(4):380–388.
50. Beck AT, Dozois DJA. Cognitive therapy: current status and future directions. *Annu Rev Med*. 2011;62:397–409.
51. Lebow J. Overview of psychotherapies. In: Skodol A, Schwenk TL, eds. *UpToDate*. Wolters Kluwer.
52. Hayes SC, Strosahl KD, Wilson KG. *Acceptance and Commitment Therapy: The Process and Practice of Mindful Change*. Guilford Press; 2012.

53. Weiss RD, Najavits LM, Greenfield SF. A relapse prevention group for patients with bipolar and substance use disorders. *J Subst Abuse Treat.* 1999;16(1):47–54.
54. Weiss RD, Griffin ML, Greenfield SF, et al. Group therapy for patients with bipolar disorder and substance dependence: results of a pilot study. *J Clin Psychiatry.* 2000;61(5):361–367.
55. Fantuzzi C, Mezzina R. Dual diagnosis: a systematic review of the organization of community health services. *Int J Soc Psychiatry.* 2020;66(3):300–310.
56. American Psychiatric Association. *Diagnostic and Statistical Manual of Mental Disorders.* 5th ed. American Psychiatric Association; 2013.
57. Freudenreich OFA, Fricchione GL. Psychosis, mania, and catatonia. In: Levenson JL, ed. *The American Psychiatric Association Publishing Textbook of Psychosomatic Medicine and Consultation-Liaison Psychiatry.* 3rd ed. American Psychiatric Association Publishing; 2019:249–279.
58. Baker WL, Silver D, White CM, et al. Dopamine agonists in the treatment of early Parkinson's disease: a meta-analysis. *Parkinsonism Relat Disord.* 2009;15(4):287–294.
59. Niebrzydowska A, Grabowski J. Medication-induced psychotic disorder: a review of selected drugs side effects. *Psychiatr Danub.* 2022;34(1):11–18.
60. Dailey MW, Saadabadi A. Mania. StatPearls Publishing. Updated July 17, 2023. Accessed January 7, 2025. https://www.ncbi.nlm.nih.gov/books/NBK493168/
61. Calabrese J, Al KhaliliY. Psychosis. StatPearls Publishing. Updated May 1, 2023. Accessed January 7, 2025. https://www.ncbi.nlm.nih.gov/books/NBK546579/
62. Fraser S, Hides L, Philips L, Proctor D, Lubman DI. Differentiating first episode substance induced and primary psychotic disorders with concurrent substance use in young people. *Schizophr Res.* 2012;136(1–3):110–115.
63. Wilson L, Szigeti A, Kearney A, Clarke M. Clinical characteristics of primary psychotic disorders with concurrent substance abuse and substance-induced psychotic disorders: a systematic review. *Schizophr Res.* 2018;197:78–86.
64. Grewal RS, George TP. Cannabis-induced psychosis: a review. *Psychiatric Times.* 2017;34(7). July 14, 2017. Accessed January 20, 2025. www.psychiatrictimes.com/view/cannabis-induced-psychosis-review
65. Kivlichan AE, Praecht A, Wang C, George TP. Substance-induced mood disorders: a scoping review. *Curr Addict Rep.* 2024;11:1–18.
66. Martinotti G, De Risio L, Vannini C, Schifano F, Pettorruso M, Giannantonio MD. Substance-related exogenous psychosis: a postmodern syndrome. *CNS Spectr.* 2021;26(1):84–91.
67. Baldacchino A, Arvapalli V, Shun A, Tolomeo S. Substance-induced mental disorders. In: el-Guebaly N, Carrà G, Galanter M, eds. *Textbook of Addiction Treatment: International Perspectives.* Springer; 2014:1–17.
68. Adan A, Benaiges I. Comorbidity between substance use disorder and severe mental illness. In: Preedy VR, ed. *Neuropathology of Drug Addictions and Substance Misuse.* Vol 3. Academic Press; 2016:65–74.
69. Revadigar N, Gupta V. Substance-induced mood disorders. StatPearls Publishing. Updated November 14, 2022. Accessed January 8, 2025. https://www.ncbi.nlm.nih.gov/books/NBK555887/
70. Hollister LE. Toxicity and adverse consequences of benzodiazepine use. *Psychiatr Ann.* 1995;25(3):158–165.
71. Ritvo AD, Foster DE, Huff C, Finlayson AJR, Silvernail B, Martin PR. Long-term consequences of benzodiazepine-induced neurological dysfunction: a survey. *PLoS One.* 2023;18(6):e0285584.
72. Peng L, Meeks TW, Blazes CK. Complex persistent benzodiazepine dependence- when benzodiazepine deprescribing goes awry. *JAMA Psychiatry.* 2022;79(7):639–640.
73. Ashton CH. *Benzodiazepines: How They Work and How to Withdraw (aka the Ashton Manual).* Benzodiazepine Information Coalition; 2002.
74. Stewart SA. The effects of benzodiazepines on cognition. *J Clin Psychiatry.* 2005;66 Suppl 2:9–13.
75. Martinotti G, Santacroce R, Pettorruso M, et al. Hallucinogen persisting perception disorder: etiology, clinical features, and therapeutic perspectives. *Brain Sci.* 2018;8(3):47.
76. Baldaçara L, Ramos A, Castaldelli-Maia JM. Managing drug-induced psychosis. *Int Rev Psychiatry.* 2023;35(5–6):496–502.
77. Griswold KS, Del Regno PA, Berger RC. Recognition and differential diagnosis of psychosis in primary care. *Am Fam Physician.* 2015;91(12):856–863.
78. University of Florida. National Drug Early Warning System (NDEWS). Accessed January 26, 2025. https://ndews.org/
79. Rocky Mountain Poison and Drug Safety. The Researched Abuse, Diversion, and Addiction-Related Surveillance (RADARS) System. https://radars.org/
80. Hasin DS, Trautman KD, Miele GM, Samet S, Smith M, Endicott J. Psychiatric Research Interview for Substance and Mental Disorders (PRISM): reliability for substance abusers. *Am J Psychiatry.* 1996;153(9):1195–1201.
81. Hasin D, Trautman K, Endicott J. Psychiatric research interview for substance and mental disorders: phenomenologically based diagnosis in patients who abuse alcohol or drugs. *Psychopharmacol Bull.* 1998;34(1):3–8.
82. Hasin D, Samet S, Nunes E, Meydan J, Matseoane K, Waxman R. Diagnosis of comorbid psychiatric disorders in substance users assessed with the Psychiatric Research Interview for Substance and Mental Disorders for DSM-IV. *Am J Psychiatry.* 2006;163(4):689–696.
83. Bruijnen CJWH, Dijkstra BAG, Walvoort SJW, et al. Prevalence of cognitive impairment in patients with substance use disorder. *Drug Alcohol Rev.* 2019;38(4):435–442.
84. Filley CM, Kleinschmidt-DeMasters BK. Toxic leukoencephalopathy. *N Engl J Med.* 2001;345(6):425–432.
85. Folstein MF, Folstein SE, McHugh PR. "Mini-mental state." A practical method for grading the cognitive state of patients for the clinician. *J Psychiatr Res.* 1975;12(3):189.
86. Nasreddine ZS, Phillips NA, Bédirian V, et al. The Montreal Cognitive Assessment, MoCA: a brief screening tool for mild cognitive impairment. *J Am Geriatr Soc.* 2005;53(4):695–699.
87. Carton C, Calafiore M, Cauet C, et al. Montreal Cognitive Assessment (MoCA) use in general practice for the early detection of cognitive impairment: a feasibility study. *BJGP Open.* 2025;9(1):BJGPO.2024.0039.
88. Tariq SH, Tumosa N, Chibnall JT, Perry MH, Morley JE. Comparison of the Saint Louis University mental status examination and the mini-mental state examination for detecting dementia and mild neurocognitive disorder—a pilot study. *Am J Geriatr Psychiatry.* 2006;14(11):900–910.
89. Szcześniak D, Rymaszewska J. The usefulness of the SLUMS test for diagnosis of mild cognitive impairment and dementia. *Psychiatr Pol.* 2016;50(2):457–472.
90. Morley JE, Tumosa TN. Saint Louis University Mental Status Examination (SLUMS). APA PsycTests; 2002.
91. Larson EB. Evaluation of cognitive impairment and dementia. In: Dekosky ST, Schmader KE, Mendez MF, Tung GA, eds. *UpToDate.* Wolters Kluwer.
92. Mendez MF. Mental status scales to evaluate cognition. In: DeKosky ST, ed. *UpToDate.* Wolters Kluwer.
93. Ting SA, Sullivan AF, Miller I, et al; Emergency Department Safety and Follow-up Evaluation (ED-SAFE) Investigators. Multicenter study of predictors of suicide screening in emergency departments. *Acad Emerg Med.* 2012;19(2):239–243.

94. Lejoyeux M, Gastal D, Bergeret A, Casalino E, Lequen V, Guillermet S. Alcohol use disorders among patients examined in emergency departments after a suicide attempt. *Eur Addict Res.* 2012;18(1):26–33.
95. Holmstrand C, Bogren M, Mattisson C, Brådvik L. First and subsequent lifetime alcoholism and mental disorders in suicide victims with reference to a community sample—the Lundby Study 1947–1997. *Front Psychiatry.* 2018;9:173.
96. Lee DJ, Kearns JC, Wisco BE, et al. A longitudinal study of risk factors of suicide attempts among Operation Enduring Freedom and Operation Iraqi Freedom veterans. *Depress Anxiety.* 2018;35(7):609–618.
97. Oquendo MA, Currier D, Liu S-M, Hasin DS, Grant BF, Blanco C. Increased risk for suicidal behavior in comorbid bipolar disorder and alcohol use disorders: results from the National Epidemiologic Survey on Alcohol and Related Conditions (NESARC). *J Clin Psychiatry.* 2010;71(7):902–909.
98. Wiener CD, Moreira FP, Zago A, et al. Mood disorder, anxiety, and suicide risk among subjects with alcohol abuse and/or dependence: a population-based study. *Revista Brasileira de Psiquiatria.* 2018;40(1):1–5.
99. SAFE-T. (Suicide Assessment) Handout. SAMHSA; Accessed January 25, 2025. https://library.samhsa.gov/product/safe-t-suicide-assessment-five-step-evaluation-and-triage/pep24-01-036
100. Warden S, Spiwak R, Sareen J, Bolton JM. The SAD PERSONS scale for suicide risk assessment: a systematic review. *Arch Suicide Res.* 2014;18(4):313–326.
101. Columbia-Suicide Severity Rating Scale. (CSSR-S) Handout. CMS; Accessed January 25, 2025. https://www.cms.gov/files/document/cssrs-screen-version-instrument.pdf
102. Stanley-Brown Safety Plan Template. Suicide Prevention Resource Center; Accessed January 25, 2025. https://sprc.org/online-library/stanley-brown-safety-plan/
103. 988 Suicide & Crisis Lifeline. https://www.samhsa.gov/mental-health/988
104. Patterson WM, Dohn HH, Bird J, Patterson GA. Evaluation of suicidal patients: The SAD PERSONS scale. *Psychosomatics.* 1983;24(4):343–349, 348–349.
105. Simpson SA. A survey of clinical approaches to suicide risk assessment for patients intoxicated on alcohol. *Psychosomatics.* 2019;60(2):197–203.
106. Olson KN, Smith SW, Kloss JS, Ho JD, Apple FS. Relationship between blood alcohol concentration and observable symptoms of intoxication in patients presenting to an emergency department. *Alcohol Alcohol.* 2013;48(4):386–389.
107. Cui C, Koob GF. Titrating tipsy targets: the neurobiology of low-dose alcohol. *Trends Pharmacol Sci.* 2017;38(6):556–568.
108. Brennan DF, Betzelos S, Reed R, Falk JL. Ethanol elimination rates in an ED population. *Am J Emerg Med.* 1995;13(3):276–280.
109. Micromedex. Accessed April 4, 2025. https://www.micromedexsolutions.com/
110. ClinicalKey Drug Monographs. Accessed April 4, 2025. https://www.clinicalkey.com/
111. Marder S. Psychosis in adults: Initial management. In: Stein MB, ed. *UpToDate.* Wolters Kluwer.
112. Press D. Management of neuropsychiatric symptoms of dementia. In: DeKosky ST, Schmader KE, Mendez MF, eds. *UpToDate.* Wolters Kluwer.
113. Jibson MD. Second-generation and other antipsychotic medications: pharmacology, administration, and side effects. In: Marder S, ed. *UpToDate.* Wolters Kluwer.
114. de Silva VA, Suraweera C, Ratnatunga SS, Dayabandara M, Wanniarachchi N, Hanwella R. Metformin in prevention and treatment of antipsychotic induced weight gain: a systematic review and meta-analysis. *BMC Psychiatry.* 2016;16(1):341.
115. Pillinger T, McCutcheon RA, Vano L, et al. Comparative effects of 18 antipsychotics on metabolic function in patients with schizophrenia, predictors of metabolic dysregulation, and association with psychopathology: a systematic review and network meta-analysis. *Lancet Psychiatry.* 2020;7(1):64–77.
116. Du W, Ge M-W, Hu F-H, et al. QTc prolongation in patients with schizophrenia taking antipsychotics: prevalence and risk factors. *J Psychopharmacol.* 2023;37(10):971–981.
117. Beach SR, Celano CM, Noseworthy PA, Januzzi JL, Huffman JC. QTc prolongation, torsades de pointes, and psychotropic medications. *Psychosomatics.* 2013;54(1):1–13.
118. Funk MC, Beach SR, Bostwick JR, et al. *Resource Document on QTc Prolongation and Psychotropic Medications.* 2018. http://psychiatry.org/getattachment/f94e1ce6-abcf-4f78-8510-4f0375c8142a/Resource-Document-2018-QTc-Prolongation-and-Psychotropic-Med.pdf
119. Funk MC, Beach SR, Bostwick JR, et al. QTc prolongation and psychotropic medications. *Am J Psychiatry.* 2020;177(3):273–274.
120. Marcus SC, Zummo J, Pettit AR, Stoddard J, Doshi JA. Antipsychotic adherence and rehospitalization in schizophrenia patients receiving oral versus long-acting injectable antipsychotics following hospital discharge. *J Manag Care Spec Pharm.* 2015;21(9):754–769.
121. Garriga M, Pacchiarotti I, Kasper S, et al. Assessment and management of agitation in psychiatry: expert consensus. *World J Biol Psychiatry.* 2016;17(2):86–128.
122. Devlin JW, Skrobik Y, Gélinas C, et al. Clinical practice guidelines for the prevention and management of pain, agitation/sedation, delirium, immobility, and sleep disruption in adult patients in the ICU. *Crit Care Med.* 2018;46(9):e825–e873.
123. Lukens TW, Wolf SJ, Edlow JA, et al; American College of Emergency Physicians Clinical Policies Subcommittee (Writing Committee) on Critical Issues in the Diagnosis and Management of the Adult Psychiatric Patient in the Emergency Department. Clinical policy: critical issues in the diagnosis and management of the adult psychiatric patient in the emergency department. *Ann Emerg Med.* 2006;47(1):79–99.
124. Williams AM. Coadministration of intramuscular olanzapine and benzodiazepines in agitated patients with mental illness. *Ment Health Clin.* 2018;8(5):208–213.
125. Marder SR, Sorsaburu S, Dunayevich E, et al. Case reports of postmarketing adverse event experiences with olanzapine intramuscular treatment in patients with agitation. *J Clin Psychiatry.* 2010;71(4):433–441.
126. Banham L, Gilbody S. Smoking cessation in severe mental illness: what works? *Addiction.* 2010;105(7):1176–1189.
127. Bakouni H, Sharafi H, Bahremand A, et al. Bupropion for treatment of amphetamine-type stimulant use disorder: a systematic review and meta-analysis of placebo-controlled randomized clinical trials. *Drug Alcohol Depend.* 2023;253:111018.
128. Dilts SL, Keleher DL, Hoge G, Haglund B. Hydroxyzine in the treatment of alcohol withdrawal. *Am J Psychiatry.* 1977;134(1):92a–93.
129. Schuckit MA. Treatment of opioid-use disorders. *N Engl J Med.* 2016;375:357–368.
130. Kampman K, Jarvis M. American Society of Addiction Medicine (ASAM) National practice guideline for the use of medications in the treatment of addiction involving opioid use. *J Addict Med.* 2015;9(5):358–367.
131. Reus VI, Fochtmann LJ, Bukstein O, et al. The American Psychiatric Association practice guideline for the pharmacological treatment of patients with alcohol use disorder. *Am J Psychiatry.* 2018;175(1):86–90.
132. Ahmed S, Stanciu CN, Kotapati PV, et al. Effectiveness of gabapentin in reducing cravings and withdrawal in alcohol

use disorder: a meta-analytic review. *Prim Care Companion CNS Disord.* 2019;21(4):19r02465.
133. McCord JJH, Hollander JE, de Lemos JA, et al. American Heart Association Acute Cardiac Care Committee of the Council on Clinical Cardiology. Management of cocaine-associated chest pain and myocardial infarction: a scientific statement from the American Heart Association Acute Cardiac Care Committee of the Council on Clinical Cardiology. *Circulation.* 2008;117(14):1897–1907.
134. Kampman KM, Dackis C, Lynch KG, et al. A double-blind, placebo-controlled trial of amantadine, propanolol, and their combination for the treatment of cocaine dependence in patients with severe cocaine withdrawal symptoms. *Drug Alcohol Depend.* 2006;85(2):129–137.
135. Boon M, van Dorp E, Broens S, Overdyk F. Combining opioids and benzodiazepines: effects on mortality and severe adverse respiratory events. *Ann Palliat Med.* 2020;9(2):542–557.
136. Brower KJ. Assessment and treatment of insomnia in adult patients with alcohol use disorders. *Alcohol.* 2015;49(4):417–427.
137. Scharf MB, Sachais BA. Sleep laboratory evaluation of the effects and efficacy of trazodone in depressed insomniac patients. *J Clin Psychiatry.* 1990;51(Suppl):13–17.
138. Geoffroy PA, Lejoyeux M, Rolland B. Management of insomnia in alcohol use disorder. *Expert Opin Pharmacother.* 2020;21(3):297–306.
139. Alimoradi Z, Jafari E, Broström A, et al. Effects of cognitive behavioral therapy for insomnia (CBT-I) on quality of life: A systematic review and meta-analysis. *Sleep Med Rev.* 2022;64:101646.
140. Koffel E, Bramoweth AD, Ulmer CS. Increasing access to and utilization of cognitive behavioral therapy for insomnia (CBT-I): a narrative review. *J Gen Intern Med.* 2018;33:955–962.
141. Baldassano CF. Illness course, comorbidity, gender, and suicidality in patients with bipolar disorder. *J Clin Psychiatry.* 2006;67(11):8–11.
142. Hunt GE, Malhi GS, Cleary M, Lai HMX, Sitharthan T. Prevalence of comorbid bipolar and substance use disorders in clinical settings, 1990-2015: systematic review and meta-analysis. *J Affect Disord.* 2016;206:331–349.
143. Rakofsky JJ, Dunlop BW. Do alcohol use disorders destabilize the course of bipolar disorder? *J Affect Disord.* 2013;145(1):1–10.
144. Salloum IM, Thase ME. Impact of substance abuse on the course and treatment of bipolar disorder. *Bipolar Disord.* 2000;2(3 pt 2):269–280.
145. Goldberg JF, Garno JL, Leon AC, Kocsis JH, Portera L. A history of substance abuse complicates remission from acute mania in bipolar disorder. *J Clin Psychiatry.* 1999;60(11):733–740.
146. George TP, Ziedonis DM, Feingold A, et al. Nicotine transdermal patch and atypical antipsychotic medications for smoking cessation in schizophrenia. *Am J Psychiatry.* 2000; 157(11):1835–1842.
147. Perugi G, Toni C, Frare F, et al. Effectiveness of adjunctive gabapentin in resistant bipolar disorder: is it due to anxious-alcohol abuse comorbidity? *J Clin Psychopharmacol.* 2002;22(6):584–591.
148. Sonne SC, Brady KT. Naltrexone for individuals with comorbid bipolar disorder and alcohol dependence. *J Clin Psychopharmacol.* 2000;20(1):114–115.
149. Naglich A, Adinoff B, Brown ES. Pharmacological treatment of bipolar disorder with comorbid alcohol use disorder. *CNS Drugs.* 2017;31(8):665–674.
150. Murthy P, Mahadevan J, Chand PK. Treatment of substance use disorders with co-occurring severe mental health disorders. *Curr Opin Psychiatry.* 2019;32(4):293–299.
151. Kelly TM, Daley DC, Douaihy AB. Treatment of substance abusing patients with comorbid psychiatric disorders. *Addict Behav.* 2012;37(1):11–24.
152. Smelson DA, Dixon L, Craig T, et al. Pharmacological treatment of schizophrenia and co-occurring substance use disorders. *CNS Drugs.* 2008;22(11):903–916.
153. Lubman DI, King JA, Castle DJ. Treating comorbid substance use disorders in schizophrenia. *Int Rev Psychiatry.* 2010;22(2):191–201.
154. Murthy P, Chand P. Treatment of dual diagnosis disorders. *Curr Opin Psychiatry.* 2012;25(3):194–200.
155. Bennett ME, Bradshaw KR, Catalano LT. Treatment of substance use disorders in schizophrenia. *Am J Drug Alcohol Abuse.* 2017;43(4):377–390.
156. Azorin J-M, Simon N, Adida M, Belzeaux R. Pharmacological treatment of schizophrenia with comorbid substance use disorder. *Expert Opin Pharmacother.* 2016;17(2): 231–253.
157. Green AI. Treatment of schizophrenia and comorbid substance abuse: pharmacologic approaches. *J Clin Psychiatry.* 2006;67(Suppl 7):31–35.
158. George TP, Vessicchio JC, Termine A, et al. A placebo controlled trial of bupropion for smoking cessation in schizophrenia. *Biol Psychiatry.* 2002;52(1):53–61.
159. Mehta DD, Praecht A, Ward HB, et al. A systematic review and meta-analysis of neuromodulation therapies for substance use disorders. *Neuropsychopharmacology.* 2024;49(4): 649–680.
160. Johnstone S, Sorkhou M, Al-Saghir N, et al. Neuromodulation to treat substance use disorders in people with schizophrenia and other psychoses: a systematic review. *Front Psychiatry.* 2022;13:793938.
161. Nelson JC, Spyker DA. Morbidity and mortality associated with medications used in the treatment of depression: an analysis of cases reported to U.S. poison control centers, 2000–2014. *Am J Psychiatry.* 2017;174(5):438–450.
162. Malekshahi T, Tioleco N, Ahmed N, Campbell ANC, Haller D. Misuse of atypical antipsychotics in conjunction with alcohol and other drugs of abuse. *J Subst Abuse Treat.* 2015;48(1):8–12.
163. Martinotti G, Chiappini S, Mosca A, et al. Atypical antipsychotic drugs in dual disorders: current evidence for clinical practice. *Curr Pharm Des.* 2022;28(27):2241–2259.
164. Kurtz SP, Buttram ME, Margolin ZR, Wogenstahl K. The diversion of nonscheduled psychoactive prescription medications in the United States, 2002 to 2017. *Pharmacoepidemiol Drug Saf.* 2019;28(5):700–706.
165. Schifano F, Chiappini S. Is there a potential of misuse for venlafaxine and bupropion? *Front Pharmacol.* 2018;9:239.
166. Benz MB, Epstein-Lubow G, Weinstock LM, Gaudiano BA. Polypharmacy among patients with major depressive disorder and co-occurring substance use disorders in a psychiatric hospital setting: prevalence and risk factors. *J Clin Psychopharmacol.* 2023;43(3):273–277.
167. Jarlenski M, Krans EE. Co-occurring substance use disorders identified among delivery hospitalizations in the United States. *J Addict Med.* 2021;15(6):504–507.
168. Substance Abuse and Mental Health Services Administration. The Management of Pregnant People Who Have Opioid Use Disorder. *Advisory.* 2023.
169. Prince MKDS, Ayers D. Substance use in pregnancy. *StatPearls [Internet].* StatPearls Publishing; 2023.
170. MotherToBaby. The organization of teratology information specialists. Accessed January 29, 2025. https://mothertobaby.org
171. Gynecologists TACoOa. Educational resources for providers, patients, and families. https://www.acog.org/programs/perinatal-mental-health/educational-resources-for-providers-patients-and-families
172. Andersson HW, Mosti MP, Nordfjaern T. Inpatients in substance use treatment with co-occurring psychiatric disorders:

a prospective cohort study of characteristics and relapse predictors. *BMC Psychiatry.* 2023;23(1):152.

173. Yule AM, Kelly JF. Integrating treatment for co-occurring mental health conditions. *Alcohol Res.* 2019;40(1):arcr.v40.1.07.
174. McGovern MP, Lambert-Harris C, Gotham HJ, Claus RE, Xie H. Dual diagnosis capability in mental health and addiction treatment services: an assessment of programs across multiple state systems. *Adm Policy Ment Health.* 2014;41(2): 205–214.
175. Division USDoJCR. File a complaint. Accessed April 3, 2025. https://www.ada.gov/file-a-complaint/
176. Illness NAoM. What is mental health parity? https://www.nami.org/your-journey/individuals-with-mental-illness/understanding-health-insurance/what-is-mental-health-parity/
177. O'Connor PG, Nyquist JG, McLellan AT. Integrating addiction medicine into graduate education in primary care: the time has come. *Ann Intern Med.* 2011;154(1):56–59.
178. Coles AS, Kozak K, George TP. A review of brain stimulation methods to treat substance use disorders. *Am J Addict.* 2018;27(2):71–91.
179. Foad W, Aziz KA, Agour M, et al. Repetitive transcranial magnetic stimulation (rTMS) is associated with increased abstinence in substance use disorders and comorbid depression. *Ann Clin Psychiatry.* 2023;35(1):31–38.
180. Mahoney JJ, Hanlon CA, Marshalek PJ, Rezai AR, Krinke L. Transcranial magnetic stimulation, deep brain stimulation, and other forms of neuromodulation for substance use disorders: review of modalities and implications for treatment. *J Neurol Sci.* 2020;418:117149.
181. Luigjes J, Segrave R, de Joode N, Figee M, Denys D. Efficacy of invasive and non-invasive brain modulation interventions for addiction. *Neuropsychol Rev.* 2019;29(1):116–138.
182. Gaudreault P-O, Sharma A, Datta A, et al. A double-blind sham-controlled phase 1 clinical trial of tDCS of the dorsolateral prefrontal cortex in cocaine inpatients: craving, sleepiness, and contemplation to change. *Eur J Neurosci.* 2021;53(9):3212–3230.
183. Kochanowski B, Kageki-Bonnert K, Pinkerton EA, Dougherty DD, Chou T. A review of transcranial magnetic stimulation and transcranial direct current stimulation combined with medication and psychotherapy for depression. *Harv Rev Psychiatry.* 2024;32(3):77–95.
184. Bormann NL, Oesterle TS, Arndt S, Karpyak VM, Croarkin PE. Systematic review and meta-analysis: combining transcranial magnetic stimulation or direct current stimulation with pharmacotherapy for treatment of substance use disorders. *Am J Addict.* 2024;33(3):269–282.
185. Minzenberg MJ, Leuchter AF. The effect of psychotropic drugs on cortical excitability and plasticity measured with transcranial magnetic stimulation: Implications for psychiatric treatment. *J Affect Disord.* 2019;253:126–140.
186. Rezai AT, Thompson-Lake DGY, D'Haese PF, et al. Focused ultrasound neuromodulation: exploring a novel treatment for severe opioid use disorder. *Biol Psychiatry.* 2025;98(1): 56–64.
187. Shi Yu, Wu W. Advances in transcranial focused ultrasound neuromodulation for mental disorders. *Prog Neuropsychopharmacol Biol Psychiatry.* 2025;136:111244.
188. Matt E, Radjenovic S, Mitterwallner M, Beisteiner R. Current state of clinical ultrasound neuromodulation. *Front Neurosci.* 2024;18:1420255.
189. Henn MC, Smith HD, Lopez Ramos CG, et al. A systematic review of focused ultrasound for psychiatric disorders: current applications, opportunities, and challenges. *Neurosurg Focus.* 2024;57(3):E8.
190. Lähteenvuo M, Tiihonen J, Solismaa A, Tanskanen A, Mittendorfer-Rutz E, Taipale H. Repurposing semaglutide and liraglutide for alcohol use disorder. *JAMA Psychiatry.* 2025; 82(1):94–98.
191. Hendershot CS, Bremmer MP, Paladino MB, et al. Once-weekly semaglutide in adults with alcohol use disorder: a randomized clinical trial. *JAMA Psychiatry.* 2025;82(4):395–405.
192. Yammine L, Green CE, Kosten TR, et al. Exenatide adjunct to nicotine patch facilitates smoking cessation and may reduce post-cessation weight gain: a pilot randomized controlled trial. *Nicotine Tob Res.* 2021;23(10):1682–1690.
193. Lee S, Li M, Le GH, et al. Glucagon-like peptide-1 receptor agonists (GLP-1RAs) as treatment for nicotine cessation in psychiatric populations: a systematic review. *Ann Gen Psychiatry.* 2024;23(1):45.

15

Behavioral and Psychosocial Treatments in the Hospital Setting

Payel Jhoom Roy, Emily E. Beahm, Sheria Y. Francis, O. Trent Hall

In September 2022, I met Ms. M, who broadened my outlook and care on patients diagnosed with comorbid opioid use disorder and infective endocarditis.

I was working at a tertiary care hospital as a social worker on our substance use care team when we first met. I was still feeling new in this position and navigating how best to support this patient population. I always felt anxious when meeting patients for the first time, uncertain of how they would respond to my services. There have been times when patients have a negative response when I introduce myself. A memory of a patient saying, "I don't need your help; it was social workers that took my kids away," did not help that anxiety.

Upon entering her room, Ms. M was lying in bed, looking disheveled with knotted hair. I introduced myself and the reason for my visit. Unprompted, she openly shared some of her trauma including being sexually abused and raped as a young teenager, experiencing domestic violence in past relationships, and being sexually and physically exploited to have her basic needs met. She appeared to disassociate when sharing these details, tears streaming down her face. After meeting with her, I felt surprised that she freely shared her traumas without much encouragement, and she was accepting of my return. I realized a foundation had begun, but there was still much progress to be made. Unfortunately, Ms. M was administratively discharged days later, and I was left wondering where she had gone. This doesn't happen in all hospitals but can happen in some hospitals if a patient is unwilling to follow expectations set by the unit and/or care team as they feel they cannot safely manage a patient. In her situation, she showed physical aggression toward staff (throwing food trays) and was not adhering to medical recommendations.

Eventually finding her way back to the hospital, she was referred to our team again, endorsing active fentanyl use and opioid withdrawal. Our team assessed her interest in treatment with methadone or buprenorphine; however, it was challenging to have a conversation with Ms. M about recovery goals due to uncontrolled opioid withdrawal and pain. It was important to make her more comfortable, so that she stayed for her infectious workup and we would have the opportunity to engage her in substance use treatment. We started her on scheduled, high-dose oxycodone to manage withdrawal symptoms, but Ms. M was more guarded with me during this admission—initially not wanting my services. I decided to make her a priority on my case list—attempting to see her often, bringing her items that would make her more comfortable such as candy, clothing, shoes, etc. When she allowed me to stay, I grabbed a chair, sat down, and listened. I couldn't solve her problems, but I was there to show compassion, empathize, and understand her needs. I was able to do actionable tasks to help her; ordered a government cell phone, made referrals to community programs, assisted with her disposition, even switching her insurance to a different coverage plan to help aid her transition of care. Tasks aside, Ms. M eventually trusted me, and started asking for me by name and valuing my opinion on her care. I learned she was an artist who loved to paint and draw, so I ensured she had art supplies so she could showcase her art around her hospital room.

Despite our therapeutic alliance, she remained guarded with her care team, inconsistently engaged in medical care, and displayed intermittent outbursts toward staff. *Why was she responding this way?* In her case, it was important to consider how social determinants of health influence treatment-seeking (ie, housing, transportation, education, discrimination/violence, food insecurity, social and economic opportunities, and access to health care). For example, Ms. M took a while to eat, even hoarding food in her room and not allowing aides to take her trays away. Her family later explained that this behavior was likely due to the fact she had limited access to food as a child.

Due to nonadherence and outbursts with staff, her care teams prioritized collaboration to effectively provide care. Our psychiatry and palliative care teams were also involved to assess capacity and delirium and to ensure staff education on trauma-informed care (ie, timing of medication administration, speaking at eye level, asking to examine with explanations, providing choices/validation, and including positive family supports in decision-making).

Ms. M was recommended for medication management of her infective endocarditis over a much-needed heart valve replacement surgery due to a lack of motivation to remain abstinent and struggle to complete preoperative work-up. Surgeons agreed to re-evaluate her once she demonstrated abstinence and commitment to her recovery. However, finding a safe facility to complete her treatment was challenging because Ms. M had been previously administratively discharged from most skilled nursing facilities and the medical respite program due to behaviors toward staff and not adhering to the program's expectations. Eventually, Ms. M was offered a tricuspid valve replacement with supportive decision-making from family.

Ms. M was a complex case for everyone involved. But as a social worker, navigating her needs was a challenging task. She had limited support from family, insecure housing, inadequate coping skills, no resources to meet her basic needs, unresolved trauma, and little insight into her disease. Could she really remain abstinent? Did she have the tools to achieve this? Was I working harder than she was? How can I help someone who has learned to be helpless related to their life circumstances?

Social workers are sometimes called miracle workers, but we quickly learn we can't solve others' problems. We can, however, teach our patients the skills they need, ensure they have the tools and resources to build a robust toolbox, and when they're ready, they can reach into their toolbox and grab what they need to make a positive change.

—Emily Beahm

Key Points

- **Creating a team mindset with open communication is key to building a cohesive and successful multidisciplinary hospital-based substance use disorder (SUD) treatment team.**
- **Motivational interviewing is a powerful tool that can engage patients with SUD during the reachable moment of hospitalization.**
- **A trauma-informed care approach should be employed as universal precautions among all patients to reduce the risk of retraumatization during hospitalization.**
- **Behavioral and psychosocial therapies in the hospital setting can be employed by all members of the hospital-based SUD treatment team.**
- **Nonmedical clinicians, including social workers and peer navigators, can assist patients with recovery support tools and smooth transitions of care post-discharge.**

There are multiple different models to provide hospital-based SUD evaluation and treatment. A common model utilizes a multidisciplinary care team that provides management of the medical needs of patients with SUD from medical clinicians, along with providing behavioral and psychosocial care by nonmedical clinicians, including social workers and/or peer recovery specialists. This chapter will describe components of the multidisciplinary team, with a focus on nonmedical clinicians, and then present ways to develop a team mindset among colleagues from different training backgrounds and expertise. The chapter conceptualizes the multidisciplinary team as an addiction consultation service, though it is recognized that not all hospitals will have this discreet service. Next, the chapter describes behavioral and psychosocial treatments that can be successfully provided in the hospital setting. Lastly, the chapter describes the roles of nonmedical clinicians providing SUD care in the hospital setting, with a specific focus on social workers and peer navigators.

The Multidisciplinary Hospital-Based SUD Treatment Team

Multidisciplinary hospital-based SUD treatment teams vary across the United States (US). Teams can include members such as addiction medicine or addiction psychiatry physician specialists, coordinators (including a social worker or case manager), persons focused on engagement (including a peer navigator or counselor), and/or other roles such as nurses and pharmacists.[1] Some services may be offered through psychiatry consult liaison services while others are offered by individual addiction medicine physicians or advanced practice providers.[1] Other models include general clinicians offering medications for SUD treatment without an addiction service (hospital-based treatment) and in-reach from community providers.[1] This chapter will describe the interprofessional model of addiction consultation services and the role of nonmedical clinicians like social workers and peer navigators in them.

Understanding the role of each individual team member and discipline, including responsibilities that can be delegated and areas of expertise, ensures every member of the team can provide the highest quality of care at the maximum level of their expertise. This requires recognizing one's own limitations, delegating appropriately, and dividing workload fairly. Table 15.1 shows different roles of nonphysicians who contribute to successful addiction consultation services. This list is not comprehensive but demonstrates the general clinician and role types that can be considered for inclusion on an addiction consultation service.

Building a Team Mindset

Assembling a group of people to work on an interprofessional addiction team is only the first step in building an effective service line. Groups of individuals with their own goals, measures of success, and viewpoints may ultimately lead to artificial harmony, lack of accountability, and poor results. Examples of disparate goals between team members may be lack of agreement on services provided by the addiction team, such as medication treatment versus non–medication-based treatment; involvement in pain management; discussions about harm reduction; and the extent to which the team participates in discharge planning. As a result, it is important to build a team mindset, where all members of the team trust each other and work toward similar goals, considering the team before individual goals and aspirations.

TABLE 15.1

Type and Credentials of Nonphysician Team Members for a Multidisciplinary Hospital-based SUD Treatment Team

Team member	Common credentials[a]	Education level[a]
Case manager	Registered Nurse (RN)	Bachelor of Science in Nursing (BSN)
	Health Promotion Advocate (HPA)	Associate Degree in Nursing (ADN)
		High school diploma
		Receive training In Brief Intervention and Referral to Treatment
Clinical pharmacist	Pharmacist (PharmD)	Pharmacy degree
Counselor	Licensed professional counselor (LPC)	Master of Counseling
	Licensed mental health counselor (LMHC)	Bachelor in related field
	Certified alcohol and drug counselor (CADC)	
Peer/patient navigator	Certified peer specialist (CPS)	No degree requirement; specialty board certifications offered
	Certified recovery specialist (CRS)	
	Community health worker (CHW)	
Social worker	Licensed social worker (LSW)	Master of Social Work (MSW)
	Licensed clinical social worker (LCSW)	
	Licensed independent clinical social worker (LICSW)	

[a]Credentials and Degrees provided as an example; required education level may be state- or hospital-specific.

TABLE 15.2

Characteristics of Dysfunctional and High-Performing Teams[3]

Dysfunctional teams	Dysfunction	High-performing teams
Frequent turnover, focus on individual over team	Lack of results	Motivated and stable team focused on team results
Lack of ownership over key issues, poor performance is tolerated	Avoidance of accountability	People understand their roles, no tolerance of poor performance
Unclear objectives and follow-through, relitigating same conflicts	Lack of commitment	Clear objectives with buy-in from a fully engaged team
Avoiding confrontation and voicing concerns	Fear of conflict	Healthy debates, develop solutions together, correct poor behavior
Assuming the worst, hiding mistakes	Lack of trust	Asking for help, assume the best in each other, assume everyone is trying their best

First, let's define what is meant by "team." Patrick Lencioni, author of The Five Dysfunctions of a Team, argues that a team is a group of 3 to 12 people who share common goals, share the rewards and responsibilities for achieving those goals, and readily set aside individual/personal needs for the good of team.[2]

Lencioni outlines five common dysfunctions among teams: Absence of *trust*, which leads to fear of *conflict*, which leads to lack of *commitment*, which leads to avoidance of *accountability*, which leads to inattention to *results*.[2] Conversely, when *trust* is established, teams can vigorously debate important topics, which ensures all voices are heard without fear of *conflict*. Thus, *commitment* can be reached, which forces clarity and closure. Commitment is not the same as consensus; in order to achieve commitment, all voices and opinions must be heard and considered when a final decision is made, usually by the leader. A team mindset requires a commitment to decisions made after group discussion, because the individual members trust that their opinion was considered and recognize that they will not "win" every discussion. Once commitment is reached, team members can then hold each other *accountable* for following through on their roles. Accountability requires each team member to confront potentially difficult issues. As a result, each individual has the buy-in necessary to achieve the *results* agreed upon by the team, where the team can focus on outcomes rather than individual gains. These concepts are outlined in Table 15.2.

Note this scheme does not imply that teams all share the same perspectives, hold the same beliefs, or agree with every decision. It does, however, mean teams trust each other to vigorously debate. To ensure healthy debate, we propose all team members understand the five dysfunctions of a team, or similar leadership/team-building schema, as well as understand conflict style modes. Conflict is common, whether among like-minded team members, between different specialty services, or between patients and their care teams. Understanding a conflict-based framework can help team members understand their own personal conflict negotiating styles, while understanding others' styles and how to reach commitment. This can be accomplished through a variety of means, including monthly team meetings, group exercises, an annual retreat, or shared mission or vision statement.

The Thomas Kilmann Conflict Mode Instrument is a tool that can help identify and understand default conflict negotiation styles. It centers on the idea that negotiating occurs on a continuum of assertiveness and cooperation. Online diagnostic tools can assist team members in identifying where they fall on this spectrum in terms of default style.[4] Figure 15.1 shows the five conflict negotiation styles and their characteristics.

Note that no one negotiation style is "correct" or best. Each has its unique role in managing conflict. For instance, for decisions that must be made quickly, a competitive approach may be needed. Conversely, for projects with long-term goals and objectives in mind, a collaborative approach may be best. Alternatively, for heated conflicts where a party may need some time to "cool off," avoiding may be most appropriate. Understanding default conflict negotiation styles among team members can facilitate conversation and debate.

Communication

Successful teams have open communication. Team members on an addiction service need to trust that they can make suggestions and ask for help without fear of being judged, all with the goal of taking better care of patients. This can occur via multiple different mechanisms.

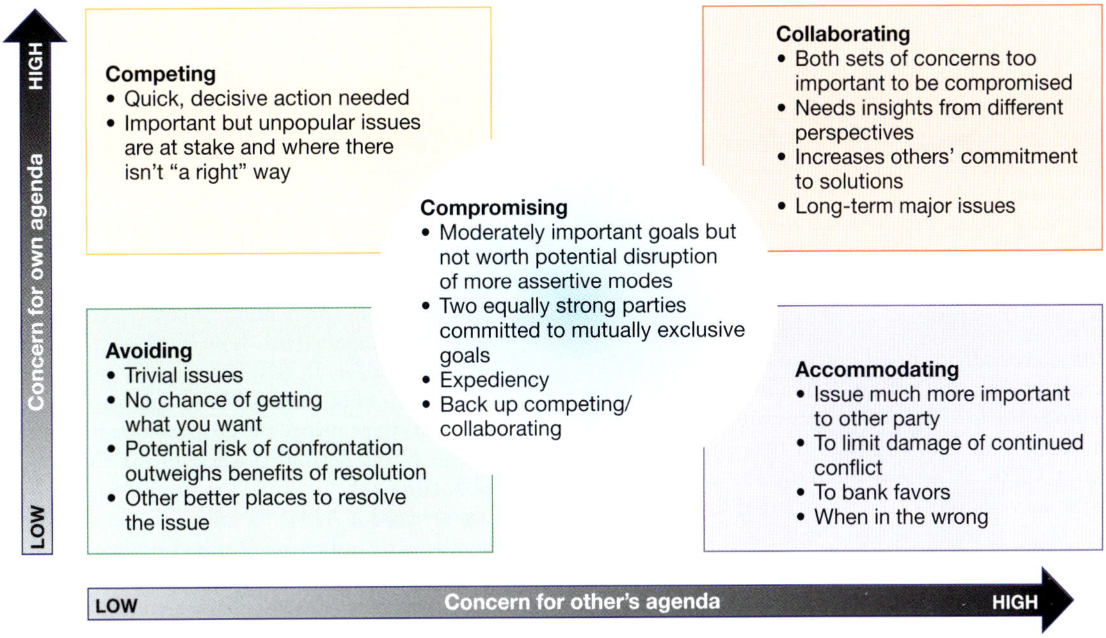

Figure 15.1: Conflict negotiation styles adapted from the Thomas Kilmann conflict mode instrument. (This figure is adapted/modified from the TKI Conflict Model that is Copyright © 2009–2023 by Kilmann Diagnostics LLC. All rights reserved. Original figure is available at https://kilmanndiagnostics.com/overview-thomas-kilmann-conflict-mode-instrument-tki/)

Within team: having regular team-based meetings and/or rounding on patient care plans are helpful. This can occur on a daily or weekly basis, to ensure all members of the team have the same goals in mind for each patient and are updated with information. HIPAA-compliant communication tools can be employed to keep team members updated throughout the day of what intervention each member is offering to patients. Larger, monthly or quarterly meetings among all team members (including all rotating attendings and addiction fellows) assist to ensure a sense of camaraderie, and to negotiate "big picture"-type issues. Periodic meetings to debrief challenging cases with difficult outcomes can also be important to maintain team morale and prevent burnout. Team-building retreats or social interactions outside of work may also help to prevent burnout and promote team cohesiveness.

Individual: it is important for each member of the team to have some time with team leadership, for instance: weekly or biweekly meetings between the team leader and each social worker, peer navigator, etc. These meetings allow time for mentorship, supervision hours (for instance, for Licensed Social Workers [LSWs] seeking Licensed Clinical Social Worker [LCSW] accreditation), questions, and an open space to discuss problems. Proactively setting regular meetings also ensures meetings are not set *only* during times of crisis or when problems arise, leading to otherwise negative connotations associated with meeting with leadership. These meetings are times that can be productive in terms of developing academic projects, evolving practice, and debriefing difficult cases.

Hospital-Based Behavioral and Psychosocial Treatment

All members of the team are responsible for providing high-quality encounters with deft communication skills. Adequate behavioral and psychosocial supports while in the hospital will complement and enhance the care patients receive from medication management of their SUD. This section discusses the principles of motivational interviewing (MI) and different behavioral and psychosocial treatments that can be implemented in the hospital setting.

Motivational Interviewing for Hospitalized Patients With SUD

Context and Rationale

An important difference between patients seen by an addiction consultation team and patients who present to specialty or outpatient SUD treatment settings is that most hospitalized patients are admitted to the hospital for reasons other than a personal desire for SUD treatment. However, even patients who have not yet begun to consider changing their relationship with substances often possess their own deeply personal reasons for change; as well as unique strengths and characteristics to empower this change. Hospital-based SUD treatment should approach ambivalent patients in a way that centers what is most valuable to them and brings to bear their own inner strengths to help them process the mixed feelings they have about change. MI is one such approach.

Definition

MI is an evidence-based practice for promoting personal growth and change.[5] Building upon a foundation provided by the person-centered counseling movement of Carl Rogers, MI first emerged in the early 1980s as a new approach for working with patients with alcohol use disorder (AUD).[5–7] According to MI founders William Miller and Stephen Rollnick, at its inception MI stood in "stark contrast to the authoritarian confrontational style in vogue for treating addictions at the time."[5] Some readers may observe similar confrontational styles in conversations between staff and patients with SUD in contemporary hospitals. MI offers "a particular way of talking with people about change and growth to strengthen their own motivation and commitment" which may not only improve patient outcomes, but might also reduce clinician burnout.[5,8,9]

Guiding Spirit of MI

Hospital clinicians are trained to diagnose and treat patients who come to the hospital with medical problems. MI teaches that the orientation of heart and mind brought to the work of helping others may be as important as the medical treatment itself.[5,10] The guiding spirit of MI encompasses a genuine interest in the patient, and careful respect for their goals, values, and expertise in their own lives.[11,12] Four essential elements inform the guiding spirit of MI: partnership, acceptance, compassion, and empowerment.[5]

- **Partnership**—Surprisingly, the role of the clinician as a motivational interviewer is not to motivate anyone. Instead, the clinician should aim to partner with their patient in a way that helps the patient find their own inherent motivation.[13] An often-repeated phrase in MI is that MI should "feel more like a dance than a wrestling match."[5] Partnership does not attempt to coerce or persuade patients. Instead, clinicians collaborate with patients on a goal that is theirs—the goal must be the patients', not the clinicians'—by guiding the patient toward a greater appreciation of their own inner strengths and reasons for change.
- **Acceptance**—In MI, acceptance is the understanding that all people have inherent worth. Clinicians can demonstrate acceptance by avoiding casting judgments, criticism, or disapproval toward patients. Notably, acknowledgment of someone's inherent worth can be accomplished without agreeing with everything the patient says or approving of all actions.[5] Acceptance is also not enabling. In fact, the experience of being accepted is thought to facilitate behavioral change.[14]
- **Compassion**—The concept of compassion in MI might be different than how clinicians are used to thinking of it. In MI, compassion is cognitive rather than emotional. To have compassion simply means to prioritize the goals, values, ideas, and feelings of the person with whom the clinician is conducting MI.[12]
- **Empowerment**—MI recognizes that lasting personal growth and change comes from within. Clinicians often experience a strong urge to compel patients to change their behavior. In MI, this urge is called the *"fixing reflex."*[5] While the fixing reflex is well-intentioned, clinicians who lack introspection into their own fixing reflex risk reducing their patients' feelings of empowerment. Advocating too strongly for change with an ambivalent patient is like shoving on a pendulum. It might seem to the clinician that they are pushing the patient in the right direction, but just like a pendulum, the patient's ambivalence is likely to shift just as strongly the opposite way. By supporting patients' autonomy to make their own decisions and openly acknowledging that only they can decide what is right for them, clinicians empower patients toward personal growth and change.[15]

Four Tasks of MI

In any motivational interview, the interviewer and patient work together on four tasks: **Engaging, Focusing, Evoking, and Planning** (Figure 15.2).[5,12] These tasks are often represented as a stairway with Engaging as the foundational step and Planning as the highest step. The metaphor of a stairway is important for two reasons. First, each task of MI represents

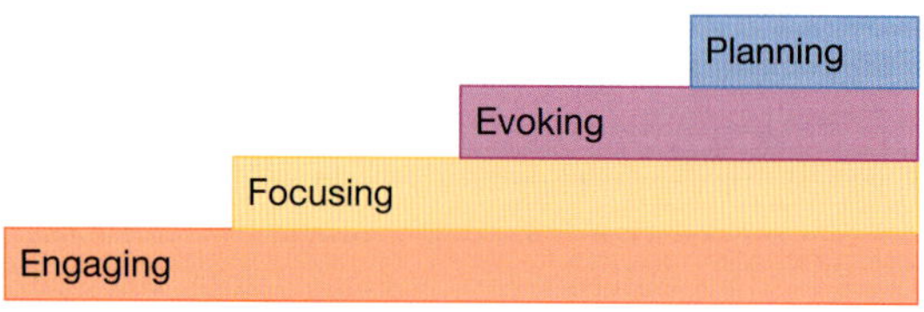

Figure 15.2: Four tasks of motivational interviewing. (Miller WR, Rollnick S. *Interviewing: Helping People Change and Grow.* 4th ed. Guilford Press; 2023.)

a necessary platform for all subsequent tasks. For example, the clinician cannot *focus* the conversation without first *engaging* the patient. Second, it is often necessary during the course of a motivational interview to back up a step and return to a previous task. For example, if the clinician begins planning before the patient feels ready for that step, the patient may disengage from the conversation, requiring the clinician to return to the engagement task. Not all motivational interviews progress through all four tasks of MI. For example, the clinician might complete a consult for a patient in the hospital, form a trusting partnership (engaging), identify that the patient has a goal of stopping alcohol (focusing), elicit from them the patient their own personal reasons for desiring this change (evoking), only for the patient to decide they do not feel ready to consider a medication for AUD or go to AUD counseling (planning). Nevertheless, this motivational interview has likely increased the patient's chances of changing their alcohol use.[16]

- **Engaging**—This task involves using empathic listening to create an atmosphere of trust, collaboration, and mutual respect. This atmosphere becomes a safe place for the patient to think out loud about conflicting feelings they might have toward personal growth and change. Clinicians should try to give about 20% of the time they expect to spend in a patient's room to the engaging task, especially for a new consultation. Less time may be required for follow-up consultations.
- **Focusing**—Focusing involves gaining an understanding of the patient's goal and then using MI skills described later in this section to guide the patient in a meaningful conversation about this goal. When focusing the conversation, it is important to guide the patient, rather than to lead them along using your own agenda or follow them wherever their stream of thought might go.[5]
- **Evoking**—Ambivalence is a normal starting point for behavioral change, particularly for hospitalized patients who are less likely to be seeking SUD treatment as the main reason they seek hospitalization.[17] The clinician will likely hear a mixture of statements that are pro-change (aka "Change Talk") and anti-change (aka "Sustain Talk") if they listen carefully to any given patient.[18] Evoking involves guiding the conversation so that patients can hear themselves say what their goal is, why it is important to them, and what steps they might take to achieve it. Evoking can be accomplished using the skills described later in this section. In general, clinician should explore why a patient might want to change their relationship with substances before diving into a plan about how to do so.
- **Planning**—When partnering with a patient on a plan, it is important to remember that they are the person who will have to take the new medicine, or go to the residential treatment program, not you. Therefore, the plan must belong to them. It should be rooted in their personal reasons for change, engage their unique strengths, and be informed by the special expertise they have about themselves. In other words, MI planning respects patients' agency.[5] Each clinician can and should provide advice. However, advice should be offered only with permission. For example, you might say something like "Would it be okay if I told you about some things other people in this situation have found helpful?" before launching into the details of a 12-step program or the benefits of medication treatment for AUD.

OARS Skills

OARS skills are helpful in ensuring the principles of MI are followed during conversations with patients (Table 15.3). OARS is an acronym for: **Open-ended questions, Affirmations, Reflections, and Summaries.**

- **Open-ended versus Closed-ended Questions**—Open-ended questions invite patients to answer however they wish.[5] In MI, open-ended questions are preferred rather than closed-ended questions which are structured in such a way as to constrain possible answers.[12] An example of this difference is illustrated by the following two questions:
  - **Closed-ended Question:** "Tony, you haven't had any alcohol since the last time you were admitted to the hospital, have you?"
  - **Open-ended Question:** "How have things been going with alcohol, Tony?"

The open-ended question invites Tony to respond however he wishes, whereas the closed-ended question implies Tony should answer that he has not returned to alcohol, even if he has. Not only are open-ended questions more likely to yield more accurate responses, they are also very useful to the evoking task of MI. Examples of evocative open-ended questions are "How would things be different if you never returned to alcohol?" "What do you think your family admires about you?" "What else is important to you in life?"

- **Affirmations**—Clinicians should listen intently to what patients say for clues about their inner strengths and resources. An affirmation is when you notice something positive about a patient and comment on it. Examples might include "You were brave coming to the hospital when you did."

TABLE 15.3

Motivational Interviewing Tasks and OARS Skills

Motivational interviewing (MI) tasks	Motivational interviewing (MI) skills
Engaging—Involves empathic listening to create an atmosphere of trust, collaboration, and mutual respect. Demonstrating genuine interest in the patient's perspective increases engagement.	**Open-ended Questions**—Cannot be answered with yes or no and do not imply that a certain answer is preferred by the questioner. Open questions are especially handy for **Evoking**.
Focusing—After gaining an understanding of the patient's goal, focusing requires thoughtful use of MI skills to guide a meaningful conversation about that goal without becoming overly directive (leading) or passive (following).	**Affirmations**—Notice something positive about the patient and comment on it. Leave the word "I" and any reference to the questioner out of affirmations to avoid perceptions of moralization. Affirmations build the self-efficacy patients need to create and enact a change plan.
Evoking—Conversing with patients in a way that draws out from them their inner strengths, reasons for change, and what they might be willing to do toward that change.	**Reflections**—Reflections involve offering back to the patient an interpretation of what they are thinking, feeling, or doing at that moment.
Planning—Partnering with patients in a way that supports their autonomy, increases their self-efficacy, while developing a change plan. Advice should be offered with permission.	**Summaries**—Large reflections combining several things a patient has said.

Note: All OARS skills are useful and important to each MI task. The table above is not intended to suggest certain skills are more important than others for achieving any particular MI task.

"It was hard for you to open up about that, and you did it."

- **Reflections**—These are perhaps the most important of the OARS skills. A reflection is when the clinician offers back to the patient a statement about what the clinician interprets the patient is thinking, feeling, or doing at that moment. In MI, the goal is to use at least twice as many reflections as questions.[12] Reflections can be simple, complex, or double-sided. The choice of what to reflect and which type of reflection to use is determined by which of the four tasks of MI the clinician is trying to achieve, and whether what the patient has communicated tilts the conversation toward or away from change. High-quality reflections convey accurate empathy or demonstrate a sincere attempt to understand what the patient has conveyed. Below are descriptions of the different types of reflections with examples.
  - **Simple Reflections**—Simple reflections involve repeating what has been said, or simply paraphrasing it.[12] They are typically brief and lack embellishments that might increase the emotion behind what the patient has said. Simple reflections are most appropriate for reflecting statements that tilt the conversation away from change (aka "sustain talk"). They are not well-suited for responding to emotional statements (whether for or against change) because they may not convey accurate empathy. An example of when a simple reflection might be appropriate would be if the clinician were working on an MI task other than engaging (ie, focusing, evoking, planning) and the patient were to suddenly say "There really isn't anything better than a cold beer on a hot day." You might respond with a simple reflection "You like that."
  - **Complex Reflections**—Complex reflections use metaphor or emotional language to convey accurate empathy.[12] They are most often used to amplify the emotion behind a patient's pro-change statements ("change talk") with the aim of eliciting more change talk. Patients are most convinced by what they hear themselves say, so complex reflections are an effective tool for promoting personal growth and change. When the clinician is working on the engagement task of MI, it may sometimes be appropriate to use a complex reflection in response to sustain talk to convey accurate empathy and establish rapport. In general, though, complex reflections are best suited for responding to change talk. Complex reflections may also be used to advance the conversation by filling in an unspoken message, deeper meaning, or anticipating what the patient might say next.[12] An example might be if a patient who recently lost her daughter to Child Protective Services said, "She's gone, and I miss her so much." and you replied "There's a gaping hole in your heart and you'd do anything to fill it." This reflection uses metaphor to convey accurate empathy,

amplify the emotion behind the patient's statement, and subtly advance the conversation toward change by implying that there might be something she could do to regain custody (ie, enter substance use treatment).

- **Double-sided Reflections**—It is normal for patients to feel ambivalent about change and double-sided reflections capture both sides of this internal debate while subtly guiding the patient toward change.[12,17] When formulating a double-sided reflection, the first part of the sentence should be a simple reflection of the sustain talk and the second part should be a longer and more complex reflection of their change talk. It is important to connect the two parts of this sentence with an "and" instead of a "but" to avoid seeming dismissive. For example, if a patient says, "They cost a lot, but these pills I buy off the street are the only thing that helps me sleep." You might respond "Now you can sleep at night, and these pills are burning a hole right through your pocket."
- **Summaries**—Are essentially larger reflections combining several pieces of information the patient has shared.[5] Summaries are particularly helpful when transitioning between MI tasks. For example, you may summarize a patient's change talk before moving into the planning task.

MI Traps

When performing MI with a patient, there are a few potential traps to be avoided, discussed below.[5,12]

- **Expert Trap**—Clinicians may have years of clinical training and perhaps even lived experience with addiction. All this knowledge will best benefit the patient depending on how the expertise is presented. Clinicians become ensnared in the Expert Trap when perceived as having special authority to identify and solve patients' problems. Patients may lose the agency needed to enact behavioral change in these situations.[5]
- **Persuasion Trap**—The clinician risks stepping into the persuasion trap when attempting to convince the patients to change. Paradoxically, the more clinicians lean into a pro-change stance, the more the patient may tilt toward not changing.[5]
- **Time Trap**—The hospital is a busy place, and clinicians must be careful to manage time during the day. However, the clinician may encounter the time trap if attempting to rush toward planning with a patient without engagement, focusing, and evoking. These tasks can be achieved efficiently and rushing through planning with a reluctant patient might end up costing more time.[5]
- **Wandering Trap**—Empathic listening is at the core of MI. Nevertheless, if the clinician follows the patient wherever their stream of thought takes them you risk losing focus.[5] When you find yourself in the Wandering Trap, try using a reflection or summary to ensure the patient feels heard followed by a change-oriented open question to guide them back toward the motivational interview's previous focus.

Example of MI on an Addiction Medicine Team

Below is an example of Dr. Hall practicing the use of MI for a patient who injects substances.

Hello, I am Dr. Hall and this is the Addiction Medicine team. We want to make sure our patients get good, respectful *care while they are here and that any withdrawal symptoms they might have are well taken care of. Some of our patients tell us they don't like how substances fit into their lives anymore. If that is the case, we want to* partner *with them on a plan that feels good to them for when they leave the hospital.* ***Having heard these things about us, how can we be helpful to you while you are here?***

Right away, we have exhibited **partnership, acceptance, compassion** and have begun to **evoke** from the patient what is important to them by asking an open question about what they might like us to address in our visit.

Many patients express that stopping substances is not a realistic or desirable goal for them in the immediate future. If that is the case, we can use MI to offer harm reduction. Consider the MI techniques used in the following example (patient responses implied but not written for brevity):

I'm hearing that stopping injecting fentanyl is not something you feel is possible for you right now **[reflection]**. *Would it be alright if we talked about some things other people who inject substances have told me are helpful for staying safe and healthy* **[asking permission/avoiding expert trap]**? *What have you already heard about harm reduction* **[open-ended question]**? *You really know a lot about safer injection* **[affirmation/acknowledgment of the patient's expertise]**. *Would it be alright if I asked you what steps you go through when you inject fentanyl* **[asking permission]**? *How do you normally inject* **[open-ended question]**? *Thank you for sharing. I can tell this is something that is difficult for you to talk about* **[reflection/demonstrating accurate empathy]**. *It takes a lot of strength to open up about such a private part of your life* **[affirmation]**. *Would it be okay if I gave you some feedback on what you've told me* **[asking permission]**? *It sounds like there is a difference between all the knowledge* *you have about safer injection practices and how you are actually injecting on a daily basis* **[developing a discrepancy]**. *It's clear from how knowledgeable you are about harm reduction, that it's important to you to stay safe and healthy* **[reflection/affirmation]**. *What do you think is holding you back from doing safer injection practices more consistently* **[open-ended question]**? *You've just moved here from out of town, and you haven't found a way to get sterile injection equipment here yet* **[reflection]**. *You feel that if you had the sterile supplies you needed, you wouldn't have to share equipment with other people* **[reflection]**. *Is it okay if I share with you how to get sterile equipment from our local Syringe Service Program* **[asking permission/avoiding persuasion trap]**? *Besides using sterile equipment each time you inject, what other things have you heard can reduce your health risks* **[open-ended question]**? *You're curious what else might help* **[reflection]**. *Would it be alright if I shared some information with you about a medication called PrEP people can take to reduce their risk of getting HIV* **[asking permission]**? *This is the first time you've heard of PrEP* **[reflection]**. *It sounds like you're concerned about potential side effects* **[reflection]**. *You want to know more about the pluses and minuses* **[reflection]**. And so on…

Summary

Patients with SUD seen in the hospital setting frequently differ from patients seen in outpatient addiction treatment centers as their primary motivator to seek medical treatment is often not a desire for SUD treatment. MI is a powerful tool that can engage these patients during the reachable moment of hospitalization. Key tasks of MI include engaging, focusing, evoking, and planning and key skills include open-ended questions, affirmations, reflections, and summaries. Avoiding the expert, persuasion, time, and wandering traps will lead to more fruitful discussions. MI skills will be the key foundation to employing the psychosocial and behavioral treatment approaches described next.

Psychosocial and Behavioral SUD Treatment Approaches

Hospitalization is a reachable moment for people who use substances to change their behaviors, whether to quit using a substance, engage in treatment, or employ harm-reduction strategies. However, hospitalization is also a time of severe medical and surgical morbidity and can be physically and psychologically overwhelming. In the US, the hospital is generally considered an abstinence-based space, with alcohol and other substance use not only not permitted but considered illegal. In this environment, patients must choose between medical treatment and continued use of substances. Those who choose medical treatment lose access to their substance of choice as a coping mechanism, as well as access to regular interactions with family and friends, often leading to poor distress tolerance and coping in the hospital setting. The psychosocial and behavioral approaches discussed here provide a framework for improving the supportive environment that patients who use substances experience in the hospital, to ensure patient engagement and improved outcomes.

There are certain challenges associated with providing psychotherapy in the hospital setting. Hospitalizations can be short, thus patient–clinician relationships are short. Semiprivate rooms, beeping cardiac monitors, and medication dosing schedules can make it challenging to create a peaceful environment and thus successful therapy session. The recommendations in this chapter are mindful of these challenges and seek to adapt psychosocial and behavioral treatment approaches to the unique medical–surgical hospital environments.

This chapter starts from general therapeutic approaches, including trauma-informed care (TIC), brief cognitive behavioral therapy (CBT), and harm reduction, and then discusses more specific approaches, including seeking safety, addressing high-risk nonadherent behaviors, and complementary therapies. Table 15.4 provides an overview of interventions and their associated purposes.

Trauma-Informed Care

TIC refers to a model of employing universal precautions for trauma, assuming that all patients may have experienced trauma and are at risk of retraumatization during hospitalization. A TIC model ensures all patients feel safe and empowered during their interaction with the medical system. This is particularly important for patients with a history of SUD and should be employed in hospital settings.

The TIC model presents a unique opportunity for fostering rapport, engagement, and increased trust within the therapeutic relationship. A TIC approach involves recognizing the widespread impact of trauma, identifying the signs and symptoms of a traumatized individual, and making a concerted effort to avoid retraumatization. A universal approach to TIC may start with clinicians who are providing SUD care but needs buy-in from hospital staff and leadership to change systemic policies and practices to have the greatest effectiveness. Principles to consider for providing TIC can be grouped into the following

TABLE 15.4

Summary Table of Psychosocial and Behavioral Interventions That Can Be Deployed in the Hospital Setting

Interventions	Purpose of intervention	Resources/websites for additional information
Framework of care		
Trauma-informed care	To provide care that is sensitive to the patient's past trauma experiences and avoid retraumatization.	■ https://www.traumainformedcare.chcs.org ■ https://www.samhsa.gov/mental-health/trauma-violence/trauma-informed-approaches-programs ■ https://www.traumainformedcare.chcs.org/resources-for-becoming-trauma-informed/
Cognitive approaches and skill-building		
Brief cognitive behavioral therapy	To help patients identify and change negative thought patterns and behaviors.	■ https://www.mirecc.va.gov/visn16/docs/therapists_guide_to_brief_cbtmanual.pdf ■ https://depts.washington.edu/dbpeds/therapists_guide_to_brief_cbtmanual.pdf ■ https://www.mirecc.va.gov/visn16/docs/mybriefcbt-patient-workbook-fillable.pdf
Behavioral chain analysis	To examine the sequence of events leading to an unhealthy behavior to identify points of intervention.	■ https://cls.unc.edu/wp-content/uploads/sites/3019/2014/10/Behavior-Chain-Analysis-Information-1.pdf ■ https://psychotherapyacademy.org/courses/inside-the-therapy-room-dbt-unveiled/modules/implementing-dbt-in-practice/section/dbt-behavioral-chain-analysis-triggers-and-solutions/
The 5Ws	To analyze and understand the who, what, when, where, and why of a situation or behavior.	■ https://comm.gatech.edu/resources/writers/5ws
Seeking Safety	To help individuals attain safety from posttraumatic stress disorder (PTSD) and substance use.	■ https://www.treatment-innovations.org/seeking-safety.html
Contingency management	Reinforces positive behaviors with the use of motivational incentives.	■ https://www.recoveryanswers.org/resource/contingency-management/ ■ https://pubmed.ncbi.nlm.nih.gov/37788613/
Behavior activation	To increase engagement in positive activities to improve mood and functioning.	■ https://www.psychologytoday.com/us/therapy-types/behavioral-activation ■ https://pmc.ncbi.nlm.nih.gov/articles/PMC6461437/pdf/CD013305.pdf ■ https://www.therapistaid.com/therapy-worksheet/behavioral-activation
Activity planning	To organize and plan daily activities to enhance structure and motivation.	■ https://store.extension.iastate.edu/product/Activity-Planning-Worksheet ■ https://www.cci.health.wa.gov.au/~/media/CCI/Mental-Health-Professionals/Depression/Depression-Worksheets/Depression-Worksheet—03—Weekly-Activity-Schedule.pdf
Activity scheduling	To plan and structure daily activities to enhance routine and reduce depressive symptoms.	■ https://positivepsychology.com/activity-scheduling-worksheets/ ■ https://pmc.ncbi.nlm.nih.gov/articles/PMC4852920/pdf/pone.0154248.pdf ■ https://www.apaservices.org/practice/business/technology/tech-column/cbt-app-depression

(*continued*)

TABLE 15.4

Summary Table of Psychosocial and Behavioral Interventions That Can Be Deployed in the Hospital Setting (*Continued*)

Interventions	Purpose of intervention	Resources/websites for additional information
Activity monitoring	To track and analyze daily activities to identify patterns and areas for intervention.	■ https://www.mirecc.va.gov/visn5/EBT/CBT-D/CBT-D-Activity-Monitoring-Form-508.pdf ■ https://pmc.ncbi.nlm.nih.gov/articles/PMC10424774/pdf/nihms-1808573.pdf
Skills training	To teach practical skills for coping with stress, emotions, and interpersonal situations.	■ https://www.ncbi.nlm.nih.gov/books/NBK551500/
Regulating and calming techniques		
Mindfulness	To promote relaxation and mindfulness through focused attention and awareness.	■ https://healthlibrary.stanford.edu/books-resources/mindfulness-meditation.html ■ https://www.freemindfulness.org/download ■ https://health.cornell.edu/resources/health-topics/meditation
Box breathing	To reduce stress and improve focus through controlled breathing techniques.	■ https://www.bsu.edu/-/media/www/departmentalcontent/counseling-practicum-clinic/pdfs-new-website/square-breathing.pdf ■ https://extension.umn.edu/two-you-video-series/box-breathing ■ https://health.clevelandclinic.org/box-breathing-benefits
Relaxation techniques (music, water)	To reduce stress and promote relaxation using soothing stimuli.	■ https://www.youtube.com/watch?v=1ZYbU82GVz4 ■ https://www.unr.edu/counseling/virtual-relaxation-room/releasing-stress-through-the-power-of-music ■ https://www.ncbi.nlm.nih.gov/books/NBK513238/
Guided imagery	To use visualization to reduce stress and promote mental and emotional well-being.	■ https://www.mentalhealth.com/library/visualization-and-guided-imagery-for-stress-reduction ■ https://www.hopkinsmedicine.org/health/wellness-and-prevention/imagery
Safety planning		
Return to use ("relapse") prevention skills	To develop strategies to prevent return to substance use or other unhealthy behaviors. Includes recognizing cognitive distortions, urge surfing, and implementing above strategies together.	■ https://www.va.gov/WHOLEHEALTHLIBRARY/tools/reducing-relapse-risk.asp ■ https://www.ncbi.nlm.nih.gov/books/NBK551500/?report=printable ■ https://pmc.ncbi.nlm.nih.gov/articles/PMC4553654/pdf/yjbm_88_3_325.pdf ■ https://www.hazeldenbettyford.org/relapse-prevention ■ https://www.therapistaid.com/therapy-article/10-tips-for-avoiding-relapse

categories: **Safety, Transparency, Collaboration, Empowerment, and Diversity Awareness.**[19]

- **Safety.** This principle involves ensuring physical, psychological, and emotional safety in the hospital setting. Examples of actions that promote safety may include speaking to patients at eye level, being aware of body language (not towering over patients), and providing clear and consistent messaging regarding anticipated medical treatments.
- **Transparency.** In general, this principle seeks to build and maintain trust by ensuring all care decisions are made with transparency. Actionable ways to promote transparency include ensuring patients understand the need for a particular task or procedure, narrating procedures so patients understand what to expect, and maintaining eye contact and engagement when talking to a patient.

- **Collaboration.** It is important to recognize and minimize the power imbalance between the clinician and the patient. This can be accomplished by inviting patients to ask questions and actively participate in decisions made about their care, allowing flexibility in those decisions, and understanding patients' strengths and the resources needed to accomplish their goals.
- **Empowerment.** It is important for patients to speak up and have a voice in their care. This can be encouraged by keeping patients well informed about their care, respecting their rights to accept or decline treatment (even if this is contrary to medical advice), and providing options whenever possible (ie, "Would you like the door open or closed?").
- **Diversity Awareness.** Patients' cultural and social factors impact their trauma response; ensuring culturally sensitive interventions can promote healing. These may include using language interpretation to provide care in the patient's preferred language if not English and asking patients their pronouns and avoiding misgendering.

Trauma-Informed Care Tips in the Hospital Setting

- Introduce new care clinicians when possible—including at change of shift and change of rotation. Let patients know when clinicians will go off-service and who will take over for care.
- Inform patients of which clinicians are on their care team. For instance, patients should understand why certain consultants are seeing them. Provide explanations of different roles for team members, especially trainees.
- Provide step-by-step explanations for all procedures, even routine ones. Discuss expectations before, during, and after these procedures.
- Proactively manage escalating behavior, recognizing this may be a trauma response. Consider a formal team huddle with representation from different clinicians to discuss approaches.

The TIC model facilitates positive rapport with patients, which is an antidote to the moral distress and compassion fatigue hospital staff frequently feel when caring for patients who use substances. Employing the TIC model as a universal precaution to engage authentically, communicate challenging topics with compassion, and managing body language ultimately improves both patient and clinician wellness in the hospital setting.

Brief Cognitive Behavioral Therapy

Brief CBT is widely regarded as a highly effective intervention for the treatment of SUD and is a version of CBT that can be offered in the hospital setting. Brief CBT is designed to address a specific set of problems that patients may encounter and provide two therapeutic approaches that are known as "cognitive" and "behavioral" interventions. Brief CBT can be provided by social workers, counselors, or clinicians, but is most times provided by social workers. A fundamental aspect of Brief CBT is the establishment of a strong therapeutic relationship. This relationship is characterized by the following elements[20]:

- *Empathy:* This involves validating the patient's experiences and placing oneself "within" the current experience to understand and empathize with their feelings.
- *Genuineness:* Transparent communication of information and an authentic presentation of oneself are fundamental principles in health care. This entails treating patients as individuals rather than merely as consumers of the hospital system. Furthermore, it involves adhering to one's commitments, maintaining consistent nonverbal expressions and feelings, and demonstrating integrity in all interactions.
- *Unconditional Positive Regard:* Demonstrating unwavering commitment to patient care involves adhering to timeliness, aiding in navigating the health care system, and maintaining a nonjudgmental approach when addressing challenges. Recognizing that disagreements are inevitable presents an opportunity to demonstrate acceptance of patient autonomy, self-determination, and displaying warmth with any patient engagement.
- *Active Listening:* This refers to the way an individual receives, processes, and subsequently transmits a message. Clarifying a message can entail verbally repeating the patient's statement, thereby fostering rapport and enhancing the sense of being understood.

The implementation of Brief CBT within the context of hospital-based SUD care can vary. The clinician can introduce this model to the patient as transparent, collaborative, time-limited, and future-oriented. This involves tasks to enhance skill development.[21] Brief CBT can assist with unhelpful thinking patterns, emotional management, setting realistic expectations, and many other challenges that patients face in the hospital. The brief interventions should be personalized and offered in a supportive, nonjudgmental manner. Providing education about the connection between one's thoughts, feelings, and emotions is essential for the patient to understand helpful and unhelpful thinking patterns and how to challenge these unhelpful thoughts. Identifying a specific problem or goal allows for a targeted intervention that can be utilized in real time.

Example of Developing a Problem Statement and Goals for Brief CBT

Problem: Increased stress associated with a 7-day hospitalization on a trauma unit

Goal: Learn one cognitive and one behavioral strategy for coping with stress associated with being in a hospital.

Cognitive Strategy:

Learn and reteach one stress management coping skill such as:

Thinking, "I'll get through this. I have a team behind me," "I can ask questions if I don't understand," "I have a choice here," "No one is out to hurt me," "I can do this; I've got this, this isn't forever," etc.

Behavioral Strategy:

Complete one self-care routine daily such as:

- Taking a shower (can be exchanged with requesting a bed bath because of ambulatory limitations)
- Brushing my teeth and hair
- Applying lotion to my skin
- Playing (comforting) music while closing my eyes (with the lights off)
- Using my stress ball

A variety of interventions are associated with the Brief CBT Model. Described below are helpful interventions to educate, practice, and reinforce with patients. These may be used in the hospital or outpatient setting, though in the hospital setting may be utilized for patients with longer length of hospital stay.

Behavioral Chain Analysis

Behavioral Chain Analysis[22] facilitates exploration of the underlying reasons behind behavioral patterns. It enables patients to delve into the "how" and "why" of a behavior, thereby gaining insights into its development. Simplified components of a behavioral chain analysis are described below. See additional resources in Table 15.4 for more information.

- Describe the specific **behavior** including what was done, said, thought, or felt
- Describe the specific **prompting event** and **vulnerabilities** that started the chain of behavior including environment, timing, accompanying thoughts or feelings, and other precipitating events
- Describe in detail the **links** in the chain of events that connected the promoting event to the behavior
- What specific **consequences** occurred because of the behavior?
- What **solutions** and prevention strategies can be identified to avoid the behavior in the future?
- Describe a plan for **solving** the prompting event, thinking through **harmful consequences**, and **repairing** consequences.

This detailed introspection can lead to a deeper understanding of problem formation and facilitate personalized safety plan or prevention of return to use plan. Through behavioral chain analysis, a patient may identify vulnerabilities that may lead to unhealthy behaviors and subsequent patient-specific prevention strategies (Table 15.5).

TABLE 15.5

Examples of Patient-Specific Vulnerabilities and Prevention Strategies With Associated Implementation Recommendations

Patient-specific vulnerability	Patient-specific prevention strategy
Low distress tolerance	■ Include supportive person (via phone or in person) when communicating treatment recommendations ■ Consider oral antianxiety medications ■ Stress ball for physical tension relief/anxiety relief ■ Coloring books/pencils for distractions ■ Puzzles and/or word search books ■ Support staff debrief after medical team update
Pain control expectations	■ Expectation setting at initial admission and reinforced by all team members ■ Education about nonopioid pain management ■ Work with team for treatment of SUD and substance withdrawal that contributes to increased pain

TABLE 15.6

Example Usage of the 5Ws and Associated Sample Questions for Patients

Who	What	When	Where	Why
The people that a person spends time with can be triggering. Asking questions related to who the patient uses substances with can be helpful in identifying the "who" related to triggers.	Certain activities can have an association with substance use. In addition, boredom can also be a trigger for substance use. Wondering or ruminating on past activities can trigger urges or cravings for substance(s).	Identifying what situations are particularly triggering can be valuable information for patients. Exploring these scenarios with patients can be helpful in gaining awareness about return to use patterns.	Location, location, location. Identifying areas of risk for patients are particularly important.	Many patients may not understand the "why" of their use; identifying triggering feelings, sensations, people, times, and locations provide information for the patient and the clinician/SUD team.
Questions to consider				
Whom (specifically) were you thinking about? Who did you feel needed to be there in the moment?	What effect do you receive from using substance(s)? What relief might you feel? What mental pain might you temporarily have relief from?	When do you feel the urge to use? Do you have the highest cravings before, during, or after a particular feeling or experience?	Where do you buy or use substances? Where do the most intense feelings start?	What things outside of yourself trigger you to use substances? What internal emotional states trigger use for you? (guilt, hurt, anger, shame, embarrassment, loneliness, grief, etc)

The 5Ws

The 5Ws, or *Who, What, When, Where, and Why questions,* can play a critical role in identifying situations that may involve risk for return to use for patients. Patients may not fully understand how emotionally overwhelming a hospitalization can become. One important role of an SUD clinician in the hospital can be to help a patient navigate these scenarios with compassion, curiosity, and unconditional positive regard. Table 15.6 has examples scenarios and responses using the 5Ws.

Seeking Safety

Seeking Safety[23] is a present-focused and client-centered approach to help individuals attain safety from posttraumatic stress disorder (PTSD) and substance use. This model is highly flexible and can be used in a variety of settings such as hospitals, mental health, criminal justice, veteran, and schools, and can be conducted in a group or as a one-on-one session. It can also be delivered by licensed professionals, peers, and paraprofessionals. Several studies have demonstrated the effectiveness of Seeking Safety. A 2016 meta-analysis showed that Seeking Safety is more effective in treating PTSD symptoms than no or many alternative treatments and was highly associated with decreased substance use.[24]

Seeking Safety is rooted in five principles including *safety* as the core goal; *integrated treatment* that incorporates both trauma and SUD simultaneously; a *focus on ideals* to counteract the loss of ideals in trauma and SUD; *four content areas* (see below); and *attention to counselor processes,* such as self-care and emotional responses for counselors.

Seeking Safety offers 25 therapy topics that specialize in the four content areas: *Interpersonal, Cognitive, Behavioral,* and *Case Management.* Each topic revolves around a safe coping skill, such as asking for help, setting boundaries, compassion, or healing from anger. It is not a requirement for participants to complete them in order or even complete all of them if not relevant to their goals. A general overview for a session is provided in the box inset below.

Seeking Safety Topic: Healing from Anger

Check-in

Quotation: Ask participants to reflect on the following quote from Charles Dickens, "A loving heart is the truest wisdom." What does this mean to the participant?

Review handouts. Titles are "Exploring Anger"; "Understanding Anger"; "Before, During, and After: Three Ways to Heal Anger"; and "Safety Contract: Protecting Yourself and Others."

Check-out and develop commitment

Similar to the structure of CBT, Seeking Safety sessions begin with a check-in to ask participants about their mood, coping skills they have recently used, unsafe behaviors they may have engaged in, and if they completed the previous assigned commitment. It moves on to discuss the inspiring quotation that typically relates to the main topic. Next, handouts are given and discussed at length, and it ends with a check-out that involves a thought from participating in the session and formulating a commitment for next time.

Prior to beginning a session with a patient in the hospital setting, best practice would be to (1) ensure the patient is able to meaningfully engage in therapy and not too ill or experiencing withdrawal, (2) confirm there are no medications due or immediate plans to be transferred for a procedure/test, and (3) ensure communication with the bedside nurse to eliminate any interruptions (consider placing a note on the door). The patient can choose a topic that speaks to them, something that can be easily relatable to their specific goals. Sometimes sessions must be shortened or modified if a patient becomes too fatigued given their current clinical situation. After sessions are complete, it is always best to discuss a commitment, which is something for the patient to work on or think about before your next visit.

Overall, Seeking Safety provides a framework for delivering TIC and CBT to address comorbid PTSD and substance use that can effectively reduce PTSD symptoms without retraumatization or the need for longitudinal treatment over weeks, months, or years, making this a great approach in the hospital setting.

Contingency Management

Contingency management (CM) is an evidence-based tool based on operant conditioning to promote specific behavior changes, including abstinence from stimulant use. CM uses motivational incentives such as vouchers, gift cards, or other rewards for positive behaviors. CM has been found to be the most effective in the treatment of stimulant use disorders and has been employed in the hospital setting, particularly for stimulant use disorders.[25] CM can be used to promote abstinence and treatment adherence in the hospital or outpatient setting.[26]

Behavioral Strategies to Promote Change

Hospitalization can be an opportunity for individuals to plan for recovery during a time of stability away from substances, particularly during prolonged hospitalizations. Behavioral strategies such as behavioral activation and activity monitoring and scheduling can be used to help promote recovery activities during and post-hospitalization.

Behavioral Activation

While CBT allows patients to understand the connection between thoughts and emotions, behavioral activation allows patients to understand the connection between behaviors and emotions. Individuals experiencing major depressive episodes may lose interest in previously enjoyable activities, leading to inactivity, which itself can contribute to depressive symptoms. This cycle results in a perpetual state of depression and resulting inactivity. Behavioral activation, through meaningful action and purposeful choice, breaks this cycle by interrupting this downward spiral.

Activity Monitoring

Activity monitoring is a tool within Behavioral Activation. It involves tracking any activities that the patient is currently engaging in without intervention in the hospital. For example, if the patient takes hot showers in the morning and finds this enjoyable, this can be used as a proactive tool for coping at the beginning or end of the day. This activity is tracked to provide baseline data and explore the level of pleasure the patient is experiencing from the shower activity. Another example is coloring in a coloring book with quiet music playing. This activity can also be a proactive coping tool or a coping tool during a difficult moment to distract from distressing feelings. A discussion surrounding effectiveness of the coping tool can be facilitated by a clinician or other SUD team member. Because the patient is hospitalized, there may be constraints regarding movement. However, using available spaces, such as requesting use of vacant rooms as a "calming space" for a prearranged period, is one way for patients to have 1 to 2 hours to themselves for relaxation and privacy for completion of exercises.

Activity Scheduling

Another tool within behavioral activation is activity scheduling, which involves purposefully scheduling enjoyable and meaningful activities during the day.[27] Individuals who use substances may be engaged in patterns of behavior that support their substance use rather than their recovery, so it is important to relearn and re-experience these enjoyable and meaningful activities.

TABLE 15.7

Example of Activity Monitoring and Scheduling Template

	Sunday	Monday	Tuesday	Wednesday	Thursday	Friday	Saturday
6:00 AM							
7:00 AM							
8:00 AM							
9:00 AM							
10:00 AM							
11:00 AM							
12:00 PM							
1:00 PM							
2:00 PM							
3:00 PM							
4:00 PM							
5:00 PM							
6:00 PM							
Overall mood (0–10):							

Instructions: Please write down all the activities you are doing in a day and rate (0–10) the level of Pleasure (P) you felt when engaging in that activity (eating breakfast, watching TV, walking the dog, talking to mom on the phone, shopping for groceries, etc). Then rate your overall mood (0–10) at the end of the day for EACH DAY.

During hospitalization, these activities might include reading or listening to music, putting on make-up or shaving, spending time with family, conversations with other patients or staff, or going for a walk. Post-hospitalization, these might include rekindling an old hobby, exercising or spending time in nature, and having family get-togethers. These suggestions are by no means exhaustive and should be developed by individual patients. Some patients may benefit from creating a schedule for their activities (Table 15.7).

Skills Training

Skills Training[28] aims to address skill deficits by providing patients with the necessary guidance and support to learn, practice, and apply specific skills. A lack of coping, problem-solving, and social skills can hinder effective coping strategies. The training process involves modeling, rehearsing, and gradually implementing the learned skills in small, manageable steps. See box inset.

Relaxation Techniques

There are multiple different types of relaxation techniques that can be considered to help hospitalized patients cope with the stress of hospitalization. After developing rapport with the patient, consider offering the patient a menu of options to help with relaxation and stress reduction. These techniques are best integrated into the care of the patient whose acute substance withdrawal has been effectively managed.

Mindfulness

Mindfulness is a training rooted in Buddhist meditation practice and philosophy. It is also integrated into a Dialectical Behavioral Therapy framework. The objective of mindfulness is to assist patients in disentangling themselves from unproductive thought patterns and enhancing their focus on the present moment. This involves practicing intentional concentration and observation to fully immerse in the present. Table 15.8 includes different applications that provide guided meditations to increase mindfulness.

Box Breathing

Box Breathing can be described as an effective regulating, relaxation technique that can assist with stress reduction, improve focus and regulate one's breathing, and calm feelings of panic.[29,30] This can be easily implemented in the hospital setting and takes little time. A 5-minute exercise is helpful for improvement in symptoms. See box inset.

Example of Facilitating a Skills Training Intervention

Social Worker: So, what I'm hearing is that when you get a call from your mom an argument starts and you can't take it and it messes up the rest of your day, is that correct? You also mentioned it gets in the way of you being able to hear what the doctors say when they round in the evening. Did I get that right?

Patient: Exactly! She calls me and talks about the bills, what my dad isn't doing and how it's just her taking care of my daughter and I just can't take it!! It just makes me so frustrated that I just want to leave.

Social Worker: Ok, I hear you. That certainly sounds very frustrating. Is it ok if we go over some tips that you might find helpful?

Patient: Yes, I guess. At this point I'll try anything!

Social Worker: Okay, so it seems like talking to your mom later in the day is very overwhelming. Would you say so?

Patient: Yes, yes. That's what it is. I just get so overwhelmed with everything. I know I can't do anything because I'm in here and I feel guilty.

Social Worker: Ok, so I hear that feeling guilty is in a part of how you feel as well. So, how about this? Maybe switching the time you talk to your mom and creating some boundaries around the conversation. It might go something like this, "Hey mom, I just called to check in. I know things have been stressful at times. However, I only have 15 minutes to talk as I'm expecting the doctor to come in around that time, and I need to listen to what's said." What do you think about that? We can even practice a few times and try it out.

Box Breathing

Step 1: Breathe in through your nose, counting to four slowly. Feel the air enter your lungs.

Step 2: Hold your breath for 4 seconds. Try to avoid inhaling or exhaling for 4 seconds.

Step 3: Slowly exhale through your mouth for 4 seconds.

Step 4: Wait for another 4 seconds before you breathe in again.

Step 5: Repeat above

Examples of Box Breathing

- https://www.youtube.com/watch?v=tEmt1Znux58
- https://www.youtube.com/watch?v=G25IR0c-Hj8
- https://www.youtube.com/watch?v=n6RbW2LtdFs

Progressive Muscle Relaxation

Progressive muscle relaxation is a relaxation technique that involves tensing and releasing different muscle groups in a sequential order to reduce physical tension associated with stress, anxiety, and panic.[31] This technique is easily implemented in the hospital setting, and its efficacy can be improved when relaxation is guided by a clinician (Table 15.9).

Music

Music[32] can suppress stress-related elevation in cortisol. Listening to nature sounds or rippling water can also elicit relaxation. Hospitalized patients may benefit from utilizing different sounds or music to help cope with stressful situations in the hospital setting.

Guided Imagery

Guided imagery[33] involves using one's mind to develop a relaxing scene, image, or person to assist with managing

TABLE 15.8

Examples of Free Apps for Mindfulness and Guided Imagery

- Insight Timer: has a free library of guided meditations, music tracks, and a timer for silent meditation, no required subscription.
- Headspace: includes a variety of guided meditation sessions.
- Calm: has guided meditations, calming exercises, and sleep stories.
- Smiling mind: designed to encourage mindfulness and offers free guided meditations and exercises.
- 100% happier: offers free access to guided meditations through their podcast.
- Healthy minds program: provides meditation training and podcast-style lessons.
- UCLA mindful: promotes stress management through guided meditations and a timer, with podcast-style lessons.
- Buddhify: offers guided meditations for various situations and moods.
- Aura: offers meditations, sleep stories, and CBT techniques.
- Simple habit: provides short, guided meditations for various situations and moods.
- Waking up: offers meditations and wisdom teachings.

TABLE 15.9

Helpful Examples of Progressive Muscle Relaxation

- https://www.youtube.com/watch?v=SNqYG95j_UQ
- https://www.youtube.com/watch?v=ihO02wUzgkc
- https://www.cci.health.wa.gov.au/-/media/CCI/Mental-Health-Professionals/Panic/Panic—Information-Sheets/Panic-Information-Sheet—05—Progressive-Muscle-Relaxation.pdf

anxiety and stress (Table 15.8). There are two techniques related to imagery:

- **Palming**[33]: Palming is the act of visualizing colors to promote relaxation. By covering one's eyes and mentally perceiving the "color" associated with stress (for instance, red), followed by visualizing its transformation into a more calming hue (such as blue), this process has been demonstrated to induce a state of relaxation.
- **Guided Imagery**[33]: Engaging in mental visualization involves creating a mental image of a preferred relaxation destination. This could encompass a beach, a forest, a cherished childhood retreat, or a serene meadow.

Relapse Prevention Training

An essential intervention to assist patients in prevention of return to substance use involves developing a return to use (also known as "relapse") prevention plan or safety plan, identifying return to use triggers, developing effective craving management strategies, establishing activities in their daily lives that support recovery, learning to effectively manage stress, and identifying and prioritizing self-care. While this is not an exhaustive list of tools to aid in prevention of return to substance use, mastering these strategies can yield substantial benefits. Bedside education and brief interventions are especially useful for patients who are receiving other hospital-based SUD services. All members of a hospital-based SUD team have a vital role in providing education, reteaching behavioral strategies, reinforcing skills, and providing supportive practice for prevention of return to substance use. The structured nature of daily hospital routines provides ample opportunities to reinforce skills and create teachable moments.

A crucial aspect of initiating and maintaining recovery involves the development of a diverse set of coping skills to address anticipated triggers and unforeseen challenges that may hinder abstinence. Conversely, when patients experience successful

My Substance Use Prevention Plan

Introduction: A substance use prevention plan is a crucial tool in supporting your recovery journey. This document outlines triggers, cravings, sensations, and emotional states that can make you vulnerable to a return to substance use situation.

In addition, this plan identifies social, internal, and external support systems, as well as your personal strengths and coping skills useful during your hospital stay.

Identifying My Common Triggers:
- People: ____________________
- Places: ____________________
- Things: ____________________

Managing My Cravings:
- Recognize and acknowledge cravings without judgment.
- Practice "urge surfing" to ride out the craving wave.
  - https://www.therapistaid.com/therapy-worksheet/urge-surfing-handout
- Engage in distraction techniques such as hobbies, exercise, or social activities.
- Use mindfulness and relaxation techniques to reduce the intensity of cravings.

Sensations and Emotional States: Certain physical sensations and emotional states can increase the risk of relapse.

Identifying My Vulnerable Sensations/Emotional States:
- ____________________
- ____________________

Identifying various support systems can provide encouragement and reduce feelings of isolation.

Social Support Systems
- Family and friends.
- 12-step mutual support groups or other peer support groups.
- Spiritual or religious communities.

My Internal/External Support Systems: __________

My Personal Strengths to use while Hospitalized:

____

Coping Skills List:

Effective coping skills are essential for managing stress and preventing relapse in a hospital setting.

Stress Management Techniques: __________
- Deep breathing
- Progressive muscle relaxation (YouTube).
- Use of Stress ball

recovery endeavors, it fosters enhanced self-efficacy and self-esteem to support recovery and overall well-being.[34] Return to use prevention strategies can include building awareness about what harmful use entails, potential negative consequences associated with active use behaviors, and distortions of thought which can influence poor decision-making ("cognitive distortions"). In addition, identifying high-risk situations that typically result in return to use is also important.[34]

Cognitive Distortions

Cognitive Distortions refer to unhelpful thinking patterns, which are developed over time, and are associated with repetitive, negative thought patterns.[35] When ruminated upon, these thoughts develop into unhelpful patterns that can be self-defeating. Identifying cognitive distortions can aid patients with recognizing how their thinking leads to unhealthy actions or feelings. Developing strategies to recognize and modify these thinking errors requires education, reteaching, practice, modeling, and role-playing. Table 15.10 provides examples of cognitive distortions and their explanations, although this is not an exhaustive list.

Cognitive distortions can be addressed with a thought record. A thought record serves as a tool to assist patients with stepping back and identifying the unhelpful thought and creates increased awareness of personal patterns of unhelpful thinking (Table 15.11). These thought patterns are often automatic in nature, pervasive, and assumed to be valid. Helping patients to question their thoughts in real time provides a valuable teachable moment.

TABLE 15.10

Examples of Cognitive Distortions

Cognitive distortion	Explanation
Jumping to conclusions[36]	Assuming something negative without proof. For example, thinking a friend is mad at you without asking them.
Personalization[37]	Blaming yourself for things beyond your control. For example, thinking you caused someone's bad mood when you didn't.
Mental filter[38]	Only focusing on the negative parts of a situation and ignoring the positives. For example, dwelling on a small mistake during a great presentation.
Catastrophizing[37]	Expecting the worst possible outcome. For example, thinking a minor health symptom is a serious illness.

Other Strategies to Promote Recovery

Ceasing or reducing substance use takes time, skills, practice, and support, which is sustained by patient readiness for change. Using bedside teaching strategies with patients is a vital learning opportunity as patients have significant potential to be captive audiences. Some skills that can be taught including avoiding triggers, urge surfing, and play the tape forward.

- ***Avoiding triggers:*** Triggers are internal cues developed from an association between a substance and cues in the environment and ultimately motivate substance-seeking behaviors.[39] For example, a patient could see someone selling drugs (a "dealer") across from the hospital when going outside briefly to get some fresh air, triggering memories of purchasing substances. Or they see a spoon on their tray when the phlebotomist came in to complete a blood draw for labs. The sight of the spoon and the sensation of a blood draw can trigger memories of injection substance use. Identifying and talking about these triggers creates awareness and helps the patient consider other reactions. A transparent and compassionate dialogue can facilitate patients in exploring their personal experiences and identifying potential triggers.[40] Table 15.12 presents common triggers and proposed coping skills.
- ***Urge surfing***[41]: Urge surfing is applying a coping mechanism when a strong desire or impulse is experienced in the body or mind to use a substance. An example that could trigger an urge or craving may be a television commercial or seeing a lighter or spoon. Surfing the urge involves distracting, enduring, and letting the intense urge to use a substance to pass. Conversely, *fighting* the urge will allow it to intensify. Urges to use often peak within the 20- to 30-minute range and then subside in intensity. An intense urge may feel like it will last for a much longer time than it does. In addition, when one succumbs to a craving or urge, the feeling is reinforced, and the intensity of a craving will strengthen over time. Some patients find it helpful to set a timer for 20 minutes when they are practicing urge surfing.
- ***Play the tape forward:*** When confronted with a potentially unhealthy decision, this is a technique that can help envision the potential consequences of that decision. See box inset.

TABLE 15.11

Examples of Challenging Cognitive Distortions With a Thought Record

Situation	Automatic thought	Feeling	What evidence supports or opposes the automatic thought?	Balanced alternative thought
My mom won't let me come home after my hospital discharge for 4 wk of IV antibiotics	"I should have known she wouldn't care" "she's done this before; I shouldn't even have asked her"	■ Disappointed ■ Hurt ■ Rejected ■ Ashamed ■ Embarrassed ■ Angry ■ Alone	"I don't know if mom cares or not because I haven't asked her" "she's allowed me to come home before"	"Just because mom won't let me come home doesn't mean she doesn't love me."

Clinical Example:

Patient: So, you'll never guess what my mom said when I called her….

Clinician: What do you mean? Oh, you called her to ask about going home for a bit for the 4 wk of IV antibiotics, is that right?

Patient: Yes, So, she said NO!!! I can't believe it! She said she wanted to support me and everything when I got here, and she was all worried that I was gonna die. Now it's like she doesn't give a crap!

Clinician: Ok, I'm so sorry to hear that. I'm sure that conversation with your mom was hard.

Patient: For sure! What am I gonna do now? I KNEW she was lying about caring about me. That's what she does!

Clinician: I'm sure the conversation upset you. What I hear you say is that your mom isn't allowing you to come home for the antibiotics and because of that you think she lied and doesn't care about you? Am I describing that right?

Patient: Yeah, exactly!

Clinician: Ok, is it ok if we slow down what happened on the phone with mom and take a look at where your mind went?

Patient: Umm, ok. I don't know how that's gonna help, but ok.

Clinician: Sure, I'll explain that and thank you for considering another way to look at this situation.

TABLE 15.12

Descriptions of Common Triggers and Proposed Coping Skills

Common triggers	Proposed coping skills
Personal experiences (running into a dealer on the street, seeing people you used to use with, etc)	■ Talking openly about what triggers you and learning to avoid them ■ Removing oneself from the situation
Stressful situations (eg, physical pain, arguments with family, anxiety about being in the hospital alone)	■ Getting support from family, friends, or support groups ■ Listening to music ■ Coloring ■ Taking a hot shower ■ Asking for a water ice ■ Having a small conversation/laugh with my nurse
Negative thoughts	■ Writing in a journal to understand and improve thoughts
Fear and anxiety about the future	■ Using mindfulness to stay in the present moment (eg, What goal can I focus on for right now? I can take a small walk with the nurse. I just had surgery, and my team talked about me needing to move around)
Cravings for substance use	■ Using urge surfing to ride out the craving
Trauma triggers (examinations that one needs to be undressed for, a male physician in the room during an examination, being strapped to a bed due to delirium, someone entering the room at night, etc)	■ Box breathing ■ Asking for a female nurse ■ Asking for a female in the room if the clinician is a male ■ Using a blanket to cover one's body; only exposing the needed body part for examination ■ Asking for the curtain to be closed (if sharing a room) ■ Asking for night rounding nurses to call out my name instead of touching me.

Play the Tape Forward Coaching

- Think of the consequences that would occur if you used versus if you did not use.
- Be as specific as possible in your visualization. The more detailed you are, the more powerful the exercise will be.
- Focus on the negative consequences of giving in to your cravings. This will help you to stay motivated to resist.
- Practice the exercise regularly. The more you use it, the more effective it becomes.
- Once you've played the tape forward, reflect on what you've imagined for a few minutes. How did it make you feel?

Computer-Based Programs that Deliver Behavioral Treatments

There are multiple different computer-based training programs or apps to address SUD that may facilitate patient insight into their triggers and risks for ongoing SUD. These programs may be helpful in settings without trained clinicians to deliver behavioral treatments. A rigorously tested computer-based program is called Computer-Based Training for Cognitive Behavioral Therapy (CBT4CBT). CBT4CBT is a low-cost computer-based program with core skill topics (12 modules) that teach patients generalizable CBT strategies for avoiding alcohol and substance use via video, graphics, audio instruction, and interactive exercises. CBT4CBT has an English and Spanish version and has focused CBT that applies to alcohol use and substance use. Like brief CBT, it is an evidence-based treatment for SUD.[42] While CBT4CBT has been previously studied in the outpatient setting, a trial is ongoing for its use in hospitalized individuals with AUD.[43]

Hospital-Based Harm Reduction

Harm reduction refers to a comprehensive set of interventions designed to mitigate the adverse consequences of behaviors without necessarily eliminating them entirely. In the health care context, harm reduction encompasses not only tools aimed at reducing the harm associated with substance use and other risky behaviors but also provides valuable insights into setting realistic expectations for patient engagement and interaction.

A harm-reduction model implemented within hospital-based SUD care fosters a pragmatic and supportive approach to clinical interventions. Exploring practices that promote trust, retention, and self-determination in patient care reduces conflicts for both patients and clinicians. Components and principles of harm reduction are discussed in depth in Chapter 19.

Management of High-Risk, Nonadherent Behaviors

High-risk, nonadherent (HRNA) behavior is an overarching term to encompass behaviors in the hospital that may pose significant harm to the patient or staff. HRNA behaviors can contribute to staff burnout and poor patient outcomes but may be mitigated by proactively anticipating and addressing patient needs in a timely manner. Addressing HRNA behaviors requires a harm-reduction and trauma-informed lens. Some examples of HRNA behaviors include leaving the hospital before medically advised, smoking in bathrooms, verbal or physical abuse toward staff, declining blood draws needed for monitoring or therapeutic treatments like physical therapy, frequently leaving the unit, and in-hospital illicit substance use. This section further describes these and then delves into ways to mitigate these risks.

- ***Early discharge:*** This may be referred to as leaving "against medical advice," "before medically advised," or as a "patient-directed discharge." These all connote a situation where the patient leaves the hospital before the medical clinician deems their discharge to be medically appropriate. The term "against medical advice" has fallen out of favor as it shifts clinicians' views on patients, making them appear difficult and careless about their health. The "against" piece describes a conflict between patient and clinician rather than a preferred collaborative approach. A developing term is "before medically advised," as it is a nonjudgmental and nonconfrontational term that can be incorporated more into medical training. Leaving the hospital before medically advised increases risk for a return to substance use, unsafe substance use, exacerbation of medical problems, and not receiving appropriate medications (ie, antibiotics, medications for SUD).[44]
- ***Declining care:*** Patients with SUD are at higher risk of mental health disorders, poor coping, and poor distress tolerance, as discussed in the TIC section. The hospital environment can be overwhelming, and patients may withdraw from care, represented by declining exams (invasive or noninvasive), sleeping during interviews, declining early morning blood draws, and declining other necessary tests and procedures.
- ***Patient movement***[45]***:*** Patients who leave their floor or unit frequently while admitted risk missing necessary treatment (ie, IV antibiotics), consultation (ie, meeting specialists), and monitoring

(ie, telemetry for arrhythmias). The risk of elopement with or without hospital equipment (ie, with a peripherally inserted central catheter line still in place) also increases when patients leave the unit for extended periods of time. The hospital is not a prison, and patients do have freedom of movement; however, this autonomy can often conflict with the role that staff are responsible for the well-being of their patients. When staff are not informed of patient whereabouts, they can appropriately become concerned about their patients.

- ***In-hospital substance use:*** Patients may be at high risk of illicit substance use during hospitalization for multiple reasons, including uncontrolled cravings, substance withdrawal, pain, ambivalence around cessation, and temptations from visitors.

For any of the above situations, there should be a discussion between the patient and care teams to approach these situations from a trauma-informed perspective, address any unmet needs, and set expectations for the safe provision of medical care. An effective tool for communication is the "Patient Safety Care Plan" (PSCP) described below.

- ***Transparent communication:*** The TIC approach entails using simple language, waiting for approval before conducting an exam, and providing anticipatory guidance and full transparency in all medical procedures recommended.
- ***Address unmet needs:*** Pain and withdrawal are typical triggers for in-hospital substance use. Ensure the patient is offered medications to treat their withdrawal, if appropriate, and adequate analgesia to manage acute pain they may be experiencing.
- ***Review expectations:*** Ensure patients understand expectations such as not to bring illicit substances to the hospital and informing staff of any time the patient spends off the unit. Staff should similarly inform patients that an assessment, urine drug screening or room searches may be completed if there is concern for substance use.
- ***Develop a Patient Safety Care Plan:*** A PSCP can be an incredibly effective trauma-informed tool for patients who display ongoing disruptive or HRNA behaviors during hospitalization.[46] A PSCP facilitates an open and transparent collaboration between patients and the care team and aims to set clear expectations and norms for safe provision of medical care. The primary goal is to address unsafe behaviors and reduce conflict while supporting patient goals. Components of the PSCP should be developed in collaboration with the patient by the multidisciplinary care team. The PSCP should be individualized to each patient and setting, and be consistent with hospital policies and procedures. Components of the PSCP may include (but not limited to) any of the following: when and for how long a patient can safely leave the medical floor, if and when visitors may be restricted, if and when drug testing may be requested. Importantly, the PSCP also addresses expectations the patient has of the care team and ways the care team can support them. The PSCP should be placed in the patient's room for the patient and all care members to view. This shared agreement can reduce conflict and improve patient engagement. An example PSCP is provided below.

Hospital-Based Twelve-Step Facilitation and Mutual Support Groups

Alcoholics Anonymous/Narcotics Anonymous

Twelve-Step facilitation (TSF) through mutual support groups (MSG) like Alcoholics Anonymous (AA) and Narcotics Anonymous (NA) can assist in recovery by offering structured social and emotional support. While individual therapy can be effective, MSG allow people to share in a common experience and thus develop close bonds. MSG offer social support and act as a protective barrier against isolation, provide direction and structure for goal setting, enhance self-assurance and promote more effective coping strategies, and provide opportunities for engaging in fulfilling activities, such as substance-free social interactions and assisting others who also grapple with substance use.[47] Table 15.13 reviews the Twelve Steps[48] taught through TSF from AA as well as the Twelve Traditions.[49]

AA/NA Virtual Meetings

AA and NA offer a variety of virtual meetings that can be accessed from anywhere in the world; we recommend offering this to patients during hospitalization. Meetings are available in different languages and time zones. For more information, visit the following websites: https://www.aa.org/find-aa and https://virtual-na.org/meetings/.

Self-Management and Recovery Training

An alternative to traditional TSF is Self-Management and Recovery Training, or SMART Recovery. SMART Recovery offers additional resources focused on self-empowerment and is grounded in a CBT model of recovery. While its primary support network is online, SMART Recovery also provides in-person meetings, albeit with limited availability and a higher concentration in urban and suburban areas.

Patient Safety Care Plan

[Insert hospital name] maintains a safe environment for all patients, staff, and visitors. Your medical team wants to partner with you to keep everyone healthy and safe. Here's what you can do:

- *Tell us your needs*, especially around cravings, triggers, anxiety, and/or pain. A member of your care team will check in approximately once per hour. Keep a list of your questions and requests to help get your needs addressed (doctors and advanced practice providers come once a day).
- *We request you do not inject, smoke, or consume any nonprescribed substances or alcohol.* Using substances in the hospital can interfere with medical treatment and put you and others at risk for injury.
- *Alcohol, tobacco, or other substances and paraphernalia may not be brought into the hospital.* If you have a change in behavior or are off unit for an extended time, a urine drug screen may be requested, and your belongings may be searched.
- *Procedure for leaving off the unit, if approved*: We want you here for your treatments. Time off the unit is at the discretion of your care team and limited to between 8 am and 5 pm. You may need to be accompanied by a member of your care team and only when they are able to accompany you.
- *IV pumps need to be unhooked by nursing staff before leaving.*
- *Visitors can provide support, or they can be disruptive to your health or care.* Let us know if you would like to restrict visitors for any reason. Visitors need to check in at nurses' station before entering your room. We reserve the right to monitor visitors, search visitors and their belongings, or prohibit visitors who are interfering with care or are under the influence. Due to infection issues and patient privacy, never enter another patient's room.
- The hospital will securely hold the personal belongings you brought to the hospital on admission.
- Outside items may only be brought to you once per week during the hours of 8 am to 5 pm (unless planned and agreed by staff) and are subject to search
- [*If needed*] The visitor restriction will be re-evaluated next week after the above boundaries are maintained. Supervised visitation during business hours 1 to 2 times per week will be considered.

Thank you for agreeing to partner with us in your care!

This may be a more appealing option for patients who decline AA/NA or want a less religious or spiritual focus. In-person and virtual meetings can be found here: https://smartrecovery.org/meeting. In addition to meetings, SMART Recovery has an active online community where members can engage in discussions, share experiences, and access resources.

Hospital-based SUD treatment has an opportunity to facilitate engagement in MSG using tools from traditional TSF, SMART Recovery, or other behavioral therapies like Seeking Safety in the hospital setting. Evidence is mixed as to whether MSG like AA, NA, or SMART Recovery are effective. A 2020 Cochrane review of 27 studies found that TSF and AA appeared to significantly improve abstinence from alcohol in comparison to other clinical interventions such as CBT.[50] Other studies have found no benefit once adjusting for confounders like motivation.[51] We support the use of open MSG in the hospital setting without the structure of TSF, given its rigidity and contradictory evidence, and favor utilizing principles from Seeking Safety and CBT instead.

Complementary and Alternative Approaches

Patients with SUD hospitalized for long periods of time can easily get bored, distracted, or return to negative behaviors. A best practice is to offer a variety of activities that can keep patients engaged in their care, including diversionary activities like arts and crafts, music therapy and pet therapy, and mind–body treatments like yoga, reiki, and acupuncture.

Many health systems have a volunteer or other patient-centered department that can offer an array of supports for admitted patients. Volunteers can provide magazines, coloring books, pencils, pens, or novels to keep patients busy and reduce any stress or anxiety related to their admission. Diversionary materials give patients a chance to shift focus from thoughts of use to positive activities. Examples of such activities may be reading, doing crafts or puzzles, writing, drawing in coloring books, watching entertainment, listening to music or podcasts, or planning to return to a previously enjoyed hobby such as working out. These activities could be offered by the hospital or brought in by patient families. Art therapy has been found to help patients with SUD decrease denial, reduce resistance to treatment for alcohol, reduce shame, and provide an outlet for communication.[52]

Music therapy has also been shown to benefit patients with SUD. In the hospital setting, music therapy may include staff playing instruments in the hallways or meeting patients at bedside to perform. Music has also been shown to benefit patients with SUD as lyrics can be inspiring and lead to positive changes; drumming is useful for patients who have repeated relapses; and music therapy overall has been

TABLE 15.13

The Twelve Steps and Twelve Traditions of AA

Twelve steps	Twelve traditions
1. We admitted we were powerless over alcohol—that our lives had become unmanageable.	1. Our common welfare should come first; personal recovery depends upon AA unity.
2. Came to believe that a Power greater than ourselves could restore us to sanity.	2. For our group purpose there is but one ultimate authority—a loving God as He may express Himself in our group conscience. Our leaders are but trusted servants; they do not govern.
3. Made a decision to turn our will and our lives over to the care of God as we understood Him.	3. The only requirement for AA membership is a desire to stop drinking.
4. Made a searching and fearless moral inventory of ourselves.	4. Each group should be autonomous except in matters affecting other groups or AA as a whole.
5. Admitted to God, to ourselves, and to another human being the exact nature of our wrongs.	5. Each group has but one primary purpose—to carry its message to the alcoholic who still suffers.
6. Were entirely ready to have God remove all these defects of character.	6. An AA group ought never endorse, finance, or lend the AA name to any related facility or outside enterprise, lest problems of money, property, and prestige divert us from our primary purpose.
7. Humbly asked Him to remove our shortcomings.	7. Every AA group ought to be fully self-supporting, declining outside contributions.
8. Made a list of all persons we had harmed, and became willing to make amends to them all.	8. Alcoholics Anonymous should remain forever nonprofessional, but our service centers may employ special workers.
9. Made direct amends to such people wherever possible, except when to do so would injure them or others.	9. AA, as such, ought never be organized; but we may create service boards or committees directly responsible to those they serve.
10. Continued to take personal inventory and when we were wrong promptly admitted it.	10. Alcoholics Anonymous has no opinion on outside issues; hence the A.A. name ought never be drawn into public controversy.
11. Sought through prayer and meditation to improve our conscious contact with God as we understood Him, praying only for knowledge of His will for us and the power to carry that out.	11. Our public relations policy is based on attraction rather than promotion; we need always maintain personal anonymity at the level of press, radio, and films.
12. Having had a spiritual awakening as the result of these Steps, we tried to carry this message to alcoholics, and to practice these principles in all our affairs.	12. Anonymity is the spiritual foundation of all our traditions, ever reminding us to place principles before personalities.

Alcoholics Anonymous. *The Twelve Traditions.* 2025. Accessed January 28, 2025. https://www.aa.org/the-twelve-traditions

positively related to a willingness to participate in substance use treatment.[52]

Mind–body methods may include yoga, reiki, and acupuncture. In Western medicine, yoga generally encompasses a combination of physical postures, breathing techniques, and meditation that together target a variety of psychologic and physiologic processes. Yoga may be employed in the hospital setting[53] and has the potential to address SUD and risk of return to substance use.[54] Reiki is a noninvasive form of healing that began in Japan, which focuses on a universal life force energy that flows through all living things. A reiki session may involve a practitioner placing their palms on or just above different areas of the body in different positions and for various amounts of time based on the flow of energy perceived. Reiki has also been found to be beneficial in SUD.[55] Acupuncture is a traditional Chinese medicine that involves inserting thin needles into specific points of the body to stimulate natural healing processes. These methods play a notable role in complementing traditional SUD treatment as it facilitates emotional stability and resilience,[56] which are core elements in the journey of recovery, and may assist with pain.[57] We recommend these approaches as complements to standard acute care therapies.

Additional services offered by various health systems may include a video game cart, nail or hair care services, and having emotional support animals. These gestures contribute to patients feeling valued, comfortable, and cared for during their hospitalization. Patients with SUD commonly experience unstable housing, comorbid mental health issues, and limited support or resources, so these acts of kindness can have a much bigger impact than expected and can potentially increase the chance of patients staying in the hospital to receive necessary medical care.

Role of the Social Worker and Behavioral Support Professionals

Social workers and behavioral support professionals, including peer navigators, contribute vital roles to hospital-based SUD care. Case managers, counselors, and health promotion advocates can also provide many of the services of a social worker, though may need additional training to provide these services. These care team members help to address the social determinants of health (SDOH) that frequently are unable to be managed by clinicians and aid patients in connecting to care following discharge. This section describes the role of the social worker and discusses support services offered from peer navigators or other team members.

Social Work

Social workers are professionals who assist patients in managing disability, life-threatening disease, mental health, or social problems, the latter of which may include unstable housing, substance use, and domestic conflict. A patient's experiences influence their perspective about their environment and the care they receive. Within the context of hospital-based SUD care, social workers comprehensively assess the patient in the context of the "whole person."[58]

Social workers in acute care settings generally have three roles: offering behavioral treatments, screening for SDOH, and assisting with disposition planning. This section focuses on SDOH screening and disposition planning.

Screening for Social Determinants of Health

A comprehensive assessment for a social worker can include screening for functional status, cultural and spiritual beliefs, employment and educational history, living arrangements and family structure, language proficiency and literacy levels, social and economic support, risk of neglect or exploitation, life-span planning, and the patient's own perception of their ability to improve their situation and barriers to care.[58] Social workers engaged in hospital-based SUD care can benefit patients by focusing on food and housing insecurity; transportation difficulties; and safety, including intimate partner violence, sex/human trafficking, and child protective service reporting.

Disposition Planning

Disposition planning involves helping to transition patients to the next appropriate level of care. It could be transferring patients to a postacute facility, such as a skilled nursing home, inpatient physical rehab, or a long-term acute care hospital. For patients directly returning home, it may involve ensuring the appropriate in-home supports are in place, such as home health care. This can be a time-consuming process as patients frequently have complex medical and social needs that must be addressed prior to discharge, often in a short amount of time. Effective discharge planning starts on the day of admission because once medical needs are satisfied, after-care plans must quickly solidify to reduce discharge delays. Social workers can assist in disposition planning by providing risk assessments and working with discharge facilities and home health care agencies to create safety plans and prevention of return to substance use plans prior to discharge.

Disposition planning also involves seamless linkage to care for SUD treatment. This may include facilitating intake appointments as quickly as possible and completing necessary paperwork and assessments during hospitalization rather than postdischarge. Other factors such as patients' health insurance status, living environment, health condition, proper identification, and reliable transportation may also need to be addressed to facilitate safe and effective disposition.

Disposition planning and linkage to care may also require drug and alcohol (D&A) assessments and level of care assessments (LOCAs) from social workers to determine appropriate referrals to licensed SUD treatment programs along the American Society of Addiction Medicine (ASAM) levels of care. Discharge planning is discussed further in Chapter 20.

Drug and Alcohol Assessment

The D&A assessment is a formalized way of obtaining a SUD-specific history. The goal of the D&A assessment is to understand how a patient's physical, social, spiritual, and cultural environments interplay and ultimately influence a patient's SUD and related behaviors.[58] It may not be feasible for all social workers providing hospital-based SUD care to complete a full assessment; however, for patients with prolonged length of stay or severe SUD, performing an assessment may assist with complex discharge planning and facilitation of ongoing SUD care. Figure 15.3 is an example D&A form that can be completed in the hospital setting and includes most if not all of the information needed to assist in appropriate discharge planning and linkage to care.

Level of Care Assessment

The ASAM Continuum of Care, Level of Care Assessment (LOCA) is another specialized assessment used to facilitate referral to the appropriate licensed SUD treatment program.[59] This should not be confused

SW D&A Assessment Form

Substance Use:

	Current Use	Last Use	Frequency	Route	Comments
Alcohol	Yes ☐ /No ☐				
Heroin	Yes ☐ /No ☐				
Methadone	Yes ☐ /No ☐				
Buprenorphine	Yes ☐ /No ☐				
Pill Opioids	Yes ☐ /No ☐				
Cocaine	Yes ☐ /No ☐				
Amphetamines	Yes ☐ /No ☐				
Benzos/Barbiturates	Yes ☐ /No ☐				
Hallucinogens	Yes ☐ /No ☐				
Cannabis	Yes ☐ /No ☐				
Inhalants	Yes ☐ /No ☐				
Other Substances	Yes ☐ /No ☐				
Gambling	Yes ☐ /No ☐				
Other Addictions	Yes ☐ /No ☐				

Additional Hx: Trauma Hx Description (If Applicable):

Increased Tolerance: Yes ☐ /No ☐
Details: ____

Impact on Family/Social/Job:

MH/D&A Treatment History:

Facility(s)	Date(s)	Outpt/Inpt	Outcome(s)
		Outpt ☐ /Inpt ☐	
		Outpt ☐ /Inpt ☐	
		Outpt ☐ /Inpt ☐	
		Outpt ☐ /Inpt ☐	

12-step Programs

AA Involvement: Yes ☐ /No ☐ Abstinence Time: Yes ☐ /No ☐, If Yes how long? ____

NA Involvement: Yes ☐ /No ☐ Sponsor: Yes ☐ /No ☐ /Homegroup: Yes ☐ /No ☐

Hx/Current Legal Involvement: Yes ☐ /No ☐

Current Parole/Probation: Yes ☐ /No ☐ Ph: ____ Active Court Date(s): ____

Hx/Current Military Involvement: Yes ☐ /No ☐ Branch: ____ VA Benefits: ____

Living Situation PTA: Street Homeless ☐, Housed (permanent) ☐, Housed (temporary) ☐, Shelter ☐

CM/Community Supports: ____ / Ph: ____

Stressors: ____ /Triggers: ____

Goals for Recovery: ____

Plan for Recovery: ____

Figure 15.3: Social work drug and alcohol assessment form.

with a D&A Assessment, which can be completed for any patients with a concern of substance use. Instead, the LOCA provides a framework for a comprehensive examination of a patient's biopsychosocial circumstances, which may have precipitated their need for hospitalization. The results of the LOCA inform the appropriate level of SUD treatment to which a patient should be referred upon hospital discharge. See Chapter 1 for more information about ASAM levels of care.

Performing this assessment will not be feasible or necessary for all hospital-based social workers because an understanding of the ASAM LOCA requires specific training. However, for hospitals that have dedicated SUD social workers, obtaining this training and understanding how to perform the LOCA can be helpful to ensure that patients are receiving the most appropriate post–hospital-based SUD care. The training can be accessed online from ASAM.[60] The six dimensions of a LOCA are provided in Figure 15.4 and inform the appropriate level of care for referral.

The six dimensions of the LOCA represent areas in which a patient's level of risk of complications from SUD and risk of return to use should be evaluated. This assessment helps determine the most clinically appropriate treatment intervention. Following the completion of a LOCA assessment, the ASAM Continuum of Care table is utilized to provide a clinically justified placement recommendation based on the assessment findings. For instance, a patient's risk of seizures from alcohol withdrawal may be assessed in Dimension 1, while an unstable living situation may be assessed in Dimension 5, ultimately suggesting they be referred to a Level 4 or hospital-based SUD level of care. Though not mandatory, performing a LOCA can facilitate transitions to posthospital-based SUD care. Most SUD programs prefer a fax or email to review clinical history, medical history, insurance, and demographics prior to considering admission.

Social workers can also assist by compiling lists of resources and SUD treatment programs in their areas. Having a strong awareness of these resources helps ensure patients receive both adequate and appropriate SUD care after hospitalization. A common misunderstanding is that all individuals who are hospitalized for SUD require "rehab," or inpatient specialty SUD treatment (ASAM LOC 3.5, or 3.7). Training staff on the various LOC and resources is therefore of paramount importance. Resources can be compiled from the free SAMHSA Treatment Locator website[61] and state-based SUD treatment services. For example, in the state of Pennsylvania, the Department of Drug and Alcohol Programs provides information on local treatment, harm reduction, and funding for any licensed program on the continuum of care.[62] Every county in the

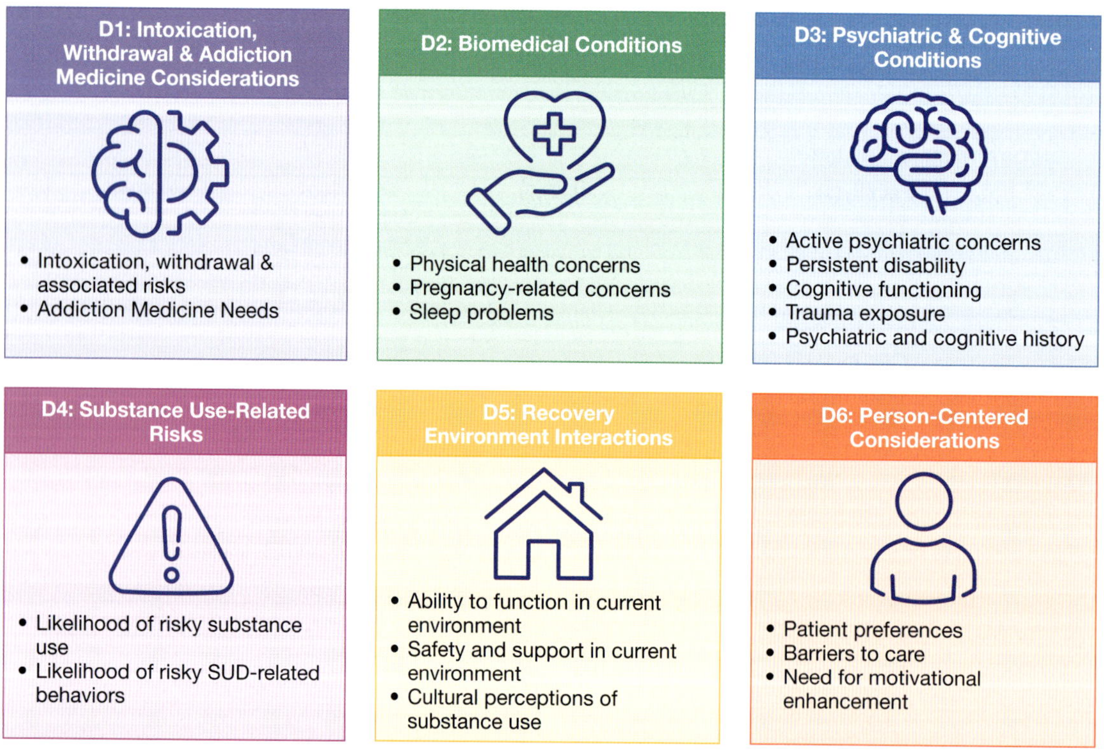

Figure 15.4: The six dimensions of an ASAM assessment.[59]

Commonwealth of Pennsylvania has a single county authority office that can assist with treatment funding, assessments, and referrals to treatment. To build a list of these programs as well as relationships with these programs, the social worker may reach out to each of these programs for more information or to introduce themselves. Having a connection with these programs can greatly facilitate discharge planning and referrals.

Daily Role of the Social Worker

It can be challenging to navigate the hospital setting as a social worker. Caseloads can fluctuate depending on the size of the health system and hospital priorities. Ideally, every patient who is receiving hospital-based SUD care should be assessed by the social worker—not only for SUD linkage to care but also to assess SDOH and provide resources for SUD recovery and prevention of return to substance use.

Templates can ease social work documentation. Most health systems are accredited by organizations such as the Joint Commission who is the official reviewer for regulatory requirements and standards.[63] Often, there are documentation requirements for SUD, trauma, and transplant assessments in a hospital setting. Below are template examples for consideration. Each state may have different regulations on what is required for social work documentation.

Peer Support

Peer support can play a key role in providing excellent care for people with SUD who receive hospital-based SUD care. This chapter uses the term "peer navigators" to refer to any persons whose role is to improve patient engagement in SUD treatment and not otherwise represented as traditional medical and nonmedical clinicians (including physicians and social workers, respectively). Other terms that may be used interchangeably include patient navigators, recovery specialists, recovery coaches, and peer mentors. While there are slight differences, the overarching similarity is their roles as people who fall outside of the traditional health care hierarchy, often having lived and living experience, and typically being more distant from medical culture.[64]

Benefits of peer navigators in the literature include assistance with system navigation, behavior change, harm reduction, and relationship building.[65] It is in this last role that peer navigators can offer some of their greatest benefits in providing hospital-based SUD care. Many people with SUD may lack trust in the health care system, limiting their ability to engage and receive recommended treatment. Peer navigators can break down these barriers by gaining patient trust and empowering patients to voice concerns. To ensure the longevity of anyone in the peer navigation role, it is vital to assist them in maintaining healthy boundaries

Substance Treatment and Recovery Services (STARS), formerly called Addiction Medicine Consult Service

Social Work Initial Drug & Alcohol Assessment

Reason for Consult:

Substance of Choice:

Urine Drug Screen/Blood Alcohol Level:

Length/Frequency/Amount Used:

Method: Oral/Intranasal/Smoke/Intravenous/Boofing/Skin-Popping

Withdrawal Symptoms/Cravings/Tolerance:

Overdose Survivor: Yes/No

Triggers:

Behavioral Addiction: Gambling/Sex/Shopping/Food/Exercise:

Treatment History for SUD:

Negative Consequences: Legal/Relationships/Job/Income/Health:

Living/Social Support:

Coping:

Period of Abstinence:

Intervention/Recommendations:

Treatment Motivation:

Recovery/Diversion Materials Offered:

Harm-Reduction Counseling: Yes/No

Disposition:

Note:

STARS, formerly called Addiction Medicine Consult Service

Social Work Follow-up Drug and Alcohol Assessment

Level of Care: Partial Hospitalization, Intensive Outpatient, Outpatient

Facility Name:

Facility Contact Name/Phone/Fax:

Releases of information Completed: Yes/No

Intake Assessment Appointment Date/Time:

Items Required at First Intake Assessment:

Updated Depart: Yes/No

Transportation:

Note:

STARS, formerly called Addiction Medicine Consult Service

Social Work MOUD/Buprenorphine Follow-Up Note

Clinician Contact Information:

Releases of information Completed: Yes/No

Type of Medication:

- buprenorphine-naloxone sublingual
- buprenorphine sublingual
- long-acting injectable buprenorphine

State Issued ID: Yes/No
Appointment Date/Time:
Transportation Type:
Rx needed: Yes/No
Updated Depart: Yes/No
Note:

STARS, formerly called Addiction Medicine Consult Service

Social Work Medication for OUD Follow-Up Note
Clinician Contact Information:
Releases of information Completed: Yes/No
(2) Forms of ID: Yes/No
Appt/Intake Date/Time:
Dosing Hours:
Need to Guest Dosing: Yes/No
Transportation Type:
Updated Depart: Yes/No
DC Summary/Dosing History Sent: Yes/No
Note:

STARS, formerly called Addiction Medicine Consult Service

Social Work Medication for AUD Follow-Up Note
Type of Medication: Acamprosate Disulfiram Naltrexone XR Naltrexone
Provider Contact Information:
Releases of information Completed: Yes/No
Appointment Date/Time:
Prescription Needed: Yes/No
Updated Depart: Yes/No
Note:

STARS, formerly called Addiction Medicine Consult Service

Social Work Progress Note
Engagement Reason:
Continued Social Support/Coping:
Treatment Follow-up:
Disposition:

with patients and supporting them through risks associated with caring for vulnerable patients with SUD.

Conclusion

People with SUD benefit from integrated medical, psychosocial, and behavioral treatments during hospitalization, using MI and a trauma-informed lens to promote engagement, reduce harm, and treat SUD. It takes a multidisciplinary hospital-based team to address all these needs and improve the care that hospitalized patients with SUD receive. Promoting a team mindset builds a strong addiction service line that can effectively provide evidence-based and trauma-informed care.

REFERENCES

1. Englander H, Jones A, Krawczyk N, et al. A taxonomy of hospital-based addiction care models: a scoping review and key informant interviews. *J Gen Intern Med.* 2022;37(11):2821–2833.
2. Lencioni P. *The Five Dysfunctions of a Team: A Leadership Fable.* Jossey-Bass; 2002.
3. Agile Mastery Ltd. *The 5 Dysfunctions of a Team.* Teams. 2024. Accessed January 28, 2025. https://agilemastery.co.uk/teams#049221d7-31c9-4a66-9ee9-69fb3abfb4a4
4. Kilmann Diagnostics. *Take the Thomas-Kilmann Conflict Mode Instrument (TKI).* Accessed January 3, 2024. https://kilmanndiagnostics.com/overview-thomas-kilmann-conflict-mode-instrument-tki/
5. Miller WR, Rollnick S. *Motivational Interviewing: Helping People Change and Grow (Applications of Motivational Interviewing Series).* 4th ed. The Guilford Press; 2023.
6. Kirschenbaum H. *Life and Work of Carl Rogers.* Amer Counseling Assn; 2008.
7. Miller WR, Moyers TB. Motivational interviewing and the clinical science of Carl Rogers. *J Consult Clin Psychol.* 2017;85(8):757–766.
8. Berman AH, Forsberg L, Durbeej N, Källmén H, Hermansson U. Single-session motivational interviewing for drug detoxification inpatients: effects on self-efficacy, stages of change and substance use. *Subst Use Misuse.* 2010;45(3):384–402.
9. Hershberger P, Flowers S, Bayless S, Conway K, Crawford TN. Interface between motivational interviewing and burnout. *Adv Med Educ Pract.* 2024;15:181–187.
10. Rollnick S, Miller WR, Butler CC, Aloia MS. Motivational interviewing in health care: helping patients change behavior. *Int J Chron Obstruct Pulmon Dis.* 2008;5(3):203.
11. Hohman M. *Motivational Interviewing in Social Work Practice (Applications of Motivational Interviewing Series).* 2nd ed. The Guilford Press; 2021.
12. Rosengren DB. *Building Motivational Interviewing Skills: A Practitioner Workbook (Applications of Motivational Interviewing Series).* 2nd ed. The Guilford Press; 2017.
13. Wood A. *The Motivational Interviewing Workbook: Exercises to Decide What You Want and How to Get There.* Rockridge Press; 2020.
14. Rogers C. *On Becoming A Person: A Therapist's View on Psychotherapy, Humanistic Psychology, and the Path to Personal Growth.* 2nd ed. Houghton Mifflin; 1995.
15. Douaihy A, Kelly TM, Gold MA. *Motivational Interviewing: A Guide for Medical Trainees.* 2nd ed. Oxford University Press; 2023.
16. Vasilaki EI, Hosier SG, Cox WM. The efficacy of motivational interviewing as a brief intervention for excessive drinking: a meta-analytic review. *Alcohol Alcohol.* 2006;41(3):328–335.

17. Miller WR. *On Second Thought: How Ambivalence Shapes Your Life*. The Guilford Press; 2021.
18. Dempsey KL, Stout DD. *The Harm Reduction Workbook for Addiction: Motivational Interviewing Skills to Create a Personalized Recovery Plan and Make Lasting Change*. New Harbinger Publications; 2024.
19. Center for Violence Prevention and Recovery. *Trauma-Informed Care Tips Sheet for Healthcare Providers*. 2021. Accessed January 16, 2025. https://bidmc.org/-/media/files/bidmc/bidmc-trauma-informed-care-tip-sheet.pdf
20. Cully JA, Dawson DB, Hamer J, Tharp AT. *A Provider's Guide to Brief Cognitive Behavioral Therapy*. Department of Veterans Affairs, South Central Mental Illness Research, Education, and Clinical Center (MIRECC). 2021. Accessed January 16, 2025. https://www.mirecc.va.gov/visn16/docs/therapists_guide_to_brief_cbtmanual.pdf
21. Institute for Quality and Efficiency in Health Care (IQWiG); 2006-. *In Brief: Cognitive Behavioral Therapy (CBT)*. [Updated 2025 Aug 21]. https://www.ncbi.nlm.nih.gov/books/NBK279297/
22. Kiluk BD, Benitez B, DeVito EE, et al. A digital cognitive behavioral therapy program for adults with alcohol use disorder. *JAMA Netw Open*. 2024;7(9):e2435205.
23. Najavits LM. *Seeking Safety: A Treatment Manual for PTSD and Substance Abuse*. The Guilford Press; 2002.
24. Lenz AS, Henesy R, Callender K. Effectiveness of seeking safety for co-occurring posttraumatic stress disorder and substance use. *J Couns Dev*. 2016;94(1):51–61.
25. Peng L, Titus H, Roellich P, Englander H. Adapting contingency management for hospitalized patients with stimulant use disorder. *J Addict Med*. 2023;17(5):580–586.
26. Appa A, Baral S, Stein B, et al. The IMPACT (Infection Management Plus Addiction Care Together) pilot: a case series of combined contingency management for substance use disorders and antibiotic adherence in the hospital setting. *J Addict Med*. 2024;18(2):138–143.
27. Edelman EJ, Rojas-Perez OF, Nich C, et al. Promoting alcohol treatment engagement post-hospitalization with brief intervention, medications and CBT4CBT: protocol for a randomized clinical trial in a diverse patient population. *Addict Sci Clin Pract*. 2023;18(1):55.
28. American Recovery Center. *Behavior Chain Analysis and Addiction Treatment*. 2023. Accessed January 16, 2025. https://americanrecoverycenter.net/behavior-chain-analysis-and-addiction-treatment/
29. University of Michigan Medicine. *Behavioral Activation for Depression*. https://medicine.umich.edu/sites/default/files/content/downloads/Behavioral-Activation-for-Depression.pdf
30. Cognitive Behavioral Therapy Los Angeles. *Cognitive Behavioral Therapy Techniques*. Accessed January 16, 2025. https://cogbtherapy.com/cognitive-behavior-therapy-techniques
31. Vetter VM, Kurth T, Konigorski S. Evaluation of easy-to-implement anti-stress interventions in a series of N-of-1 trials: study protocol of the anti-stress intervention among physicians study. *Front Psychiatry*. 2024;15:1420097.
32. Cleveland Clinic Health Essentials. *How Box Breathing Can Help You Destress*. https://health.clevelandclinic.org/box-breathing-benefits
33. Toussaint L, Nguyen QA, Roettger C, et al. Effectiveness of progressive muscle relaxation, deep breathing, and guided imagery in promoting psychological and physiological states of relaxation. *Evid Based Complement Alternat Med*. 2021;2021:5924040.
34. Hohmann L, Bradt J, Stegemann T, Koelsch S. Effects of music therapy and music-based interventions in the treatment of substance use disorders: a systematic review. *PLoS One*. 2017;12(11):e0187363.
35. Johns Hopkins Medicine. *Imagery*. Accessed January 17, 2025. https://www.hopkinsmedicine.org/health/wellness-and-prevention/imagery
36. Recovery Research Institute. *Relapse Prevention (RP) (MBRP)*. Accessed January 17, 2025. https://www.recoveryanswers.org/resource/relapse-prevention-rp/
37. Ota M, Takeda S, Pu S, et al. The relationship between cognitive distortion, depressive symptoms, and social adaptation: a survey in Japan. *J Affect Disord*. 2020;265:453–459.
38. Dinar AB, Peddireddy SR, Nazery D, Mastrangelo L, Opler DJ. Recognizing cognitive distortions in post-traumatic stress disorder using popular media. *Acad Psychiatry*. 2023;47(3):316–320.
39. Özparlak A, Karakaya D. The associations of cognitive distortions with internet addiction and internet activities in adolescents: a cross-sectional study. *J Child Adolesc Psychiatr Nurs*. 2022;35(4):322–330.
40. Özdemir İ, Kuru E. Investigation of cognitive distortions in panic disorder, generalized anxiety disorder and social anxiety disorder. *J Clin Med*. 2023;12(19):6351.
41. Compton WM, Wargo EM, Volkow ND. Neuropsychiatric model of addiction simplified. *Psychiatr Clin North Am*. 2022;45(3):321–334.
42. Mayo Clinic Staff. *Quitting Smoking: 10 Ways to Resist Tobacco cravings. Healthy Lifestyle: Quit Smoking*. 2022. Accessed January 17, 2025. https://www.mayoclinic.org/healthy-lifestyle/quit-smoking/in-depth/nicotine-craving/art-20045454
43. Bowen S, Marlatt A. Surfing the urge: brief mindfulness-based intervention for college student smokers. *Psychol Addict Behav*. 2009;23(4):666–671.
44. Thakrar AP, Lowenstein M, Greysen SR, Delgado MK. Trends in before medically advised discharges for patients with opioid use disorder, 2016–2020. *JAMA*. 2023;330(23):2302.
45. Stream S, Alfandre D. "Just getting a cup of coffee"—considering best practices for patients' movement off the hospital floor. *J Hosp Med*. 2019;14(11):712–715.
46. Englander H, Mahoney S, Brandt K, et al. Tools to support hospital-based addiction care. *J Addict Med*. 2019;13(2):85–89.
47. Burzinski CA, Zgierska A. *Recovery-Oriented Mutual Self-Help Groups*. Whole Health Library. Accessed January 28, 2025. https://www.va.gov/WHOLEHEALTHLIBRARY/tools/recovery-based-mutual-self-help-groups.asp
48. Alcoholics Anonymous. *The Twelve Steps*. 2025. Accessed January 28, 2025. https://www.aa.org/the-twelve-steps
49. Alcoholics Anonymous. *The Twelve Traditions*. 2025. Accessed January 28, 2025. https://www.aa.org/the-twelve-traditions
50. Kelly JF, Humphreys K, Ferri M. Alcoholics Anonymous and other 12-step programs for alcohol use disorder. *Cochrane Database Syst Rev*. 2020;3(3):CD012880.
51. Kaskutas LA. Alcoholics anonymous effectiveness: faith meets science. *J Addict Dis*. 2009;28(2):145–157.
52. Aletraris L, Paino M, Edmond MB, Roman PM, Bride BE. The use of art and music therapy in substance abuse treatment programs. *J Addict Nurs*. 2014;25(4):190–196.
53. Dangel AR, Demtchouk VO, Prigo CM, Kelly JC. Inpatient prenatal yoga sessions for women with high-risk pregnancies: a feasibility study. *Complement Ther Med*. 2020;48:102235.
54. Khanna S, Greeson JM. A narrative review of yoga and mindfulness as complementary therapies for addiction. *Complement Ther Med*. 2013;21(3):244–252.
55. Prasad K, Dyer NL, St Sauver J, et al. Effect of reiki on measures of well-being in low-income patients with mental health diagnoses. *Glob Adv Integr Med Health*. 2025;14:27536130251323581.
56. Kitzman JM, Bowman LC, Lin YC. Acupuncture in addiction medicine: its history, evidence, and possibilities. *Med Acupunct*. 2023;35(3):111–116.
57. Nielsen A, Dusek JA, Taylor-Swanson L, Tick H. Acupuncture therapy as an evidence-based nonpharmacologic strategy for

comprehensive acute pain care: the academic consortium pain task force white paper update. *Pain Med.* 2022;23(9):1582–1612.
58. National Association of Social Workers. *NASW Standards for Social Work Practice in Health Care Settings.* NASW Practice Standards & Guidelines. 2016. Accessed January 28, 2025. https://www.socialworkers.org/Practice/NASW-Practice-Standards-Guidelines/NASW-Standards-for-Social-Work-Practice-in-Health-Care-Settings
59. American Society of Addiction Medicine. *About the ASAM Criteria.* https://www.asam.org/asam-criteria/about-the-asam-criteria
60. American Society of Addiction Medicine. *ASAM eLearning.* 2025. Accessed January 28, 2025. https://elearning.asam.org/
61. Substance Abuse and Mental Health Services Administration. Accessed January 28, 2025. https://findtreatment.gov/
62. Commonwealth of Pennsylvania. *Department of Drug and Alcohol Programs.* 2025. Accessed January 28, 2025. https://www.pa.gov/agencies/ddap.html
63. The Joint Commission. *Hospital Accreditation. Health Care Settings.* 2025. Accessed January 28, 2025. https://www.jointcommission.org/what-we-offer/accreditation/health-care-settings/hospital/
64. Englander H, Gregg J, Gullickson J, et al. Article commentary: recommendations for integrating peer mentors in hospital-based addiction care. *Subst Abus.* 2020;41(4):419–424.
65. Incze MA, Kelley AT, James H, et al. Post-hospitalization care transition strategies for patients with substance use disorders: a narrative review and taxonomy. *J Gen Intern Med.* 2024;39(5):837–846.

16

Cultural Humility, Social Determinants of Health, and Structural Competency

Max Jordan Nguemeni, Ethan Manelin

During residency, we were both involved in the care of an older Black gentleman hospitalized with heart failure. He was a veteran but struggled to access the benefits he was entitled to. His medical history included depression, cocaine use disorder, and homelessness. He had family, but they had distanced themselves from him because of his substance use. His life had been shaped not just by illness but by isolation—by systems and relationships that had failed him when he needed them most.

Like many patients we have cared for with a history of substance use, his struggles were not just with his physical health. His body carried the burden of chronic disease, but the weight of his social conditions was just as heavy. He was suicidal—a combination of his untreated depression and the crushing reality of life on the margins. Because of that, during this hospitalization, he required constant monitoring. That meant either a chaperone sitting in his room 24 hours a day or a camera watching him. He hated both.

He antagonized the in-person chaperone verbally, pushing back against the forced company. When we switched to the camera, thinking it might give him a greater sense of space, that did not help either. *"I can't even piss in peace without y'all watching me!"* he shouted, frustrated that even his most basic bodily functions were under surveillance. His resistance was not welcomed by all staff. He was thought of as "difficult" and "disruptive." But to him, It was not about being defiant for the sake of defiance. It was about dignity: about feeling like a person instead of an organism under constant watch; about having some sense of privacy in a place where every other choice had been taken from him.

But during that admission, there was one thing he wanted even more than to be left alone. He wanted a haircut. He asked everyone who walked into his room, from those who brought his meals to the custodial staff who emptied the trash, if they could cut his hair. It seemed small in the grand scheme of things. But when you have been stuck in a hospital bed for weeks, unable to care for yourself, unable to control even the smallest parts of your life, something as simple as a haircut can mean the world. Having served in the military, keeping a low cut had become ingrained in his hygiene routine.

So, we made it happen. One of us (E.M.) bought the clippers, and the other (M.J.N.) cut his hair. I (M.J.N.) had years of experience cutting my own, and we had come to know how much a clean cut would mean to him. When I showed him the mirror afterward, his whole face lit up. He was so happy with how he looked that he asked me to update his profile picture in his medical chart. He wanted to be seen like this—clean, put together, more like himself than he had felt in a long time.

He stabilized medically and was transferred to an inpatient psychiatric facility. But when he left our service, he had to leave the clippers behind due to risk concerns. It was another small thing, but it crushed him. Those clippers had been a rare token of control, something that belonged to him in a world where so much had been taken away.

About a year later, he was back in the emergency department. In the time since I had last seen him, he had lost what little stability he had. He had been staying on a friend's couch for a while, but eventually, he was back on the streets. Then he was robbed. His medications were stolen. And he was done. So, he attempted suicide after using a large amount of cocaine, which tipped him into another heart failure exacerbation. When I walked into his room, we immediately recognized each other. His eyes brightened. "Yeah, I remember you. Can you give me another cut this time too?" he said, as if that moment—one brief act in a long, painful life—had stayed with him. After completing the admission, I ran upstairs to our old workroom from the year before. The clippers were still there! So, I did it again—I cut his hair once he was medically stable. And this time, when he left, I made sure he could take the clippers with him.

For a man with nothing, the hospital was one of the safest places he had. Here, at least, he had food. He had a bed. He was seen. And while the medical interventions we provided were necessary, it was the small things—the haircut, the clippers, the brief sense of dignity—that made the difference to him.

His story reminded us of a truth that is easy to forget in clinical practice: people's material conditions don't just shape their social networks, financial security, or access to care. They shape our patients' health in ways we rarely account for in our treatment plans. We spend so much time discussing medications, procedures, and evidence-based interventions that we risk overlooking the simplest, most human acts of care.

A haircut did not change his material conditions. It did not fix the poverty, the homelessness, or the deep fissures in the health care system that had yawned wide at his every turn. It did not bring his family back or make it easier for him to access his benefits. But it did remind him—and us—that dignity matters: that meeting people's basic needs, however small, is part of the work of healing.

—Max Jordan Nguemeni and Ethan Manelin

Key Points

- **Substance use disorders (SUDs) are deeply intertwined with social determinants of health (SDOH) such as housing, income, education, incarceration, and health care access.**
- **Hospitalized patients with SUD often experience stigma, undertreated pain, poorly managed withdrawal, and barriers to addressing their health-related social needs.**
- **Punitive hospital policies toward in-hospital substance use and patient-directed discharges undermine trust and engagement in care; harm-reduction and patient-centered approaches are critical alternatives.**
- **Trauma-informed care, relationship building, and structural competency are essential skills for clinicians caring for hospitalized individuals with SUD.**
- **Addressing patients' social needs during hospitalization and at discharge, including through linkages to community-based services, is crucial to improving long-term health outcomes.**
- **Future efforts must focus on reducing stigma, integrating harm reduction into hospital care, strengthening hospital-to-community transitions, and advocating for systemic reforms that better serve people with SUD.**

Social and cultural factors profoundly shape the nature of substance use disorders (SUDs). Moreover, those who suffer from SUD often have a markedly different experience of social life. The effects of a SUD on social life—consequences for jobs, family life, carceral status, and so on—may in fact clinch the diagnosis of the disorder. The social world has a wide array of effects on health status and disease states in general, but SUDs are especially, and perhaps even uniquely, interdigitated with SDOH.

From the clinician's standpoint, social and cultural factors that affect their patients may range from being invisible to taking over every conversation. Health professional schools and training programs have increased their coverage of these topics in recent years, but often this education is relatively abstracted from patient experience and the applied skills of addressing such issues in clinical practice. Given the special salience of social and cultural factors in the context of SUDs, it is crucial for clinicians treating these disorders to have a good working understanding of conceptual and practical approaches. Furthermore, hospitalization presents unique challenges, circumstances, and opportunities in relation to the social and cultural factors that affect patients with SUDs. This chapter reviews key concepts, literature, and practical techniques at the complex intersection of social life and hospital-based SUD care.

Key Definitions

Social determinants of health (SDOH) are economic, cultural, political, and emotional–psychological factors that affect health status and health outcomes throughout the life course. Examples include early childhood experiences, education, literacy, housing, food access, financial resources, and experiences of discrimination and stigma. The health effects of some of these factors begin very early in life, even during gestation. Many stem from complex and large-scale social processes and consequently may not be easily addressed by patient-level interventions.[1]

Health-related social needs are discrete areas where a specific disadvantage or lack of resources harms a person's health. Examples include housing instability or being unhoused, lack of access to food, lack of access to transportation, and lack of employment or financial resources. Most of these areas can be addressed by patient-level interventions, though resources are often limited.[2]

Cultural humility is a conceptual framework developed by Melanie Tervalon and Jann Murray-Garcia, two physicians and medical educators, to prompt a shift to a more authentically patient-centered clinical approach to culture.[3] The preceding movement for "cultural competency" in health care did important work in making visible how cultural difference can affect care and outcomes. However, its positioning of "competence" on a wide array of distinct cultures as something desirable or even attainable often had the unintended consequence of prompting the creation of oversimplified or even stereotyped versions of specific cultures to be consumed in a brief training or booklet. Cultural humility, in contrast, asks the clinician to maintain an orientation toward the individual patient and a curiosity about what may be important to that person as far as their cultural influences.

Structural competency is a conceptual framework developed by physician–social scientists Helena Hansen and Jonathan Metzl to prompt a shift in focus by health systems and medical educators from cultural to structural factors as the most salient aspects of social life for health.[4] It is far more often things like housing costs, immigration status, income inequality, or racial discrimination, and much less frequently cultural misunderstanding, which have the largest effect on patients' health. Structural competency, then, is aimed at developing health workers' competencies in dealing with such factors—for example, through educational efforts to help with recognition of institutional racism, or provision of key resources such as housing navigation or medicolegal partnerships.

Racism is the stratification of power and advantage based on racial classification. Race is a socially constructed category often defined in terms of physical characteristics and/or putative ancestry. Race is typically incorporated into a social system in which there is a hierarchy of racial groups, with access to power and resources partially determined by racial identity. In Euro-American contexts, this has historically featured white populations at the top of the hierarchy, Black and/or Indigenous populations at the bottom, and other racial groupings (such as Asian, Middle Eastern, and Latine/Mestizo populations) in intermediate positions.

Stigma is a form of belief or stereotype associated with a particular condition or status and typically characterized by negative perception and ostracism. Examples of stigmatized conditions in US society include HIV, severe mental illness, and SUD.

Overview of Chapter

The remainder of this chapter is divided into five sections. The first section focuses on cultural humility, emphasizing its importance in clinical practice by encouraging clinicians to recognize the fluid, individualized nature of culture, avoid assumptions, and engage in respectful, reflective, and adaptive approaches to patient care. The second section addresses SDOH such as income, employment, housing, and transportation. The focus is on how SDOH shape people's experiences of substance use, including substance initiation, escalation, and SUD, access to treatment, and recovery, and how substance use reciprocally shapes SDOH. The third section describes common issues that arise during hospitalization, including stigma and discrimination against people with SUD, addressing these patients' complex needs, substance use in the hospital, and patients leaving before it is medically advised. The fourth section shares a structural competence approach to providing care for people with SUD during hospitalization, including trauma-informed care, relationship and trust building, and conflict resolution. The fifth section focuses on addressing patients' social needs at critical points of transition including perioperative planning, patient-directed discharges, and discharge planning.

Cultural Humility in Clinical Practice

The nature of culture has been the subject of debates by social scientists for more than a century. Originally construed as a static, external body of beliefs and practices, extensive work by anthropologists and sociologists has revealed culture to be fluid and often highly local.[5] While larger-scale patterns and groupings are identifiable, it has been increasingly understood that labels like "Mexican culture" or "Chinese culture" work primarily as either nationalist tools (usually within a certain national community) or as stereotypes (usually outside that community). For any given person of a particular heritage or ethnicity, it is common to find that local or regional practices, religious beliefs, class identity, racial identity, political affiliation, or other factors are at least as important as the supposed culture to which they belong. In other words, culture is anything but monolithic—how any one person experiences culture at any particular time is dependent on their life history, recent experiences, and current social circumstances.

As defined earlier in the chapter, cultural humility puts this understanding into practice. Rather than pursuing "detached mastery of a theoretically finite body of knowledge," cultural humility dictates that clinicians approach each patient with minimal preconceived notions.[3] The aim is especially to avoid assuming their own superiority and correctness in the face of difference, but also to avoid making assumptions about the nature of that difference. Two patients who ostensibly belong to the same culture may have entirely different orientations and priorities due to relatively more subtle distinctions in background or social situation. Clinicians must be alert to this possibility rather than anchoring on a single broad-stroke aspect of a patient's identity.

Because culture is not only attached to features like "being from Laos" or "being African American" (for example), but also to being from a particular subregion, or characteristics like belonging to a certain church or a labor union, or having a certain sexual or gender identity, it follows that *everyone* has a matrixed cultural makeup that must be accounted for in practicing cultural humility. Culture is not only relevant in the context of caring for immigrants or members of ethnic minorities, but for all patients. Moreover, clinicians themselves also bring their own culture to their work, which necessarily includes influences from the culture of biomedicine that has trained and shaped their professional practice. Cultural humility is not a set of lenses to be slipped on when dealing with a patient who is obviously "other," but rather a universal principle to be embedded in all clinical care by all members of the health care team for all patients.

There are several key techniques or habits of mind that can help clinicians to translate this principle from theory to practice.

- **Respect for difference:** This is the most essential element of cultural humility—it is necessary but not sufficient. Respect for difference means recognizing that a difference exists, acknowledging it, and not denigrating or blaming the difference for problems.
- **Curiosity:** Building upon respect, practitioners of cultural humility must want to understand something about their patient's culture. As outlined above, culture necessarily has highly individualized nuances. Cultural humility asks for an effort to learn about the influences, beliefs, context, and relationships that comprise a given person's cultural makeup.
- **Active listening:** Developed by psychologists Carl Rogers and Richard Farson, active listening is a tool that can be used for the type of respectful individual learning that constitutes the practice of cultural humility. There are three main elements in active listening:
  - *Listen for total meaning*—attempt to understand the overall message and context, not just the plain sense of the words.
  - *Respond to feelings*—reply to affirm or address emotions rather than content, so that the speaker feels understood and may continue to share.
  - *Note all cues*—attend to subtle verbal hints and nonverbal cues, which may reveal an otherwise undetectable aspect of what someone is trying to say.[6]
- **Self-reflection and self-critique:** This is the heart of cultural humility. In the course of practicing the above techniques, a clinician must devote some attention inward to understanding their own biases, their own cultural makeup, and to reflect on what effects their efforts are having. Then, having reflected, they can try to adapt and improve what they are doing. In other words, the aim of cultural humility is not just to serve as an antiethnocentric value system but to inculcate an actual practice of *personal* humility in the face of difference.[3]

An example is useful to illustrate how these techniques can be applied in the course of hospital-based care of patients with SUD.

Mr. M is a 49-year-old man who presented to the Emergency Department with abdominal pain, nausea, and vomiting, and was found to have acute pancreatitis. He has received very little medical care, especially since immigrating to the United States from Guatemala approximately 15 years ago. He is predominantly Spanish-speaking and works in construction. He reports drinking a 6-pack of beer every night and 12 or more beers on most weekend days.

Adapting the techniques of cultural humility in this example is primarily in service of detecting nuances in this case that may complicate or enrich a fairly common clinical scenario. If we presume that the clinician maintains respect for difference, the next step is curiosity. How does Mr. M's drinking relate to his immigration history? What about how it relates to his most frequent social milieux, whether family, roommates, or coworkers? Is he religious, nonreligious, lapsed, or something else? Does he have experiences of trauma? Was he a refugee from a particular threat, or did he come to the United States primarily for economic reasons? All of these questions and more certainly bear on Mr. M's cultural makeup and may well affect his alcohol use.

Perhaps the culturally humble clinician asks Mr. M whether he has any religious or faith tradition. He responds that he does not but looks uncomfortable and averts his eyes. A follow-up question reveals that he used to attend a Pentecostal church but does not anymore, and he again looks uncomfortable. Using the techniques of active listening, the clinician then responds to and names his discomfort, asking about it directly. Mr. M discloses that he used to go to church with his wife until a few years ago and only occasionally used alcohol at that time. However, he and his wife have now separated, and he lives with multiple male roommates and does not attend church anymore. This discussion may offer additional opportunities to respond to emotions, such as sadness or guilt, and ultimately their connection to his alcohol use.

Ultimately, taking a history in this way can reveal the many cultural influences that bear on a patient's substance use. Whatever the outcome, though, self-reflection and critique after the fact are just as essential to a continuing practice of cultural humility. Perhaps Mr. M's clinician realizes that they made an assumption, or that they noted negative feelings toward something about the patient as they worked with him. These realizations may prompt additional self-investigation or caution in speaking with patients and can be highly valuable in improving care not only for patients with SUD but for all patients.

Social Determinants of Health in Hospitalized Individuals With SUD

The various stages and aspects of substance use, including initiation, escalation into frequent or high-risk use, progression to SUD, access to treatment, cessation, return to use, and overdose are all tied to the structural, cultural, and socioeconomic contexts within which individuals live. In particular, race, gender, and class are some key structural determinants of individuals' life course and health outcomes. Many hospitalized people with SUDs have complex social histories that shape not only their substance use, but also their overall health, and substance use itself may in turn affect their social functioning. This section describes how health-related social needs and risks shape the health of people with SUDs, and how substance use may impact those social needs and risks concerning their overall health.

Identifying patients with the needs discussed below is a problem unto itself. A wide variety of screening tools are available for use by clinicians and researchers. Many of these tools have been catalogued by the Social Interventions Research and Evaluation Network at University of California San Francisco and are available for comparison on their website.[7] In clinical practice, it is unlikely that a busy hospital-based clinician will sit down with a patient to complete an entire screening tool, but it is useful for clinicians to know the types of questions they might ask to elicit information about a specific need (Table 16.1).

Housing

Substance use often co-occurs with unhoused or housing-unstable status.[8] The interplay between these factors is likely heterogeneous, and in some cases their co-occurrence is more likely due to a third factor driving both such as severe mental illness, trauma, poor coping abilities, or disordered personality traits. However, there is a consensus that in many cases substance use and becoming unhoused are direct mutual risk factors.[9,10] Unhoused status is also a risk factor for overdose, though paradoxically, this risk, and especially risk of fatal overdose, is thought by many clinicians to increase immediately following being housed, as people are more likely to use substances alone and out of sight.[11] Data across multiple studies suggest that alcohol use disorder (AUD) may have a different interaction with housing more than other substances. For example, recovery in cocaine use disorder was observed to be associated with attainment of housing while AUD recovery had no effect compared to persistent use—possibly because of the relatively modest cost of alcohol compared to cocaine.[12] Conversely, a randomized trial of a Housing First intervention found significant decreases in alcohol intake, but no effect on other types of substance use. The mechanism of this difference is not known, and the authors do not propose any hypotheses, though alcohol's easy availability, legality, and relatively low cost might suggest it as the optimal self-coping strategy of necessity that could be tapered down in a more tolerable housing situation.[13]

TABLE 16.1

Examples of Social Need Screening Questions

Social determinant of health need	Example screening question	Source
Housing	Do you think you are at risk of becoming homeless?	THRIVE[14]
Financial strain	Do you have trouble paying your heating or electricity bill?	THRIVE[14]
Employment	What is your current work situation?	Protocol for Responding to & Assessing Patients' Assets, Risks & Experiences (PRAPARE)[15]
Social connectedness	Overall, how often do you feel lonely or socially isolated?	Accountable Health Communities Screening Tool (AHC)[16]
Food security	Within the past 12 mo, were you worried whether your food would run out before you got money to buy more?	THRIVE[14]
Education	What is the highest level of school that you have finished?	THRIVE[14]
Literacy	How often do you need to have someone help you read instructions, pamphlets, or other written materials from your doctor or pharmacy?	Single Item Literacy Screener[17]
Incarceration	In the past year, have you spent more than 2 nights in a row in a jail, prison, detention center, or juvenile correctional facility?	PRAPARE[15]
Transportation	Has lack of transportation kept you from medical appointments, meetings, work, or from getting things needed for daily living?	PRAPARE[15]
Health care access	Do you have trouble paying for medical care (eg, co-pays, medical services, medical equipment)?	THRIVE[14]
Immigration	Are you an immigrant or refugee?	PRAPARE[15]

Finances, Income, and Class

Finances, income, and class significantly influence substance use behaviors and recovery outcomes. Lower-income and working-class individuals often experience systemic biases in the diagnosis and treatment of SUDs, with overdiagnosis in those living in poverty and underdiagnosis in wealthier individuals. Socioeconomic status also impacts access to treatment, as financial instability makes sustained recovery programs more difficult to engage with. Entitlement programs can offer some protection; for instance, larger state-level earned income tax credits have been linked to lower rates of binge alcohol use, particularly among women with only a high school education.[18] In addition, substance use can lead to financial consequences, such as job loss or divorce, which disproportionately harm those without strong financial support networks. Being mindful of and addressing such financial disparities is crucial for improving substance use prevention and recovery outcomes.

Employment

People's working conditions significantly impact their mental health and their ability to cope with stress without turning to substance use. Those in low-wage jobs are more likely to use substances as a coping mechanism, and job loss often leads to escalating substance use. For example, deindustrialization and the rise of automation have been linked to a sharp increase in opioid use and overdose deaths in Appalachian states.[19] Similarly, retirement, an often-overlooked life change in the context of substance use, has been associated with increased alcohol consumption.[20] Conversely, substance use itself can lead to job loss due to missed work or impairment while on the job. The Centers for Disease Control recommends that employers establish Workplace Supported Recovery Programs to reduce stigma and assist workers with SUDs because two-thirds of individuals with a SUD are employed.[21] Relatedly, employment opportunities contribute to the well-being of people with SUD.

One randomized controlled trial of job skill training and workplace vouchers for unemployed adults in Baltimore methadone treatment programs (ie, opioid treatment programs, or OTPs) who also use cocaine led to a significant decrease in cocaine use.[22] Other studies have linked baseline employment and employment before abstinence respectively to a shorter time to cessation of injection and longer abstinence durations.[23] Furthermore, treatment modalities can influence employment opportunities. Access to treatment enables individuals to stabilize their lives, allowing them to maintain employment or pursue new job opportunities. For example, buprenorphine treatment for OUD has been associated with improved employment outcomes, with patients more likely to secure new jobs after starting treatment.[24] However, certain treatment methods, such as methadone treatment for opioid use disorder (OUD), may create barriers to maintaining employment due to near-daily medication supervision requirements at OTPs. Overall, addressing employment-related barriers in SUD treatment is crucial for supporting long-term recovery and workforce participation.

Social Connectedness

Social connectedness plays a critical role in substance use initiation, recovery, relapse, overdose, and mortality. Strong social ties—whether through family, friends, or supportive communities like places of worship—are protective against substance use by providing emotional support, reducing isolation, and offering alternative coping mechanisms. Conversely, a lack of social connectedness, including social isolation or rejection, is linked to higher risks of substance initiation and use, as individuals may turn to substance use to cope with loneliness or stress.[25,26] Social connectedness may also influence individuals' motivation to limit their substance use and seek treatment. A study found that having a healthy peer network with minimal substance use among peers helped adolescents living in socioeconomically disadvantaged neighborhoods limit their substance use. Another study found that an increase in social support over time was strongly associated with a decline in problems related to substance use.[24–26] In terms of seeking treatment for SUD, one study found that among people with OUD, a greater number of direct support network connections were associated with a higher likelihood of taking medications for OUD.[27] In recovery, maintaining social connections with supportive peers can significantly improve outcomes, helping individuals navigate challenges and reinforcing positive behaviors.[28] However, in the absence of such networks, individuals are at greater risk of returning to substance use, as they may struggle to manage stressors without healthy social support. Social connectedness is also crucial among people with SUD because shared experiences can foster mutual support, reduce stigma, and help individuals access resources. Unfortunately, for many, lack of connectedness can contribute to fatal outcomes, with isolation exacerbating vulnerability to overdose and increasing mortality rates. Building and maintaining social networks, especially for those in recovery or actively using substances, is essential to improving overall health and reducing the harms associated with substance use.

Food Security

Food insecurity is highly prevalent among people living in poverty, a group that is at increased risk of substance use initiation, has a high prevalence of substance use, and has a high substance-related mortality rate. One study of US high school students found that binge alcohol use, cannabis use, and lifetime use of substances was higher among students experiencing food insecurity.[29] In a national longitudinal cohort study of women with or at risk of HIV, food insecurity was associated with higher odds of cannabis, stimulant, and opioid use.[30] People experiencing food insecurity may rely on substances as a coping mechanism, or because of their appetite/hunger suppressing effects (eg, stimulants, tobacco).

Education

Education has a great impact on people's health. Regardless of substance use, for instance, literacy and numeracy both affect patients' ability to read and follow written medical instructions. More specifically, education plays a significant role in the experience of people with SUD across the lifespan. First, school environments contribute to adolescents' substance use initiation. Structural factors, social norms, and interpersonal experiences alike are contributors. For instance, racially segregated schools, particularly those with tracking systems (separating students based on their perceived academic ability, and assigning each group to classes with different levels of curriculum, instruction, and rigor), create environments where marginalized adolescents face higher stress, lower academic expectations, and increased exposure to substance-using peers.[31] These factors contribute to a higher likelihood of substance use initiation, since students in these settings may use substances as a coping mechanism or due to peer influence. For minority students, experiences of discrimination in schools are another factor associated with substance use.[32,33] Beyond adolescence, educational achievement significantly impacts substance use initiation, recovery, and relapse. Lower educational attainment is associated with a higher likelihood of substance use and its downstream consequences, as adults with less education may face increased stress and are more likely to live in poverty. Studies show that people with lower educational attainment are significantly more likely to experience overdose across substances, and substance-related mortality is much higher among people without any college education.[34] Education helps individuals earn higher wages and shape their health literacy, which are both protective against substance use initiation as well as overdose and mortality.

Health Literacy

Health literacy is defined as the ability to obtain, process, and understand basic health information. Low health literacy is highly prevalent among people with SUD compared to the general population. Individuals with low health literacy are more likely to misperceive the risks associated with substance use and be more easily influenced by peer pressure due to lower ability to evaluate health-related information critically.[27,34] People with low health literacy have worse outcomes, due to poorer engagement and retention in treatment, and more difficulty following instructions, as well as navigating the health care system and social services, which may be critical in assisting them with accessing treatment and resources that may facilitate successful and consistent treatment, such as transportation and housing.[35]

Incarceration

Individuals with prior incarceration have a much higher risk of experiencing poor health outcomes, including overdoses, due to disrupted access to health care. Because of the criminalization of substance use, people with SUD are at increased risk of being incarcerated. One study found that among individuals undergoing OUD treatment with methadone, those who had early-age arrests were less likely to decrease opioid use. Individuals with severe SUD also had the earliest average age of first arrest and the longest duration of incarceration.[36] Once released from carceral settings, individuals' risk of overdose death is extremely high, especially in the first 2 weeks following release, but this risk remains elevated throughout the first year after release.[37]

Transportation

Lack of reliable transportation is a major barrier to accessing health care services, leading to missed appointments and interruptions in treatment. For people with OUD receiving methadone treatment, required near-daily visits to their OTP requires reliable transportation. Several studies highlight the impact of long travel times on accessing OTPs, particularly in rural areas. Some patients travel 50 to 200 miles or cross state borders for methadone treatment, with average driving times around 20 minutes but longer in rural counties.[38] Distance can significantly affect treatment adherence—patients traveling shorter distances are more likely to be retained in treatment, while those living over 10 miles away are more likely to miss methadone treatment doses and fall out of treatment.[39] Racial disparities in travel times exist, influenced by access to public transit. Even post–COVID-19, transportation barriers persist, with low-income individuals facing lengthy commutes. Ultimately, inadequate transportation options can deter individuals from starting or continuing treatment.[40]

Access to Health Care

Implementation of "medication first" approaches, meaning rapid, sustained low-barrier access to medications for SUD have been shown to increase retention in SUD treatment, notably among people with OUD.[41,42] Geographic disparities in access to medication treatments for OUD (MOUD), like buprenorphine and methadone, remain an issue. For instance, rural areas have low access to MOUD.[43] In addition, racial segregation shapes access to both in metropolitan and adjacent settings such that areas with a greater share of White residents have greater access to buprenorphine, while access to methadone through OTPs is concentrated in urban settings with a greater proportion of Black residents.[44,45]

Health Insurance

Among individuals with SUD but are not in SUD treatment, those with health insurance are more likely to have a visit for SUD treatment in the years that follow. Individuals with high deductibles are less likely to seek primary care and psychiatric care.[46] Some health insurance plans, to control costs, create barriers to treatment in various ways including prior authorization requirements and required stepped therapy. The passage of the Affordable Care and mental health and addiction parity laws sought to increase access to SUD treatment.[47] However, there remains wide variation in states' Medicaid and commercial insurance coverage of different types of SUD treatment. Few states provide all the levels of care recommended by the American Society of Addiction Medicine (ASAM). One study found that Medicaid insurance plans' prior authorization requirements for buprenorphine sometimes included requirements inconsistent with clinical practice guidelines, such as mandated dose maximums or tapers of medication after a specified period, required participation in group therapy, frequent, random urine drug screenings, and pill counts.[48] Patients who use nonprescribed buprenorphine to treat their OUD or withdrawal symptoms report a burdensome treatment apparatus (including such aforementioned requirements) as a reason not to seek SUD treatment.[49,50]

Immigration Concerns, Language Barriers

Migrant patients face significant barriers to SUD treatment due to language and legal challenges. For example, a lack of language-concordant care limits access for monolingual non-English speakers, with funding priorities often neglecting linguistic needs. Beyond language, culturally appropriate care—including familiar cultural references and regional dialects—enhances SUD engagement. Legal barriers further restrict access, as individuals who have undocumented immigration status fear deportation and often avoid public programs, instead seeking faith-based or community recovery programs that do not require social security numbers.[51,52] Some SUD treatment programs exclude undocumented individuals. In addition, many community recovery programs serving undocumented individuals are concerned about potential shutdowns, though authorities often tolerate them due to their crucial role in serving marginalized communities. Given these challenges, community recovery programs and faith-based program directors often choose to avoid bureaucratic burdens to maintain autonomy.[52]

Addressing the complex social needs that shape SUD is essential to providing effective care for hospitalized patients with SUDs. Each factor—housing instability, financial insecurity, unemployment, social isolation, food insecurity, education gaps, low health literacy, incarceration history, transportation barriers, insurance coverage gaps, and immigration concerns—can profoundly affect patients' engagement with care, adherence to treatment, and recovery trajectories. Hospitalization offers a unique opportunity to assess and begin addressing these barriers. Clinicians can screen for social needs and refer patients to concrete resources such as United Way's 211 network, FindHelp.org, and FindTreatment.gov. Specific interventions may include linkage to harm-reduction services such as Next Distro and Safe Spot overdose prevention, food assistance programs, housing support referrals, virtual mutual support groups, and culturally tailored recovery services like Latino Recovery Advocacy. Recognizing and addressing these needs during hospitalization and at discharge planning is critical to improving patient outcomes, reducing avoidable readmissions, and supporting long-term recovery.

The next section explores specific SDOH that most directly shape substance use and recovery for hospitalized patients.

Common Social Issues That Arise During Hospitalization

Stigma and Discrimination

People with SUD face pervasive stigma that affects every aspect of their lives, from health care access to employment opportunities and social relationships. This stigma is rooted in deeply entrenched moral narratives that portray substance use as a personal failing rather than a complex health issue influenced by structural and biologic factors. As a result, people with SUD are often blamed for their condition, subjected to discrimination, and denied compassionate, evidence-based care. In the legal system, substance use is disproportionately criminalized in ways that target marginalized communities, reinforcing cycles of poverty, incarceration, and systemic neglect. Socially, people with SUD may be ostracized by family and friends, limiting their support networks, and making it harder to access medical and SUD treatment or harm-reduction services. Stigma not only exacerbates harm but also deters individuals from seeking care, perpetuating poor health outcomes, and increasing the risk of overdose and other preventable complications. In health care settings, stigma manifests as clinicians dismissing their pain, attributing all health concerns to substance use, or refusing to prescribe necessary medications. To address this, society must shift away from punitive and judgmental frameworks toward approaches that recognize substance use as a public health issue, emphasizing dignity, harm reduction, and access to comprehensive support services.

Tolerance of Complex Needs

Studies have consistently shown that physicians, nurses, and other health care workers often harbor significant stigma toward people with SUD, which directly influences hospital policies and bedside care. Surveys of medical professionals reveal that many associate using substances with personal irresponsibility, dishonesty, and criminality rather than viewing SUD as a medical condition. This bias leads to reluctance to prescribe opioids for acute pain, hesitancy to offer evidence-based treatments like buprenorphine to treat opioid withdrawal, and punitive hospital policies that prioritize control over compassionate care. Many hospitals have restrictive policies that enforce rigid abstinence-based approaches, criminalize in-hospital use of substances, or discharge patients prematurely if they are suspected of ongoing substance use—all of which disproportionately harm people with SUD, particularly those with complex medical and psychosocial needs. These policies are not purely driven by clinical concerns but are shaped by clinician discomfort, misconceptions about SUDs, and the moralization of substance use in medical settings. As a result, people with SUD often encounter an unwelcoming and punitive environment when hospitalized, making it harder for them to receive the care they need.

At the same time, people with SUD may struggle to fully participate in their own care, a response that is often interpreted as defiance or irresponsibility rather than a reflection of past trauma and negative health care encounters. Patients with histories of incarceration, homelessness, or forced substance withdrawal in medical settings may exhibit distrust toward clinicians, leading them to refuse blood draws, leave the hospital prematurely, or struggle to adhere to restrictive hospital policies (such as being confined to a room). Instead of recognizing these behaviors as understandable reactions to systemic harm, health care workers often reinforce the cycle of stigma by labeling these patients as "noncompliant" or "difficult," which can influence how future clinicians approach their care. The intersection of complex medical and psychosocial needs—such as pain management, withdrawal symptoms, unstable housing, and untreated psychiatric conditions—demands a deeper understanding about SUD as a medical disease and a higher level of flexibility, patience, and harm-reduction–based care than many hospitals are structured to provide. Until hospitals shift toward models that proactively treat SUD, acknowledge the impact of trauma, prioritize patient autonomy, and actively combat clinician bias, people with SUD will continue to receive substandard care, further reinforcing their alienation from the very systems that are meant to support them.

Substance Use in the Hospital

In-hospital substance use is an issue that often causes conflict between patients and the medical team, and such conflicts can disrupt medical care. Studies show that many patients hospitalized for causes related to their SUD report using illicit substances during their hospital stay. Patients hospitalized with SUD often experience overwhelming urges to use substances, even within the hospital setting. Some patients actively seek substance use to manage withdrawal and boredom, while others find the hospital environment emotionally distressing, which heightens their urges to use substances.

A common experience of patients who use illicit substances during hospitalization is inadequate pain management. Many feel their reports of pain are not believed, and their opioid tolerance is ignored, resulting in accusations of substance-seeking behavior. Some patients describe going outside the hospital to purchase substances to self-medicate their pain, while others rely on friends to bring substances to them. Some patients may abstain from substance use while hospitalized due to barriers such as being too ill to use, lacking money to buy substances, or being physically restricted from leaving their rooms.

To avoid reprimands or potential discharge, many patients describe concealing their substance use. Some use substances in bathrooms, at night when fewer staff are present, or in ways that do not leave visible evidence. Others, particularly those using stimulants, find it more difficult to hide due to the noticeable effects of the drug. Some patients conceal their substance use out of respect for others in the hospital rather than fear of repercussions.

Health care clinicians vary in their awareness of in-hospital substance use. While some claim never to have witnessed it, others acknowledge it occurs but is often well hidden. Some clinicians note that certain substances, such as cannabis, are easier to conceal, while others, like stimulants, are more apparent due to their behavioral effects.

Hospitals often lack formal policies on in-hospital substance use, leaving responses to the discretion of individual health care clinicians. This results in a wide spectrum of approaches, from enforcing abstinence through threats of discharge and increased monitoring to more harm-reduction–oriented strategies to prevent early departures.

Many patients are unaware of any hospital policies until they are found using substances. Responses to detected substance use varied widely, with some clinicians calling security, confiscating substances, or reducing pain medications. In contrast, others allow patients to leave the floor for substance use, or they turn a blind eye to avoid escalating conflicts.

In contrast, a small number of clinicians and hospitals have policies and procedures that focus on harm reduction, advocating for managing withdrawal symptoms and ensuring patients remain hospitalized for necessary medical treatment. Some argue that hospitals should apply the same standards to opioid use as they do for tobacco, offering alternatives like methadone or buprenorphine rather than forcing abstinence, and implementing nonpunitive substance use disclosure policies. In addition to navigating substance use during hospitalization, clinicians must also prepare for situations where patients may choose to leave before medical discharge is advised.

Patient-Directed Discharges

Patient-directed discharges also known as "before medically advised" or "against medical advice" occur when patients leave the hospital before their treating medical or surgical team recommends discharge. This phenomenon accounts for 1% to 2% of all hospital discharges. The reasons patients choose to discharge prematurely are varied and can include dissatisfaction with care, personal obligations, feeling better, or frustration with hospital policies. Notably, among people with SUD, factors such as unmanaged withdrawal symptoms, mistrust of the health care team due to prior negative experiences, and the desire to use substances can significantly contribute to the decision to prematurely discharge.

Leaving the hospital prematurely is associated with several risks. Studies have shown that prematurely discharged patients have higher rates of hospital readmission and increased mortality compared to those who follow medical advice. For people with SUD, these risks are compounded by the potential for untreated infections, complications from substance use, and the lack of continuity in SUD treatment. In response to premature discharges, health care clinicians often request that patients sign a so-called "AMA" (Against Medical Advice) form. The practice of requiring patients to sign this form when they choose to leave the hospital prematurely can sometimes be wielded coercively by clinicians. This approach may convey to patients that their decision is considered defiant or irresponsible, reinforcing feelings of stigma and shame. Such forms are intended to document that the patient has been informed of the potential risks associated with leaving the hospital before it is medically advised. However, their implementation can sometimes be confusing and coercive, potentially undermining the patient's autonomy and trust in the health care system. It is essential to note that while obtaining a patient's signature on this form serves as documentation of the informed consent process, it does not absolve health care clinicians or institutions from legal responsibility. The critical aspect is ensuring that the patient comprehensively understands the potential risks of leaving and that their decision is voluntary and informed. Coercing a patient into signing such a form undermines the ethical standards of patient care. It may have limited legal significance if the patient's consent was not genuinely informed and voluntary.

Practicing With Structural Competence

Building on the challenges outlined in prior sections, this section shifts toward practical frameworks and techniques clinicians can use to improve hospital-based care for people with SUD. Most hospitalized people with SUD, regardless of their medical, social, and psychological backgrounds, are under significant stress merely by virtue of their illness and dislocation from daily life. For people with SUD, this stress can be compounded by experiences of substance withdrawal, stigma, social isolation, and shame. Caring for people under these circumstances can be difficult at best and can lead to moral injury for clinicians and medical trauma for patients if not done well. Such outcomes are not always avoidable at the level of a patient and clinician, as they are determined in part by factors beyond the control of any individual. However, while there is no panacea, certain relational skills and techniques can be usefully applied to caring for patients in these difficult circumstances to improve the potential for positive outcomes. The following are best practices to employ in the care of complex patients with SUD and likely other SDOH that contribute to their care needs.

Trauma-Informed Care

Trauma occurs when a person is exposed to an event or circumstances that they experience as severely harmful or potentially life threatening and that, for developmental, environmental, or psychological reasons, they cannot integrate in order to move on from the experience.[53] As a result, they remain in a stress-response state linked to that unresolved trauma, which manifests as a constellation of symptoms such as hypervigilance, intrusive re-experiencing, negative emotions, and avoidance.[54] Substance use and trauma have a very high co-occurrence rate, with one study finding that 92.9% of people with SUD had had at least two traumatic experiences. Many studies estimate that at least 20% to 30% of people with SUD also have active co-occurring PTSD.[55–57] There are mechanisms that work in both directions—that is, each condition is a risk factor for the other. The hyperaroused stress response of trauma leads people to cope with substances, while both the pursuit of substances and the actual effects of intoxication put people with SUD at risk for traumatic experiences such as physical or sexual violence.

Hospitalized people with SUD are therefore quite likely to have experienced trauma. Due to the stressful context of an acute hospitalization—not to mention those whose primary trauma may have been medical in nature—many patients with SUD in the hospital may feel the impulse toward avoidance, hypervigilance, and irritability. It is immensely difficult to build a therapeutic alliance under such conditions. However, the paradigm of trauma-informed care

TABLE 16.2

Six Core Principles of Trauma-Informed Care[58]

Core principles	Practice examples
Safety	Do not touch patients without asking permission first
	Talk through each exam maneuver prior to doing it
	Help patients to keep track of their belongings and who is responsible for storing them
Trustworthiness and transparency	Follow through on commitments—do not say "I'll swing back in the afternoon" if you are unlikely to do it
	Do not give overly optimistic estimates for timing of studies, procedures, or discharge
	Be honest about uncertainty
Peer support	Health systems should engage recovery coaches or other staff with lived experience
	Offer virtual mutual support (eg, Alcoholics Anonymous, Narcotics Anonymous, Smart Recovery, etc) opportunities
Collaboration and mutuality	Sit down when speaking to the patient
	Explicitly conduct shared decision making for all major decisions
Empowerment, voice, and choice	Offer patients options—for example, if weaning opioids, the patient can select between decreasing dose or decreasing frequency
	Ask patients for input on their goals for a hospitalization
Cultural, historical, and gender issues	Acknowledge stigma faced by people with SUD
	Acknowledge racial or cultural biases that may impact patients

offers some best practices in caring for traumatized patients. The six core principles of trauma-informed care according to the Substance Abuse and Mental Health Services Administration are presented below, along with practical tips for implementation in the hospital context (Table 16.2).[58]

Relationship and Trust Building

Even for patients without trauma histories, trust is crucial to building a therapeutic alliance. Much of the medical literature on trust focuses on the outpatient setting, predominantly in primary care and to a lesser extent in specialty care such as oncology.[59,60] Extant literature on hospital-based trust is largely focused on the relationship between the patient and the bedside nurse.[61] One study that explored general population attitudes toward hospitals at the institutional level identified three key areas that mattered for patients in developing trust: competence, caring, and communication.[62] The same study also noted that patients' experiences of hospital billing practices or perceptions of financial interests tended to erode trust.

In the specific context of caring for hospitalized patients with SUDs, trust is complicated by trauma, stigma, and the specialized but not always widely available nature of addiction medicine expertise. A mixed-methods study of trust in hospital physicians by patients with SUD found four themes that promoted trust, which appear like a hybrid of the general population's hospital trust themes with the principles of trauma-informed care below.[63] This study also found that consultation of an addiction consult service tended to raise patients' trust in their hospital physicians overall.

- **Humanizing care**—for example, by tailoring a plan to individual preferences or simply being physically and emotionally present with a patient
- **Demonstrating addiction expertise**—such as by knowing slang terms or demonstrating an element of successful management
- **Reliability**—as above in the "Trustworthiness and Transparency" element of trauma informed care
- **Granting agency**—as above in the "Empowerment, Voice, and Choice" element of trauma informed care

Conflict Resolution

Many of the common sources of conflict between clinicians and hospitalized patients with SUD are covered elsewhere in this chapter and Chapter 15. This section lists specific practical techniques to apply in a variety of situations that can create conflict between the patient and the care team.

- **Prevent, prevent, prevent**—The best way to resolve a conflict is to keep it from happening in the first place. Application of the core principles of trauma-informed care as well as the additional trust-building principles outlined above may help with preventing conflict. For an individual patient with a history of conflicts around a certain issue, this should be anticipated and planned for in subsequent hospitalizations. In practice, this could entail treating substance withdrawal symptoms proactively starting in the ED.

- **Listen actively**—As discussed in an earlier section, active listening can be a very helpful technique in caring for patients, and all the more so in the context of a conflict. Many times, patients simply want to be heard and understood, and then ultimately align with their clinical team. To review, in active listening, the goals are to listen for the full meaning, respond to feelings, and note all cues. For example, rather than responding to a specific allegation, one could reply to an irate patient by saying, *"Help me understand—what was the thing that made you the angriest?"* Mirroring the patient's language also demonstrates that you are listening carefully, so one might instead say *"What was the thing that pissed you off the most?"* if that is the language the patient is using. Motivational interviewing frameworks are also effective tools to use for active listening.
- **Turn down the temperature**—During a conflict, people tend to raise their voices, use imposing or threatening body language, and perhaps even prepare for a literal fight-or-flight situation. Acting counter to these tendencies can, by itself, help to move a conflict toward resolution. Speaking relatively softly forces the other person to lower their own voice slightly to hear. Turning one's body sideways, leaning against a wall, or even sitting down are all ways to appear less threatening. And finally, a temporary exit after calmly giving a timeframe for one's return can be an effective way to give a patient the space they need to cool off. If the hospital has nonclinical areas that patients can access, spending time in this area with the patient or allowing them to go there (if it is safe) may also help. Eliciting the help of nonmedical staff such as social workers can also help in these situations. Those individuals may use distraction, alternative coping mechanisms, relaxation techniques, and support that the medical team is not able to provide.
- **Roll with the punches**—Patients in conflict with their health care teams often make accusations that are not strictly relevant to the conflict at hand. Common topics include financial interest, negligent or incompetent care, and bias or discrimination. It is tempting to become angry, and either to dispute the statement or end the conversation. However, in most cases, the patient is testing limits or attempting to provoke rather than laying a serious charge. The most effective response is to smile, treat it like a joke (especially if—as in many cases—the patient has made some effort to be funny), and redirect the conversation to a more productive topic. For example, if a patient makes an accusation that something is being done in their care so that the hospital can bill for and profit from it, a clinician could respond, "*You would think that if they were doing that kind of thing, they could afford to serve better food in the cafeteria!*"
- **Return to common ground**—In most cases, the best way to frame a conflict is as a shared problem that can be solved by cooperation between the patient and their clinicians. Patients will not always accept it, but this framing can be promoted by using "we" language, asking the patient for substantive input in an open-ended way, and summarizing shared action items. For instance, in the situation of a patient upset in the context of poorly controlled pain, one could say, "*It seems like the most important thing we are working on here is getting your pain to a manageable level. Is there anything that has worked well in the past that we could try?*" and then summarize any action items that result. It often helps to use this technique as a counterpoint, bringing it back in regularly to balance other components of the conflict.
- **"Focus on interests, not positions"**—This phrase is drawn from the widely read book on negotiations, *Getting to Yes*.[64] The underlying idea is that negotiations break down when the parties become fixated on certain positions—for example, that there is a gap between the amounts a buyer and seller are willing to pay and accept respectively. What the authors of *Getting to Yes* argue is that usually a negotiation has been boiled down to positions for simplicity's sake, but that the actual interests of the parties are not limited to the positions. For example, a conflict over a certain opioid dose is not actually over the dose—for the patient, it is about achieving adequate pain control, and for the clinician it is about maintaining safety and progress toward discharge. These interests might all be served by adding one or more additional multimodal pain agents and sidestepping the issue of the opioid dosage.
- **Set boundaries**—Not every conflict can be managed away through the techniques described above. Sometimes there is an irreconcilable difference. Sometimes a patient is being truly inappropriate or unsafe. And sometimes clinicians simply need to cut their losses and protect themselves from further moral injury. In these cases, the right conflict management strategy is to calmly, firmly, and clearly set a boundary and outline the consequences or next steps if the boundary is crossed. Then if the boundary is in fact crossed, the consequences should be calmly, firmly, and clearly implemented as previously stated. For instance, if a patient began yelling at the team during rounds, one could say "*Mr. X, it is okay to be angry, but it is*

not acceptable to shout at us. If you can't lower your voice, we are going to have to leave and come back when you have calmed down." If the patient continues yelling, or stops temporarily and then resumes yelling, then the clinician would say, *"Alright Mr. X, we are going to leave now. I will be back in a few hours once you have had a chance to calm down."*

As described in Chapter 15, Patient Safety Care Plans utilize many of these components in their development, creation, and maintenance.

Addressing Social Needs and Health Risks at Critical Transitions

Building on the challenges outlined in prior sections, this section shifts toward practical frameworks and techniques clinicians can use to improve hospital-based care for individuals with SUDs. Critical transition points in hospitalization—such as the perioperative period, patient-directed discharges, and hospital discharge planning—represent key moments when people with SUD face heightened vulnerability. These transitions often determine whether people with SUD receive continued care, experience complications, or disengage from the health care system entirely. Given the increased risks of untreated pain, withdrawal, overdose, and postdischarge morbidity in this population, an approach based on harm-reduction principles is necessary to ensure that social needs and health risks are adequately addressed. This section outlines strategies for improving care for people with SUD at these crucial junctures.

Perioperative Planning

After addressing the hospital stay itself, it is equally important to focus on high-risk transition points such as surgery and hospital discharge. The perioperative period presents unique challenges for people with SUD, particularly those with OUD or chronic pain. Traditional perioperative care often focuses on opioid minimization without adequately considering the unique pharmacologic and psychosocial needs of patients who have opioid tolerance, dependence, or are receiving MOUD.

One major challenge in perioperative care is the undertreatment of pain due to stigma and clinician concerns about opioid misuse. People with OUD—especially those on buprenorphine or methadone—frequently require modified pain management strategies to account for their opioid tolerance. Standard opioid-sparing protocols may be insufficient, leading to inadequate pain control, distress, and even premature discharge. Best practices include continuing MOUD perioperatively (rather than abruptly stopping buprenorphine or methadone), utilizing multimodal analgesia, and dosing opioids appropriately for opioid-tolerant patients rather than applying uniform, one-size-fits-all prescribing restrictions. This is addressed further in Chapter 17.

In addition, perioperative care should incorporate harm-reduction principles, such as early engagement with peer recovery coaches or social workers, screening for withdrawal risk, and ensuring naloxone is available for postdischarge use. For patients with SUD, early consultation with addiction medicine specialists can facilitate safer perioperative planning, thereby reducing complications and improving surgical outcomes. By prioritizing these tailored strategies, clinicians can prevent inadequate pain control, withdrawal, and unnecessary escalation to opioid-related complications, improving both the patient experience and clinical outcomes.

Patient-Directed Discharges

Responding to patients' intention to leave before it is medically advised is recommended by their clinical team requires planning. When a patient expresses a desire to leave before it is medically advised, the priority should not be to simply document their decision but to understand the reasons behind it and address modifiable barriers to continued care. Too often, the premature discharge process is treated as a rigid, bureaucratic event—clinicians may feel frustrated, assume the patient is making an irrational choice, and push them to sign an "AMA form" that serves more as a deterrent than a tool for shared decision making. Instead of approaching patient-directed discharges as a failure of patient compliance, clinicians should shift toward harm-reduction–based, patient-centered strategies that keep the door open for ongoing care.

The first step is engaging the patient in an open, nonjudgmental conversation about their reasons for wanting to leave. For people with SUD, common drivers of patient-directed discharges include unmanaged withdrawal, inadequate pain relief, restrictive hospital policies, and past negative health care experiences. A simple but essential approach is to ask, "*What would need to happen for you to feel comfortable staying?*" This can reveal barriers that are solvable, such as modifying pain regimens, allowing movement outside the hospital room, adjusting visitor policies, or ensuring that withdrawal symptoms are managed appropriately. Even if a patient still decides to leave, this conversation builds trust and increases the likelihood they will return for care when needed.

If a patient remains intent on leaving, providers should avoid using "AMA" forms as a punitive

TABLE 16.3

Components of a "Soft Exit" Approach to Patient-Directed Discharges

Components	
Ensure understanding of their medical condition	Ensure they leave with a clear understanding of their condition and when to return for care.
Establish outpatient resources	Offer harm-reduction resources, including naloxone, wound care kits, or safe-use supplies, if appropriate.
	Offer peer support and connection to ongoing treatment outside of the hospital.
	Prescribe bridge medications for withdrawal, pain, or infection treatment to minimize immediate risk postdischarge.
Establish contact information	With patient's permission, obtain a phone number to call them in the next few days to check on them and offer additional referrals or address care needs.
Offer alternative medical care resources	Give a warm handoff to community partners such as street medicine teams, primary care, or case management who may check on the patient in the community.
Outline return to hospital plan	Leave the "hospital door open" and ensure they know that they can return when they are ready without judgment.
	Facilitate an easy return by avoiding stigmatizing labels like "frequent flyer" in medical records.

measure or to shame patients into staying. Instead, the focus should be on providing a "soft exit" approach (Table 16.3).

The goal is not to force compliance but to create an environment where patients feel respected and supported—even when they choose to leave. A harm-reduction approach to patient-directed discharges recognizes that engagement in care is a process, not a one-time event. Patients are far more likely to return for treatment if their autonomy and dignity are preserved in these critical moments.

Discharge Planning

For hospitalized people with SUD, discharge planning is a critical transition point that determines health outcomes posthospitalization. Without a structured plan that accounts for both medical and SDOH, patients often fall through the cracks, leading to avoidable complications, readmissions, and overdose risk. Effective discharge planning for people with SUD requires a harm-reduction framework, addressing SDOH, prioritizing continuity of care, safe medication access, and linkage to community-based services.

A fundamental challenge in discharge planning is the high burden of housing instability, incarceration history, and lack of primary care access among people with SUD. Many patients are discharged to the street or unstable environments, where wound care, medication adherence, and follow-up appointments become nearly impossible to maintain. Hospitals should actively coordinate with medical respite programs, harm-reduction organizations, and housing services to offer patients leaving the hospital a safe place to recover, if possible. These programs may not always be available but creating a list of community resources that can help meet patients' needs and informing them of these resources prior to discharge can be helpful. Failing to do so often leads to recurrent hospitalizations for preventable complications, such as infected injection sites, recurrent endocarditis, or acute withdrawal episodes.

Medication continuity is another crucial component of discharge planning. Many people with SUD, particularly those with OUD, chronic pain, or stimulant use disorders, may face barriers in accessing prescriptions posthospitalization. Patients on MOUD should have continued access without delay, ideally with warm handoffs to community providers before discharge. In addition, patients with pain syndromes benefit from connection to ongoing services to address their pain.

Finally, harm-reduction strategies should be embedded into discharge planning to prevent overdose and other complications. Every hospitalized patient with OUD should receive naloxone on discharge, and all people with SUD should receive education on safer substance use practices. Hospital-based harm-reduction navigators or peer recovery coaches can play a key role in ensuring patients are discharged with practical tools (eg, clean syringes, fentanyl test strips, wound care kits) that reduce their risk of immediate posthospitalization harm. Connecting patients to syringe service programs, overdose prevention sites, or street outreach teams can improve engagement with care even after they leave the hospital. See Chapter 20 for more information about transitions of care.

Summary

To promote positive outcomes for hospitalized individuals with SUD, it is important to shift the paradigm of care toward recognizing hospitalization as a key opportunity for intervention, engagement, and harm reduction. Effective hospital-based care for people with SUD includes understanding SUD as a medical condition, trauma-informed practices, trust building, and conflict-resolution strategies to improve patient engagement. Structural and cultural humility frameworks highlight the importance of recognizing systemic barriers rather than attributing challenges solely to individual behavior. Moving forward, integrating harm reduction into hospital settings, reducing stigma, and strengthening hospital-to-community transitions are essential for improving both health outcomes and the overall experience of care for people with SUD.

REFERENCES

1. Social Determinants of Health—Healthy People 2030 | odphp.health.gov. Accessed April 22, 2025. https://odphp.health.gov/healthypeople/priority-areas/social-determinants-health
2. Renaud J, McClellan SR, Depriest K, et al. Addressing health-related social needs via community resources: lessons from accountable health communities. *Health Aff.* 2023;42(6):832–840.
3. Tervalon M, Murray-García J. Cultural humility versus cultural competence: a critical distinction in defining physician training outcomes in multicultural education. *J Health Care Poor Underserved.* 1998;9(2):117–125.
4. Metzl JM, Hansen H. Structural competency: theorizing a new medical engagement with stigma and inequality. *Soc Sci Med.* 2014;103:126–133.
5. Kuper A. *Culture.* Harvard University Press; 1999.
6. Rogers CR, Farson RE. *Active Listening.* Mockingbird Press; 2021.
7. Research on Integrating Social & Medical Care | SIREN: Social Interventions Research & Evaluation Network. Accessed April 21, 2025. https://sirenetwork.ucsf.edu
8. Barry R, Anderson J, Tran L, et al. Prevalence of mental health disorders among individuals experiencing homelessness: a systematic review and meta-analysis. *JAMA Psychiatry.* 2024;81(7):691–699.
9. McVicar D, Moschion J, van Ours JC. From substance use to homelessness or vice versa? *Soc Sci Med.* 2015;136–137:89–98.
10. Vangeest JB, Johnson TP. Substance abuse and homelessness: direct or indirect effects? *Ann Epidemiol.* 2002;12(7):455–461.
11. Yamamoto A, Needleman J, Gelberg L, Kominski G, Shoptaw S, Tsugawa Y. Association between homelessness and opioid overdose and opioid-related hospital admissions/emergency department visits. *Soc Sci Med.* 2019;242:112585.
12. North CS, Eyrich-Garg KM, Pollio DE, Thirthalli J. A prospective study of substance use and housing stability in a homeless population. *Soc Psychiatry Psychiatr Epidemiol.* 2010;45(11):1055–1062.
13. Kirst M, Zerger S, Misir V, Hwang S, Stergiopoulos V. The impact of a Housing First randomized controlled trial on substance use problems among homeless individuals with mental illness. *Drug Alcohol Depend.* 2015;146(1):24–29.
14. Buitron de la Vega P, Losi S, Sprague Martinez L, et al. Implementing an EHR-based screening and referral system to address social determinants of health in primary care. *Med Care.* 2019;57(Suppl 2):S133–S139.
15. Protocol for Responding to & Assessing Patients' Assets, Risks & Experiences (PRAPARE®)—National Association of Community Health Centers (NACHC). Accessed March 11, 2026. https://www.nachc.org/resource/prapare/
16. Billioux A, Verlander K, Anthony S, Alley D. Standardized Screening for Health-Related Social Needs in Clinical Settings: The Accountable Health Communities Screening Tool—NAM. *NAM Perpsectives.* 2017. Accessed April 21, 2025. https://nam.edu/perspectives/standardized-screening-for-health-related-social-needs-in-clinical-settings-the-accountable-health-communities-screening-tool/
17. Morris NS, MacLean CD, Chew LD, Littenberg B. The single item literacy screener: evaluation of a brief instrument to identify limited reading ability. *BMC Fam Pract.* 2006;7(1):21.
18. Xuan Z, Nelson TF, Heeren T, et al. Tax policy, adult binge drinking, and youth alcohol consumption in the United States. *Alcohol Clin Exp Res.* 2013;37(10):1713–1719.
19. Venkataramani AS, Bair EF, O'Brien RL, Tsai AC. Association between automotive assembly plant closures and opioid overdose mortality in the United States: a difference-in-differences analysis. *JAMA Intern Med.* 2020;180(2):254–262.
20. Wang X, Steier JB, Gallo WT. The effect of retirement on alcohol consumption: results from the US Health and retirement study. *Eur J Public Health.* 2014;24(3):485–489.
21. Frone MR, Chosewood LC, Osborne JC, Howard JJ. Workplace supported recovery from substance use disorders: defining the construct, developing a model, and proposing an agenda for future research. *Occup Health Sci.* 2022;6(4):475–511.
22. Silverman K, Wong CJ, Needham M, et al. A randomized trial of employment-based reinforcement of cocaine abstinence in injection drug users. *J Appl Behav Anal.* 2007;40(3):387–410.
23. Nosyk B, Anglin MD, Brecht ML, Lima VD, Hser YI. Characterizing durations of heroin abstinence in the California Civil Addict Program: results from a 33-year observational cohort study. *Am J Epidemiol.* 2013;177(7):675–682.
24. Burke MA, Sullivan R, Carman K, Wen H, Wharam JF, Yu H. *Employment Trajectories among Individuals with Opioid Use Disorder: Can Evidence-Based Treatment Improve Outcomes?* Federal Reserve Bank of Boston; 2022.
25. Christie NC. The role of social isolation in opioid addiction. *Soc Cogn Affect Neurosci.* 2021;16(7):645–656.
26. Desai R, Karim S, Freeborn J, Trivedi C, Husain K, Jain S. Contextualizing the relationship between social isolation and substance abuse. *Prim Care Companion CNS Disord.* 2024;26(5):23m03679.
27. Kumar N, Oles W, Howell BA, et al. The role of social network support in treatment outcomes for medication for opioid use disorder: a systematic review. *J Subst Abuse Treat.* 2021;127:108367.
28. Muller AE, Skurtveit S, Clausen T. Building abstinent networks is an important resource in improving quality of life. *Drug Alcohol Depend.* 2017;180:431–438.
29. Turner VE, Demissie Z, Sliwa SA, Clayton HB. Food insecurity and its association with alcohol and other substance use

among high school students in the United States. *J Sch Health.* 2022;92(2):177–184.
30. Whittle HJ, Sheira LA, Frongillo EA, et al. Longitudinal associations between food insecurity and substance use in a cohort of women with or at risk for HIV in the United States. *Addiction.* 2019;114(1):127–136.
31. Walsemann KM, Bell BA. Integrated schools, segregated curriculum: effects of within school segregation on adolescent health behaviors and educational aspirations. *Am J Public Health.* 2010;100(9):1687–1695.
32. Dai HD, Thiel G, Hafer D. Perceived racism and discrimination and youth substance use in the United States—Intersections with sex and ethnicity. *Prev Med (Baltim).* 2024;178: 107811.
33. Rogers CJ, Forster M, Vetrone S, Unger JB. The role of perceived discrimination in substance use trajectories in Hispanic young adults: a longitudinal cohort study from high school through emerging adulthood. *Addict Behav.* 2020;103: 106253.
34. Fothergill KE, Ensminger ME, Green KM, Crum RM, Robertson J, Juon HS. The impact of early school behavior and educational achievement on adult drug use disorders: a prospective study. *Drug Alcohol Depend.* 2008;92(1–3):191–199.
35. Allen-Meares P, Lowry B, Estrella ML, Mansuri S. Health literacy barriers in the health care system: barriers and opportunities for the profession. *Health Soc Work.* 2020;45(1):62–64.
36. Grella CE, Lovinger K. 30-Year trajectories of heroin and other drug use among men and women sampled from methadone treatment in California. *Drug Alcohol Depend.* 2011; 118(2–3):251–258.
37. Hartung DM, McCracken CM, Nguyen T, Kempany K, Waddell EN. Fatal and nonfatal opioid overdose risk following release from prison: a retrospective cohort study using linked administrative data. *J Subst Use Addict Treat.* 2023;147: 208971.
38. Rosenblum A, Cleland CM, Fong C, Kayman DJ, Tempalski B, Parrino M. Distance traveled and cross-state commuting to opioid treatment programs in the United States. *J Environ Public Health.* 2011;2011:948789.
39. Amiri S, Lutz R, Socías E, McDonell MG, Roll JM, Amram O. Increased distance was associated with lower daily attendance to an opioid treatment program in Spokane County Washington. *J Subst Abuse Treat.* 2018;93:26–30.
40. Labban M, Chen CR, Frego N, et al. Disparities in travel-related barriers to accessing health care from the 2017 National Household Travel Survey. *JAMA Netw Open.* 2023; 6(7):E2325291.
41. Winograd RP, Presnall N, Stringfellow E, et al. The case for a medication first approach to the treatment of opioid use disorder. *Am J Drug Alcohol Abuse.* 2019;45(4):333–340.
42. Winograd RP, Wood CA, Stringfellow EJ, et al. Implementation and evaluation of Missouri's Medication First treatment approach for opioid use disorder in publicly-funded substance use treatment programs. *J Subst Abuse Treat.* 2020;108:55–64.
43. Morenz AM, Nance RM, Mixson LS, et al. Barriers to accessing medications for opioid use disorder among rural individuals. *Int J Drug Policy.* 2025;140:104805.
44. Hansen HB, Roberts SK. Two tiers of biomedicalization: methadone buprenorphine and the racial politics of addiction treatment. *Adv Med Sociol.* 2012;14:79–102.
45. Hansen HB, Siegel CE, Case BG, Bertollo DN, DiRocco D, Galanter M. Variation in use of buprenorphine and methadone treatment by racial, ethnic, and income characteristics of residential social areas in New York City. *J Behav Health Serv Res.* 2013;40(3):367–377.
46. Schilling CJ, Eisenberg MD, Kennedy-Hendricks A, et al. Effects of high-deductible health plans on enrollees with mental health conditions with and without substance use disorders. *Psychiatr Serv.* 2022;73(5):518–525.
47. Abraham AJ, Andrews CM, Grogan CM, et al. The affordable care act transformation of substance use disorder treatment. *Am J Public Health.* 2017;107(1):31–32.
48. Nguemeni Tiako MJ, Dolan A, Abrams M, Oyekanmi K, Meisel Z, Aronowitz SV. Thematic analysis of state Medicaid buprenorphine prior authorization requirements. *JAMA Netw Open.* 2023;6(6):E2318487.
49. Allen B, Harocopos A. Non-prescribed buprenorphine in New York city: motivations for use, practices of diversion, and experiences of stigma. *J Subst Abuse Treat.* 2016;70:81–86.
50. Silverstein SM, Daniulaityte R, Miller SC, Martins SS, Carlson RG. On my own terms: motivations for self-treating opioid-use disorder with non-prescribed buprenorphine. *Drug Alcohol Depend.* 2020;210:107958–107958.
51. Derr AS. Mental health service use among immigrants in the United States: a systematic review. *Psychiatr Serv.* 2016;67(3): 265–274.
52. Pagano A. Barriers to drug abuse treatment for latino migrants: treatment providers perspectives. *J Ethn Subst Abuse.* 2014;13(3):273–287.
53. Fassin D, Rechtman R. *The Empire of Trauma: An Inquiry into the Condition of Victimhood.* Princeton University Press; 2009.
54. American Psychiatric Association. *Diagnostic and Statistical Manual of Mental Disorders.* American Psychiatric Association; 2013.
55. Bowe A, Rosenheck R. PTSD and substance use disorder among veterans: characteristics, service utilization and pharmacotherapy. *J Dual Diagn.* 2015;11(1):22–32.
56. Mills KL, Teesson M, Ross J, Peters L. Trauma, PTSD, and substance use disorders: findings from the Australian National Survey of Mental Health and Well-Being. *Am J Psychiatry.* 2006; 163(4):652–658.
57. Reynolds M, Hinchliffe K, Asamoah V, Kouimtsidis C. Trauma and post-traumatic stress disorder in a drug treatment community service. *Psychiatrist.* 2011;35(7):256–260.
58. SAMHSA's Trauma and Justice Strategic Initiative. SAMHSA's concept of trauma and guidance for a trauma-informed approach. *HHS Publication.* 2014;14(4884).
59. Merenstein Z, Shuemaker JC, Phillips RL. Measuring trust in primary care. *Milbank Q.* 2023;101(3):841–880.
60. Wu Q, Jin Z, Wang P. The relationship between the physician-patient relationship, physician empathy, and patient trust. *J Gen Intern Med.* 2022;37(6):1388–1393.
61. Ozaras G, Abaan S. Investigation of the trust status of the nurse–patient relationship. *Nurs Ethics.* 2018;25(5):628–639.
62. Greene J, Samuel-Jakubos H. Building patient trust in hospitals: a combination of hospital-related factors and health care clinician behaviors. *Jt Comm J Qual Patient Saf.* 2021; 47(12):768–774.
63. King C, Collins D, Patten A, Nicolaidis C, Englander H. Trust in hospital physicians among patients with substance use disorder referred to an addiction consult service: a mixed-methods study. *J Addict Med.* 2022;16(1):41–48.
64. Fisher R, Ury W, Patton B. Getting to yes: negotiating agreement without giving. In: *Getting to Yes: Negotiating Agreement without Giving In.* Published online January 1, 1991. Accessed April 21, 2025. https://digitalcommons.usu.edu/unf_research/47

17

Addressing Acute and Chronic Pain in Hospitalized Patients With Substance Use Disorders

Thomas R. Hickey, Dale Terasaki, Melissa B. Weimer

Ms. S is a 44-year-old woman with opioid use disorder (OUD) who presented to the emergency department (ED) with back pain, gait instability, and fever. She was found to have a thoracic spine (T8–T9) vertebral osteomyelitis, discitis, and paravertebral abscess thought to be seeded by bacteria from injection substance use. Surgical intervention and intravenous (IV) antibiotics were recommended for multiple weeks.

She was not on medications for OUD (MOUD) at the time of admission. Her substance history included starting heroin via injection around age 24, transitioning to blue fentanyl tablets (about 20 pills per day) via smoking at age 40. She also reported frequent methamphetamine use by injection. She denied any history of an overdose. She had been involved briefly in an opioid treatment program (OTP) receiving methadone during her period of heroin use many years ago which she found helpful, most of the time on a dose of about 65 mg/d. She had once tried nonprescribed buprenorphine (while off methadone) within the last year and reported feeling "more dopesick than I've ever felt" immediately afterward.

Soon after admission, she was started on methadone for treatment of opioid withdrawal by the inpatient addiction consultation team, starting with three sequential doses of 20 mg for a cumulative total of 60 mg on the first day. It was quickly increased to 80 mg. She had as-needed oral oxycodone 5 to 10 mg every 4 hours, IV hydromorphone 0.4 to 0.8 mg every 2 hours, in addition to non-opioid analgesics including acetaminophen, duloxetine, and gabapentin. For the first 48 hours, she was frequently somnolent but without signs of opioid toxicity. During periods of wakefulness, she reported excruciating "10 out of 10" pain. After 72 hours, she abruptly left the hospital, citing concerns about returning to work as a hairdresser, inadequate analgesia, and overall anxiety.

Fortunately, 1 month later she returned to the hospital "to finish treatment." She reported fentanyl use but no methamphetamine use in the interim. It was communicated to her primary team, her specialists, and nursing staff that pain control was her "biggest priority" and that our collective primary goal was to facilitate completion of her infection treatment course, even at the "expense" of very high amounts of pain and anxiety medications. She resumed methadone (starting at 40 mg but quickly increased in subsequent days) and started on a patient-controlled analgesia (PCA) system with hydromorphone. She briefly received as-needed benzodiazepines for intense anxiety as she grappled with fear of permanent spinal cord injury. Over the next week, her methadone dose was up-titrated to 100 mg daily and her IV hydromorphone PCA was increased to 4 mg per hour (basal) and 1 mg every 15 minutes (demand). She remained fully awake and alert, without hypoxemia, and expressed reasonable management of her pain.

She subsequently underwent multiple surgical procedures to treat the infection and stabilize the spine. Her IV antibiotics were continued, and her pain regimen was reduced moderately. An addiction medicine physician and rotating psychology trainee met with her semiregularly for 2 weeks to discuss pharmacotherapy as well as nonmedication pain coping strategies, respectively. Physical and occupational therapy met with her to assess and guide her level of functioning, mobility, and experience with a spinal brace. An inpatient social worker met with her frequently to arrange her posthospital discharge plan including outpatient methadone treatment. A peer support worker provided nonclinical support and helped her develop posthospital strategies for remaining in substance use disorder (SUD) treatment. At the end of 2 weeks, she was offered the chance to switch to a weekly antibiotic infusion, which could occur as an outpatient through an infusion center. She felt excited at this opportunity and her subjective and objective pain assessments showed a marked improvement. Her methadone dose was gradually increased prior to discharge to 120 mg/d in the context of reducing and stopping her hydromorphone PCA. Among other prescriptions, she was discharged with a short course of as-needed oxycodone. She followed up at the hospital-associated OTP right away and remained engaged in care, reporting persistent but tolerable pain. Unfortunately, she appeared to disengage from care a few months later.

My clinical involvement with Ms. S was impactful to my practice in several ways. Her history of transitioning between different opioids (heroin versus illicitly manufactured fentanyl) and different routes (injection versus inhalation) conferred different risks in terms of infection and the extent of opioid tolerance. Her lack of a history of opioid overdose despite relatively high amounts of high-potency synthetic opioids like fentanyl suggested a vastly high opioid tolerance. Why, then, was somnolence so prominent early on? Could this have constituted a manifestation of stimulant withdrawal (or "washout") and its accrued sleep deficit, compounded by the energy and physiologic reserves drained by infection? Her clinical presentation and what I learned from it impacted my approach to patients *early* in admission, making me careful not to reflexively ascribe any reduction in alertness to iatrogenic causes and encouraged me to consider the need for short-acting opioid analgesics at higher doses, particularly for those with high opioid tolerance.

Next, her high opioid tolerance coincided with a very high quantity of opioids required to alleviate her distress. Although calculating a morphine milligram equivalent (MME) from methadone can be imprecise, her maximum daily MME likely exceeded 2,000 per day. Her acute nociceptive and neuropathic pain represented only a portion of her overall distress, with opioid-related cravings, subtle opioid withdrawal symptoms, and context-related anxiety amplifying her suffering. The high MME administered mitigated her distress in more ways than one, ultimately facilitating the pragmatic goal of infection treatment completion. Staff communication through electronic messages, chart documentation, and in-person discussion was important to ensure a common understanding and relieve staff concerns about the potential hazards of high opioid doses. Moreover, I had to be mindful of my own negative countertransference occurring when seeing a patient in such acute suffering that seemed out of proportion to the medications administered and different than some other patients in her situation. This was an essential step to developing a cohesive and compassionate—and ultimately pragmatic—plan of care.

Notably, by the end of her admission, there appeared to be a clear link between her improving outlook and reduced "demand" (on the PCA) for opioids. And by discharge, some of the reduction in as-needed opioids was "folded" into her total methadone dose, which mitigated fear of cravings and withdrawal symptoms from both the patient and clinician standpoint.

Various staff members from other disciplines helped her greatly in this painful hospital course. Her surgical team, her primary medical team, and the addiction consultation team were instrumental in ensuring support, and adequate pharmacotherapy was available for her. Psychology trainees, social workers, and peer support workers helped with coping skills and posthospital linkage assistance. And nurses navigated difficult bedside discussions of distress plus ad hoc triaging of and advocacy for her needs. Each patient with severe pain and SUD has unique needs, requiring staff to flexibly adjust their own expectations and actions depending on what is empirically manifesting from the patient. As illustrated in this narrative, this can be done while also ensuring the patient's safety and medical stability.

I can certainly envision patients such as Ms. S presenting to a hospital without an explicit focus on SUD care, leaving (multiple times) in frustration prior to a proper course of treatment, and losing the ability to walk or even dying of sepsis. While her posthospital disengagement from care was difficult to learn about, it brought me gratitude for the privilege of doing this work and for Ms. S's good in-hospital outcome. There is much we cannot control in our patients' recovery journeys, yet we can try our best to ease the complex suffering of pain with the tools we have.

—Dale Terasaki

Key Points

- **Pain is common, complex, and highly personal.**
- **Pain and SUD commonly co-occur and result in significant health care utilization and can be challenging to treat.**
- **Individuals with pain and SUD may have other associated psychiatric and medical comorbidities that impact the treatment of their pain and SUD.**
- **SUD and pain should be treated simultaneously.**
- **Effective management of patients with comorbid pain and SUD should include a multidisciplinary approach, a multimodal analgesia strategy, an individualized plan, careful monitoring of opioid analgesics, and discharge planning including outpatient follow-up for SUD and pain.**
- **There is limited evidence to support any specific pharmacologic intervention for pain in individuals with acute pain and SUD; however, like all individuals with acute pain, multimodal treatment is the standard of care.**
- **Use of full-agonist opioids are not contraindicated in the controlled setting of the hospital and typically work well with other non-opioid pain treatments.**

Pain is among the most common reasons patients seek medical care.[1] Pain is also highly prevalent in hospital-based care and accounts for over half of emergency department (ED) visits.[2] Twenty percent of older (≥65 years individuals) admitted to a medicine service report moderate to severe pain,[3] and incidence of pain is higher on hospital discharge than admission.[4] Individuals with substance use disorder (SUD) report high levels of pain at baseline, and it is estimated that chronic pain occurs in 60% of patients with SUD.[4] Pain is also an important cause of ongoing SUD risk.[5]

Estimated associated costs of health care utilization for acute and chronic pain in the United States, including estimated surgical costs, are over $14 billion[6] and historically exceed annual costs of heart disease, cancer, or diabetes.[7] Meanwhile, a SUD diagnosis increases annual medical costs in a working-age, employer-sponsored insurance population by 2.5 times.[8]

What Is Pain?

The International Association for the Study of Pain (IASP) recently revised a definition of pain established in 1979. The revised definition, which was the product of a 2-year effort from a 14-member multinational workgroup, was that pain is "an unpleasant sensory and emotional experience associated with, or resembling that associated with, actual or potential tissue damage."[9] That such an effort was required to define this universal human experience attests to the complexity of pain, a subjective experience influenced by biologic, psychological, and social factors.

Pain terminology can be confusing, so key definitions are provided here. Acute pain is typically sudden in onset, resulting from injury to the body. Provided the injury is resolved and healing proceeds, an episode of acute pain generally resolves within minutes to weeks. Acute pain can progress to chronic pain, particularly if it is poorly treated. IASP defines chronic pain as pain lasting longer than three to six months, beyond the time normally required for healing after injury.

There are four basic processes or phases of pain: transduction, transmission, modulation, and perception (Figure 17.1). Transduction of nociceptive pain refers to the conversion of the peripheral noxious stimulus, via the involved pain receptor(s), into an

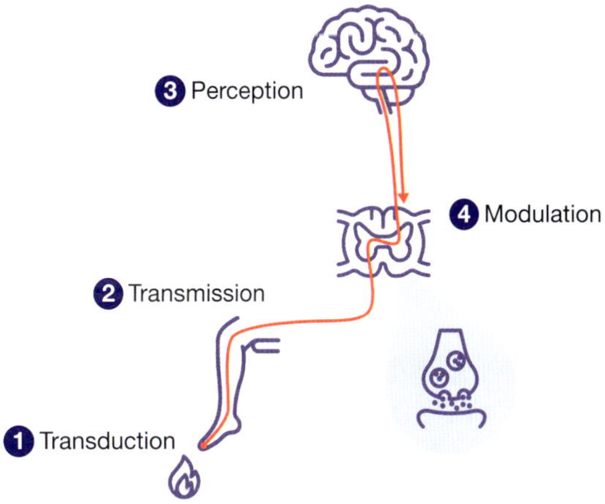

Figure 17.1: Four basic processes of pain.

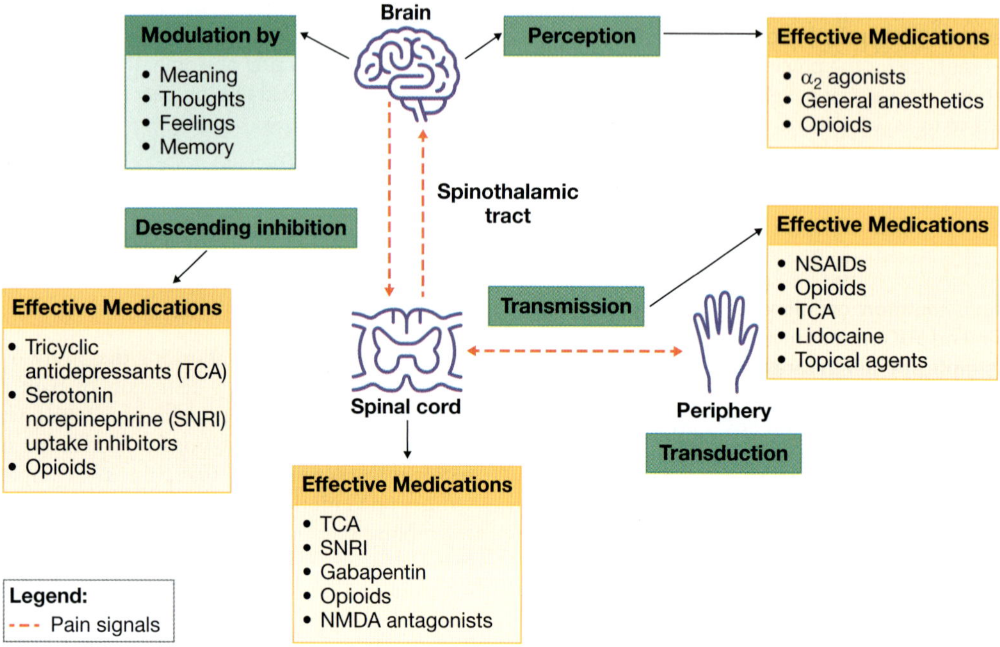

Figure 17.2: Pain pathways and different medication treatments that target these pathways.

activation of the associated nerves. The signal is then transmitted via dorsal horn spinal neurons to the brain cortex and limbic system where perception and modulation occurs. Modulation of pain signals occur in the brain and are mediated by meaning, thoughts, feelings, and memories which can amplify or inhibit pain signals. Sensitization, or increased responsiveness of these peripheral and central nociceptive pathways, contributes to pain becoming chronic and severe.

Conceptualizing these basic pain processes and what are thought to be sites of action of various analgesic medications may be helpful when considering pain treatment options and implementing multiple treatments to synergistically reduce pain (Figure 17.2). For example, treatments such as nonsteroidal anti-inflammatory drugs (NSAIDs), acetaminophen, and local anesthetics (eg, lidocaine) reduce the transduction of pain. In contrast, opioids, alpha-2-receptor agonists, and N-methyl-D-aspartate (NMDA)-receptor antagonists are thought to reduce the perception and modulation of pain. Medication treatments are further discussed in the next section.

Distinguishing Different Types of Pain

A patient's pain may involve multiple, often overlapping, pain pathologies. However, it is useful to distinguish between the three main types of pain whenever possible, particularly as these distinctions inform treatment decisions. The three main types of pain are **nociceptive**, **neuropathic**, and **nociplastic** (Figure 17.3). It is possible for individuals to have complex pain that includes all three types of pain. It is also possible for individuals have all three types of pain, while also having pain that is both acute and chronic in nature. A thorough pain evaluation is important to help differentiate and address all of the patient's pain generators as well as associated symptoms.

Nociceptive Pain

Nociceptive pain refers to pain arising from nonneural tissue injury and typically involves viscera, muscles, and bone. Nociceptive pain can be characterized as somatic pain or as visceral pain. Examples of ***somatic*** nociceptive pain include osteoarthritis, bursitis, a muscle strain or sprain, and a bone fracture. Somatic nociceptive pain arises from activation of peripheral pain receptors with transmission of pain

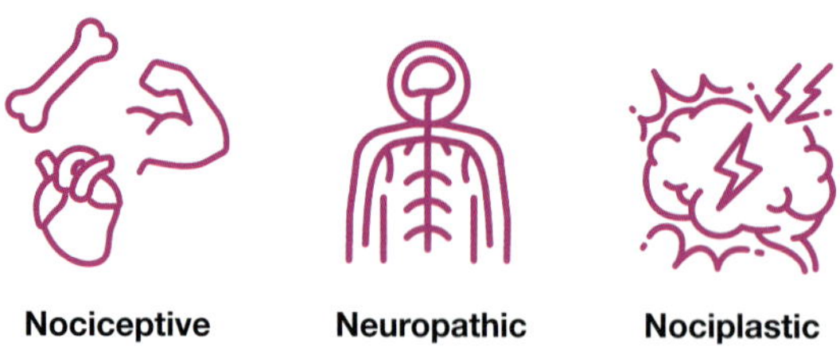

Figure 17.3: Three types of pain.

sensation to the central nervous system via large, myelinated A-δ fibers, and small, unmyelinated C fibers. These afferent fibers, that is, fibers conducting inward toward the central nervous system, result in pain that is characterized as sharp, stabbing, localized, aching, burning, or throbbing. In contrast to somatic nociceptive pain, ***visceral*** nociceptive pain arises from injury to internal organs, for example, tumor invasion, bowel, bladder, bile duct, or ureter obstruction, angina, and pancreatitis. Visceral nociceptive pain is characteristically vague, less localized than somatic pain, and more unpleasant than nociceptive somatic pain. Impulses from the injured organ travel to the associated parasympathetic ganglia, then via greater and lesser splanchnic nerves to pre- and paravertebral ganglia en route to the spinal cord.[10]

Neuropathic Pain

Neuropathic pain results from injury to the peripheral and or central nervous system, via injury (eg, trauma, surgery) or a disease process (eg, diabetes mellitus). Typical pain descriptors are burning, electric, shooting, pins/needles, or numbness/tingling. Neuropathic pain can be characterized as ***acute*** or ***chronic***. ***Acute*** neuropathic pain includes new-onset sciatic pain or herpes zoster, or pain following surgical or traumatic injury to a nerve. ***Chronic*** neuropathic pain diagnoses include diabetic peripheral neuropathy, postherpetic neuralgia, radicular pain, peripheral nerve injury, complex regional pain syndrome, phantom limb pain, and spinal cord injury. A chronic neuropathic pain diagnosis requires a history of nervous system injury or injurious disease process with a plausible corresponding pain pattern and can be supported by diagnostic testing. Chronic neuropathic pain may result in hyperalgesia (increased pain response to painful stimulus), allodynia (pain response to nonpainful stimulus), or a sensory deficit in the neuroanatomic distribution of the injured nerve. Neuropathic pain may be paroxysmal or provoked.

Nociplastic Pain

Recently, the IASP released clinical criteria and a grading system for a third pain classification: *nociplastic*.[11] Nociplastic pain refers to chronic pain that is characterized by (1) duration over 3 months, (2) a regional rather than discrete distribution, (3) lack of nociceptive or neuropathic attribution, and (4) signs of hyperalgesia. It is thought that this type of pain accounts for a large portion of chronic pain syndromes and is highly mediated by central nervous system dysfunction rather than tissue damage. Examples of nociplastic pain include fibromyalgia, tension headache, and irritable bowel syndrome. Some attribute the experience of "chronic overlapping pain conditions"—a group of at least 10 conditions including chronic migraine headache, chronic low back pain, and chronic vulvodynia—to this type of pain.[12,13] Treatment of nociplastic pain often defies conventional tissue or receptor-targeted strategies, so new modalities to treat nociplastic pain are under development. Nociplastic pain generally has other associated features such as fatigue, sleep disturbance, cognitive and memory disturbance, and mood symptoms.

Comorbid Pain and SUD

Pain and SUD are highly associated. Individuals with SUD may use substances to treat underlying pain disorders which can unfortunately lead to more complex pain due to increased risk of injury as well as substance-withdrawal–mediated pain. Individuals with SUD are also more likely to have concomitant mood disorders like depression and anxiety which mediate more complex pain.

Analysis of a large data set in a tertiary academic center found that among patients with SUD, prevalence of chronic noncancer pain was 60% compared to 45% prevalence in people without SUD.[5] There was a 71% prevalence of chronic noncancer pain in individuals with three or more concomitant SUD. Chronic pain was identified in 75% of patient with opioid use disorder (OUD), 72% sedative use disorder, 64% cannabis use disorder, 59% alcohol use disorder, and 60% tobacco use disorder. A systematic review and meta-analysis of 56 studies reported a prevalence of 60% for current pain and 44% prevalence for chronic pain in individuals receiving opioid agonist treatment for OUD.[14] There are no apparent consistent demographic or clinical differences between patients with chronic pain and SUD versus SUD alone.[15]

Comorbid pain and SUD may lead to secondary conditions, including sleep disturbance, depression, anxiety, or posttraumatic stress disorder (PTSD), physical disability, and other conditions highlighted in Figure 17.4. These resulting conditions can, in turn, exacerbate pain and SUD leading to a vicious cycle (Figure 17.4).

Pain and SUD in the Hospital Setting

SUD can increase hospital utilization and pain is likely to be a feature among hospitalized patients with SUD. Among a cohort of patients presenting to the ED with a SUD diagnosis, 36% reported severe pain and 27% moderate pain.[16]

Primary medical and surgical teams may not feel comfortable managing pain in individuals with SUD

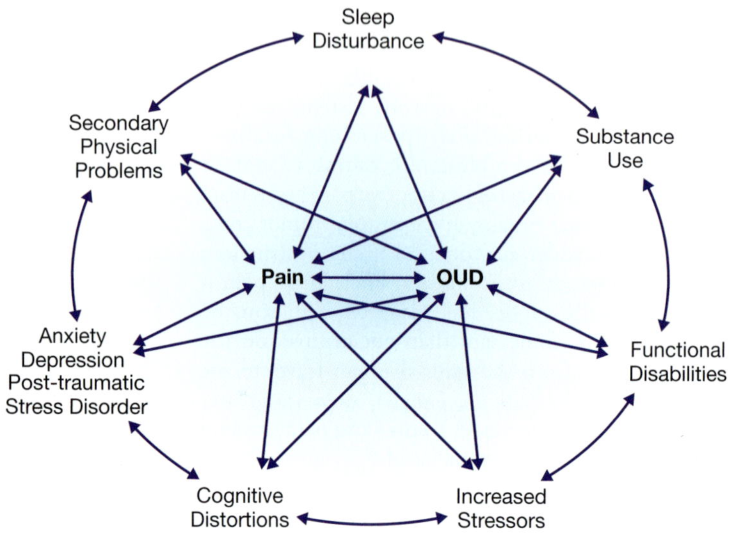

Figure 17.4: A schematic of how pain and opioid use disorder (OUD) are reinforcing and have many other associated conditions and symptoms. Treating pain and OUD simultaneously leads to improved outcomes.

and may ask for the assistance of the acute pain service, when available, to help manage complex pain. In hospitals with addiction consultation services, they may be called to advise for patients even when a diagnosis of SUD is unclear. How this is handled depends on each addiction consultative services' capacity, comfort, and scope of practice in the hospital. Some addiction consultation services limit their scope to patients with a clear or likely SUD as the primary indication for consultation, while others may feel more comfortable comanaging complex pain for individuals with opioid tolerance without SUD. The ability to differentiate complex pain with physical dependence from OUD, as an example, is a complex task which requires both an understanding of pain and OUD. Collaborating with anesthesia or an acute pain service is very helpful for perioperative pain management of patients, including those with OUD and other SUD.

Unique Pain Management Challenges in SUD

Well-known barriers to general medical care for patients with SUD include stigma, clinician biases, lack of knowledge, and mutual mistrust among patients and clinicians, all of which impact pain management.[17] Patients with comorbid pain and SUD often report inadequate pain management.[18] Fear of inadequate pain control, often informed by prior experience, is common in patients with SUD.[19] These fears are an established reason for persons with OUD to delay seeking necessary care and for leaving the hospital before completing medical treatment.[20] Patient-directed discharge, already increased among patients with SUD, is twice as likely in those hospitalized with acute pain compared to those without.[21,22] Inadequate pain management also interferes with the important goal of treating the comorbid SUD.[23] Patients with comorbid pain and SUD are at greater risk of prescription medication misuse and are more likely to be prescribed opioids and at higher doses, though the latter may vary by health care system.[15] In a population of individuals on medication for OUD (MOUD), wherein even minor disruptions in MOUD significantly increase overdose mortality,[24] the combination of hospitalization and poorly controlled pain creates particular vulnerabilities for adverse OUD outcomes such as return to unprescribed opioid use and opioid overdose.

Cancer Pain and SUD

Over half of patients with cancer experience pain.[25] Cancer pain syndromes may arise from medical intervention and disease process, and thus often have both acute and chronic components. Opioids may create particular challenges in the treatment of cancer pain among people with SUD, given their misuse potential and knowledge that SUD can worsen the pain experience.[26] Partnering with palliative care teams can be beneficial for individuals with comorbid SUD and cancer-related pain. See Chapter 18 for more information.

Common Comorbidities Associated With Pain and SUD

Psychiatric disorders are common in patients with pain and SUD, including anxiety, depression, sleep disorders, PTSD, and personality disorders. Medical comorbidities are also common in patients with pain and SUD, including cancer, heart disease, HIV,

TABLE 17.1

Common Psychiatric and Medical Comorbidities Associated With Individuals Who Have Pain and SUD

	Common comorbidities
Psychiatric disorders	Sleep disorders
	Depressive disorders
	Generalized anxiety disorders
	Personality disorders
	Posttraumatic stress disorder
Medical disorders	Cancer
	Heart disease
	Obesity
	HIV
	Hepatitis C
	Other infectious conditions

hepatitis C, and other infectious diseases. Disabilities related to chronic pain can contribute to metabolic conditions like diabetes and functional impairments that can ultimately make pain more challenging to treat. See Table 17.1.

Risk Factors for Poorly Controlled Acute Pain and Progression to Chronic Pain

There are multiple risks factors for the progression from acute pain to chronic pain. SUD itself is an independent risk factor for more severe acute pain and it may be more challenging to treat postsurgical pain in people with comorbid pain and SUD, as described earlier. Most individuals who undergo surgery, regardless of presence of SUD, will experience at least moderate acute pain.[27] The following risk factors predict poorly controlled acute postoperative pain in individuals *without* SUD: younger age, female gender, anxiety, depression, sleep disturbance, obesity, chronic pain, and baseline opioid analgesic use.[28] Risk factors for progression to chronic pain vary by surgery and study for individuals without SUD, and include younger age, female gender, anxiety, depression, pain catastrophizing, poorly controlled acute postoperative pain, preoperative pain, and preoperative opioid use.[29] Preexisting patient factors such as these are often as (or more) influential over pain outcomes than the nature of the surgery itself.[30] Individuals receiving prescribed long-term opioids will have physical opioid dependence and opioid tolerance which may complicate postoperative or acute pain. In some instances, individuals prescribed opioids may develop opioid-induced hyperalgesia which may further complicate effective pain treatment.

Hospital-Based Pain Evaluation for a Patient With SUD

The initial step to safely and effectively treating pain in the hospital setting involves a dedicated pain evaluation (Table 17.2). This evaluation will help the clinician better characterize the pain condition, differentiate acute pain from chronic pain, understand pain generators and complexity, and then determine the best treatment options for the type of pain the patient is experiencing. The mnemonic SOCRATES which stands for site, onset, character, radiation, associations, time course or pattern, exacerbating/relieving factors, and severity is one tool to use during a pain evaluation. PQRST is another mnemonic and stands for the following:

- Provocation—What triggers the pain? What makes the pain better?
- Quality—What does the pain feel like (eg, sharp, dull, throbbing)?
- Region—Where is the pain located? Does it radiate or spread?
- Severity—How intense is the pain? How does it affect your day to day?
- Timing—Is the pain constant or intermittent? When does the pain occur? How long does it last?

Acute pain intensity scales include the numeric rating scale (10-point scale), visual analog scale, and emoji-based scale.[31,32] For individuals with chronic pain, multidimensional instruments such as the Brief Pain Inventory and PEG (Pain, Enjoyment, and General Activity) Scale are recommended.[33,34]

Once you have established these components of the pain history, you can determine its time course as *acute or chronic or acute on chronic* and its classification: *nociceptive, neuropathic, nociplastic*, or a combination. If a diagnosis of SUD has not already been established, this will be important to assess during the pain evaluation. Once established, it is important to understand how SUD may be contributing to the patient's pain. Is the patient in active substance withdrawal? Does the patient have profound opioid tolerance? Does the patient use substances to help manage his or her pain? If the patient has OUD, is he or she interested in medication treatment for OUD?

Pain Evaluation Case Example

Patient is a 48-year-old female with a past medical history of severe OUD on methadone treatment, severe cocaine use disorder, tobacco use disorder, hypertension, depression, and anxiety. She presented to the hospital for pain after a fall and trouble walking. She describes her pain as follows: site:

TABLE 17.2

Pain Evaluation Components and Tools

Components of a comprehensive pain evaluation	Evaluation questions/tools
Pain evaluation	▪ **SOCRATES**—Site, onset, character, radiation, associations (signs or symptoms related to pain), time course or pattern (intermittent or constant), exacerbating/relieving factors, and severity of pain ▪ **PQRST**—provocation, quality, region, severity, and timing
Pain intensity scales	▪ Numeric rating scale ▪ Visual Analog Scale ▪ Emoji-Based Scale ▪ Brief Pain Inventory ▪ Pain, Enjoyment, and General Activity Scale (PEG)
Functional impairment and pain interference evaluation	▪ What number best describes how pain has interfered with your general activity? ▪ How much does pain interfere with your day to day activities?
Patient pain goals	▪ What are your hopes for managing your pain? ▪ What pain level (0–10) is acceptable to you?
Risk assessment for progression from acute to chronic pain	▪ STarT MSK Screening Tool[35]
Unhealthy substance use screening and substance use history	▪ AUDIT-C[36] ▪ TAPS[37] ▪ RIP TEAR[38] ▪ DSM-5[39]
Psychiatric comorbidities	▪ Depression screening—PHQ-2[40] ▪ Anxiety screening—GAD-2[41] ▪ Others as indicated
Physical exam	▪ Examine the painful area and surrounding areas ▪ Neurologic exam, as indicated ▪ Assess for underlying medical conditions ▪ Assess for allodynia and hyperalgesia
Laboratory tests	▪ Comprehensive metabolic panel ▪ Complete blood count ▪ Consider thyroid function tests, hemoglobin A1c, hepatitis panel, HIV screening, Vitamin B12, Vitamin D, Ferritin ▪ Urine drug testing

chest and back; onset: she has had severe back pain for the last 5 years but the pain in her chest started 3 hours before arrival; character: sharp and stabbing in her chest and dull and achy in her back; radiation: chest pain does not radiate but her back pain radiates down her left leg; associations: restlessness, irritability; time course or pattern: pain is constant in her back and intermittent in her chest; exacerbating/relieving factors: chest pain is worse with inspiration, back pain is worse with any movement and improved with rest; severity: 8/10 in her chest and 10/10 in her back. She shares that she previously was diagnosed with "sciatica" and her baseline pain severity in her back is 8/10.

On further evaluation, the clinician asks her about her OUD and its treatment. She states she is on a methadone dose of 80 mg/d but has missed the last 3 days of treatment for unclear reasons. She has been using opioids and cocaine over the last 3 days. She is feeling opioid withdrawal symptoms including restlessness, irritability, rhinorrhea, piloerection, sweating, and body aches. She would like to resume her methadone treatment and thinks this will also help reduce her overall body aches.

Based on the evaluation, the clinician can determine that the patient has both acute and chronic pain. She has nociceptive acute pain in the chest and nociceptive and neuropathic chronic pain in her back. The acute pain is likely attributed to the recent fall, but the chronic pain clearly preceded the fall and is likely unrelated or worsened by the fall based on her history. Acute evaluation of the pain can be focused on the chest pain because her back pain is at her baseline. X-ray of the chest reveals a 10th rib fracture. Treatment of nociceptive acute rib fracture includes NSAIDs and ice. In addition, she has opioid withdrawal, and this is likely contributing to her pain, so restarting her methadone is indicated along with recommendation to continue daily methadone treatment. With these treatments the patient now states her chest pain is 2/10 and her back pain is improved from its baseline.

This case illustrates why it is important to fully evaluate the features of the patient's pain. In the absence of this evaluation, the acute management may have included further evaluation of chronic pain that was unrelated to the presenting acute symptom. In addition, addressing the patient's opioid withdrawal was effective to better manage both her acute and chronic pain. By adequately evaluating her pain, the most safe and effective treatments were also provided for the patient.

Management of Acute Pain in a Patient With SUD

Many clinicians report they lack the clinical expertise to evaluate and adequately treat pain in individuals with SUD. Patients with pain and SUD may subsequently perceive that their pain is unseen or unheard contributing to poor outcomes. As discussed throughout this chapter, with appropriate evaluation and treatment, pain in the setting of SUD can be safely and effectively managed.

Principles for hospital-based acute pain treatment in the setting of SUD can differ depending on the type of pain that is being treated (eg, perioperative pain, nonperioperative pain, or acute-on-chronic pain). In general, however, after a detailed pain evaluation is completed, effective pain care includes coordinating a multidisciplinary approach, offering multimodal pain treatments, and connecting patients to ongoing care for both pain and SUD after hospital discharge. These practice principles are consistent with a 2024 multispecialty consensus statement resulting from input from medical, surgical, addiction medicine, anesthesia, and pain specialists and provides guiding principles for the perioperative care of patients with chronic pain, SUD, and/or preoperative opioid tolerance.[42] The consensus statement emphasized the potential need for a pain specialist or anesthesiologist to offer "personalized analgesic options, medication titration, postdischarge tapering, and timely responsiveness to episodes of inadequate analgesia or medication side effects."[42] The consensus statement also emphasized the need for effective communication and care coordination to ensure patients receive ongoing care and monitoring after hospital discharge.

The following sections outline principles and specific treatment modalities for safe and effective pain management for individuals with acute pain in the setting of SUD. Subsequent sections will describe how to comanage acute pain and SUD.

Communication Principles

When treating patients hospitalized with acute pain and SUD, clinicians ought to:

- Avoid terms like "drug seeking" or "drug seeker" when describing individuals with concomitant acute pain and SUD.
- Take the person's pain seriously and provide a thorough and complete evaluation.
- Avoid arguing with the patient about their pain. Each patient has a unique internal experience that is entirely their own, and their overall distress may increase when confronted by an overly skeptical or accusatory clinician.
- Emphasize pain as a legitimate, distressing experience with multiple contributors and manifestations. A goal of zero pain is desirable for all parties but may not be safe or feasible.
- Reflect on one's own countertransference and biases related to painful distress and coping. Acute distress expressed by another individual can sometimes elicit strong emotions in clinicians, leading to responses that are not helpful, and may be detrimental to accurately assess and address patients' pain. These emotions do not preclude working closely with the patient but should be acknowledged and understood to impact one's interpretation of the situation.
- Communicate the patient's unique pain needs with nursing staff and other clinicians.
- Seek consultation from pain specialists and addiction medicine, if available, who can collaborate and assist with safe and effective pain and SUD treatment.
- Prior to hospital discharge, ensure the patient has a safe and feasible follow-up plan, including adequate ongoing medication treatment as needed.

Pharmacotherapies for Acute Pain

Research is limited about specific pharmacotherapies for pain treatment in individuals with SUD.[43] A 2025 systematic review assessed studies addressing acute pain in people with OUD. Unfortunately, the overall quality of evidence was limited and highlighted significant research gaps.[44] The systematic review did identify single randomized controlled trials demonstrating potential benefit in pain and opioid analgesic reductions with: oral clonidine versus placebo in orthopedic fractures[45]; a combination of intramuscular (IM)

TABLE 17.3

Summary of Select Pharmacotherapies for Acute Pain[50]

Medication	Number needed to treat—medication vs placebo for 50% pain relief
Acetaminophen (1,000 mg)	3.6 (3.2–4.1)
Acetaminophen + oxycodone (325 mg/5 mg)	5.4 (3.9–8.8)
Acetaminophen + oxycodone (1 g/10 mg)	1.8 (1.6–2.2)
Celecoxib (200 mg)	4.2 (3.4–5.6)
Celecoxib (400 mg)	2.6 (2.3–3.0)
Diclofenac (50 mg)	6.6 (4.1–17)
Diclofenac (100 mg)	1.9 (1.7–2.3)
Gabapentin (250 mg)	11 (6.4–35)
Ibuprofen (200 mg)	2.9 (2.7–3.2)
Ibuprofen (400 mg)	2.5 (2.4–2.6)
Ibuprofen + acetaminophen (400 mg/1 g)	1.5 (1.4–1.7)
Naproxen (220 mg)	3.4 (2.4–5.8)
Naproxen (440 mg)	2.7 (2.2–3.5)
Oxycodone (15 mg)	4.6 (2.9–11)
Gabapentin (250 mg)	11 (6.4–35)

haloperidol, IM midazolam, and IV morphine versus IV morphine alone in limb or abdominal pain[46]; and intraoperative IV lidocaine infusion versus intraoperative IV ketamine or placebo infusion in postoperative pain after orthopedic surgery.[47] These studies were done mostly in men who were using opium in Iran, so the result may not be generalizable to other populations.

Despite limited evidence specifically in individuals with SUD, multispecialty clinical practice guidelines for the treatment of acute postoperative pain and acute musculoskeletal injury recommend multimodal analgesic regimens in most situations.[48,49] The use of multiple different analgesic modalities improves pain by targeting multiple different pain pathways and reduces overreliance on opioids. This section will review the various pharmacotherapies and behavioral interventions for acute pain (Table 17.3). The following section will focus specifically on the management of OUD and concomitant acute pain.

Acetaminophen (Paracetamol)

Acetaminophen, a non-opioid analgesic, is a mainstay in hospital-based treatment of acute pain. There is no high-level evidence assessing acetaminophen for pain in patients with SUD. However, acetaminophen in the general population is supported by high-level evidence and multidisciplinary consensus guidelines.[48] An overview of Cochrane reviews calculated numbers needed to treat (NNTs) for at least 50% maximum postoperative pain relief after a single analgesic dose over 4 to 6 hours.[50] The NNT for a 975-mg acetaminophen dose was 3.6 (95% CI 3.2 to 4.1). Acetaminophen is generally well tolerated up to 4 g/d, and typically ordered standing at 1 g every 6 hours for the treatment of acute pain. Risks and benefits should be assessed in patients with severe liver disease. Acetaminophen can be used as standalone treatment, but most commonly is used in addition to other analgesics. The use of acetaminophen with full-agonist opioids, for example, provides greater analgesic benefit than opioids used alone.

Nonsteroidal Anti-Inflammatory Drugs (NSAIDs)

Like acetaminophen, NSAIDs, such as celecoxib, ibuprofen, ketorolac, and naproxen, are mainstays in hospital-based acute pain management. There is no high-level evidence assessing NSAIDs for pain in patients with SUD. However, NSAIDs in a general population are supported by high-level evidence and multidisciplinary consensus guidelines.[48] An overview of Cochrane reviews calculated NNT for at least 50% maximum postoperative pain relief after a single analgesic dose over 4 to 6 hours.[50] The NNT for a 200-mg ibuprofen dose was 2.9 (95% CI 3.4 to 5.6); and for a 400-mg celecoxib dose was 2.6 (95% CI 2.3 to 3.0). NSAIDs should be considered more frequently in acute pain situations and can be safely used after many different surgeries.

Risks and benefits should be assessed in the elderly (age 65 or greater) or those with a history of significant cardiovascular or renal dysfunction. Like acetaminophen, NSAIDs can be scheduled (eg, celecoxib, 200 mg twice daily), often with a limited number of doses to minimize adverse effects. Risk of gastrointestinal complications should be considered, particularly if the patient is concurrently prescribed corticosteroids. Like acetaminophen, the use of NSAIDs with full-agonist opioids provides greater analgesic benefit than opioids used alone.

NSAID and Acetaminophen

Combining NSAIDs and acetaminophen can be very effective for analgesia. A combined dose of 400-mg ibuprofen and 1-g acetaminophen, for at least 50% maximum postoperative pain relief over 4 to 6 hours, resulted in an NNT of 1.5 (95% CI 1.4 to 1.7).[50] This impressively low NNT reinforces how effective these medications are for analgesia and should be administered together whenever possible. For individuals with pain and SUD, scheduling these medications together can have beneficial and synergistic effects. Scheduling these medications in addition to as needed full-agonist opioids, if used, is also very effective.

Regional and Neuraxial Blocks

Regional and neuraxial blocks involve the administration of local anesthetic around targeted nerves to produce anesthesia and/or analgesia in targeted areas of the body. For example, a preoperative supraclavicular brachial plexus block may be performed to provide complete intraoperative anesthesia for wrist surgery, and a continuous thoracic epidural may be performed to provide postoperative analgesia after abdominal and thoracic surgery. Local anesthetics (eg, bupivacaine, lidocaine, ropivacaine) are generally the principle analgesic administered in a regional or neuraxial block. They are often mixed with other analgesics (eg, alpha agonist, corticosteroid, opioid) to quicken the onset and prolong the duration of the sensory block. Use of sensory blocks for acute pain typically involves consultation by a pain specialist who is experienced in providing them.

There are no high-level studies assessing regional and neuraxial blocks in patients with SUD. However, in the perioperative setting, both interventions are supported by high-level evidence and multidisciplinary consensus guidelines.[48] It is notable that patients who are opioid tolerant may demonstrate some degree of resistance to local anesthetic effects.[51]

Lidocaine

Lidocaine is a local anesthetic. For pain management, typical use is by subcutaneous (SQ) injection to provide field block for common procedures (eg, central-line placement, minor surgery), and via intravenous (IV) infusion. Use of lidocaine for acute pain typically involves consultation by a pain specialist. There is no high-level evidence assessing continuous IV or transdermal lidocaine in patients with SUD. Perioperative IV lidocaine's benefits in early perioperative pain scores were unclear per a Cochrane review.[52]

Alpha-2-Receptor Agonists

Clonidine

Clonidine is an alpha-2-receptor agonist available in an oral and transdermal formulation. Alpha-2 agonists suppress sympathetic outflow from the central nervous system resulting in suppression of noradrenergic pathways that may result in sedation. Stimulation of dorsal horn alpha-2 receptors may directly inhibit nociceptive neurons and provide analgesia.[53] There is no high-level evidence assessing clonidine for acute pain management in patients with or without SUD. In an opioid-naïve surgical population, meta-analysis shows statistically significant, but clinically questionable, reductions in pain and opioid use.[54,55] A 7.0-cm^2 transdermal system, for example, delivers 0.2-mg clonidine per day over 7 days. A single-week therapy of the transdermal formulation makes clonidine rebound hypertension unlikely and a wean, therefore, unnecessary.

For patients with OUD and acute pain, clonidine can be used as an adjunct to opioid withdrawal treatment which may improve pain by helping to treat opioid withdrawal in individuals with OUD.[53] For patients without acute opioid withdrawal, it may provide a small, analgesic benefit.

Dexmedetomidine

Dexmedetomidine is an alpha-2-receptor agonist available in an IV formulation generally given as an infusion in a critical care area due to the possibility of hypotension, bradycardia, and sedation. There is no high-level evidence assessing dexmedetomidine for pain in patients with SUD. In opioid naïve surgical population, meta-analyses show statistically significant reductions in pain and opioid consumption but of unclear clinical significance.[56–58] Dexmedetomidine may also be used for treatment of severe agitation related to substance withdrawal or substance intoxication.

NMDA-Receptor Antagonists

Ketamine

Ketamine is an NMDA-receptor antagonist that is used in the hospital at high doses as an anesthetic and at lower doses as an analgesic. Oral, intranasal, and SQ administration is possible, but its use in the hospital for the treatment of pain is generally IV. Ketamine's mechanism of action may be effective to reduce hyperalgesia and central sensitization in individuals with opioid tolerance by promoting upregulation of mu-opioid receptors.[59] Ketamine can be effective as an adjunct to other analgesic modalities for individuals with severe pain and SUD. There is no contraindication to the use of ketamine for individuals with SUD.

A systematic review and meta-analysis demonstrated that, in an opioid-tolerant population, ketamine administration resulted in a clinically relevant decrease in opioid consumption in the perioperative setting.[60] The nine included RCTs assessed a variety of administration strategies including bolus (0.15 to 0.5 mg/kg of ideal body weight [IBW]), infusion (0.002 to 0.6 mg/kg IBW/h), and patient-controlled analgesia (PCA) (2-mg demand bolus with 10-minute lock-out interval). Two double-blind, double-dummy controlled trials in the ED reported on 15-minute IV infusions at a low dose (0.3 mg/kg), which provided similar analgesia and fewer adverse effects compared to IV push.[61,62] Based on these studies and the experience of the authors, it is very reasonable to consider a low-dose ketamine infusion (0.05 to 1 mg/kg/h) for individuals with severe pain despite use of other treatment modalities.

Low-dose ketamine infusions for pain can be safely provided, even outside of critical care areas such as general medical or surgical floors with appropriate monitoring protocols. Given its potential to render patients unresponsive, institutional policy should be developed to ensure appropriate monitoring. A typical requirement would be close nurse monitoring and appropriate clinician experience to ensure patient safety and tolerance.[63] Patients who receive ketamine for pain should be monitored for pulmonary aspiration, hypertension, tachycardia, and psychomimetic effects such as hallucinations or delirium.

Magnesium

Magnesium's analgesic effects are typically attributed to NMDA-receptor antagonism. For the treatment of perioperative pain, it is generally administered intraoperatively as a slow IV bolus and or continuous IV infusion. There is no high-level evidence assessing magnesium for pain in patients with SUD. Meta-analyses report statistically significant, but clinically questionable reductions in pain and opioid consumption in patients with acute pain.[64] A slow bolus dose of approximately 30 mg/kg and/or infusion of 15 mg/kg/h are typical. Patients receiving magnesium infusions should be monitored for flushing, hypotension, and bradycardia. It has muscle relaxant qualities and should be used with caution in neuromuscular disease (eg, myasthenia gravis).

Transdermal Analgesics

Transdermal formulations are available for many analgesics including NSAIDs, opioids (eg, fentanyl), lidocaine, clonidine, and capsaicin. In general, they have a slow onset, prolonged duration of action, and achieve stable plasma concentration in steady state. They are useful in situations where enteral administration is suboptimal (eg, nil per os) and are consistent with best practices of avoiding parenteral analgesia when possible. They are simple and, in general, result in less class-specific adverse effects compared with other formulations. There is no high-level evidence assessing any transdermal medication for pain in patients with SUD. However, given their simplicity and tolerability, it is reasonable to consider them a useful part of a multimodal analgesia strategy. A long-acting transdermal formulation may also provide a useful bridge to outpatient follow-up on discharge. Transdermal fentanyl should only be used in individuals with high opioid tolerance.

Corticosteroids

Corticosteroids such as prednisone and dexamethasone are powerful anti-inflammatory agents and can be used as an adjunct for pain treatment. They come in both oral and IV formulations. There is no high-level evidence assessing corticosteroids for acute pain in patients with SUD. In the perioperative setting, there is evidence to support decreased postoperative pain and reduced opioid consumption, though the clinical significance is unclear.[65] Corticosteroids are likely to be especially effective in inflammatory pain such as bursitis, and may be used to reduce tissue damage (and consequent pain) in various inflammatory conditions such as inflammatory bowel disease and rheumatoid arthritis. They are commonly prescribed in the treatment of cancer pain syndromes despite a mixed evidence base.[66] Similar to NSAIDs, they should be used with caution in individuals who are elderly, are on anticoagulation, have gastritis, or have poorly controlled hyperglycemia.

Gabapentinoids

Gabapentinoids decrease hyperexcitability of dorsal horn neurons and may provide analgesia via modulation of calcium-induced release of the excitatory neurotransmitter glutamate and by activation of descending modulating pathways. They have oral formulations only. There is no high-level evidence assessing gabapentin or pregabalin for acute pain in patients with SUD. 250-mg oral gabapentin resulted in an NNT, for at least 50% maximum postoperative pain relief over 4 to 6 hours, of 11 (95% CI 6.4 to 35).[50] Gabapentin can potentiate opioid adverse effects including sedation and respiratory depression prompting an FDA warning in 2019.[67] Gabapentinoids may be a home medication for the hospitalized patient, often for the indication of neuropathic pain; in general, they should be continued throughout the admission. This class of medications has misuse potential that must be considered. Gabapentin may also have some benefit as an adjunct to alcohol withdrawal treatment and alcohol use disorder treatment. It is reasonable to consider

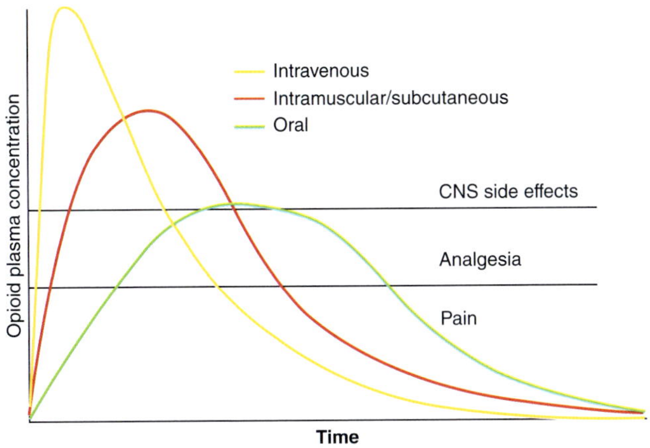

Figure 17.5: Different pharmacokinetics of opioid formulations. (Used with permission of Springer Nature BV, from Savage SR, Kirsh KL, Passik SD. Challenges in using opioids to treat pain in persons with substance use disorders. *Addict Sci Clin Pract*. 2008;4[2]:4–25; permission conveyed through Copyright Clearance Center, Inc.)

gabapentinoids for individuals with high anxiety and neuropathic or nociplastic pain. Gabapentin, for example, is typically started at a low dose and titrated to effect over days to weeks to effective doses of 600 to 900 mg oral three times a day. Caution should be exercised for elderly patients and patients with renal impairment will need dose adjustments.

Full-Agonist Opioids

Full-agonist opioids include oxycodone, hydrocodone, morphine, methadone, hydromorphone, and fentanyl, among others. Opioids provide analgesia in several ways including turning on descending inhibitory pain signals, preventing ascending transmission of pain signals, inhibiting terminals of C-fibers in the spinal cord, inhibiting activation of peripheral nociceptors, and activating opioid receptors in the midbrain involved in the reward pathway. Short-acting or immediate-release opioids are frequently provided for acute pain treatment in the hospital setting by oral, IV, IM, or SQ route. Clinicians should consider the clinical goal when choosing an opioid formulation for administration. IV opioids provide the fastest analgesic effect but have the shortest duration of action compared to IM, SQ, and oral routes of administration. In addition, IV formulations have the most central nervous system side effects like sedation and reward. Oral opioids have the slowest onset of action compared to IV, IM, and SQ opioids, but the longest duration of action (Figure 17.5). For these reasons, oral opioids are generally preferred over IV, IM, or SQ opioids when patients can take medications by mouth. For adequate acute pain relief, oral opioids may need to be given as frequently as every 3 hours. IV, IM, or SQ opioids can be combined with oral opioids for patients with severe, break through pain; however, in individuals with SUD, the use and overreliance on IV, IM, or SQ opioids should be monitored closely.

In the hospital setting, IV PCA is another option for patients with severe pain. PCAs have the added benefit of providing the patient more control of the administration of their analgesic medications and reduce periodicity of analgesic effects (see Figure 17.6). This can be particularly helpful for patients with unclear analgesic needs, who report severe pain despite frequent

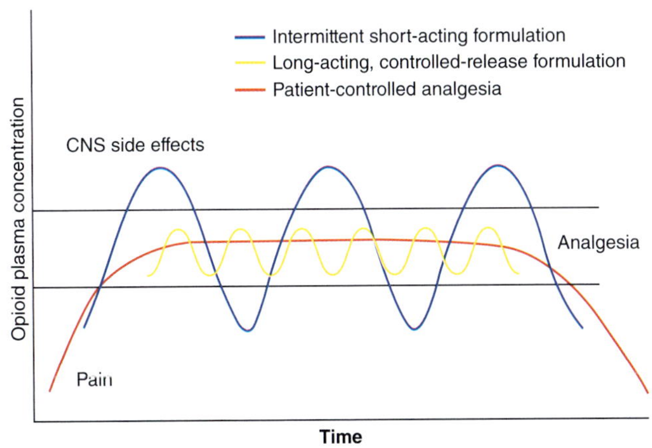

Figure 17.6: Comparison of benefits and side effects of different formulations of opioids.[68] (Used with permission of Springer Nature BV, from Savage SR, Kirsh KL, Passik SD. Challenges in using opioids to treat pain in persons with substance use disorders. *Addict Sci Clin Pract*. 2008;4[2]:4–25; permission conveyed through Copyright Clearance Center, Inc.)

TABLE 17.4

Buprenorphine Formulations[70]

Buprenorphine formulation	Route	Bioavailability[72]
FDA indication for OUD		
Sublingual buprenorphine and sublingual buprenorphine-naloxone (Suboxone®, Zubsolv®)	Sublingual	~30%
Extended-release long-acting buprenorphine (Sublocade®, Brixadi®)	Subcutaneous depot	See Table 17.6
FDA indication for pain		
Intravenous buprenorphine (Buprenex)[71]	Intravenous	100%
Buccal buprenorphine (Belbuca®)	Buccal	46–65%
Transdermal buprenorphine (Butrans®)	Transdermal	~15%

administration of opioids, or who are unable to take medications by mouth.

There is no high-level evidence assessing opioids for pain management in patients with SUD. For patients with acute pain without SUD, a 15-mg oral oxycodone resulted in an NNT, for at least 50% maximum postoperative pain relief over 4 to 6 hours compared with placebo, of 4.6 (95% CI 2.9 to 11).[50]

Patients who are opioid tolerant from long-term prescribed opioids or OUD who have acute pain will require their baseline opioid tolerance to be met and will likely need additional opioids and other pain treatments for analgesic benefit. For example, if an individual is prescribed oxycodone 10 mg orally three times a day outside of the hospital for low back pain over the last 1 year, that person will likely need additional opioids and other pain treatments provided if they are hospitalized with acute pain. In other words, their regular home dose of opioids is insufficient to treat their acute pain; though having acute pain does not always mean the person requires additional opioids. An acute ankle sprain, for example, may be best treated with an NSAID and acetaminophen versus additional opioids.[69] Management of concomitant OUD and acute pain is discussed later in the chapter.

For any patient-prescribed opioids, a bowel regimen should be concurrently prescribed or administered due to the common side effect of constipation with all opioids.

Buprenorphine—Partial-Agonist Opioids

Buprenorphine is a schedule III opioid with multiple formulations, historically categorized as a partial agonist (Table 17.4). It was initially approved by the US Food and Drug Administration (FDA) as an injectable formulation for the treatment of pain in 1981. In 2002, its sublingual (SL) formulation was approved for the treatment of OUD. Buprenorphine formulations for the treatment of OUD include SL buprenorphine and extended-release (XR) monthly and weekly SQ injections and are dosed in milligrams. Transdermal and buccal buprenorphine formulations are FDA approved for the treatment of pain in microgram doses. Buprenorphine formulations approved for pain management are available in doses much lower than buprenorphine formulations approved for the treatment of OUD and should not be used interchangeably. Transmucosal formulations are typically administered for analgesia in two to three doses per day. Transdermal formulations are also available, but have the disadvantage of a relatively slow onset for the treatment of acute pain. For continuous pain or pain that is subacute, transdermal buprenorphine can be effective once it achieves steady state.

Over 70 randomized controlled trials have compared buprenorphine to other opioids for the treatment of acute pain.[73] A 2025 systematic review and meta-analysis of RCTs comparing buprenorphine to other opioids for acute postoperative pain in adults found significantly reduced pain intensity and rescue analgesia in the buprenorphine-treated group.[74] There is increasing enthusiasm for the use of buprenorphine as a front-line opioid to manage acute pain in opioid non-dependent patients given its efficacy and safety advantages compared with full agonists. It may also be an attractive option in non-opioid dependent patients with SUD (including OUD), given its reduced abuse potential. Its potential role in the acute pain management of patients with active OUD or on MOUD is not yet clear.

Nonpharmacologic Treatments

Pain is mediated by multiple factors such as mood, expectations, and emotional distress. A component of effective multimodal acute pain treatment entails helping patients proactively understand and address how these factors impact their pain. Nonpharmacologic (NP) treatments are one way to help them do this. NP treatments for pain encompass a wide range of modalities sometimes considered "complementary" or "alternative." This section introduces NP therapies for acute pain, some of which can be utilized in the hospital setting and some that are more appropriate for referral at hospital discharge. Hospital-based pain management is often primarily focused on acute pain, as medical illnesses, injuries, and procedures are inherent to the indications for hospitalization. However, it is exceedingly evident to those practicing in hospitals that many patients suffer from chronic pain that may be exacerbated during hospitalization. Moreover, in situations of high distress, it can be difficult to distinguish between these temporal (ie, acute or chronic), etiologic (eg, distention, infection, migraine, anxiety), as well as mechanistic (eg, neuropathic, nociceptive, nociplastic, etc) categories of pain. Fortunately, many NP treatments may in part be "transdiagnostic," in that the potential effects address multiple forms of pain and distress.

These NP treatments are appealing due to their low cost, low risk of adverse events, target of a different—and perhaps more relevant—pathologic mediator or modifier of pain/distress, active, patient-centered approach to pain treatment, and lack of the need for a prescribing professional. The latter factor is less important in the hospital setting (with abundant clinicians who can place orders), but it implies a greater diversity of staff (eg, social workers, psychologists, students, etc) who can be enlisted to administer interventions.

There is a paucity of data specific to hospitalized patients or patients with SUD regarding NP interventions. However, the literature on pain includes many potential modalities that can be extrapolated to this patient population. Table 17.5 is a nonexhaustive list of interventions described in the literature that

TABLE 17.5

Selected Categories of Nonpharmacologic Pain Interventions With Examples and References

Category	Modality	Brief description	Selected evidence/comments
Brief psychotherapy/ skills training	Mindfulness-based cognitive therapy (MBCT)—brief exercises	A type of psychotherapy that combines aspects of cognitive therapy with mindfulness medication practices	Studies have suggested improvements in sleep, depressive symptoms, present pain intensity, self-efficacy, and mental quality of life among those with chronic pain.[75] A systematic review on pain treatments among cancer patients attested to this modality's effectiveness.[76] Brief exercises that could be accomplished in the hospital setting include 3-min breathing space and body scan.[77]
	Progressive muscle relaxation	A brief exercise, commonly included in dialectical behavioral therapy, of actively tensing and relaxing sequential muscle groups	It has shown beneficial effects in multiple sclerosis pain,[78] postsurgical pain,[79] chronic osteoarthritis,[80] low back pain during pregnancy,[81] and pain-related distress in terminal cancer.[82] A systematic review on pain treatments among cancer patients attested to this modality's effectiveness.[76]
	Acceptance and commitment therapy (ACT)—brief exercises	A type of psychotherapy that can include brief skill-building exercises focused on acceptance and flexible action toward values, in contrast to rigid avoidance of distressing thoughts and sensations	A systematic review suggested medium to large effects on chronic pain acceptance and psychological flexibility, smaller effects on functioning and depressive symptoms, and minimal/ no effects on quality of life and pain intensity.[83] Another synthesis of data suggested long-term beneficial effects on the psychological aspects of pain, including pain catastrophizing.[84] Brief exercises that could be accomplished in the hospital setting include *The ACT Matrix*[85] and *ACT metaphors*.[86]

(*continued*)

TABLE 17.5

Selected Categories of Nonpharmacologic Pain Interventions With Examples and References (*Continued*)

Category	Modality	Brief description	Selected evidence/comments
	Emotion and symptom focused engagement	A manualized intervention developed for patients with leukemia that provides supportive therapy based partly on trauma-focused cognitive therapy and early palliative care consultation triggered by moderate/ severe physical symptoms	A systematic review on pain treatments among cancer patients attested to this modality's effectiveness. In a phase II randomized trial, the treatment was associated with improvements in traumatic stress symptoms, pain intensity, and pain interference at various time points.[87] Application to hospitalized patients with SUD: approach the patient's condition with a recognition of the trauma of advanced illness and how that may contribute to both pain and substance cravings. Consider ordering palliative care consultation or outpatient referral when available and appropriate.
Complementary/ alternative/ integrative	Music therapy	An intervention that incorporates music within a therapeutic relationship to accomplish individualized goals	Music therapy receipt (compared to no receipt) resulted in lower pain and anxiety scores among surgical patients,[88] and a randomized trial of hospitalized patients with a palliative care consultation demonstrated effectiveness as well.[89]
	Acupuncture/ acupressure	A form of complementary medicine that involves pricking the skin (acupuncture) or manually applying pressure (acupressure) in specific anatomic locations, originating in traditional Chinese medicine	A systematic review and meta-analysis of 17 trials found that, compared with a sham intervention, acupuncture was associated with reduced pain intensity among those with cancer.[90]
	Hypnosis	A guided experience into an altered state of consciousness, focusing attention away from pain and discomfort	A systematic review and meta-analysis of 85 studies (mostly crossover trials) found analgesic effects for hypnosis, though strongly influenced by "hypnotic suggestibility" and "direct analgesic suggestion."[91] It has been specifically employed in the hospital for pain from labor,[92] major burns,[93] and minor surgical procedures.[94] A study of a 15-min session with hypnotic suggestion delivered by hospital social workers showed reduction in pain compared to psychoeducation.[95]
	Virtual reality	The use of immersive virtual environments to divert attention away from pain and its intensity	A systematic review in a gaming journal included 41 studies and suggested statistically significant differences in analgesia for both acute and chronic pain conditions.[96]

TABLE 17.5

Selected Categories of Nonpharmacologic Pain Interventions With Examples and References (*Continued*)

Category	Modality	Brief description	Selected evidence/comments
Physical therapy based	Stretching	Intentional elongation of muscle groups in a static or dynamic manner to promote flexibility and elasticity	A review article provided four take-aways: (1) acute stretching protocols have reported variable magnitude decreases in musculoskeletal and headache pain; (2) chronic stretching programs report consistent alleviation of pain; (3) mechanisms include several theories; (4) effects of stretching on delayed soreness are conflicting.[97]
	Cryotherapy or thermotherapy	The application of heat or cold (including ice) to a targeted area, generally with the intention of reducing inflammation and pain	In one comparison study, thermotherapy plus naproxen over 1 wk performed better than cryotherapy and control in treating acute low back pain.[98] Evidence for cryotherapy reducing pain after surgical procedures was classified as "moderate certainty" in a review of 34 studies.[99]
	Nerve stimulation via Transcutaneous electrical nerve stimulation (TENS)	A procedure in which electrodes placed on the skin give off an electric signal that stimulates nerve cells	A systematic review of three studies highlighted the lack of high-quality evidence to guide treatment, though one of the studies described TENS administered in emergency settings with resultant clinically worthwhile relief of low back pain.[100]
	Early therapy in emergency department	An emergency department–based intervention consisting of education, reassurance, pain management, mobility training, interferential therapy, walking training, and walking aids	Participants reported less pain intensity and greater satisfaction on discharge from the emergency department.[101]

may be relevant for treatment of pain in patients with SUD who are hospitalized.

This table lists a variety of types of NP interventions for pain covering various types of pain, various populations, and in various settings. Synthesizing the data for consideration of treatment in the hospital setting among patients with SUD may include the following:

- A trained staff member (eg, social worker or psychologist) can approach patients with severe acute pain to offer, in addition to their pharmacologic regimen, a menu of NP interventions. Brief and easily facilitated interventions for the hospital setting are mindfulness exercises, progressive muscle relaxation (see Table 17.5), and coping skills training.
- For those interested in additional, more targeted interventions, basic training in increasingly common psychotherapeutic modalities may be useful. Activities within Acceptance and Commitment Therapy such as the "ACT Matrix" can be feasibly employed to clarify values, decouple thoughts from identity and automatic actions, and brainstorm committed actions.[85] Hospital-based psychologists could utilize and implement these types of exercises as they relate to coping with pain.[102]
- Other NP interventions such as music therapy, acupuncture/acupressure, stretching, and cryotherapy or thermotherapy can be implemented in the hospital setting.
- Refer patients to outpatient resources including pain-focused psychotherapy, complementary and alternative medicine, and physical therapy. Other NP interventions after hospitalization such as yoga and massage may help with patient pain recovery as well.

Progressive Muscle Relaxation

This activity is designed to help reduce stress and some pain symptoms. Practicing multiple times per day can help patients become more aware of the feelings in their body and help the body relax. It can be administered by any clinician (including social workers or psychologists) at nearly any level of training (including students).

There are different ways to practice progressive muscle relaxation. See the text box for instructions on one method adapted from a Veterans Affairs "Whole Health" handout.[103] Patients can be seated or lying down when participating in the activity. Patients should avoid this activity if they are experiencing significant muscle spasms.

Progressive Muscle Relaxation Instructions[103]

Step 1: Inhale	Step 2: Take note	Step 3: Exhale	Step 4: Notice	Step 5: Move on
And tighten the muscles for approximately 5 s	Of how your body feels and what thoughts you have	And release the muscles for approximately 5 s	How your body and mind feel	To the next muscle group and repeat the steps

Muscle groups with instructions:

1. Hands: make fist and clench them
2. Arms (biceps): bend your elbows and tense up
3. Arms (triceps): straighten your arms and tighten the back of your arms
4. Shoulders: shrug your shoulders
5. Forehead: wrinkle your forehead
6. Eyes: close your eyes as tight as you can
7. Jaw: clench your jaw
8. Mouth: smile as big as you can
9. Neck: Move your chin down to your chest; on next breath look above your head
10. Lower back: arch your back away from the ground or chair
11. Abdomen/stomach: tighten your stomach muscles
12. Buttocks: Tighten your buttock muscles
13. Thighs: Tighten your thighs; this may cause your legs to come off the ground
14. Lower legs: Point your toes away from your head; on next breath point them toward you head

Concomitant Management of Pain and OUD

Management of Patients With OUD and Acute Pain Not Currently on OUD Treatment

Acute pain in the setting of OUD, particularly untreated OUD, is one of the most challenging clinical scenarios in hospital-based addiction treatment. It is challenging because the two conditions, pain and OUD, exacerbate each other and can cause significant distress for both the patient and the clinical team. Traditional approaches to pain treatment are generally inadequate in this population because the untreated OUD and high opioid tolerance overshadow most available pain treatments. For this reason, the approach to the treatment of acute pain and OUD must include the concomitant, simultaneous attention and treatment of both.

To treat both effectively, the clinician must understand opioid tolerance. When individuals with OUD enter the hospital, they are immediately not able to access their usual opioid supply which generally causes them to enter acute opioid withdrawal, a condition that is inherently painful and can increase existing acute pain and chronic pain syndromes. The abrupt missing opioid presence and subsequent opioid withdrawal can be understood as their "opioid debt." The opioid debt can be addressed or resolved, with the addition of high-potency opioids like methadone and buprenorphine for the treatment of OUD. Once their baseline opioid tolerance and acute withdrawal has been addressed, other pain treatment modalities can be added to address acute pain (Figure 17.7). See Chapter 7 for more information about the management of OUD and how to help patients who may not be interested to start methadone or buprenorphine.

For example, a patient with severe OUD using high doses of IV opioids per day is hospitalized with a broken femur. The patient's OUD could be addressed by starting oral methadone 50 mg/d. If the patient refuses methadone, other full-agonist opioids such as morphine or oxycodone can be used to treat their opioid withdrawal; buprenorphine could be an alternative for certain patients. The patient's acute pain can be addressed by starting scheduled acetaminophen, scheduled NSAID, full-agonist opioid such as oxycodone 15 mg every 4 hours as needed, elevation of the leg, and ice/heat as tolerated. Additional case examples can be found at the end of the chapter.

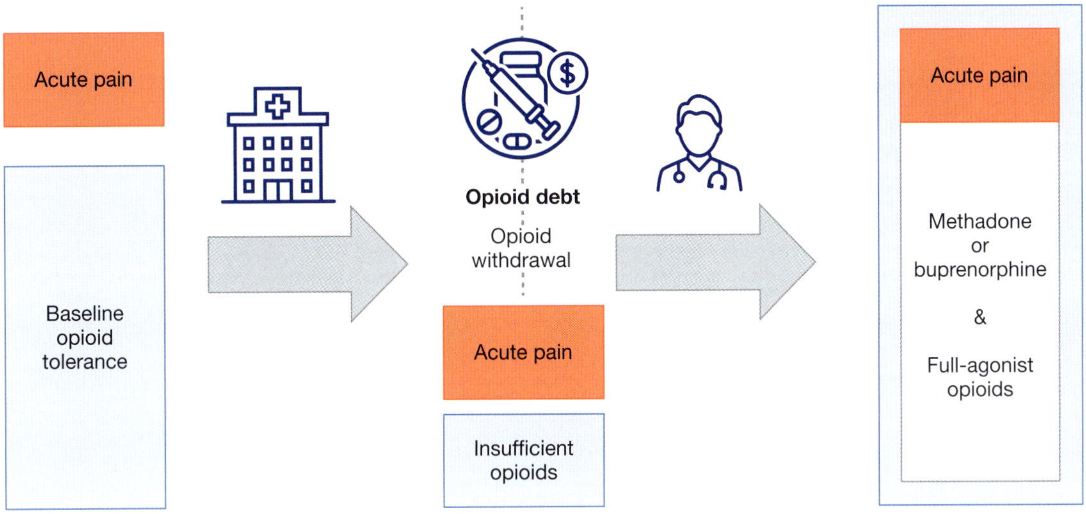

Figure 17.7: Schematic of how to address baseline opioid tolerance and acute pain in hospitalized individuals with OUD and acute pain.

Management of Patients With Acute Pain Receiving Methadone for OUD

Methadone is a full-opioid agonist indicated for both OUD treatment and pain treatment. There is limited evidence for the management of individuals with both acute pain and OUD treated with methadone.[44] Best practice based on expert opinion has always recommended continuation of methadone at the same or higher dose for individuals who have been prescribed methadone for the treatment of OUD. Methadone's duration of action for the treatment of OUD can last up to 120 hours which greatly exceeds its duration for analgesia (4 to 8 hours). Thus, when a patient with OUD is experiencing acute pain, they may benefit from divided doses of methadone into two or three doses throughout the day. However, empirical data to support this practice are lacking among patients with OUD, and the net benefit of splitting methadone doses for analgesic purposes in the hospital setting has been questioned.[104] One patient reported, "When I was on the…split methadone, first off the dose…wasn't high enough, but as soon as you guys split it on me, it made it almost ineffective completely."[104] Ultimately, whether and how to split a methadone dose should be a collaborative, patient-centered, and flexible decision. More data—particularly for those experiencing chronic pain—are being generated as of this writing.[105]

Consideration can also be given to increasing the daily methadone dose, particularly for patients who are using opioids in addition to methadone prior to hospitalization. The main purpose of methadone, however, should be to treat OUD and opioid withdrawal versus for analgesic purposes. Given the high opioid tolerance of patients with OUD, patients who are receiving methadone treatment may need higher doses of full-agonist opioids than patients without OUD. Therefore, for patients receiving methadone for OUD, patients will potentially need their methadone doses adjusted and will also need other medications and full-agonist opioids in addition to methadone to treat their acute pain.

In the operative setting and for patients who are not able to take oral intake, IV methadone can be used. The dose conversion is 2:1 oral to IV conversion (eg, 50 mg of oral methadone is 25 mg of IV methadone).

Clinicians should be aware of methadone's variable pharmacokinetics and potential for drug–drug interactions. For example, patients receiving rifampin and carbamazepine may have highly induced hepatic enzymes, resulting in faster metabolism of methadone.

Management of Patients With Acute Pain Receiving Buprenorphine Treatment for OUD

Buprenorphine formulations for the treatment of OUD include SL buprenorphine and XR monthly and weekly SQ injections; these formulations will be the focus of this section (Table 17.5).

In the setting of acute pain, multidisciplinary expert consensus and a systematic review of current literature

Preoperative period for all surgeries

- **Patient-centered discussion**
  - Discuss pain expectations and anticipated duration of pain
  - Discuss pain management goals including use of full agonist opioids
  - Discuss importance of multimodal approach to acute pain treatment
- **Address other substance use, if applicable**
  - Encourage smoking cessation or reduction
  - Manage and address any underlying concomitant substance use such as stimulant and alcohol use
  - Complete detoxification prior to surgery, if needed
  - If patient unable to abstain from other substances, offer a supportive and controlled environment before surgery
- **Advise patient to continue home dose of buprenorphine** without skipping doses or reducing buprenorphine dose
  - If patient receiving long-acting injectable buprenorphine, consider scheduling the surgery on day 21–28 of the injection
  - If patient is 28 d or more from the last injection, provide SL buprenorphine at equivalent dose during perioperative period
- **Consider a preoperative consultation with anesthesia**
  - Discuss regional anesthesia options like nerve blocks
  - Discuss intraoperative management options like IV methadone, IV infusion of ketamine, lidocaine or magnesium

Period of acute pain or day of procedure

- **Buprenorphine management**
  - Take buprenorphine dose the AM of surgery
  - Continue home dose of buprenorphine after the surgery even if patient is intubated
  - Consider buprenorphine split dosing to BID or TID after the surgery
  - If pain is poorly controlled despite multimodal treatment, consider an increase of buprenorphine (to 24–32 mg/d) OR a decrease (by 4–8 mg/d) of buprenorphine based on patient preference
  - Do not stop buprenorphine
- **Multimodal pain treatment**
  - *Maximize nonopioid analgesia*
    - If available and appropriate, consider regional anesthesia like nerve blocks
    - Schedule acetaminophen
    - Consider scheduling a nonsteroidal anti-inflammatory
    - Consider muscle relaxants (eg, tizanidine, cyclobenzaprine)
    - Consider antineuropathic agents (eg, gabapentin)
    - Avoid benzodiazepines and carisoprodol
    - Consider topical agents (eg, transdermal lidocaine)
    - For severe, refractory pain, consider ketamine infusion
  - *Full agonist opioids*
    - Offer as-needed oral opioids at higher dose (eg, oxycodone IR 10–15 mg q3–4h PRN severe pain, hydromorphone 4–6 mg q3–4h PRN severe pain)
    - Patient controlled analgesia may be an alternative option for severe pain in patient who can't tolerate oral meds
  - *Nonpharmacologic management*
    - Ice or heat, position changes, relaxation strategies, distraction, music, peer recovery

Preparing for hospital discharge

- Continue buprenorphine and resume home or increased dose
- Schedule time to resume long-acting buprenorphine and continue SL buprenorphine at equivalent dose until buprenorphine injection is obtained
- Ensure adequate pain control with oral analgesics
- Whenever possible, taper full agonist opioids prior to discharge
- If discharging with opioid prescription, provide a taper plan and warm handoff to the outpatient prescriber
- Discharge with naloxone
- Discuss family or friend support

Figure 17.8: Recommendations for perioperative buprenorphine and pain management for patients prescribed sublingual or injectable buprenorphine. (Adapted from Sandhu S, Calcaterra SL. How Do I Manage Acute Pain for Patients Prescribed Buprenorphine for Opioid Use Disorder? *NEJM Evid.* 2024;3(5). PMID: 38815158; PMCID: PMC11282871; Kohan L, Barreveld A, Potru S, Abd-Elsayed A, Viscusi ER. Narrative review: Managing buprenorphine and opioid use disorder in the perioperative setting. *Pain Pract.* 2025;25:e13427.)

support buprenorphine continuation throughout the period of acute pain, including in the perioperative setting (Figure 17.8).[42–44,106] Compared to buprenorphine discontinuation in the acute pain period, continuation of buprenorphine results in improved pain-related outcomes such as reduced pain intensity and reduced full-agonist opioid dose. Discontinuation of buprenorphine during the acute pain period causes opioid withdrawal, increased pain, and places patients at high risk for return to unprescribed opioid use. There is uncertainty if buprenorphine SL doses >16 mg/d should be reduced in the perioperative period; the theoretical rationale of this reduction would be to increase mu opioid receptor availability while maintaining therapeutic effect though the clinical benefit of this is disputed. Given the high risk for return to unprescribed opioid use as well as high risk for causing opioid withdrawal, buprenorphine doses are generally not recommended to be reduced from patient's home doses in the acute pain or perioperative setting. There are no robust prospective data to support the need for dose adjustments or down titration of buprenorphine in the perioperative period. Figure 17.8 illustrates recommendations for management of acute pain in the perioperative setting focusing on continuation of patient's usual buprenorphine dose and use of multimodal treatments.

Like methadone, buprenorphine's duration of action for the treatment of OUD exceeds its duration for analgesia. Thus, dividing a patient's daily buprenorphine dose into multiple doses throughout the day, with or without overall dose increases, may improve analgesia in the setting of acute pain. The choice to divide the buprenorphine dose should be a patient-centered, flexible decision. Importantly, the patient's baseline buprenorphine dose should be considered a home MOUD rather than as an analgesic for acute pain management. If opioids are required for additional analgesia while individuals are on buprenorphine treatment, they should be offered full-agonist opioids in doses approximately two to three times those used for opioid-naïve patients, given their opioid tolerance.[107] In general, high-affinity full agonists such as hydromorphone and fentanyl are safe and effective to be concomitantly provided in addition to buprenorphine. Many patients also receive benefit from higher doses of oxycodone over shorter time periods, that is, every 3 to 4 hours as needed.

Similarly, there is little to guide management of patient-prescribed XR-buprenorphine anticipating pain management (eg, elective surgery). For patients on XR-buprenorphine anticipating elective surgery likely to result in moderate or greater pain, it is reasonable to schedule surgery around day 20 to 28 after the injection. For patients in a steady state on XR-buprenorphine formulations, predicted median plasma concentrations are expected to stay above 2 ng/mL, a concentration at which both opioid withdrawal and subjective effects of exogenous opioids are controlled, for over 1 month

TABLE 17.6

Equivalent Doses Between SL and XR-Buprenorphine Formulations[109,110]

Dose SL buprenorphine	C_{avg} (ng/mL)[a]	Equivalent dose Brixadi® Q1Wk	Equivalent dose Brixadi® Q4Wk	C_{avg} (ng/mL)	Equivalent dose Sublocade® Q4Wk	C_{avg} (ng/mL)
2–6 mg	Not reported (NR)	8 mg	Not applicable (N/A)	N/A	N/A	N/A
8–10 mg	1.37	16 mg	64 mg	NR	100 mg	3.21
12–16 mg	1.79	24 mg	96 mg	NR	100 mg	3.21
18–24 mg	2.16	32 mg	128 mg	3.89	300 mg	6.54
26–32 mg	2.84		160 mg	5.27	300 mg	6.54

[a]C_{avg} (ng/mL) represents average concentration of buprenorphine in the plasma at steady state.

(Table 17.6).[108] Given the very long half-life, patients can be reassured that therapeutic levels of buprenorphine will be maintained for the treatment of OUD. Multimodal analgesics, including short-acting opioids, can and should be utilized per above to provide additional pain treatment.[107]

Management of Patients With Acute Pain and Naltrexone Treatment for OUD

Naltrexone is an opioid antagonist which blocks the mu-opioid receptor. It is FDA approved for the treatment of alcohol use disorder and OUD. A therapeutic naltrexone level in patients on either oral or XR naltrexone will severely limit the effect of opioid analgesia. Thus, if an acute pain episode is anticipated (eg, in case of elective surgery expected to require opioids), naltrexone should be held preoperatively.

For oral naltrexone, which has a 10-hour half-life,[111] most recommendations suggest holding naltrexone 72-hours before the procedure. For emergent acute pain scenarios in patients within that 72-hour window, a multimodal strategy prioritizing non-opioids is likely to achieve the best outcomes.

For XR naltrexone, which results in a higher plasma concentration than oral naltrexone and a 5- to 10-day half-life,[112] the ability to overcome mu-opioid receptor antagonism develops in the fourth week after the injection.[113] Thus, most recommendations are to schedule surgeries expected to require opioids at least 30 days after the most recent XR naltrexone injection. Oral naltrexone can be used as a bridge depending on the timing of the surgery and then held 72 hours before the procedure. For emergent acute pain scenarios in patients within the 4-week XR naltrexone windows, a multimodal strategy prioritizing non-opioids is likely to achieve the best outcomes. If opioids are needed, consultation with anesthesia is advised in these situations.

Multidisciplinary Approach to the Treatment of Complex Pain

A multidisciplinary approach for complex pain management allows for effective collaboration to provide the best care possible to patients with concomitant pain and SUD or OUD. This section outlines various hospital-based specialists and how they can support hospitalized patients with acute pain and SUD.

Addiction Medicine Consultation

Addiction medicine trained clinicians can assist with pain evaluation and treatment of individuals with SUD and pain by helping to treat the SUD and any associated withdrawal syndromes and facilitate treatment. In addition, by completing a full SUD history, they can help establish the patient's baseline opioid tolerance and other psychosocial factors that may mediate the patient's pain. In many instances, they can guide the primary team toward safe and effective doses of analgesic medications like opioids, recognizing that individuals with OUD may need higher opioid doses for beneficial effect than opioid-naïve patients. Addiction medicine consultation teams may have other individuals on the team such as social workers or peer recovery specialists who can support patients through the challenges of hospitalization.

Anesthesia/Acute Pain Consultation

Anesthesiologists typically comprise hospital-based "Acute Pain Services." They possess an understanding of routine analgesics including contraindications, pharmacokinetics and dynamics, and may offer less routine interventions (eg, continuous lidocaine and ketamine infusions, postoperative regional blocks). They also have special expertise in postoperative pain.

Enhanced recovery after surgery (ERAS) pathways aim to improve patient recoveries after major surgery by implementing evidence-based practices across the perioperative care period. For health care systems with such pathways, anesthesiologists will be familiar with the treatments that can be drawn upon in the management of pain for individuals with SUD. While focused on a surgical population, a key foundation of ERAS is to improve overall outcomes by improving pain management and minimizing opioid adverse effects. For example, an ERAS pathway may include protocolizing a multimodal analgesia strategy that begins in the preoperative phase (eg, oral celecoxib and acetaminophen before surgery), employment of regional/neuraxial techniques when appropriate, standing non-opioid analgesics in recovery, and early ambulation. Standardizing and targeting interventions known to be most effective for pain management improves patient outcomes. In addition, for patients on medications for OUD presenting for elective or emergent surgery, anesthesiologists should be part of a multimodal team that develops a perioperative management strategy for this population.

Interventional Pain Consultation Service

In addition to being expert in devices increasingly seen in individuals with chronic pain (eg, spinal cord stimulators, intrathecal pumps), there is enthusiasm to apply typical outpatient chronic pain interventions to the acute inpatient pain setting to improve outcomes.[114] For example, these physicians may be able to offer radiofrequency ablation, cryoneurolysis, neuromodulation, and botulinum toxin or trigger point injections. They may also offer nerve blocks that can relieve pain in the case of abdominal visceral pain often seen in malignancy (eg, celiac plexus block in pancreatic cancer).

Pharmacists

Pharmacists possess a common understanding of routine and nonroutine analgesics including contraindications, pharmacokinetics and dynamics, drug–drug interactions, and relevant order sets. Pharmacists also have knowledge of the hospital formulary and are in a unique position to provide medication reconciliation including at the time of discharge.

Psychology/Mental Health Specialists

Some hospitals have access to psychologists, psychiatrists, or other staff trained in psychotherapy, which has a robust and growing literature supporting its use for pain-related distress and coping. If they have sufficient capacity, these mental health professionals can employ brief interventions (see "Nonpharmacologic Treatments" section) and supportive therapy, in addition to pharmacologic, procedural, and other adjunctive modalities.

Nursing

Nurses are expert in routine pain assessment tools, are often the key communicator to patient and family including of any required teaching and may possess unique insights into patient's home circumstances (ie, home life, supports, etc). When treating individuals with pain and SUD, it is important to include nursing in all treatment planning and strategies because they spend the most time with the patient and may have important information to share about the patient's experience.

Other

Surgery is frequently the inciting cause for acute pain. For example, 36% of persons who inject substances presenting to the hospital with infection underwent surgery during the admission.[115] Surgeons often play a key leadership role in multidisciplinary management, including frequently being the primary admitting team. Surgeons should therefore have a strong working relationship with local resources available to assist in managing this patient population (ie, acute pain service, addiction consult services, pharmacy). Surgeons will also play a key leadership role in any hospital ERAS pathway, which as above may be drawn upon as an example of standardizing best pain practices.

Physical therapy, occupational therapy, and palliative care may also contribute to effective multimodal pain treatment for individuals with pain and SUD. See Chapter 18 for more information on the role of palliative care in individuals with SUD.

Emerging Evidence

The first new class of analgesics in decades was approved by the FDA in January 2025. Suzetrigine is a nonopioid medication that inhibits a unique sodium channel involved in pain signaling. Two phase 2 trials reported its analgesic efficacy among patients undergoing abdominoplasty and bunionectomy procedures, finding that high-dose suzetrigine was superior to placebo and equivalent to hydrocodone-acetaminophen.[116] The manufacturer has reported that suzetrigine is "without evidence of addictive potential," implying its possible utility as an analgesic among those with or at risk for a SUD.[117]

Case Examples of Acute Pain in Setting of SUD

Case 1: Patient With Acute Pain and Alcohol Use Disorder

Mr. S is a 36-year-old man with a past medical history of severe alcohol use disorder (AUD), hypertension, and severe pancreatitis complicated by necrotizing pancreatitis. He returns to the hospital due to severe, unrelenting pain (10/10) and inability to tolerate oral intake. His initial presentation for pancreatitis occurred 2 months ago and over the last 2 months he has had 2 necrosectomies. His last necrosectomy was 1 week ago. He has lost approximately 35 lb in the last 2 months. He describes the pain as unrelenting, stabbing, sharp, and burning, and located in his epigastric region. He has effectively been treated with oral oxycodone 15 mg every 4 hours, but his primary care clinician refused to continue prescribing this to him and he ran out of the medication 3 days ago. The primary clinician cited concerns about his AUD and thinking his dose of oxycodone was too high. He is not eligible for any interventional pain treatments. He has not been able to locate other outpatient pain resources or treatment.

He is seen by addiction medicine who diagnoses him with severe AUD, in early remission since his diagnosis of severe pancreatitis. This diagnosis is confirmed by his family and biomarker screening (eg, PEth) which is negative. After his last hospitalization, the patient took oxycodone as prescribed, but reported it was not effective at times and he sometimes vomited right after taking it. He presents with diaphoresis and irritability consistent with opioid withdrawal from not having his oral oxycodone for the last 3 days. His goal is to resume oral oxycodone. The addiction medicine clinician did not find any signs or symptoms of misuse of his opioid medication, and he expectedly has opioid withdrawal from abruptly running out of his oxycodone prescription. The patient is open to other modalities of effective pain treatment.

This patient has severe acute-on-chronic necrotizing pancreatitis, nausea and vomiting, poor nutrition and oral intake, severe AUD in early remission, and opioid withdrawal from abrupt cessation of prescribed opioids. Treatment includes starting standing acetaminophen 1,000 mg three times a day, gabapentin 300 mg three times a day, buprenorphine transdermal patch 10 mcg, as needed oxycodone 10 mg every 4 hours for severe pain, and as needed clonidine for opioid withdrawal symptoms. The patient stabilizes over the next 3 days and is discharged with acetaminophen, gabapentin, and the transdermal buprenorphine patch. A transdermal buprenorphine patch was an ideal choice for him because he has ongoing nausea and vomiting, he does not have high opioid tolerance, and he is expected to have this pain for the next 3 to 6 months. He is referred to mutual support for AUD, outpatient AUD treatment, and a new primary care clinician who has agreed to see him to manage his pain. He elects not to start medication for AUD due to his other medical conditions but is open to this in the future. He will continue to follow up with gastroenterology for ongoing treatment of his severe pancreatitis.

Case 2: Patient With a History of Severe OUD in Remission Presenting for Major Surgery

Mr. J is a 62-year-old man with a past medical history of non–insulin-dependent diabetes mellitus, anxiety, depression, chronic low back pain, severe OUD in sustained remission, AUD in sustained remission, presenting for total knee arthroplasty (TKA) in the setting of severe, debilitating osteoarthritis. His only home analgesic is topical diclofenac.

His OUD history is recognized during review of his chart because he has a "narcotic allergy." The patient recalls how opioids "ruined [his] life," and that he has been in sustained recovery (from OUD and AUD) for over a decade. He denies prior treatment with medications for OUD but is aware of the potential benefits of methadone and buprenorphine.

The anesthesiologist is concerned that the patient has multiple established risk factors for poorly controlled acute postoperative pain: anxiety, depression, history of SUD, and chronic pain. He is also concerned because the patient will undergo a surgery expected to result in severe pain. The anesthesiologist explains to the patient that despite the usual plan for multimodal analgesia, there is essentially a universal need for some opioid analgesics after TKA. He also explains that some commonly administered perioperative medications, for example, benzodiazepines for anxiolysis, may be evocative of the positive reinforcing effects of alcohol and opioids. The patient's overwhelming priority is accomplishment of the surgery, and he is confident that he can manage pain, whether or not management eventually includes opioids, without destabilizing his remission.

The anesthesiologist suggests buprenorphine as a reasonable option for acute perioperative pain management, in addition to a multimodal strategy. He explains its strong evidence for efficacy for this indication, and improved safety profile including reduced euphorigenic effects, and that at a minimum it should reduce the need for other full-agonist opioids. The patient, based on his prior knowledge of buprenorphine by reputation, states that "it doesn't really get you high."

Premedication is given with 1-g oral acetaminophen, 400-mg oral celecoxib, 300-mcg IV buprenorphine, a single-shot adductor canal regional block was performed using 0.5% ropivacaine with 50-mcg dexmedetomidine added to prolong the sensory block. He receives a spinal anesthetic, which is typical for TKA. For sedation, he receives propofol infusion. Early in the case, he receives a 0.1-mg/kg dose of IV dexamethasone and a subanesthetic dose of IV 0.5-mg/kg ketamine, both intended to decrease postoperative pain. Prior to surgical closure, the surgeon injects the joint with 0.2% ropivacaine.

The patient undergoes an uneventful PACU recovery, with pain remaining minimal after resolution of the spinal block. He receives a standard postoperative order set, which included standing acetaminophen and ketorolac, as needed rescue full-agonist opioids, and the addition of 450-mcg buccal buprenorphine twice daily. His pain was well controlled on the floor, with a mean numerical rating score of 2.5/10. He receives no opioids other than buprenorphine. He is discharged on postoperative day 1. He requests no opioids be prescribed at discharge, including buprenorphine and has an uneventful outpatient recovery.

Case 3: Patient With Acute Pain and Long-Term Use of Prescribed Opioids for Chronic Low Back Pain

Mr. N is a 66-year-old man with a past medical history of hypertension, insulin-dependent diabetes, treated hepatitis C, hyperlipidemia, depression, tobacco use disorder in remission, alcohol use disorder in sustained remission, and long-term use of opioids for chronic low back pain. He presents to the emergency department (ED) with worsening dyspnea.

In the ED, the patient is found to be in rapid atrial fibrillation with an elevated brain natriuretic peptide and chest x-ray findings consistent with pulmonary edema. He endorses adherence with prescribed medications including metoprolol, atorvastatin, apixaban, and oxycodone 5 to 10 mg every 3 to 4 hours as needed for pain. On exam he is found to have a diabetic foot ulcer without signs or symptoms of systemic infection, and of which he had been unaware. He is admitted for medical management.

His dyspnea rapidly improves with rate control and diuresis on the day of admission. He is continued on his home medications, including opioids. On the morning of the second day of his admission, exacerbation of his baseline low back pain becomes his chief complaint, rated as 10/10 and unbearable. He appears restless, diaphoretic, and nauseous. 1-g oral acetaminophen, 15-mg IV ketorolac, 10-mg oral oxycodone, and 0.2-mg IV hydromorphone are given, which improve his symptoms. A stat CT was performed given the apparent acute onset and severity of the pain, which showed no significant change from a recent study. His outpatient neurosurgeon confirmed a diagnosis of postlaminectomy syndrome and suggests no further interventional treatments. An acute pain consult is placed. On further questioning by the acute pain service, the patient endorses regularly taking opioids prescribed to his wife, an estimated 120-daily MME. His pain is consistent in character with his baseline pain and he is diagnosed with opioid withdrawal. A Clinical Opioid Withdrawal Scale (COWS) is initiated, and he is started on standing acetaminophen, NSAIDs, and prescribed opioids to approximate his home dose.

On the second inpatient day, the patient feels "basically back to normal." At morning rounds he asked the medicine team, "Is there anything we can do about the pain meds?" On further discussion, he expressed significant distress about taking oxycodone, in particular how it had created stress in his home as his wife had reluctantly continued filling oxycodone prescriptions for his use, which were prescribed after a routine surgery several months ago. He is diagnosed with moderate OUD. The team discusses treatment options for OUD and he chooses buprenorphine. He chooses a traditional transition to buprenorphine by stopping his oxycodone at 10 PM that evening and starting buprenorphine/naloxone SL the next morning. His pain remarkably improves, and he is able to discharge from the hospital.

Case 4: Patient With Acute Pain and Untreated OUD

Ms. H is a 36-year-old female with a past medical history of hepatitis C, tobacco use disorder, and severe OUD. She is admitted for a large abscess on her right forearm requiring incision and drainage. She has been using at least 15 to 20 bags of IV opioids prior to hospitalization. She also typically smokes crack cocaine two to three times a day. She is interested in methadone treatment for OUD and is very worried about the potential pain from the surgical procedure. She is currently scoring a 12 on the COWS consistent with mild opioid withdrawal.

To stabilize her OUD and pain, she is started on methadone 40 mg oral once. To stabilize her pain, she is given ketorolac 30 mg IV, acetaminophen 1,000 mg, and oxycodone 20 mg. After 3 hours, the patient reports a pain score of 7/10 and appears uncomfortable. She is given a dose of methadone 10 mg and reports a pain score of 5/10 after 1 hour. She stabilizes on methadone which is titrated up over her 72-hour hospitalization and a combination of NSAIDs, acetaminophen, and oxycodone 15 mg every 4 hours as needed.

REFERENCES

1. Finley CR, Chan DS, Garrison S, et al. What are the most common conditions in primary care? Systematic review. *Can Fam Physician*. 2018;64(11):832–840.
2. Cordell WH, Keene KK, Giles BK, Jones JB, Jones JH, Brizendine EJ. The high prevalence of pain in emergency medical care. *Am J Emerg Med*. 2002;20(3):165–169.

3. Deng LX, Patel K, Miaskowski C, et al. Prevalence and characteristics of moderate to severe pain among hospitalized older adults. *J Am Geriatr Soc.* 2018;66(9):1744–1751.
4. Lin LY, Hung TC, Lai YH. Pain control and related factors in hospitalized patients. *Medicine (Baltimore).* 2021;100(30): e26768.
5. John WS, Wu LT. Chronic non-cancer pain among adults with substance use disorders: prevalence, characteristics, and association with opioid overdose and healthcare utilization. *Drug Alcohol Depend.* 2020;209:107902.
6. Schoenfeld A, Geiger J, Princic N, et al. EE359 economic burden of managing acute and chronic pain in the United States: national estimates from 2022 data. *Value in Health.* 2024;27(6):S123–S124.
7. Gaskin DJ, Richard P. The economic costs of pain in the United States. *J Pain.* 2012;13(8):715–724.
8. Li M, Peterson C, Xu L, Mikosz CA, Luo F. Medical costs of substance use disorders in the us employer-sponsored insurance population. *JAMA Netw Open.* 2023;6(1):e2252378.
9. Raja SN, Carr DB, Cohen M, et al. The revised International Association for the Study of Pain definition of pain: concepts, challenges, and compromises. *Pain.* 2020;161(9): 1976–1982.
10. Boezaart AP, Smith CR, Chembrovich S, et al. Visceral versus somatic pain: an educational review of anatomy and clinical implications. *Reg Anesth Pain Med.* 2021;46(7):629–636.
11. Kosek E, Clauw D, Nijs J, et al. Chronic nociplastic pain affecting the musculoskeletal system: clinical criteria and grading system. *Pain.* 2021;162(11):2629–2634.
12. Maixner W, Fillingim RB, Williams DA, Smith SB, Slade GD. Overlapping chronic pain conditions: implications for diagnosis and classification. *J Pain.* 2016;17(9 Suppl):T93–T107.
13. Johnston KJA, Signer R, Huckins LM. Chronic overlapping pain conditions and nociplastic pain. *HGG Adv.* 2025;6(1): 100381.
14. Yang J, Jung M, Picco L, et al. Pain in people seeking and receiving opioid agonist treatment: a systematic review and meta-analysis of prevalence and correlates. *Addiction.* 2024; 119(11):1879–1901.
15. Morasco BJ, Gritzner S, Lewis L, Oldham R, Turk DC, Dobscha SK. Systematic review of prevalence, correlates, and treatment outcomes for chronic non-cancer pain in patients with comorbid substance use disorder. *Pain.* 2011;152(3): 488–497.
16. Zhang X, Wang N, Hou F, et al. Emergency department visits by patients with substance use disorder in the United States. *West J Emerg Med.* 2021;22(5):1076–1085.
17. Merrill JO, Rhodes LA, Deyo RA, Marlatt GA, Bradley KA. Mutual mistrust in the medical care of drug users: the keys to the "narc" cabinet. *J Gen Intern Med.* 2002;17(5):327–333.
18. St Marie B. Health care experiences when pain and substance use disorder coexist: "just because I'm an addict doesn't mean I don't have pain." *Pain Med.* 2014;15(12):2075–2086.
19. Morgan BD. Knowing how to play the game: hospitalized substance abusers' strategies for obtaining pain relief. *Pain Manag Nurs.* 2006;7(1):31–41.
20. Summers PJ, Hellman JL, MacLean MR, Rees VW, Wilkes MS. Negative experiences of pain and withdrawal create barriers to abscess care for people who inject heroin. a mixed methods analysis. *Drug Alcohol Depend.* 2018;190:200–208.
21. Compton P, Aronowitz SV, Klusaritz H, Anderson E. Acute pain and self-directed discharge among hospitalized patients with opioid-related diagnoses: a cohort study. *Harm Reduct J.* 2021;18(1):131.
22. Southern WN, Nahvi S, Arnsten JH. Increased risk of mortality and readmission among patients discharged against medical advice. *Am J Med.* 2012;125(6):594–602.
23. Velez CM, Nicolaidis C, Korthuis PT, Englander H. "It's been an experience, a life learning experience": a qualitative study of hospitalized patients with substance use disorders. *J Gen Intern Med.* 2017;32(3):296–303.
24. Bogdanowicz KM, Stewart R, Chang CK, et al. Excess overdose mortality immediately following transfer of patients and their care as well as after cessation of opioid substitution therapy. *Addiction.* 2018;113(5):946–951.
25. van den Beuken-van Everdingen MH, de Rijke JM, Kessels AG, Schouten HC, van Kleef M, Patijn J. Prevalence of pain in patients with cancer: a systematic review of the past 40 years. *Ann Oncol.* 2007;18(9):1437–1449.
26. Compton P, Chang YP. Substance abuse and addiction: implications for pain management in patients with cancer. *Clin J Oncol Nurs.* 2017;21(2):203–209.
27. Gan TJ, Habib AS, Miller TE, White W, Apfelbaum JL. Incidence, patient satisfaction, and perceptions of post-surgical pain: results from a US national survey. *Curr Med Res Opin.* 2014;30(1):149–160.
28. Yang MMH, Hartley RL, Leung AA, et al. Preoperative predictors of poor acute postoperative pain control: a systematic review and meta-analysis. *BMJ Open.* 2019;9(4):e025091.
29. Costelloe C, Burns S, Yong RJ, Kaye AD, Urman RD. An analysis of predictors of persistent postoperative pain in spine surgery. *Curr Pain Headache Rep.* 2020;24(4):11.
30. Brummett CM, Waljee JF, Goesling J, et al. New persistent opioid use after minor and major surgical procedures in US adults. *JAMA Surg.* 2017;152(6):e170504.
31. He S, Renne A, Argandykov D, Convissar D, Lee J. Comparison of an emoji-based visual analog scale with a numeric rating scale for pain assessment. *JAMA.* 2022;328(2): 208–209.
32. Turk DC, Melzack R, eds. *Handbook of Pain Assessment.* 3rd ed. The Guilford Press; 2011:xvii, 542-xvii, 542.
33. Krebs EE, Lorenz KA, Bair MJ, et al. Development and initial validation of the PEG, a three-item scale assessing pain intensity and interference. *J Gen Intern Med.* 2009;24(6): 733–738.
34. Tan G, Jensen MP, Thornby JI, Shanti BF. Validation of the brief pain inventory for chronic nonmalignant pain. *J Pain.* 2004;5(2):133–137.
35. Campbell P, Hill JC, Protheroe J, et al. Keele aches and pains study protocol: validity, acceptability, and feasibility of the Keele STarT MSK tool for subgrouping musculoskeletal patients in primary care. *J Pain Res.* 2016;9:807–818.
36. Bush K, Kivlahan DR, McDonell MB, Fihn SD, Bradley KA. The AUDIT alcohol consumption questions (AUDIT-C): an effective brief screening test for problem drinking. Ambulatory Care Quality Improvement Project (ACQUIP). Alcohol use disorders identification test. *Arch Intern Med.* 1998;158(16):1789–1795.
37. McNeely J, Wu LT, Subramaniam G, et al. Performance of the Tobacco, Alcohol, Prescription Medication, and Other Substance Use (TAPS) Tool for substance use screening in primary care patients. *Ann Intern Med.* 2016;165(10): 690–699.
38. Daneshvar HTJ, Stahl N, Mullins K, Morford K, Chan CA. #8 Back to Basics: A Stigma-Free History with Dr Jeanette Tetrault. *The Curbsiders Addiction Medicine Podcast.* Accessed March 11, 2026. https://thecurbsiders.com/addiction-medicine-podcast/8-back-to-basics-a-stigma-free-history
39. *Diagnostic and Statistical Manual of Mental Disorders DSM-5-TR.* 5th ed. American Psychiatric Association Publishing; 2022:lxix, 1050.
40. Kroenke K, Spitzer RL, Williams JB. The patient health questionnaire-2: validity of a two-item depression screener. *Med Care.* 2003;41(11):1284–1292.

41. Kroenke K, Spitzer RL, Williams JB, Monahan PO, Löwe B. Anxiety disorders in primary care: prevalence, impairment, comorbidity, and detection. *Ann Intern Med.* 2007;146:317–325.
42. Dickerson DM, Mariano ER, Szokol JW, et al. Multiorganizational consensus to define guiding principles for perioperative pain management in patients with chronic pain, preoperative opioid tolerance, or substance use disorder. *Reg Anesth Pain Med.* 2024;49(10):716–724.
43. Vadeghani AT, Grant M, Forget P. Perioperative pain management interventions in opioid user patients: an overview of reviews. *BMC Anesthesiol.* 2024;24(1):310.
44. Buonora MJ, Mackey K, Khalid L, et al. Acute pain management in people with opioid use disorder: a systematic review. *Ann Intern Med.* 2025;178(4):558–570.
45. Rostamipoor Z, Nazemi-Rafi M, Mirafzal A, Ilka S, Hosseininasab M. Effect of oral clonidine on pain reduction in patients with opioid use disorder in the emergency department: a randomized clinical trial. *Br J Clin Pharmacol.* 2024; 90(12):3003–3009.
46. Afzalimoghaddam M, Edalatifard M, Nejati A, Momeni M, Isavi N, Karimialavijeh E. Midazolam plus haloperidol as adjuvant analgesics to morphine in opium dependent patients: a randomized clinical trial. *Curr Drug Abuse Rev.* 2016;9(2): 142–147.
47. Sahmeddini MA, Khosravi MB, Farbood A. Comparison of perioperative systemic lidocaine or systemic ketamine in acute pain management of patients with opioid use disorder after orthopedic surgery. *J Addict Med.* 2019;13(3):220–226.
48. Chou R, Gordon DB, de Leon-Casasola OA, et al. Management of postoperative pain: a clinical practice guideline from the American Pain Society, the American Society of Regional Anesthesia and Pain Medicine, and the American Society of Anesthesiologists' Committee on Regional Anesthesia, Executive Committee, and Administrative Council. *J Pain.* 2016;17(2):131–157.
49. Hsu JR, Mir H, Wally MK, Seymour RB. Clinical practice guidelines for pain management in acute musculoskeletal injury. *J Orthop Trauma.* 2019;33(5):e158–e182.
50. Moore RA, Derry S, Aldington D, Wiffen PJ. Single dose oral analgesics for acute postoperative pain in adults—an overview of Cochrane reviews. *Cochrane Database Syst Rev.* 2015;2015(9):CD008659.
51. Marti F, Lindner G, Ravioli S. Resistance to local anaesthetics: a literature review. *Br J Anaesth.* 2022;129(2):e43–e45.
52. Weibel S, Jelting Y, Pace NL, et al. Continuous intravenous perioperative lidocaine infusion for postoperative pain and recovery in adults. *Cochrane Database Syst Rev.* 2018;6(6): CD009642.
53. Giovannitti JA Jr, Thoms SM, Crawford JJ. Alpha-2 adrenergic receptor agonists: a review of current clinical applications. *Anesth Prog.* 2015;62(1):31–39.
54. Blaudszun G, Lysakowski C, Elia N, Tramèr MR. Effect of perioperative systemic α2 agonists on postoperative morphine consumption and pain intensity: systematic review and meta-analysis of randomized controlled trials. *Anesthesiology.* 2012;116(6):1312–1322.
55. Sanchez Munoz MC, De Kock M, Forget P. What is the place of clonidine in anesthesia? Systematic review and meta-analyses of randomized controlled trials. *J Clin Anesth.* 2017;38:140–153.
56. Jessen Lundorf L, Korvenius Nedergaard H, Møller AM. Perioperative dexmedetomidine for acute pain after abdominal surgery in adults. *Cochrane Database Syst Rev.* 2016;2(2): CD010358.
57. Habibi V, Kiabi FH, Sharifi H. The effect of dexmedetomidine on the acute pain after cardiothoracic surgeries: a systematic review. *Braz J Cardiovasc Surg.* 2018;33(4):404–417.
58. Wang X, Liu N, Chen J, Xu Z, Wang F, Ding C. Effect of intravenous dexmedetomidine during general anesthesia on acute postoperative pain in adults: a systematic review and meta-analysis of randomized controlled trials. *Clin J Pain.* 2018;34(12):1180–1191.
59. Gupta A, Devi LA, Gomes I. Potentiation of μ-opioid receptor-mediated signaling by ketamine. *J Neurochem.* 2011; 119(2):294–302.
60. Meyer-Frießem CH, Lipke E, Weibel S, et al. Perioperative ketamine for postoperative pain management in patients with preoperative opioid intake: a systematic review and meta-analysis. *J Clin Anesth.* 2022;78:110652.
61. Clattenburg EJ, Hailozian C, Haro D, et al. Slow infusion of low-dose ketamine reduces bothersome side effects compared to intravenous push: a double-blind, double-dummy, randomized controlled trial. *Acad Emerg Med.* 2018;25(9):1048–1052.
62. Motov S, Mai M, Pushkar I, et al. A prospective randomized, double-dummy trial comparing IV push low dose ketamine to short infusion of low dose ketamine for treatment of pain in the ED. *Am J Emerg Med.* 2017;35(8):1095–1100.
63. Schwenk ES, Viscusi ER, Buvanendran A, et al. Consensus guidelines on the use of intravenous ketamine infusions for acute pain management from the American Society of Regional Anesthesia and Pain Medicine, the American Academy of Pain Medicine, and the American Society of Anesthesiologists. *Reg Anesth Pain Med.* 2018;43(5):456–466.
64. Puch Oernskov M, Gaspar Santos S, Sohail Asghar M, Wildgaard K. Is intravenous magnesium sulphate a suitable adjuvant in postoperative pain management?—A critical and systematic review of methodology in randomized controlled trials. *Scand J Pain.* 2023;23(2):251–267.
65. Waldron NH, Jones CA, Gan TJ, Allen TK, Habib AS. Impact of perioperative dexamethasone on postoperative analgesia and side-effects: systematic review and meta-analysis. *Br J Anaesth.* 2013;110(2):191–200.
66. Leppert W, Buss T. The role of corticosteroids in the treatment of pain in cancer patients. *Curr Pain Headache Rep.* 2012;16(4):307–313.
67. O'Neill A, Lirk P. Multimodal analgesia. *Anesthesiol Clin.* 2022;40(3):455–468.
68. Savage SR, Kirsh KL, Passik SD. Challenges in using opioids to treat pain in persons with substance use disorders. *Addict Sci Clin Pract.* 2008;4(2):4–25.
69. Jones P, Lamdin R, Dalziel SR. Oral non-steroidal anti-inflammatory drugs versus other oral analgesic agents for acute soft tissue injury. *Cochrane Database Syst Rev.* 2020;8(8): CD007789.
70. Hickey T, Abelleira A, Acampora G, Becker WC, Falker CG, Nazario M, Weimer MB. Perioperative buprenorphine management: a multidisciplinary approach. *Med Clin North Am.* 2022;106(1):169–185.
71. Reckitt Benckiser Healthcare (UK) Ltd. Buprenex [package insert]. Hull, England. December 2023.
72. Mendelson J, Upton RA, Everhart ET, Jacob P III, Jones RT. Bioavailability of sublingual buprenorphine. *J Clin Pharmacol.* 1997;37(1):31–37.
73. Hickey T, Acampora G. Buprenorphine: an anesthesia-centric review. *J Opioid Mgmt.* 2024;20(6):503–527.
74. Hickey TR, Costa GPA, Oliveira D, et al. Buprenorphine versus full agonist opioids for acute postoperative pain management: a systematic review and meta-analysis of randomized controlled trials. *Reg Anesth Pain Med.* 2026;51(1):1–16.
75. Pardos-Gascón EM, Narambuena L, Leal-Costa C, Ramos-Morcillo AJ, Ruzafa-Martínez M, van-der Hofstadt Román CJ. Effects of mindfulness-based cognitive therapy for chronic

pain: a multicenter study. *Int J Environ Res Public Health*. 2021;18(13):6951.
76. Ruano A, García-Torres F, Gálvez-Lara M, Moriana JA. Psychological and non-pharmacologic treatments for pain in cancer patients: a systematic review and meta-analysis. *J Pain Symptom Manage*. 2022;63(5):e505–e520.
77. Shapero BG, Greenberg J, Pedrelli P, de Jong M, Desbordes G. Mindfulness-based interventions in psychiatry. *Focus (Am Psychiatr Publ)*. 2018;16(1):32–39.
78. Bikmoradi A, Zafari A, Oshvandi K, Mazdeh M, Roshanaei G. Effect of progressive muscle relaxation on severity of pain in patients with multiple sclerosis: a randomized controlled trial. *HAYAT*. 2014;20:26–37.
79. Hasanpour-Dehkordi A, Solati K, Tali SS, Dayani MA. Effect of progressive muscle relaxation with analgesic on anxiety status and pain in surgical patients. *Br J Nurs*. 2019;28(3):174–178.
80. Baird CL, Sands L. A pilot study of the effectiveness of guided imagery with progressive muscle relaxation to reduce chronic pain and mobility difficulties of osteoarthritis. *Pain Manag Nurs*. 2004;5(3):97–104.
81. Akmeşe ZB, Oran NT. Effects of progressive muscle relaxation exercises accompanied by music on low back pain and quality of life during pregnancy. *J Midwifery Womens Health*. 2014;59(5):503–509.
82. De Paolis G, Naccarato A, Cibelli F, et al. The effectiveness of progressive muscle relaxation and interactive guided imagery as a pain-reducing intervention in advanced cancer patients: a multicentre randomised controlled non-pharmacological trial. *Complement Ther Clin Pract*. 2019;34:280–287.
83. Hughes LS, Clark J, Colclough JA, Dale E, McMillan D. Acceptance and commitment therapy (ACT) for chronic pain: a systematic review and meta-analyses. *Clin J Pain*. 2017;33(6):552–568.
84. Martinez-Calderon J, García-Muñoz C, Rufo-Barbero C, Matias-Soto J, Cano-García FJ. Acceptance and commitment therapy for chronic pain: an overview of systematic reviews with meta-analysis of randomized clinical trials. *J Pain*. 2024;25(3):595–617.
85. ACBS Foundation. *The ACT Matrix*. Accessed May 19, 2025. https://contextualscience.org/act_matrix
86. ACBS Foundation. *Metaphors*. Accessed May 19, 2025. https://contextualscience.org/metaphors
87. Rodin G, Malfitano C, Rydall A, et al. Emotion and symptom-focused engagement (EASE): a randomized phase II trial of an integrated psychological and palliative care intervention for patients with acute leukemia. *Support Care Cancer*. 2020;28(1):163–176.
88. Bojorquez GR, Jackson KE, Andrews AK. Music therapy for surgical patients: approach for managing pain and anxiety. *Crit Care Nurs Q*. 2020;43(1):81–85.
89. Gutgsell KJ, Schluchter M, Margevicius S, et al. Music therapy reduces pain in palliative care patients: a randomized controlled trial. *J Pain Symptom Manage*. 2013;45(5):822–831.
90. He Y, Guo X, May BH, et al. Clinical evidence for association of acupuncture and acupressure with improved cancer pain: a systematic review and meta-analysis. *JAMA Oncol*. 2020;6(2):271–278.
91. Thompson T, Terhune DB, Oram C, et al. The effectiveness of hypnosis for pain relief: a systematic review and meta-analysis of 85 controlled experimental trials. *Neurosci Biobehav Rev*. 2019;99:298–310.
92. Cyna AM, McAuliffe GL, Andrew MI. Hypnosis for pain relief in labour and childbirth: a systematic review. *Br J Anaesth*. 2004;93(4):505–511.
93. Berger MM, Davadant M, Marin C, et al. Impact of a pain protocol including hypnosis in major burns. *Burns*. 2010;36(5):639–646.
94. Kendrick C, Sliwinski J, Yu Y, et al. Hypnosis for acute procedural pain: a critical review. *Int J Clin Exp Hypn*. 2016;64(1):75–115.
95. Garland EL, Baker AK, Larsen P, et al. Randomized controlled trial of brief mindfulness training and hypnotic suggestion for acute pain relief in the hospital setting. *J Gen Intern Med*. 2017;32(10):1106–1113.
96. Goudman L, Jansen J, Billot M, et al. Virtual reality applications in chronic pain management: systematic review and meta-analysis. *JMIR Serious Games*. 2022;10(2):e34402.
97. Behm DG, Kay AD, Trajano GS, Alizadeh S, Blazevich AJ. Effects of acute and chronic stretching on pain control. *J Clin Exerc Physiol*. 2021;10(4):150–159.
98. Dehghan M, Farahbod F. The efficacy of thermotherapy and cryotherapy on pain relief in patients with acute low back pain, a clinical trial study. *J Clin Diagn Res*. 2014;8(9):LC01-4.
99. Klintberg IH, Larsson ME. Shall we use cryotherapy in the treatment in surgical procedures, in acute pain or injury, or in long term pain or dysfunction?—A systematic review. *J Bodyw Mov Ther*. 2021;27:368–387.
100. Binny J, Joshua Wong NL, Garga S, et al. Transcutaneous electric nerve stimulation (TENS) for acute low back pain: systematic review. *Scand J Pain*. 2019;19(2):225–233.
101. Lau PM, Chow DH, Pope MH. Early physiotherapy intervention in an accident and emergency department reduces pain and improves satisfaction for patients with acute low back pain: a randomised trial. *Aust J Physiother*. 2008;54(4):243–249.
102. Caprio E, Belfer K, Terasaki D. Exploring the role of psychologists on addiction consult services in acute care settings. *J Clin Psychol Med Settings*. 2025;32(3):405–411.
103. U.S. Department of Veterans Affairs. *Progressive Muscle Relaxation and Progressive Relaxation*. 2020. https://www.va.gov/WHOLEHEALTH/veteran-handouts/docs/Progress-MuscleRelax__Final508_11-13-2018.pdf
104. Terasaki D, Abts D, Ferraro K. Questioning methadone split-dosing for analgesia among hospitalized patients with opioid use disorder. *Addiction*. 2024;119(12):2044–2047.
105. McKendrick G, Davis W, Sklar M, et al. The IMPOWR Network Divided or Single Exposure Study (DOSE) protocol: a randomized controlled comparison of once versus split dosing of methadone for the treatment of comorbid chronic pain and opioid use disorder. *Subst Use Addctn J*. 2025;46(1):197–200.
106. Kohan L, Potru S, Barreveld AM, et al. Buprenorphine management in the perioperative period: educational review and recommendations from a multisociety expert panel. *Reg Anesth Pain Med*. 2021;46(10):840–859.
107. Hickey T, Abelleira A, Acampora G, et al. Perioperative buprenorphine management: a multidisciplinary approach. *Med Clin North Am*. 2022;106(1):169–185.
108. Jones AK, Ngaimisi E, Gopalakrishnan M, Young MA, Laffont CM. Population pharmacokinetics of a monthly buprenorphine depot injection for the treatment of opioid use disorder: a combined analysis of phase II and phase III trials. *Clin Pharmacokinet*. 2021;60(4):527–540.
109. Coe MA, Lofwall MR, Walsh SL. Buprenorphine pharmacology review: update on transmucosal and long-acting formulations. *J Addict Med*. 2019;13(2):93–103.
110. Invidior Inc. Sublocade [package insert]. North Chesterfield, Virginia. August 2022.
111. Duramed Pharmaceuticals Inc. Revia [package insert]. Pomona, New York. October 2013.
112. Alkermes Inc. Vitriol [package insert]. Waltham, Massachusetts. September 2022.

113. Sullivan MA, Vosburg SK, Comer SD. Depot naltrexone: antagonism of the reinforcing, subjective, and physiological effects of heroin. *Psychopharmacology (Berl)*. 2006;189(1):37–46.
114. Ye Y, Gabriel RA, Mariano ER. The expanding role of chronic pain interventions in multimodal perioperative pain management: a narrative review. *Postgrad Med*. 2022;134(5):449–457.
115. Lim J, Pavalagantharajah S, Verschoor CP, et al. Infectious diseases, comorbidities and outcomes in hospitalized people who inject drugs (PWID). *PLoS One*. 2022;17(4):e0266663.
116. Jones J, Correll DJ, Lechner SM, et al. Selective inhibition of Na(V)1.8 with VX-548 for acute pain. *N Engl J Med*. 2023;389(5):393–405.
117. Vertex Pharmaceuticals Incorporated. Vertex Announces FDA Approval of JOURNAVX™ (Suzetrigine), a First-in-Class Treatment for Adults With Moderate-to-Severe Acute Pain. January 30, 2025. https://news.vrtx.com/news-releases/news-release-details/vertex-announces-fda-approval-journavxtm-suzetrigine-first-class

18

Palliative Care and Hospice Management for Individuals With Substance Use Disorders

Reed A. Nerness, Julie W. Childers

BT was diagnosed with laryngeal squamous cell carcinoma a month before I met him. The 47-year-old was admitted to the hospital with plans for him to remain inpatient for a month while receiving curative treatment with cisplatin chemotherapy and 33 fractions of external beam radiation therapy after having a total laryngectomy. Housing and transportation limitations had necessitated admission for the duration of his treatment, one that typically proceeds in the outpatient setting. Furthermore, BT had an active substance use disorder (SUD). As a teenager, he had started using stimulants, tobacco, and heroin. In his thirties, BT developed chronic pain in his lower back and right shoulder from traumatic injuries and work-related overuse and increased his opioid use to treat his pain. He was diagnosed with stimulant use disorder and opioid use disorder (OUD) and for a time was on buprenorphine treatment before being lost to outpatient follow-up. I met BT as part of the inpatient palliative care consult service who was asked to assist with symptoms.

Radiation-related mucositis had given BT acute laryngeal inflammation and pain. Typically, this pain is managed with immediate-release (IR) opioids, which was what BT's primary team started for him. In theory, BT's pain was not different than the pain experienced by those without a history of OUD but treating BT's pain was more complicated. Earlier on in this admission, he had experienced acute opioid withdrawal symptoms, which were treated using the short-acting opioids started for his pain. Caring clinicians worried that providing opioid medications to BT for pain management could fuel his OUD and were unsure how to dose opioids appropriately to overcome his opioid tolerance. There were also concerns about BT's motives for reporting a high pain level and that prescribed medications could be diverted.

Addressing BT's suffering started with a methodical assessment of his pain. He had acute inflammatory pain that would resolve after treatment and chronic pain related to degenerative joint disease. Chronic opioid exposure and OUD had intensified BT's experience of acute pain. He had a type of cancer that was expected to be cured, but treatment he was undergoing commonly left patients with high degree of chronic symptoms including pain and mood disorders. Treatment of acute-on-chronic pain with SUD history needed to be chosen carefully, considering these factors.

I started buprenorphine for his chronic pain and OUD and immediate-release morphine as needed for his acute cancer–related pain. With these treatments, BT weathered the cancer treatment remarkably well. After receiving the final fraction of radiation in the morning, BT was discharged that afternoon. He had an appointment with a palliative care specialist who was comfortable caring for individuals with addiction, who had been in contact with the hospital team and had a plan to taper oxycodone after discharge.

Multiple factors increased BT's risk of an inequitable outcome; he identified as Black, he had low-income, he was a person experiencing housing instability, and he had SUD. The hospital had provided a stable place for him to complete curative treatment and a connection to a clinic for ongoing symptom management with buprenorphine for OUD and chronic malignant pain as he recovered from both his cancer treatment and SUD. Nurse case managers, social workers, and clinicians each provided warm handoffs to the next set of support outside of the hospital in an effort to address the social drivers of health he would continue to face.

Cancerous cells were no longer threatening BTs life, but the impact of cancer still was, and it probably always would be. For the palliative care team, BT's treatment had not ended with the cure. Our team was able to set up follow-up care tailored to his needs: chronic serious illness, chronic pain, and SUD. In this way a through line was set up, connecting the hard work BT and the hospital teams had done, to the ongoing work of maximizing quality well-being outside of the hospital. Looking back, I am proud we were taking steps with BT to treat his present suffering with an eye always looking toward future care. I am hopeful for more stories like BT's.

—Reed A. Nerness

Key Points

- **Individuals with substance use disorders (SUD) have a high prevalence of chronic serious illnesses and are increasingly requiring palliative and/or hospice care.**
- **Careful assessment of pain in those with opioid use disorder (OUD) and serious illness (including cancer) is vital to care that avoids harm *and* relieves suffering.**
- **Treatment for OUD with methadone or buprenorphine/naloxone should be continued as long as possible throughout the course of serious illness; other medications for pain can be added, including opioids after careful assessment, if needed for symptom management.**
- **Caring for those with SUD and serious illness is complex and requires increased multidisciplinary support and close attention to care coordination between inpatient and outpatient settings.**
- **For several reasons, goals of care and advanced care planning can be more difficult for those with SUD. Hospital-based clinicians should document goals, values, and surrogate decision maker as these discussions arise.**
- **Patients may continue to use substances, even with serious illnesses and at the end of life, and efforts to safely and effectively treat them can be challenging but are essential.**

Those with life-limiting serious illnesses benefit from specialty palliative care and end-of-life (EOL) care, including those with SUD. The term serious illness refers to a condition with high mortality risk and negative impact on a patient's daily quality of life. The World Health Organization defines palliative care as care that "improves the quality of life of patients and that of their families who are facing challenges associated with life-threatening illness, whether physical, psychological, social or spiritual."[1] Palliative care in the hospital setting typically is practiced by a multidisciplinary team who act as consultants to address the primary domains of palliative care. These domains include assessment and treatment of symptoms related to serious illnesses, medical decision-making support, and facilitation of transitions of care at EOL. Patients do not need to have a prognosis of less than 6 months to receive palliative care services.

The main differentiating factor between palliative care and hospice care is the patient's priorities. Palliative care is care focused on quality of life and medical decision making for those with serious illness. Those receiving palliative care are generally those who want to prioritize treatment of their serious illness to prolong life while also addressing quality of life concerns. One way that palliative care can be provided is through hospice (Figure 18.1). Hospice is a form of palliative

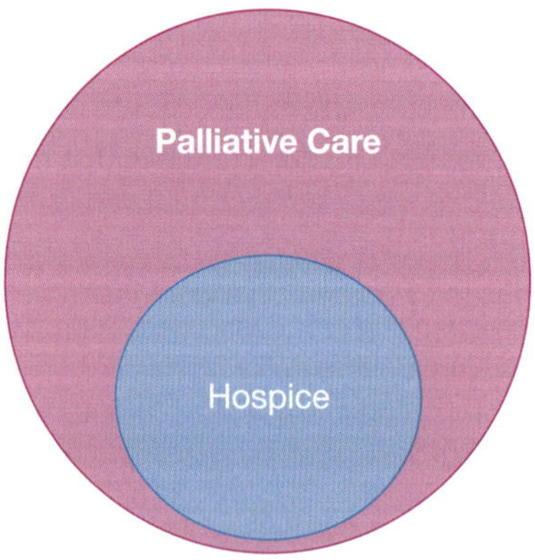

Figure 18.1: Palliative care focuses on quality of life and medical decision making. Hospice services are part of palliative care.

care that is reserved for those who have decided to prioritize quality of life and comfort over the pursuit of life prolonging interventions. Hospice is a Medicare benefit that is available to patients whose goals align with hospice and have an anticipated life expectancy of less than 6 months. Hospice services generally include care from a multidisciplinary group, typically a clinician or medical director, nurses, aids, social workers, and chaplains. Hospice services can be provided in the hospital if the patient meets certain criteria, meaning they need a high level of care to control their symptoms (eg, frequent intravenous medications for comfort). At hospital discharge, hospice services can also be provided in a nursing facility or in the home. The hospice service or agency provides medications for comfort, medical equipment, nurses and aids, and bereavement support. They are available by phone 24 hours per day, 7 days a week. Hospice does not provide caregiving.

As serious illness progresses, palliative and/or hospice care is often involved to relive suffering. Palliative care and hospice clinicians use certain categories of serious illness. These groupings, outlined in Table 18.1, can help guide care and these terms will be used throughout this chapter to refer to estimated prognoses. Special attention should be given to the different timeframe associated with the terms "limited prognosis" and "EOL." Variation in the meaning of these terms is common. The prognoses associated with each term outlined in Table 18.1 are those that will be used throughout this chapter.

For those with serious illness and SUD, the introduction and practice of palliative care and transition to hospice care often occurs in the hospital setting. This chapter aims to provide guidance on the recommended approaches to common complex situations when those with SUD require palliative and/or hospice care in the hospital.

Epidemiology/Scope of the Problem Related to the Hospital Setting

Those with SUD are increasingly in need of palliative and/or hospice care because SUDs are associated with excess morbidity and mortality compared to the general population.[2–5] Those with SUD also carry high rates of comorbid serious illness, like cancer, cardiac, pulmonary, liver, and kidney disease, and chronic infections like HIV.[6–12] Interestingly, there is also evidence that prior cancer diagnoses can increase the risk of later development of SUD.[13]

Hospital care for those with SUD and serious illness is complex and outside the scope of the traditional training of general hospitalists and palliative care specialists. There is evidence that cancer-related pain management for those with SUDs admitted to the hospital is poor.[14] Subspecialist training is also limited in the overlap between serious illness and SUD. Palliative care clinicians are generally not trained in addiction medicine and may not be comfortable with pain management for those with OUD and cancer-related pain in the hospital.[15] Palliative care trainees who frequently encounter opioid misuse during the treatment of pain may not be comfortable with its assessment and management.[16]

Follow-up posthospital discharge also has its challenges. Those with symptoms, often pain, related to their serious illness are commonly referred to palliative care clinics. Palliative care clinicians in ambulatory setting, while experts in treatment of symptoms and opioid management, report low confidence in addressing opioid misuse behavior, tapering opioids, and treating addiction.[17] There has also been limited adoption of standardized clinic procedures like urine drug testing and naloxone coprescribing to mitigate opioid misuse risk.[18] Those with SUDs and

TABLE 18.1

Outline of Stages of Serious Illness and Associated Description and Timeline

Stage	Prognosis	Description	Timeframe
Diagnosis	Life-limiting diagnosis	Relatively preserved function, low symptom burden	Years
For some: cure	Normal life expectancy	Return to normal function, no symptoms or may have chronic symptoms related to curative treatment	Years
For others: Progression of disease	Longer prognosis	Loss of function, growing symptom burden	Months to Years
End-stage disease	Limited prognosis	High degree of functional limitation, high symptom burden	Weeks to Months
End of life (EOL)	Active dying phase	Signs and symptoms of dying, high degree of symptoms	Hours to Weeks

malignancy often follow up with oncology offices who are tasked with also addressing disease-related symptoms. Studies have found that oncologists are even less comfortable managing cancer-related pain, especially in light of the opioid epidemic and related efforts to limit opioid prescriptions.[19] In addition, a qualitative study of oncologists caring for those with SUD found unresolved social challenges, active substance use, opioid complexity and pain, and stigma were the main challenges faced by clinicians and staff.[20] Hospice clinicians frequently encounter patients with SUD and report limited confidence in treatment of opioid misuse or OUD as well as management of pain in those with opioid misuse or OUD.[21]

In addition, addiction-trained clinicians may not be trained to care for those with serious illness and disease-related symptoms. Hospitalists are trained in the care of a wide range of chronic and serious illnesses including SUD, however studies have found that treatment of OUD during hospitalization, for example, is low.[22] For all of these reasons, when individuals are hospitalized with SUD and life-limiting illness, it is important for different specialties to work together to provide safe and effective care through collaboration between hospital medicine, palliative care, and addiction medicine.

Summary of Evidence

Growth and Benefits of Palliative Care

Palliative care involvement in the care of those with serious illness has been shown to improve patient's quality of life and survival.[23] The availability of hospital-based palliative care is growing. Since 2000, the number of hospitals with 50 or more beds and a palliative care service has more than tripled; in 2020, 83% of hospitals had a palliative care service.[24]

Prevalence of Pain

Symptom management is a core domain of palliative care. Pain is one of the most prevalent symptoms encountered in serious illness. A systematic review and meta-analysis from 2016 found over half of those with cancer undergoing cancer-directed therapies had pain. This percentage increased to over 66% in those with advanced disease.[25] Unfortunately, pain did not appear to resolve with curative treatment, and this study found that nearly 40% of those who had been cured of their cancer lived with persistent pain.[25] Those with serious illness other than cancer also experience chronic pain which may or may not be related to their serious illness.[26] For many, chronic pain can become a primary condition itself (called primary chronic pain, see section on assessment of pain for details). Those with SUD carry a high burden of chronic pain and this can be particularly pronounced in the setting of serious illness.[27,28]

Heightened Pain Perception in Those With SUD

There is evidence of higher sensitivity to pain in those with SUD, particularly in those with OUD and alcohol use disorder (AUD). This heightened sensitivity can persist even after individuals go into remission from their SUD.[29,30]

A recent systematic review and meta-analysis confirmed those with opioid use and OUD have lower pain thresholds than those without OUD.[31] The question has been raised whether treatment of OUD with opioids could induce a state of hyperalgesia; however, this was not supported by the study.[31] Understanding the altered pain responses in those with OUD is important when assessing and managing pain in those with OUD.

Those with AUD also have high pain sensitivity and a higher prevalence of chronic pain. Expert theories have been proposed that link the cycle of alcohol use to self-treatment of pain leading to acute withdrawal and associated hyperalgesia.[30]

Other SUDs like stimulant use disorder, benzodiazepine use disorder, or cannabis use disorder, for example, can increase the potential for both acute and chronic pain related to increased risk for traumatic injury, accident, and infection. Tobacco use disorder is also related to higher risk of chronic pain and can delay healing from surgical interventions and infections.[32,33] Therefore, whenever treating pain in individuals with SUD, it is of the utmost importance to offer them evidence-based treatment for their SUD while simultaneously providing adequate pain and symptom management.

Importance of Interdisciplinary Approach to Care

As has been mentioned, the care of those with SUDs and serious illness is complex, and psychosocial factors associated with having a SUD add to this complexity. Interdisciplinary collaboration is important when providing care for this population. Studies of interdisciplinary interventions, including social work, chaplains, pharmacists, and nurses, have been found to be feasible and have a positive impact on the care of individuals with SUD and serious illness.[34–36]

Limitations in Care for Those With Advanced Disease

Hospice care is a program that is available to those with advanced disease with a limited prognosis (estimated less than 6-month prognosis; Table 18.1) through Medicare or other health insurance. As serious illness progresses, function declines and symptoms build. For those with co-occurring SUD, providing hospice care has added complexity. Psychosocial factors like housing instability, comorbid mental illness, and physiologic factors like ongoing substance use add to this complexity. A narrative review described some of the challenges of providing hospice care to those with SUD in the United States. The review found that those with SUD and limited social support often don't have those who are able to provide caregiving and support as function declines.[37] When loved ones are not available to provide care in the home with hospice services, this often means patients are discharged to a nursing facility with hospice services. Stigma, facility structure, and expectations of nursing facilities can place added stress on those with SUD and prevent quality care. Other barriers to high quality hospice care noted in the review were the limited hospice and palliative care clinician comfort with identifying, assessing, and treating SUD as well as difficulties with pain management.[37]

Clinical Guidance

The complexity of care for individuals with serious illness and SUD necessitates a personalized and, at times, creative approach. There is a high degree of variability between practice settings and available resources making development of guidelines for providing hospice and palliative care to those with SUD nearly impossible—in fact, no comprehensive resources exist.

The clinical guidance in this chapter aims to highlight several common complex situations faced by hospital-based clinicians caring for individuals with SUD and serious illness. For information on the assessment and management of pain in a patient without serious illness, see Chapter 17 on pain management.

Pain, SUDs, and Serious Illness

The following steps in assessing pain are informed by expert opinion and a modified Delphi panel aimed at providing a consensus statement on the management of cancer-related pain in those with opioid misuse and OUD.[38–40] This section should be used to guide the assessment of pain for those with cancer and/or noncancer serious illnesses, and co-occurring SUD. Key recommendations from this section will be summarized with cases in Table 18.6, including an assessment and recommended plan for each case. These cases will be referred to throughout this section.

Assessment of Pain

While prone to being overlooked, a careful assessment of pain prior to initiating treatment is crucial to providing quality pain management, especially for those who have been diagnosed with SUD. For people who have pain and suspected SUD, it is important to establish a SUD diagnosis, if present, during the assessment and treatment of pain. There are six recommended steps to a complete pain assessment in someone with a previously diagnosed SUD. These six steps are: (1) evaluation of pain etiology, (2) review opioid responsiveness of pain, (3) explore how substance use has impacted the patient's life and their pain including assessment for withdrawal symptoms, (4) gain understanding of prognosis, (5) focus on patient goals for SUD and pain treatment, (6) explore outpatient follow-up options. These steps are summarized in Table 18.2.

The **first step** is to characterize the patient's pain. Categories to assess include chronicity, etiology, and quality. Acute pain related to trauma or clinical decompensation of serious illness can be resolved by addressing the underlying cause of pain. Chronic pain is less likely to be curable and requires a more sustainable management plan. It is also helpful to define if pain is malignancy related or not. Malignancy-related pain is often best managed postdischarge by an outpatient palliative care clinician, if available. Patients with cancer and SUD can also have pain that is not related to their malignancy or that predates their serious illness (Case 7). It is important to differentiate and describe the patients' pain as acute, acute-on-chronic, or chronic and identify the location of the pain the person is experiencing which could be related or unrelated to their serious illness. See Chapter 17 for more information.

All of these factors can impact postdischarge follow-up availability. In addition, malignancy-related pain can be chronic but can still sometimes be reduced or resolved with disease-specific therapies (eg, chemotherapy, radiation, etc) The pathophysiology behind the pain can provide clues toward effective treatment. For example, pain related to local inflammation (eg, nociceptive pain) responds differently to therapies than pain caused by compression or damage of a nerve (eg, neuropathic pain) or organ distortion (eg, visceral pain). It is also important to identify when pain has become a disease itself. Sometimes called "pathologic pain" or simply "chronic

TABLE 18.2

Summary of Steps in Assessment of Pain in Those With Cancer and SUD

Step 1	Characterize the pain—chronicity, type, location, etiology, factors that worsen or improve pain (eg, PQRST assessment model)
Step 2	Assess for medication and opioid responsiveness—previous medication trials, previous opioid exposure, perceived benefit
Step 3	Explore substance use and its impact ■ Use validated unhealthy substance use screening tools such as AUDIT, DAST, TAPS ■ Perform substance use history for patients who screen positive for unhealthy substance use ■ Explore social factors, prior or current use, triggers ■ Provide diagnosis via DSM-5, if one is not previously provided
Step 4	Estimate prognosis—understanding treatment options, using online tools
Step 5	Understand patient goals—values, priorities, hopes for SUD treatment
Step 6	Coordinate with outpatient clinicians—identify clinic for follow-up, handoff. Ensure ongoing treatment for SUD is maintained. Address social determinants of health.

pain," this type of pain lasts longer than 3 months and manifests as a complex syndrome defined as "pain that persists past the normal time of healing."[41] This type of pain often requires a bio-psycho-social approach to treatment.

The **second step** is to assess the medication and opioid responsiveness of pain. Helpful details of the individual's history include if opioids have been used in the past to treat this pain and if pain was improved. Patients with chronic or relapsing pain often have rich experience with various modalities and medications which can be vital to building a pain management plan.

The **third step** is to understand how SUD has impacted the patient and what role SUD currently has in their lives, including their experience of withdrawal symptoms. Over time SUD often impact people's housing, social network, and finances. Having an understanding of these factors helps hospital-based clinicians make a feasible and sustainable plan for discharge. For individuals with AUD, as an example, exploring their ability to manage medications safely and avoid alcohol will be important when developing a plan. For individuals with OUD, exploring details of opioid use will provide valuable information on their individual opioid tolerance and be necessary when determining appropriate doses and developing a plan for ongoing management after discharge. Acute withdrawal symptoms are common among those in the hospital. The need for treatment of these symptoms will be important to include as an appropriate plan to address pain is built. Whether the patient's SUD is active or in remission also influences the plan (Case 3). For instance, the level of vulnerability to harms of prescribed opioids is very different for those with active OUD versus those with treated OUD in remission.

The **fourth recommended step** is to gain an understanding of the patient's prognosis. While inaccuracy of prognostic estimation exists, determining an estimated prognosis aids in guiding choice of pain therapy. The stage of disease helps determine goals and priorities as well as risks and benefits of pain treatment, including opioid therapy. For patients with pain who are at EOL comfort and quality of life frequently become priorities. People with advanced disease who may have a limited prognosis may have a high burden of pain related to their serious illness and SUD requiring frequent reassessment and management of pain. For those with longer prognosis and/or viable disease-specific treatment options, initiation of opioid therapy can carry greater consequences, including triggering or worsening current SUD.

Traditionally, prognostication for individuals with cancer has been clearer because of the trajectory of malignant disease; generally conceptualized as a period of stable decline with a rapid decline at EOL. However, with improvements in cancer-directed therapies, those diagnosed with cancer are living longer and this previously more predictable trajectory is becoming more variable. For some, this has resulted in cancer-related pain that is chronic (Case 5). Over a third of patients with cancer continue to have pain after curative treatment.[25] When caring for those with SUD and cancer it is important to work closely with oncology colleagues to gain an understanding of the available therapies and whether they are of curative or palliative intent.

Prediction of prognosis for individuals with nonmalignant serious illness like chronic heart, liver, kidney, lung disease and chronic infections like hepatitis C and HIV/AIDS can be more difficult. Disease trajectories for these noncancer serious illnesses are characterized by progressive decline with episodes of acute illness and relative recovery, making prognostication particularly challenging. In addition, they have a high burden of symptoms with no curative options and can still live for many years.

The **fifth recommended step**, to explore the patient goals for treatment of their serious illness and/or SUD (if not already getting treatment), should be incorporated into the entire process. Partnering with the patient on the plan for pain management is vital, particularly if part of the plan includes the possibility of continuing or starting treatment for SUD. Their goals for SUD will also impact the final step which is coordination of the care started during the hospital stay to ensure safe and sustainable follow-up.

It is important to recognize that some patients with SUD may not be interested in SUD treatment, particularly those with a limited prognosis. Balancing the benefits and risks of SUD treatment in this situation becomes complex because ongoing SUD will likely worsen symptoms and/or hasten death. In this situation assessment of goals regarding symptom management, especially pain management, can be very challenging. For example, a patient admitted to the hospital with chronic cancer-related pain and active OUD may express a goal of discharging home with a prescription for intravenous hydromorphone; however, this may not be an option that the treating clinicians are willing or able to offer. In addition, establishing the goals of care of those with active, untreated SUD may be more challenging. The values and wishes of someone with active SUD may be framed by the SUD itself and lead to an expression of different priorities than they would have otherwise shared. See a later section on goals of care conversations for more information.

The last step is to plan for pain management follow-up after hospital discharge. Special attention to care coordination between hospital-based interdisciplinary teams as well as between hospital and outpatient teams is key to addressing the complexity of care faced by patients with serious illness and SUD. Prior to hospital initiation of opioid therapy for people with SUD, serious illness, and pain, it is important to identify availability of an outpatient clinician to manage this therapy. Opioid regimens should be cocreated with the outpatient clinician who will be responsible for monitoring and prescription refills. Due to complexity, higher risk of prescribed opioid misuse, and need for frequent follow-up, options can be limited as primary care clinicians can be uncomfortable or unable to accommodate the level of monitoring necessary to provide safe opioid treatment. For patients taking methadone for OUD via an outpatient treatment program (OTP), it is best practice to partner with the OTP about the ongoing methadone treatment and any adjustments that are made. Similarly, for individuals who are receiving buprenorphine therapy for OUD, this should be continued, and efforts made to coordinate care with the outpatient clinician who is managing that treatment. For patients discharging to nursing facilities and long-term care facilities, it is unfortunately common that they do not accept patients on methadone or with history of recent substance use. The presence of serious illness also places limits on options for SUD treatment. Many SUD inpatient treatment programs do not have staff who can provide the level of care needed to someone with a serious illness and often are unable to accommodate certain modes of therapy, for example, dialysis. For patients at EOL whose goals align with a hospice plan of care, postdischarge follow-up prescribing will be done via hospice team. Partnering with the hospice medical director may be necessary to create a plan of care that is safe and effective for those with current or recent substance use.

Treatment of Pain

After pain is assessed, this information can be used to guide treatment decisions and plan for hospital discharge and follow-up. This section will outline guidance on the treatment of pain in those with SUD and compare differences in management for those with cancer-related pain and those with non–cancer-related pain. It will also highlight some differences in pain treatment for those with OUD versus non-OUDs.

Nonopioid Pharmacotherapy and Nonpharmacologic Options

For all patients with pain, including those with SUD and serious illness, treatment of the underlying process resulting in pain should first be explored. If resolution of pain is not feasible or will take time, initiation of therapies targeting pain relief is often necessary. Nonpharmacologic modalities and nonopioid pharmacotherapy should be considered first. Please see Chapter 17 for more details. Some causes of pain are more commonly seen in patients receiving hospice or palliative care and have specific treatment options available. One of these is metastatic bone pain. It can be most effectively treated with a low number of fractions of palliative radiation therapy.[42,43] Anti-inflammatory medications like corticosteroids and nonsteroidal anti-inflammatory drugs (NSAIDS) are also effective. Radiation therapy followed by a short course of dexamethasone is regularly used to prevent a flare of pain in the days to weeks following radiation therapy before reduction in pain is seen.[44] Bone pain can also occur with administration of granulocyte-colony stimulating factor (G-CSF) medications like filgrastim and a combination of loratadine and famotidine have been found to be preventive.[45] Nociceptive visceral pain related to capsular stretch of an organ like the liver or kidney can also be treated using anti-inflammatory medications like corticosteroids and NSAIDs.[46] Another form of pain commonly encountered in the hospice and palliative population is chemotherapy-induced peripheral neuropathy for which evidence supports the use of duloxetine.[47] Osteoporosis is common in those with serious illness and can result in painful compression fractures. In the case of acute compression fracture, intranasal calcitonin has been shown to be effective at reducing pain in as soon as 1 week.[48]

Those living with serious illness, especially those with SUD with heightened pain perception, often develop complex pain that becomes a syndrome itself. The experience of pain can be triggered by both physical and psychological factors and develop into chronic pain which is defined as "pain lasting over 3 months associated with emotional distress and/or functional disability that cannot be explained by another diagnosis" (in which case it would be called secondary chronic pain).[49] Complex pain like this requires a whole-person approach, which can benefit from nonpharmacologic approaches such as cognitive behavioral therapy, guided imagery, mindfulness therapy, and progressive muscle relaxation.[50]

Principles of Opioid Therapy for Those With SUD

After exploring all options for nonopioid medications and treatments to relieve pain, opioid therapy may become necessary. The term "full-agonist opioids" will be used to refer to all opioids (eg, morphine, oxycodone, hydromorphone, fentanyl, etc) used for pain that are not buprenorphine nor once-daily methadone for OUD.

For those with SUD, understanding the anticipated duration of pain is key to providing safe and effective pain management with opioids. A careful, interdisciplinary approach is essential in considering opioid therapy. While details of opioid selection are outlined below, ultimately the choice of agent to start in the hospital frequently is determined by what makes sense for outpatient follow-up and monitoring. This is why generating the hospital-based plan in collaboration with the outpatient provider is so important to providing quality symptom management.

Acute Pain

Resolvable pain with an anticipated endpoint, like perioperative pain or acute traumatic pain from a fracture, is appropriately treated with short-term full-agonist opioids (Case 3). Effective multimodal pain management in this setting is no different for those with concurrent SUD, though doses for effective analgesia in those with OUD may be higher and more frequent to overcome higher opioid tolerance. In this situation, the benefits of addressing suffering and promotion of engagement in care outweigh the risks because the amount of time opioids will be prescribed is short and therefore limits risk of development of opioid-related harms. It is important to discuss goals of opioid therapy, anticipated duration of therapy, and plan for discontinuation. It is recommended to continue buprenorphine and methadone for the treatment of OUD at their respective outpatient doses throughout the treatment of acute pain. It is recommended that full-agonist opioid therapy not be continued at discharge, if possible. For those requiring ongoing full-agonist opioid therapy at discharge, the plan for opioid and pain management should be cocreated with the clinician who will be responsible for monitoring and follow-up after discharge.

Nonmalignant Chronic Pain

Many patients with SUD and noncancer serious illness have nonmalignant chronic pain. People with cancer also experience nonmalignant chronic pain. Studies estimate between 19% and 34% of those with cancer also report nonmalignant chronic pain.[51] Safe and effective nonopioid analgesics and other therapeutic options should be offered to all patients to treat chronic pain (Table 18.3). If there is an underlying process that is causing or exacerbating the nonmalignant chronic pain, interventions to reduce or resolve that process should be investigated and offered. Any treatment of chronic pain will likely be unsuccessful if the patient's SUD goes untreated. For those with OUD, it is recommended to start OUD treatment with either methadone or buprenorphine in addition to addressing pain.

Treatment of nonmalignant chronic pain with long-term full-agonist opioids is not recommended for anyone with a longer prognosis, with or without SUD (Cases 1, 4, and 7). There is substantial evidence that use of long-term opioid therapy (LTOT) (defined as >3 months of LTOT) for chronic pain can result in more harm than benefit over time.[52] Cases should be assessed individually as LTOT can rarely become necessary and should be paired with close clinic follow-up, especially in those with SUD. The preferred agent for those with SUD and a serious illness requiring opioid analgesia for nonmalignant chronic pain is buprenorphine.[53] This may mean that buprenorphine is used to address both OUD and chronic pain. Buprenorphine is recommended for pain in those with limited and longer prognoses because it is an effective analgesic with unique characteristics (Case 1). See the section on buprenorphine for more information. When those with nonmalignant chronic pain are at EOL it

TABLE 18.3

Opioid-Sparing Interventions for Specific Types of Cancer-Related Pain

Type of pain	Opioid-sparing interventions
Metastasis-related bone pain	Radiation NSAIDs Corticosteroids
G-CSF–associated bone pain	Loratadine with famotidine
Stretch of encapsulated viscera	NSAIDs Corticosteroids
Chemotherapy-induced peripheral neuropathy	Duloxetine
Primary nociceptive chronic pain	Guided imagery Mindfulness-based therapy Cognitive behavioral therapy SNRI NSAID Acetaminophen Topical treatments Physical therapy modalities
Primary neuropathic chronic pain	Gabapentin or pregabalin SNRI Guided Imagery Mindfulness-based therapy Cognitive behavioral therapy
Regional pain	Nerve blocks
Compression fracture pain	Intranasal calcitonin

is recommended to use full-agonist opioids to relieve pain. In this setting, buprenorphine can be continued, but generally should not be initiated to address pain at the immediate EOL. Please see section on symptom management at EOL for more information. Remember, the recommended treatment approaches are influenced by the patient's prognosis and terminology referring to different prognoses can differ. Please review definitions of prognostic terminology used in this chapter (eg, limited prognosis vs EOL) outlined in Table 18.1.

As cancer therapies improve, more people are surviving for many years after completing treatment. While obviously a welcome outcome, many people experience chronic pain as the result of the cancer-directed therapies.[23] Examples include chemotherapy-related neuropathy and chronic back pain related to pathologic compression fractures. Treatment of chronic pain experienced by cancer survivors is understudied but likely has similar risks and can be approached in a similar way to nonmalignant chronic pain.[52]

Malignant Pain

Malignant pain is pain related to destruction or displacement of tissue due to the spread of cancer. Opioid therapy is indicated for those with moderate to severe cancer-related pain according to National Comprehensive Cancer Network (NCCN) guidelines.[54] Malignant pain frequently can be reduced or resolved with disease-specific therapies (chemotherapy, radiation, etc) and other nonopioid medications (Table 18.3). In conjunction with exploring these options, opioid therapy may be needed. Effective opioid analgesic treatment plans will depend on the patient's prognosis as well as hospital discharge follow-up. As is true in nonmalignant chronic pain, use of full-agonist opioid therapy for malignant pain without treating the patient's OUD with buprenorphine or methadone is not recommended due to risks of overdose, diversion, and exacerbation of existing OUD. Notably, it has been found the risk of opioid overdose for individuals receiving full-agonist LTOT is similar when prescribed to those with and without malignancy-related pain.[55]

For those with active SUD with moderate to severe cancer-related pain who have either curable disease or a longer anticipated prognosis, buprenorphine is recommended (Case 2). For those with active SUD and episodes of severe malignant pain or those with limited prognosis starting buprenorphine plus a full-agonist opioid as needed could be considered (Case 1). People with SUD and malignant pain who need buprenorphine plus an as-needed full-agonist opioid will require clinic follow-up equipped to provide close monitoring, often with weekly office visits.

Although it is outside of the scope of the hospital clinician, it can be helpful to understand the goal of treatment plans started in the hospital. The aim of buprenorphine plus full-agonist therapy for someone with OUD is to provide stability from withdrawal and cravings using sublingual buprenorphine with the expectation that non-prescribed opioid use is reduced over time (ideally days to weeks). It is very unlikely that prescribed as-needed full-agonist opioids, for example, 30 mg of immediate-release oxycodone, will be an effective analgesic for someone using intravenous illicit fentanyl due to high opioid tolerance. However, as nonprescribed opioid use is heavily reduced or stopped, prescribed opioid analgesics will be more effective at controlling malignant pain. Pain management for people with OUD already on methadone or buprenorphine who develop malignant pain will be discussed in a future section. Those with

SUD other than OUD are at higher risk of developing OUD (see step three in assessment of pain). Buprenorphine as the first-line opioid analgesic for malignant pain is recommended for those with other SUD like AUD or stimulant use disorder.

As those with malignant pain progress to EOL, use of short-acting full-agonist opioids becomes the most appropriate choice in addition to their SUD treatment (Case 6). A later section will review symptom management, including pain management, for those with SUD at EOL.

Recommendations Regarding Specific Opioids

Morphine

Morphine is available in a variety of formulations that may have an advantage in individuals with serious illness and SUD. Oral formulations include extended-release and immediate-release options. For individuals with SUD and pain requiring outpatient full-agonist opioid treatment, morphine is the recommended choice (Cases 1 and 3). Morphine is preferred over oxycodone for short-acting pain relief because there is evidence it has less "drug-liking" potential than oxycodone.[56] The pharmacokinetic differences and unique analgesic profile of morphine are thought to be a protective factor, making it less commonly diverted and/or sold than oxycodone. Morphine should not be used in those with renal impairment due to the risk of accumulation of a toxic morphine metabolite which can result in neurotoxicity.

Fentanyl

Prescribed fentanyl is a high-potency opioid with transdermal, oral, and intravenous formulations. In the hospital, intravenous fentanyl is an effective analgesic, especially for those with acute and/or periprocedural pain. Using fentanyl as part of a pain management plan for a patient leaving the hospital requires some additional consideration. The transdermal formulation of fentanyl can be helpful for individuals with high opioid tolerance who require around-the-clock opioid treatment and are unable to tolerate oral formulations. For those with SUD and pain, clinicians should consider if urine drug testing will be part of the patient's follow-up care before recommending fentanyl for pain. Fentanyl is the predominant opioid in the illicit supply of substances and has been found in opioid and nonopioid illicit substances. Interpretation of tests monitoring for nonprescribed substance use is more challenging when the patient is also taking prescribed fentanyl. Some patients, like those with AUD, have a lower risk of using nonprescribed fentanyl, therefore, prescribing fentanyl for pain management may be an appropriate option for them. Generally, it is recommended to use other opioids rather than fentanyl in the treatment of pain in those with a SUD.

Oxycodone

Oxycodone is more potent than morphine and comes in multiple different immediate-release and extended-release formulations. Certain high-dose immediate-release formulations of oxycodone (eg, 30-mg tablets) carry a high value if diverted or sold. Prescribing these can add to stressors to someone with OUD. Oxycodone may be a necessary alternative to morphine for individuals with renal impairment.

Buprenorphine

Buprenorphine is a potent, partial opioid agonist with two formulation categories: low-dose formulations used for acute and chronic pain and high-dose formulations for OUD. Both low- and high-dose formulations of buprenorphine can be used in the treatment of pain in patients without SUD. See Table 18.4 for a summary of buprenorphine formulations, indications, dose ranges, oral morphine equivalents, and indications which are based on a guide to buprenorphine for chronic pain by Case et al[57] High-dose formulations are reserved for patients with higher opioid tolerance. For patients with co-occurring OUD and pain, high-dose buprenorphine formulations are recommended to treat both OUD and chronic pain, including primary chronic pain, malignant pain, and nonmalignant chronic pain. There is evidence for improved safety and efficacy of buprenorphine for the treatment of chronic pain over other opioids.[58–61] Buprenorphine is an effective analgesic for neuropathic pain and can be safely used in those with renal and hepatic impairment including dialysis.[62]

For patients with malignant pain and OUD, twice or three times daily dosing of buprenorphine is a safe and effective option regardless of prognosis.[39] For those with SUD requiring a short-acting opioid for severe episodic malignant pain, nonopioid analgesics can be added. If short-acting full-agonist opioids are required to control malignant pain, this should be done with close outpatient follow-up. Hospital clinicians should use caution in starting full-agonist opioids for malignant pain in those with SUD whose cancer may be cured or who have a longer prognosis due to the potential harms of LTOT.[38]

Hospitalizations can sometimes reveal evidence patients are experiencing harms of LTOT or a new diagnosis of SUD. Transition to buprenorphine for the ongoing treatment of chronic pain as well as SUD, if present, is recommended. For those on LTOT, opioid doses greater than 100 mg of oral morphine (or other equivalent opioid) per day or those with OUD, transition to a high-dose formulation of

TABLE 18.4

Summary of Buprenorphine Formulations, Brand Names, Oral Morphine Equivalents, and Indications

Formulation	Buprenorphine formulation (brand name)	Indication	Daily oral morphine equivalents								
			12	24	48	60	80	100	150	300	>300
Low dose	Transdermal patch (Butrans)	Chronic pain	5 mcg/h q7d	10 mcg/h q7 d	20 mcg/h q7d						
	Buccal patch (Belbuca)	Chronic pain	75 mcg daily	75 mcg q12h	150 mcg q12h		300 mcg q12h		450 mcg q12h		
High dose	Sublingual tablets or films (suboxone, Zubsolv or Subutex)	Chronic pain with opioid tolerance and/or OUD					1 mg BID		1 mg TID	2 mg TID	Typical daily doses 5–32 mg[a]

[a]See chapter on treatment of OUD.

BID, twice daily; TID, three times daily; mcg, micrograms; mg, milligrams.

Adapted from Case AA, Kullgren J, Anwar S, Pedraza S, Davis MP. Treating chronic pain with buprenorphine—The practical guide. *Curr Treat Options Oncol.* 2021;22(12):116. Springer Nature.

buprenorphine is recommended to achieve affective analgesia in the setting of opioid tolerance. For those with opioid misuse or who are at high risk of development of opioid-related harms but who are not taking more than an equivalent of 100 mg of oral morphine per day, low-dose formulations of buprenorphine are typically initially used and can be titrated up to high-dose formulations over time to achieve analgesia, if needed (Case 5).

Starting high-dose formulations of buprenorphine requires extra planning because administration of higher doses of buprenorphine to someone taking full-agonist opioids can cause acute opioid withdrawal. When low-dose buprenorphine formulations are indicated for patients already on full-agonist opioids, these formulations can be started while the patient continues to take full-agonist opioids without the risk of inducing acute opioid withdrawal. Therefore, there is no need for an overlapping initiation plan when starting low-dose buprenorphine formulations.

Traditional approaches to starting high-dose formulations of buprenorphine for patients already taking full-agonist opioids, prescribed or nonprescribed opioids, is to stop all opioids and allow the patient to progress to mild withdrawal before initiating buprenorphine. In those with pain, stopping opioids is not an option as this would result in uncontrolled symptoms. It is safe and effective to continue full-agonist opioids to control pain while simultaneously starting buprenorphine via a buprenorphine initiation technique called "low-dose overlapping transition." There are multiple different strategies for low-dose overlapping buprenorphine transitions that have been described in observational studies and expert opinion.[63] The method outlined in Table 18.5 is used to start high-dose buprenorphine and taper off a full-agonist opioid. This process takes about 5 days and avoids opioid withdrawal symptoms and uncontrolled pain.

Methadone

Methadone is a high-potency, long-acting opioid with unique pharmacologic and policy-related factors. Pharmacologically distinct from other opioid medications, methadone requires experience and expertise for safe initiation and titration. Also, unlike other opioids, methadone can significantly prolong the QTc and requires additional monitoring. From a regulatory perspective, outpatient prescriptions of methadone for OUD, dosed once per day, are limited to OTPs by law. Comparatively, prescriptions for methadone for pain management, dosed twice or three times daily, can be prescribed by outpatient clinicians with expertise who are not associated with an OTP. Hospital clinicians can start and continue methadone prescriptions for OUD or pain during hospital admission. Starting methadone in the hospital must be done with careful attention to who will be monitoring and prescribing it after discharge, for example, an OTP or an outpatient palliative care clinician.

Starting methadone for OUD for individuals with serious illness in the hospital is recommended for patients who are able to and agree to follow up with an OTP for treatment of OUD. Limitations are mainly present in discharge planning and can include the patient's physical ability to follow up for daily dosing at an OTP, especially those with advanced serious illness. Those with functional decline often

TABLE 18.5

Low-Dose, Overlapping Initiation of High-Dose Formulation of Buprenorphine

	Option 1—sublingual		Option 2—buccal and sublingual	
	Buprenorphine	**Full-agonist opioid**	**Buprenorphine**	**Full-agonist opioid**
Day 1	0.5 mg SL once	Continue baseline opioid dose	225 mcg buccal once	Continue baseline opioid dose
Day 2	0.5 mg SL BID	Continue baseline opioid dose	225 mcg buccal twice daily	Continue baseline opioid dose
Day 3	1 mg SL BID	Continue baseline opioid dose	450 mcg buccal twice daily	Continue baseline opioid dose
Day 4	2 mg SL BID	Continue baseline opioid dose	2 mg SL BID	Continue baseline opioid dose
Day 5	4 mg SL BID	Continue baseline opioid dose	4 mg SL BID	Continue baseline opioid dose
Day 6	4 mg SL TID	Continue baseline opioid dose	4 mg SL TID	Continue baseline opioid dose
Day 7	8 mg SL BID	Discontinue	8 mg SL BID	Discontinue
Day 8 and beyond	Titrate buprenorphine dose to symptoms by 4–8 mg SL daily		Titrate buprenorphine dose to symptoms by 4–8 mg SL daily	

require discharge to nursing facilities and taking methadone for OUD can be a barrier to acceptance at many facilities.

Methadone can also be an effective treatment for pain, especially pain with neuropathic components. Some experts report improved efficacy in pain management with methadone compared to buprenorphine; however, head-to-head trials are lacking.[38] Methadone for malignant pain is typically managed by outpatient palliative care clinicians. While many palliative care clinics have expertise in the management of methadone, a much more limited number of palliative care clinicians are comfortable managing methadone for pain for individuals with SUD. Those with SUD may be at a higher risk of impulsively taking methadone differently than prescribed or experience barriers to careful dosing multiple times. Taking methadone differently than prescribed, intentionally or unintentionally, poses serious safety risks because of the long half-life and biphasic elimination. For these reasons, the use of methadone for pain outside the hospital is not a recommended initial choice for those with active SUD.

Urine Toxicology Monitoring

Urine drug tests are used in the hospital setting on admission when substance use is suspected to be contributing to current condition. In clinics, periodic urine drug testing is used to monitor use of nonprescribed substances and prescribed medications. Various types of urine drug testing are available.[64] Immunoassay tests use antibodies to detect a drug or metabolite and are used in initial screening test and require confirmation if positive. The confirmatory testing is done with gas or liquid chromatography mass spectrometry. Any urine test will only detect substances it is designed to capture. For example, some institutions had to redesign their urine drug tests to detect fentanyl as this has become more common.

Patients With OUD Already on MOUD

Buprenorphine or methadone for OUD should be continued for patients taking them prior to hospital admission. For patients with pain, nonopioid and opioid analgesics can be used in addition to buprenorphine or methadone (Case 3). See the section on EOL symptom management for information on management of buprenorphine and methadone at EOL.

Methadone

For patients in the hospital on stable doses of once daily methadone for OUD through an OTP prior to admission, it is recommended to continue methadone after confirming the patient's methadone dose with the OTP. Stopping methadone should only be considered if there are safety concerns such as encephalopathy, persistently prolonged QTc (>500 ms), or other adverse effects related to methadone. Treating pain experienced by those already on methadone for OUD can be challenging. It is not recommended to stop methadone and replace it with another opioid (including buprenorphine) in an effort address uncontrolled pain.[38] Stopping methadone for OUD results in untreated OUD, opioid withdrawal, and can cause patients to lose connection to the OTP, which serves as a support system in many people's recovery. Changing methadone to twice or three times daily dosing (or "split dosing") may be a way to use methadone to control both pain and OUD and limit polypharmacy but should be discussed with the patient for input and collaborative care planning. Split dosing can be feasibly done in the hospital; however, split dosing may not be feasible outside the hospital due to OTP restrictions. Generally, it is recommended to continue methadone for OUD once daily and use other as needed analgesics to address pain unless there are compelling patient factors or other factors that support split dosing of methadone.

Hospital clinicians should use caution in initiating full-agonist opioids to be continued after hospital discharge in those on methadone with longer prognosis or potential for cure due to possibility for harm from longer-term use of full-agonist opioids. For patients with limited prognosis and uncontrolled pain it may be appropriate to add full-agonist opioid analgesics in addition to methadone for OUD while communicating closely with the patient's OTP and follow-up prescriber.[38]

In some instances, ongoing methadone for OUD via an OTP may no longer be feasible. In the serious-illness population, this can be the result of progression to advanced disease limiting functional ability which makes daily clinic attendance unrealistic. Some clinicians outside of an OTP may feel comfortable prescribing methadone for pain in these situations. Careful documentation will be needed from the clinician that the methadone being prescribed is being used for pain. Another option is transition to high-dose formulations of buprenorphine for ongoing treatment of OUD. It is important to recognize that doses of methadone higher than 60 mg will be challenging to "replace" with full-agonist opioids due to the high potency of methadone. These transitions, if needed, should be done carefully to minimize the risk of causing opioid withdrawal and destabilization of OUD. See Chapter 17 for more information.

Buprenorphine

Similarly, high-dose buprenorphine for OUD should be continued for patients in the hospital unless there is a compelling safety reason it should be discontinued. Adjustments in buprenorphine doses can be made to address pain and should be done in coordination with the outpatient clinician responsible for follow-up. For example, someone admitted on buprenorphine/naloxone 8 mg sublingual two times daily for OUD could be offered sublingual buprenorphine three times daily or a higher dose (Case 9). Full-agonist opioids in addition to buprenorphine may be needed for pain. Though data are limited, higher starting doses of full-agonist opioid for those on doses of buprenorphine greater than 16 mg/d may be needed. The idea is that higher doses of full-agonist opioid are sometimes needed to overcome the partial agonism of high-dose formulations of buprenorphine to achieve effective analgesia. For example, prescribing 10 mg of immediate-release oxycodone rather than 5 mg of oxycodone in addition to sublingual buprenorphine. See Chapter 17 for more information.

Naltrexone

Naltrexone is an opioid-receptor antagonist used to treat OUD and AUD with oral and intramuscular formulations. Naltrexone for SUD should be continued on admission unless there is evidence of adverse effects or patients require opioid analgesia. The need for opioid analgesics should be anticipated, if possible, as oral naltrexone and intramuscular naltrexone will need to be stopped prior to starting opioid analgesics for at least 3 days or 30 days, respectively. Because of this, naltrexone for SUD is less commonly used in those with serious illness, particularly cancer, due to the higher likelihood of pain related to their disease or treatments requiring opioid analgesics. If a patient taking naltrexone requires immediate acute pain treatment, a consultation to anesthesia is recommended. See Chapter 17 for more information.

Palliative Care and Untreated SUD

Treatment of SUD is an important part of providing palliative care to those with serious illness and some patients will not be ready to receive treatment for their SUD. In these cases, hospital clinicians can continue to provide primary palliative care in an effort to maintain clinician–patient rapport and trust, reduce harm, and manage symptoms. Luckily, the practice of palliative care and treatment of SUD is highly overlapping.[65] Application of palliative care skills and approaches outlined below can be meaningful tools to facilitate treatment of SUD, even when patients are not ready for addressing SUD directly.

Symptom Management

Effective SUD treatment and palliative care both prioritize assessment and treatment of the patient's

TABLE 18.6

Summary Cases for Pain Management in Those With SUD and Serious Illness[66,67]

	Brief case	Assessment	Co-created plan
Case 1	▪ 65-y-old ▪ Active, untreated OUD ▪ Chronic pain ▪ Admitted for acute lower back pain and dyspnea ▪ Diagnosed with metastatic lung cancer with malignant pleural effusion and bone lesions in lumbar spine	▪ Cancer-related pain ▪ Chronic nonmalignant knee osteoarthritis ▪ Chronic housing instability, limited transportation ▪ Poor functional status ▪ Severe OUD; Daily nonprescribed intranasal fentanyl use ▪ Prognosis of weeks to months ▪ Discussed with outpatient palliative care clinician ▪ Patient open to OUD treatment	▪ Radiation oncology referral for palliative radiation ▪ Start sublingual buprenorphine 8 mg three times daily for pain and OUD ▪ Start dexamethasone daily for 1 wk for pain ▪ Start IR morphine 30 mg every 6 h for severe pain not relieved by buprenorphine (oxycodone or hydromorphone can also be used) ▪ Office visit with outpatient palliative care clinician within 1 wk with plan for frequent visits
Case 2	▪ 52-y-old ▪ Active, untreated OUD ▪ Localized hepatocellular cancer ▪ Admitted for right upper quadrant pain	▪ Cancer-related pain ▪ Severe OUD; intravenous heroin use ▪ Previously on methadone for OUD, self-discontinued ▪ Prognosis likely years ▪ Patient is agreeable to follow up with outpatient palliative care clinic ▪ Patient open to OUD treatment	▪ Start as needed NSAIDs for pain related to liver capsule stretch (if preserved liver function) ▪ Start sublingual buprenorphine 3 mg three times daily for OUD and pain in coordination with outpatient palliative care clinician
Case 3	▪ 48-y-old ▪ History of OUD in sustained remission on methadone ▪ Admitted for surgical resection of colorectal mass	▪ Acute cancer–related rectal and abdominal pain ▪ Severe OUD in sustained remission; Urine drug testing positive for methadone only ▪ Discussed care with outpatient palliative care clinician ▪ Likely curable cancer, prognosis of years	▪ Continue once daily methadone for OUD unchanged at OTP ▪ Start IR morphine as needed for abdominal and rectal pain with plan to taper and stop ▪ Communicated plan with OTP and outpatient palliative care clinician
Case 4	▪ 62-y-old ▪ Liver cirrhosis ▪ Chronic progressive abdominal pain ▪ Ascites ▪ Admitted for sepsis ▪ Urine test positive for methamphetamines	▪ Chronic abdominal pain related to ascites ▪ Severe stimulant use disorder; using inhaled methamphetamine ▪ Prognosis of months to years	▪ Paracentesis ▪ Diuretics for ascites ▪ Referral to outpatient SUD treatment program ▪ Start buccal buprenorphine for pain after discussion with primary care clinician and SUD treatment program ▪ Close outpatient monitoring
Case 5	▪ 42-y-old ▪ History of breast cancer s/p cure with mastectomy and radiation ▪ Chronic cancer–related pain on oxycodone ▪ Admitted with pulmonary embolism ▪ Urine drug testing with +cocaine, benzodiazepines, and oxycodone	▪ No history of prescribed benzodiazepines, only intermittent use with no harms ▪ Meets criteria for unhealthy substance use but not substance use disorder at this time based on history ▪ Anxiety disorder ▪ Follows with outpatient palliative care clinician ▪ Cured cancer, no evidence of recurrent disease	▪ Counsel on risks of nonprescribed substance use and harms of cocaine use ▪ Plan to monitor and re-evaluate substance use in the outpatient setting ▪ Communicate findings with outpatient palliative care clinician and discuss plan to taper oxycodone ▪ Start transdermal buprenorphine and taper off oxycodone ▪ Treat anxiety

TABLE 18.6

Summary Cases for Pain Management in Those With SUD and Serious Illness[66,67] (*Continued*)

	Brief case	Assessment	Co-created plan
Case 6	■ 68-y-old ■ End-stage heart failure ■ Active opioid, stimulant, and alcohol use disorders ■ Admitted to intensive care with cardiogenic shock	■ Acute-on-chronic bilateral lower extremity pain ■ Acute-on-chronic anxiety and dyspnea ■ Severe opioid use disorder, alcohol use disorder, stimulant use disorder ■ Active opioid and alcohol withdrawal ■ Patient and family goals are aligned with comfort measures only ■ Prognosis is hours to days ■ Due to high level of care to maintain comfort, plan is made to remain admitted through EOL	■ Start intravenous hydromorphone and lorazepam for symptom management ■ If ongoing symptoms appear related to opioid withdrawal, can give IV methadone[a] to treat opioid withdrawal symptoms ■ Titrate medications to maintain comfort ■ If using more than four doses of as needed medication in a 12-h period, consider starting continuous infusion
Case 7	■ 58-y-old ■ Active methamphetamine, cannabis, and tobacco use disorders ■ Diagnosed with metastatic pancreatic adenocarcinoma after incidental finding of mass on imaging	■ Chronic nonmalignant lower back and bilateral shoulder pain ■ Severe methamphetamine use disorder ■ Moderate cannabis use disorder ■ Tobacco use disorder ■ Prognosis of weeks to months	■ Start buccal buprenorphine for pain in the setting of nonopioid SUDs after discussion with outpatient palliative care clinician ■ Advise about harms of ongoing methamphetamine use and cannabis use ■ Offer nicotine replacement therapy ■ If patient continues to use substances, may need to revisit the plan
Case 8	■ 67-y-old ■ Active alcohol and cocaine use disorders ■ Relapsed multiple myeloma ■ Admitted with acute pathologic pelvic fracture related to lytic lesion	■ Acute right-sided pelvic pain, worse with transfers and turning in bed ■ Chronic bone pain related to lytic lesions ■ Severe alcohol use disorder ■ Severe cocaine use disorder ■ Impaired renal function ■ Prognosis of weeks to months ■ Follows with outpatient palliative care clinic	■ Discuss pain and limited prognosis with outpatient palliative care clinician, together make a plan to address acute cancer–related pain ■ Start transdermal buprenorphine for pain ■ Start oral hydromorphone as needed for severe pain ■ Provide treatment options for alcohol use and cocaine use ■ Treat acute alcohol withdrawal ■ Monitor patient closely and may need to revisit plan if ongoing cocaine and alcohol use
Case 9	■ 50-y-old ■ OUD in remission on SL buprenorphine ■ Generalized anxiety disorder ■ Admitted with neck pain and dysphagia ■ Diagnosed with squamous cell carcinoma with region lymphadenopathy	■ Chronic pain (bilateral knees) and acute pain of neck related to malignancy ■ OUD stable on 8 mg BID of SL buprenorphine/naloxone from primary care doctor ■ Plan for curative treatment with surgery, chemotherapy, and radiation ■ Referred to outpatient palliative care clinic for symptom management	■ Discussed with primary care and outpatient palliative care clinician, together made plan for increase to 8 mg TID of SL buprenorphine for pain and OUD ■ SL buprenorphine to be prescribed by palliative care clinician ■ Continue buprenorphine at raised dose through the perioperative period ■ Provide full-agonist opioids and other pain treatments for multimodal pain care ■ Started duloxetine for pain and anxiety ■ Referred to counseling for those with cancer for anxiety in setting of new diagnosis

(*continued*)

TABLE 18.6

Summary Cases for Pain Management in Those With SUD and Serious Illness[66,67] (*Continued*)

	Brief case	Assessment	Co-created plan
Case 10	■ 64-y-old ■ Polysubstance use (opioids, alcohol, benzodiazepines) ■ Alcohol-related liver disease ■ Admitted to the ICU with sepsis ■ Transitioned to comfort focused care after goals of care conversation with family	■ Encephalopathic ■ Bilateral upper extremity tremors, diaphoresis, restlessness, grimacing unresponsive to multiple doses of IV lorazepam and hydromorphone over last 8 h ■ Estimated prognosis is hours to days	■ Start monitoring with RDOS and CPOT[66,67] ■ Start continuous infusion of IV hydromorphone based on last 24 hr use ■ Start IV hydromorphone 2 mg every 1 h as needed for RDOS >2 and CPOT >2 ■ Start scheduled IV lorazepam 1 mg every 8 h with as needed dose for restlessness, second line for RDOS and/or CPOT >2 ■ If ongoing symptoms appear related to opioid withdrawal, can give IV methadone[a] to treat opioid withdrawal symptoms

[a]Methadone PO to IV methadone has a 2:1 dosing ratio. For example, 40 mg of oral methadone is equal to 20 mg of IV methadone.

RDOS, Respiratory Distress Observation Scale; CPOT, Critical care Pain Observation Tool.

symptoms. Patients in the hospital should be assessed for symptoms like pain, nausea, fatigue, and mood disorders related to their serious illness and offered treatment. Close attention is required as the patient will likely be experiencing a combination of heightened pain perception, high degree of pain interference, substance withdrawal symptoms, and acute symptoms related to their serious illness. See the section on EOL symptom management for information on treating withdrawal at EOL. Promptly treating symptoms can facilitate a therapeutic alliance and be the first step in addressing SUD.

Preferably those with SUD and serious illness will be ready to receive treatment for their SUD. However, often offers of in-hospital and postdischarge SUD treatment are declined. If controlled medications (often opioids) are required at hospital discharge to manage symptoms related to a serious illness, patients are typically referred to an outpatient palliative care clinician, however, untreated SUD can be a barrier to this follow up. In most communities there are not clinics or clinicians equipped to provide outpatient palliative care for those with active SUD. Ideally this complexity necessitates follow up with a clinic equipped to provide close follow up (weekly visits) and monitoring, especially when the patient requires medications which may be higher risk for possibly exacerbating ongoing substance use (eg, opioid analgesics, benzodiazepines, stimulants). Instead, hospital clinicians may be able to effectively treat the patient's symptoms during the hospital admission, promote and encourage engagement in SUD treatment, and provide a prescription for opioid or other medications needed to control symptoms at discharge. Unfortunately, coordination of follow up may not always be possible. In this situation patients should continue to be offered standard serious illness care including aggressive symptom management and SUD treatment. The patient may have multiple admissions before they can be effectively connected to outpatient care and their SUD treated. Hospital clinicians can be key to helping patients break out of patterns of SUD because hospitals can become people's primary source of care until a degree of stability is achieved to facilitate outpatient follow-up. Though it may require more than one hospital admission, compassion and repeated offers of treatment can facilitate individuals engaging with SUD care.

Individualized Care

Providing palliative care for those with untreated SUD and serious illness requires an individualized approach. Hospital clinicians should gain an understanding of the patient's goals in the setting of their unique biopsychosocial context. Integration of psychological, social, spiritual, and physical support using a tailored approach can alleviate suffering and minimize harms of continued substance use. When available, social workers, chaplains, peer specialists, and case managers can provide support for patients in a holistic, individualized way. Connection to available resources to address multiple dimensions of care is part of treating SUD, even if the patient declines to start medications or other treatments for SUD.

The practice of palliative care includes careful assessment of the patient's social and cultural environment. Attention to the social and structural factors impacting the patient's serious illness can also be used to guide trauma-informed care and help maintain the patient's connection to care until they are ready for treatment of their SUD.

Harm Reduction

Offering treatment for SUD is a key part of effective palliative care in this population of people. Treatment for SUD can provide stability and promote well-being, without the patient necessarily ending all substance use. Rather than focusing on complete cessation, attention should be focused on clinical care that reduces harm and recognizes the impact of social drivers of health. For example, in the serious-illness population, treating pain and other symptoms aggressively can be an effective form of harm reduction.

Care Coordination

As highlighted in the summary of evidence section, the use of a multidisciplinary team while hospitalized and in transitions of care is vital. Communication between pharmacy staff and the hospital-based prescriber can prevent confusion regarding concomitant prescriptions for both partial and full-agonist opioids. In addition, prior authorizations are often needed for opioid medications. Ideally, before initiating a full-agonist opioid for pain in addition to buprenorphine, the inpatient team would have discussed the plan of care with the outpatient clinician who will be responsible for management and refills. Lack of identification of an outpatient prescriber can obviously prevent this communication. If available palliative care clinician are a good option for patients' cancer-related symptoms. Palliative care clinics are typically not equipped to follow-up on management of opioid therapy for nonmalignant chronic pain. For those without access to a palliative care clinic for patients without malignancy, the responsibility can fall to primary care or addiction medicine clinicians. As mentioned above, palliative care, primary care, oncologists, and addiction medicine clinicians may not be adequately prepared to manage complex situations involving opioids. In some academic centers there are clinics specializing in the care of those with chronic pain, serious illness, and SUD but these are not widely available.

Goals of Care

As individuals age and serious illness progresses, decisions about next steps in care need to be made. Goals of care conversations, sometimes called serious illness conversations, can be helpful touchpoints to share information, provide support, and gain insight into patient and loved one's values. Exploration of values helps clinicians match available therapeutic and supportive options with patient goals and make recommendations. These conversations are often challenging. Adding the complexity of a diagnosis of SUD can make prognostication more difficult, in turn decision making also gets more difficult. On top of those challenges, there are layers of stigma and structural barriers which can add to patient needs and detract from available resources.

Utilizing conversation guides like REMAP (reframe, expect emotion, map values, align, plan), a framework used in palliative care as part of VitalTalk, can provide practical guidance on language and topics to discuss with patients and their loved ones.[68] The Serious Illness Conversation Guide through Ariadne Labs is another helpful resource.[69] If conversations are had while in the hospital, these should be documented in a clear way (in an advance directive [AD] or other form if appropriate, see next paragraph) to help guide future care and ongoing discussions.

Advance Care Planning

Advance care planning (ACP) is different from goals of care conversations because ACP aims to help patients outline their wishes regarding medical care in the future. Goals of care conversations aim to talk about the present situation. ACP has been defined as a process that helps patients develop and share their "personal values, life goals, and preferences regarding future medical care. The goal of ACP is to help ensure that people receive medical care that is consistent with their values, goals, and preferences during serious and chronic illness."[70] Wishes expressed during ACP conversations are communicated to surrogates and clinicians in the future via an AD. An AD often refers to the documentation of a person's future wishes, typically in state-disseminated AD forms, living wills, or physician order for life-sustaining therapy (POLST) or medical order for life-sustaining treatment (MOLST) forms. These documents also designate a surrogate decision maker, sometimes called a medical power of attorney. For people who may have more social complexity, having documentation of the person's wishes regarding any limitations on future care (resuscitation, artificial hydration and nutrition, dialysis, etc) and preferred surrogate decision maker is particularly beneficial. Several resources are available to facilitate ACP and AD completion; some include websites like, "The Conversation Project" and "Prepare for Your Care."[71,72]

Challenges of Goals of Care Conversations for Those With SUD

Rates of AD completion in the general adult population in the United States are low.[73] AD completion by those with SUD has not been studied. Studies of several vulnerable populations, including those with vulnerabilities that have been associated with SUD, have found AD completion rates are even lower.[74–76] Multiple factors are thought to limit ACP discussions and AD creation for those with SUD.

Strained Relationships

Any serious illness can add strain to relationships. SUD can have a similar negative impact on relationships and degrade a person's support network over time. By the time a person with SUD has aged and the burden of serious illness has built up, it can be difficult to identify a trusted medical surrogate decision maker.

Fragmentation of Care

The guidelines on ACP by the American College of Physicians recommend that ACP conversations be start in the outpatient setting.[77] Generating outpatient continuity for patients with any illness is difficult, even more so for those with SUD. In theory, an outpatient clinician has a longer therapeutic relationship with patients and is therefore better positioned to discuss sensitive topics like declining health and what that could mean for future care. In addition, inpatient clinicians often meet patients in periods of health crisis when patients' imaginations are more closed to planning for future declines. Hospital stays for those with serious illness with or without SUDs are common and can lead to fragmented care that disrupts the recommended pattern of ACP discussions.

Delay Discounting

Delay discounting is defined as a viewpoint that the value of something decreases as more time passes before one receives that thing. It is termed delay discounting because the thing that is delayed (ie, in the future) is perceived to have a discounted value simply because that thing is in the future. This psychological phenomenon can be increased for individuals with SUD.[78,79] Devaluation of future events or rewards can artificially reduce patients' ability to envision the future. As a result, the value we assign to future events now may differ from the value we would assign to that event in a future moment. This viewpoint has the potential to impair decision making around hypothetical future medical events, like a cardiac arrest, critical care admission, or need for a feeding tube.

Psychological Comorbidities

Severe mental illness contributes to the fragmentation of outpatient care and therefore can limit effective ACP as mentioned above. In addition, severe mental illness can lead to clinician concerns about patient capacity to have serious-illness conversations.[80] Psychosocial comorbidities and associated systemic structural inequities can also push those with SUDs to develop mistrust of the medical system and clinicians. Mistrust in medicine and impulsive thinking can similarly prevent engagement in ACP altogether.

Social Drivers of Health

Socioeconomic status, race, ethnicity, and geography are known to be significant factors impacting a person's health and longevity, including access and quality of SUD treatment and palliative care.[81–90] These barriers can prevent people from getting the medical care they need and deserve. A qualitative study of ACP with those with limited income found that acknowledgment of hardships, continuity, and feeling their story was heard were important ways to facilitate effective ACP.[91] Barriers to ACP in individuals experiencing housing instability include focus on present needs rather than future needs (housing, SUD recovery), emotional burden of ACP discussion while person is in a vulnerable state (early recovery, unhoused), and uncertainty around prognosis.[92]

Stigma

Stigma is an unfortunately common source of health care disparity for individuals with SUD. Those with serious illness and SUD face stigma related to their serious illness as well. SUDs and pain are additional sources of stigma in health care. By the time people with SUD and serious illness require palliative care and/or hospice care, they have almost certainly encountered these barriers. Someone with this prior experience may not be ready or able to accept the idea of placing limits on future medical care; the care they had previously worked so hard to gain.

Hospice

Some hospital admissions are used to connect patients with serious illness and SUD with limited prognosis to hospice care. After using goals of care conversations to establish that the patient's values align with comfort as a priority over attempting to gain longevity, consideration of discharge with hospice services is appropriate. See the introduction for a review of hospice services.

For those with SUD, there can be limitations to receiving the hospice care they deserve. Some hospice agencies have regulations that may prevent enrollment of those with SUD. Other agencies may be apprehensive about their ability to provide effective comfort to someone actively using substances. Regardless of SUD or not, it is common for people to have difficulty finding a place to discharge where they can receive hospice services. Again, hospice is a service, not a place. Many people with end-stage serious illness require frequent, if not around-the-clock caregiver support, and this often makes discharge home not feasible. Discharge to a nursing facility can be expensive because Medicare only covers hospice services, it does not include room and board. Those with SUD may face additional barriers. Social networks have often been fragmented by substance use or other social disparities leaving the patient without trusted family and friends to care for them. Nursing facilities can have regulations on the types of medications they will or will not administer or intolerance of ongoing substance use.

Prognostication

Determination of prognosis is necessary for those whose goals align with hospice care because an estimated prognosis of less than 6 months is required by Medicare to qualify for the hospice benefit. Prognostication is challenging. For those with cancer, recognizing when the patient has entered the end stage of their disease is more straightforward than those with other chronic serious illnesses. Clinicians commonly have a more difficult time identifying when those with noncancer serious illnesses have entered this stage of their disease because of difference in disease trajectories. Those with chronic heart failure, for example, may have recurrent admissions for acute decompensations, where they will receive diuresis and possibly inotropic therapy, stabilize, feel better, and discharge. Identifying the one admission when they will not stabilize and not feel better, no matter the intervention offered (ventricular assist devices, home inotropic therapy, dialysis, etc) is more difficult. Prognostication in these patients, as well as those with cancer, can be aided using prognostic tools. In palliative and hospice care, one of the most common tools is called the Palliative Performance Scale (PPS). The PPS is a validated tool, commonly accessed through the ePrognosis website, and uses readily available historical information like nutritional intake and functional status.[93–95] Several disease-specific scoring symptoms have been developed to aid prognostication, see Table 18.7 for a list of some of the available tools for patients in the hospital.[96–101]

TABLE 18.7

Summary of Available Scores to Aid in Prognostication for Patients Admitted to the Hospital With Common Noncancer Serious Illnesses

Decompensated Heart Failure	EFFECT (Enhanced Feedback for Effective Cardiac Treatment) Risk Score[96]
COPD	ADO (Age, Dyspnea, Airflow obstruction) index
	BODE (Body mass index, Airflow obstruction, Dyspnea, Exercise capacity) Score[97]
Decompensated Cirrhosis	Model for end-stage liver disease (MELD)
	Child–Pugh–Turcotte Score[98]
End-Stage Renal Disease on Dialysis	Charlson Comorbidity Index[99]
Cancer	Eastern Cooperative Oncology Group (ECOG) Performance Status[100,101]

End-of-Life Care

The EOL stage is defined as having likely hours to days to live (Table 18.1). At this stage of serious illness, prognostication is informed more by physical exam and vital signs than earlier stages. Increased somnolence, delirium, being bedbound are all indicators that time may be short. At the EOL, a patient's temperature typically rises and blood pressure lowers. Extremities become cool and there is mottling of the skin, often initially the palms and soles. In those with PPS less than or equal to 20%, those without drooping of nasolabial fold have 42% of 3-day mortality rate, while those with drooping of nasolabial fold have 94% of 3-day mortality rate.[102]

After a patient has been identified as being at EOL and goals of care conversations have determined that the patient and/or their surrogate values prioritizing comfort over life extension, aggressive symptom management becomes the focus. For those requiring a higher level of care than can be achieved outside the hospital and/or those with hours to days of life, continuing hospital admission for EOL care is appropriate. Otherwise EOL care often ends up occurring with hospice services, either at home or in a nursing facility.

Approach to Symptom Management at EOL

At EOL, full-agonist opioids should be used as comfort and quality of remaining life become the highest priorities. Those with long-term substance exposure, especially benzodiazepines and opioids, generally require higher doses of comfort-focused medications at shorter intervals to control symptoms and overcome baseline tolerance. In this situation, it is especially important to use the patient's symptoms to guide dosing and frequency of medications. Frequent reassessment of symptoms is important and often challenging in the hospital setting, depending on nursing demands.

Medications for comfort are best given via oral, sublingual, buccal, or intravenous routes. As people near the EOL, it is common for the oral route to no longer be available and medications are converted to sublingual concentrated solutions or intravenous formulations. Transdermal routes are typically not started for those at EOL because of the delayed onset of action (days) and limited titratability. If a patient is already on a transdermal medication such as transdermal fentanyl before they transition to comfort-focused care, this can be continued or converted to another formulation taking care to avoid underdosing and causing opioid withdrawal. Many medications commonly used for comfort are available in subcutaneous formulations and underutilized, mainly due to lack of familiarity or supplies for subcutaneous administration. Rectal administration of medications can be done, however should be limited to less frequently required medications. Intramuscular medications can cause unnecessary discomfort and should be avoided.

Pain

Pain at the EOL is common. It can be assessed directly via patient report or through information from a caregiver or loved one. Frequently patients at EOL are not able to report symptoms including pain. In this situation, the use of the critical care pain observation tool (CPOT) as well as nonverbal cues like grimacing, moaning, and withdrawing from touch are helpful.[66] The first-line medications for pain are short-acting full-agonist opioids. Long-acting formulations are not the first line because of their slow onset of action, limited titratability, and potential to build up resulting in toxicities. If a patient requires more than four or five doses of an as-needed mediation in a 12-hour period, it is recommended to consider starting a continuous infusion. Choice of opioid can be individualized to the patient. Morphine products should be avoided in those with pre-existing renal dysfunction.

Medications for SUD at EOL

Methadone or buprenorphine for OUD should be continued, if possible. Naltrexone and other medications for AUD like disulfiram and acamprosate should be stopped. Clinicians should anticipate the potential loss of oral access and the need to transition methadone to another full-agonist opioid or converted to intravenous methadone. The ratio of intravenous methadone to oral methadone is 1:2 (eg, 100 mg of oral methadone is equal to 50 mg of IV methadone). If the hospital or hospice agency does not have intravenous methadone, other full-agonist opioids can be used but the dose will likely be very high. For example, those on 100 mg of daily methadone could be appropriately transitioned to an intravenous or sublingual equivalent of about 300 mg/d of oral morphine using a 1:3 ratio for oral methadone to oral morphine.[103] This conversion ratio is conservative, meaning the resulting oral morphine dose after converting from oral methadone may underestimate what the patient will ultimately require for analgesia and prevention of opioid withdrawal.

Rarely, patients at EOL are no longer able to take buprenorphine sublingually and conversion to an intravenous, subcutaneous, or transdermal opioid is required. Please use Table 18.4 to guide conversion of low-dose and high-dose buprenorphine formulations to their approximate oral morphine equivalent. For people previously taking a high-dose formulation of buprenorphine a ratio of about 1:30 for *milligrams* of buprenorphine to oral morphine is recommended, however, this may not be appropriate in all cases. Conversion from buprenorphine products to full-agonist opioids has little supporting literature and published ratios vary widely (from 1:10 to 1:110).[104] All conversions from buprenorphine or methadone to full-agonist opioids should be done in close consultation with a pharmacist. Once the appropriate full-agonist dose in oral morphine equivalents is determined, this should be used to calculate the appropriate dose of a long-acting formulation or continuous intravenous infusion. In this way, the new long-acting full agonist is effectively replacing the buprenorphine or methadone, while other short-acting medications target EOL symptoms.

Substance Withdrawal at EOL

At EOL, all symptoms, including symptoms related to withdrawal, should be frequently assessed and aggressively managed. The complexity and overlap of symptoms related to tolerance, withdrawal, and EOL will require additional attention to ensure comfort during the dying process. If possible, use prior medication doses (eg, oral morphine equivalents over last 24 hours, reported prior benzodiazepine use) to guide starting doses of comfort-focused medications.

Obtaining information from the patient or caregiver about how much of a substance the patient was using just prior to being EOL can also help guide symptom management. Effectiveness of medications should be frequently reassessed, often multiple times an hour initially. Patients at EOL may not be able to report symptoms using typical scales for assessing opioid, alcohol, and benzodiazepine withdrawal. Clinicians should monitor for physical signs such as diaphoresis, tremor, hypertension, and tachycardia to guide dosing of medications for withdrawal treatment. If a dose of a medication is ineffective, the dose should be increased by 50% to 100% until symptoms are controlled. If substance withdrawal syndrome is a dominant driver of symptoms, scheduled short-acting medications or long-acting medications can be considered, such as scheduled benzodiazepines or phenobarbital for alcohol withdrawal or a higher dose of scheduled short-acting opioid for opioid withdrawal. Dosing and frequency can be guided by using the total medication usage over the last 12 or 24 hours to guide dosing and frequency (Case 10). Additional medications should be used in addition to medications for withdrawal to treat EOL symptoms. All symptoms at EOL should be treated aggressively favoring use of more medications rather than risk undertreating in last hours to days of life.

Breathlessness

Dyspnea or breathlessness is another commonly encountered symptom for those in the dying process. This can be assessed using patient-reported breathlessness and/or information from someone at the bedside. For patients unable to give a verbal description, use the Respiratory Distress Observation Scale (RDOS) to quantify breathlessness and guide medication administration.[67] First-line therapy for dyspnea at the EOL is a short-acting full-agonist opioid that is titrated to symptom relief similar to the approach to pain management. Breathlessness can lead to anxiety, and anxiety can exacerbate breathlessness, generating a positive feedback loop. To address this, often anxiolytics like benzodiazepines are used in conjunction with opioids. Like in the treatment of pain, doses and/or frequency of medications may be elevated in those with long-term opioid and/or benzodiazepine exposure. Nonpharmacologic therapies have also been found to be effective for breathlessness and include repositioning, air humidification, and/or using a fan directed at the face.[105,106] A trial of oxygen therapy is appropriate. However, if oxygen is not beneficial to relieve symptoms or not tolerated, this should be discontinued.

Anxiety

Anxiety can be evident by patient report at EOL, but more commonly it is observed as restlessness or agitation. Benzodiazepines are the medication of choice to treat anxiety at EOL. Clinicians should pay careful attention to the possibility that anxiety (or its manifestation) is not due to an untreated or undertreated substance withdrawal syndrome. If present, withdrawal should be treated with effective medications as described in the section on substance withdrawal at EOL.

Deprescribing Other Medications

Stopping medications at EOL can be challenging and should be assessed on case-by-case basis. Decisions regarding the benefit of continuing antidepressants, stimulants, muscle relaxers, and antipsychotics should be individualized with attention to those medications associated with withdrawal syndrome (eg, venlafaxine and baclofen). More generally, it is recommended to stop medications intended for primary or secondary prevention (statins, anticoagulation). For those with hyperglycemia or diabetes who can eat or drink, it is recommended to continue limited glucose monitoring and insulin administration with the goal of avoiding serum glucose >200, which can result in glucosuria, dehydration, and discomfort.

Emerging Evidence and Future Directions

Pain is a common but understudied area, especially in those at the intersection of SUD and serious illness. Future research is needed to expand our understanding of appropriate assessment and treatment of pain with research that includes those with SUD and cancer-related pain.

Improving pain management for those with OUD on methadone and serious illness will require revision of policies and laws regulating methadone which can complicate this care. Ongoing advocacy is needed to address stigma faced by those with SUD and that can limit care options, especially regarding care facilities.

A greater availability of outpatient clinicians trained in the care of SUD and palliative care is needed to meet the needs of a growing population of those aging with SUD and serious illness. As outpatient follow-up options emerge, care can be optimized through increased multidisciplinary coordination from hospital to outpatient settings.

REFERENCES

1. Palliative care. Accessed October 3, 2024. https://www.who.int/news-room/fact-sheets/detail/palliative-care
2. Roerecke M, Rehm J. Cause-specific mortality risk in alcohol use disorder treatment patients: a systematic review and meta-analysis. *Int J Epidemiol.* 2014;43(3):906–919.
3. Degenhardt L, Singleton J, Calabria B, et al. Mortality among cocaine users: a systematic review of cohort studies. *Drug Alcohol Depend.* 2011;113(2–3):88–95.
4. Degenhardt L, Bucello C, Mathers B, et al. Mortality among regular or dependent users of heroin and other opioids: a systematic review and meta-analysis of cohort studies. *Addiction.* 2011;106(1):32–51.
5. Singleton J, Degenhardt L, Hall W, Zabransky T. Mortality among amphetamine users: a systematic review of cohort studies. *Drug Alcohol Depend.* 2009;105(1–2):1–8.
6. Jones KF, Osazuwa-Peters OL, Des Marais A, Merlin JS, Check DK. Substance use disorders among US adult cancer survivors. *JAMA Oncol.* 2024;10(3):384–389.
7. Yusufov M, Braun IM, Pirl WF. A systematic review of substance use and substance use disorders in patients with cancer. *Gen Hosp Psychiatry.* 2019;60:128–136.
8. Aldridge RW, Story A, Hwang SW, et al. Morbidity and mortality in homeless individuals, prisoners, sex workers, and individuals with substance use disorders in high-income countries: a systematic review and meta-analysis. *Lancet.* 2018;391(10117):241–250.
9. Callaghan RC, Gatley JM, Sykes J, Taylor L. The prominence of smoking-related mortality among individuals with alcohol- or drug-use disorders. *Drug Alcohol Rev.* 2018;37(1):97–105.
10. Fitzgerald Jones K, Ho JJ, Merlin J, Childers J. Chapter 11: How does the opioid epidemic impact palliative medicine practice? In: Goldstein N, Woodrell C, Morrison RS, eds. *Evidence-Based Practice of Palliative Medicine.* 2nd ed. Elsevier; 2023:85–93.
11. Degenhardt L, Randall D, Hall W, Law M, Butler T, Burns L. Mortality among clients of a state-wide opioid pharmacotherapy program over 20 years: risk factors and lives saved. *Drug Alcohol Depend.* 2009;105(1–2):9–15.
12. Hser YI, Mooney LJ, Saxon AJ, et al. High mortality among patients with opioid use disorder in a large healthcare system. *J Addict Med.* 2017;11(4):315–319.
13. Crump C, Stattin P, Brooks JD, et al. Risks of alcohol and drug use disorders in prostate cancer survivors: a national cohort study. *JNCI Cancer Spectr.* 2023;7(4):pkad046.
14. Singh SA, Moreland RA, Fang W, et al. Compassion inequities and opioid use disorder: a matched case-control analysis examining inpatient management of cancer-related pain for patients with opioid use disorder. *J Pain Symptom Manage.* 2021;62(3):e156–e163.
15. Vipler E, Nowels MA, Youngwerth J. Differences in inpatient management of cancer-related pain among patients with opioid use disorder. *J Palliat Med.* 2024;27(9):1200–1203.
16. Childers JW, Arnold RM. "I feel uncomfortable 'calling a patient out'": educational needs of palliative medicine fellows in managing opioid misuse. *J Pain Symptom Manage.* 2012;43(2):253–260.
17. Merlin JS, Young SR, Arnold R, et al. Managing opioids, including misuse and addiction, in patients with serious illness in ambulatory palliative care: a qualitative study. *Am J Hosp Palliat Care.* 2020;37(7):507–513.
18. Merlin JS, Patel K, Thompson N, et al. Managing chronic pain in cancer survivors prescribed long-term opioid therapy: a national survey of ambulatory palliative care providers. *J Pain Symptom Manage.* 2019;57(1):20–27.
19. Schenker Y, Hamm M, Bulls HW, et al. This is a different patient population: opioid prescribing challenges for patients with cancer-related pain. *JCO Oncol Pract.* 2021;17(7):e1030–e1037.
20. Kale SS, Rush LJ, Eramo JL, et al. Care for patients with cancer and substance use disorders: a qualitative study of oncology team experiences. *Support Care Cancer.* 2025;33(2):146.
21. Langmann GA, Childers J, Merlin JS. Caring for patients with opioid misuse or substance use disorders in hospice: a national survey. *J Palliat Med.* 2024;27(2):209–215.
22. Calcaterra SL, Martin M, Bottner R, et al. Management of opioid use disorder and associated conditions among hospitalized adults: a consensus statement from the Society of Hospital Medicine. *J Hosp Med.* 2022;17(9):744–756.
23. Zanghelini F, Zimmermann IR, Souza de Andrade CA, Wu O. Early palliative care for improving quality of life and survival in patients with advanced cancer: a systematic review and meta-analysis. *J Palliat Care Med.* 2018;08(05).
24. *Growth of Palliative Care in U.S. Hospitals: 2022 Snapshot.* Center to Advance Palliative Care; 2022.
25. van den Beuken-van Everdingen MHJ, Hochstenbach LMJ, Joosten EAJ, Tjan-Heijnen VCG, Janssen DJA. Update on prevalence of pain in patients with cancer: systematic review and meta-analysis. *J Pain Symptom Manage.* 2016;51(6):1070–1090.e9.
26. Viderman D, Tapinova K, Aubakirova M, Abdildin YG. The prevalence of pain in chronic diseases: an umbrella review of systematic reviews. *J Clin Med.* 2023;12(23):7302.
27. Rosenblum A, Joseph H, Fong C, Kipnis S, Cleland C, Portenoy RK. Prevalence and characteristics of chronic pain among chemically dependent patients in methadone maintenance and residential treatment facilities. *JAMA.* 2003;289(18):2370–2378.
28. John WS, Wu LT. Chronic non-cancer pain among adults with substance use disorders: prevalence, characteristics, and association with opioid overdose and healthcare utilization. *Drug Alcohol Depend.* 2020;209:107902.
29. Ren ZY, Shi J, Epstein DH, Wang J, Lu L. Abnormal pain response in pain-sensitive opiate addicts after prolonged abstinence predicts increased drug craving. *Psychopharmacology (Berl).* 2009;204(3):423–429.
30. De Aquino JP, Sloan ME, Nunes JC, et al. Alcohol use disorder and chronic pain: an overlooked epidemic. *Am J Psychiatry.* 2024;181(5):391–402.
31. Trøstheim M, Eikemo M. Hyperalgesia in patients with a history of opioid use disorder: a systematic review and meta-analysis. *JAMA Psychiatry.* 2024;81(11):1108–1117.
32. Dev R, Kim YJ, Reddy A, et al. Association between tobacco use, pain expression, and coping strategies among patients with advanced cancer. *Cancer.* 2019;125(1):153–160.
33. Khan JS, Hah JM, Mackey SC. Effects of smoking on patients with chronic pain: a propensity-weighted analysis on the Collaborative Health Outcomes Information Registry. *Pain.* 2019;160(10):2374–2379.
34. Given SH, Reid Ponte P, Lally K, Chua IS. Interdisciplinary pain board for managing patients with palliative care needs and substance use disorder: a pilot study. *J Palliat Med.* 2024;27(9):1171–1176.
35. Arthur JA, Edwards T, Lu Z, et al. Interdisciplinary intervention for the management of nonmedical opioid use among patients with cancer pain. *Cancer.* 2022;128(20):3718–3726.
36. Kale SS, Tosto GD, Rush LJ, et al. Creating a palliative care clinic for patients with cancer pain and substance use disorder. *J Pain Symptom Manage.* 2024;68(2):e138–e145.

37. Rudy L, Lacroix E. Substance use disorders in hospice palliative care: a narrative review of challenges and a case for physician intervention. *Palliat Support Care.* 2024:1–9.
38. Merlin JS, Khodyakov D, Arnold R, et al. Expert panel consensus on management of advanced cancer-related pain in individuals with opioid use disorder. *JAMA Netw Open.* 2021;4(12):e2139968.
39. Fitzgerald Jones K, Khodyakov D, Arnold R, et al. Consensus-based guidance on opioid management in individuals with advanced cancer-related pain and opioid misuse or use disorder. *JAMA Oncol.* 2022;8(8):1107–1114.
40. Ho JJ, Fitzgerald Jones K, Merlin J, Childers J. Chapter 12: how does one approach the patient with an opioid use disorder? In: Goldstein N, Goodrell C, Morrison RS, eds. *Evidence-Based Practice of Palliative Medicine.* 2nd ed. Elsevier Inc.; 2023:94–107.
41. Raffaeli W, Arnaudo E. Pain as a disease: an overview. *J Pain Res.* 2017;10:2003–2008.
42. Sze WM, Shelley MD, Held I, Wilt TJ, Mason MD. Palliation of metastatic bone pain: single fraction versus multifraction radiotherapy—a systematic review of randomised trials. *Clin Oncol (R Coll Radiol).* 2003;15(6):345–352.
43. Alcorn S, Cortés ÁA, Bradfield L, et al. External beam radiation therapy for palliation of symptomatic bone metastases: an ASTRO clinical practice guideline. *Pract Radiat Oncol.* 2024;14(5):377–397.
44. Chow E, Meyer RM, Ding K, et al. Dexamethasone in the prophylaxis of radiation-induced pain flare after palliative radiotherapy for bone metastases: a double-blind, randomised placebo-controlled, phase 3 trial. *Lancet Oncol.* 2015;16(15): 1463–1472.
45. Gavioli E, Abrams M. Prevention of granulocyte-colony stimulating factor (G-CSF) induced bone pain using double histamine blockade. *Support Care Cancer.* 2017;25(3):817–822.
46. Barghi K, Edmonds KP, Ajayi TA, Atayee RS. Prescribing trends of palliative care team's use of dexamethasone for cancer-related pain. *J Pain Palliat Care Pharmacother.* 2018; 32(1):37–43.
47. Loprinzi CL, Lacchetti C, Bleeker J, et al. Prevention and management of chemotherapy-induced peripheral neuropathy in survivors of adult cancers: ASCO guideline update. *J Clin Oncol.* 2020;38(28):3325–3348.
48. Knopp JA, Diner BM, Blitz M, Lyritis GP, Rowe BH. Calcitonin for treating acute pain of osteoporotic vertebral compression fractures: a systematic review of randomized, controlled trials. *Osteoporos Int.* 2005;16(10):1281–1290.
49. Definitions of chronic pain syndromes—International Association for the Study of Pain (IASP). Accessed January 25, 2025. https://www.iasp-pain.org/advocacy/definitions-of-chronic-pain-syndromes/
50. Ruano A, García-Torres F, Gálvez-Lara M, Moriana JA. Psychological and non-pharmacologic treatments for pain in cancer patients: a systematic review and meta-analysis. *J Pain Symptom Manage.* 2022;63(5):e505–e520.
51. Kernick L, Glare P, Hosie A, Chiu A, Kissane DW. Prevalence and management of chronic nonmalignant pain in palliative care populations: a systematic review. *Palliat Support Care.* 2024;22(4):840–846.
52. Chou R, Turner JA, Devine EB, et al. The effectiveness and risks of long-term opioid therapy for chronic pain: a systematic review for a National Institutes of Health Pathways to Prevention Workshop. *Ann Intern Med.* 2015;162(4): 276–286.
53. Wong SSC, Chan TH, Wang F, Chan TCW, Ho HC, Cheung CW. Analgesic effect of buprenorphine for chronic noncancer pain: a systematic review and meta-analysis of randomized controlled trials. *Anesth Analg.* 2023;137(1):59–71.
54. Swarm R, Youngwerth J, Agne J. National comprehensive cancer network: adult cancer pain. Accessed December 24, 2024. https://www.nccn.org/professionals/physician_gls/pdf/pain.pdf
55. Merlin JS, Black AC, Midboe AM, et al. Long-term opioid therapy trajectories and overdose in patients with and without cancer. *BMJ Oncol.* 2023;2(1):e000023.
56. Kibaly C, Alderete JA, Liu SH, et al. Oxycodone in the opioid epidemic: high "liking", "wanting", and abuse liability. *Cell Mol Neurobiol.* 2021;41(5):899–926.
57. Case AA, Kullgren J, Anwar S, Pedraza S, Davis MP. Treating chronic pain with buprenorphine-the practical guide. *Curr Treat Options Oncol.* 2021;22(12):116.
58. Lazaridou A, Paschali M, Edwards RR, Gilligan C. Is buprenorphine effective for chronic pain? A systematic review and meta-analysis. *Pain Med.* 2020;21(12):3691–3699.
59. Webster L, Gudin J, Raffa RB, et al. Understanding buprenorphine for use in chronic pain: expert opinion. *Pain Med.* 2020;21(4):714–723.
60. Aiyer R, Gulati A, Gungor S, Bhatia A, Mehta N. Treatment of chronic pain with various buprenorphine formulations: a systematic review of clinical studies. *Anesth Analg.* 2018; 127(2):529–538.
61. Gudin J, Fudin J. A narrative pharmacological review of buprenorphine: a unique opioid for the treatment of chronic pain. *Pain Ther.* 2020;9(1):41–54.
62. Davis MP. Twelve reasons for considering buprenorphine as a frontline analgesic in the management of pain. *J Support Oncol.* 2012;10(6):209–219.
63. Ho JJ, Jones KF, Merlin JS, Sager Z, Childers J. Buprenorphine initiation: low-dose methods #457. *J Palliat Med.* 2023; 26(6):867–869.
64. Moeller KE, Lee KC, Kissack JC. Urine drug screening: practical guide for clinicians. *Mayo Clin Proc.* 2008;83(1):66–76.
65. Jones KF, Ho JJ, Sager Z, Childers J, Merlin J. Adapting palliative care skills to provide substance use disorder treatment to patients with serious illness. *Am J Hosp Palliat Care.* 2022;39(1):101–107.
66. Asadi-Noghabi AA, Gholizadeh M, Zolfaghari M, Mehran A, Sohrabi M. Nurses use of critical care pain observational tool in patients with low consciousness. *Oman Med J.* 2015; 30(4):276–282.
67. Murphy MC, Simonis J. Assessment tools for dyspnea and respiratory distress at the end of life #453. *J Palliat Med.* 2023;26(4):582–583.
68. Quick Guides—VitalTalk. Accessed January 7, 2025. https://www.vitaltalk.org/resources/quick-guides/
69. Serious Illness Conversation Guide – Ariadne Labs. Accessed January 7, 2025. https://www.ariadnelabs.org/resources/downloads/serious-illness-conversation-guide/
70. Rosa WE, Izumi S, Sullivan DR, et al. Advance care planning in serious illness: a narrative review. *J Pain Symptom Manage.* 2023;65(1):e63–e78.
71. The Conversation Project—Have You Had The Conversation? Accessed January 7, 2025. https://theconversationproject.org/
72. PREPARE. Accessed January 7, 2025. https://prepareforyourcare.org/en/welcome
73. Yadav KN, Gabler NB, Cooney E, et al. Approximately one in three US adults completes any type of advance directive for end-of-life care. *Health Aff (Millwood).* 2017; 36(7):1244–1251.
74. Sangarlangkarn A, Merlin JS, Tucker RO, Kelley AS. Advance care planning and HIV infection in the era of antiretroviral therapy: a review. *Top Antivir Med.* 2016;23(5):174–180.
75. Leung AK, Nayyar D, Sachdeva M, Song J, Hwang SW. Chronically homeless persons' participation in an advance

directive intervention: a cohort study. *Palliat Med.* 2015;29(8):746–755.
76. Hubbell SA. Advance care planning with individuals experiencing homelessness: literature review and recommendations for public health practice. *Public Health Nurs.* 2017;34(5):472–478.
77. Fleshner MJ, Kennedy AJ, Veldkamp PJ, Childers JW. Would you be surprised if this patient died this year? Advance care planning in substance use disorders. *J Gen Intern Med.* 2019;34(11):2630–2633.
78. Weinsztok S, Brassard S, Balodis I, Martin LE, Amlung M. Delay discounting in established and proposed behavioral addictions: a systematic review and meta-analysis. *Front Behav Neurosci.* 2021;15:786358.
79. Mitchell SH. Linking delay discounting and substance use disorders: genotypes and phenotypes. *Perspect Behav Sci.* 2019;42(3):419–432.
80. Gill RK, Droney J, Owen G, Riley J, Stephenson L. Digital advance care planning with severe mental illness: a retrospective observational cohort analysis of the use of an electronic palliative care coordination system. *BMC Palliat Care.* 2024;23(1):56.
81. Acevedo A, Panas L, Garnick D, et al. Disparities in the treatment of substance use disorders: does where you live matter? *J Behav Health Serv Res.* 2018;45(4):533–549.
82. Mennis J, Stahler GJ. Racial and ethnic disparities in outpatient substance use disorder treatment episode completion for different substances. *J Subst Abuse Treat.* 2016;63:25–33.
83. Ward E, Jemal A, Cokkinides V, et al. Cancer disparities by race/ethnicity and socioeconomic status. *CA Cancer J Clin.* 2004;54(2):78–93.
84. Fiscella K, Franks P, Gold MR, Clancy CM. Inequality in quality: addressing socioeconomic, racial, and ethnic disparities in health care. *JAMA.* 2000;283(19):2579–2584.
85. Islami F, Baeker Bispo J, Lee H, et al. American Cancer Society's report on the status of cancer disparities in the United States, 2023. *CA Cancer J Clin.* 2024;74(2):136–166.
86. Gilmore N, Grant SJ, Bethea TN, et al. A scoping review of racial, ethnic, socioeconomic, and geographic disparities in the outcomes of older adults with cancer. *J Am Geriatr Soc.* 2024;72(6):1867–1900.
87. Magesh S, John D, Li WT, et al. Disparities in COVID-19 outcomes by race, ethnicity, and socioeconomic status: a systematic-review and meta-analysis. *JAMA Netw Open.* 2021;4(11):e2134147.
88. Kardashian A, Serper M, Terrault N, Nephew LD. Health disparities in chronic liver disease. *Hepatology.* 2023;77(4):1382–1403.
89. Jones T, Luth EA, Lin SY, Brody AA. Advance care planning, palliative care, and end-of-life care interventions for racial and ethnic underrepresented groups: a systematic review. *J Pain Symptom Manage.* 2021;62(3):e248–e260.
90. Nelson KE, Wright R, Peeler A, Brockie T, Davidson PM. Sociodemographic disparities in access to hospice and palliative care: an integrative review. *Am J Hosp Palliat Care.* 2021;38(11):1378–1390.
91. Kimpel CC, Frechman E, Chavez L, Maxwell CA. Essential advance care planning intervention features in low-income communities: a qualitative study. *J Pain Symptom Manage.* 2025;69(1):e46–e52.
92. Hudson BF, Shulman C, Low J, et al. Challenges to discussing palliative care with people experiencing homelessness: a qualitative study. *BMJ Open.* 2017;7(11):e017502.
93. Bischoff KE, Patel K, Boscardin WJ, O'Riordan DL, Pantilat SZ, Smith AK. Prognoses associated with palliative performance scale scores in modern palliative care practice. *JAMA Netw Open.* 2024;7(7):e2420472.
94. Wilner LS, Arnold RM. The palliative performance scale #125. *J Palliat Med.* 2006;9(4):994.
95. Anderson F, Downing GM, Hill J, Casorso L, Lerch N. Palliative performance scale (PPS): a new tool. *J Palliat Care.* 1996;12(1):5–11.
96. Heidenreich PA, Bozkurt B, Aguilar D, et al. 2022 AHA/ACC/HFSA guideline for the management of heart failure: a report of the American College of Cardiology/American Heart Association Joint Committee on clinical practice guidelines. *Circulation.* 2022;145(18):e895–e1032.
97. Guerra B, Haile SR, Lamprecht B, et al. Large-scale external validation and comparison of prognostic models: an application to chronic obstructive pulmonary disease. *BMC Med.* 2018;16(1):33.
98. Rogal SS, Hansen L, Patel A, et al. AASLD practice guidance: palliative care and symptom-based management in decompensated cirrhosis. *Hepatology.* 2022;76(3):819–853.
99. Cohen LM, Ruthazer R, Moss AH, Germain MJ. Predicting six-month mortality for patients who are on maintenance hemodialysis. *Clin J Am Soc Nephrol.* 2010;5(1):72–79.
100. Buccheri G, Ferrigno D, Tamburini M. Karnofsky and ECOG performance status scoring in lung cancer: a prospective, longitudinal study of 536 patients from a single institution. *Eur J Cancer.* 1996;32A(7):1135–1141.
101. Oken MM, Creech RH, Tormey DC, et al. Toxicity and response criteria of the Eastern Cooperative Oncology Group. *Am J Clin Oncol.* 1982;5(6):649–655.
102. Hui D, Dos Santos R, Chisholm G, Bansal S, Souza Crovador C, Bruera E. Bedside clinical signs associated with impending death in patients with advanced cancer: preliminary findings of a prospective, longitudinal cohort study. *Cancer.* 2015;121(6):960–967.
103. McPherson MLM. *Demystifying Opioid Conversion Calculations: A Guide for Effective Dosing.* 2nd ed. American Society of Health-System Pharmacists; 2018.
104. Neale KJ, Weimer MB, Davis MP, et al. Top ten tips palliative care clinicians should know about buprenorphine. *J Palliat Med.* 2023;26(1):120–130.
105. Kako J, Morita T, Yamaguchi T, et al. Fan therapy is effective in relieving dyspnea in patients with terminally ill cancer: a parallel-arm, randomized controlled trial. *J Pain Symptom Manage.* 2018;56(4):493–500.
106. Tsai JJ, Chen KH, Fang HF, Huang TW. Relieving from breathlessness in the wind: a meta-analysis and subjective report of effectiveness of fan blowing in patients with cardiorespiratory diseases or cancer. *Am J Hosp Palliat Care.* 2022;39(8):977–985.

19 Harm Reduction in Hospital Settings

Raagini Jawa, Margaret Shang, Ilana Hull

I first met JK while interviewing her for a research study about her experiences with xylazine and caring for xylazine wounds. She recounted stigmatizing interactions she had with health care workers, legal involvement due to in-hospital substance use, difficulties with accessing wound care and harm reduction supplies, and inadequate inpatient pain and withdrawal management. However, among these things, what stood out to me the most was when she commented matter-of-factly that she would have rather died than seek care at a hospital again.

Fortunately, her friends convinced her to come about an hour and a half northwest of where she was living to our hospital. She sought treatment once more for her superinfected bilateral forearm wounds, a result of regular xylazine use, now complicated by osteomyelitis. JK had these wounds for 2 years, initially unaware they were the result of unintentional xylazine exposure from the unregulated fentanyl supply. She found juggling her wound care and a busy work schedule to be challenging, further complicated by cost of the wound care supplies and a lack of information about how to best care for her wounds. JK continued to use fentanyl due to the pain, sometimes injecting into her wound when she had difficulty with venous access. She also tried switching from injecting to snorting, but her wounds progressively worsened. JK reported feeling isolated and hid her wounds from others. "Nobody talks about it," she said, only becoming aware of xylazine after seeing it on the news. With syringe service programs still illegal in her state, JK lacked access to harm reduction services, including safer use equipment like sterile needles and substance checking equipment like xylazine test strips.

During JK's hospitalization, our addiction consultation service prescribed short-acting opioids for withdrawal management and pain control with adequate doses to account for her opioid tolerance. We provided JK education on the effects of xylazine on her body and self-care strategies to support wound healing. Through continued engagement and rapport building, JK expressed a desire to stop using fentanyl but also acknowledged that her living environment and arm pain would make it difficult to fully abstain. She was hesitant about starting medications for opioid use disorder (OUD), but was receptive to discussing strategies to support her health and to keep her safe from fentanyl-related harms. Over JK's hospitalization, we explored harm-reduction strategies related to overdose prevention, substance checking, and safer substance use. Due to unforeseen personal circumstances, JK left the hospital before completing medical treatment. Our addiction consultation service ensured she was discharged with oral antibiotics, naloxone, xylazine test strips, wound care supplies, and had a follow-up appointment scheduled at a low-barrier OUD treatment and primary care clinic. Upon leaving the hospital, JK expressed relief that she had finally found a team of clinicians who cared for her with dignity and respect.

Following hospital discharge, JK connected with the low-barrier clinic for methadone treatment and primary care clinic where she continues to receive wound care today. JK has periods when she returns to fentanyl use; she shares these instances openly, recognizing that she is able to continue to receive health care without the expectation of abstinence from her medical team.

JK's case highlights how hospitalizations are an important opportunity to engage people who use substances to build trust with the health care system. This is done by respecting their autonomy, acknowledging their personal experiences, providing them with compassionate, nonjudgmental care, and empowering them to make personal decisions to support their health and to reduce harms. Through normalization of harm reduction education, provision of harm reduction supplies, and adequate treatment of opioid withdrawal and pain management, hospital-based clinicians have an opportunity to create a supportive environment that fosters collaboration, reduces stigma, and promotes the health of people with substance use disorder.

—Margaret Shang

Key Points

- **Due to the increasingly toxic unregulated substance supply in the United States (US), people with substance use disorder (SUD) are facing unprecedented rates of substance use–related morbidity and mortality and associated hospitalizations.**
- **Harm reduction is an evidence-based patient-centered approach that encompasses both *relational* and *structural* aspects that promote the health and dignity of people with SUD.**
- ***Relational harm reduction* includes six principles (humanism, pragmatism, autonomy, individualism, incrementalism, accountability without termination) that underpin the clinician–patient relationship to foster trust, respect, and collaboration.**
- ***Structural harm reduction* is a set of practical strategies that complement *relational harm reduction* to minimize substance use–related complications and includes laboratory screening, immunizations, safer substance use counseling and equipment, overdose prevention and education, substance checking, and overdose prevention centers.**
- **Historically, hospitals and hospital-based clinicians emphasized an abstinence-based approach when caring for hospitalized people with SUD. To reduce patient-directed discharge and associated morbidity and mortality, hospitals and hospital-based clinicians must undergo a paradigm shift to embrace a harm reduction model to support their patients to remain in the hospital to receive life-saving care.**
- **Integration of *relational* and *structural harm reduction* within hospital settings through clinician–patient communication, supportive and collaborative hospital policies, and risk mitigation education and tools can enhance patient outcomes, reduce health disparities, and promote a more inclusive and compassionate hospital care environment.**

This chapter on harm reduction explores the philosophy, strategies, and implementation of harm-reduction practices in the context of substance use, public health, and the hospital setting. It begins by defining harm reduction as a pragmatic approach that prioritizes minimizing the negative consequences associated with substance use rather than insisting on abstinence. This chapter highlights the historical evolution of harm reduction, its grounding in public health principles, and its alignment with human rights. It outlines how harm reduction challenges traditional punitive models by focusing on compassion, autonomy, and meeting individuals "where they are" without judgment. Next, a key portion of the chapter discusses practical interventions used in harm reduction, such as syringe service programs (SSPs), overdose prevention centers (OPCs), naloxone distribution, and medication treatment for substance use disorders (SUDs). These interventions are framed not only as tools to reduce overdose deaths and the spread of infectious diseases but also as gateways to building trust with marginalized populations. This chapter also addresses common misconceptions and critiques of harm reduction, such as concerns that it enables substance use, countering by providing data and ethical arguments emphasizing the value of saving lives and fostering engagement with health care. Finally, the chapter examines the systemic and policy challenges facing harm reduction efforts, including stigma, criminalization, and funding limitations both within and outside of the hospital setting. Lastly, this chapter emphasizes the importance of advocacy, interdisciplinary collaboration, and community-led initiatives to advance harm reduction work in the context of hospitalized people who use substances or who have SUD.

Definition and Principles of Harm Reduction

Harm reduction encompasses three major concepts: a philosophy of practice, a bundle of practical strategies to reduce the harmful consequences of substance use, and a larger public health and social justice movement.[1] These three concepts center around promoting the health and dignity of people with SUD. The philosophy of the practice of harm reduction in health care settings, also described as *relational harm reduction*, is defined by six principles grounded in the clinician–patient relationship: humanism, pragmatism, individualism, autonomy, incrementalism, and accountability without termination.[2] The practical implementation of harm reduction, also described as *structural harm reduction*, includes a set of strategies that minimizes harms associated with substance use including substance checking, immunizations, overdose education and prevention, safer substance use supplies, human immunodeficiency (HIV) and hepatitis C viral (HCV) testing, wound care, safe sex supplies, and linkage to SUD treatment.[2] Together, *relational harm reduction* and associated *structural harm reduction strategies* benefit the health and dignity of people with SUD, thereby benefiting society as a whole.[1,2]

Substance use occurs on a spectrum from no use at all to occasional use to regular use to SUD as defined by the DSM-5 criteria.[3] Harm reduction interventions are equally applicable to those with a diagnosed SUD, to those who use substances sporadically, and to those who use substances just once.

History and Current State of Harm Reduction in the US

The term "harm reduction" was popularized in 1987 and was born from a global movement in response to the growing HIV and AIDS epidemic in the 1980s. Early harm reduction efforts in the United States (US) included syringe exchanges where used syringes were exchanged for new ones and HIV educational campaigns like BleachMan which promoted using household bleach to disinfect syringes to decrease transmission of HIV. This strategy is still sometimes recommended in areas with limited access to syringe services. Figure 19.1 includes directions for cleaning injection supplies with bleach when access to new syringes is limited.

Later, in the 1990s, grassroots harm reduction activists worked to expand efforts related to overdose education and prevention through public health campaigns to raise awareness and targeted distribution of naloxone to higher-risk populations and syringe

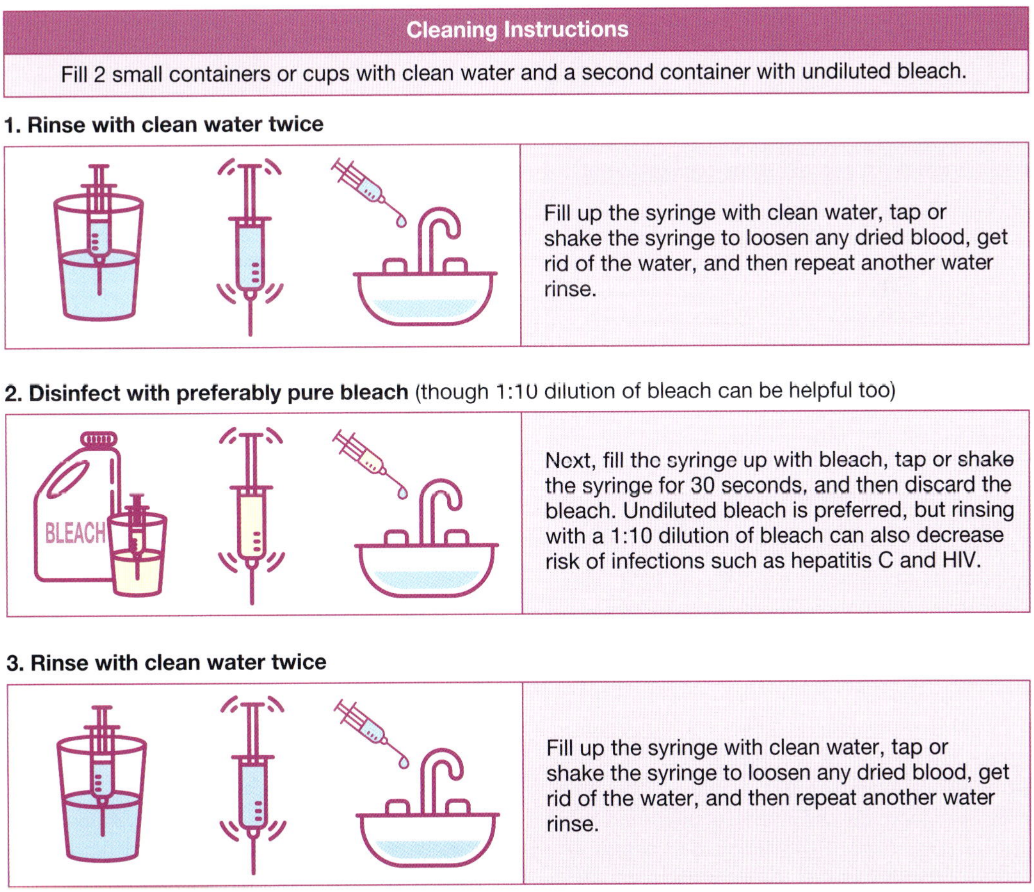

Figure 19.1: Patient handout: Cleaning equipment with bleach. (Resources for safer injection and substance use. Yale Program in Addiction Medicine in affiliation with the Yale New Haven Hospital Multidisciplinary Endocarditis Evaluation Team [MEET]. Accessed November 12, 2025. https://safersubstanceuse.org/cleaning-equipment-with-bleach/)

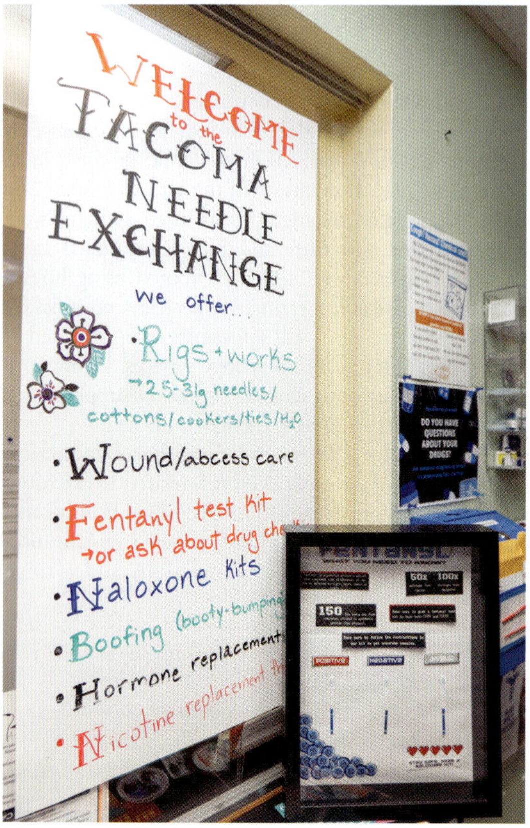

Figure 19.2: Tacoma needle exchange. Sign at the services window at Tacoma Needle Exchange, a syringe services program, showing a list of available community health and safer use supplies. Next to the sign is a framed display titled "Fentanyl: What You Need to Know" that shows three different fentanyl test strip results: positive, negative, and invalid. (Source: https://empathylens.org/photo/tne008/). Accessed November 12, 2025.

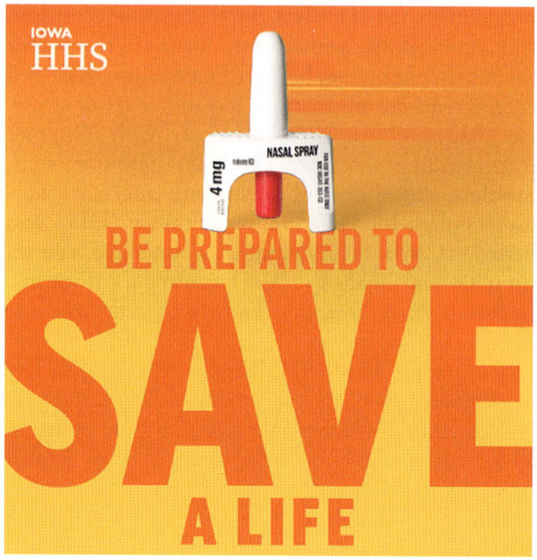

Figure 19.3: Naloxone campaign. Iowa Health and Human Programs and Services. Save a life with naloxone. (Naloxone Bus Shelter Ad. Centers for Disease Control and Prevention. Overdose Research Exchange. September 23, 2024. Accessed March 6, 2026. https://www.cdc.gov/overdose-resources/files/naloxone-bus-shelter-ad.html)

exchanges. These programs aimed to humanize people by reducing stigma and providing harm reduction supplies. Figure 19.2 depicts a welcoming sign for a community needle exchange program that dispenses fentanyl test strips (FTS), wound care supplies, and naloxone to people who use drugs. Figure 19.3 depicts a state educational campaign to increase awareness and access to naloxone for overdose reversal.

In the US, staunch opposition to these efforts arose among community members and politicians who viewed that proponents of harm reduction were encouraging or enabling substance use. Moreover, prohibitionist policies throughout the 1900s in the US were founded on the moral condemnation of the use of psychoactive substances and stigmatization of certain racial and ethnic minorities (eg, use of smoking opium among Chinese immigrants, crack cocaine use among Black individuals, and cannabis use among Mexican immigrants).[4] As a result, a "War on Drugs" ideology was formulated, centered around generation of fear and anger around substance use, criminalization for substance use over treatment, and abstinence-based care models, which starkly opposed the foundational principles of harm reduction.[5] In the years since its inception, discourse surrounding the "War on Drugs" in the US, has been critical of its disproportionate impact on certain communities.

In 1988, use of US federal funds for harm-reduction efforts was temporarily prohibited by Congress on the basis that more evidence was needed to demonstrate that harm reduction was safe and effective.[6] Even though the Human Health and Services Secretary deemed that syringe exchange was indeed safe and effective, in 1998, Congress passed an unconditional ban on use of federal funds for harm reduction.[4] The federal funding ban was repealed in 2009, reinstated in 2011, and repealed again in 2015. Finally, under the 2021 Biden–Harris administration American Rescue Plan Act, an unprecedented 30 million US federal dollars were allocated for harm reduction.[7]

Today, harm reduction efforts are primarily funded privately or at the state or local levels and delivered through community-based organizations called syringe service programs (SSPs). SSPs have evolved over time from offering syringe exchange to providing broad services including substance checking, other forms of safer substance use supplies, immunizations, laboratory screening and testing, and linkage to SUD and infectious disease treatment.[8,9]

As of 2023, SSPs remain illegal in 12 US states; however, due to local or county exceptions and grassroot efforts, only 4 of them do not have operational SSPs.[10] The current state of SSP legality and their slow uptake, despite strong evidence for harm reduction, largely reflects the effects of the US federal funding ban and other prohibitionist policies. As the protection of public health is traditionally a state-level and not a federal-level domain, individual state representatives can authorize and prohibit SSPs. However, banning of US federal funds for SSPs symbolizes disapproval, leading to reluctance from states to operate SSPs without federal support.

Furthermore, health care settings traditionally embrace an abstinence-based approach to SUD treatment, further limiting access to life-saving evidence-based harm reduction services.[11] Due to rising morbidity and mortality associated with use of the unregulated US drug supply, it is critical to integrate harm reduction practices in health care settings. This chapter focuses on describing both *structural* and *relational harm reduction* considerations in the hospital setting to ensure the promotion of the health and dignity of people who use drugs.

Scope of the Problem

People with SUD experience increased rates of health care utilization, with emergency department visits five times higher, and hospitalizations seven times higher, than the general population.[12] Fentanyl adulteration in the unregulated drug substance marketed increased hospitalizations related to overdose.[13] High-risk injection practices with fentanyl use led to outbreaks of HIV and HCV, as well as infectious complications related to injection, such as endocarditis and cellulitis.[13,14] These trends contribute to higher mortality and health care costs.[15] Projections suggest that by 2030, over a quarter-million people who inject substances will die from endocarditis, and 40% of new HCV infections will occur in this population.[16] Given the rise in hospitalizations among people with SUD, these moments present an opportunity to address overdose and infectious risks.

Despite medical harms associated with substance use, many people with SUD avoid or delay seeking medically necessary health care due to stigma, lack of SUD treatment services, inadequate withdrawal and pain management, legal concerns, or ambivalence toward their substance use.[17] Furthermore, hospitals can be high-risk environments.[18,19] In the US, approximately one-third of hospitalized patients with an injection-related infection engages in in-hospital nonprescribed substance use.[20,21] This places patients at risk for syringe sharing or using substances alone in hospital bathrooms, both of which are associated with adverse health outcomes like infectious disease transmission, overdose, and death.[22] Furthermore, in-hospital substance use may lead to involuntary hospital discharge, room searches, in-hospital arrest, or patient bans from hospitals.[23,24] Negative staff attitudes and inadequate management of pain and withdrawal further exacerbate health disparities and lead to patient-directed discharges.[19,25] Unsurprisingly, people with SUD are four times more likely to leave the hospital as a patient-directed discharge compared to people without SUD, and leaving before completing medical treatment is a strong predictor of frequent and costly hospital readmissions.[26] These challenges underscore the urgent need for compassionate, patient-centered, and harm reduction–informed care models for people with SUD.

To effectively integrate harm reduction into hospitals, it is crucial to recognize the philosophical differences between the harm reduction and the traditional medical model (see Table 19.1).[27] The medical model is a hierarchical, high-threshold system that demands patient adherence with treatments and leaves little room for patient autonomy. In contrast, the harm

TABLE 19.1

Differences Between the Harm Reduction and Medical Models

	Harm reduction model	Medical model
Structural philosophy	Inclusive	Hierarchical
System design	Low threshold	High threshold
Clinician's role	Collaborative decision making	Expert knowledge
Patient's role	Understand options, make choices, reduce harms	Accept and comply with treatment
Locus of control	Patient centered	Clinician centered

Adapted from Heller D, McCoy K, Cunningham C. An invisible barrier to integrating HIV primary care with harm reduction services: philosophical clashes between the harm reduction and medical models. *Public Health Rep*. 2004;119(1):32–39. Copyright © 2004 US Surgeon General's Office. Reprinted by Permission of Sage Publications.

reduction model is more inclusive, patient centered, and respectful of individual autonomy. Historically, the medical model has perpetuated systemic issues such as racism, colonialism, ableism, criminalization, and discrimination, which has understandably led to mistrust of the health care system among people with SUD.[28] Recognizing that people with SUD are more likely to be rehospitalized, hospital leaders and hospital-based clinicians must implement new approaches when caring for people with SUD that address the risk environment within hospitals and ensure that all patients receive high-quality, equitable, and compassionate care, regardless of their substance use history. In turn, this will support people with SUD to remain in the hospital to complete medical treatment and reduce future rehospitalizations.[24]

While harm reduction has long been central to community-based support for people with SUD, hospitals have been slower to adopt these strategies. Decades of evidence links harm reduction to improved patient outcomes, such as reduced overdose deaths, fewer infectious complications, and better engagement in medical and SUD treatment.[29–32] Although research on integrating *structural harm reduction* strategies into the hospital settings is limited, both US and international models show promise.[33–36]

Naloxone education and distribution in US health care settings is strongly linked to a decrease in fatal overdoses, though most programs have focused on emergency settings.[37,38] A pilot project at Massachusetts General Hospital demonstrated the feasibility of inpatient naloxone education and distribution, significantly increasing patient access to naloxone for overdose prevention.[39] Increasingly, hospitals offer employee educational workshops with standardized curricula on naloxone administration to expand in-hospital overdose prevention.[40] More hospitals support cost-effective multidisciplinary addiction consultation services with trained clinicians and team members with lived experience with SUD who integrate harm reduction–oriented discussions into routine clinical care.[41]

Case Study 1

Perera et al. describe the implementation of a hospital intervention to provide harm reduction, education, and equipment to hospitalized people with SUD.[42] At Zuckerberg San Francisco General Hospital, the Addiction Care Team (ACT) partnered with the San Francisco AIDS Foundation, a community-based organization that serves people with SUD and people living with HIV, to obtain harm reduction equipment for in-hospital distribution. Next, ACT team members obtained buy-in from the hospital's executive leadership and the Director of Regulatory Affairs. ACT engaged and partnered with nursing leadership to implement the program in a way that was both supportive of nursing staff and of people with SUD. Following these activities, ACT successfully created a program to educate hospitalized people with SUD about harm reduction strategies and provide harm reduction kits for various substances. Their harm reduction intervention improved access to SUD treatment, reduced stigma, and improved trust, particularly among racially and ethnically marginalized populations.[42,43] Figure 19.4 includes the three primary goals of developing an in-hospital harm reduction program recommended by Perera et al.[42]

Relational Harm Reduction

Relational harm reduction focuses on the importance of trust, respect, and collaboration in health care relationships to reduce the harms of substance use. People with SUD often face stigma and judgment in interactions in health care settings, leading to suboptimal care and patient-directed discharge. Incorporation of *relational harm reduction* into health care involves the use of nonstigmatizing, patient-centered communication and creating supportive environments that foster trust and collaboration between patients and all clinical team members (including clinicians, nurses, social workers, peer recovery specialists). *Relational harm reduction* health care promotes patient autonomy, acknowledging that individual choices are shaped by social factors, access to resources, and past experiences. Importantly, *relational harm reduction* is most effective when combined with *structural harm-reduction* strategies but can still improve outcomes in the absence of supportive policies.[2,44]

In 2017, Hawk et al. developed six principles of harm reduction for the health care setting based on

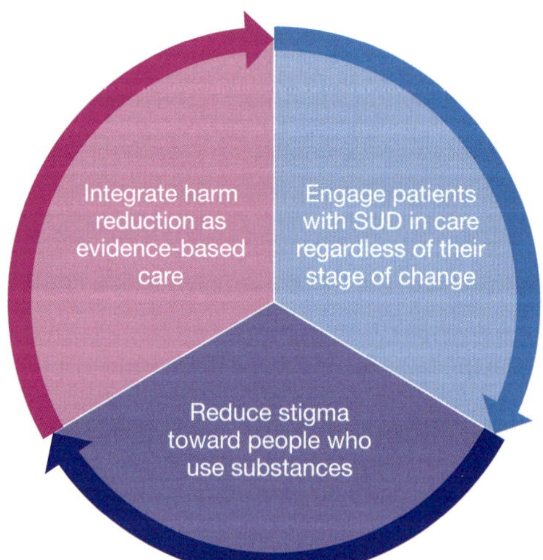

Figure 19.4: Goals of developing an in-hospital harm reduction program.[42]

qualitative work with people with SUD and clinicians in an HIV clinic: humanism, pragmatism, individualism, autonomy, incrementalism, and accountability without termination.[2] These tenants provide an effective framework for health care clinicians to use in all communication with patients but have specific utility when working with individuals who make choices that the clinician may see as having negative health consequences. The six principles are further defined and applied to the role of the hospital-based clinician aiming to integrate *relational harm reduction* in caring for people with SUD in Table 19.2.

Approaches to Talking About Harm Reduction in the Hospital Setting

The use of proven communication strategies between hospital-based clinicians and hospitalized people with SUD will build trust, reduce stigma, and create a more supportive environment that encourages open dialogue.[45] Communication strategies and example script are listed below.

Use Nonstigmatizing, Person-First Language

Hospital-based clinicians and hospital staff should use nonstigmatizing language to avoid perpetuating negative stereotypes, discrimination, or moral judgment. While patients should be given the freedom to use terms that best describe their personal practices, beliefs, and experiences, clinicians should use precise and accurate medical terminology that focuses the conversation to be objective, compassionate, and clinical. Clinicians should use person-first language in which the individual is always put before the diagnosis (eg, "a person with a substance use disorder" rather than "substance abuser" or "addict") to acknowledge their full identity and humanity and to avoid labeling a person by a single diagnosis or behavior.[46] Clinicians should use nonstigmatizing, person-first language in clinical documentation and in discussions with patients and care team members. By doing so, clinicians model best practices for the entire care team.[47]

Normalize Discussions About Substance Use and Harm Reduction

Hospital-based clinicians should ask questions about substance use in the same neutral manner that other health conditions and behaviors are discussed.[48] They should acknowledge that substance use is common among hospitalized patients and that discussions about substance use are a routine part of hospital care. They should convey to patients and to the medical team that they are comfortable working with patients with a range of goals related to their substance use and that they are interested and open to discussing harm-reduction strategies that align with the patient's goals.

Example Language

- I ask all of my patients about substance use because it is very common and may impact people's well-being, health, and hospitalization. I know people use substances for many different reasons. My goal is for you to receive the medical care you need during this hospital stay. What, if anything, would you like me to know about your substance use and how it impacts your life? How can I support you during this hospital stay?
- I often meet people in the hospital who are concerned that their substance use is impacting their health. Some of these people want to make changes and reduce or stop using substances. Other people plan to continue using substances, but may want to do so in a safer way to reduce their risk of overdose and infections. Are you concerned about your substance use? Do you have any goals around your substance use?

Practice Trauma-Informed Care

Hospital-based clinicians should recognize that many people with SUD have experienced trauma, both in the community and within health care settings. A trauma-informed approach acknowledges the effects of past trauma, ensuring that interactions are safe, empowering, and not retraumatizing. This includes asking for permission before discussing substance use or potential harms and before a physical examination, respecting patient boundaries and providing clear explanations before any exams or procedures to create and maintain a calm and safe care environment.[49]

Example Language

- It sounds like you felt very stigmatized the last time you were in the hospital, making it difficult to be here and to share your story. We want you to feel comfortable in the hospital so you can stay to receive the care you need and deserve. What are some things our team can do to make this a better experience for you?
- I want to make sure you are as safe as possible when you leave the hospital. It sounds like you plan to continue using substances, and I have some information that I think might help prevent future infections. Are you open to hearing about this?

Use Open-Ended Questions and Motivational Interviewing Techniques

Using open-ended questions when discussing substance use allows patients to share their experiences in

TABLE 19.2

Summary of Relational Harm Reduction Principles, Definitions, and Approaches in Caring for People With SUD in the Hospital Setting

Principles	Definition of clinician role	Approaches
Humanism	■ Value, care, respect, and dignify people with SUD as individuals ■ Aim to understand why patients make decisions and what drives their decisions about substance use ■ Aim to understand the balance between harms and benefits of patient's substance use	■ Approach conversations about substance use without judgment ■ Be curious about your patient's choices around substance use ■ Do not hold previous choices or behaviors against someone
Pragmatism	■ Appreciate the real-world experiences of people with SUD ■ Recognize that patients may not desire to stop using substances ■ Recognize that life circumstances may make it difficult for patients to meet their goals ■ Do not view substance use or return to use as failure	■ Do not assume that long-term abstinence is the patient's goal or prioritize abstinence above other goals ■ Provide support and choice regardless of patient's goals ■ Focus on actual harms of substance use as opposed to moral or societal standards ■ Address harm reduction even in those with stated goals of abstinence ■ Address social drivers of health
Individualism	■ Understand that people with SUD have different reasons for using substances and goals related to their substance use ■ Acknowledge individual needs and strengths ■ Accept that treatment approaches need to be adapted for spectrums of harm and receptivity to change	■ Do not assume a one-size-fits-all approach ■ Recognize that people with SUD are their own experts and approach conversations with cultural humility ■ Explore individual goals and priorities ■ Tailor messages and interventions to individual patients
Autonomy	■ Acknowledge and accept that people with SUD have agency to make choices about their treatment and health behavior	■ Provide education and offer suggestions while utilizing shared decision-making ■ Accept patient choices ■ Be open to reciprocal learning ■ Do not implement coercive or punitive action when patient choice differs from recommendations made by medical team
Incrementalism	■ Acknowledge that any positive change can improve health ■ Accept that positive change takes time ■ Understand and plan for backward movement	■ Celebrate any positive changes ■ Provide positive reinforcement ■ Recognize that plateaus or negative trajectories are part of life
Accountability without termination	■ Reflect on personal responsibility for choices and behaviors ■ Acknowledge that people with SUD have the right to make personal harmful health decisions while aiming to educate about the consequences of these choices ■ Communicate willingness and responsibility to care for individuals regardless of their choices	■ Avoid punitive approaches including administrative discharges ■ Do not make decisions about current treatment plan based on choices patients made during previous hospital admissions ■ Have open and honest conversations with patients when there are concerns current choices are impacting personal or staff safety during their hospitalization and engage patient in planning for safe hospitalization

Adapted from Hawk M, Coulter RWS, Egan JE, et al. Harm reduction principles for healthcare settings. *Harm Reduct J*. 2017;14(1):70. https://creativecommons.org/licenses/by/4.0/

their own words, leading to more detailed and nuanced responses. Unlike rigid or accusatory questions that can reinforce stigma, open-ended questions demonstrate empathy and curiosity, fostering collaboration and a sense of partnership in care. This approach is central to motivational interviewing (MI), a patient-centered technique that helps resolve ambivalence about behavior change.[50] MI emphasizes collaboration, guiding patients to explore their motivations for change rather than imposing decisions. Key MI techniques, such as reflective listening, affirmations, and summaries, support patients in examining their substance use and its impact on health. The Substance Abuse and Mental Health Services Administration (SAMHSA), a US federal agency, offers a helpful advisory for providers on MI with further details in Chapter 15.[51]

Example Language

- What role do substances play in your life?
  - What do you like about substance use?
  - Are there aspects of your substance use that you don't like?
  - Are there aspects of your substance use that you would like to change or modify?
- What are some of the things you do to keep yourself safe when you are using substances?
  - What are some of the things you've seen others do to keep themselves safe?
- How have your substance use goals changed over time?
  - Why have your goals changed over time?

Demonstrate Cultural Humility

Cultural humility is adopting a respectful, open-minded, and self-reflective approach to patient care.[52] It acknowledges the diverse cultural, social, and historical contexts that influence an individual's experiences with substance use and health. Rather than assuming expertise based on general knowledge or stereotypes, cultural humility requires clinicians to actively listen, learn from their patients, and adapt health care to meet the unique needs and values of each individual.[53]

Example Language

- You are the expert on your life. I want to learn about what is most important to you and walk alongside you, not to tell you what to do. What is most important to you when it comes to your health and well-being?
- I am sorry you had experiences where you felt judged. I recognize that I might not fully understand everything about your experiences or the challenges you've faced. If I say something that does not feel like it aligns with your experiences or values, please let me know. I am here to listen and learn from you.

Use a Strength-Based Approach

Hospital-based clinicians and other team members can help the patient identify their strengths, resources, and capabilities through open-ended questioning and active listening, rather than focusing on what is lacking or are deficits.[54] By focusing on the positives of what an individual is doing well, the team can help the patient recognize and build confidence in their abilities to overcome challenges and achieve their goals.

Example Language

- I can tell that you really care about other members of your community and take a lot of steps to keep each other as safe as possible. Where are some areas you feel you could use additional support?
- It took a lot of courage to come in today, and I appreciate you being so open and willing to share. What else do you think is important for us to know about you? What is most important to you while you are in the hospital?

Trauma-Informed, Nonpunitive Hospital Policies to Support Harm Reduction

Hospital-based clinicians should prioritize compassionate, evidence-based care for people with SUD, avoiding punitive measures that can worsen health outcomes. Punitive actions, like denying care, unnecessary involvement of security or law enforcement, increased surveillance, loss of privileges, discontinuing medications, and threats of discharge undermine trust and discourage people with SUD from seeking medical care. These measures are linked to negative outcomes, such as patients hiding their substance use, engaging in high-risk behaviors, and patient-directed discharge, which increases the likelihood of readmission, adverse health outcomes, and death.[55–57] A qualitative analysis identified reasons for patient-directed discharge, such as poorly managed symptoms, pain, stigma, discriminatory treatment, and restrictive policies.[20,58,59] Such punitive experiences can also lead people with SUD to delay or avoid care in the future, even in life-threatening situations.[19,20,60,61]

In-hospital substance use is common among people with SUD, with over 40% of people using substances to cope with untreated or undertreated withdrawal symptoms, untreated pain, emotional stress, boredom, isolation, and stigma.[24] Many hospitals lack clear and official policies on in-hospital use, and those that do often adopt abstinence-based, punitive approaches, which have proven ineffective and often result in patient-directed discharges.[19,61] While in-hospital substance use can lead to adverse outcomes such as overdose, punitive measures ignore the underlying reasons for in-hospital substance use and miss the opportunity for patient-centered care, safety planning, and better patient, clinician, and staff experiences. These approaches ignore the complex, multifaceted nature of substance use and reflect the "War on Drugs" carceral policies that worsen health disparities, especially for marginalized groups, and undermine healing-centered care.[22]

Best Practices in Harm Reduction Policy Development and Implementation

Hospital-based care teams should take all possible steps to reduce in-hospital substance use. This begins with adequate substance withdrawal management and pain management and involves maximizing patient safety during hospitalization.

Role of Hospital-Based Clinicians

Hospital-based clinicians should familiarize themselves with their hospital's policies addressing in-hospital substance use (if one exists), and when necessary, revise them to be patient-centered with a focus on supporting patients to remain in the hospital to receive essential medical care. If no policy exists, hospital-based clinicians should work with hospital leadership to develop an evidence-based policy with input from interdisciplinary team members, including nurses, physicians, advanced practice professionals, pharmacists, social workers, and people with lived experience with substance use. The goal of the policy should be to standardize the hospital's approach to in-hospital substance use rather than leaving individual team members to apply their personal beliefs and inconsistent or informal strategies to address in-hospital substance use.

Role of Hospital Administration

Hospital administration should identify and fund multidisciplinary teams of clinicians and staff champions to lead the development and revision of in-hospital substance use policies. These efforts should be complemented by comprehensive staff education that includes the rationale behind the policies, patient-reported reasons for in-hospital substance use, the harms caused by stigmatizing and punitive responses, and best practices for evidence-based SUD and pain management. Additionally, training should focus on harm reduction strategies, fostering empathetic, nonjudgmental communication, and enhancing de-escalation skills to ensure compassionate, effective care for all patients. Policies about in-hospital substance use should be communicated upfront to all patients and visitors to normalize these discussions, avoid bias, and set expectations.

Best Practices for Communication and Patient Care

Clinicians should explore substance use with hospitalized patients to help identify their needs, allowing for proactive management of concerns like withdrawal and pain. While in-hospital substance use concerns should not be ignored, they can be used to enhance patient–clinician communication and strengthen the therapeutic alliance. In the case of an in-hospital overdose, immediate coordinated action is required—assessing the situation, calling for help, supporting breathing and circulation, continuously monitoring vital signs, evaluating the cause, notifying relevant health care teams for follow-up care, and documenting the event thoroughly. Naloxone should be administered if there is high clinical suspicion for an opioid overdose (eg, pinpoint pupils, respiratory depression, or apnea). However, if a patient is somnolent but responsive or without respiratory depression, administering naloxone may cause unnecessary harm, including precipitating opioid withdrawal symptoms, causing discomfort for the patient. In such cases, the care team should first assess safety measures, such as pulse oximetry, repositioning, and oxygen therapy, and wait until the patient can engage in conversation before proceeding with further interventions.

In the Event of In-Hospital Substance Use: Clinician Response

When addressing concerns for in-hospital substance use, hospital-based clinicians should meet with the patient to discuss the facts, that is, a syringe was found in the room or the nurse witnessed in-hospital substance use, while expressing concern for the patient's and staff's safety: "an important aspect of your care is ensuring that you are safe while in the hospital." It is best to ask the patient open-ended questions to determine if any un- or undertreated symptoms, such as withdrawal or pain, may be driving their in-hospital substance use while using shared decision making to develop a plan to mitigate these symptoms. Remind patients of any support services available in the hospital for people with SUD and, if the patient has an opioid use disorder (OUD), the hospital-based clinician should offer buprenorphine or methadone to address opioid withdrawal. If available, addiction consultation services can be utilized for difficult to manage pain in the setting of OUD or complicated withdrawal syndromes. Hospital-based clinicians should remember that simply being in the hospital can be traumatizing for many patients and explore other supports that can be provided (ie, books/diversionary materials, pastoral support).

In the Event of In-Hospital Substance Use: Multidisciplinary Response

Hospital leadership should explore establishing multidisciplinary response teams that may include the primary team, nurses, pharmacists, pain management specialists, social workers, peer specialists, etc, to guide management strategies and ensure uniformity in practice. The multidisciplinary response and/or primary team should review the hospital policies regarding in-hospital substance use with the patient and discuss concerns about how use of nonprescribed substances can be dangerous and impede provision of appropriate hospital care.

In the Event of In-Hospital Substance Use: Considering Other Approaches

Calling security, performing room searches, and increasing surveillance (eg, sitters) should only be considered if there are imminent safety risks for patients and/or health care workers. Such practices undermine patient autonomy and may be reminiscent of prior experiences of incarceration or institutionalization. Whenever possible, hospital staff and clinicians should avoid calling security unless there is a potential for physical harm to the hospital staff or other patients.

Urine drug testing may be helpful to provide qualitative data to clarify the patient's clinical presentation, that is, acute encephalopathy or somnolence, and whenever possible, the clinician should obtain the patient's consent. In general, given the potential for false positives with the urine drug immunoassay testing, they are more useful to rule out a diagnosis, that is, in-hospital fentanyl use as a cause of a patient's acute encephalopathy is unlikely in the absence of fentanyl in the urine. Similar to any laboratory test, a hospital-based clinician should be prepared to accurately interpret the urine drug tests and consult their laboratory or toxicology specialists, if needed. If any of these actions are taken, the patient should be informed first, along with an explanation of the reason for doing so.

Structural Harm Reduction Strategies

Structural harm reduction refers to practical strategies and considerations to minimize risks associated with substance use. These strategies range from laboratory testing for viral bloodborne infections, vaccinations, medications for HIV prevention, overdose prevention and education, safer substance use strategies and equipment, and substance checking. All of these strategies can be implemented in the hospital setting.

Case Study 2

Martin et al. outline the processes and procedures undertaken to revise one hospital's substance use policy. After identifying harms their current in-hospital substance use policies had on patient care, key partners at the Zuckerberg San Francisco General Hospital and Trauma Center (ZSFG) convened an interprofessional workgroup of administrators, nurses, and physicians, including addiction specialists, who aimed to revise their policies.[24] The team began by examining the literature to clarify common reasons for in-hospital substance use. Next, the group agreed on best practices for responding to in-hospital substance use and staff safety concerns through nonpunitive approaches.[19–21,61] Such approaches included ensuring adequate pain control, offering evidence-based medications for cravings and withdrawal, providing snacks, books, journals, phone chargers, etc, to counter the hours of downtime in the hospital.[24] The team also provided training for hospital staff and received endorsement of the policy by legal, security, regulatory, leadership, and other hospital committees to ensure successful implementation of the revised policy and buy-in from health care workers. The authors include eight recommendations for in-hospital substance use policies listed in Table 19.3.

Prevention, Screening, and Immunizations

People with SUD are disproportionately impacted by infectious complications including bloodborne viral infections like HIV and HCV, skin and soft tissue infections (SSTIs), and other preventable health outcomes.[62–64] However, due to numerous barriers like stigma and various social and structural conditions, people with SUD frequently avoid health care settings, rely on self-care, and delay seeking treatment until they require acute medical and surgical interventions.[65–67] Thus, while preventative services are best delivered in primary care settings, due to low engagement with primary care[68] and high rates of acute care utilization among people with SUD,[12,69,70] hospitalizations present as an opportunity for hospital-based clinicians to address infectious risk and prevention, including offering screenings for infectious complications. Despite this, screening rates for sexually transmitted infections (STIs), HIV, and HCV among people with SUD across US hospitals are suboptimal.[71,72]

Hospital-based clinicians should familiarize themselves with the Centers for Disease Control and Prevention (CDC) recommendations for laboratory screening and testing among people with SUD and

TABLE 19.3

Recommendations for Developing an In-Hospital Substance Use Policy

1. Convene an interprofessional group that includes people with SUD and patients to create or review an existing policy
2. Ensure the policy is patient centered without punitive measures, including security as first responders; security should always be the last resort
3. Evaluate the policy with an equity lens to identify who will be disproportionately affected and how
4. Obtain legal, security, regulatory, nursing, and leadership buy-in; ensure consistent messaging of policy to staff
5. Educate hospital staff about the policy, evidence-based SUD care, harms of stigma, and SUD-related inequities (especially around race/ethnicity)
    a. Provide best-practice scripts for responding to in-hospital substance use
6. Involve hospital staff in policy implementation and ongoing improvement processes
7. Inform all patients of the policy, regardless of substance use history
8. Offer patients adequate pain control, evidence-based SUD treatment, and supportive care that helps them tolerate hospitalization, ie, books, movies, phone charger, colored pencils.

Adapted with permission from Wolters Kluwer Health, Inc.: Martin M, Snyder HR, Otway G, Holpit L, Day LW, Seidman D. In-hospital Substance Use Policies: An Opportunity to Advance Equity, Reduce Stigma, and Offer Evidence-based Addiction Care. *J Addict Med.* 2023;17(1):10–12. https://journals.lww.com/journaladdictionmedicine/fulltext/2023/01000/in_hospital_substance_use_policies__an_opportunity.4.aspx

offer these interventions, including vaccinations, to hospitalized people with SUD (Table 19.4).

This includes screening for STIs, HIV, viral hepatitis, and tuberculosis and discussing prevention (ie, HIV post- or preexposure prophylaxis [PrEP]) and treatment options. For hepatitis A viral infections (HAV) and hepatitis B viral infection (HBV), and tetanus, for those with evidence of nonimmunity based on bloodwork, incomplete vaccination status, no prior vaccine documentation, or need for boosters, hospital-based clinicians should discuss and offer immunization. For HAV and HBV, immunization series can be initiated in the hospital and completed in outpatient follow-up. For vaccines requiring multiple doses, providing a single dose in the hospital can be more beneficial than no doses at all. For example, a single dose of the HAV vaccine can produce protective antibody levels for up to 11 years.[73]

Improving rates of screening, testing, and immunizations in hospital settings requires system-level changes, and hospital-based clinicians should explore strategies to implement these evidence-based practices at their hospital. Such strategies include encouraging a routine opt-out testing approach, implementing bundled or packaged testing orders,[74,75] using clinical decision support systems like electronic health record reminders,[71] performing reflex testing when appropriate, establishing workflows that include referral to treatment pathways, and utilizing standing orders for screening tests that can be initiated by nurses.[76]

Hepatitis C Treatment

Due to substantial advancements in HCV treatment, there are now highly effective, well-tolerated oral direct-acting antivirals (DAA) with cure rates higher than 95%.[77] For treatment-naive patients, two FDA-approved daily pan-genotypic regimens glecaprevir/pibrentasvir (Mavyret) and sofosbuvir/velpatasvir (Epclusa) are given over a course of 8 or 12 weeks, respectively. These therapies are dosed once daily, have minimal toxicity, and do not require ongoing laboratory monitoring, which simplifies treatment and improves adherence.[78] Moreover, as treatment algorithms have become more simplified and straightforward, HCV infections can also be managed by generalists, including hospital-based clinicians, thereby increasing capacity for treatment and lowering barriers to care.[79] Despite this, treatment initiation for HCV remains low,[80] with even lower rates among people with SUD.[81,82] More information about HCV and its treatment is discussed in Chapter 11.

Several structural barriers to HCV treatment remain, including cost.[83] State Medicaid programs vary in access to DAAs and include conditions such as prior authorization requirements, substance use restrictions, and prescriber constraints (limits prescribers to designated specialists). As of August 2024, seven states have some form of sobriety restrictions for DAA therapy.[84]

Per 2023 Hepatitis C Guidance from the American Association for the Study of Liver Diseases-Infectious Diseases Society of America (AASLD-IDSA), active or recent substance use is not a contraindication for initiating treatment for chronic HCV.[85] For people with SUD who do receive HCV treatment, they are able to similarly achieve sustained virologic response compared to the general population.[86,87] Given the wide HCV treatment gap among people with SUD, hospitalizations represent an opportunity for treatment discussion and initiation.[88,89] Prior qualitative work suggests that people with SUD are willing to discuss HCV treatment during hospitalizations and complete any necessary work-up inpatient as per AASLD-IDSA guidelines (hcvguidelines.org) to facilitate outpatient care.[90,91] As such, in addition to HCV screening, hospital-based clinicians should discuss positive results with

TABLE 19.4

Recommendations on Routine Screening for People With SUD and Practical Considerations to Minimize Infectious Risks

	Screening recommendations[a]	Type of testing	Practical considerations
HIV	At least annual testing if ongoing risk factors	HIV-1/2 antigen and antibody test with reflexes	If at risk (eg, sharing drug equipment), discuss and consider initiating HIV PrEP. Start PEP if suspected HIV exposure.
Hepatitis A	If no evidence of past completed series, screening at least once	Immunoglobulin G antibodies to HAV (IgG anti-HAV)	If hepatitis A nonimmune, offer hepatitis A vaccination: ■ Hepatitis A single-antigen vaccine: two doses 6 mo apart ■ Twinrix (combination hepatitis A and B vaccine): three doses at 0, 1, and 6 mo
Hepatitis B	At least one-time screening in lifetime, particularly if no documented prior immunizations or unclear vaccination status	Hepatitis B surface antigen (HBsAg) Hepatitis B surface antibody (anti-HBs) Total antibody to hepatitis B core antigen (total anti-HBc)	If hepatitis B nonimmune, offer hepatitis B vaccination: ■ Heplisav-B: two doses 1 mo apart ■ Twinrix (combination hepatitis A and B vaccine): three doses at 0, 1, and 6 mo If evidence of acute or chronic hepatitis B infection, link to treatment
Hepatitis C	At least one-time testing in lifetime Annual testing if ongoing injection and/or sharing drug-use equipment Anyone requesting	Hepatitis C antibody with reflex HCV RNA PCR	If evidence of chronic hepatitis C infection, discuss treatment options. If appropriate, obtain additional lab work needed for HCV treatment per AASLD-IDSA guidelines (hcvguidelines.org). Consider initiating treatment in hospital if possible and/or provide linkage to outpatient care.
Sexually transmitted infection	At least annually, or every 3–6 mo if increased sexual risk behaviors Anyone requesting	Gonorrhea (GC) NAAT Chlamydia trachomatis (CT) NAAT RPR	If positive, provide treatment and offer expedited partner treatment. If elevated risk and prior STI in past 12 mo, consider prescribing HIV PrEP and doxy PEP (taking doxycycline 200 mg PO once within 72 h after sexual encounter)
Tuberculosis	Annually if active risk factors (eg, incarceration, unhoused)	Tuberculin skin test or interferon-gamma release assay blood test	If positive symptoms and positive test, consult ID. If negative symptoms and positive test with concern for latent TB, ensure follow-up with local public health clinics
Tetanus	–	–	Tdap at least once as an adult, then Tdap or Td every 10 y
Pneumococcal	–	–	Pneumococcal vaccine (PCV20 or PCV21): one-time dose for individuals aged 19–49 if have tobacco and/or alcohol use disorder and for all individuals aged 50 or greater

[a]Recommendations for screening and immunizations are tailored for people with SUD and are adapted from the CDC and do not include other potential indications for testing and immunizations. For complete immunization recommendations, follow the Advisory Committee on Immunization Practices (ACIP) guidelines.

HIV, human immunodeficiency virus; HAV, hepatitis A virus; HCV, hepatitis C virus; ID, infectious diseases; STI, sexually transmitted infections; NAAT, nucleic acid amplification test; PrEP, pre-exposure prophylaxis; PEP, postexposure prophylaxis; TB, tuberculosis; Tdap, tetanus, diphtheria, and pertussis.

patients, determine eligibility for treatment, inform patient of treatment options, complete additional work-up needed, and provide appropriate linkage to outpatient care.

Furthermore, some hospital settings have explored novel methods to increase access to HCV treatment including inpatient initiation of DAAs with telehealth follow-up. Two programs at different US institutions found in-hospital HCV treatment to be feasible and effective in curing HCV.[92,93] Moreover, a 2023 stepped wedge cluster randomized trial in Norway (OPPORTUNI-C) found that in-hospital HCV treatment compared to usual care was associated with significantly higher rates of treatment initiation and completion.[94] While sustained viral response at 4 weeks and 2 years was similar between groups, time to virologic cure was shorter in the intervention group.[94,95]

Safer Sex Considerations

People with SUD are also at an increased risk for HIV, HCV, and other STIs due to higher-risk sexual practices compounded by many structural barriers related to testing and treatment. Moreover, people with SUD with intersecting social identities related to gender, sexuality, and sex work experience multiple forms of stigma and are subject to overlapping systems of oppression.

Sex work, sometimes described as "dates" by people who provide this service, refers to the exchange of sexual services for goods or money and can fall on a spectrum from choice to circumstance to coercion.[96] Approximately 1 in 5 people who use injection substances in North America engaged in past-year sex work, with higher prevalence rates among women.[64] Women sex workers who inject substances are disproportionately affected by HIV compared to male sex workers who inject substances and to sex workers who do not inject substances. These gender disparities may be from several factors, including increased rates of sexual violence and potential for exploitation such as human trafficking and higher likelihood of injection by others.[97] In addition to harm reduction strategies related to substances and sex in general (eg, use of condoms, contraception, regular screening for STIs), ways to mitigate harms for individuals engaging in both include avoiding using someone else's substances, avoiding having others inject for them, developing a buddy system, and having an exit strategy.

Another intersection of substance use and sex is "chemsex," which refers to the use of substances to enhance or facilitate sexual experiences and is also known colloquially as "Party and Play" (PNP). Common substances used in this practice include cocaine, methamphetamines, ecstasy, ketamine, gamma-hydroxybutyrate (GHB), mephedrone, and alkyl nitrites (poppers), which are often used in combination. Chemsex is most common among men who have sex with men and is associated with multiple sexual partners, casual sex, condomless anal sex, and nonconsensual sex, placing participants at higher risk for STI acquisition.[98] In addition to regular use of condoms, use of PrEP and postexposure prophylaxis (PEP), and engaging in safer substance use practices (eg, not mixing substances like poppers with oral erection medications), individuals engaging in chemsex should also try to avoid anonymous parties and stay within the same sex network.

Thus, hospital-based clinicians should explore opportunities to screen hospitalized people with SUD for higher-risk sexual practices and STIs, offer condoms, provide treatment or PEP if necessary (Table 19.4), and discuss harm reduction and prevention strategies including PrEP and other forms of contraception.

Box 19.1 Example Language to Assess Sexual Risk

- In the last year, approximately how many sexual partners have you had?
- Who do you typically have sex with? What is/are the gender(s) of your sex partner(s)?
- Do you ever use substances during sexual encounters? Do any of your sexual partners use substances?
- How do you talk to partners about their HIV status? Do you discuss STI and HIV prevention with your partners? What forms do you use?
- How often do you have vaginal or anal sex without a condom?
- Do you ever trade sex for your needs, such as money, drugs, a place to stay, or something else? Who organizes your dates? Are you being or have you been pimped, trafficked, or forced to have sex?

Family Planning Considerations

Individuals of reproductive age (15 to 50 years old) who use substances are less likely to access regular primary and reproductive health care and less likely to use contraception.[99,100] This leads to high rates of unintended pregnancies, with as many as 9 of 10 pregnancies in women who use opioids being unintended, a rate 2 to 3 times higher than the general public.[99] Those who use contraception are more likely to use condoms but are less likely to have access to the most effective forms including long-acting reversible contraception (LARC; eg, implants and intrauterine devices).[100]

Unintended pregnancies have far-reaching physical, mental health, and social implications. In this population, they also carry additional fetal and infant risks.[99] Expanding access to contraception should be viewed as a harm reduction strategy, which is especially important as access to abortion care is now limited in many parts of the US.[101] Hospitalizations should be seen as an opportunity to engage people with SUD in discussions about their fertility goals without judgment and provide education about contraception options if the patient does not desire pregnancy. Resources such as Bedsider (https://www.bedsider.org/) help patients obtain evidence-based information about contraception options, many of which can be prescribed on hospital discharge.[102] Partnerships with reproductive health clinicians should be explored to consider hospital administration of LARC or facilitate follow-up with clinicians who can provide these services in a low-barrier setting in the community. More information on this topic is discussed in Chapter 12.

HIV Prevention

Injection substance use is responsible for 1 in 10 HIV infections globally and in the US. People who use injection substances experience a higher risk of HIV acquisition, particularly with sharing needles and other injection equipment.[103] Sharing injection equipment can contribute to acute HIV outbreaks,[104] with the highest rates, over 40%, observed among those under 30 years old.[105]

Indications for PrEP

HIV PrEP involves the use of antiretroviral medication to prevent HIV infection among individuals without HIV but who have a high risk of exposure through sex or injection substance use. While PrEP has been shown to be effective in decreasing HIV acquisition by 99% from sex and at least 74% from injection substance use, uptake of PrEP among people who inject substances has been relatively low.[106,107] Based on 2021 CDC guidelines, PrEP is indicated for people who inject substances in the past 6 months, without acute or established HIV infection, with either risk of sexual acquisition, any sharing of substance use equipment, or for anyone who requests it. However, despite a high willingness to use PrEP among people who inject substances, few report discussing PrEP with a clinician.[108] Facilitators of these discussions include being tested for HIV, having a clinician recommend HIV testing, and receiving free condoms from a prevention program.[103] Evidence suggests that barriers to PrEP prescription involve limited clinician knowledge on PrEP and stigma around substance use.[109,110]

PrEP Formulations

PrEP formulations include daily oral pills and long-acting injections. FDA-approved daily oral options include tenofovir disoproxil fumarate and emtricitabine (TDF/FTC, Truvada) and tenofovir alafenamide and emtricitabine (TAF/FTC, Descovy). Cabotegravir is a form of injectable PrEP given every 2 months following two initial injections a month apart. More recently, lenacapvair, a long-acting injectable multistage HIV-1 capsid inhibitor given every 6 months, was FDA-approved. All forms of PrEP can be prescribed to adolescents and adults weighing at least 35 kg (77 lb). Promising alternatives not yet FDA approved include dapivirine, a monthly nonsystemic silicone vaginal ring for cisgender women.[111,112]

The most suitable PrEP regimen depends largely on patient preference for improved adherence. For most patients with sexual and injection-related risk factors, once-daily TDF-FTC is recommended. TDF-FTC also has been best studied among people who inject substances, individuals engaging in vaginal sex, and men who have sex with men. However, for those with reduced kidney function (eGFR <60 mL/min/1.73 m^2) or have osteoporosis, alternatives include once-daily TAF-FTC and for those with eGFR <30 mL/min/1.73 m^2, cabotegravir and lenacapavir are preferable. Of note, cabotegravir and lenacapavir has not been well-evaluated among people who inject substances with studies ongoing.

PrEP Initiation

Before starting PrEP, clinicians must ensure the patient has a negative HIV antigen/antibody test within 1 week of initiating medication. If the patient shows symptoms consistent with an acute HIV infection or has had a known exposure to HIV in the past 4 weeks, an HIV RNA test should be performed. Additionally, laboratory studies assessing kidney function, HBV, and HCV should be conducted. Clinicians can initiate patients on PrEP in the hospital, similar to HCV treatment initiation.[113] Patients should be educated on adherence, signs of acute HIV infection, and the need for prompt medical attention if symptoms arise. Potential side effects include initial mild gastrointestinal upset, hepatitis B flare upon discontinuation (if HBV positive), decreased renal function, or reduced bone mineral density (if on TDF/FTC). Oral PrEP is covered by Medicaid and most private health plans, and clinicians can prescribe a 90-day supply upon hospital discharge and assist with follow-up no later than 3 months.

Postexposure Prophylaxis

HIV PEP is indicated for people with SUD if HIV exposure is suspected either through unprotected sexual intercourse or through sharing of substance use equipment with a person who is HIV positive or status unknown. Patients should have a baseline HIV test. For adults, TDF/FTC plus raltegravir twice daily or dolutegravir once daily should be initiated as soon as possible, ideally within 72 hours of the suspected exposure and continued for 28 days. Hospital-based clinicians should ensure follow-up upon hospital discharge to assess symptoms, adherence, and subsequent HIV testing at 4 to 6 weeks and 3 months following exposure. Additional HIV prevention and treatment details are discussed in Chapter 11.

Safer Use Practices and Counseling

It is critical for hospital-based clinicians to engage in conversations with people with SUD on how they use substances to recognize infectious and other risks to guide treatment strategies, risk mitigation counseling, and anticipatory guidance. While harm reduction counseling can be delivered by peers or addiction medicine specialists, hospital-based clinicians should also feel comfortable having these conversations. A patient- and clinician-informed website can aid in these conversations (www.safersubstanceuse.org).[114]

There are various routes of administration for substances including oral, intranasal, inhalation, injection (intravenous, subcutaneous, intramuscular), and rectal. The next sections discuss *structural harm-reduction* strategies associated with each type of route of administration.

Safer Injection Use

Injecting substances carries the highest risk of morbidity and mortality, including overdose, wounds, vascular injury, and infectious complications, including HIV, HBV, HCV, SSTIs, and endocarditis. Increased injection frequency carries higher risks of these complications. Hospital-based clinicians should be knowledgeable about safer injection practices to appropriately counsel patients on how to reduce risks of infections. A variety of substances can be injected including opioids, methamphetamines, cocaine, and steroids and can be prepared from different forms including powder, pills, liquid, and rock crystals. Injection can be intravenous, subcutaneous (also known as skin popping), and intramuscular (also known as muscling).

Drug Preparation

The first step of safer injection substance use is having a clean and unused syringe and needle. Patients should be counseled to only use their own syringes and needles and to always use a new syringe and needle for each injection use. Needles become very dull after each injection use and can increase the risk for infection.

In general, the injection process can be divided into two major steps: preparation of the substance and injection. Preparing the substance depends on the type and form of the substance. If the substance does not come as a liquid preparation, it has to be dissolved into a solution in order to be injected. This can be done by crushing and mixing the substance with sterile water or saline. Some substances like crack cocaine and brown heroin, sometimes referred to as "black tar" heroin, require an acidifier to dissolve. Vitamin C is a safe acidifier for cocaine; vinegar should be avoided. Heat may be applied to help dissolve the substance and is generally recommended to help decrease the microbial burden. The dissolved substance is then drawn up through the needle using a filter into the syringe.

Substance Injection

Injection involves identifying the injection site using a tourniquet, if possible, and cleaning the site with an alcohol wipe or soap and water. The injection site ideally should be located on the upper extremities (see Figure 19.5). Veins are preferred to arteries. The site of injection should be rotated to allow prior injection sites to rest and heal. When injecting substances, the needle should be inserted at around a 45-degree angle with the bevel up toward the heart. If possible, venous access can be optimized by ensuring hydration, warmth, good lighting, and clenching the fist. See Table 19.5 for a summary of safer injection supplies and practices.

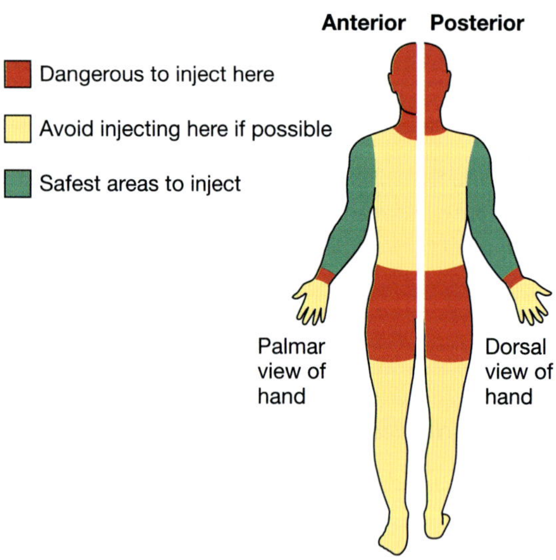

Figure 19.5: Hierarchy of places to inject substances.

TABLE 19.5

Summary of Safer Injection Supplies and Practices

Supply	Purpose
Alcohol wipe	■ Clean area of skin before injecting
Ascorbic acid (vitamin C) 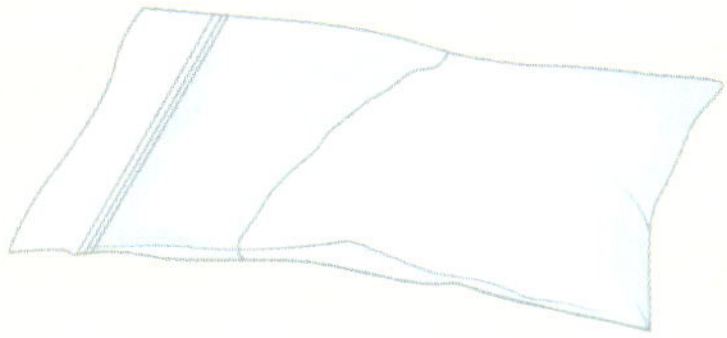	■ Helps dissolve certain substances like crack cocaine or brown heroin ■ Use as little as possible to decrease damage to veins ■ Avoid using vinegar or citrus fruits (eg, lemon), which can increase damage to veins and risk for fungal infections (*Candida* spp.)
Cooker 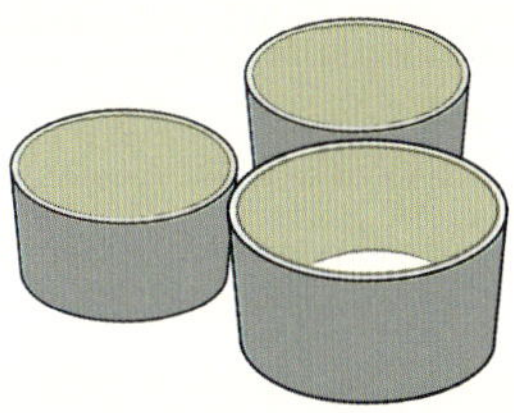	■ Used to prepare substance for injection ■ Apply heat for at least 10 seconds to decrease the burden of bacteria and fungi ■ Avoid sharing or reuse
Filters 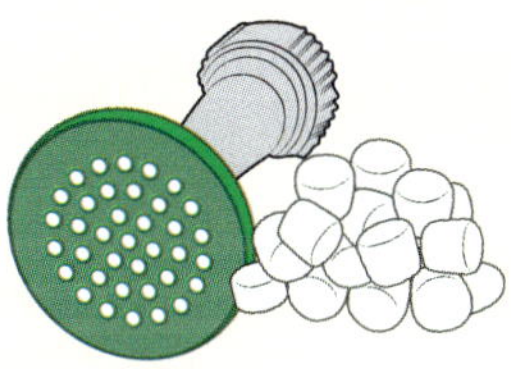	■ Removes undissolved solid particles (eg, pill coating) ■ Can be single-use syringe/wheel filter or dental cottons ■ Avoid sharing or reuse and using other items (eg, q-tips, cigarette filters)
Sterile saline or water	■ Medium to dissolve substance for injection ■ Avoid boiled, bottled, or tap/well water
Syringe/needle 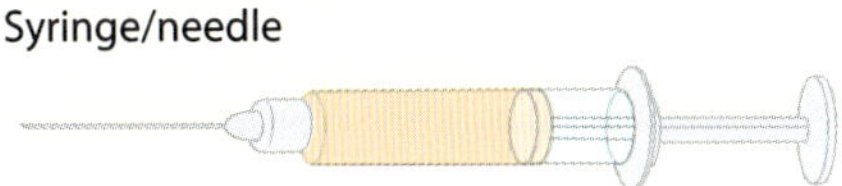	■ Syringe size: 0.5–1 cc ■ Needle length: 1/2, 5/8, 5/16 inch (IV), 1–1.5 inch (IM) ■ Needle gauge: 27–31 G (IV), 21–25 G (IM) ■ Generally, larger gauges (smaller the size of the needle hole) are preferred due to smaller puncture holes which reduces risk of infection ■ Avoid sharing and reuse of needles, licking needles before injecting
Tourniquet 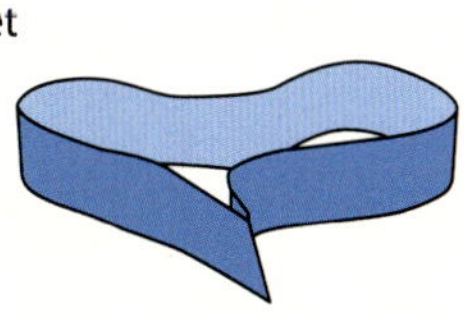	■ Allows for better visualization and palpation of veins to reduce multiple attempts at vein access ■ Decreases potential risk of vein damage and infection
Sharps disposal container 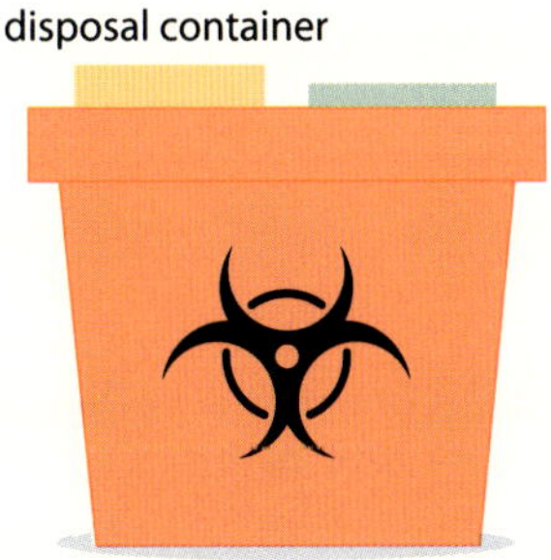	■ Reduces community presence of needles by allowing for safe disposal

Box 19.2 Example Language to Assess Injection Risk

- Walk me through how you inject your substances. Which substances do you typically inject and how often?
- Where/how do you get your injection equipment?
- Do you ever share or reuse your needles, works, or equipment? How often? If you share or reuse, how do you clean equipment between uses?
- When was the last time you shared injection equipment?
- Does anyone you share with have HIV or hepatitis C?
- Where on your body do you typically inject?

Subcutaneous and Intramuscular Injection

Some people inject subcutaneously or intradermally (ie, skin popping) or intramuscularly (ie, muscling) either intentionally or accidentally if they miss a vein. While they may use these methods of injecting due to difficulty with venous access, some substances like hormones and steroids can only be given intramuscularly. These injection practices carry higher risks of developing SSTI and deep abscesses.

Preparation of the substance and the site of injection is the same as for intravenous injection. For both methods, filtering is extremely important to ensure the solution is free of particles to decrease the risk of infection.[115] For skin popping, individuals should insert the needle at 15 to 45 degrees to the skin and inject no more than 0.5 cc of the solution in one site. Generally, the arms or upper thigh are preferred locations for skin popping. For intramuscular injections, individuals may need to use a longer (1 to 1.5 inches) and a lower gauge (22 to 25 G) needle. Harm reduction techniques include relaxing the muscle prior to injecting, injecting at 90 degrees to the skin, retracting the needle shaft to look for a flash of blood to ensure the needle is not in a blood vessel, and utilizing larger muscles, including the deltoid, vastus lateralis, and ventrogluteal muscles.[116]

Wounds

People with SUD who inject substances are at increased risk of developing various types of dermatologic complications, including SSTIs such as cellulitis and abscesses, as well as chronic wounds linked to vein damage, direct drug toxicity, and other injection practices. Among individuals who primarily inject substances, previous studies report that the prevalence of wounds ranges from 29% to 36%, while the prevalence of injection-related SSTIs is between 55% and 68%.[117–119] Up to three-quarters of people who inject substances have experienced lifetime infections, and up to half have had a recent infection.[119] SSTIs impose a significant burden on health care systems and are the leading reason for people with SUD to seek care in emergency departments.[120] The rate of hospitalizations for drug use-related SSTIs nearly doubled between 2000 and 2010.[121] Xylazine, a veterinary-grade sedative, contaminated various regions of the US drug supply, leading clinicians in regions with high levels of xylazine adulteration to observe a growing number of patients presenting with chronic wounds. Consulting wound care services in the hospital, providing appropriate self-care education, supplies for care, and linkage to outpatient treatment is critical for people with SUD who are hospitalized with substance-related wounds.

Syringe/Needle Prescriptions

Given the limited availability and accessibility of SSPs, it is important to consider how to ensure people with SUD access safer use supplies beyond community referrals. One tangible method for hospital-based clinicians is to prescribe sterile syringes to patients on discharge, as is done for patients prescribed insulin. See Table 19.5 for suggested syringe and needle sizes. An example prescription would be "insulin needles 28 G × 1/2″, 1 cc, quantity 100, use as directed, substitutions allowed." Associated ICD-10 codes include Z20.6 (contact with and [suspected] exposure to HIV), Z20.2 (contact with and [suspected] exposure to infection with a predominantly sexual mode of transmission), or Z77.21 (contact with and [suspected] exposure to potentially hazardous body fluids). Moreover, hospital-based clinicians can partner with their institutional or local outpatient pharmacy to ensure that certain common syringe sizes are in stock and dispensed without question.

Laws on possession of syringes for use in injecting illegal substances and pharmacist dispensing of syringes for this purpose vary from state to state. All US states allow individuals to purchase syringes at a pharmacy without a prescription, and all US states except Kansas do not prohibit prescribing syringes to people with SUD.[122] In US states with active substance paraphernalia laws, it is important to counsel patients who receive these prescriptions that possession of syringes is still considered illegal. The Legislative Analysis and Public Policy Association (LAPPA) is a good resource that summarizes US state laws on paraphernalia.[123]

Changing Routes

As injection carries the highest infection risks, encouraging people with SUD to consider other routes of administration is a form of harm reduction counseling. This is particularly salient in cases in which people with SUD have a current SSTI or wound and giving their skin a holiday from injection will facilitate healing. Other reasons to encourage route rotation include difficulty with venous access or an inability to obtain sterile needles. "Boofing" (per rectal administration) as described later can be another viable route of use if the sample is already prepared (ie, dissolved and drawn up in the syringe), but the individual is unable to find a vein for injection.

Safer Smoking

Various substances can be used via inhalation, including crack cocaine, methamphetamines, and opioids. Different *structural harm reduction* tools are used depending on the substance, including foils and pipes (Table 19.6). See Figure 19.6 for types of pipes used.

Unique risks associated with smoking substances involve damage to the respiratory system: oral mucosal burns, thermal airway injury, pulmonary edema and hemorrhage, hypersensitivity reactions, interstitial lung disease, and chronic obstructive pulmonary disease.[124,125] Unsafe smoking practices such as sharing equipment are common because many SSPs do not provide safer smoking equipment; when this equipment is available, people with SUD engage in fewer risk behaviors and have improved health outcomes.[126–128] Currently, there is active research on developing, implementing, and evaluating safer smoking equipment and training interventions in England.[129] General harm-reduction strategies include avoiding sharing pipes as transmission of bloodborne viruses like HCV is still possible, using high-quality pipes from US-based harm-reduction organizations such as Smoke Works,[130] rubber mouthpieces with pipes to prevent lip burns or cuts, and practicing good lip care. Pipes with cracks, chips, or scratches should be discarded in a sharps container. In general, substances should be inhaled slowly followed by immediate exhalation as holding the vapor in the lungs can cause burns and does not lead to a better high.

Box 19.3 Example Language of How to Assess Smoking Risk

- Where do you get your smoking equipment?
- How often do you smoke your substances, and do you share your pipes or mouthpieces?
- When was the last time you shared your smoking equipment? If you share or reuse, how do you clean your equipment?
- Has smoking made it harder for you to breathe or keep up with your day-to-day activities?

TABLE 19.6

Summary of Safer Smoking Supplies and Practices

Supply	Purpose
Alcohol wipe	■ Clean supplies like mouthpiece and pipe
Brass screen or chore 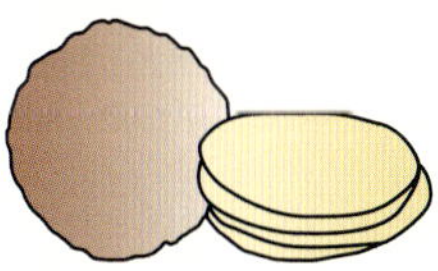	■ Used to hold crack rock in place in straight stem ■ Blocks small hot particles from entering mouth/lungs and causing burns ■ Preferred over steel wool, which is coated with toxic chemicals and can break apart into smaller hot pieces that can damage the respiratory tract
Glass pipe (see Figure 19.6 for types)	■ Quality glassware decreases risk of pipe exploding when heated and increases durability for use over time ■ Avoid sharing ■ Replace pipe if cracked, scratched, or chipped. Discard old pipe in sharps container
Foils	■ Foil sheets that are made for substance use are thicker and create a more stable surface when heated compared with household aluminum foil (which has an oil coating that will burn off) ■ Avoid sharing and discard after use
Lip balm	■ Keeps lips moisturized
Mouthpiece 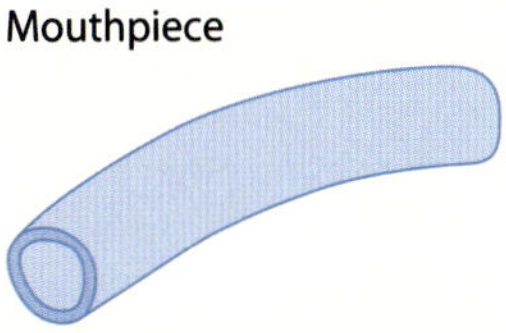	■ Prevents cuts or burns from hot pipe ■ Avoid sharing
Wooden push stick	■ Pushes screen or chore into place in straight stem ■ Preferred over metal which can scratch the pipe

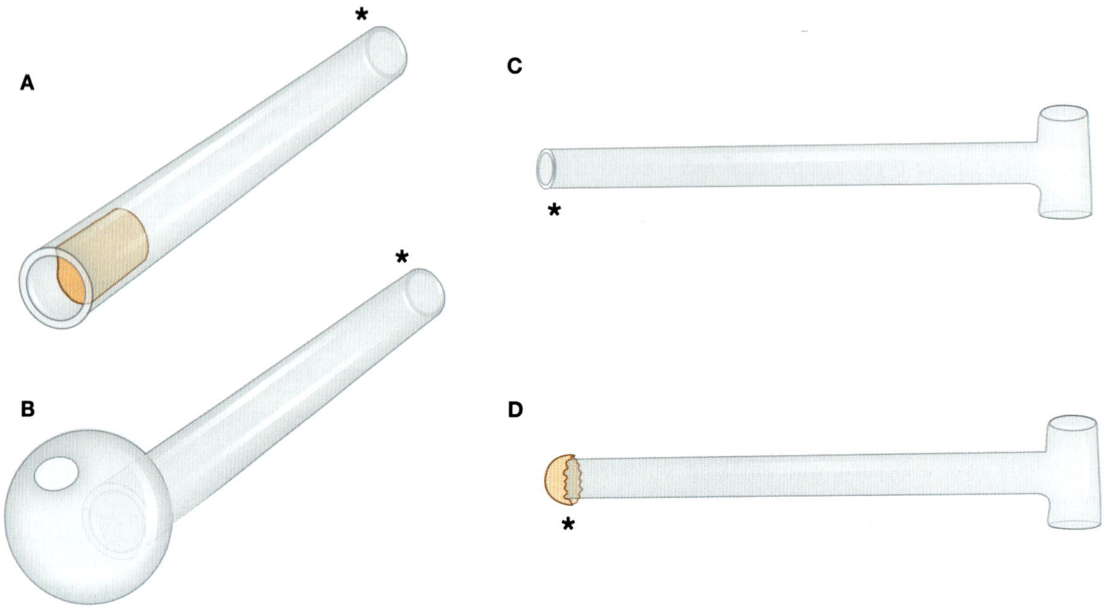

Figure 19.6: Types of pipes used for smoking. **A:** Straight stem typically used for smoking crack cocaine. Push folded brass screens or chore into place at one end of the pipe, leaving about 1 cm at the end where the crack rock is placed. Place mouthpiece at the other end. Apply heat to stem end with crack rock. **B:** Bowl pipe used for smoking methamphetamines. Crystals placed in bowl while mouth piece placed on the other end. Apply heat over bowl. **C:** Hammer pipe used for smoking opioids. Opioids can also be smoked using foil. Hammer pipes are designed to contain the drug better than foil. **D:** Wrap the screen around the pipe end and then put on the mouthpiece. Place tar or powder in the hammer head end. Apply heat with a torch (a lighter will not work given the thickness of the glass).

Safer Snorting

Many substances can be used intranasally (also known as snorting, sniffing, or nasal insufflation). Unique risks associated with this method of use include sinusitis and damage to the nasal mucosa, such as septal perforation. General harm reduction strategies for snorting include replacing daily household items which carry higher bacterial burden with single-use supplies (see Table 19.7), avoiding sharing supplies as transmission of bloodborne viruses like HCV is still possible, alternating nostrils with use, flushing the nose with saline or water after use, which can move any residual drug along the nasal passageway, and applying a water-based lubricant after use.

Box 19.4 Example Language to Assess Risks from Intranasal Substance Use

- How do you sniff the [substance]?
- How often do you use a bill/paper/straw after someone else?
- When is the last time you shared a bill or straw? How often do you share this item?

Safer Rectal Use

"Boofing" refers to the rectal administration of substances and is also known as "plugging" or "booty bumping." This method of administration offers a more similar rush compared to injection than

TABLE 19.7

Summary of Safer Snorting Supplies and Practices

Supply	Purpose
Alcohol wipe	▪ Cleans supplies
Blank card	▪ Clean surface to prepare and use substance from
Plastic razor	▪ Crushes substance into a finer powder to reduce damage to nasal mucosa
Scoop	▪ Avoid use of keys or fingernails
Straw (plastic or paper)	▪ Avoid sharing or using other items like dollar bills ▪ Kits often distribute different color straws to allow individuals to keep track of their own

TABLE 19.8

Summary of Safer Boofing Supplies and Practices

Supply	Purpose
Cooker	■ Used to prepare the substance for use
Lubricant	■ Facilitates syringe insertion into the rectum ■ Decreases risk of damage to rectal mucosa
Sterile water/saline	■ Used to dissolve substances for use
Syringe	■ Usually 1 cc syringe, preferably luer slip tip or oral syringe ■ Avoid sharing

smoking or intranasal routes, given higher bioavailability of the substance via the rectum. Preparation of the substance for rectal administration typically involves dissolving it into a solution in the same process as for injection (Table 19.8). The solution is then drawn up into a syringe without a needle. With lubricant applied, the syringe is inserted around 1 to 2 cm into the rectum while standing, squatting, or laying on one side.

Overdose Prevention and Safer Use Strategies

The following sections discuss the *structural harm-reduction strategies* involving general overdose education and safer use strategies, recognizing that the presentation and management of overdoses vary depending on the substances involved.

General Overdose Prevention Strategies

General overdose prevention strategies include the avoiding mixing substances, using tester shots, and concept of "never using alone." "Test" or "tester shots," which can also be described as "start low, go slow," involve using small quantities of the substance to check its potency before using subsequent doses. While using substances with someone else who can respond in the event of an overdose is ideal, it is important to recognize that not all people with SUD may be in situations or have social circles in which this regularly occurs. Virtual overdose monitoring services, also called virtual spotting services, serve as an alternative in these situations and include 24/7 hotlines like SafeSpot,[131] which allows the client to access their support services anonymously. For these support services, the hotline operator and client develop an emergency safety plan before the client uses the substance. The emergency safety plan is activated by the operator if the client stops responding over the telephone. Such virtual spotting or overdose monitoring services are an effective harm reduction strategy to ensure timely emergency support for people with SUD.[132]

Safer Stimulant Use

"Overamping" is a term used to describe effects of stimulant toxicity, signs, and symptoms of which are less well-defined but may include extreme anxiety or panic, hallucinations, paranoia, hypervigilance, headache, chest pain/tightness, tachycardia/palpitations, shortness of breath, hyperthermia, and hypertension.[133,134] Severe cases of overamping can lead to more serious outcomes such as seizures, stroke, heart attack, and cardiac arrest, described in Chapter 10. Harm reduction strategies to prevent overamping involve staying hydrated with water, eating, resting adequately, taking breaks from using, avoiding using multiple stimulants at once (including caffeine), and doing test doses. In cases of overamping, management is generally supportive, including going somewhere calm and quiet, lying down, drinking water, eating, and cooling down with ice packs, cold towels, or a fan.[135] For signs and symptoms of stroke, myocardial infarction, seizure, or hyperthermia (>104 °F), individuals should seek emergency services.

Overdose Prevention Centers

OPCs also known as supervised consumption/injection sites are facilities in which people with SUD can use their preobtained substances in a private but monitored setting. In addition to having trained personnel respond in the event of an overdose, OPCs may also provide safer use supplies and refer people with SUD to additional resources including treatment options. OPCs are a *structural harm reduction* strategy that have existed since the mid-1980s in Europe with now almost 200 of them operating in at least 17 countries, including Canada which has a hospital-based OPC.[22] In the US, underground OPCs have existed since 2014. The first US city-sanctioned OCP is OnPoint NYC, operating in New York City since November 2021. The first US state-sanctioned OCP is Project Weber/RENEW, operating in Rhode Island since December 2024. San Francisco operated a temporary 11-month OPC via HealthRIGHT 360 in 2022.[136] In May 2023, Minnesota passed an omnibus appropriations bill that included funding for OPCs. In June 2024, Vermont legislators overrode their governor's veto that authorizes OPCs and provides pilot funding through opioid settlement money.[136]

Decades of research on OPCs domestically and internationally demonstrate that they prevent overdose deaths, decrease spread of bloodborne viral infections, increase connection to care, reduce costs by decreasing emergency response service usage, and improve public safety by decreasing public substance use without increasing crime.[9,137–139] Despite strong evidence supporting OPCs, many barriers remain in their implementation including public support and punitive substance use policies that stem from stigmatizing and discriminatory attitudes toward people with SUD.[140] Political opponents cite that OPCs violate the federal statute 21 U.S.C. Section 856 passed in 1986 (also known as the "crack house statute") that states it is "illegal for individuals or organizations to maintain or open any place for the purpose of using any controlled substance." However, this argument ignores the context in which this statute was passed and its purpose in preventing substance use facilitation.[141] OPCs do not enable substance use as supported by evidence[138,142,143]; rather, they provide safer substance use and reduce preventable overdose deaths.

Overdose Education and Naloxone Distribution

The following sections discuss the *structural harm-reduction strategies* involving overdose education and naloxone distribution for opioid-related overdose events.

Naloxone

Naloxone is a high-affinity mu-opioid receptor antagonist used for rapid reversal of opioid overdoses. Naloxone can be given via different routes of administration including intravenous, intramuscular, and intranasal (Table 19.9). Subcutaneous autoinjectors were discontinued. Both intramuscular and intranasal formulations are distributed for bystander use, though the nasal spray is most frequently prescribed and/or distributed due to its ease of use, particularly by laypersons. This formulation was approved by the FDA for over-the-counter (OTC) use in 2023.

Naloxone Effectiveness

With the emergence of higher-potency opioids including illicitly manufactured fentanyl, fentanyl analogs, and other novel synthetic opioids, some pharmaceutical companies developed alternative formulations of opioid reversal agents including high-dose naloxone and nalmefene, which has a higher opioid receptor affinity and half-life to naloxone. While some research suggests a trend of increasing cumulative doses of naloxone given for overdoses in clinical and community settings,[144,145] current evidence demonstrates that fentanyl-associated overdoses can typically be reversed using standard dosing of naloxone.[146–148] A comparative study in 2024 demonstrated that high-dose naloxone formulations do not provide additional benefit in patient-related outcomes and instead lead to many more side effects from precipitated opioid withdrawal like vomiting.[149] From a patient-centered perspective, the standard of care for management of opioid overdoses should be administering the lowest effective naloxone dose to reverse respiratory depression. As such, particularly for opioid-tolerant individuals, high-dose formulations of reversal agents, which are also more expensive, should be avoided.[146,147]

In-Hospital Naloxone Distribution

Hospital-based clinicians should always offer in-hand naloxone or a naloxone prescription to patients at risk of opioid-related overdoses upon hospital discharge. Hospital-based clinicians or hospital staff,

TABLE 19.9

Summary of FDA-Approved Opioid Reversal Agents

Agent/Route	Dose	Brand	Over the counter	Notes
Naloxone (IV, IM)	0.4 mg/mL	Generic	No	Given IV or IM. Usually comes as a kit of two 1 mL vials. Also comes as a 10 mL vial though not as commonly distributed.
	5 mg/0.5 mL	Zimhi	No	Given IM via preloaded autoinjector of 0.5 mL. Gives 25 times higher dose than generic IM.
Naloxone (IN)	3 mg/0.1 mL	ReVive	Yes	All formulations packaged in boxes with two doses.
	4 mg/0.1 mL	Naloxone Generic	Yes	
	8 mg/0.1 mL	Kloxxado	No	
Nalmefene (IN)	2.7 mg/0.1 mL	Opvee	No	Half-life of ~11 h (compared to 60–90 min of naloxone)

that is, discharging hospital nurses or pharmacists, should ensure that the patient and any potential bystanders (ie, family members, friends, roommates) are provided education on naloxone administration. As of 2024, all US states including the District of Columbia, except for Wyoming, have overdose Good Samaritan Laws that provide some level of immunity for bystanders and/or the person who overdosed.[150] US state laws vary, either providing protection from charge, prosecution, or arrest for possession of controlled substances and/or drug paraphernalia, with laws protecting from arrest associated with lower rates of overdose deaths.[151]

Patients Who May Benefit from Naloxone

Given widespread fentanyl adulteration in other substances like cocaine and methamphetamine, naloxone should be given both to individuals using the unregulated opioid supply and/or with an OUD and to those who use cocaine, methamphetamines, pressed pills (ie, counterfeit pills sold as prescription opioids, benzodiazepines, and stimulants), or other street substances. Additionally, patients prescribed long-term opioids and anyone who requests naloxone should receive a prescription.

Routes of Distribution and Payer Source

Hospital-based clinicians should ensure that their hospital's outpatient pharmacy and/or local community pharmacies have naloxone in stock. Delivering naloxone "meds to bed" prior to discharge can ensure patients receive naloxone in hand before discharge. All state Medicaid programs provide financial coverage for some formulation of naloxone.[152] For patients who are uninsured, unable to afford a copay, or have an insurance plan that does not cover naloxone, hospitals should have a supply of free naloxone to distribute. This can be done by partnering with local harm reduction organizations, county and US state-level health departments, or local pharmacies. Patients can also access naloxone through local or mail-order harm reduction organizations (ie, NEXT Distro),[153] vending machines, or local pharmacies via statewide standing orders or over the counter (OTC).

Implementation of In-Hospital Naloxone Distribution

Many hospitals have adopted standardized protocols to distribute take-home naloxone kits in inpatient and emergency department settings.[38] Implementation strategies vary but generally include multidisciplinary teams of clinicians, pharmacists, nurses, and peer specialists, use of order sets through the electronic health record, and storage of naloxone for distribution in secure units (eg, Pyxis, Omnicell). Kits include intramuscular or intranasal forms of naloxone, syringes for intramuscular injection (eg, 3 mL, 25 G, 1-inch syringe), and patient instructions on naloxone use. Providing these kits upon hospital admission rather than discharge is preferable due to the potential for unanticipated discharges.

Overview of Substance Checking Services and Awareness of Local Substance Supply

Substance checking is a *structural harm reduction* strategy in which nonpharmaceutical or nonprescription substances are analyzed to identify their chemical composition or the presence of any adulterants.

The unregulated US substance supply has evolved significantly over time, with the emergence of new adulterants with unique clinical implications. Since the mid-2010s, the opioid supply has shifted from predominantly heroin to nonpharmaceutical, illicitly manufactured fentanyl, fentanyl analogs, and other novel high-potency synthetic opioids. Moreover, increasing fentanyl adulteration in the nonopioid supply, including cocaine and methamphetamines accounts for a significant rise in unintentional fatal overdoses. Since 2019, xylazine, which is an alpha-2-adrenergic agonist and kappa opioid receptor agonist, FDA approved as a veterinary sedative, has become increasingly prevalent in the unregulated opioid supply. Other substances like nitazenes (potent synthetic opioids), designer benzodiazepines (eg, etizolam), and medetomidine (veterinary sedative) have also emerged on the illicit market.

Benefits to Checking Substances

Substance checking empowers people with SUD to make informed decisions about the substances they use and can inform harm reduction organizations, the broader community, and public health surveillance efforts. Substance checking has the potential to increase engagement, serve as quality control in an unregulated market by increasing accountability and shifting power to people who use substances, and influence policymaking around substance use and SUD.[154] Studies identified that the vast majority of people with SUD are interested and would utilize these services if accessible to them.[155,156]

Substance Checking Modalities

Substance checking can range from simpler forms, such as liquid reagent–based testing and immunoassay test strips to more advanced laboratory techniques like mass or infrared spectrometry. Liquid reagent–based testing and immunoassay test strips are easier to use, lower cost, and more accessible, but are only able to detect whether a substance is present or absent. More sophisticated technologies can provide more comprehensive qualitative and quantitative data. While test strips give real-time at-hand results, they provide qualitative information, are subject to error, and do not test for all compounds within a substance, underscoring the importance of more comprehensive and accurate detection methods.[157] There are many other forms of substance checking as *structural harm-reduction* strategies including Fourier-transform infrared (FTIR) spectroscopy, Raman spectroscopy, high-pressure mass spectrometry (HPMS), thin-layer chromatography (TLC), high-performance liquid chromatography (HPLC), gas-chromatography-mass spectrometry (GC-MS), and liquid chromatography-mass spectrometry (LC-MS).[158]

Test Strips

Test strips utilize lateral flow immunoassays, a diagnostic technique using antibodies to detect the presence or absence of a substance in a liquid sample, typically through competitive binding. If the substance being tested for is present in the sample, the substance (ie, antigen) will bind to the color-tagged antibody, preventing it from binding to the test line but not the control line, resulting in only one line present (ie, a positive test). This is the opposite of sandwich binding immunoassays utilized in pregnancy or COVID-19 tests, in which two lines indicate a positive test. Fentanyl and xylazine test strips (XTSs) are most utilized and distributed by the harm reduction community, but test strips for other substances exist, including benzodiazepines, nitazines (potent synthetic opioid), and medetomidine (veterinary alpha-2 agonist).[156] Use of test strips involve (1) diluting the substance (or drug residue) in water; (2) holding the test strip by the end with the solid color and dipping the other end in the diluted substance for 10 to 15 seconds (depending on the brand); (3) laying the strip flat and waiting for 3 to 5 minutes (depending on the brand); and finally, (4) interpreting the results (see Figure 19.7).

Fentanyl Test Strips

Fentanyl test strips (FTS) were first developed to test for fentanyl in urine samples but have now been widely adopted "off-label" as a harm reduction strategy to test samples for fentanyl adulteration. Since then, there are several commercially available brands for which validation studies demonstrate a sensitivity of 87.5% to 98.5%, a specificity of 89.2% to 95.2%, a false-negative rate of 1.5% to 12.5%, and a false positive rate of 5% to 10.9%.[159,160] Detection limits range between 100 and 200 ng/mL. These ranges of FTS performance may be due to inaccurate sample preparation, sample heterogeneity, and brand-to-brand and lot-to-lot variability.[161] As of 2024, some commercially available FTS brands (Rapid Response, BTNX Inc, Pickering, ON, Canada) cross reacted with methamphetamines, 4-methylenedioxymethamphetamine (MDMA), and diphenhydramine, which is a commonly used cutting agent, potentially leading to false positives[162] while others do not (DanceSafe/WHPM). FTS also vary in their ability to detect various fentanyl analogs, with some detected more reliably.[163]

Because the unregulated opioid market is predominantly fentanyl, FTS testing is helpful when the individual is opioid naive to assess for fentanyl

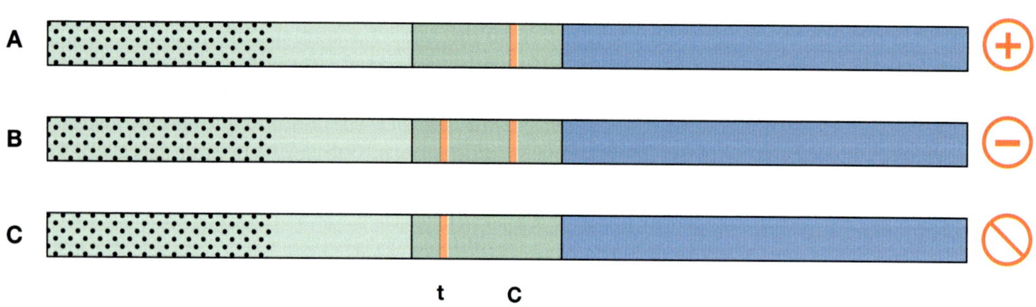

"t" indicates the test line and "c" indicates the control line.

A. If only the control line is present, then the test is positive.

B. If the test line is present (even faintly) along with the control line, then the test is negative.

C. If only the test line is present, then the test is invalid.

Figure 19.7: Generic instructions for test strip interpretation.

adulteration in methamphetamines, cocaine, pressed pills (ie, counterfeit pills sold as prescription opioids, benzodiazepines, and stimulants), and other non-opioid street substances. Harm reduction strategies, if substances test positive for fentanyl, include not using the sample, switching dealers, changing route of administration, and other overdose prevention strategies (eg, using less, using with someone else). Even for negative tests, individuals should be counseled to proceed with caution due to potential false negatives from undetected fentanyl analogs, fentanyl concentrations below the detection limit, and the presence of fentanyl in parts of the sample that were not tested.

Xylazine Test Strips

In early 2023, xylazine test strips (XTS) became commercially available. To date, there are limited validation studies, particularly ones done in real-world settings. Two studies noted a limit of detection of 2,000 to 2,500 ng/mL (2.0 to 2.5 μg/mL), higher than the limit of detection of 1,000 ng/mL advertised by manufacturers.[164] False-positive results were mostly caused by lidocaine cross reactivity and, to a lesser degree, other common cutting agents such as levamisole (described in Chapter 10).[165] There was no cross reactivity with other alpha-2-agonists like medetomidine.[165] Thus, due to XTS cross reactivity with cutting agents frequently used in stimulants, XTS should only be used to test opioid samples. While one study demonstrated a sensitivity of 0.974 and specificity of 1.00 for XTS in testing drug residue samples,[165] a subsequent study on real-world performance of XTS in residue samples demonstrated a high rate of false negatives with XTS, particularly when xylazine was present in smaller quantities.[157] This highlights the importance of further research in this area and for pairing XTS testing with other substance checking modalities.

Evidence for Test Strips

There are numerous studies examining the use of FTS among various populations of people with SUD, including those who predominantly use opioids or stimulants, many of which demonstrate the acceptability and feasibility of FTS.[166–169] Positive FTS results are associated with theoretical or actual behavioral changes to decrease the risk of overdose, including discarding the substance, using with someone else, and doing a test shot.[167,170–175] While there are less studies examining the actual impact of FTS on overdose-related outcomes, limited data suggests that use of FTS decreases rates of overdose or fatal overdose.[167,176] There is limited literature on the acceptability, feasibility, interest in using, and the impact of XTS use among people who use drugs.[177,178]

Practical Considerations for Test Strip Distribution in Hospital Settings

While data supports the use of test strips, there are a variety of barriers that impede their use in the hospital. Barriers include lack of awareness about adulterants[179]; knowledge of test strips, their use, and interpretation; limited access to test strips; potential for false-positive or negative results; structural conditions that limit test strip use (eg, lack of a private place to test) or behavioral changes (eg, ubiquity of adulterant in samples in geographic region); and legality of substance checking equipment.[168]

Laws Regarding Substance Checking in the US

US laws around drug checking supplies vary from state to state depending on their definition of substance paraphernalia. In many states, this definition includes "testing equipment used, intended for use, or fashioned specifically for use in identifying, or in analyzing the strength, effectiveness or purity of controlled substances," based on the DEA's 1979 Model Drug Paraphernalia Act adopted by many states.[180] Through advocacy, some states removed this language from their paraphernalia definition, while others included clauses that allow for specific substance checking equipment, including test strips. A summary of these US laws by state can be found through the LAPPA website.[123]

Expanding access to test strips aligns well with the 2022 and 2024 US White House National Drug Control Strategy, and hospitals serve as an optimal setting for doing so. Various hospitals in the US have implemented distribution of test strips to patients who are admitted to the hospital or presenting to the emergency department. North American hospitals exploring test strip distribution should consider providing prepackaged kits that include test strips, cookers (or other containers for dilution), sterile water, a microscoop, instructions on test strip use and interpretation, and harm reduction strategies.[169] Before doing so, implementors should verify their state or provincial laws to ensure they are in compliance.

Identify a Test Strip Supplier

Prices for test strips vary based on the brand, distributor, and quantity purchased. As of 2024, based on wholesale pricing for the most common commercially available brands, the cost of FTS ranged from $0.65 to 0.75 per strip, while the cost of XTS ranged from $0.89 to 1.75 per strip.[181–183] Following the passage of the US American Rescue Plan Act that allocated

$30 million for evidence-based harm reduction services, in April 2021, the CDC and SAMHSA announced that US federal funds could be used to purchase FTS.[184] Several US state and county health departments enacted programs that provided test strips for free to various entities for distribution.

Community Drug Checking

Drug checking services (DCS), often run by community organizations or in partnership with a university or health department, involve testing samples submitted by individuals or harm reduction organizations. Information from DCS directly inform individuals, their networks, and organizations about their local substance supply and can be used for broader public health surveillance purposes.

Different DCS Modalities

Many harm reduction organizations use hand-held Raman spectroscopy or portable FTIR spectrometry as low-barrier methods of checking substances.[185] While these devices provide more comprehensive information about the presence and quantity of various compounds in samples, they are less sensitive than rapid immunoassay test strips, particularly for trace detection.[158,186] Thus, many organizations use a combination of onsite test strips (described above) and Raman/FTIR spectroscopy while sending samples offsite for confirmatory testing with mass spectrometry (also described above and in Chapter 10).[187] Some DCS, like the Street Drug Analysis Lab at the University of North Carolina provide services nationally.[188] The Harm Reduction Innovation Lab houses a directory of DCS in North America.[189]

Building Awareness of the Evolving Local Substance Supply

As there is no standardized public health approach to surveillance of the unregulated substance supply, significant investments are needed to support real-time monitoring. Identification of real-time changes and experiences often relies on the reported experiences of people with SUD, forensic reports from law enforcement seizures, and overdose mortality records. At the expense of the health and well-being of people with SUD, this delay in recognition leads to a reactive model, such that public health and medical community responses occur well beyond the optimal window for determining and implementing effective interventions. This was particularly exemplified with the increasing prevalence of xylazine and identification of clinical harms among people with SUD, including severe chronic skin ulcerations. Despite its steady appearance and rise in the opioid supply since 2019, there are still significant gaps in current literature, research efforts, and clinical responses related to xylazine, highlighting the need for better public health approaches to navigate the changing drug supply.

Talk to Hospitalized People With SUD to Become Aware of the Local Substance Supply

To best understand how to care for people with SUD, hospital-based clinicians should be knowledgeable about emergent adulterants and substances used most frequently in their geographic region. Hospital-based clinicians can gain understanding of current experiences through discussions with hospitalized people with SUD by utilizing the communication strategies described in the *relational harm reduction* section and open dialogue and partnerships with their local SSP or DCS. People with SUD are experts on their own bodies and in their personal experience with substance use, making it essential for hospital-based clinicians to actively listen to their concerns, especially regarding new or unusual clinical manifestations. This collaborative approach not only enhances patient care but also helps in better understanding the nuances of substance use and its impact on health.

Treatment Approaches for Hospital-Based Management of SUD

Always offer and provide hospitalized people with SUD adequate withdrawal and pain management if appropriate, offer and initiate SUD treatment, facilitate posthospital discharge treatment linkage, and connect them with resources to address any social needs. Hospital-based clinicians, with the support of pharmacists, can offer medications to reduce withdrawal and treat SUD, while social workers, peers, and care managers are responsible for linkage to postdischarge appointments and community resources.

Adequate Pain Management

From a harm reduction perspective, particularly for patients with opioid tolerance and regardless of whether a person is on medications for OUD (MOUD) or interested in initiating MOUD, full-agonist opioids for acute pain management should not be withheld if considered standard of care (eg, acute fracture, postoperative management). Moreover, due to high opioid tolerance and the potency of the unregulated opioid supply, patients with OUD generally need higher doses of opioids to achieve adequate analgesia.

Hospital-based clinicians may hesitate to initiate or escalate opioid therapy for fear of worsening the patient's OUD. On the contrary, inadequate inpatient pain management for people with SUD increases the risk of self-management of pain (ie, in-hospital use), patient-directed discharge, and avoidance of future health care utilization. Hospital-based clinicians should optimize non-opioid analgesia with the support of their inpatient pain management team, if needed or available. See Chapter 17 for more details on pain management.

Adequate Withdrawal Management

Inadequate withdrawal treatment places people with SUD at-risk of in-hospital substance use and patient-directed discharge. Many hospitals have standardized protocols for management of withdrawal from opioid and GABAergic agents through nurse-driven protocols and symptom-triggered medications (see Chapter 8).

Medications for Opioid Use Disorder and Adjunctive Therapy

MOUD, including buprenorphine and methadone, are considered first-line therapies for treatment of opioid withdrawal with as-needed adjunct opioid withdrawal medications (eg, clonidine, ondansetron, loperamide, hydroxyzine).

Short-Acting Opioids

In addition to MOUD, hospital-based clinicians should consider providing full agonist short-acting opioids for withdrawal management.[190] Reasons for this are twofold: (1) to improve treatment of opioid withdrawal symptoms to prevent in-hospital use and patient-directed discharge and (2) to maintain opioid tolerance. Opioid withdrawal is not generally considered life-threatening, but symptoms can be severe and difficult to manage. While MOUD can be effective in treating withdrawal, challenges include precipitated opioid withdrawal with buprenorphine, concerns about achieving effective analgesia, need for titration over several days to achieve therapeutic doses, and patient disinterest.

Maintenance of Opioid Tolerance

Studies demonstrate that patients with OUD who experience a period of abstinence are at higher risk of overdose after returning to opioid use due to a loss of opioid tolerance.[191] For patients who are uninterested in MOUD and/or are not interested in stopping their opioid use, providing full agonist opioids is also a harm reduction strategy to maintain opioid tolerance. Providing full agonist opioids to reduce the risk of patient-directed discharge due to inadequate withdrawal management allows for an opportunity to build rapport, engage with the patient about their recovery goals, and maintain the chance to initiate MOUD later during the hospitalization.

Planning Contingencies for Patient-Directed Discharges

People with SUD admitted to the hospital may leave as a patient-directed discharge for a variety of reasons. In addition to inadequate withdrawal and/or pain management, patient-directed discharges can occur due to stigma including negative interactions with staff and security searches, boredom and isolation, social consequences (eg, loss of housing or employment, childcare needs), and restrictive hospital policies (eg, visitor restrictions) discussed in detail earlier in this chapter.[19,23,192,193]

Discharge Planning

Patient-directed discharges are prone to suboptimal follow-up treatment plans, including incomplete referrals to outpatient follow-up, lack of linkage to SUD treatment, and inappropriate discharge medications, including a lack of antibiotic provision. Consequently, patient-directed discharges, particularly among people with SUD, are associated with higher rates of rehospitalization, decreased treatment completion, and increased mortality.[57,60,194–196]

In the event of a patient-directed discharge, contingency planning is important for individuals requiring coordination of care, follow-up, and long-term therapies, such as those with invasive infections like infective endocarditis, which requires extended antibiotics. Provision of partial oral antibiotic therapy for patients leaving as a patient-directed discharge leads to better outcomes than no antibiotics at all.[195,197] In the case of a life-threating infection, hospital-based clinicians must work with infectious disease specialists, addiction specialists, when available, social workers, and care managers to develop contingency plans ensuring that patients are not discharged without antibiotics and appropriate follow-up plans. This practice is supported by the 2022 statement from the American Heart Association on management of infective endocarditis in people who use injection substances.[198] These plans should include a specific antibiotic regimen (ie, oral antibiotic or long-acting lipoglycopeptide antibiotic, dose, duration), MOUD plan (ie, buprenorphine bridge prescription), naloxone, and follow-up information with infectious disease, cardiology, and addiction. Another consideration for patients at high-risk of leaving as a patient-directed discharge is offering and providing long-acting injectable buprenorphine during their hospitalization.[199] Hospital-based clinicians should document contingency plans in their daily progress notes so that all care team members involved are aware of them.[200] These topics are covered in detail in Chapters 11 and 20.

Future Directions

In-Hospital Syringe Service Programs

In-hospital SSPs and harm reduction initiatives have been implemented in North America to improve outcomes for people with SUD. In the US, some hospitals have adjacent SSPs or distribute supplies upon patient discharge, while Canada has integrated SSPs into acute and subacute care facilities and emergency departments. A Toronto hospital serving patients living with HIV implemented a program offering safer use injection and smoking kits, resulting in yearly increases in the number of kits accepted and improved communication between patients and clinicians about drug-related harms.[201,202] These programs help reduce harm, prevent early discharge, improve patient care, and warrant further expansion across the US.

In-Hospital Overdose Prevention Centers

Another promising intervention is hospital-based OPCs, where individuals can use preobtained nonprescribed substances in a designated, supervised space without the risk of criminal prosecution.[138,203,204] A notable example, implemented in Western Canada in 2018, provides overdose monitoring, sterile supplies, and safe disposal of used equipment.[203] Patients attending the in-hospital OPC complete an intake and consent process, disclose their substance type and consumption method, and provide their name to confirm hospital registration.[22] Patients use the service to access sterile supplies, reduce infection risks, and engage in safer consumption practices while avoiding overdose and potentially confrontational discussions with staff. The OPC also ensures safe disposal of used supplies and offers protection from stigma and social violence associated with substance use in the hospital, particularly in the context of criminalization. Models for in-hospital OPCs can be nurse led or managed by the addiction medicine consultation team, and while the program has shown promise in improving safety and engagement, further research is needed to assess its long-term effectiveness and broader implementation.[205]

In-Hospital Overdose Detection Technologies

An innovative and acceptable hospital-based strategy is to install overdose detection technologies, such as an antimotion alarm system, in public restrooms where overdose fatalities are at risk of occurring.[206,207] Research shows that people with SUD may prefer to use their substances in single occupancy restrooms.[208] These systems activate when the restroom door is closed and locked, triggering an alarm to local public safety personnel after 4 minutes of motionlessness. While several are in the early stages of development, the Brave Sensor is an example of a contactless radar sensor device that has been commercially available since 2018 that hospitals can consider installing to mitigate in-hospital overdose.[209]

Harm Reduction Education and Training

Implementation research highlights several effective strategies for increasing the adoption of in-hospital harm reduction services, including communication and educational strategies, engagement of champions, and adapting infrastructure.[210] However, foundational education on *structural* and *relational harm reduction* remains underrepresented in medical curricula and should be expanded.[211,212]

To build capacity and enable future hospital-based clinicians to champion in-hospital harm reduction initiatives, medical trainees must gain experience in understanding harm reduction principles and receive interprofessional education using evidence-based tools to minimize harms associated with substance use through a nonabstinence lens.[213] For example, when Internal Medicine trainees at an urban institution serving a large population of people with SUD received harm reduction education, their compassion satisfaction in caring for this population increased with time, potentially improving care.[214]

Models for hospital champions include harm reduction nurses who address stigma and support patient-centered care by bridging the harm reduction and medical model.[215] Additionally, integrated health programs, located near hospitals—offering services like harm reduction–focused day health programs, 24-hour specialized nursing care residences, and enhanced supported housing can reduce patient-directed discharge.[216] Programs like Project TRUST at Boston Medical Center, which uses community health workers to connect people to SUD and urgent care, exemplify how integrating community-based harm reduction programs into the hospital setting can improve clinical outcomes and provide a comprehensive approach to patient care.[217]

Sustaining In-Hospital Harm Reduction: Structural Changes, Policy Reform, and Funding

The future of in-hospital harm reduction must reconcile the philosophical differences between harm-reduction and the medical model, striving for synergy that prioritizes the well-being, respect, and autonomy of patients. Health care systems should focus on meeting the needs of individuals rather than imposing mandatory engagement, recognizing that people with SUD may have valid reasons for mistrusting the system and that hospitals are obligated to keep patients and staff safe. Thus, meaningful collaboration and partnership among patients,[185] hospital staff, hospital-based clinicians, and other interested partners is necessary to ensure that all perspectives are considered to develop an inclusive and trauma-informed health care environment that embraces harm reduction. Addressing barriers such as institutional policies, stigma, and gaps in SUD education is vital. Bold, decisive action from all relevant stakeholders (ie, hospital leadership, hospital-based clinicians, payers) is required to reduce preventable deaths, ensure adequate reimbursement for harm reduction services, and promote trauma-informed care that rebuilds trust with people with SUD.

There is also a need to prioritize allocated funding for research from the National Institutes of Health and SAHMSA into health care stigma reduction, harm reduction education, innovative programs such as hospital-based harm reduction services, safe supply, and the integration of community-based harm reduction organizations. Finally, there is a critical need to understand how to sustainably fund hospital-based harm reduction services by exploring billing and reimbursement models.

REFERENCES

1. https://www.waukeshacounty.gov/media/lp3hyerk/harm-reduction-framework.pdf
2. Hawk M, Coulter RWS, Egan JE, et al. Harm reduction principles for healthcare settings. *Harm Reduct J.* 2017;14(1):70.
3. American Psychiatric Association. *Diagnostic and Statistical Manual of Mental Disorders.* 5th ed. Author; 2013.
4. Des Jarlais DC. Harm reduction in the USA: the research perspective and an archive to David Purchase. *Harm Reduct J.* 2017;14(1):51.
5. Hari J. *Chasing the Scream: The First and Last Days of the War on Drugs.* Bloomsbury Publishing USA; 2015.
6. H.R.5210—Anti-Drug Abuse Act of 1988. https://www.congress.gov/bill/100th-congress/house-bill/5210
7. Showalter D. Federal funding for syringe exchange in the US: explaining a long-term policy failure. *Int J Drug Policy.* 2018;55:95–104.
8. Des Jarlais DC, Feelemyer J, LaKosky P, Szymanowski K, Arasteh K. Expansion of syringe service programs in the United States, 2015–2018. *Am J Public Health.* 2020;110(4):517–519.
9. Levengood TW, Yoon GH, Davoust MJ, et al. Supervised injection facilities as harm reduction: a systematic review. *Am J Prev Med.* 2021;61(5):738–749.
10. LAAPP Association. Syringe services programs: summary of state laws. 2023.
11. Dineen KK, Pendo E. Ending the war on people with substance use disorders in health care. *Am J Bioeth.* 2021;21(4):20–22.
12. Lewer D, Freer J, King E, et al. Frequency of health-care utilization by adults who use illicit drugs: a systematic review and meta-analysis. *Addiction.* 2020;115(6):1011–1023.
13. Hodder SL, Feinberg J, Strathdee SA, et al. The opioid crisis and HIV in the USA: deadly synergies. *Lancet.* 2021;397(10279):1139–1150.
14. Moorman AC, Bixler D, Teshale EH, et al. Hepatitis C Virus-HIV coinfection in the United States among people who inject drugs: data needed for ending dual epidemics. *Public Health Rep.* 2023:333549231181348.
15. Ronan MV, Herzig SJ. Hospitalizations related to opioid abuse/dependence and associated serious infections increased sharply, 2002–12. *Health Aff (Millwood).* 2016;35(5):832–837.
16. Barocas JA, Eftekhari Yazdi G, Savinkina A, et al. Long-term infective endocarditis mortality associated with injection opioid use in the united states: a modeling study. *Clin Infect Dis.* 2021;73(11):e3661–e3669.
17. Gilbert AR, Hellman JL, Wilkes MS, Rees VW, Summers PJ. Self-care habits among people who inject drugs with skin and soft tissue infections: a qualitative analysis. *Harm Reduct J.* 2019;16(1):69.
18. Grewal HK, Ti L, Hayashi K, Dobrer S, Wood E, Kerr T. Illicit drug use in acute care settings. *Drug Alcohol Rev.* 2015;34(5):499–502.
19. McNeil R, Small W, Wood E, Kerr T. Hospitals as a 'risk environment': an ethno-epidemiological study of voluntary and involuntary discharge from hospital against medical advice among people who inject drugs. *Soc Sci Med.* 2014;105:59–66.
20. Eaton EF, Westfall AO, McClesky B, et al. In-hospital illicit drug use and patient-directed discharge: barriers to care for patients with injection-related infections. *Open Forum Infect Dis.* 2020;7(3):ofaa074.
21. Parmar GS, Hayashi K, Nolan S, et al. Non-medical prescription opioid use and in-hospital illicit drug use among people who use drugs. *Drug Alcohol Rev.* 2021;40(6):959–963.
22. Nolan S, Kelian S, Kerr T, et al. Harm reduction in the hospital: an overdose prevention site (OPS) at a Canadian hospital. *Drug Alcohol Depend.* 2022;239:109608.
23. Simon R, Snow R, Wakeman S. Understanding why patients with substance use disorders leave the hospital against medical advice: a qualitative study. *Subst Abus.* 2020;41(4):519–525.
24. Martin M, Snyder HR, Otway G, Holpit L, Day LW, Seidman D. In-hospital substance use policies: an opportunity to advance equity, reduce stigma, and offer evidence-based addiction care. *J Addict Med.* 2023;17(1):10–12.

25. Pauly BB, McCall J, Browne AJ, Parker J, Mollison A. Toward cultural safety: nurse and patient perceptions of illicit substance use in a hospitalized setting. *ANS Adv Nurs Sci.* 2015;38(2):121–135.
26. Anis AH, Sun H, Guh DP, Palepu A, Schechter MT, O'Shaughnessy MV. Leaving hospital against medical advice among HIV-positive patients. *CMAJ.* 2002;167(6):633–637.
27. Heller D, McCoy K, Cunningham C. An invisible barrier to integrating HIV primary care with harm reduction services: philosophical clashes between the harm reduction and medical models. *Public Health Rep.* 2004;119(1):32–39.
28. Hall OT, Jordan A, Teater J, et al. Experiences of racial discrimination in the medical setting and associations with medical mistrust and expectations of care among black patients seeking addiction treatment. *J Subst Abuse Treat.* 2022;133:108551.
29. Emmanuelli J, Desenclos JC. Harm reduction interventions, behaviours and associated health outcomes in France, 1996–2003. *Addiction.* 2005;100(11):1690–1700.
30. Dunleavy K, Munro A, Roy K, et al. Association between harm reduction intervention uptake and skin and soft tissue infections among people who inject drugs. *Drug Alcohol Depend.* 2017:174:91–97.
31. Drucker E, Lurie P, Wodak A, Alcabes P. Measuring harm reduction: the effects of needle and syringe exchange programs and methadone maintenance on the ecology of HIV. *AIDS.* 1998;12:S217–S230.
32. Hawk KF, Vaca FE, D'Onofrio G. Reducing fatal opioid overdose: prevention, treatment and harm reduction strategies. *Yale J Biol Med.* 2015;88(3):235–245.
33. Hagan H, McGough JP, Thiede H, Hopkins S, Duchin J, Alexander ER. Reduced injection frequency and increased entry and retention in drug treatment associated with needle-exchange participation in Seattle drug injectors. *J Subst Abuse Treat.* 2000;19(3):247–252.
34. Macias-Konstantopoulos W, Heins A, Sachs CJ, Whiteman PJ, Wingkun NG, Riviello RJ. Between emergency department visits: the role of harm reduction programs in mitigating the harms associated with injection drug use. *Ann Emerg Med.* 2021;77(5):479–492.
35. Jawa R, Tin Y, Nall S, et al. Estimated clinical outcomes and cost-effectiveness associated with provision of addiction treatment in us primary care clinics. *JAMA Netw Open.* 2023;6(4):e237888.
36. Shang M, Thiel B, Liebschutz JM, Kraemer KL, Freund A, Jawa R. Implementing harm reduction kits in an office-based addiction treatment program. *Harm Reduct J.* 2023;20(1):163.
37. Wheeler E, Davidson PJ, Jones TS, Irwin KS; Centers for Disease Control and Prevention (CDC). Community-based opioid overdose prevention programs providing naloxone—United States, 2010. *MMWR Morb Mortal Wkly Rep.* 2012; 61(6):101–105.
38. Sindhwani MK, Friedman A, O'Donnell M, Stader D, Weiner SG. Naloxone distribution programs in the emergency department: a scoping review of the literature. *J Am Coll Emerg Physicians Open.* 2024;5(3):e13180.
39. Nguyen TT, Applewhite D, Cheung F, Jacob S, Mitchell E. Implementation of a multidisciplinary inpatient opioid overdose education and naloxone distribution program at a large academic medical center. *Am J Health Syst Pharm.* 2022;79(24):2253–2260.
40. Jawa R, Luu T, Bachman M, Demers L. Rapid naloxone administration workshop for health care providers at an Academic Medical Center. *MedEdPORTAL.* 2020;16:10892.
41. Barocas JA, Savinkina A, Adams J, et al. Clinical impact, costs, and cost-effectiveness of hospital-based strategies for addressing the US opioid epidemic: a modelling study. *Lancet Public Health.* 2022;7(1):e56–e64.
42. Perera R, Stephan L, Appa A, et al. Meeting people where they are: implementing hospital-based substance use harm reduction. *Harm Reduct J.* 2022;19:14.
43. Fraimow-Wong L, Martín M, Thomas L, et al. Patient and staff perspectives on the impacts and challenges of hospital-based harm reduction. *JAMA Netw Open.* 2024;7(2):e240229.
44. Hawk M, Kay ES, Jawa R. Relational harm reduction for internists: a call to action. *J Gen Intern Med.* 2024;39(9): 1746–1748.
45. Hawk M, Jawa R, Kay ES. Communication about harm reduction with patients who have opioid use disorder. *JAMA.* 2025;333(2):163–164.
46. Kowalchuk A, Gonzalez SJ, Zoorob RJ. Substance misuse in adults: a primary care approach. *Am Fam Physician.* 2024;109(5):430–440.
47. Calcaterra SL, Buresh M, Weimer MB. Better care at the bedside hospitalized patients with opioid use disorder. *J Hosp Med.* 2023;18(12):1134–1138.
48. Callon W, Beach MC, Saha S, et al. Assessing problematic substance use in HIV care: which questions elicit accurate patient disclosures? *J Gen Intern Med.* 2016;31(10):1141–1147.
49. Administration SAMHSA. Substance Abuse and Mental Health Services Administration: Practical Guide for Implementing a Trauma-Informed Approach. Publication No PEP23-06-05-005. 2023.
50. Hettema J, Steele J, Miller WR. Motivational interviewing. *Annu Rev Clin Psychol.* 2005;1(1):91–111.
51. Administration SAMHSA. Using Motivational Interviewing in Substance Use Disorder Treatment. Advisory. Publication No PEP20-02-02-0142021.
52. Hook JN, Davis DE, Owen J, Worthington EL, Utsey SO. Cultural humility: measuring openness to culturally diverse clients. *J Couns Psychol.* 2013;60(3):353–566.
53. Tham SS, Solomon P. Practicing cultural humility will achieve recovery-oriented mental health practice and service delivery. *Adm Policy Ment Health.* 2024;51(1):10–13.
54. Ezell JM, Pho M, Jaiswal J, et al. A systematic literature review of strengths-based approaches to drug use management and treatment. *Clin Soc Work J.* 2023;51:294–305.
55. Weingart SN, Davis RB, Phillips RS. Patients discharged against medical advice from a general medicine service. *J Gen Intern Med.* 1998;13:568–571.
56. Glasgow JM, Vaughn-Sarrazin M, Kaboli PJ. Leaving against medical advice (AMA): risk of 30-day mortality and hospital readmission. *J Gen Intern Med.* 2010;25(9):926–929.
57. Southern WN, Nahvi S, Arnsten JH. Increased risk of mortality and readmission among patients discharged against medical advice. *Am J Med.* 2012;125(6):594–602.
58. Compton P, Aronowitz SV, Klusaritz H, Anderson E. Acute pain and self-directed discharge among hospitalized patients with opioid-related diagnoses: a cohort study. *Harm Reduct J.* 2021;18:131.
59. Alrawashdeh M, Rhee C, Klompas M, et al. Association of early opioid withdrawal treatment strategy and patient-directed discharge among hospitalized patients with opioid use disorder. *J Gen Intern Med.* 2023;38(10):2289–2297.
60. Appa A, Adamo M, Le S, et al. Patient-directed discharges among persons who use drugs hospitalized with invasive staphylococcus aureus infections: opportunities for improvement. *Am J Med.* 2022;135(1):91–96.
61. Strike C, Robinson S, Guta A, et al. Illicit drug use while admitted to hospital: patient and health care provider perspectives. *PLoS One.* 2020;15(3):e0229713.
62. Walker ER, Pratt LA, Schoenborn CA, Druss BG. Excess mortality among people who report lifetime use of illegal drugs in the United States: a 20-year follow-up of a nationally representative survey. *Drug Alcohol Depend.* 2017;171:31–38.

63. Lake S, Kennedy MC. Health outcomes associated with illicit prescription opioid injection: a systematic review. *J Addict Dis*. 2016;35(2):73–91.
64. Degenhardt L, Peacock A, Colledge S, et al. Global prevalence of injecting drug use and sociodemographic characteristics and prevalence of HIV, HBV, and HCV in people who inject drugs: a multistage systematic review. *Lancet Glob Health*. 2017;5(12):e1192–e1207.
65. Biancarelli DL, Biello KB, Childs E, et al. Strategies used by people who inject drugs to avoid stigma in healthcare settings. *Drug Alcohol Depend*. 2019;198:80–86.
66. van Boekel LC, Brouwers EP, van Weeghel J, Garretsen HF. Stigma among health professionals towards patients with substance use disorders and its consequences for healthcare delivery: systematic review. *Drug Alcohol Depend*. 2013; 131(1–2):23–35.
67. Figgatt MC, Salazar ZR, Vincent L, et al. Treatment experiences for skin and soft tissue infections among participants of syringe service programs in North Carolina. *Harm Reduct J*. 2021;18(1):80.
68. Khandor E, Mason K, Chambers C, Rossiter K, Cowan L, Hwang SW. Access to primary health care among homeless adults in Toronto, Canada: results from the Street Health survey. *Open Med*. 2011;5(2):e94–e103.
69. Moallef S, Dale L, Homayra F, et al. Suboptimal nonmedical qualities of primary care linked with care avoidance among people who use drugs in a Canadian setting amid an integrated health care reform. *J Subst Abuse Treat*. 2022;139:108784.
70. Kendall CE, Boucher LM, Mark AE, et al. A cohort study examining emergency department visits and hospital admissions among people who use drugs in Ottawa, Canada. *Harm Reduct J*. 2017;14(1):16.
71. Westgard LK, Sato T, Bradford WS, et al. National HIV and HCV screening rates for hospitalized people who use drugs are suboptimal and heterogeneous across 11 US hospitals. *Open Forum Infect Dis*. 2024;11(5):ofae204.
72. Srivastava P, Modi V, Lier AJ. Sexually Transmitted Infection (STI) incidence, STI screening, and human immunodeficiency virus preexposure prophylaxis uptake in united states veterans with opioid use disorder in long island, New York. *Open Forum Infect Dis*. 2024;11(8):ofae429.
73. Ott JJ, Wiersma ST. Single-dose administration of inactivated hepatitis A vaccination in the context of hepatitis A vaccine recommendations. *Int J Infect Dis*. 2013;17(11): e939–e944.
74. Marks LR, Reno H, Liang SY, et al. Value of packaged testing for sexually transmitted infections for persons who inject drugs hospitalized with serious injection-related infections. *Open Forum Infect Dis*. 2021;8(11):ofab489.
75. D Grussing E, Pickard B, Khalid A, et al. Implementation of a bundle to improve HIV testing during hospitalization for people who inject drugs. *Implement Res Pract*. 2023;4:26334895231203410.
76. NASTAD. Viral Hepatitis Testing: Health System Assessment Toolkit. https://nastad.org/resources/viral-hepatitis-testing-health-system-assessment-toolkit
77. Falade-Nwulia O, Suarez-Cuervo C, Nelson DR, Fried MW, Segal JB, Sulkowski MS. Oral direct-acting agent therapy for hepatitis C virus infection: a systematic review. *Ann Intern Med*. 2017;166(9):637–648.
78. Brown A, Welzel TM, Conway B, et al. Adherence to pangenotypic glecaprevir/pibrentasvir and efficacy in HCV-infected patients: A pooled analysis of clinical trials. *Liver Int*. 2020;40(4):778–786.
79. Dieterich DT. A simplified algorithm for the management of hepatitis C infection. *Gastroenterol Hepatol (N Y)*. 2019; 15(5 Suppl 3):1–12.
80. Yehia BR, Schranz AJ, Umscheid CA, Lo Re V III. The treatment cascade for chronic hepatitis C virus infection in the United States: a systematic review and meta-analysis. *PLoS One*. 2014;9(7):e101554.
81. Jiang X, Parker RL, Vouri SM, et al. Cascade of hepatitis C virus care among patients with substance use disorders. *Am J Prev Med*. 2021;61(4):576–584.
82. Corcorran MA, Tsui JI, Scott JD, Dombrowski JC, Glick SN. Age and gender-specific hepatitis C continuum of care and predictors of direct acting antiviral treatment among persons who inject drugs in Seattle, Washington. *Drug Alcohol Depend*. 2021;220:108525.
83. Bredenberg E, Callister C, Dafoe A, Holliman BD, Rowan SE, Calcaterra SL. Subspecialty physicians' perspectives on barriers and facilitators of hepatitis C treatment: a qualitative study. *Harm Reduct J*. 2024;21(1):140.
84. Hepatitis C State of Medicaid access. *2024 National Snapshot Report*. https://stateofhepc.org/2024-national-snapshot-report/
85. Bhattacharya D, Aronsohn A, Price J, Lo Re V; AASLD-IDSA HCV Guidance Panel. Hepatitis C guidance 2023 update: AASLD-IDSA recommendations for testing, managing, and treating hepatitis C virus infection. *Clin Infect Dis*. 2023;25:ciad319.
86. Norton BL, Fleming J, Bachhuber MA, et al. High HCV cure rates for people who use drugs treated with direct acting antiviral therapy at an urban primary care clinic. *Int J Drug Policy*. 2017;47:196–201.
87. Grebely J, Dalgard O, Conway B, et al. Sofosbuvir and velpatasvir for hepatitis C virus infection in people with recent injection drug use (SIMPLIFY): an open-label, single-arm, phase 4, multicentre trial. *Lancet Gastroenterol Hepatol*. 2018; 3(3):153–161.
88. Valerio H, Alavi M, Law M, et al. Opportunities to enhance linkage to hepatitis C care among hospitalized people with recent drug dependence in New South Wales, Australia: a population-based linkage study. *Clin Infect Dis*. 2021;73(11):2037–2044.
89. Rowan SE, Wyles DL. Don't put off until tomorrow what you can do today: hospital admissions as an opportunity to treat hepatitis C. *Clin Infect Dis*. 2024;78(3):591–593.
90. Levander XA, Vega TA, Seaman A, Korthuis PT, Englander H. Utilising an access to care integrated framework to explore the perceptions of hepatitis C treatment of hospital-based interventions among people who use drugs. *Int J Drug Policy*. 2021;96:103356.
91. Levander XA, Vega TA, Seaman A, Korthuis PT, Englander H. Exploring how hospitalization can alter hepatitis c virus treatment prioritization and trajectories in people who use drugs: a qualitative analysis. *Subst Abus*. 2022;43(1):245–252.
92. McCrary LM, Roberts KE, Bowman MC, et al. Inpatient hepatitis C treatment coordination and initiation for patients who inject drugs. *J Gen Intern Med*. 2023;38(15):3428–3433.
93. Babiarz J, Ryu H, Williams C, Ham Y, Rivera Sarti J, Levander XA. Slicing through silos: development and evaluation of a hospital-based telehealth hepatitis C virus treatment program. *Int J Drug Policy*. 2024;127:104396.
94. Midgard H, Malme KB, Pihl CM, et al. Opportunistic treatment of hepatitis C infection among hospitalized people who inject drugs (OPPORTUNI-C): a stepped wedge cluster randomized trial. *Clin Infect Dis*. 2024;78(3):582–590.
95. Malme KB, Stene-Johansen K, Klundby I, et al. Virologic response and reinfection following HCV treatment among hospitalized people who inject drugs: follow-up data from the OPPORTUNI-C trial. *Viruses*. 2024;16(6):858.
96. NHR Coalition. *Sex Work and Harm Reduction*. https://harmreduction.org/issues/sex-work/harm-reduction-facts/

97. Emanuel E, Slater L, Croxford S, et al. Adverse health outcomes among people who inject drugs who engaged in recent sex work: findings from a national survey. *Public Health*. 2023; 225:79–86.
98. Ivey K, Bernstein KT, Kirkcaldy RD, et al. Chemsex drug use among a national sample of sexually active men who have sex with men, American men's internet survey, 2017–2020. *Subst Use Misuse*. 2023;58(5):728–734.
99. Heil SH, Jones HE, Arria A, et al. Unintended pregnancy in opioid-abusing women. *J Subst Abuse Treat*. 2011;40(2): 199–202.
100. Terplan M, Hand DJ, Hutchinson M, Salisbury-Afshar E, Heil SH. Contraceptive use and method choice among women with opioid and other substance use disorders: A systematic review. *Prev Med*. 2015;80:23–31.
101. Grossman D, Perritt J, Grady D. The impending crisis of access to safe abortion care in the US. *JAMA Intern Med*. 2022;182(8):793–795.
102. Bedsider.org. https://www.bedsider.org/
103. Vincent W, McFarland W. Missed opportunities for healthcare providers to discuss HIV preexposure prophylaxis with people who inject drugs. *Int J Drug Policy*. 2022;110:103873.
104. Ball LJ, Puka K, Speechley M, et al. Sharing of injection drug preparation equipment is associated with HIV infection: A cross-sectional study. *J Acquir Immune Defic Syndr*. 2019;81(4): e99–e103.
105. Centers for Disease Control and Prevention (CDC). HIV and People Who Inject Drugs. 2022.
106. Suprasert B, Tate M, Reagan D, et al. Continuing low awareness and use of pre-exposure prophylaxis (PrEP) for HIV among people who inject drugs (PWID), San Francisco, 2022. *AIDS Behav*. 2024;28(6):2089–2100.
107. Centers for Disease Control and Prevention (CDC). PrEP Effectiveness. 2022.
108. Mistler CB, Copenhaver MM, Shrestha R. The pre-exposure prophylaxis (PrEP) care cascade in people who inject drugs: a systematic review. *AIDS Behav*. 2021;25(5):1490–1506.
109. Dubov A, Krakower DS, Rockwood N, Montgomery S, Shoptaw S. Provider implicit bias in prescribing HIV preexposure prophylaxis (PrEP) to people who inject drugs. *J Gen Intern Med*. 2023;38(13):2928–2935.
110. Pleuhs B, Mistler CB, Quinn KG, et al. Evidence of potential discriminatory HIV pre-exposure prophylaxis (PrEP) prescribing practices for people who inject drugs among a small percentage of providers in the U.S. *J Prim Care Community Health*. 2022;13:21501319211063999.
111. Baeten JM, Palanee-Phillips T, Mgodi NM, et al. Safety, uptake, and use of a dapivirine vaginal ring for HIV-1 prevention in African women (HOPE): an open-label, extension study. *Lancet HIV*. 2021;8(2):e87–e95.
112. Bekker LG, Das M, Karim QA, et al. Twice-yearly lenacapavir or daily F/TAF for HIV prevention in cisgender women. *N Engl J Med*. 2024;391(13):1179–1192.
113. Flynn S, Adamo M, Kochanska M, Garcia-Grossman I. Initiating pre-exposure prophylaxis in the inpatient setting: a quality improvement project. *BMJ Open Qual*. 2024; 13(1):e002416.
114. Chan CA, Minahan-Rowley R, Biegacki ET, Sue KL, Weimer MB. Development of a patient and clinician informed website on injection drug use related infective endocarditis. *Subst Use Addctn J*. 2025;46(2):280–290.
115. NHR Coalition. *Getting off right: A safety manual for injection drug user*. https://harmreduction.org/issues/safer-drug-use/injection-safety-manual/safer-injection-basics/
116. Next Distro. *Introduction to Common Wounds for PWID*. https://nextdistro.org/resources-collection/introduction-to-common-wounds-for-pwid
117. Hope VD, Marongiu A, Parry JV, Ncube F. The extent of injection site infection in injecting drug users: findings from a national surveillance study. *Epidemiol Infect*. 2010; 138(10):1510–1518.
118. Takahashi TA, Baernstein A, Binswanger I, Bradley K, Merrill JO. Predictors of hospitalization for injection drug users seeking care for soft tissue infections. *J Gen Intern Med*. 2007;22(3):382–388.
119. Phillips KT, Stein MD. Risk practices associated with bacterial infections among injection drug users in Denver, Colorado. *Am J Drug Alcohol Abuse*. 2010;36(2):92–97.
120. Palepu A, Tyndall MW, Leon H, et al. Hospital utilization and costs in a cohort of injection drug users. *CMAJ*. 2001;165(4):415–420.
121. Ciccarone D, Unick GJ, Cohen JK, Mars SG, Rosenblum D. Nationwide increase in hospitalizations for heroin-related soft tissue infections: associations with structural market conditions. *Drug Alcohol Depend*. 2016;163:126–133.
122. Chatterjee A, Bannister M, Hill LG, Davis CS. Prescribing syringes to people who inject drugs: advancing harm reduction in primary care. *J Gen Intern Med*. 2023; 38(8):1980–1983.
123. LAAPP Association. Drug checking equipment, needles/syringes, and drug paraphernalia: summary of state laws. 2024.
124. Harris M. An urgent impetus for action: safe inhalation interventions to reduce COVID-19 transmission and fatality risk among people who smoke crack cocaine in the United Kingdom. *Int J Drug Policy*. 2020;83:102829.
125. Laposata EA, Mayo GL. A review of pulmonary pathology and mechanisms associated with inhalation of freebase cocaine ("crack"). *Am J Forensic Med Pathol*. 1993;14(1):1–9.
126. Applewhite D, Regan S, Mackin S, et al. Individuals reporting past 3-month smoked stimulant use are placed at risk for infection and injury amid COVID-19. *J Addict Med*. 2023;17(2):e129–e131.
127. Tapper A, Ahern C, Graveline-Long Z, Newberger NG, Hughto JMW. The utilization and delivery of safer smoking practices and services: a narrative synthesis of the literature. *Harm Reduct J*. 2023;20(1):160.
128. Prangnell A, Dong H, Daly P, Milloy MJ, Kerr T, Hayashi K. Declining rates of health problems associated with crack smoking during the expansion of crack pipe distribution in Vancouver, Canada. *BMC Public Health*. 2017;17(1):163.
129. Harris M, Scott J, Hope V, et al. Safe inhalation pipe provision (SIPP): protocol for a mixed-method evaluation of an intervention to improve health outcomes and service engagement among people who use crack cocaine in England. *Harm Reduct J*. 2024;21(1):19.
130. *Smoke Works*. https://smokeworks.org/
131. Safe Spot Overdose Hotline. https://safe-spot.me/
132. Matskiv G, Marshall T, Krieg O, Viste D, Ghosh SM. Virtual overdose monitoring services: a novel adjunctive harm reduction approach for addressing the overdose crisis. *CMAJ*. 2022;194(46):E1568–E1572.
133. Harding RW, Wagner KT, Fiuty P, Smith KP, Page K, Wagner KD. "It's called overamping": experiences of overdose among people who use methamphetamine. *Harm Reduct J*. 2022;19(1):4.
134. Mansoor M, McNeil R, Fleming T, et al. Characterizing stimulant overdose: a qualitative study on perceptions and experiences of "overamping." *Int J Drug Policy*. 2022;102: 103592.
135. Next Distro. *Overamping: Stimulant Overdose*. https://nextdistro.org/resources-collection/overamping-stimulant-overdose
136. DF Alliance. *Overdose Prevention Centers: State of the Law*. https://drugpolicy.org/wp-content/uploads/2024/04/DPA-OPC-Legal-Risk-Analysis-Updated-December-2024.pdf

137. Harocopos A, Gibson BE, Saha N, et al. First 2 months of operation at first publicly recognized overdose prevention centers in US. *JAMA Netw Open*. 2022;5(7):e2222149.
138. Potier C, Laprevote V, Dubois-Arber F, Cottencin O, Rolland B. Supervised injection services: what has been demonstrated? A systematic literature review. *Drug Alcohol Depend*. 2014;145:48–68.
139. Kral AH, Lambdin BH, Wenger LD, Davidson PJ. Evaluation of an unsanctioned safe consumption site in the United States. *N Engl J Med*. 2020;383(6):589–590.
140. Koehm K, Rosen JG, Yedinak Gray JL, Tardif J, Thompson E, Park JN. "Politics versus policy": qualitative insights on stigma and overdose prevention center policymaking in the United States. *Subst Use Addctn J*. 2024;45(4):682–689.
141. *United States v. Safehouse*. https://www.sciencedirect.com/science/article/pii/S0091743520300943
142. Kerr T, Stoltz JA, Tyndall M, et al. Impact of a medically supervised safer injection facility on community drug use patterns: a before and after study. *BMJ*. 2006;332(7535):220–222.
143. Kerr T, Tyndall MW, Zhang R, Lai C, Montaner JS, Wood E. Circumstances of first injection among illicit drug users accessing a medically supervised safer injection facility. *Am J Public Health*. 2007;97(7):1228–1230.
144. Geiger C, Smart R, Stein BD. Who receives naloxone from emergency medical services? Characteristics of calls and recent trends. *Subst Abus*. 2020;41(3):400–407.
145. Faul M, Lurie P, Kinsman JM, Dailey MW, Crabaugh C, Sasser SM. Multiple naloxone administrations among emergency medical service providers is increasing. *Prehosp Emerg Care*. 2017;21(4):411–419.
146. Hill LG, Zagorski CM, Loera LJ. Increasingly powerful opioid antagonists are not necessary. *Int J Drug Policy*. 2022;99:103457.
147. Lemen PM, Garrett DP, Thompson E, Aho M, Vasquez C, Park JN. High-dose naloxone formulations are not as essential as we thought. *Harm Reduct J*. 2024;21(1):93.
148. Moe J, Godwin J, Purssell R, et al. Naloxone dosing in the era of ultra-potent opioid overdoses: a systematic review. *CJEM*. 2020;22(2):178–186.
149. Payne ER, Stancliff S, Rowe K, Christie JA, Dailey MW. Comparison of administration of 8-milligram and 4-milligram intranasal naloxone by law enforcement during response to suspected opioid overdose—New York, March 2022–August 2023. *MMWR Morb Mortal Wkly Rep*. 2024;73(5):110–113.
150. TNDPH Law. *Legal Interventions to Reduce Overdose Mortality: Overdose Good Samaritan Laws*. https://www.networkforphl.org/wp-content/uploads/2024/11/Legal-Interventions-to-Reduce-Overdose-Mortality_Overdose-Good-Samaritan-Laws.pdf
151. Hamilton L, Davis CS, Kravitz-Wirtz N, Ponicki W, Cerda M. Good Samaritan laws and overdose mortality in the United States in the fentanyl era. *Int J Drug Policy*. 2021;97:103294.
152. TNDPH Law. *Naloxone Insurance Coverage Mandates*. https://www.networkforphl.org/wp-content/uploads/2023/05/Naloxone-Insurance-Coverage-Mandates.pdf
153. Next Distro. Naloxone. https://nextdistro.org/naloxone
154. Wallace B, van Roode T, Pagan F, Hore D, Pauly B. The potential impacts of community drug checking within the overdose crisis: qualitative study exploring the perspective of prospective service users. *BMC Public Health*. 2021;21(1):1156.
155. Sherman SG, Morales KB, Park JN, McKenzie M, Marshall BDL, Green TC. Acceptability of implementing community-based drug checking services for people who use drugs in three United States cities: Baltimore, Boston and Providence. *Int J Drug Policy*. 2019;68:46–53.
156. Reed MK, Borne E, Esteves Camacho T, Kelly M, Rising KL. Recommendations from people who use drugs in Philadelphia, PA about structuring point-of-care drug checking. *Harm Reduct J*. 2024;21(1):26.
157. Thompson E, Tardif J, Ujeneza M, et al. Pilot findings on the real-world performance of xylazine test strips for drug residue testing and the importance of secondary testing methods. *Drug Alcohol Depend Rep*. 2024;11:100241.
158. Gozdzialski L, Wallace B, Hore D. Point-of-care community drug checking technologies: an insider look at the scientific principles and practical considerations. *Harm Reduct J*. 2023;20(1):39.
159. Park JN, Sherman SG, Sigmund V, Breaud A, Martin K, Clarke WA. Validation of a lateral flow chromatographic immunoassay for the detection of fentanyl in drug samples. *Drug Alcohol Depend*. 2022;240:109610.
160. Ti L, Tobias S, Lysyshyn M, et al. Detecting fentanyl using point-of-care drug checking technologies: a validation study. *Drug Alcohol Depend*. 2020;212:108006.
161. Lieberman M, Badea A, Desnoyers C, Hayes K, Park JN. An urgent need for community lot testing of lateral flow fentanyl test strips marketed for harm reduction in Northern America. *Harm Reduct J*. 2024;21(1):115.
162. Lockwood TE, Vervoordt A, Lieberman M. High concentrations of illicit stimulants and cutting agents cause false positives on fentanyl test strips. *Harm Reduct J*. 2021;18(1):30.
163. Hayes KL, Lieberman M. Assessment of two brands of fentanyl test strips with 251 synthetic opioids reveals "blind spots" in detection capabilities. *Harm Reduct J*. 2023;20(1):175.
164. Krotulski AJ, Shinefeld J, Teixeira da Silva D, Logan BK. *Evaluation of Xylazine Test Strips (BTNX) for Drug Checking Purposes*. https://www.cfsre.org/images/content/reports/drug_checking/Evaluation_of_BTNX_Xylazine_Test_Strips_for_Drug_Checking_230322.pdf
165. Sisco E, Nestadt DF, Bloom MB, et al. Understanding sensitivity and cross-reactivity of xylazine lateral flow immunoassay test strips for drug checking applications. *Drug Test Anal*. 2024;16(9):942–947.
166. Mistler CB, Rosen AO, Eger W, Copenhaver MM, Shrestha R. Fentanyl test strip use and overdose history among individuals on medication for opioid use disorder. *Austin J Public Health Epidemiol*. 2021;8(5):1117.
167. Kutscher E, Barber Grossi M, LaPolla F, Lee JD. Fentanyl test strips for harm reduction: a scoping review. *J Addict Med*. 2024;18(4):373–380.
168. Reed MK, Roth AM, Tabb LP, Groves AK, Lankenau SE. "I probably got a minute": Perceptions of fentanyl test strip use among people who use stimulants. *Int J Drug Policy*. 2021; 92:103147.
169. Reed MK, Salcedo VJ, Guth A, Rising KL. "If I had them, I would use them every time": Perspectives on fentanyl test strip use from people who use drugs. *J Subst Abuse Treat*. 2022; 140:108790.
170. Allen ST, O'Rourke A, White RH, Sherman SG, Grieb SM. Perspectives on fentanyl test strip use among people who inject drugs in rural Appalachia. *Subst Use Misuse*. 2020;55(10):1594–1600.
171. Klaire S, Janssen RM, Olson K, et al. Take-home drug checking as a novel harm reduction strategy in British Columbia, Canada. *Int J Drug Policy*. 2022;106:103741.
172. Krieger MS, Goedel WC, Buxton JA, et al. Use of rapid fentanyl test strips among young adults who use drugs. *Int J Drug Policy*. 2018;61:52–58.
173. Goodman-Meza D, Arredondo J, Slim S, et al. Behavior change after fentanyl testing at a safe consumption space for women in Northern Mexico: a pilot study. *Int J Drug Policy*. 2022;106:103745.

174. Goldman JE, Waye KM, Periera KA, Krieger MS, Yedinak JL, Marshall BDL. Perspectives on rapid fentanyl test strips as a harm reduction practice among young adults who use drugs: a qualitative study. *Harm Reduct J.* 2019;16(1):3.
175. Oh H, Kim K, Miller D, Veloso D, Lin J, McFarland W. Fentanyl self-testing in a community-based sample of people who inject drugs, San Francisco. *Int J Drug Policy.* 2020;82:102787.
176. Karamouzian M, Dohoo C, Forsting S, McNeil R, Kerr T, Lysyshyn M. Evaluation of a fentanyl drug checking service for clients of a supervised injection facility, Vancouver, Canada. *Harm Reduct J.* 2018;15(1):46.
177. Quijano T, Crowell J, Eggert K, et al. Xylazine in the drug supply: emerging threats and lessons learned in areas with high levels of adulteration. *Int J Drug Policy.* 2023;120:104154.
178. Reed MK, Imperato NS, Bowles JM, Salcedo VJ, Guth A, Rising KL. Perspectives of people in Philadelphia who use fentanyl/heroin adulterated with the animal tranquilizer xylazine; Making a case for xylazine test strips. *Drug Alcohol Depend Rep.* 2022;4:100074.
179. Aronson ID, Ardouin-Guerrier MA, Baus JE, Bennett AS. Barriers to, and facilitators of, checking drugs for adulterants in the era of fentanyl and xylazine: qualitative study. *JMIR Form Res.* 2024;8:e56755.
180. U.S. Department of Justice Criminal Division Office of Professional Development and Training. *Drug Paraphernalia Federal Prosecution Manual.* https://www.ojp.gov/pdffiles1/Digitization/134764NCJRS.pdf
181. *Fentanyl Test Strip.* https://dancesafe.org/fentanyl/
182. *Fentanyl Test Strips.* https://www.lochnessmedical.com//product/fentanyl-test-strips
183. *Xylazine Test Strip.* https://dancesafe.org/xylazine-test-strips/
184. SAMHSA Administration. *Federal Grantees May Now Use Funds to Purchase Fentanyl Test Strips.* Published April 7, 2021. Accessed July 2, 2023. https://www.samhsa.gov/newsroom/press-announcements/202104070200
185. Adams A, Ferguson M, Greer AM, et al. Guideline development in harm reduction: considerations around the meaningful involvement of people who access services. *Drug Alcohol Depend Rep.* 2022;4:100086.
186. Green TC, Park JN, Gilbert M, et al. An assessment of the limits of detection, sensitivity and specificity of three devices for public health-based drug checking of fentanyl in street-acquired samples. *Int J Drug Policy.* 2020;77:102661.
187. Park JN, Tardif J, Thompson E, Rosen JG, Lira JAS, Green TC. A survey of North American drug checking services operating in 2022. *Int J Drug Policy.* 2023;121:104206.
188. UNC Street Drug Analysis Lab. *Public Health Drug Checking by Mail.* https://www.streetsafe.supply/
189. HRI Labs. Directory of North American Drug Checking Programs. 2024.
190. Stern SJ, D'Orazio JL, Work BD, Calcaterra SL, Thakrar AP. Point/counterpoint: Should full agonist opioid medications be offered to hospitalized patients for management of opioid withdrawal? *J Hosp Med.* 2024;19(4):339–343.
191. Morgan JR, Wang J, Barocas JA, et al. Opioid overdose and inpatient care for substance use disorder care in Massachusetts. *J Subst Abuse Treat.* 2020;112:42–48.
192. Pollini RA, Paquette CE, Drvar T, et al. A qualitative assessment of discharge against medical advice among patients hospitalized for injection-related bacterial infections in West Virginia. *Int J Drug Policy.* 2021;94:103206.
193. Ti L, Ti L. Leaving the hospital against medical advice among people who use illicit drugs: a systematic review. *Am J Public Health.* 2015;105(12):e53–e59.
194. Choi M, Kim H, Qian H, Palepu A. Readmission rates of patients discharged against medical advice: a matched cohort study. *PLoS One.* 2011;6(9):e24459.
195. Marks LR, Liang SY, Muthulingam D, et al. Evaluation of partial oral antibiotic treatment for persons who inject drugs and are hospitalized with invasive infections. *Clin Infect Dis.* 2020;71(10):e650–e656.
196. Kumar N. Burden of 30-day readmissions associated with discharge against medical advice among inpatients in the United States. *Am J Med.* 2019;132(6):708–717.e4.
197. Lewis S, Liang SY, Schwarz ES, et al. Patients with serious injection drug use-related infections who experience patient-directed discharges on oral antibiotics have high rates of antibiotic adherence but require multidisciplinary outpatient support for retention in care. *Open Forum Infect Dis.* 2022;9(2):ofab633.
198. Baddour LM, Weimer MB, Wurcel AG, et al. Management of infective endocarditis in people who inject drugs: a scientific statement from the American Heart Association. *Circulation.* 2022;146(14):e187–e201.
199. Shah R, Hendrickson S, Fanucchi L, Lofwall M, Platt T, Rhudy C. Utility of an integrated health system specialty pharmacy in provision of extended-release buprenorphine for patients with opioid use disorder. *Am J Health Syst Pharm.* 2023;80(1):e59–e66.
200. Thakarar K, Appa A, Abdul Mutakabbir JC, et al. Frame shift: focusing on harm reduction and shared decision making for people who use drugs hospitalized with infections. *Clin Infect Dis.* 2024;78(2):e12–e26.
201. Brooks HL, O'Brien DC, Salvalaggio G, Dong K, Hyshka E. Uptake into a bedside needle and syringe program for acute care inpatients who inject drugs. *Drug Alcohol Rev.* 2019;38(4):423–427.
202. Brooks HL, Speed KA, Dong K, et al. Perspectives of patients who inject drugs on a needle and syringe program at a large acute care hospital. *PLoS One.* 2024;19(2):e0297584.
203. Kosteniuk B, Salvalaggio G, McNeil R, et al. "You don't have to squirrel away in a staircase": Patient motivations for attending a novel supervised drug consumption service in acute care. *Int J Drug Policy.* 2021;96:103275.
204. Dong KA, Brouwer J, Johnston C, Hyshka E. Supervised consumption services for acute care hospital patients. *CMAJ.* 2020;192(18):E476–E479.
205. Dogherty E, Patterson C, Gagnon M, et al. Implementation of a nurse-led overdose prevention site in a hospital setting: lessons learned from St. Paul's Hospital, Vancouver, Canada. *Harm Reduct J.* 2022;19(1):13.
206. Buchheit BM, Crable EL, Lipson SK, Drainoni ML, Walley AY. "Opening the door to somebody who has a chance." The experiences and perceptions of public safety personnel towards a public restroom overdose prevention alarm system. *Int J Drug Policy.* 2021;88:103038.
207. Rioux W, Kilby K, Jones S, Joshi P, Vandenberg S, Ghosh SM. Perspectives of healthcare workers on the integration of overdose detection technologies in acute care settings. *Addict Sci Clin Pract.* 2024;19(1):4.
208. Fozouni L, Buchheit B, Walley AY, Testa M, Chatterjee A. Public restrooms and the opioid epidemic. *Subst Abus.* 2020; 41(4):432–436.
209. Lombardi AR, Arya R, Rosen JG, et al. Overdose detection technologies to reduce solitary overdose deaths: a literature review. *Int J Environ Res Public Health.* 2023;20(2):1230.
210. Harvey LH, Sliwinski SK, Flike K, et al. The integration of harm reduction services in the Veterans Health Administration (VHA): a qualitative analysis of barriers and facilitators. *J Addict Dis.* 2024;42(4):326–334.
211. Watts T, Bane C, Brandley J, Schmidt E, Tucker M. Nursing harm reduction education and care for people who use drugs or who engage in sex work. *Public Health Nurs.* 2023;40(5):762–765.

212. Smith KR, Shah NK, Adamczyk AL, Weinstein LC, Kelly EL. Harm reduction in undergraduate and graduate medical education: a systematic scoping review. *BMC Med Educ.* 2023;23(1):986.
213. Gugala E, Briggs O, Moczygemba LR, Brown CM, Hill LG. Opioid harm reduction: A scoping review of physician and system-level gaps in knowledge, education, and practice. *Subst Abus.* 2022;43(1):972–987.
214. Jawa R, Laks J, Saravanan N, Demers L, Wishik-Miller G. Physician trainees' compassion satisfaction, burnout, and self-efficacy when caring for people who inject drugs. *Subst Abus.* 2022;43(1):675–681.
215. Goff A, Lujan-Bear S, Titus H, Englander H. Integrating hospital-based harm reduction care-harnessing the nursing model. *Subst Use Addctn J.* 2024;45(2):307–313.
216. Ti L, Milloy MJ, Turje RB, Montaner J, Wood E, Kerr T. The impact of an HIV/AIDS adult integrated health program on leaving hospital against medical advice among HIV-positive people who use illicit drugs. *J Public Health (Oxf).* 2017;39(2):e33–e39.
217. Khan GK, Harvey L, Johnson S, et al. Integration of a community-based harm reduction program into a safety net hospital: a qualitative study. *Harm Reduct J.* 2022;19(1):35.

20

Care Transitions and Postacute Care for People With Substance Use Disorders

Michael A. Incze, Soraya Azari

"Hello? Are you the doctor?" The disembodied voice sounded thin through the speaker of our care manager's cell phone. A wave of relief washed over me. The voice belonged to Richard, a man in his mid-30s who had recently been hospitalized with vertebral osteomyelitis most likely resulting from injection drug use. Richard was scheduled to see us for hospital discharge follow-up in an integrated primary care and substance use disorder (SUD) treatment clinic a few miles from the hospital, but was nowhere to be found at the time of the appointment. After an hour and a half of dedicated outreach from our peer support specialist and nurse care manager, we had him on the telephone.

Richard received excellent care during his hospitalization, including a buprenorphine initiation to treat opioid use disorder (OUD) by the Addiction Consultation Service and a tailored antibiotic regimen of intravenous daptomycin chosen following a hypersensitivity reaction to first-line antibiotic treatment. At discharge, the hospital team prescribed a week's worth of buprenorphine, ensured a follow-up appointment was scheduled at our clinic, and placed a peripherally inserted central catheter (PICC) after arranging for home health to oversee ongoing antibiotic therapy.

The patient left the hospital, and the hospital team turned their attention to their new admissions. That's when things started to fall apart. Richard lived in a rural community about 45 minutes away from the hospital. The solitary home health agency that served the area made one visit before deciding that the patient's home was too unsanitary to continue providing services. Richard, left with a PICC and a small pile of daptomycin vials, was unsure how to administer his antibiotics, and had no one to contact for contingency planning. Plans for wound care and weekly blood draws to monitor the safety of his antibiotic were also suddenly up in the air.

Moreover, Richard was accustomed to a higher dose of buprenorphine than prescribed at hospital discharge and was using buprenorphine to treat acute pain in addition to opioid cravings. For these reasons, he had been using more buprenorphine than was prescribed. By the time we spoke to him, Richard had been out of his buprenorphine for 2 days and was experiencing significant pain and opioid withdrawal symptoms.

In addition to these significant treatment barriers, Richard lacked transportation to attend his scheduled clinic follow-up appointment. Richard did not have a car and relied on a small group of family and friends to help with travel when they were available. Taking public transit to our clinic was not an option from his rural town, and a cab ride was prohibitively expensive. He resigned himself to a return visit to the local emergency department before we finally reached him by telephone.

We were able to prevent that emergency department visit, but it took a concerted effort from our multidisciplinary team, including nursing, social work, peer support, and clinicians. We located a pharmacy near Richard's home that carried buprenorphine and prescribed a higher dose. We conferred with his infectious disease doctors about alternative antibiotic regimens that might be more conducive to Richard's current situation, but given the recent hypersensitivity reaction and the nature of the infection, they advised continuing the daptomycin. Our care managers arranged transportation support and scheduled appointments at our local infusion center. Our peer support specialists provided near-daily outreach to help with Richard with care navigation and OUD recovery support. Then, the day before Richard's first infusion appointment, we learned that his insurance was not accepted within our health care system.

It was Richard who informed us—the infusion center called him directly advising him to go elsewhere for his care after reviewing his insurance information. All his specialist follow-up visits and infusions would have to be cancelled and made anew within a different regional health care system. Our nurses and peer support specialists worked tirelessly to facilitate the transition without delaying essential medical care. We continued to provide OUD treatment and overarching medical care via telehealth while the patient sought to re-establish in a new system. Eventually, Richard was able to find a local physician who agreed to prescribe his buprenorphine and oversee his care in a new health care system. After experiencing some gaps in antibiotic treatment due to the infeasibility of ongoing intravenous treatments, Richard was switched to an oral alternative. We lost touch with Richard after that; his phone number abruptly stopped working, visits within his new health care system were not visible in our electronic health record, and other attempts to contact him were unsuccessful.

Stories like this are far too common among patients representing marginalized groups such as people with SUD. Medical, psychosocial, geographic, structural, and other factors synergize into formidable barriers to access continuity of care in the community after hospital discharge—barriers that are often faced by the patient alone while physically and emotionally depleted from a recent hospitalization. Typical models for hospital follow-up care involve scheduled appointments in brick-and-mortar clinics like ours, sometimes with a plethora of specialists. These models are ill equipped to overcome the barriers to care faced by many during care transitions, and patients often fall through the cracks. Diverse skills and expertise are needed to provide the intensive, holistic support required to ensure equitable access to treatment. It takes a village to care for patients during times of transition, when so many societal and systems-level factors are aligned against them.

As primary care and addiction medicine physicians, we have the great joy and privilege of helping patients recover their health and achieve their goals over time. But we also see how tenuous the bridge is between hospital and community care, even when excellent SUD care is provided in the hospital. Health care systems and payment systems must create stronger, more flexible, and more holistic supports for patients during transitions of care, informed by multidisciplinary wisdom and guided by patient priorities. Fortunately, growing leadership and expertise in addiction treatment across the spectrum of hospital-to-community care provides a strong foundation for innovation in this area. Through building stronger bridges across care settings, we promote access to care for all in need.

—Michael A. Incze

Key Points

- **Care transitions represent high-risk times for people with substance use disorders (SUDs) but also opportunities to engage people into long-term medical and SUD care. Careful planning around the time of discharge is necessary to facilitate care linkage and continuity of care.**
- **Treatment initiation for SUD in the hospital is central to strengthening linkage to care after hospital discharge. Titrating medications to an effective dose prior to discharge and ensuring continuity of SUD care in the community is necessary to facilitate treatment linkage and retention.**
- **Implementing hospital-based protocols that facilitate care linkage (eg, remote opioid treatment program enrollment) and partnerships with community treatment programs can strengthen care linkage around the time of hospital discharge.**
- **Clear communication with the patient and continuity clinicians is key to ensuring that a thorough and patient-centered care plan is realized after discharge. Contingency planning including low-barrier/walk-in options and telehealth can help strengthen care linkage and retention after discharge.**
- **Implementing interdisciplinary care transition supports for patients with SUD is feasible in most health care systems. Several models have shown early evidence of effectiveness.**

- **Understanding patient rights through the American Disabilities Act can help to support continuity of medication treatment of SUD at skilled nursing facilities and/or long-term care programs after hospital discharge.**
- **Developing a patient-centered contingency plan that is clearly documented in the hospital note can help to support continuity of care during patient-directed discharge.**

Transitions of care after a medical hospitalization represent a fundamental and challenging aspect of hospital-based substance use disorder (SUD) care. **Care transitions** are defined by Coleman as "the movement patients make between health care practitioners and settings as their condition and care needs change during the course of a chronic or acute illness."[1,2] Patients with SUD who are leaving the hospital after an acute illness may transition to a variety of care settings, ranging from subacute inpatient care at skilled nursing facilities (SNF) to vastly under-resourced environments for individuals who are undomiciled like shelters. Each patient's situation outside of the hospital is unique, and a significant challenge for hospital teams is anticipating barriers to ongoing care and creating a postdischarge care plan that supports patients as they transition their medical and SUD treatment to community settings.[3]

Patients with SUD face similar psychosocial barriers to successful care transitions as other vulnerable groups in addition to unique challenges related to a SUD diagnosis. Overarching factors complicating care transitions potentially include a lack of stable housing, inadequate transportation, insufficient means of communication (eg, internet, telephone), insurance limitations, pain and physical debilitation from recent acute illness, and lack of social supports.[4–6] Patients with SUD may also disproportionately experience stigma at community medical facilities, denial of evidence-based medical treatments, cravings and withdrawal symptoms, environmental triggers for substance use, and more.[7] Further, for individuals with opioid use disorder (OUD), reduced opioid tolerance from inconsistent access to opioids while hospitalized may increase the risk for overdose in the immediate postdischarge period, particularly if they are not treated with medications for OUD.[8–10]

Prior research has examined interventions to support posthospitalization care transitions for select medically and socially vulnerable groups, such as individuals with severe chronic medical illness (eg, congestive heart failure, chronic obstructive pulmonary disease [COPD]) and older adults.[11–15] Interventions include enhanced teaching prior to discharge,[16,17] postdischarge telephone outreach,[18,19] caregiver education,[11] and direct linkage to community programs.[13] Results of previous studies have been mixed. For example, a single-site randomized clinical trial (RCT) of a 3 month community-based care transition intervention for hospitalized patients with COPD demonstrated *increased* rates of hospitalization and emergency department (ED) usage without improving quality of life in the intervention group.[11] Conversely, a small RCT of a nurse-led hospital-to-community intervention for older adults undergoing open heart surgery demonstrated improved quality of life and reduced hospitalizations over 9 weeks postdischarge.[13] The discrepancy in these findings highlights the complexity of care transitions, where the target population, the care setting (eg, these trials were performed in the United States and Turkey, respectively), and underlying health conditions all play significant roles in determining the effectiveness of a given intervention. While some care transition models for common chronic medical diseases have shown promise in reducing hospital readmission and improving quality of life after hospital discharge, there is no definitive evidence from which to extrapolate models for patients with SUD. However, a small body of research has evaluated SUD-specific posthospitalization care transition interventions.[20–22] These models will be covered in detail later in the chapter.

The primary goal of this chapter is to help prepare hospital-based clinicians to promote safe, patient-centered, and successful care transitions for their patients with SUD. The paradigm of orchestrating successful posthospitalization care transitions for patients with SUD starts with hospital-based SUD interventions but must also include a vision that extends beyond the hospital walls. Optimally, diverse professional expertise, including social work, nursing, pharmacy, peer support, addiction specialty care, and partnerships with outpatient clinicians is included. Some fundamental aspects of SUD care transitions, such as offering initiation and stabilization of pharmacotherapy for SUD and harm reduction counseling prior to discharge, are covered in detail elsewhere in this book. This chapter provides in-depth considerations of best practices to support transitions of care among hospitalized patients with SUD, including ensuring continuity of SUD treatment when arranging postdischarge level of care (eg, subacute or skilled nursing facilities, home health care services), creating flexible and patient-centered follow-up plans (eg, transportation support, walk-in or telehealth options), and shared decision-making to facilitate contingency planning during patient-directed discharge events, historically described as "leaving against medical advice."[23]

Epidemiology and Barriers to Care Transitions

SUDs are highly prevalent among hospitalized patients. National estimates suggest that one in nine hospitalized patients has a SUD.[24] For the vast majority of these patients, there is an inevitable discharge event and transition to follow-up care. This amounts to thousands of care transition events for people with SUD every day. Despite how commonplace these events are, there are gaps in both research and implementation regarding how to best support patients with SUD during and after their departure from the hospital.

Observational studies demonstrate that the period immediately following hospitalization is one of elevated risk for both SUD-related and all-cause mortality. For example, among a cohort of hospitalized Oregon Medicaid patients with an OUD diagnosis, 7.8% died within a year following an index discharge event. Nearly 60% of these deaths were directly related to OUD, followed by cardiovascular and pulmonary causes.[10] In another single-site study, nearly one-third of a cohort of hospitalized patients with OUD, in addition to other substance use (ie, polysubstance use), died within a 5.5 year postdischarge observation window, with 53% of deaths attributable to overdose.[9] Patients with SUD often enter the posthospitalization period physically debilitated from their acute illness and faced with life-altering disruptions in community support and treatment (eg, missed methadone doses while hospitalized, stolen possessions, lost income, eviction). Additionally, people with SUD may experience cravings, withdrawal, and a lower opioid tolerance stemming from a period of reduced or absent exposure to substances while hospitalized. These factors can synergize to increase the risk of rehospitalization and death, underscoring the importance of intensive and multipronged supports in the immediate posthospitalization period.

Compounding the physiologic factors that place patients with SUD at high risk for adverse outcomes in the posthospitalization period are multifarious environmental barriers to accessing care. These barriers may be insurance related, including a lack of insurance access or underinsurance and coverage exclusions for medications to treat SUD. They may be geographic, such as a dearth of opioid treatment programs (OTP) providing methadone access, a particular barrier in the United States.[25] They may be policy driven, including policies that require daily in-person methadone dosing that potentially conflict with employment and parenting responsibilities. They may also include a lack of transportation access and unreliable communication methods (eg, internet and telephone access). Each of these factors impact access to follow-up care and increase risk for patients in the posthospitalization period.

Stigma and outright discrimination further impact care transitions among patients with SUD. SNF and long-term acute care hospital (LTACH) facilities have, at times, employed discriminatory policies toward patients with SUD, including refusal to continue medications for SUD treatment and outright denial of care on the grounds of a co-occurring SUD diagnosis.[26–31] While discriminatory policies at medical facilities against patients with well-controlled SUD (ie, not actively using) constitute a violation of the Americans with Disabilities Act (ADA), leveraging the ADA to improve practices at SNF and LTACHs has been a challenge across the United States.[26] This has profound implications for posthospitalization care transitions because limiting access to SNF and LTACH disproportionately impacts patients with the most acute and complex medical needs. Resources, education, and accountability measures directed toward empowering SNF and LTACH to provide high-quality SUD treatment integrated with medical care are needed. Compiling and sharing information pertaining to the rights of patients with SUD under the ADA can help prepare health care systems and clinicians to effectively advocate for their patients when faced with discrimination in community medical settings. Legal and educational resources to aid this process are discussed later in the chapter. Table 20.1 provides an overview of different levels of posthospitalization care available to patients after hospitalization.

Another systemic factor that impedes successful care transitions for patients with SUD is an increasingly siloed health care system. For example, while the hospitalist movement has led to a shortened length of hospital stay, stable and improved quality of care, and decreased costs in hospital systems compared to the traditional hospital care model, the expansion of the hospitalist movement also led to a greater division between hospital and outpatient care teams.[32] While there are benefits to specializing care in this way, they come at the cost of limiting clinical perspective to a discrete "slice" of the patient's care experience. This care "siloing" may affect care transitions specifically by slowing the development of care transition models that span care settings and integrate the perspectives of relevant experts (including people with lived and living SUD experience first and foremost) on both sides of the care transition spectrum. The impacts of this care gap are perhaps most acutely felt during unexpected patient-directed discharges, where follow-up arrangements must be made urgently, and when patients are at highest risk of negative outcomes, including death.[33] Developing models that iteratively solicit and leverage the expertise of key partners from diverse disciplines,

TABLE 20.1

Common Terms and Definitions

Term	Abbreviation	Definition/characteristics
Skilled nursing facility/ subacute rehabilitation center	SNF or SAR	Residential setting with 24-h nursing care, medication administration, physician oversight, and rehabilitation services. Can administer medications for substance use disorders, but cannot dispense methadone for OUD (ie, patients receiving methadone must be enrolled in a partnering opioid treatment program)
Home health care		Nursing, social work, and rehabilitation services provided in a patient's home temporarily after hospital discharge. Typically, a menu of health care services available including wound care, intravenous medication administration, bathing/meal preparation, and physical/occupational therapy.
Long-term acute care hospital	LTACH	Medical hospitals that are designed to provide prolonged acute care, usually over a duration of weeks. Because of their designation as a hospital, they can dispense methadone without a partnering opioid treatment program.
Opioid treatment program	OTP	Also known as "methadone clinics," these are federally licensed outpatients centers that provide methadone and other substance use disorder care. While these clinics often have embedded psychosocial services, there is typically no medical care offered.
Medical respite	N/A	A short-term postacute care facility typically designed to facilitate ongoing medical and/or SUD treatment for people experiencing homelessness who are too ill or frail to heal in the community but not ill enough to remain in the hospital.
Residential substance use treatment program/ intensive residential treatment	IRT	Substance use disorder treatment programs that offer temporary housing along with provision of intensive behavioral treatments for substance use disorders (eg, groups, individual counseling). There is wide variability between programs. Many do not offer certain types of medical care such as intravenous antibiotics. Some do not allow medications to treat substance use disorders. Corresponds to ASAM Level of Care 3.5 or 3.7.

care settings, and life experiences pertaining to care transitions is key to developing effective, comprehensive, and acceptable models of care.

Care transitions are exceedingly common and high-risk events for people with SUD. Multiple physiologic and environmental factors may synergize to increase the risk of harm and even death in the posthospitalization period. Fortunately, there are several emerging models to support patients with SUD during care transitions.[20,21] Next, we review the evidence on existing care transition models for hospitalized patients with SUD, followed by a summary of best practices and clinical guidance.

Evidence for and Models of SUD-Specific Care Transitions

By definition, posthospitalization care transitions span multiple care domains. These may include the hospital, community-based clinics, telehealth, home care, homeless health care, SNF/LTACH, carceral settings, and more. Innovative care models exist within several of these settings to improve care transitions for patients with SUD.[21,20,34] Broadly speaking, existing interventions may be hospital based, embedded in community settings, designed specifically to intervene during the transition from hospital to outpatient care, or encompass any combination of the three. Many of these care models were developed by local champions in response to perceived clinical need while utilizing available resources. Most of the supporting evidence comes from single-site studies and program evaluations. Taken together, research provides an important bedrock of evidence to guide program innovation for health care systems and clinicians, as well as future larger-scale studies. Figure 20.1 summarizes several current care transition models for individuals with SUD.

Setting	Model	Core Components	Core Activities	Citations
Inpatient	***Addiction Consultation Teams***	Addiction specialists, care managers, social workers, peer navigators, pharmacists, nurses	Initiate medications for SUD, facilitate connection to post-discharge care, provide support to hospital medical teams, lead institutional SUD care	36–45, 111
Inpatient	***Inpatient Protocol Development and Implementation***	Adaptable to local resources. Often hospitalist-led and intended for broad adoption by hospital care teams.	Typically a focused goal, such as improving treatment initiation for alcohol use disorder in the hospital, improving buprenorphine initiation by hospital teams, or improving referral processes to post-discharge care.	50–53, 114, 116, 122, 142, 143
Inpatient	***SBIRT***	Adaptable to local resources. A dedicated team often led by nursing, peer support specialists, or pharmacists	Screen for unhealthy substance use/SUD, conduct a brief intervention and assessment, and orchestrate a referral to post-discharge SUD care.	47–48
Transitional	***Transitional Care Management***	Nurse care manager or social worker; may be embedded into addiction consult teams	Meet patients in the hospital, then provide outreach and ongoing support after discharge to facilitate linkage to SUD and medical care.	18, 22, 46, 69–76
Transitional	***Care Transition Models for SNF and LTACH***	Requires coordination between inpatient social work, SNF/LTACH staff, +/–community SUD treatment programs	Careful coordination to ensure that SNF/LTACH are able to provide SUD treatment and needed medical care after discharge. May require further action to link to community care after SNF/LTACH discharge.	82–84
Transitional	***Peer Navigation***	People with lived/living experience with SUD; may be embedded into addiction consult teams	Meet patients in the hospital, then provide outreach and ongoing support after discharge to facilitate linkage to SUD and medical care.	46, 71–74, 79–80
Transitional	***Models for People Experiencing Homelessness***	Adaptable to local resources. May include physicians, pharmacists, social workers, etc	Ensure discharge protocols that address barriers such as housing, ID requirements, employment/insurance, and transportation. Prioritize flexible follow-up options with contingency planning	53, 54, 56, 58, 61, 67, 68, 83
Outpatient	***Bridge Clinic***	Addiction specialists, nurses, medical assistants, care managers	Outpatient clinic that provides low-barrier access (eg, walk-in availability, telehealth access) to continuity of SUD and medical care.	55–66, 86, 110
Outpatient	***In-reach Models***	Outpatient clinicians, social workers, care managers, or peer navigators	Outpatient-based care teams meet hospitalized patients with SUD in the hospital and provide outreach after discharge to facilitate linkage to follow-up care.	49, 67
Outpatient	***Post-discharge Outreach***	Adaptable to local resources. May include physicians, pharmacists, social workers, etc	Identify hospitalized patients with SUD and provide outreach after discharge to facilitate connection to care and interim treatment access.	68–70

Figure 20.1: Select posthospitalization care transition models focused on individuals with SUD.

Addiction Consultation Teams

Effective care transitions uniformly start in the realm of hospital-based SUD care. Careful discharge planning, ensuring adequate medication treatment if desired, harm-reduction counseling, shared decision-making, and thorough patient-centered communication are all hospital-based interventions that are essential elements of effective care transitions. Several hospital-based SUD treatment models have been developed to improve care in these domains. Most notably, the rise of addiction consultation teams has dramatically impacted predischarge SUD care and care transitions across North America.[6,35–44] Covered in detail in Chapter 4, addiction consultation teams typically include multidisciplinary expertise and focus on engaging individuals with SUD in the hospital, optimizing SUD care during the hospitalization, and facilitating linkage to community-based SUD care after hospital discharge. Addiction consultation teams are diverse in composition and activities, with some offering ongoing postdischarge support through interventions like peer navigation,[45] care management,[22] and partnering with low-barrier outpatient clinics.[41] Addiction consultation teams also play a key care transition role through the initiation and titration of medications to treat SUD in the hospital and provision of an adequate supply of medication to facilitate transitions to follow-up care at the time of hospital discharge.

Hospital-based Protocol Development and Implementation

For hospitals and health care systems which do not currently have the resources or staff to implement an addiction consultation team, developing protocols around SUD screening, counseling, treatment initiation, and discharge care planning using existing infrastructure can be a feasible and adaptable intervention to improve SUD care transitions and hospital-based SUD care more broadly.

For example, Screening, Brief Intervention, and Referral to Treatment (SBIRT) is an established protocol that can be implemented in a variety of general medical settings, including hospitals. In this model, a team of health care professionals (eg, licensed vocational nurses, social workers, peer navigators) screens hospitalized patients for unhealthy substance use and/or SUD, intervenes using techniques like motivational interviewing to explore interest in treatment, then orchestrates a referral to SUD care after hospital discharge for interested individuals. While a 2015 meta-analysis of RCTs found that SBIRT models did not lead to improved linkage to care,[46] programs administered in hospital settings and/or combined with other care transition models may be more effective.[47,48]

Other hospital-based protocols seek to improve care transitions by facilitating hospital initiation of medications for SUD[49–52] and enhancing discharge planning using existing staff and care teams[52] in diverse community and academic hospitals. Evidence for these interventions is limited; however, they show promise toward improved care linkage and reduced hospital readmissions. While the results of these program evaluations and quality improvement initiatives should be confirmed through clinical trials, current evidence and expert consensus suggest that health care systems should feel empowered to design and implement systems to improve SUD care transitions using locally available resources.[34,53]

Outpatient Clinics

In addition to hospital-based models, there are a number of community-based strategies designed to support patients with SUD during posthospitalization care transitions. Flexibility, outreach, and interdisciplinary care are each hallmarks of existing outpatient-based models. For example, outpatient "bridge clinics" represent a growing outpatient care model to facilitate care transitions from acute care settings such as the hospital or the ED to the outpatient setting.[54] Bridge clinics are community-based clinics that serve as flexible and low-barrier entry points to SUD treatment. While clinic models vary, bridge clinics often accommodate walk-in appointments, offer telehealth care, provide both medical and SUD treatment, and are staffed by interdisciplinary teams that can provide intensive support and wrap-around services.[54–64] The ultimate goal is typically facilitating linkage to long-term community medical and SUD treatment once patients are stable from a medical, SUD, and psychosocial perspective. Evidence suggests that bridge clinics effectively improve linkage to and retention in SUD care after acute care utilization,[54,57,59,60,65] as well as serving as stigma-free hubs for patients to receive harm-reduction services and medical care.[58,63]

Hospital In-Reach Models

Similar to bridge clinics, "in-reach" into hospitals from partnering outpatient clinics is an emerging community-based model to improve care transitions for people with SUD. In this model, a partnering clinic, SUD treatment program (eg, OTP), or community organization (eg, local peer support organizations) is consulted by the hospital-based clinician while a patient is hospitalized. The outpatient entity sends representatives into the hospital to meet with the patient, develop rapport, schedule follow-up appointments, and exchange contact information to facilitate ongoing communication to support successful SUD treatment linkage posthospital discharge. After the patient leaves the hospital, the in-reach team continues to follow the patient in the community and support linkage to, and retention in, care at their clinic or through other community-based options. While research on this model is nascent, at least two studies demonstrated improved linkage to community care following hospitalization.[48,66]

With any medical treatment decision and care transition plan, it is important to ensure that patients can exercise autonomy to make decisions about their preferred follow-up destination, rather than feeling forced to follow-up at a specific clinic. Furthermore, implementation factors including finding a partnering outpatient clinic who can facilitate flexible scheduling, as well as training and supporting staff to work across care settings, require more resources than some other models.

Postdischarge Outreach

Postdischarge outreach is another important community-based model to support care transitions, which can take many forms. These models involve teams that specialize in identifying people with SUD who have recently discharged from the hospital and providing outreach to support linkage to community care. Some of these models are relatively low intensity, such as a program that enlisted clinical pharmacists within the Veterans Health Administration to conduct phone outreach to recently discharged patients with SUD.[67] Other programs involve interdisciplinary teams that conduct street outreach to locate and provide clinical care on-site to recently hospitalized patients, including those with complex medical problems such as serious injection drug use-related infections.[68,69] While these programs are typically outpatient-based, close collaboration with hospital teams is integral to their function through identification of patients who might be in greatest need of additional support after discharge. In locations where these programs are available, hospital-based clinicians play an important role in identifying patients who are most in need of intensive postdischarge follow-up for referral.

Transitional Care Management

Another subset of SUD care transition models is designed specifically to help patients during the period following hospital discharge as they navigate linkage to community care. These models include peer navigation (ie, individuals with lived or living experience with SUD),[45,70–73] transitional care management (eg, nurses or social workers),[22] and leveraging community health workers/health promotion advocates (ie, community members who provide support with care linkage and who may or may not have personal experience with SUD).[74,75] These interventions may operate as stand-alone programs or be integrated into other care models such as addiction consultation teams or partnering outpatient clinics. They may also leverage partnerships with community organizations or utilize staff hired by health care systems to fill these roles depending on local resources. The breadth of disciplines and backgrounds that can serve in these roles makes this type of transition model highly adaptable to different care settings, including rural environments.[75–78] Furthermore, results from single-site clinical studies and program evaluations consistently demonstrate effectiveness in linkage to community treatment after acute care utilization.[45,70–72,79,80] For example, an RCT of 400 hospitalized adults with SUD demonstrated that integrating postdischarge transitional care management into an addiction consultation team model improved linkage to community SUD treatment and reduced 30-day hospital readmissions compared to addiction consultation team care alone.[22]

Care Transition Models for SNF and LTACH

In between community and medical hospital levels of care are inpatient facilities such as SNF, LTACH, and residential SUD treatment facilities (ie, American Society of Addiction Medicine [ASAM] Level of Care 3.1, 3.5, or 3.7). Integrating comprehensive medical and SUD care into these posthospitalization destinations is an important model to support care transitions. Consolidating postdischarge medical and SUD treatment under one care team can improve efficiency, reduce communication errors, strengthen care coordination, and add convenience for patients and their loved ones. Historically, barriers limited integration of SUD and medical care at postacute care facilities[26,29–31]; however, innovative medical and SUD treatment models address these obstacles. For example, hospital-based groups in Oregon and Utah, respectively, implemented programs for patients to receive ongoing parenteral antibiotics, which are typically administered in the hospital setting for people with SUD, at residential SUD treatment programs. Administration of parental antibiotics at a residential SUD treatment program facilitates a hospital discharge (with associated cost savings) to a setting that provides *both* medical treatment for the infection and comprehensive psychosocial SUD treatment.[81,82] Based in part on the success of these clinical innovations, the 4th Edition of the ASAM Criteria recommends that Level 3.7 (eg, medically managed residential level of care) SUD treatment facilities offer basic postacute medical care, including continuation of parenteral antibiotics.[83,84]

Care Transition Models for People Experiencing Homelessness

Individuals who are experiencing homelessness or other forms of social instability face especially profound barriers to receiving follow-up medical and SUD care in traditional primary care settings, such as scheduled appointment times, insurance requirements, and geographic accessibility. To address this care gap, more counties are innovating care systems that flex to the needs of vulnerable patients. "Low-barrier" or "low-threshold" primary care and SUD treatment clinics are growing in number. In general, these clinics have drop-in hours, will see patients regardless of insurance status, and employ clinicians who have expertise in SUD care.[54,55,57,59,62,85] Some programs are co-located within harm-reduction centers, while others provide street-level outreach and care, including direct outreach to tents, encampments, and shelters.[68,69]

For people experiencing homelessness with more complex medical needs, arranging for temporary supportive shelter or medical respite is an evidence-based and cost-effective intervention.[86,87] Medical respites are a form of congregate shelter, but with on-site medical personnel to help with medication adherence, transportation to follow-up appointments, and applying for entitlements. Further investment by health care systems and state and local governments are needed to make this resource more widely available to patients.

Models That Facilitate Postdischarge Medical Care for People With SUD

While not specifically related to care transitions models, there is emerging evidence on various treatment modalities that have great relevance to the postdischarge care of hospitalized individuals with SUD. For example, research on switching from intravenous to oral antibiotics at discharge for infections such as bacteremia, infective endocarditis, and osteomyelitis that disproportionately affect people with SUD has challenged longstanding paradigms related to infectious disease management.[88–97] While landmark trials in this area had stringent selection criteria that may not be generalizable to all people with SUD (eg, excluding right-sided endocarditis),[97] they provide clinicians and patients with important oral antibiotic options for methicillin-susceptible and methicillin-resistant *Staphylococcus aureus* infections during events like unexpected patient-directed discharge to continue treatment while linking to community care. An American Heart Association (AHA) Scientific Statement provides specific antibiotic treatment recommendations for injection-related endocarditis while highlighting evidence to support step down from intravenous to oral antibiotic therapy as being superior to incomplete intravenous antibiotic treatment with lower all-cause readmissions.[92,98] Emerging research on long-acting injectable lipoglycopeptides (dalbavancin and oritavancin) represent another promising development to facilitate effective antimicrobial coverage during posthospitalization transitions to community care.[99–108] Home and infusion center administration of lipoglycopeptides has been used in the treatment of infective endocarditis with clinical success. To date, there are no clinical trial data to support lipoglycopeptides to treat infective endocarditis, but their use may be individualized with input from the infectious disease team and the patient.[92]

Taken in sum, there is a growing body of research to guide clinical practice related to care transitions for people with SUD. This includes evaluations of diverse care transitions models as well as specific interventions (eg, tailored antibiotic strategies) to improve care for people with SUD around hospital discharge. At least two studies have asked panels of interdisciplinary experts to evaluate a variety of posthospitalization care transition interventions for patients with SUD according to evidence and personal experience, and there has been a consensus of support for all approaches.[34,53] This implies that health care systems can choose from a menu of different care transition models based on local resources and likely improve care in the near term for people with SUD compared to the status quo. Clinical research on the effectiveness and implementation of various care transition models will undoubtedly lead to stronger and more nuanced guidance regarding a hierarchy of different approaches in the future.

Clinical Guidance for SUD Care Transitions

Because all posthospitalization care transitions begin in the hospital setting, general medical inpatient clinicians, hospitalists, and other inpatient care team members including social workers, pharmacists, and nurses all play crucial roles in shaping patients' postdischarge care experience. There are several best practices that hospitalists can employ to improve care for patients around the time of discharge (Figure 20.2). Many of these are rooted in basic tenets of patient-centered care, such as clear communication, proactive linkage to follow-up care, and shared decision-making. In other cases, there are specific strategies focused on linkage to SUD care, such as leveraging flexibilities in methadone policy (eg, federal rules that permit dispensing up to 3 days of methadone to a patient at discharge)[109] and providing harm-reduction counseling and supplies (eg, Safersubstanceuse.org[110]) at hospital discharge as permitted by local laws and ordinances.

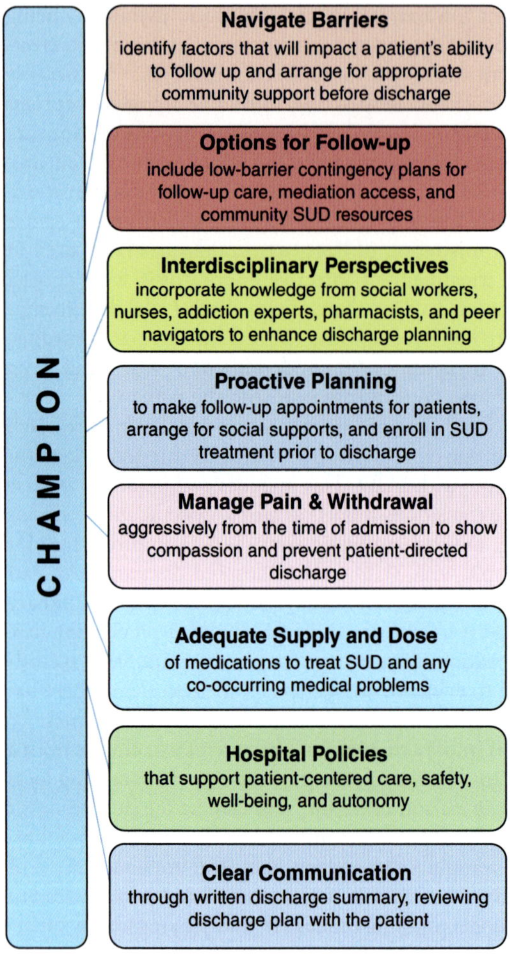

Figure 20.2: CHAMPION model of best practices for hospital teams related to posthospitalization care transitions.

Prior to Discharge

One pillar of effective discharge planning in the hospital setting is clearly communicating and facilitating a mutually agreed-upon discharge plan. This includes thoroughly reviewing with the patient new medications, upcoming appointments, and any other counseling related to changes in health status and SUD treatment, identifying factors that may affect safety, healing, SUD management, and following through with a care plan after discharge. Hospitalists are uniquely positioned to lead these conversations with patients given their overarching knowledge of the postdischarge treatment plan. Optimally, interdisciplinary care team members such as pharmacists, physical therapists, addiction specialists, and social workers each incorporate their expertise related to specific medical, psychosocial, SUD-related, and functional discharge needs either by directly counseling the patient or through coordinating with the primary hospital care team. One cannot overstate the importance of discharge planning conversations between patients and their medical teams, which can elicit key preferences, questions, and barriers to postdischarge care prior to patients leaving the hospital. They can also provide an opportunity to compromise on parts of the discharge plan where there may not be complete agreement, such as timing of discharge and discharge medications.

Once a clear plan has been created and barriers to follow-up care have been identified, hospital teams can facilitate individualized interventions to strengthen postdischarge care transitions. For example, social workers may be able to access programs that provide prepaid cell phones at discharge to patients without telephone access.[111] Many insurance plans include a benefit for transportation to medical appointments, which can be arranged by hospital-based social workers or care managers. Social workers can also offer information about local resources for shelters or discounted hotels for patients who lack stable housing. Some hospitals have used or donated clothes that they provide patients who may lack sufficiently warm clothes for winter weather. Connecting patients to home health, adaptive transportation resources, insurance linkage, supportive housing, residential SUD treatment, peer navigation, and/or community agencies are other interventions that may be prompted by identifying factors affecting patients' respective abilities to safely recover from illness and access ongoing medical and SUD after discharge.

Another facet of care transition management that falls within the purview of hospital care teams is connection to continuity of medical and SUD care after hospital discharge. Hospitalists should ask their patients early in the course of hospitalization about primary care access and insurance status, with subsequent consultation of social work, case management, and/or eligibility workers for assistance as needed. Some patients can identify a continuity clinic that they attend, but many will not. Traditional primary care practices, either in private practice, federally qualified health centers (FQHCs), academic medical centers, or tribal clinics, usually require patients to be enrolled before making a follow-up appointment. Some centers may be accepting new patients. Available clinics can be searched by zip code (https://findahealthcenter.hrsa.gov/). Clinic access may be contingent on insurance status. For patients that may be eligible for Medicaid, or have lapsed insurance, the person may be required to re-present at the local Medicaid field office (https://www.medicaid.gov/about-us/contact-us/index.html). States that did not expand Medicaid through the Affordable

Care Act may have a network of free or sliding-scale clinics that peers, case managers, and/or social workers will have expertise in accessing.

It bears special mention that immigration status may have especially profound impacts on a patient's ability to access community care.[112] Working with social workers in the hospital, who can engage community organizations on behalf of patients before discharge, is crucial to ensuring adequate support and access to treatment in the posthospitalization period.

Qualitative research has demonstrated that patients with SUD value the hospital care teams "taking the first step" with them to proactively schedule follow-up appointments, orchestrate warm hand offs to community supports, communicate with outpatient clinicians in primary care and SUD treatment facilities, and provide material support to help patients connect to continuity of care in the outpatient setting. These proactive efforts are generally more effective than passive efforts by hospital-based teams such as providing patients with pamphlets or handouts.

At the Time of Discharge

When the patient is medically cleared to discharge from the hospital, the patient's discharging nurse should review the posthospitalization follow-up plan documented on a printed after visit summary with the patient. This includes describing the reason for the patient's hospitalization, reviewing any procedures or imaging the patient had during their hospitalization, highlighting medication changes, upcoming appointments, and offering to answer any remaining questions the patient may have. This predischarge step is an important strategy to ensure that no parts of the care plan are overlooked or poorly understood by the patient. Optimally, the written discharge instructions should be in the patient's native language and should include contingency planning if unexpected circumstances arise that interrupt the care transition plan. Specific to SUD treatment, this may include a list of local walk-in clinics, low-barrier SUD treatment programs, and community-based bridge clinics where available.[54,59,61,62,85] A hospital, clinic, or clinician phone number should be included in the after-visit summary to contact members of the care team if there are further questions, unanticipated complications with follow-up care, or other discharge-related issues. Patient contact information and emergency contact information should be updated in the medical record providing that the patient is amenable to sharing that information.

Specific considerations are warranted for patients who are experiencing homelessness at discharge. These include providing a paper copy of their discharge summary and discharge medications in bottles, if possible. The discharge summary should include a description of current medical problems, a summary of the inpatient treatment course, a current medication list, a list of all follow-up appointments, and a clearly demarcated list of all necessary action items to facilitate comprehensive follow-up care. If medication dispensing is not available, medications can be sent to an external pharmacy of the patient's choosing, but a member of the pharmacy team should confirm that the patient has acceptable payment (eg, insurance coverage) for the medication. Some pharmacies will require a patient to present an identification card to pick up controlled medications such as buprenorphine. If the patient does not have an identification card, the medical team can call the pharmacy to preemptively inform them and request permission to dispense.

Best Practices Related to Medication Treatment for SUD

Ensuring all patients with SUD are offered appropriate medication-based treatment that has been titrated to an effective dose prior to leaving the hospital is critical to ensuring a safe and effective transition to community-based SUD care. Patients should be prescribed an adequate supply of medications such as buprenorphine, acamprosate, and naltrexone at discharge to last at minimum until their scheduled follow-up appointment. All patients with opioid or stimulant use disorder should be provided with naloxone and drug checking materials such as fentanyl testing strips at discharge as permitted by local laws. Whenever possible, these medications and supplies should be brought to the patient's bedside prior to leaving the hospital. Delivering these medications to the bedside both provides an opportunity for patient counseling regarding their use and circumvents any potential problems that patients may encounter picking medications up at external pharmacies, such as insurance coverage problems, pharmacy supply chain issues, and identification requirements.

Initiating long-acting injectable buprenorphine or naltrexone prior to hospital discharge is an emerging strategy that holds promise to improve consistent SUD medication access during transitions from acute care to community settings.[113] While there have traditionally been insurance-related, clinical, and administrative barriers to administering long-acting injectable medications for SUD in the hospital, several innovative programs have engineered workflows to facilitate the practice. These include developing in-hospital initiation protocols for injectable buprenorphine utilizing both low-dose sublingual and "direct-to-inject" approaches tailored to avoid precipitated withdrawal.[114] They also include protocols designed to circumvent insurance coverage restrictions on in-hospital administration of long-acting injectable buprenorphine through partnerships with outpatient pharmacies who are capable of delivering the medication to hospital pharmacies,[114,115] as well as through partnerships with insurers themselves.[116] A growing evidence base has demonstrated similar protocols for facilitating the administration of extended-release naltrexone in hospital settings.[117–120] By modeling workflows on these published examples, many hospitals can integrate long-acting injectable medications for SUD into inpatient care.

Facilitating Methadone Access During Care Transitions

Because community methadone treatment for OUD is currently restricted to highly regulated OTP settings, posthospitalization care transitions for individuals taking methadone in the United States are often imbued with an extra level of complexity. Fortunately, there are several ways that hospitalists can make transitions from hospital to community methadone treatment stronger and easier for patients. For example, in March 2022, the Drug Enforcement Administration (DEA) created an exception to 21 CFR 1306.07(b), allowing hospitals to dispense up to a 72-hour supply of methadone to patients at discharge to continue treatment during care transitions.[121] This flexibility is especially important given that OTPs are commonly closed on weekends and/or offer limited daily opportunities for new intakes, which can delay establishing follow-up care. Hospitals are increasingly leveraging the "72 hour rule" to ensure continuity of OUD treatment while patients are awaiting intake at a community OTP after discharge (see Chapter 3 for more information). Importantly, federal law does not currently allow methadone to be prescribed for OUD or dispensed from an outpatient pharmacy; rather, it must be dispensed directly to the patient from the hospital (ie, inpatient) pharmacy prior to discharge. Working with hospital pharmacy leadership to implement methadone dispensing at discharge as allowed by state laws can greatly improve transitions to community-based methadone treatment, especially if patients are discharged close to the weekend or holidays when many OTPs are closed to new enrollments. Developing partnerships with local OTPs and communicating with them directly about patients who are transitioning from the hospital to their care is another way to strengthen care transitions for patients. Federal law now allows for remote OTP enrollment, which can be conducted while patients are admitted to the hospital and further strengthen linkage to postdischarge methadone treatment.[6,122]

For hospitalists, there are several important considerations to discuss together with patients taking methadone before discharge. If the patient is a new enrollee to the OTP, they will often be required to present a form of ID during their intake process. Several forms of ID may be accepted, including a hospital ID bracelet, jail ID bracelet, a photo of their ID, a hospital face sheet, or a public benefit card. The OTP will need to know the timing and strength of the last dose of methadone, which can be communicated through a "Last Dose Letter" given to the patient while hospitalized and through a telephone "warm hand-off" from the inpatient team to the OTP. There is no maximum hospital dose for methadone and OTPs can accept patients who are already stabilized on methadone.

OTP intake will need to be arranged for patients who have newly initiated methadone during hospitalization. Prior to discharge, a team member should call to inquire if the OTP is accepting new patients for intake and set up the intake process. Recent updates to federal regulations may allow the OTPs to accept the hospital history and physical in their intake process, which can greatly facilitate the speed of the admission. It will be helpful for the hospital to establish agreed-upon processes to most effectively collaborate with local OTPs and understand their admission criteria and intake process. Most OTPs, for instance, will need lab work such as HIV screening and hepatitis screening and may want to have a screening electrocardiogram. If these labs and tests can be obtained in the hospital and shared with the OTP, it can greatly facilitate OTP admission (Table 20.2).

Due to changes in federal regulations, OTP providers have increased flexibility in granting take-home methadone bottles to patients, which means that if a patient is recuperating from illness, the hospital medical team can advocate via letter for the patient to receive early take-home methadone doses to facilitate their physical recovery.[123] Pregnant people can also more easily receive split dosing of methadone with new federal regulations.

Patients who present to the hospital already on methadone and are continued on it after hospital admission should be easily able to return to their OTPs within 30 days. If the patient has been hospitalized longer than 30 days, they may need to be fully readmitted to the OTP. A warm hard off such as a phone call or "Last Dose Letter" can facilitate a seamless transition back to the OTP for the patient. If the patient is provided new medications that may affect the patient's methadone dose, this would also be important to share.

TABLE 20.2

Common Criteria for Opioid Treatment Program Admission for Methadone Care

Age and identification requirements

- Age ≥18 y
- Age <18 y may be admitted to an OTP with written consent of a parent, legal guardian, or responsible adult designed by the relevant State authority: see 42 CFR § 8.12(e)(2)
- A picture ID is required in some states and by several OTPs to obtain methadone treatment, though this does not have to be state issued.
  - Some states allow any documentation with the patient's name or photo (ie, a hospital bracelet + face sheet with a photo may suffice in some OTPs)
- Assisting the patient with clarifying these requirements locally and facilitating the acquisition of necessary identification can be started during the hospitalization

Criteria for OTP Admission[a]

- Meets diagnostic criteria for moderate to severe OUD; or
- Has active, moderate to severe OUD or OUD in remission; or
- Is at high risk for recurrence of use or overdose
- Clinician ensures patient provides informed consent to treatment after the clinician outlines the relevant factors concerning use of MOUD
  - [a]A 1-y history of OUD is no longer required by federal regulations for enrollment, but each state differs and should be discussed with the local OTP

Medical admission process

- Screening examination (can be completed by <u>any</u> licensed clinician)
  - Done to determine if the patient meets the criteria for OTP admission and if there are contraindications to receipt of medications for OUD (MOUD).
  - Patients can receive MOUD immediately following the screening examination.
  - If a non–OTP-affiliated clinician completes this exam (ie, a hospital-based clinician), the patient must present to the OTP within 7 d for the full OTP admission
  - Screening exam should include:
    - Substances used and severity (mild, moderate, severe) (ie, OUD, severe)
    - Selected MOUD, rationale, and titration plan
    - Co-occurring medical/psychiatric conditions requiring care coordination (ie, syphilis)
    - Cardiac conditions, family history of sudden cardiac death
    - Urine toxicology results and treatment plan
    - Preventive care planning
    - Overdose education, naloxone
    - Patient education about health conditions and potential complications with MOUD
- Full history, psychosocial assessment, and examination (must be completed by an OTP-affiliated clinician or an authorized health care professional under the supervision of an OTP physician)
  - In-depth history and physical exam that must be completed within 14 d of the patient's OTP admission
  - Laboratory studies must be completed within 30 d of the OTP admission
  - Must include a care plan that addresses the patient's goals and actions for the patient to meet these goals
  - Must Include the recommended frequency of care to be provided to the patient

Laboratory testing

- Recommended studies include HIV, hepatitis B and C, syphilis, tuberculosis, pregnancy, comprehensive metabolic panel, comprehensive blood count, and an electrocardiogram
- If done in the hospital, fax the test results to the OTP and ensure that there is a plan and accurate contact information to follow-up test results requiring action
- Ultimately, laboratory testing is determined by OTP clinicians informed by their history and physical examination

What a hospital-based clinician can do to facilitate an OTP intake

- Partner with local OTPs to identify a point of contact, an email address, and a fax number to send completed in-hospital exams and laboratory studies
- Clarify the OTP's ID requirements and provide any helpful documents to the patient that may meet the ID requirement
- Clarify the OTP's dosing and intake hours
  - Create an in-hospital program[146] to dispense (not prescribe) up to 72-h of methadone to support the patient's hospital to OTP linkage; refer to 21 CFR §1306.07(b)

Substance Abuse and Mental Health Services Administration. Federal Guidelines for Opioid Treatment Programs. HHS Publication No. PEP24-02-011. Rockville, MD: Substance Abuse and Mental Health Services Administration, 2024.

Medications for SUD Treatment and Postacute Care Facilities

Fortunately, most medications used to treat SUD can be easily prescribed at hospital discharge and continued in the postacute facility setting, though it is important to ensure that the postacute facility is accepting of the medication and has it on their formulary. Buprenorphine, for example, can be prescribed without any restrictions, but some postacute facilities may not accept patients on this medication or may not have it on their formulary. Use of extended-release injectable buprenorphine may be helpful in those types of situations because it can be given prior to hospital discharge and lasts up to 30 days.

Unfortunately, methadone treatment in the postacute setting can be quite complicated due to the federal regulations restricting its use. When a hospitalized patient on methadone for OUD is referred to an SNF after hospital discharge, it is incumbent upon the hospital's case manager or social worker to identify an SNF and OTP that will partner to continue methadone for OUD treatment. With changes to federal law (42 CFR, part 8), any SNF that is registered with the DEA as a hospital or clinic is authorized to dispense methadone to a patient for OUD without OTP involvement.[124] In this scenario, the SNF provides the patient their daily methadone dose, similarly to how methadone is provided to hospitalized patients for OUD treatment. Many SNFs do not have this DEA designation, but securing it can be feasible.[125] If the SNF is not registered with the DEA as a hospital or clinic, the patient must either go to the OTP daily or the patient's methadone must be delivered from the OTP to the SNF as individual bottles of liquid methadone. The methadone bottles are transported and stored at the SNF and then dispensed to the patient on a daily basis. If the person is on a stable dose of methadone, the SNF can request up to 28 bottles of methadone be delivered from the OTP at a time through a process called "chain of custody" (Table 20.3). To facilitate this, a staff member from the SNF can go to the OTP, sign a form to confirm they have received the methadone, and will ensure the medication is safely secured, handled, and dispensed.

In the case that a patient is initiated on methadone during their hospitalization and they are not currently enrolled in an OTP, the patient will need to complete an in-hospital OTP intake or immediately posthospital OTP intake before they will be able to receive methadone dosing at the SNF (if the SNF is not registered as a clinic or hospital with the DEA). Per updated federal regulations, an OTP intake can be completed in the hospital via a telehealth OTP appointment.[123] Scheduling this appointment may be logistically challenging and requires in-hospital case management support to schedule the virtual appointment with the OTP and then provide the patient with a tablet to complete the face-to-face encounter. Once this appointment is completed and the patient is enrolled in the OTP, the SNF can legally accept methadone deliveries from the OTP and dispense it to the patient each day. Even though federal regulations allow this, some state regulations may prohibit it. It is important to check with your state opioid treatment authority about their OTP regulations.

Some OTPs may dispense take-home bottles of methadone directly to the patient in the SNF. In this case, the patient would authorize the SNF to hold and dispense their daily methadone to them while they are at SNF (eg, following the "patient taking own medication" workflow). In this case, the OTP provider manages the dose and the SNF provider is encouraged to communicate directly with the OTP doctor to advocate for a dose increase if, for example, the person is having cravings for the drug, or having opioid analgesics weaned off.

Once the patient is medically ready for SNF discharge, the SNF clinician will contact the OTP to let them know the patient's last methadone dose date and milligrams of dosage. The patient will then follow-up with the OTP per usual to resume methadone dosing.

LTACHs have a different designation and regulations than SNFs.[126] Regarding the provision of methadone, LTACHs are regulated in a similar fashion to medical hospitals. Methadone can generally be dispensed to patients residing at an LTACH without a partnering OTP; however, it is necessary to facilitate intake with a local OTP prior to LTACH discharge to ensure uninterrupted treatment once the patient leaves. Each state may have different regulations for LTACHs or SNFs, so it is important to know your state-specific regulations.

Unfortunately, denial of patient admission to an SNF and/or LTACH because they are taking methadone or buprenorphine is common. For any patient who is denied access to an SNF or LTACH because of their SUD treatment, this qualifies as a violation of the American Disabilities Act. These cases can be reported to the Department of Justice online.[127] In Massachusetts, the attorney general sent a warning letter to SNFs about this issue, reminding the facilities of the civil penalties for ADA violations with financial consequences.[128]

Patient-Directed Discharge

Patient-directed discharge occurs when a patient decides to leave the hospital during an acute treatment episode, often before they have completed the hospital portion of their treatment. Patient-directed discharges disproportionately affect people with SUD,

TABLE 20.3

Methadone Chain of Custody (COC) for Skilled Nursing Facilities

Task	Responsible person(s)	Timeframe	Note
Verify that patient is on methadone for opioid use disorder (OUD) and they were previously going to an opioid treatment program (OTP)	Medical or surgical team	7 d prior to discharge	Report to social worker or case manager: (1) name of methadone clinic; (2) current dose; and (3) is the dose stable
Patient must sign a 2-way release of information (ROI) that is HIPAA and 42-CFR part II compliant and fax to opioid treatment program (OTP)	Social work or case management team	4–6 d prior to discharge	See contact list ROI must be for communication between: OTP, SNF, and hospital (list on ROI)
Inform OTP of date of expected discharge to SNF and need for COC methadone (14–28 d)	Social work or case management team	4–6 days prior to discharge	Allows the OTP to give the methadone to a staff member from the SNF for administration to the patient
Request state exception for COC methadone	OTP	2–4 d prior to discharge	
Patient receives morning methadone and is discharged to SNF	Patient	Day of discharge	
SNF must designate staff member to be COC for methadone, and release the staff member to pick up the patient's methadone medication	SNF, Staff member	Day of discharge	Staff member will need to: ▪ Wear ID ▪ Bring copy of ID ▪ Sign COC form (see appendix) ▪ Receive education about safe methadone storage and administration ▪ Bring a container for safe storage
OTP prepares individually labeled prepoured take-home daily doses of methadone in childproof containers	OTP	Day of discharge	
Staff member brings methadone to nursing station and stores medication	SNF, Staff member	Day of discharge	Store the medication in a double-locked secure area (same as other controlled medications)
Provider writes order for daily methadone ("patient's own med")	SNF, Medical Provider	Day of discharge	
Patient receives ongoing daily methadone and this is documented in medical record and COC form	SNF and patient	Daily	SNF staff member will administer and observe the patient ingesting their medication daily. Do not leave the dose at bedside. The patient should be at baseline prior to med administration and should exhibit no signs of sedation or impairment. *If dose is not administered or there are questions about methadone, call the dispensary nurse in the OTP (see directory)
SNF documents receipt of methadone on the COC form and faxes form to OTP or brings the log to the clinic when they next pick up the next supply of methadone	SNF	Daily notation that dose of methadone taken on COC form	

(continued)

TABLE 20.3

Methadone Chain of Custody for Skilled Nursing Facilities (*Continued*)

Task	Responsible person(s)	Timeframe	Note
SNF contacts OTP by phone or email to confirm whether patient will continue to be at SNF and whether to prepare additional COC methadone	SNF	Every 1–4 wk	SNF should communicate with the OTP regarding the patient's overall well-being and convey pertinent information to the OTP regarding new medication(s) or updates or concerns regarding their health
If patient requests a change in methadone dose, the SNF will contact the OTP to arrange an in-person or telehealth appointment	SNF	As needed	
If patient directs their own discharge or leaves before methadone used, the SNF contacts the OTP to document wasting of bottles	SNF and OTP	Time of patient-directed discharge or authorized discharge from SNF	Follow SNF protocol for wasting of controlled medications. Patient does NOT take leftover bottles with them at time of discharge.
Inform the OTP of date that patient is discharged from or has left the SNF	SNF	Day of discharge from SNF	Fax COC form indicating last dose patient received

including individuals with severe and complex health issues resulting from substance use.[33,129] They occur in as many as 11% of hospitalizations among people with SUD, and among people who inject substances the estimated rate is 25% to 30%.[130,131] These events can happen unexpectedly and are often a source of frustration and confrontation between hospital care teams and patients. Moreover, patient-directed discharge is associated an increased risk of mortality and hospital readmission. There are multifarious reasons why patients may choose to leave the hospital prior to completing hospital treatment. Listening to patients and working with them to address these factors may help to prevent patient-directed discharge in some instances. In other cases, shared decision-making and collaborative contingency planning can help to mitigate some of the risks of leaving the hospital prior to treatment completion.

Understanding common reasons that patients with SUD leave the hospital via patient-directed discharge allows hospital teams to proactively address these issues. Prior qualitative research has identified undertreated withdrawal, stigma from health care team members, and behavioral restrictions (eg, unable to leave the hospital ward) as common reasons for patient-directed discharge.[132] For patients with a history of incarceration in particular, hospital restrictions on movement and visitation can be retraumatizing. In other instances, competing priorities such as work, caregiving, paying the rent, or caring for pets can be reasons that prompt all patients, regardless of SUD, to leave the hospital prematurely. Identifying these factors early during the hospital stay, and anticipating things like pain and withdrawal at hospital admission, can increase patient comfort, build therapeutic relationships, and may reduce the likelihood of patient-directed discharge.

Interdisciplinary care team members play important roles to prevent patient-directed discharge. Social workers should educate patients about community resources such as temporary pet sheltering services (eg, humane societies, https://www.ruffhaven.org), facilitate communication with employers and landlords, and work with eligible patients to apply for entitlements (eg, general assistance or social security) or low-cost phone access (eg, https://oclawin.org/be-informed/cell-phones-homelessness/). Physical therapists can help with mobility and pain management. Nurses should be trained to use tools such as the Clinical Opioid Withdrawal Scale (COWS) to identify signs of withdrawal early and notify medical teams so they can initiate medications for OUD. All care team members can participate in training related to nonstigmatizing communication and patient care.

Hospital policies also play an important role in preventing patient-directed discharge. "Zero tolerance" policies for in-hospital substance use, involuntary search and seizure of personal belongings, and restricting visitation and movement off of the hospital wards all likely contribute to patient-directed

TABLE 20.4

Best Practices for Creating Hospital Policies That Promote Person-Centered and Equitable Care for Individuals With SUD

Principle	Example
Engage multiple partners including people with lived/living SUD experience when creating or reviewing hospital policies that affect people with SUD	Convene an interprofessional group that includes patients to create or review the policy
Ensure the policy is patient centered and does not include punitive measures, including security as a first responder. If security is included, confirm they are a last resort.	Review existing policies related to suspected in-hospital substance use, visitation, and other scenarios that affect patients with SUD to ensure that they are not punitive.
Ensure that policies are designed and implemented in a way that promotes compassion, equity, and anti-racism.	Review existing policies that affect patients with SUD with an equity lens to determine who will be disproportionately affected and how, based on policy implementation trends across race/ethnicity and substance use.
Ensure that policies are mutually agreed upon and clearly understood by all partners in the hospital setting.	Obtain legal, security, regulatory, nursing, and leadership sponsorship of the policy to ensure consistent messaging and support
Ensure that policies are paired with appropriate education and training for hospital staff, leadership, security, clinicians, and other relevant partners.	Educate health care workers about the policy, evidence-based addiction care, harms of stigma, and SUD-related inequities, especially around race/ethnicity. Provide best-practice scripts of how to respond to in-hospital substance use concerns
Ensure that policies are adaptable based on the needs of patients with SUD and hospital employees.	Involve health care workers in policy implementation and a continual improvement process.
Ensure that policies are clearly communicated.	Inform all patients, regardless of substance use history, of the policy on admission.
Set patients with SUD up for success in the hospital through patient-centered care practices.	Offer patients adequate pain control, evidence-based addiction treatment, and supportive care that helps them tolerate hospitalization.

Adapted with permission from Wolters Kluwer Health, Inc.: Martin M, Snyder HR, Otway G, Holpit L, Day LW, Seidman D. In-hospital Substance Use Policies: An Opportunity to Advance Equity, Reduce Stigma, and Offer Evidence-based Addiction Care. *J Addict Med.* 2023;17(1):10–12. https://journals.lww.com/journaladdictionmedicine/fulltext/2023/01000/in_hospital_substance_use_policies__an_opportunity.4.aspx

discharge. Implementing more patient-centered, least-restrictive policies for patients with SUD should be a goal of all health care systems, balancing patient autonomy with safety (Table 20.4).[133] Standardizing a patient-centered approach to care for hospitalized patients with SUD can be a tool to reduce stigmatizing and/or discriminatory behavior by clinicians and staff. In instances where patients are unable to comply with institutional rules (eg, in-hospital substance use), it should lead to a conversation with the patient about how to better address the factors underlying the behavior. Ensuring the safety of staff, while addressing patient needs, is often attainable. Hospital-based contingency management is an emerging strategy that may also promote engagement with hospital care among patients with stimulant use disorder.[134,135] Every effort should be made to partner with the patient and provide a safe and therapeutic environment for them.

The Effect of Uncontrolled Pain and Withdrawal on Patient-Directed Discharge

Addressing pain and withdrawal is of paramount importance in preventing patient-directed discharge. For patients with a history of OUD, offering methadone and buprenorphine as first-line agents to treat opioid withdrawal reduces rates of patient-directed discharge and should be protocolized as a part of routine hospital care.[136] These protocols must take into account the high prevalence of fentanyl in the illicit drug supply, which has increased the risk of precipitated opioid withdrawal during buprenorphine initiation owing to fentanyl's lipophilicity (see Chapter 7).[129] Other agents to manage opioid withdrawal symptoms such as clonidine, hydroxyzine, and ondansetron should be offered as medically appropriate. Finally, hospital teams should strongly consider the use of short-acting opioids such as hydromorphone and immediate-release oxycodone to manage pain and withdrawal symptoms in cases where first-line treatments are not desired or insufficient to address symptoms. For people with OUD, required opioid analgesic doses are expected to be high due to opioid tolerance, and clinicians should consider scheduled doses of analgesics while hospitalized to avoid gaps in treatment.[137] The practice of administering or dispensing opioids to mitigate opioid withdrawal symptoms among hospitalized patients is legal and can be found in Title 21 Code of Federal Regulations Part 1306.07 section "Administering or dispensing of narcotic drugs" which specifically calls out hospitalized patients with experiencing withdrawal[121]:

> *"This section is not intended to impose any limitations on a physician or authorized hospital staff to administer or dispense narcotic drugs in a hospital to maintain or detoxify a person as an incidental adjunct to medical or surgical treatment of conditions other than addiction, or to administer or dispense narcotic drugs to persons with intractable pain in which no relief or cure is possible or none has been found after reasonable efforts."*

Thus, in the United States, physicians and hospital staff members are permitted by law to treat withdrawal syndromes with scheduled (ie, controlled medications), to manage intractable pain and opioid withdrawal. This rule is not limited to opioid withdrawal management. Consider the well-established practice to administer long-acting benzodiazepines or phenobarbital to manage benzodiazepine withdrawal. This federal regulation allows for use of scheduled medications to manage withdrawal symptoms among hospitalized patients.

In cases where efforts to prevent patient-directed discharge fail, contingency planning is necessary to preserve access to needed treatment after discharge. Provide the patient with in-hand harm-reduction supplies, including naloxone, a supply of buprenorphine, and list of OUD clinics and a map of local syringe service program. Whenever possible, administer long-acting injectable medications for OUD or alcohol use disorder. This is an emerging approach that can offer another useful option for patients.[138,139] For patients receiving intravenous antibiotics for bacteremia, endocarditis, or osteomyelitis, long-acting injectable (eg, dalbavancin) and oral alternatives can be safe and effective in many cases.[88,90,91,95,96,140] Ask the infectious disease specialist to provide oral antibiotic treatment recommendations if there is concern that a patient is at risk of a patient-directed discharge. Proactively engaging in contingency planning and documenting detailed instructions in clinical notes for future clinicians can help facilitate rapid and appropriate care in the event of patient-directed discharge.

Recommendations to support a patient leaving prior to treatment completion include:

1. Provide an adequate supply of medications to treat SUD such as buprenorphine or naltrexone; long-acting injectable formulations (extended release [XR]-buprenorphine or XR-naltrexone) may be helpful in these instances
2. Provide the remaining course of oral antibiotics to treat a skin and soft tissue, bone, or valvular infection
   a. Utilize "meds to bed" programs to ensure the medications are in-hand before the patient leaves
3. Provide in-hand harm-reduction supplies like naloxone and drug checking materials
4. Provide a list and map of community resources, including syringe service programs, shelters, and warms locations
5. Make sure the patient is aware of any upcoming medical or SUD appointments
   a. Issue printed instructions with appointment times and walk-in options for follow-up SUD and medical care

Emerging Evidence and Future Directions

Care for hospitalized people with SUD is rapidly evolving, driven by a changing policy landscape and innovative care models being developed and disseminated around the world. In this section, we highlight emerging models of care that may shape the care transition process for individuals with SUD in the future. Through sharing cutting-edge developments in SUD care transition management, we hope to inspire clinicians and health care systems to adapt promising care models based on local resources and needs.

Innovations in Methadone Delivery

Methadone provision during and immediately after hospitalization is among the areas where the most rapid and meaningful changes to clinical practice are taking place. One such innovation involves implementing rapid inpatient titration protocols for methadone to more efficiently and effectively address withdrawal and other OUD symptoms. Quickly achieving a therapeutic dose of methadone is especially important in the fentanyl era, as traditional dosing and titration schedules for medications to treat OUD have frequently proven to be insufficient.[129] Several hospitals have reported rapid methadone titration protocols to methadone-naïve patients with appropriate monitoring and frequent assessment.[141–144] Titrating medications for OUD to an effective dose prior to discharge has been identified as a key element of supporting transitions to community care.[34,53]

Some US policy changes have paved the way for innovation in facilitating OTP intake for hospitalized patients with OUD, which has traditionally been a laborious and tenuous process affecting transitions of care. In April 2024, the US Substance Abuse and Mental Health Systems Administration (SAMHSA) made key changes to 42 CFR part 8, codifying many methadone delivery flexibilities granted temporarily during the COVID-19 public health emergency.[123] These include increased use of telehealth-based OTP assessments, reducing federal requirements for biologic specimen testing in methadone care, and allowing non-OTP clinicians to complete remote OTP enrollment for patients.

As outlined in "*Medications for SUD Treatment and Post-Acute Care Facilities*," in addition to the completion of a virtual OTP intake in the hospital using telehealth, under the final provision in SAMHSA's CFR part 8, hospitalists can complete an intake screening and physical examination in the hospital and fax it to a local OTP to initiate the OTP intake process required by the US federal government.[123] Once the initial intake screening and physical examination is completed, the patient is required to present to the OTP within 14 days to complete a full psychosocial assessment. The benefit of this process is that the patient is partially enrolled in the OTP at the time of hospital discharge and can continue to receive a methadone dose at the OTP while they arrange for the psychosocial assessment. While still somewhat cumbersome, these changes are an improvement. Previous federal regulation required that a person present to the OTP in opioid withdrawal before receiving their first methadone dose, increasing a risk of return to opioid use before OTP linkage. This federal change facilitates hospital to OTP linkage, wherein a person can avoid a period of opioid withdrawal and engage in medical and SUD treatment following hospital discharge.

Example Cases

Case Example 1: Telehealth to Support Hospital to SNF Linkage

A health care system in Seattle has piloted a program where hospitalized patients taking methadone who are discharging to a skilled nursing facility are able to complete an intake to a partnering OTP via telehealth while in the hospital, with methadone doses from the OTP subsequently transported to the skilled nursing facility to seamlessly continue OUD care after discharge (personal communication, Addiction Medicine colleague at University of Washington, Sarah Leyde, MD).

Case Example 2. Hospital-Based OTP Enrollment

One Addiction Consultation Service (ACS) in Colorado partnered with a local OTP to complete federally compliant in-hospital OTP enrollments. This process required that the ACS team members become affiliated with their partnering OTP and allows them to document a history and physical examination, results of HIV, hepatitis C, syphilis testing, and an electrocardiogram directly into the OTP's electronic health record. An OTP nurse visits patients in the hospital to complete the federally required psychosocial assessment. During hospitalization, the ACS clinician titrates the patient's methadone dose to comfort. At the time of hospital discharge, the OTP nurse ensures the patient has transportation to the OTP, a Medicaid benefit. When the patient is discharged from the hospital, their OTP enrollment is complete and their methadone dose is continued and titrated as needed at the OTP.[145]

Case Example 3. Leveraging the 72-Hour Rule

Some health care systems have begun to implement the 72-hour rule in certain hospitals, emergency departments, and bridge clinics to facilitate low-barrier access to methadone treatment during care transitions. This allows for the hospital, the emergency department, or the bridge clinic clinician to dispense up to three take-home methadone doses to the patient at one time. In order to remain compliant with the US federal government, the methadone doses must be prepared in an inpatient pharmacy and dispensed, not prescribed, to the patient. US federal regulations prohibits methadone for OUD treatment to be prescribed from an outpatient pharmacy.[85,109,122] These programs can facilitate weekend hospital discharges by providing patients with take-home methadone doses when the OTPs are closed to facilitate weekday hospital to OTP linkage.[146]

Finally, a proposed policy that has potential to redefine methadone delivery in the United States, with substantial implications for posthospitalization care transitions, is the Modernizing Opioid Treatment Access Act (M-OTAA).[147] This federal bill contains several provisions to expand and facilitate access to methadone in community settings. Notably, it would allow Board-certified addiction specialists to prescribe office-based methadone for OUD outside of the OTP system. While M-OTAA's enactment remains uncertain, the bill has the potential to greatly expand access to community-based methadone, giving patients and hospital care teams more options for continuity of care after hospitalization.

Innovations in Buprenorphine Initiation

Innovative care models for people choosing buprenorphine are also rapidly emerging. For example, both low-dose and high-dose buprenorphine initiation protocols are being increasingly adopted to facilitate hospital-based buprenorphine initiation.[129,148,149] New "direct-to-inject" protocols have also been developed in hospitals and EDs to give people rapid access to long-acting injectable buprenorphine, which can provide weeks of continued therapeutic benefit after hospital discharge.[114,150]

Innovations in Hospital Collaborative Care Models

Beyond medications, several novel and creative interventions to support care transitions are emerging. These include embedded addiction medicine services within organ transplant teams, co-staffed cardiology and addiction medicine clinics for people with stimulant-associated heart failure,[151,152] multidisciplinary interventions focused on individuals with overlapping SUD and severe infections,[68,153] pharmacist-led management of buprenorphine in low-resource settings,[154] and mobile low-barrier primary care and addiction services for people experiencing homelessness.[68,69] Care transition teams are increasingly co-led by people with lived experience with SUD who can provide unique and powerful care transition support as well as critical guidance on future research and implementation priorities related to improving care transitions for people with SUD. Finally, there is increasing collaboration between community organizations, such as syringe service programs and community mental health clinics, with traditional medical services. Payors are also innovating to address the social needs of their patients, with more access to food support, housing assistance, transportation, and caregiving needs—all of which helps bend the curve of health disparities toward justice and meaningfully improve quality of life for patients.

The important gains and promising opportunities related to posthospitalization care transitions described here are the result of local innovation and tireless advocacy by countless individuals around the world who are dedicated to improving the health of people with SUD. While current evidence does not point to a single model that is superior in its ability to support care transitions after hospitalization, the cumulative body of research indicates that a wide variety of models are feasible and likely to improve care transitions for people with SUD compared to the status quo. Put another way, there is a menu of existing models that can be readily adapted to improve care in any health care system based on local resources and needs. As frontline clinicians and leaders in hospital-based care, hospitalists can serve as local champions to teach, advocate, and facilitate the adoption of innovative care models to support patients with SUD in the hospital and beyond.

REFERENCES

1. Labson MC. Innovative and successful approaches to improving care transitions from hospital to home. *Home Healthc Now.* 2015;33(2):88–95.
2. Coleman EA. The care transitions program. *Division of Health Care Policy and Research.* University of Colorado Denver; 2026.
3. Incze MA, Huebler S, Chen D, et al. Hospitalists' attitudes and experiences with posthospitalization care transitions for patients with substance use disorders: a cross-sectional analysis. *J Addict Med.* 2024;18(4):425–431.
4. Bell J, Turbow S, George M, Ali MK. Factors associated with high-utilization in a safety net setting. *BMC Health Serv Res.* 2017;17(1):273.
5. Calcaterra SL, Beaty B, Mueller SR, Min SJ, Binswanger IA. The association between social stressors and drug use/hazardous drinking among former prison inmates. *J Subst Abuse Treat.* 2014;47(1):41–49.
6. Calcaterra SL, Lockhart S, Callister C, Hoover K, Binswanger IA. Opioid use disorder treatment initiation and continuation: a qualitative study of patients who received addiction consultation and hospital-based providers. *J Gen Intern Med.* 2022;37(11):2786–2794.
7. Greysen SR, Allen R, Lucas GI, Wang EA, Rosenthal MS. Understanding transitions in care from hospital to homeless shelter: a mixed-methods, community-based participatory approach. *J Gen Intern Med.* 2012;27(11):1484–1491.
8. Bogdanowicz KM, Stewart R, Chang CK, et al. Excess overdose mortality immediately following transfer of patients and their care as well as after cessation of opioid substitution therapy. *Addiction.* 2018;113(5):946–951.
9. Hochstatter KR, Nordeck C, Mitchell SG, Schwartz RP, Welsh C, Gryczynski J. Polysubstance use and post-discharge mortality risk among hospitalized patients with opioid use disorder. *Prev Med Rep.* 2023;36:102494.
10. King C, Cook R, Korthuis PT, Morris CD, Englander H. Causes of death in the 12 months after hospital discharge among patients with opioid use disorder. *J Addict Med.* 2022;16(4):466–469.
11. Aboumatar H, Naqibuddin M, Chung S, et al. Effect of a hospital-initiated program combining transitional care and long-term self-management support on outcomes of patients hospitalized with chronic obstructive pulmonary disease: a randomized clinical trial. *JAMA.* 2019;322(14):1371–1380.
12. Corsino L, Padilla BI. A transition of care model from hospital to community for Hispanic/Latino adult patients with diabetes: design and rationale for a pilot study. *Pilot Feasibility Stud.* 2022;8(1):246.
13. Coskun S, Duygulu S. The effects of Nurse Led Transitional Care Model on elderly patients undergoing open heart surgery: a randomized controlled trial. *Eur J Cardiovasc Nurs.* 2022;21(1):46–55.

14. Li M, Li Y, Meng Q, et al. Effects of nurse-led transitional care interventions for patients with heart failure on healthcare utilization: a meta-analysis of randomized controlled trials. *PLoS One*. 2021;16(12):e0261300.
15. McAiney C, Markle-Reid M, Ganann R, et al. Implementation of the Community Assets Supporting Transitions (CAST) transitional care intervention for older adults with multimorbidity and depressive symptoms: a qualitative descriptive study. *PLoS One*. 2022;17(8):e0271500.
16. Blumer V, Gayowsky A, Xie F, et al. Effect of patient-centered transitional care services on patient-reported outcomes in heart failure: sex-specific analysis of the PACT-HF randomized controlled trial. *Eur J Heart Fail*. 2021;23(9):1488–1498.
17. Mitchell J, Probst J, Li X. The association between hospital care transition planning and timely primary care follow-up. *J Rural Health*. 2022;38(3):660–667.
18. Snyder ME, Krekeler CE, Jaynes HA, et al. Evaluating the effects of a multidisciplinary transition care management program on hospital readmissions. *Am J Health Syst Pharm*. 2020;77(12):931–937.
19. Boggan JC, Sankineni S, Dennis PA, et al. Effectiveness of synchronous postdischarge contacts on health care use and patient satisfaction: a systematic review and meta-analysis. *Ann Intern Med*. 2025;178(2):229–240.
20. Incze MA, Kelley AT, James H, et al. Post-hospitalization care transition strategies for patients with substance use disorders: a narrative review and taxonomy. *J Gen Intern Med*. 2024;39(5):837–846.
21. James H, Morgan J, Ti L, Nolan S. Transitions in care between hospital and community settings for individuals with a substance use disorder: a systematic review. *Drug Alcohol Depend*. 2023;243:109763.
22. Gryczynski J, Nordeck CD, Welsh C, Mitchell SG, O'Grady KE, Schwartz RP. Preventing hospital readmission for patients with comorbid substance use disorder: a randomized trial. *Ann Intern Med*. 2021;174(7):899–909.
23. Kleinman RA, Brothers TD, Morris NP. Retiring the "against medical advice" discharge. *Ann Intern Med*. 2022;175(12):1761–1762.
24. Suen LW, Makam AN, Snyder HR, et al. National prevalence of alcohol and other substance use disorders among emergency department visits and hospitalizations: NHAMCS 2014–2018. *J Gen Intern Med*. 2022;37(10):2420–2428.
25. Joudrey PJ, Edelman EJ, Wang EA. Drive times to opioid treatment programs in urban and rural counties in 5 US states. *JAMA*. 2019;322(13):1310–1312.
26. Bann M, Cullen R, de Boer C, Hrachovec D, Rozler A, Blume G. A Climate of stigma, uncertainty, and distrust: stakeholder perception of barriers to SNF placement for patients with opioid use disorder treated with methadone. *J Gen Intern Med*. 2025;40(9):2116–2123.
27. Dineen KK. Disability discrimination against people with substance use disorders by postacute care nursing facilities: it is time to stop tolerating civil rights violations. *J Addict Med*. 2021;15(1):18–19.
28. Kimmel SD, Rosenmoss S, Bearnot B, Larochelle M, Walley AY. Rejection of patients with opioid use disorder referred for post-acute medical care before and after an anti-discrimination settlement in Massachusetts. *J Addict Med*. 2021;15(1):20–26.
29. Nishar S, Soske J, Vanjani R, Kimmel SD, Roma C, Dow PM. Access and care for people with opioid use disorder in U.S. skilled nursing facilities: a policy commentary. *Int J Drug Policy*. 2024;133:104607.
30. Parkhideh A, Beiting KJ, Yang M, Landi AJ, Levine S. Substance use disorder care in skilled nursing facilities: characterizing resident experiences. *J Addict Med*. 2024;18(5):533–539.
31. Waters K, Handa L, Caballero B, Telahun A, Bann M. Substance use disorder as a predictor of skilled nursing facility referral failure. *J Gen Intern Med*. 2022;37(13):3506–3508.
32. Kulkarni SA, Wachter RM. The hospitalist movement 25 years later. *Annu Rev Med*. 2024;75:381–390.
33. Thakrar AP, Lowenstein M, Greysen SR, Delgado MK. Trends in before medically advised discharges for patients with opioid use disorder, 2016–2020. *JAMA*. 2023;330(23):2302–2304.
34. Incze MA, Huebler S, Szczotka K, Grant S, Kertesz SG, Gordon AJ. Expert panel consensus on the effectiveness and implementation of models to support posthospitalization care transitions for people with substance use disorders. *J Addict Med*. 2024;18(6):696–704.
35. Callister C, Lockhart S, Holtrop JS, Hoover K, Calcaterra SL. Experiences with an addiction consultation service on care provided to hospitalized patients with opioid use disorder: a qualitative study of hospitalists, nurses, pharmacists, and social workers. *Subst Abus*. 2022;43(1):615–622.
36. Englander H, Dobbertin K, Lind B, et al. Inpatient addiction medicine consultation and post-hospital substance use disorder treatment engagement: a propensity-matched analysis. *J Gen Intern Med*. 2019;34(12):2796–2803.
37. Englander H, Jones A, Krawczyk N, et al. A taxonomy of hospital-based addiction care models: a scoping review and key informant interviews. *J Gen Intern Med*. 2022;37(11):2821–2833.
38. Marks LR, Munigala S, Warren DK, Liang SY, Schwarz ES, Durkin MJ. Addiction medicine consultations reduce readmission rates for patients with serious infections from opioid use disorder. *Clin Infect Dis*. 2019;68(11):1935–1937.
39. Salvalaggio G, Dong KA, Hyshka E, et al. Impact of an addiction medicine consult team intervention in a Canadian inner city hospital on acute care utilization: a pragmatic quasi-experimental study. *Subst Abuse Treat Prev Policy*. 2022;17(1):20.
40. Trowbridge P, Weinstein ZM, Kerensky T, et al. Addiction consultation services—Linking hospitalized patients to outpatient addiction treatment. *J Subst Abuse Treat*. 2017;79:1–5.
41. Wakeman SE, Metlay JP, Chang Y, Herman GE, Rigotti NA. Inpatient addiction consultation for hospitalized patients increases post-discharge abstinence and reduces addiction severity. *J Gen Intern Med*. 2017;32(8):909–916.
42. Weinstein ZM, Cheng DM, D'Amico MJ, et al. Inpatient addiction consultation and post-discharge 30-day acute care utilization. *Drug Alcohol Depend*. 2020;213:108081.
43. Weinstein ZM, Wakeman SE, Nolan S. Inpatient addiction consult service: expertise for hospitalized patients with complex addiction problems. *Med Clin North Am*. 2018;102(4):587–601.
44. Wilson JD, Altieri Dunn SC, Roy P, Joseph E, Klipp S, Liebschutz J. Inpatient addiction medicine consultation service impact on post-discharge patient mortality: a propensity-matched analysis. *J Gen Intern Med*. 2022;37(10):2521–2525.
45. Jack HE, Denisiuk ED, Collins BA, et al. Peer providers and linkage with buprenorphine care after hospitalization: a retrospective cohort study. *Subst Abus*. 2022;43(1):1308–1316.
46. Glass JE, Hamilton AM, Powell BJ, Perron BE, Brown RT, Ilgen MA. Specialty substance use disorder services following brief alcohol intervention: a meta-analysis of randomized controlled trials. *Addiction*. 2015;110(9):1404–1415.
47. Cooper L, Donald B, Osborne K, et al. The effect of inpatient addiction screening and intervention on readmissions. *Appl Nurs Res*. 2022;65:151573.
48. Schwarz A-S, Nielsen B, Søgaard J, Søgaard Nielsen A. Making a bridge between general hospital and specialised community-based treatment for alcohol use disorder—A pragmatic randomised controlled trial. *Drug Alcohol Depend*. 2019;196:51–56.

49. Terasaki D, Loh R, Cornell A, Taub J, Thurstone C. Single-dose intravenous ketamine or intramuscular naltrexone for high-utilization inpatients with alcohol use disorder: pilot trial feasibility and readmission rates. *Addict Sci Clin Pract.* 2022;17(1):64.
50. Wang SJ, Wade E, Towle J, et al. Effect of inpatient medication-assisted therapy on against-medical-advice discharge and readmission rates. *Am J Med.* 2020;133(11):1343–1349.
51. Stephens JR, Moore C, Stepanek KV, et al. Implementation of a process for initiating naltrexone in patients hospitalized for alcohol detoxification or withdrawal. *J Hosp Med.* 2018;13(4):221–228.
52. Wei J, Defries T, Lozada M, Young N, Huen W, Tulsky J. An inpatient treatment and discharge planning protocol for alcohol dependence: efficacy in reducing 30-day readmissions and emergency department visits. *J Gen Intern Med.* 2015;30(3):365–370.
53. Krawczyk N, Miller M, Englander H, et al. Toward a consensus on strategies to support opioid use disorder care transitions following hospitalization: a modified Delphi process. *J Gen Intern Med.* 2025;40(5):1048–1058.
54. Taylor JL, Wakeman SE, Walley AY, Kehoe LG. Substance use disorder bridge clinics: models, evidence, and future directions. *Addict Sci Clin Pract.* 2023;18(1):23.
55. Tofighi B, McNeely J, Yang J, et al. Outcomes of a NYC public hospital system low-threshold tele-buprenorphine bridge clinic at 1 year. *Subst Use Misuse.* 2022;57(8):1337–1340.
56. Aronowitz SV, Holliday-Davis M, French R, et al. Barriers and facilitators to implementing CareConnect: a telehealth, low-barrier buprenorphine bridge clinic in Philadelphia. *Int J Drug Policy.* 2024;133:104569.
57. Casey SK, Howard S, Regan S, et al. Linkage to care outcomes following treatment in a low-threshold substance use disorder bridge clinic. *Subst Use Addctn J.* 2025;46(2):247–255.
58. Chirunomula S, Muscarella A, Whelchel K, et al. Hepatitis C cascade of care in a multidisciplinary substance use bridge clinic model in Tennessee. *Open Forum Infect Dis.* 2024;11(5):ofae205.
59. Lynch MJ, Houck P, Meyers J, Schuster J, Yealy DM. Use of a telemedicine bridge clinic to engage patients in opioid use disorder treatment. *J Addict Med.* 2022;16(5):584–587.
60. Lynch MJ, Vargas D, Winger ME, et al. A telemedicine bridge clinic improves access and reduces cost for opioid use disorder care. *Drug Alcohol Depend Rep.* 2024;11:100227.
61. Snow RL, Simon RE, Jack HE, Oller D, Kehoe L, Wakeman SE. Patient experiences with a transitional, low-threshold clinic for the treatment of substance use disorder: a qualitative study of a bridge clinic. *J Subst Abuse Treat.* 2019;107:1–7.
62. Sullivan RW, Szczesniak LM, Wojcik SM. Bridge clinic buprenorphine program decreases emergency department visits. *J Subst Abuse Treat.* 2021;130:108410.
63. Braun HM, Walter C, Farrell N, Biello KB, Taylor JL. HIV exposure prophylaxis delivery in a low-barrier substance use disorder bridge clinic during a local HIV outbreak at the onset of the COVID-19 pandemic. *J Addict Med.* 2022;16(6):678–683.
64. Zhang A, Spiegel T, Bundy A, et al. Evaluation of a transitions clinic to bridge emergency department and primary care. *J Hosp Med.* 2023;18(3):217–223.
65. Incze MA, Sehgal SL, Hansen A, Garcia L, Stolebarger L. Evaluation of a primary care-based multidisciplinary transition clinic for patients newly initiated on buprenorphine in the emergency department. *Subst Abus.* 2023;44(3):220–225.
66. Shanahan CW, Beers D, Alford DP, Brigandi E, Samet JH. A transitional opioid program to engage hospitalized drug users. *J Gen Intern Med.* 2010;25(8):803–808.
67. Smith A, Hansen J, Colvard M. Impact of a pharmacist-led substance use disorder transitions of care clinic on postdischarge medication treatment retention. *J Subst Abuse Treat.* 2021;130:108440.
68. Serota DP, Rosenbloom L, Hervera B, et al. Integrated infectious disease and substance use disorder care for the treatment of injection drug use-associated infections: a prospective cohort study with historical control. *Open Forum Infect Dis.* 2023;10(1):ofac688.
69. Serota DP, Tookes HE, Hervera B, et al. Harm reduction for the treatment of patients with severe injection-related infections: description of the Jackson SIRI Team. *Ann Med.* 2021;53(1):1960–1968.
70. Byrne KA, Roth PJ, Merchant K, et al. Inpatient link to peer recovery coaching: results from a pilot randomized control trial. *Drug Alcohol Depend.* 2020;215:108234.
71. Lennox R, Lamarche L, O'Shea T. Peer support workers as a bridge: a qualitative study exploring the role of peer support workers in the care of people who use drugs during and after hospitalization. *Harm Reduct J.* 2021;18(1):19.
72. Magidson JF, Regan S, Powell E, et al. Peer recovery coaches in general medical settings: changes in utilization, treatment engagement, and opioid use. *J Subst Abuse Treat.* 2021; 122:108248.
73. McGuire AB, Powell KG, Treitler PC, et al. Emergency department-based peer support for opioid use disorder: emergent functions and forms. *J Subst Abuse Treat.* 2020;108:82–87.
74. D'Onofrio G, Degutis LC. Integrating Project ASSERT: a screening, intervention, and referral to treatment program for unhealthy alcohol and drug use into an urban emergency department. *Acad Emerg Med.* 2010;17(8):903–911.
75. Heetderks-Fong E, Bobb A. Community mental health workers: their workplaces, roles, and impact. *Community Ment Health J.* 2024;60(8):1547–1556.
76. Bogan C, Jennings L, Haynes L, et al. Implementation of emergency department-initiated buprenorphine for opioid use disorder in a rural southern state. *J Subst Abuse Treat.* 2020;112S:73–78.
77. Seliski N, Madsen T, Eley S, et al. Implementation of a rural emergency department-initiated buprenorphine program in the mountain west: a study protocol. *Addict Sci Clin Pract.* 2024;19(1):63.
78. Hamilton J, Ti L, Korchinski M, Nolan S. Peer support specialists: an underutilized resource in the criminal justice system for opioid use disorder management? *J Addict Med.* 2022;16(2):132–134.
79. Eddie D, Hoffman L, Vilsaint C, et al. Lived experience in new models of care for substance use disorder: a systematic review of peer recovery support services and recovery coaching. *Front Psychol.* 2019;10:1052.
80. Upadhyaya A, Marks LR, Schwarz ES, Liang SY, Durkin MJ, Liss DB. Care cascade for patients with opioid use disorder and serious injection related infections. *Toxicol Commun.* 2021;5(1):6–10.
81. Englander H, Wilson T, Collins D, et al. Lessons learned from the implementation of a medically enhanced residential treatment (MERT) model integrating intravenous antibiotics and residential addiction treatment. *Subst Abus.* 2018;39(2):225–232.
82. Gelman SS, Stenehjem E, Foster RA, Tinker N, Grisel N, Webb BJ. A novel program to provide drug recovery assistance and outpatient parenteral antibiotic therapy in people who inject drugs. *Open Forum Infect Dis.* 2022;9(2):ofab629.
83. Padwa H, Mark TL, Wondimu B. What's in an "ASAM-based assessment?" Variations in assessment and level of care determination in systems required to use ASAM patient placement criteria. *J Addict Med.* 2022;16(1):18–26.
84. American Society of Addiction Medicine. The ASAM criteria 4th edition treatment criteria for addictive, substance-related, and co-occurring conditions. 2023.
85. Taylor JL, Laks J, Christine PJ, et al. Bridge clinic implementation of "72-hour rule" methadone for opioid

withdrawal management: impact on opioid treatment program linkage and retention in care. *Drug Alcohol Depend.* 2022;236:109497.
86. Doran KM, Ragins KT, Gross CP, Zerger S. Medical respite programs for homeless patients: a systematic review. *J Health Care Poor Underserved.* 2013;24(2):499–524.
87. Bring C, Kruse M, Ankarfeldt MZ, et al. Post-hospital medical respite care for homeless people in Denmark: a randomized controlled trial and cost-utility analysis. *BMC Health Serv Res.* 2020;20(1):508.
88. Okumura N, Hayakawa K, Yamamoto K, Yamada G, Mezaki K, Ohmagari N. Effectiveness of oral cephalexin in antibiotic-course completion for methicillin-susceptible Staphylococcus aureus-induced bacteremic vertebral osteomyelitis. *BMC Infect Dis.* 2023;23(1):307.
89. Marconi L, Tedeschi S, Zamparini E, et al. Oral versus standard antimicrobial treatment for pyogenic native vertebral osteomyelitis: a single-center, retrospective, propensity score-balanced analysis. *Open Forum Infect Dis.* 2022;9(8): ofac366.
90. Schechter MC, Sax PE, Cortes-Penfield N. What is the best oral therapy for *Staph aureus* osteomyelitis? *NEJM Evid.* 2022;1(11):EVIDtt2200119.
91. Spellberg B, Chambers HF, Musher DM, Walsh TL, Bayer AS. Evaluation of a paradigm shift from intravenous antibiotics to oral step-down therapy for the treatment of infective endocarditis: a narrative review. *JAMA Intern Med.* 2020;180(5):769–777.
92. Baddour LM, Weimer MB, Wurcel AG, et al. Management of infective endocarditis in people who inject drugs: a scientific statement from the American Heart Association. *Circulation.* 2022;146(14):e187–e201.
93. Tingsgard S, Bastrup Israelsen S, Jorgensen HL, Ostergaard C, Benfield T. Early switch from intravenous to oral antibiotics for patients with uncomplicated gram-negative bacteremia. *JAMA Netw Open.* 2024;7(1):e2352314.
94. Eleftheriotis G, Marangos M, Lagadinou M, Bhagani S, Assimakopoulos SF. Oral antibiotics for bacteremia and infective endocarditis: current evidence and future perspectives. *Microorganisms.* 2023;11(12):3004.
95. Lee TC, Spellberg B, McDonald EG. Oral antibiotics for Staphylococcus aureus bacteremia including endocarditis: sauce for the goose is sauce for the gander. *Clin Infect Dis.* 2025;80(6):e96–e98.
96. Chowdhury J, Patel R, Chambers H. Oral versus intravenous antibiotics for endocarditis. *N Engl J Med.* 2021; 385(12):1141–1143.
97. Iversen K, Ihlemann N, Gill SU, et al. Partial oral versus intravenous antibiotic treatment of endocarditis. *N Engl J Med.* 2019;380(5):415–424.
98. Marks LR, Liang SY, Muthulingam D, et al. Evaluation of partial oral antibiotic treatment for persons who inject drugs and are hospitalized with invasive infections. *Clin Infect Dis.* 2020;71(10):e650–e656.
99. Van Hise NW, Petrak RM, Shah K, Diaz M, Chundi V, Redell M. Oritavancin versus daptomycin for osteomyelitis treatment after surgical debridement. *Infect Dis Ther.* 2024;13(3):535–547.
100. Texidor WM, Miller MA, Molina KC, et al. Oritavancin as sequential therapy for Gram-positive bloodstream infections. *BMC Infect Dis.* 2024;24(1):127.
101. Moenster RP, Wallace-Lacey A, Western H, et al. Oritavancin vs standard of care for treatment of nonendovascular gram-positive bloodstream infections. *Open Forum Infect Dis.* 2023;10(11):ofad411.
102. Giuliano G, Benedetti S, Sambo M, Pierguidi F, Tumbarello M. Successful treatment of complicated infective endocarditis due to Enterococcus faecium in a patient with substance use disorder using oritavancin as sequential maintenance therapy. *Clin Microbiol Infect.* 2024;30(4):556–557.
103. Buonomo AR, Cattaneo L, Viceconte G, et al. Long-term oritavancin therapy for shoulder prosthetic joint infection: a case guided by therapeutic drug monitoring (TDM). *IDCases.* 2024;38:e02105.
104. Bongiovanni M, Thoueille P, Barda B, et al. Oritavancin use in patients with recurrent bone infections by methicillin-resistant Staphylococcus aureus with monitoring of concentrations. *Eur J Clin Microbiol Infect Dis.* 2024;43(7): 1503–1504.
105. Salinas-Botran A, Olmos-Blanco C, Fernandez de Velasco-Perez D, Guzman-Carreras A, Morales-Rosas A, Gomez-Ramirez D. Dalbavancin as consolidation antibiotic treatment in infective endocarditis, cardiac implantable electronic devices infection and bacteremia: clinical experience of 7 years. *Enferm Infecc Microbiol Clin (Engl Ed).* 2025;43(2):71–79.
106. Leanza GM, Rando E, Frondizi F, et al. A systematic review of dalbavancin efficacy as a sequential therapy for infective endocarditis. *Infection.* 2025;53(1):15–23.
107. Crapis M, Venturini S, Callegari A, et al. Usefulness of dalbavancin in early discharge and nonhospitalization. It's time to throw your heart over the obstacle? *Glob Reg Health Technol Assess.* 2024;11(Suppl 2):18–21.
108. Almangour TA, Alrasheed MA. Dalbavancin for the treatment of bone and joint infections: a meta-analysis. *J Infect Chemother.* 2025;31(1):102473.
109. Shahlapour M, Singh S, Christine PJ, et al. Novel Uses of methadone under the "72-hour rule" to facilitate transitions of care and low-dose buprenorphine induction in an outpatient bridge clinic. *J Addict Med.* 2024;18(3):345–347.
110. Chan CA, Minahan-Rowley R, Biegacki ET, Sue KL, Weimer MB. Development of a patient and clinician informed website on injection drug use related infective endocarditis. *Subst Use Addctn.* 2025;46(2):280–290.
111. Harris MTH, Peterkin A, Bach P, et al. Adapting inpatient addiction medicine consult services during the COVID-19 pandemic. *Addict Sci Clin Pract.* 2021;16(1):13.
112. DeFries T, Kelley J, Martin M, Kimball SL. Immigration status matters: the intersectional risk of immigration vulnerability and substance use disorder. *Addiction.* 2022; 117(7):1827–1829.
113. D'Onofrio G, Herring AA, Perrone J, et al. Extended-release 7-day injectable buprenorphine for patients with minimal to mild opioid withdrawal. *JAMA Netw Open.* 2024;7(7):e2420702.
114. O'Conor C, Farhi S, Cowan E, Fitzgerald R. Inpatient ini tiation of long-acting injectable buprenorphine at a community hospital: a retrospective case series. *J Addict Dis.* 2025;43(4):338–344.
115. Shah R, Hendrickson S, Fanucchi L, Lofwall M, Platt T, Rhudy C. Utility of an integrated health system specialty pharmacy in provision of extended-release buprenorphine for patients with opioid use disorder. *Am J Health Syst Pharm.* 2023;80(1):e59–e66.
116. Ganetsky VS, Salzman M, Carroll G, et al. Hospital-initiated extended-release injectable buprenorphine using a novel real-location initiative from an outpatient addiction medicine clinic. *J Addict Med.* 2023;17(1):108–110.
117. Busch AC, Denduluri M, Glass J, et al. Predischarge injectable versus oral naltrexone to improve postdischarge treatment engagement among hospitalized veterans with alcohol use disorder: a randomized pilot proof-of-concept study. *Alcohol Clin Exp Res.* 2017;41(7):1352–1360.
118. Calcaterra SL, Mann S, Grimm E, Keniston A, Saunders S. Perspectives of in-hospital intramuscular naltrexone and

oral medications for alcohol use disorder: a study of addiction clinicians and hospitalized patients. *J Gen Intern Med.* 2025;40(12):2981–2988.
119. Kirchoff RW, Mohammed NM, McHugh J, et al. Naltrexone initiation in the inpatient setting for alcohol use disorder: a systematic review of clinical outcomes. *Mayo Clin Proc Innov Qual Outcomes.* 2021;5(2):495–501.
120. Tigh J, Daniel K, Balasanova AA. Impact of hospital-administered extended-release naltrexone on readmission rates in patients with alcohol use disorder: a pilot study. *Prim Care Companion CNS Disord.* 2022;24(6):22m03213.
121. Drug Enforcement Administration. § 1306.07 Administering or dispensing of narcotic drugs. 2022.
122. Bowman LA, Berger O, Nesbit S, Stoller KB, Buresh M, Stewart R. Operationalizing the new DEA exception: a novel process for dispensing of methadone for opioid use disorder at discharge from acute care settings. *Am J Health Syst Pharm.* 2024;81(6):204–218.
123. US Substance Abuse and Mental Health Systems Administration. 42 CFR Part 8. In: US Department of Health and Human Services, ed2024.
124. Department of Health and Human Services. Medications for the Treatment of Opioid Use Disorder. In. Vol 42 CFR 82024:7528-7563.
125. Health JHUBSoP. Providing Methadone in Jails and Prisons: An explanation of a new approach to increase access to methadone in carceral settings FAQ. https://opioidprinciples.jhsph.edu/wp-content/uploads/2023/05/Methadone-Fact-Sheet.pdf.
126. Drug Enforcement Administration. 21 CFR 1306.07, Administering or dispensing of narcotic drugs. In: Department of Justice, ed2025.
127. Department of Justice. https://civilrights.justice.gov/report/?utm_campaign=499a0d26-884a-47aa-9afc-70094d92e6f5
128. United States Attorney's Office, District of Massachusetts. U.S. Attorney's Office Warns Skilled Nursing Facilities Not to Refuse Treatment to People with Opioid Use Disorder [press release]. 2022.
129. Englander H, Thakrar AP, Bagley SM, Rolley T, Dong K, Hyshka E. Caring for hospitalized adults with opioid use disorder in the era of fentanyl: a review. *JAMA Intern Med.* 2024;184(6):691–701.
130. Foster K, Caswell A, James L, et al. The risk factors, consequences, and interventions of discharge against medical advice—A narrative review. *Am J Med Sci.* 2023;366(1):16–21.
131. Zhu H, Wu LT. Discharge against medical advice from hospitalizations for substance use disorders: the potential impact of the Affordable Care Act. *Drug Alcohol Depend.* 2019;197:115–119.
132. Simon R, Snow R, Wakeman S. Understanding why patients with substance use disorders leave the hospital against medical advice: a qualitative study. *Subst Abus.* 2020;41(4):519–525.
133. Martin M, Snyder HR, Otway G, Holpit L, Day LW, Seidman D. In-hospital substance use policies: an opportunity to advance equity, reduce stigma, and offer evidencebased addiction care. *J Addict Med.* 2023;17(1):10–12.
134. Appa A, Baral S, Stein B, et al. The IMPACT (Infection Management Plus Addiction Care Together) pilot: a case series of combined contingency management for substance use disorders and antibiotic adherence in the hospital setting. *J Addict Med.* 2024;18(2):138–143.
135. Peng L, Titus H, Roellich P, Englander H. Adapting contingency management for hospitalized patients with stimulant use disorder. *J Addict Med.* 2023;17(5):580–586.
136. Kays LB, Steltenpohl ED, McPheeters CM, Frederick EK, Bishop LB. Initiation of buprenorphine/naloxone on rates of discharge against medical advice. *Hosp Pharm.* 2022;57(1):88–92.
137. Thakrar AP. Short-acting opioids for hospitalized patients with opioid use disorder. *JAMA Intern Med.* 2022;182(3): 247–248.
138. Hansen ER, South AM, Lofwall MR, Fanucchi LC. Extended-release buprenorphine administered at discharge in hospitalized persons with opioid use disorder: a case series. *J Addict Med.* 2024;18(1):65–67.
139. De Vito A, Fiore V, Colpani A, et al. The current and future off-label uses of dalbavancin: a narrative review. *Eur Rev Med Pharmacol Sci.* 2023;27(3):1222–1238.
140. Gill AS, Gorski M, Strage KE, Dunn JT, Jerabek M, Hoffman KM. Oral versus intravenous antibiotics for residual osteomyelitis after amputation in the diabetic foot. *J Foot Ankle Surg.* 2022;61(4):735–738.
141. Casey S, Regan S, Gale E, et al. Rapid methadone induction in a general hospital setting: a retrospective, observational analysis. *Subst Abus.* 2023;44(3):177–183.
142. Klaire S, Fairbairn N, Ryan A, Nolan S, McLean M, Bach P. Safety and efficacy of rapid methadone titration for opioid use disorder in an inpatient setting: a retrospective cohort study. *J Addict Med.* 2023;17(6):711–713.
143. Racha S, Patel SM, Bou Harfouch LT, Berger O, Buresh ME. Safety of rapid inpatient methadone initiation protocol: a retrospective cohort study. *J Subst Use Addict Treat.* 2023;148:209004.
144. Liu P, Chan B, Sokolski E, Patten A, Englander H. Piloting a hospital-based rapid methadone initiation protocol for fentanyl. *J Addict Med.* 2024;18(4):458–462.
145. Calcaterra SL, Saunders S, Grimm E, et al. In-hospital methadone enrollment: a novel program to facilitate linkage from the hospital to the opioid treatment program for vulnerable patients with opioid use disorder. *J Gen Intern Med.* 2024;39(3):385–392.
146. Calcaterra SL, Weimer MB, Grimm E, et al. Leveraging the 72-hour rule change to support transition from hospital to opioid treatment program. *JAMA Netw Open.* 2025;8(11):e2544996.
147. S.644—Modernizing Opioid Treatment Access Act, 118th Cong. 2023. https://www.congress.gov/bill/118th-congress/senate-bill/644
148. Spadaro A, Faude S, Perrone J, et al. Precipitated opioid withdrawal after buprenorphine administration in patients presenting to the emergency department: a case series. *J Am Coll Emerg Physicians Open.* 2023;4(1):e12880.
149. Thakrar AP, Faude S, Perrone J, et al. Association of urine fentanyl concentration with severity of opioid withdrawal among patients presenting to the emergency department. *J Addict Med.* 2023;17(4):447–453.
150. Perdue M, Hosseini Ghomi R, Rees P, Arzubi E. 5-Day injectable extended-release buprenorphine initiation in non-opioid-tolerant individuals in a carceral setting: a case series. *J Addict Med.* 2025;19(2):227–229.
151. Davis J, Bepo L, Suen LW, et al. Implementing heart plus: design and early results of a novel co-management clinic for patients with stimulant-associated cardiomyopathy. *J Card Fail.* 2024;30(7):869–876.
152. Leyde S, Abbs E, Suen LW, et al. A Mixed-methods evaluation of an addiction/cardiology pilot clinic with contingency management for patients with stimulant-associated cardiomyopathy. *J Addict Med.* 2023;17(3):312–318.
153. Fanucchi LC, Walsh SL, Thornton AC, Nuzzo PA, Lofwall MR. Outpatient parenteral antimicrobial therapy plus buprenorphine for opioid use disorder and severe injection-related infections. *Clin Infect Dis.* 2020;70(6):1226–1229.
154. Green TC, Serafinski R, Clark SA, Rich JD, Bratberg J. Physician-delegated unobserved induction with buprenorphine in pharmacies. *N Engl J Med.* 2023;388(2):185–186.

Index

Note: Page numbers followed by "f" indicate figures and "t" indicate tables.